WF 140 ALB £126

CLINICAL RESPIRATORY MEDICINE

CLINICAL RESPIRATORY MEDICINE

THIRD EDITION

RICHARD K. ALBERT

Professor of Medicine, University of Colorado
Adjunct Professor of Engineering and Computer Science, University of Denver
Chief, Department of Medicine
Denver Health
Denver, Colorado
United States

STEPHEN G. SPIRO

Professor of Respiratory Medicine
Consultant Physician, General and Thoracic Medicine
University College London Hospitals NHS Trust
London
United Kingdom

JAMES R. JETT

Professor of Medicine
Mayo Clinic College of Medicine
Consultant in Pulmonary Medicine and Medical Oncology
Rochester, Minnesota
United States

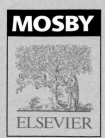

MOSBY

ELSEVIER

MOSBY
ELSEVIER

1600 John F. Kennedy Blvd.
Ste 1800
Philadelphia, PA 19103-2899

CLINICAL RESPIRATORY MEDICINE, THIRD EDITION   ISBN: 978-0-323-04825-5

Library of Congress Cataloging-in-Publication Data
Clinical respiratory medicine / [edited by] Richard K. Albert, Stephen G. Spiro,
  James R. Jett. — 3rd ed.
      p. ; cm.
  Includes bibliographical references and index.
  ISBN-13: 978-0-323-04825-5

  1. Respiratory organs—Diseases.   I. Albert, Richard K.   II. Spiro, Stephen G.   III. Jett, James R.
[DNLM: 1. Respiratory Tract Diseases. 2. Lung Diseases. WF 140 C641 2008]
RC731.C65 2008
616.2—dc22

                                                                    2007024654

Senior Acquisitions Editor: Dolores Meloni
Developmental Editor: Adrianne Brigido
Editorial Assistant: Kimberly DePaul
Project Manager: Bryan Hayward
Design Direction: Ellen Zanolle

Printed in China

Last digit is the print number: 9 8 7 6 5 4 3 2 1

To our teachers

Contributors

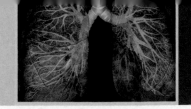

RICHARD K. ALBERT, MD
Professor of Medicine, University of Colorado, Adjunct Professor of Engineering and Computer Science, University of Denver, Chief, Department of Medicine, Denver Health, Denver, Colorado
CHEST PAIN

MARK S. ALLEN, MD, FACS
Professor of Surgery, Division of General Thoracic Surgery, Chair, Division of General Thoracic Surgery, Mayo Clinic, Rochester, Minnesota
DIAGNOSTIC THORACIC SURGICAL PROCEDURES

CHARLES W. ATWOOD, JR, MD, FCCP, FAASM
Associate Professor of Medicine, Director, Sleep Medicine Fellowship Program, Division of Pulmonary, Allergy, and Critical Care Medicine, University of Pittsburgh, Medical Director, Sleep Laboratory, Pulmonary and Critical Care Medicine, VA Pittsburgh Healthcare System, University Drive Division, Pittsburgh, Pennsylvania
CENTRAL SLEEP APNEA AND OTHER FORMS OF SLEEP-
   DISORDERED BREATHING

MARIE CHRISTINE AUBRY, MD
Consultant and Associate Professor, Department of Laboratory Medicine and Pathology, Mayo Clinic, Rochester, Minnesota
MALIGNANT PLEURAL MESOTHELIOMA

ALAN F. BARKER, MD
Professor of Medicine, Division of Pulmonary and Critical Care, Department of Internal Medicine, Oregon Health and Science University, Portland, Oregon
BRONCHIECTASIS

PETER J. BARNES, DM, DSc, FRCP, FMedSci
Professor of Thoracic Medicine, National Heart and Lung Institute, Imperial College, London, United Kingdom
β_2-AGONISTS, ANTICHOLINERGICS, AND OTHER NONSTEROID DRUGS

THOMAS BENFIELD, MD, DMSci
Clinical Associate Professor, Department of Surgery and Internal Medicine, University of Copenhagen, Copenhagen, Denmark, Senior Physician, Department of Infectious Diseases, Hvidovre University Hospital, Hvidovre, Denmark
NONINFECTIOUS CONDITIONS

SURINDER S. BIRRING, MD, MRCP
Honorary Senior Lecturer, Allergy, Asthma and Lung Biology, King's College London, University of London, Consultant Respiratory Physician, Respiratory Medicine, King's College Hospital, London, United Kingdom
COUGH

CHRIS T. BOLLIGER, MD, PhD
Professor, Division of Pulmonology, Department of Medicine, Director, Respiratory Research Unit, University of Stellenbosch, Principle Medical Specialist, Division of Pulmonology, Department of Medicine, Tygerberg Academic Hospital, Cape Town, Western Cape, South Africa
PREOPERATIVE PULMONARY EVALUATION

LUKAS BRANDER, MD
Department of Intensive Care Medicine, University Hospital – Inselspital, Bern, Switzerland
INVASIVE MECHANICAL VENTILATION

ROY G. BROWER, MD
Professor of Medicine, Medical Director, Medical Intensive Care Unit, John Hopkins University School of Medicine, Baltimore, Maryland
PULMONARY CIRCULATION

JEREMY BROWN, MBBS, PhD, FRCP
Senior Lecturer, Centre for Respiratory Research, Department of Medicine, University College London, Consultant Respiratory Physician, Department of Medicine, University College London Hospital, London, United Kingdom
PNEUMONIA IN THE NON-HIV IMMUNOCOMPROMISED HOST

TODD M. BULL, MD
Associate Professor of Medicine, Division of Pulmonary Sciences and Critical Care Medicine, University of Colorado at Denver Health Sciences Center, Denver, Colorado
PULMONARY EMBOLISM

PHILIPPE CAMUS, MD
Chairman, Division of Pulmonary and Intensive Care, Hôpital du Bocage; Faculté de Médecine, Université Bourgogne, Centre Hospitalier Universitaire de Dijon, Dijon, France
INFLAMMATORY BOWEL DISEASE; DRUGS AND THE LUNGS

CHRISTOPHER CARLSTEN, MD, MPH
Senior Fellow, Division of Pulmonary and Critical Care Medicine, Occupational and Environmental Medicine Program, Department of Medicine, University of Washington, Seattle, Washington
AIR POLLUTION

STEPHEN D. CASSIVI, MD, MSc, FRCSC, FACS
Associate Professor of Surgery, Division of General Thoracic Surgery, Surgical Director of Lung Transplantation, William J. von Liebig Transplant Center, Mayo Clinic, Rochester, Minnesota
CHEST TUBE INSERTION AND MANAGEMENT; DIAGNOSTIC THORACIC
   SURGICAL PROCEDURES

MOIRA CHAN-YEUNG, MB, FRCPC
Emeritus Professor, Department of Medicine, University of British Columbia, Vancouver, British Columbia, Canada
OCCUPATIONAL ASTHMA

JESSICA Y. CHIA, MD
Fellow in Pulmonary, Allergy, and Critical Care, Department of Medicine, Duke University Medical Center, Durham, North Carolina
PULMONARY COMPLICATIONS OF HEMATOPOIETIC STEM CELL
   TRANSPLANTATION

CHUNG-WAI CHOW, MD, PhD, FRCP(C)
Assistant Professor, Department of Medicine, University of Toronto, Toronto, Ontario, Canada
HOST DEFENSES

THOMAS V. COLBY, MD
Professor of Pathology, Mayo Clinic Arizona, Scottsdale, Arizona
INFLAMMATORY BOWEL DISEASE

CHRISTOPHER D. COLDREN, PhD
Assistant Professor, Department of Medicine, University of Colorado at Denver and Health Sciences Center, Denver, Colorado
BASIC SCIENCE OF GENETICS APPLIED TO LUNG DISEASES

JEAN-FRANÇOIS CORDIER, MD
Professor of Respiratory Medicine, Department of Respiratory Medicine, Reference Center for Orphan Pulmonary Diseases, Hôpital Louis Pradel, Université Claude Bernard, Lyon, France
EOSINOPHILIC LUNG DISEASE; ORGANIZING PNEUMONIA

ULRICH COSTABEL, MD, FCCP
Professor of Medicine, Medicine Faculty, University of Duisburg-Essen, Chief, Pheumology and Allergy, Ruhrlandklinic, Essen, Germany
IDIOPATHIC PULMONARY FIBROSIS AND OTHER IDIOPATHIC INTERSTITIAL PNEUMONIAS

VINCENT COTTIN, MD, PhD
Professor of Respiratory Medicine, Université Claude Bernard, Department of Respiratory Medicine Reference Center for Orphan Pulmonary Disease, Hôpital Louis Pradel, Lyon, France
EOSINOPHILIC LUNG DISEASE; ORGANIZING PNEUMONIA

GERARD J. CRINER, MD
Professor of Medicine, Director of Pulmonary & Critical Care Medicine, Temple University School of Medicine, Temple University Hospital, Pulmonary & Critical Care Medicine, Temple University, Director, Temple Lung Center, Temple University Hospital, Philadelphia, Pennsylvania
OXYGEN THERAPY

BRUCE H. CULVER, MD
Associate Professor of Medicine, Division of Pulmonary and Critical Care, University of Washington School of Medicine, Seattle, Washington
RESPIRATORY MECHANICS; GAS EXCHANGE IN THE LUNG; PULMONARY CIRCULATION; ACID–BASE BALANCE AND CONTROL OF VENTILATION; PULMONARY FUNCTION TESTING

CHARLES L. DALEY, MD
Professor of Medicine, Division of Pulmonary and Critical Care Medicine, University of Colorado Health Sciences Center, Head, Division of Mycobacterial and Respiratory Infections, Department of Medicine, National Jewish Medical and Research Center, Denver, Colorado
TUBERCULOSIS AND NONTUBERCULOUS MYCOBACTERIAL INFECTIONS

HELEN E. DAVIES, MB, BS, MRCP
Research Fellow, Oxford Centre for Respiratory Medicine and University of Oxford, Churchill Hospital, Oxford, United Kingdom
PLEURAL EFFUSION, EMPYEMA, AND PNEUMOTHORAX

MARC DECRAMER, MD, PhD
Professor, Respiratory Division, Katholieke Universiteit, Department of Pneumology, UZ Gasthuisberg, Leuven, Belgium
PULMONARY REHABILITATION

CLAUDE DESCHAMPS, MD, FACS
Professor of Surgery, Division of General Thoracic Surgery, Chair, Department of Surgery, Mayo Clinic, Rochester, Minnesota
CHEST TUBE INSERTION AND MANAGEMENT

ANDREAS H. DIACON, MD, PhD
Senior Lecturer, Division of Pulmonology, Department of Medicine, University of Stellenbosch, Part-Time Specialist, Division of Pulmonology, Department of Medicine, Tygerberg Academic Hospital, Cape Town, Western Cape, South Africa
PREOPERATIVE PULMONARY EVALUATION

CHRISTOPHE DOOMS, MD
Deputy Head of Clinic, Respiratory Oncology Unit, University Hospital Gasthuisberg, Leuven, Belgium
PET IMAGING

RYAN H. DOUGHERTY, MD
Clinical Fellow, Medicine – Pulmonary & Critical Care, University of California, San Francisco, San Francisco, California
ASTHMA: CELL BIOLOGY

NEIL J. DOUGLAS, MD, FRCP, FRCPE
Professor of Respiratory & Sleep Medicine, Department of Respiratory Medicine, University of Edinburgh, Director, Scottish National Sleep Centre, Edinburgh, United Kingdom
OBSTRUCTIVE SLEEP APNEA

GREGORY P. DOWNEY, MD, FRCP(C)
Professor, Medicine and Immunology, University of Colorado, Executive Vice President, Academic Affairs, Professor, Department of Medicine, Pediatrics, and Immunology, National Jewish Medical and Research Center, Denver, Colorado
HOST DEFENSES

SCOTT E. EVANS, MD
Assistant Professor, Department of Pulmonary Medicine, University of Texas-M.D. Anderson Cancer Center, Houston, Texas
PULMONARY FUNCTION TESTING

TIMOTHY W. EVANS, BSc, MD, PhD, DSc, FRCP, FRCA, FMedSci
Professor of Intensive Care Medicine, Critical Care Unit, Imperial College School of Medicine, Consultant in Intensive Care and Thoracic Medicine, Intensive Care Unit Royal Brompton Hospital, London, United Kingdom
PULMONARY HYPERTENSION

JEAN-WILLIAM FITTING, MD
Associate Professor, Service de Pneumologie, Centre Hospitalier Universitaire Vaudois, Lausanne, Switzerland
DISEASES OF THE THORACIC CAGE AND RESPIRATORY MUSCLES

RODNEY J. FOLZ, MD, PhD
Professor and Chief, Division of Pulmonary, Critical Care, and Sleep Disorders Medicine, University of Louisville Health Sciences Center, Louisville, Kentucky
PULMONARY COMPLICATIONS OF HEMATOPOIETIC STEM CELL TRANSPLANTATION

EDWARD R. GARRITY, JR, MD, MBA
Professor of Medicine, Section of Pulmonary and Critical Care, Vice-Chair, Clinical Operations, Department of Medicine, University of Chicago, Chicago, Illinois
LUNG TRANSPLANTATION

BRIAN K. GEHLBACH, MD
Assistant Professor of Medicine, Section of Pulmonary and Critical Care, University of Chicago, Chicago, Illinois
OBESITY

MARK W. GERACI, MD
Professor of Medicine, Head, Division of Pulmonary Sciences and Critical Care Medicine, Department of Medicine, University of Colorado Health Sciences Center, Denver, Colorado
BASIC SCIENCE OF GENETICS APPLIED TO LUNG DISEASES

RIK GOSSELINK, PT, PhD
Professor, Department of Rehabilitation Sciences, Katholieke Universiteit Leuven, Department of Pneumology, UZ Gasthuisberg, Leuven, Belgium
PULMONARY REHABILITATION

E. BRIGITTE GOTTSCHALL, MD, MSPH
Assistant Professor, Division of Pulmonary and Critical Care Medicine, Department of Medicine, Department of Preventive Medicine and Biometrics, University of Colorado at Denver and Health Sciences Center, Denver, Colorado
ASBESTOSIS

MICHAEL P. GRUBER, MD
Division of Pulmonary Sciences and Critical Care Medicine, University of Colorado Health Sciences Center, Denver, Colorado
PULMONARY EMBOLISM

J.C. GRUTTERS, MD, PhD
Heart Lung Center Utrecht, Department of Pulmonology, St. Antonius Hospital, Niewegein, the Netherlands
CONNECTIVE TISSUE DISORDERS

JESSE B. HALL, MD
Professor of Medicine, Anesthesia, and Critical Care, Section Chief, Pulmonary and Critical Care, University of Chicago, Chicago, Illinois
OBESITY

DAVID M. HANSELL, MD, FRCP, FRCR
Professor of Thoracic Imaging, Department of Radiology, Royal Brompton Hospital, London, United Kingdom
IMAGING TECHNIQUES

INDERJIT K. HANSRA, MD, MS
Clinical Associate, Department of Pulmonary and Critical Care, Tufts University, Boston, Massachusetts
NONINVASIVE MECHANICAL VENTILATION

FELIX J.F. HERTH, MD, PhD, FCCP
Professor of Medicine, Pneumology and Critical Care Medicine, Thoraxklinik, University of Heidelberg, Heidelberg, Germany
TRANSBRONCHIAL AND ESOPHAGEAL ULTRASOUND-GUIDED BIOPSY OF THE MEDIASTINUM

NICHOLAS S. HILL, MD
Professor of Medicine, Chief, Division of Pulmonary, Critical Care, and Sleep Medicine, Tufts-New England Medical Center, Tufts University School of Medicine, Boston, Massachusetts
NONINVASIVE MECHANICAL VENTILATION

STELLA E. HINES, MD, FACP
University of Colorado Health Sciences Center, Denver, Colorado
EXTRINSIC ALLERGIC ALVEOLITIS

RICHARD HUBBARD, MSc, DM
Professor of Respiratory Epidemiology, Epidemiology, and Public Health, University of Nottingham, Consultant Chest Physician, Respiratory Medicine, Nottingham City Hospital, Nottingham, United Kingdom
ASTHMA: EPIDEMIOLOGY AND RISK FACTORS

GÉRARD J. HUCHON, MD
Head of Service de Pneumologie et Réanimation, Hôpital de l'Hôtel-Dieu, Professor of Respiratory Medicine, Université René Descartes, Paris, France
BACTERIAL PNEUMONIA; NONBACTERIAL PNEUMONIA

LEONARD D. HUDSON, MD
Professor, Division of Pulmonary and Critical Care Medicine, Department of Medicine, Seattle, Washington
ACUTE RESPIRATORY DISTRESS SYNDROME

JOHN R. HURST, PhD, MRCP
Senior Lecturer, Academic Unit of Respiratory Medicine, Royal Free & University College Medical School, University College London, Honorary Consultant in Respiratory and Acute Medicine, Royal Free Hampstead NHS Trust, London, United Kingdom
MANAGEMENT OF ACUTE EXACERBATIONS OF CHRONIC OBSTRUCTIVE PULMONARY DISEASE

MICHAEL C. IANNUZZI, MD, MBA
Division of Pulmonary, Critical Care, and Sleep Medicine, Department of Medicine, Mount Sinai School of Medicine, New York, New York
SARCOIDOSIS

JAMES R. JETT, MD
Professor of Medicine, Mayo Clinic College of Medicine, Consultant in Pulmonary Medicine and Medical Oncology, Rochester, Minnesota
LUNG TUMORS; MALIGNANT PLEURAL MESOTHELIOMA

JOEL D. KAUFMAN, MD, MPH
Professor, Department of Medicine, Department of Environmental and Occupational Health Sciences, Department of Epidemiology, University of Washington, Seattle, Washington
AIR POLLUTION

VICTOR KIM, MD
Assistant Professor of Medicine, Division of Pulmonary and Critical Care Medicine, Department of Internal Medicine, Temple University School of Medicine, Philadelphia, Pennsylvania
OXYGEN THERAPY

COENRAAD F.N. KOEGELENBERG, MBChB, FCP(SA), MRCP(UK)
Senior Specialist, Division of Pulmonology, Department of Medicine, University of Stellenbosch, Senior Specialist, Division of Pulmonology, Department of Medicine, Tygerberg Academic Hospital, Cape Town, Western Cape, South Africa
PREOPERATIVE PULMONARY EVALUATION

JOHN W. KREIT, MD
Associate Professor of Medicine, Division of Pulmonary, Allergy, and Critical Care Medicine, University of Pittsburgh School of Medicine, Pittsburgh, Pennsylvania
HEMOPTYSIS

MICHAEL J. KROWKA, MD
Professor of Medicine, Pulmonary and Critical Care, Mayo Clinic, Rochester, Minnesota
HEPATIC AND BILIARY DISEASE

DANIEL LANGER, MSc
Department of Rehabilitation Sciences, Katholieke Universiteit Leuven, Respiratory Division, UZ Gasthuisberg, Leuven, Belgium
PULMONARY REHABILITATION

STEPHEN E. LAPINSKY, MB BCh, MSc, FRCPC
Associate Professor of Medicine, Department of Medicine, University of Toronto, Site Director, Intensive Care Unit, Department of Medicine, Mount Sinai Hospital, Toronto, Ontario, Canada
PREGNANCY

STEPHEN C. LAZARUS, MD
Professor of Medicine, Director, Fellowship Program in Pulmonary & Critical Care Medicine, Associate Director, Adult Pulmonary Laboratory, Senior Investigator, Cardiovascular Research Institute, Division of Pulmonary and Critical Care Medicine, University of California, San Francisco, San Francisco, California
ASTHMA: CELL BIOLOGY

Y.C. GARY LEE, MBChB, PhD, FRACP, FCCP
Consultant Chest Physician and Senior Lecturer, Oxford Centre for Respiratory Medicine, University of Oxford, Churchill Hospital, Oxford, United Kingdom
PLEURAL EFFUSION, EMPYEMA, AND PNEUMOTHORAX

SYLVIE LEROY, MD
Medical Doctor - Practitioner, Department of Pulmonology, Hospital Calmette, Lille, France
SILICOSIS AND COAL WORKER'S PNEUMOCONIOSIS

MARC C.I. LIPMAN, MD, FRCP
Cunsultant Physician, Department of Respiratory & HIV Medicine, Royal Free Hospital, London, United Kingdom
PULMONARY INFECTIONS

WILLIAM MACNEE, MBChB, MD, FRCP(Glas), FRCP(Edin)
Professor of Respiratory & Environmental Medicine, MRC Centre for Inflammation Research, University of Edinburgh, Honorary Consultant Physicians, Respiratory Medicine, Royal Infirmary of Edinburgh, Edinburgh, Scotland, United Kingdom
CHRONIC OBSTRUCTIVE PULMONARY DISEASE: EPIDEMIOLOGY, PHYSIOLOGY, AND CLINICAL EVALUATION

JEAN-LUC MALO, MD
Professor, Department of Medicine, Faculté de Médecine, Université de Montréal, Chest physician, Medicine, Hôpital du Sacré.-Coeur de Montréal, Montréal, Québec, Canada
OCCUPATIONAL ASTHMA

RYAN M. MCGHAN, MD, MSPH
Instructor in Medicine, Division of Pulmonary Sciences and Critical Care, Department of Medicine, University of Colorado at Denver and Health Sciences Center, Denver, Colorado
CORTICOSTEROIDS

SARAH MCKINLEY, MD
University of Colorado Health Sciences Center, Denver, Colorado
BASIC SCIENCE OF GENETICS APPLIED TO LUNG DISEASES

DAVID E. MIDTHUN, MD
Associate Professor of Medicine, Pulmonary and Critical Care Medicine, Mayo Clinic College of Medicine, Rochester, Minnesota
LUNG TUMORS

ROBERT F. MILLER, MB, BS, FRCP
Professor, Centre for Sexual Health and HIV Research, University College London, Honorary Consultant, University College London Hospitals, London, United Kingdom
PULMONARY INFECTIONS

THEO J. MORAES, MD, FRCPC
Fellow, Division of Respirology, The Hospital for Sick Children, Toronto, Ontario, Canada
HOST DEFENSES

JEFFREY L. MYERS, MD
A. James French Professor of Diagnostic Pathology, Department of Pathology, University of Michigan Medical School, Director, Division of Anatomic Pathology, Department of Pathology, University of Michigan Health System, Ann Arbor, Michigan
LAM AND OTHER DIFFUSE LUNG DISEASES

MARGARET J. NEFF, MD
Associate Professor of Medicine, Division of Pulmonary and Critical Care Medicine, Department of Medicine, University of Washington, Seattle, Washington
ACUTE RESPIRATORY DISTRESS SYNDROME

LEE S. NEWMAN, MD, MA
Professor, Department of Preventive Medicine and Biometrics, Department of Medicine, University of Colorado at Denver and Health Sciences Center, Denver, Colorado
ASBESTOSIS; TOXIC INHALATIONAL LUNG INJURY

ERIC J. OLSON, MD
Associate Professor of Medicine, Mayo Clinic College of Medicine, Division of Pulmonary and Critical Care Medicine, Mayo Clinic, Rochester, Minnesota
LAM AND OTHER DIFFUSE LUNG DISEASES

SIMON P.G. PADLEY, BSc, MB.BS, FRCP, FRCR
Honorary Senior Lecturer, Imperial College School of Medicine, Imperial College, Consultant, Radiology Department, Chelsea and Westminster Hospital, Royal Brompton Hospital, London, United Kingdom
IMAGING TECHNIQUES

MARTYN R. PARTRIDGE, MD, FRCP
Professor of Respiratory Medicine, National Heart and Lung Institute Division, Charing Cross Hospital, Honorary Consultant Physician, Department of Respiratory Medicine, Imperial College London, London, United Kingdom
ASTHMA: CLINICAL FEATURES, DIAGNOSIS, AND TREATMENT

IAN D. PAVORD, DM, FRCP
Honorary Professor of Medicine, Department of Respiratory Medicine, Allergy and Thoracic Surgery, Glenfield Hospital, Leicester, United Kingdom
COUGH

JOANNA C. PORTER, MA, BM, BCh, FRCP, PhD
Honorary Senior Lecturer in Respiratory Medicine, Laboratory for Molecular Cell Biology, University College London, Honorary Consultant in Respiratory and General Internal Medicine, Department of Respiratory Medicine, University College London Hospitals NHS Trust, Clinical Research Fellow, MRC Laboratory for Molecular Cell Biology, University College London, London, United Kingdom
DYSPNEA

ANTOINE RABBAT, MD
Praticien Hospitalier, Assistance Publique Hôpitaux de Paris, Pneumologie and Réanimation, Hôtel-Dieu, Paris, France
BACTERIAL PNEUMONIA; NONBACTERIAL PNEUMONIA

FELIX RATJEN, MD, PhD, FRCPC
Professor, Department of Pediatrics, University of Toronto, Division Head, Department of Respiratory Medicine, The Hospital for Sick Children, Toronto, Ontario, Canada
CYSTIC FIBROSIS

ANNA K. REED, MB, ChB, MRCP
Clinical Research Fellow in Pulmonary Vascular Disease, Unit of Critical Care, Imperial College School of Medicine and National Heart Lung Institute, Royal Brompton Hospital, London, United Kingdom
PULMONARY HYPERTENSION

MELISSA L. ROSADO-DE-CHRISTENSON, MD, FACR
Adjunct Professor of Radiology, Department of Radiology and Nuclear Medicine, Uniformed Services University of the Health Sciences, Bethesda, Maryland
DISORDERS OF THE MEDIASTINUM

CECILE S. ROSE, MD, MPH
Associate Professor of Medicine, University of Colorado Health Sciences Center, Director, Occupational Lung Disease Clinic, National Jewish Medical and Research Center, Denver, Colorado
EXTRINSIC ALLERGIC ALVEOLITIS

CHARIS ROUSSOS, MD, PhD
Professor and Chairman, Pulmonary and Critical Care, University of Athens, Medical School, Athens, Greece
PHYSIOLOGY AND TESTING OF RESPIRATORY MUSCLES

LUIS G. RUIZ, MD
Fellow, Section of Pulmomary and Critical Care Department of Medicine, University of Chicago, Chicago, Illinois
LUNG TRANSPLANTATION

JAY H. RYU, MD
Professor of Medicine, Division of Pulmonary and Critical Care Medicine, Mayo Clinic College of Medicine, Rochester, Minnesota
LAM AND OTHER DIFFUSE LUNG DISEASES

GLENIS K. SCADDING, MA, MD, MRCP
Honorary Senior Lecturer, Department of Immunology, University College, Consultant Allergist/Rhinologist, Department of Allergy/Medical Rhinology, Royal National Throat, Nose, and Ear Hospital, London, United Kingdom
RHINITIS AND SINUSITIS

PAUL D. SCANLON, MD
Professor of Medicine, Division of Pulmonary and Critical Care Medicine, Mayo Clinic, Rochester, Minnesota
PULMONARY FUNCTION TESTING

REBECCA E. SCHANE, MD
Clinical Research Fellow, General and Internal Medicine, Division of Pulmonary/Critical Care Medicine, Center for Tobacco Control Research and Education, General and Internal Medicine, Cardiovascular Research Institute, University of California, San Francisco, San Francisco, California
CHRONIC OBSTRUCTIVE PULMONARY DISEASE: MANAGEMENT
   OF CHRONIC DISEASE

MARVIN I. SCHWARZ, MD
University of Colorado Health Sciences Center, James C. Campbell Professor of Pulmonary Medicine, Division of Pulmonary Sciences and Critical Care Medicine, University of Colorado, Denver, Colorado
PULMONARY VASCULITIS AND HEMORRHAGE

FABIAN SEBASTIAN, MD, FRCR
Radiology Registrar, Department of Radiology, University College Hospital, London, United Kingdom
PERCUTANEOUS BIOPSY PROCEDURES

JONATHAN E. SEVRANSKY, MD
Assistant Professor of Medicine, Medical Director, JHMBC ICU, Division of Pulmonary and Critical Care Medicine, Johns Hopkins Asthma and Allergy Center, Baltimore, Maryland
PULMONARY CIRCULATION

LORI SHAH, MD
Assistant Professor of Medicine, Associate Director, Lung Transplantation Program, Department of Medicine, Mount Sinai School of Medicine, New York, New York
SARCOIDOSIS

PENNY SHAW, MBBS, DMRD, MRCP, FRCR
Consultant Radiologist with Thoracic Subspecialty Interest, Department of Radiology, University College London Hospitals NHS Trust, London, United Kingdom
PERCUTANEOUS BIOPSY PROCEDURES

DAVID W. SHIMABUKURO, MDCM
Assistant Professor, Department of Anesthesia and Perioperative Care, University of California, San Francisco, San Francisco, California
AIRWAY MANAGEMENT

KATHY E. SIETSEMA, MD
Professor of Medicine, Department of Medicine, David Geffen School of Medicine at UCLA, Los Angeles, California, Chief, Division of Respiratory & Critical Care Physiology and Medicine, Department of Medicine, Harbor-UCLA Medical Center, Torrance, California
EXERCISE TESTING

ANITA K. SIMONDS, MD
Consultant in Respiratory Medicine, Royal Brompton
Hospital, London, United Kingdon
SCOLIOSIS AND KYPHOSCOLIOSIS

ARTHUR S. SLUTSKY, MD, PhD
Professor, Department of Medicine, Surgery and
Biomedical Engineering, University of Toronto,
Vice President, Research, St. Michael's Hospital, Toronto,
Ontario, Canada
INVASIVE MECHANICAL VENTILATION

STEPHEN G. SPIRO, MD, FRCP
Professor of Respiratory Medicine, Consultant Physician,
General and Thoracic Medicine, University College
London Hospitals NHS Trust, London, United Kingdom
THORACENTESIS AND CLOSED PLEURAL BIOPSY

DANIEL H. STERMAN, MD
Associate Professor of Medicine, Department of Medicine,
University of Pennsylvania, Director of Interventional
Pulmonology, Pulmonary, Allergy, and Critical Care Division,
University of Pennsylvania School of Medicine, Philadelphia,
Pennsylvania
BRONCHOSCOPY

KAYLAN E. STINSON, MSPH
Professional Research Assistant, Department of Preventive
Medicine and Biometrics, University of Colorado at Denver
and Health Science Center, Denver, Colorado
TOXIC INHALATIONAL LUNG INJURY

DIANE C. STROLLO, MD, FACR
Associate Professor, Department of Radiology, University of
Pittsburgh Medical Center, Pittsburgh, Pennsylvania
DISORDERS OF THE MEDIASTINUM

PATRICK J. STROLLO, JR, MD, FCCP, FAASM
Associate Professor of Medicine, Medical Director, UPMC
Sleep Medicine Center, Division of Pulmonary, Allergy, and
Critical Care Medicine, University of Pittsburgh, Pittsburgh,
Pennsylvania
CENTRAL SLEEP APNEA AND OTHER FORMS OF SLEEP-DISORDERED
  BREATHING

DARRYL Y. SUE, MD
Professor of Clinical Medicine, Department of Medicine,
David Geffen School of Medicine at UCLA, Los Angeles,
California, Associate Chair and Program Director, Department
of Medicine, Harbor-UCLA Medical Center, Torrance,
California
EXERCISE TESTING

ALVIN S. TEIRSTEIN, MD
Professor of Medicine, Department of Medicine,
Mout Sinai School of Medicine, New York, New York
SARCOIDOSIS

ANTONI TORRES, MD
Professor, Facultat de Medicina, Universitat de Barcelona,
Chief, Department of Pulmonology, Hospital Clinic,
Barcelona, Spain
NOSOCOMIAL PNEUMONIA

THIERRY TROOSTERS, PhD
Professor Respiratory Division, Katholieke Universiteit
Leuven, Department of Pneumology, UZ Gasthuisberg,
Leuven, Belgium
PULMONARY REHABILITATION

ELIZABETH TULLIS, MD, FRCPC
Associate Professor, Department of Respirology, University of
Toronto, Medical Director, Adult Cystic Fibrosis Clinic,
Division Head, Department of Respirology, St. Michael's
Hospital, Toronto, Ontario, Canada
CYSTIC FIBROSIS

ANIL VACHANI, MD
Assistant Professor of Medicine, Department of Medicine,
University of Pennsylvania, Philadelphia, Pennsylvania
BRONCHOSCOPY

MAURICIO VALENCIA, MD
Senior Researcher, Respiratory Intensive Care Medicine,
Hospital Clinic de Barcelona, Barcelona, Spain
NOSOCOMIAL PNEUMONIA

J.M.M. VAN DEN BOSCH, MD
Heart Lung Center Utrecht, Department of Pulmonology,
St. Antonius Hospital, Niewegein, The Netherlands
CONNECTIVE TISSUE DISORDERS

JOHAN VANSTEENKISTE, MD, PhD
Associate Professor, Internal Medicine, Catholic
University, Head of Clinic, Respiratory Oncology Unit
(Pulmonology), University Hospital Gasthuisberg, Leuven,
Belgium
PET IMAGING

THEODOROS VASSILAKOPOULOS, MD
Assistant Professor, Critical Care Department,
University of Athens, Medical School,
Athens, Greece
PHYSIOLOGY AND TESTING OF RESPIRATORY MUSCLES

BENOIT WALLAERT, MD
Professor of Medicine, University Lille, Head, Clinique
des Maladies Respiratoirses, Hospital Calmette, Lille,
France
SILICOSIS AND COAL WORKER'S PNEUMOCONIOSIS

JADWIGA A. WEDZICHA, MD, FRCP
Professor of Respiratory Medicine, Academic Unit of
Respiratory Medicine, Royal Free & University College
Medical School, University College London, Royal Free
Hampstead NHS Trust, London, United Kingdom
MANAGEMENT OF ACUTE EXACERBATIONS OF CHRONIC OBSTRUCTIVE
  PULMONARY DISEASE

ATHOL WELLS, MBChB, FRACP, MD
Consultant Physician, Royal Brompton Hospital, London,
United Kingdom
APPROACH TO DIAGNOSIS OF DIFFUSE LUNG DISEASE

DOROTHY A. WHITE, MD
Assistant Professor of Medicine, Memorial Sloan-Kettering
Cancer Center, New York, New York
DRUGS AND THE LUNGS

JEANINE P. WIENER-KRONISH, MD
Professor of Anesthesia and Medicine, Department of
Anesthesia and Perioperative Care, University of California,
San Francisco, San Francisco, California
AIRWAY MANAGEMENT

MARK A. WOODHEAD, MBBS, BSc, DM, FRCP
Consultant in General and Respiratory Medicine, Department
of Respiratory Medicine, Manchester Royal Infirmary,
Honorary Senior Lecturer, Faculty of Medical and Human
Sciences, University of Manchester, Manchester, United
Kingdom
AN APPROACH TO THE DIAGNOSIS OF PULMONARY INFECTION

PRESCOTT G. WOODRUFF, MD, MPH
Assistant Professor of Medicine in Residence, Department
of Medicine, Division of Pulmonary Critical Care Medicine,
University of California, San Francisco, California
CHRONIC OBSTRUCTIVE PULMONARY DISEASE: MANAGEMENT
    OF CHRONIC DISEASE

STEPHEN J. WORT, MA (OXON), MBBS, MRCP, PhD
Clinical Senior Lecturer, Pulmonary Hypertension and Critical
Care, Imperial College, Consultant, Pulmonary Hypertension
and Critical Care, Royal Brompton and Harefield NHS Trust,
London, United Kingdom
PULMONARY HYPERTENSION

JOKKE WYNANTS, MD
Resident, Respiratory Oncology Unit (Pulmonology),
University Hospital Gasthuisberg, Leuven, Belgium
PET IMAGING

Preface

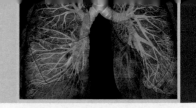

The second edition of this book was published in 2004, 5 years after its initial launch. The intent of both editions was (a) to bring the ideas of the world community of respiratory medicine together into a single publication, (b) to utilize the extraordinary advances in computer graphics and publishing to emphasize a visual, as opposed to a textual, presentation of material, and (c) to combine detailed presentations of lung structure and physiology with clinical material. We were gratified by the resulting product, the continuing praise given to the book by its reviewers, the comments we received from numerous readers, and its acceptance by our colleagues around the world.

This third edition maintains this same focus, emphasizing highly visual presentation including numerous figures, graphics, and tables. One third of the chapters are written by new contributors. Each chapter that retains the same authorship has been rewritten and rereviewed. There are new chapters on PET Imaging, the Basic Science of Genetics, Exercise Testing, Mediastinal Noninvasive Biopsy, Oxygen Therapy, and Rehabilitation. The book was extensively reorganized for the second edition and this system remains. Additional emphasis has been placed on controversial issues and on a limited number of "selected readings" rather than exhaustive reference lists.

This third edition remains directed at trainees in respiratory medicine, physicians practicing general medicine, and all respiratory medicine clinicians. Once again, the editors have been greatly supported by the development editors at Elsevier. In particular, Adrianne Brigido has kept the project on schedule and encouraged all contributors to deliver. Her guidance is pivotal and we are most grateful to her. We hope readers enjoy and profit from this volume and that it provides a step forward in the management of common respiratory problems.

Contents

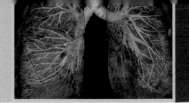

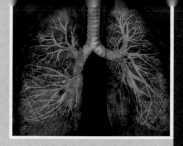

1 Imaging Techniques

SIMON P.G. PADLEY • DAVID M. HANSELL

Today, clinicians have two main imaging techniques at their disposal for the investigation of patients with chest disease—the chest radiograph, which produces a projectional image, and computed tomography (CT), which provides a cross-sectional view. Other techniques, such as magnetic resonance imaging (MRI), radionuclide scanning, and ultrasonography, can provide valuable additional information but are rarely performed without prior chest radiography or CT. Because imaging is an integral part of the practice of respiratory medicine, an understanding of the strengths and weaknesses of these various techniques is vital. The advent of high-resolution and spiral CT has lent further precision to the investigation of patients with suspected chest disease, but the use of such sophisticated tests should not be indiscriminate; accurate interpretation of the chest radiograph remains the mainstay of thoracic imaging.

PLAIN CHEST RADIOGRAPHY

Technical Considerations

The views of the chest most frequently performed are the erect posteroanterior (PA) and lateral projections, taken with the patient's breath held at total lung capacity. On a frontal PA chest radiograph, just under half the lung is free from overlying structures, such as the ribs or diaphragm. Many technical factors, notably the kilovoltage and film-screen combination used, determine how well the lungs are shown. The characteristics of radiographic film make it impossible to obtain perfect exposure of the least and most dense parts of the chest in a single radiograph. Methods to overcome this handicap of radiographic film include the use of high-kilovoltage techniques, asymmetric film-screen combinations, and sophisticated devices that control regional X-ray exposure.

Because the coefficients of X-ray absorption of bone and soft tissue approach one another at high kilovoltage, the skeletal structures do not obscure the lungs on a higher kilovoltage radiograph to the same degree as on low-kilovoltage radiographs. The high-kilovoltage radiograph thus demonstrates much more of the lung. Improved penetration of the mediastinum also allows some of the central airways to be seen. Although high-kilovoltage radiographs are preferable for routine examinations of the lungs and mediastinum, low-kilovoltage radiographs provide good detail of unobscured lung because of the improved contrast between lung vessels and surrounding lung (Figure 1-1). Furthermore, dense lesions, for example, calcified pleural plaques, are particularly well demonstrated on low-kilovoltage films.

One of the most important major advances in plain-film radiography in recent times was the introduction of more sensitive phosphorescent screens. Screens luminesce when an X-ray beam falls on them, are housed in a film cassette, and

are in contact with the radiographic film, which records the image. The improved light emission from the latest rare-earth phosphors compared with older calcium screens results in shorter exposure times and thus sharper images. A significant advance in film-screen combinations for chest imaging was the development of an asymmetric combination of a thin front screen and high-contrast film emulsion and, on the reverse side of the film base, a thicker back screen and a low-contrast film emulsion. In this way, the wide spectrum of transmission of X-rays through the thorax can be accommodated. Such a film-screen combination shows significantly more detail in the mediastinum and lung obscured by the diaphragm and heart.

To overcome the considerable density differences between the mediastinum and lungs, attempts have been made to produce a more uniformly exposed chest radiograph (Figure 1-2). One of the most widely used was the advanced multiple beam equalization radiography (AMBER) system. However, the advent of the digital chest radiograph, both as an image stored on a phosphor plate and then digitally scanned, or as an images captured directly onto a detector plate, have largely superseded the AMBER radiograph. This is largely because of the much wider latitude of digital systems that allow the image to be postprocessed to provide optimum visualization of the relevant structures (see Figure 1-2).

The frontal and lateral projections are sufficient for most purposes in chest radiography. Other radiographic views are less frequently required, but they should not be overlooked because they may solve a particular problem quickly and cheaply. The lateral decubitus view is not, as its name implies, a lateral view. It is a frontal view taken with a horizontal beam and the patient lying on his or her side. Its main purpose is to demonstrate the movement of fluid in the pleural space (Figure 1-3). An adaptation of this is the "lateral shoot-through" sometimes used in bed-bound patients—a lateral radiograph of the supine patient is taken to show an anterior pneumothorax behind the sternum (not always visible on a frontal chest radiograph; Figure 1-4). If a pleural effusion is not loculated, it gravitates, to some extent, to the dependent part of the pleural cavity. If the patient lies on his or her side, the fluid layers between the chest wall and the lung edge. This view may also be useful for demonstrating a small pneumothorax, because the visceral pleural edge of the lung falls away from the chest walls in the nondependent hemithorax.

The lordotic view, now rarely performed, is taken by angling the X-ray beam 15 degrees cranially, either by positioning the patient upright and angling the beam up or by leaving the beam horizontal and leaning the patient backward. In this way, the lung apices are demonstrated free from the superimposed clavicle and first rib. It may be useful to differentiate pulmonary

FIGURE 1-1 The effect of low and high kilovoltage on the chest radiograph. **A,** Low-kilovoltage chest radiograph showing good detail of the bones. Note the calcified fibroadenoma within the right breast (*arrow*). **B,** A high-kilovoltage radiograph of the same patient shows better soft tissue detail within the mediastinum but less definition of bony structures. Note the loss of visualization of the calcified fibroadenoma in the right breast.

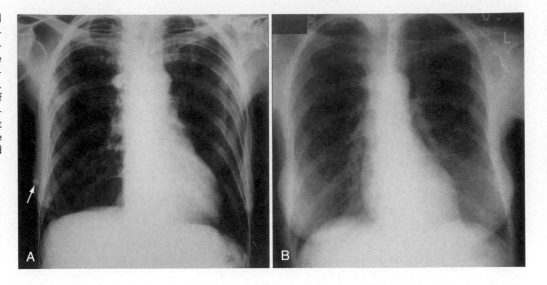

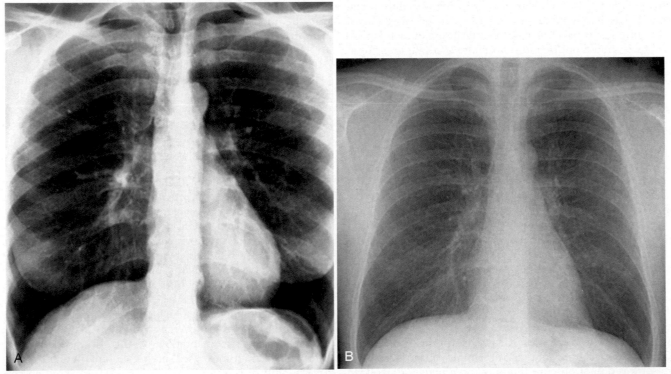

FIGURE 1-2 Comparison of conventional and advanced multiple beam equalization radiographs. **A,** Advanced multiple-beam equalization radiograph (scanning equalization radiograph) revealing detail behind the heart and right hemidiaphragm. **B,** Typical digital chest radiograph.

shadows from incidental calcification of the costochondral junctions (Figure 1-5).

Portable Chest Radiography

Portable or mobile chest radiography has the obvious advantage that the examination can be carried out without moving the patient from the ward. However, the portable radiograph has many disadvantages. The shorter-focus film distance results in undesirable magnification, and high-kilovoltage techniques cannot be used because most portable machines are unable to deliver high kilovoltage. Furthermore, the maximum current is limited so that long exposure times are needed, which potentially increases blurring of the image. Portable lateral radiographs are even less likely to be successful because of the extremely long exposure times required.

To position patients for portable radiography is difficult, and the resultant radiographs are often suboptimal. Even in the so-called erect position, in which the patient sits up, the chest is rarely as vertical as it is in a standing patient. Because many patients are unable to move to the radiography department

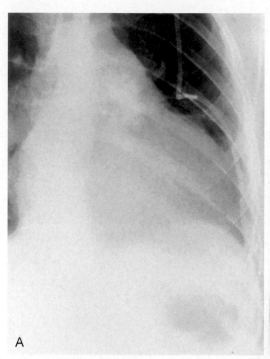
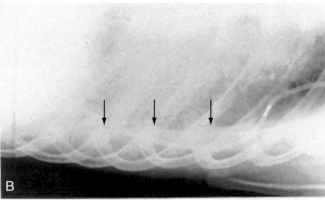

FIGURE 1-3 Demonstration of small effusions. **A,** Posteroanterior chest radiograph of a patient who has a ventriculoperitoneal shunt. More soft tissue than usual occurs between the gastric air bubble and the base of the lung because of a subpulmonic effusion. **B,** Decubitus film shows redistribution of fluid to the dependent part of the chest (*arrows*).

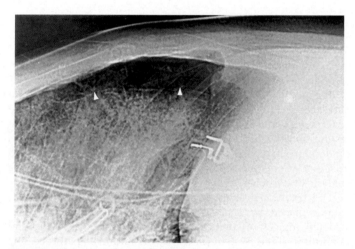

FIGURE 1-4 Lateral shoot-through digital radiograph of a patient in the intensive care unit. The anterior pneumothorax (note the visceral pleural edge—*arrowheads*) was not obvious on the anteroposterior portable radiograph.

for a formal radiograph, any method of improving the quality of a portable chest radiograph, such as digital radiography, represents a significant advance.

Digital Chest Radiography

Digital technology is integral to techniques such as CT and MRI. Conventional film radiography as a means of image capture, storage, and display represents something of a compromise, and it has become apparent that digital image acquisition, transmission, display, and storage can, with advantage, be applied to chest radiography.

The most widely employed systems use conventional radiographic equipment but use a reusable photostimulatable plate instead of conventional film. The reusable phosphor plate is housed in a cassette and stores some of the energy of the incident X-ray as a latent image. On scanning the plate with a laser beam, the stored energy is emitted as light that is detected by a photomultiplier and converted into a digital signal. The digital information is then manipulated, displayed, and stored in whatever format is desired. The phosphor plate can be reused once the latent image has been erased by exposure to light. Most currently available computed radiography systems produce a digital radiograph with a resolution of more than 10 line pairs per millimeter. The fundamental requirement to segment the image into a finite number of pixels has resulted in much work to determine the relationship between pixel size, which affects spatial resolution, and the detectability of focal abnormalities. Although it might seem desirable to aim for an image composed of pixels of the smallest possible size, an inverse relationship occurs between pixel size and the cost and speed of data handling. Thus, pixel size is ultimately a compromise between image quality and ease of data processing and storage.

An unequivocal advantage of digital computed radiography over conventional film radiography is the linear photoluminescence-dose response, which is much greater than that of conventional film. This extremely wide latitude coupled with the facility for image processing produces diagnostic images over a wide range of exposures.

Observer performance studies have shown that computed radiography could equal conventional film radiography in virtually any task. However, postprocessing of the digital image has to be used to match the digital radiograph to the specific task. Enhancement of the image for one purpose often degrades it for another. Reports conflict as to whether digital chest

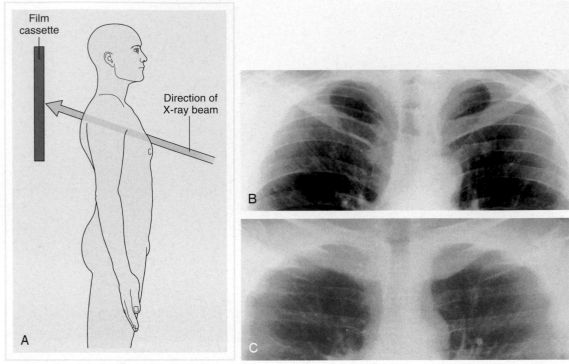

FIGURE 1-5 The value of lordotic views. **A,** Method of obtaining a lordotic view of the lung apices: the X-ray beam is angled upward. **B,** Selective view of the upper zones of a patient who presented with hemoptysis, with a suggestion of a small opacity projected over the anterior end of the left first rib. **C,** A lordotic view confirms that the small opacity is intrapulmonary (rather than calcified costochondral cartilage).

radiographs can be satisfactorily interpreted on television monitors, as opposed to laser-printed film, but it is increasingly apparent that high-resolution monitors are adequate for making primary diagnoses from digital chest radiographs.

COMPUTED TOMOGRAPHY

The same basic principles as for film radiography apply to CT, namely the absorption of X-rays by tissues that contain constituents of different atomic number. By use of multiple projections and computed calculations of radiographic density, slight differences in X-ray absorption are displayed as a cross-sectional image. The components of a CT scanner include an X-ray tube, which rotates around the patient, an array of X-ray detectors opposite the tube, together contained within the gantry. The patient lies on the examination couch, and this moves the patient through the aperture of the CT gantry. The data acquired are then processed by the CT computer, resulting in the final images, displayed on the CT monitor, and traditionally printed onto film.

There has been an impressive and rapid improvement in CT hardware capability in the past decade. Most particularly, the advent of multiple-channel CT scanners results in the ability to acquire simultaneous helical data sets. An accompanying increase in gantry rotation speed coupled with the reduction in the size of the individual detectors has resulted in extremely detailed images being acquired in very short scan times. On the current top specification scanners from the major manufacturers, there are 64 channels available, each with a detector size of as little as 0.5 mm. An entire thorax can now be scanned at submillimeter resolution in 6–10 sec. Thus, spiral (also known as volume or helical) scanning entails continuous scanning and table movement

into the CT gantry (Figure 1-6). The information is reconstructed into axial sections, perpendicular to the long axis of the patient, identical to conventional CT sections.

Temporal resolution has been further improved, because data reconstruction algorithms now allow CT images to be generated from a partial rotation of the gantry. Thus, temporal resolution of as little as 125 msec is now possible and enables modern multichannel CT scanners to acquire cardiac gated images that effectively freeze cardiac motion. This then allows analysis of coronary artery and cardiac anatomy.

The traditional analysis of printed film has, by necessity, been replaced by analysis of axial and multiplanar reconstructed images on dedicated CT or Picture Archiving and Communications System (PACS) workstations. Postprocessing of these thin sections also allows the production of surface-rendered images that mimic the appearances familiar to bronchoscopists. These virtual bronchoscopic images are visually pleasing and allow an exquisite appreciation of the endoluminal anatomy. They also have a role in the planning of interventional procedures, including transbronchial needle biopsy and endoluminal stent insertion (Figure 1-7).

Technical Considerations

The CT image is composed of a matrix of picture elements (pixels). A fixed number of pixels make up the matrix, so the size of each pixel varies according to the diameter of the circle to be scanned. A typical matrix in a modern CT system would be 512 × 512 pixels. The smaller the circle size, the smaller the area represented by a pixel and the higher the spatial resolution of the image. In practical terms, the field of view size is adjusted to the size of area of interest, usually the chest diameter.

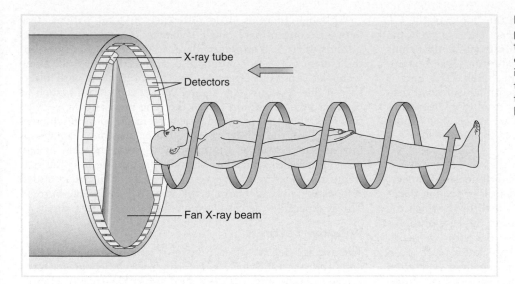

FIGURE 1-6 The principle of spiral computed tomography. The patient moves into the scanner with the X-ray tube continuously rotating and the detectors acquiring information. The rapidity of data acquisition allows a complete examination of the thorax to be performed in a single breath hold.

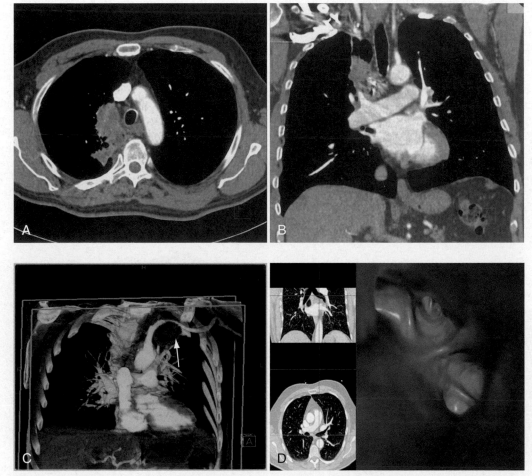

FIGURE 1-7 Data set from a multi-detector CT. **A,** This axial image demonstrates a bronchogenic carcinoma lying in a right paratracheal position. **B,** A reformat from the same data demonstrates the same abnormality in the coronal plane without loss of image resolution. **C,** A coronal volume rendered image of a different patient demonstrating a left superior sulcus tumour encasing the left subclavian artery (*arrow*). **D,** Virtual bronchoscopy image from a normal patient.

Often a marked difference occurs in the "look" of the CT images obtained on different CT scanners. This is largely the result of differences in the software reconstruction algorithms used to smooth the image, to a greater or lesser extent, by averaging the density of neighboring pixels. The lung is a high-contrast environment, so less smoothing is needed than in other parts of the body. Higher spatial-resolution algorithms (which make image noise—a granular appearance—more conspicuous) are generally more desirable for lung work.

Section Thickness

Although a CT section is viewed as a two-dimensional image, it has a third dimension of depth. The depth, or section thickness, is determined by the width of the slit through which the X-ray beam passes (beam collimation) or in the case of multichannel systems by the width of the detector elements. Because a section has a predetermined thickness, each pixel has a volume, and this three-dimensional element is referred to as a voxel. The computer calculates the average radiographic density of tissue within each voxel, and the final CT image consists of a representation of the numerous voxels (not individually visible without magnification) in the section. The single attenuation value of a voxel represents the average of the attenuation values of all the various structures within the voxel. The thicker the section, the greater the chance that different structures will be included within the voxel and so the greater the averaging that occurs. This is known as the partial volume effect; the easiest way to reduce this effect is to use thinner sections (Figure 1-8).

When the entire chest is examined, contiguous sections 5-mm thick are usually reconstructed for analysis. If the study is undertaken on a multichannel system, the data set may be reconstructed at thinner intervals predetermined by the thickness of the detector rows, and these thinner sections may be used for reporting or multiplanar reconstructions. Thinner sections are also used to study fine detail and complex areas of anatomy, such as the aortopulmonary window and subcarinal regions. Another specific example for which narrow sections may be useful to display differential densities (which would otherwise be lost because of the partial volume effect) is the small foci of fat or calcium that are sometimes seen within a hamartoma.

Although there is little difference in total patient dose between conventional single-channel CT and multichannel systems, there is a striking difference in the radiation dose to the patient between contiguous sections and interspaced fine sections. Thus, the effective dose to the patient with interspaced fine sections (e.g., 1 or 2 mm) every 10 mm, such as used for high-resolution CT of the lung parenchyma, is 5–10 times less than that imposed by single-channel or multichannel spiral CT of the entire chest volume. The disadvantage of interspaced sections is the inability to view the data in any plane, but for the purposes of assessment of the lung interstitium, this added refinement is not usually of sufficient added diagnostic value to warrant the increased radiation burden. This is especially the case in the relatively younger patient.

Window Settings

The average density of each voxel is measured in Hounsfield units (H); the units have been arbitrarily chosen so that zero is water density and −1000 is air density. The span of Hounsfield units in the thorax is wider than in any other part of the body, ranging from aerated lung (approximately −800 H) to ribs (+700 H). Two variables are used that allow the operator to select the range of densities to be viewed—window width and window center (or level).

The window width determines the number of Hounsfield units to be displayed. Any densities greater than the upper limit of the window width are displayed as white, and any below the limit of the window are displayed as black. Between these two limits, the densities are displayed in shades of gray. The median density of the window chosen is the center or level, and this center can be moved higher or lower at will, thus moving the window up or down through the range. The narrower the window width, the greater the contrast discrimination within the window. No single window setting can depict the wide range of densities encountered in the chest on a single image. For this reason, at least two sets of images are required to demonstrate the lung parenchyma and soft tissues of the mediastinum, respectively (Figure 1-9). Standard window widths and centers for thoracic CT vary between departments, but generally for the soft tissues of the mediastinum a window width of 400–600 H and a center of +30 H is appropriate. For the lungs, a wide window of 1500 H and

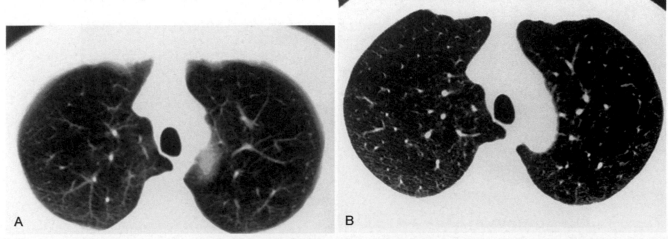

FIGURE 1-8 The partial volume effect on computed tomography. **A,** This 10-mm computed tomography section shows a poorly defined opacity, adjacent to the left superior mediastinum, apparently within the lung. **B,** The 1.5-mm section through the same region reveals that the appearance in **(A)** results from a partial volume effect, that is, the aortic arch is partially included in the 10-mm-thick sections.

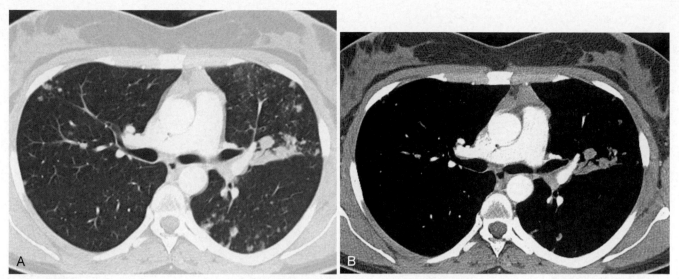

FIGURE 1-9 The effect of window settings on computed tomography scans. A 5-mm-thick computed tomography section displayed on different window settings. **A,** On lung windows (center 500 H, width 1500 H), nodules in the lungs and pulmonary vessels are clearly visible. **B,** On soft-tissue windows (center 35 H, width 400 H), the contrast-enhanced vessels in the mediastinum and the soft tissue structures are delineated, but the lung detail is lost.

a center of approximately −500 H is usually satisfactory. For bones, the widest possible window setting at a center of 30 H is best.

Window settings have a profound influence on the size and conspicuity of normal and abnormal structures. Nonetheless, it is impossible to prescribe precise window settings, because there is an element of observer preference, and there are differences between machines. The most accurate representation of an object seems to be achieved if the value of the window level is half way between the density of the structure to be measured and the density of the surrounding tissue. For example, the diameter of a pulmonary nodule, measured on soft tissue settings appropriate for the mediastinum, will be grossly underestimated. When inappropriate window settings are used, smaller structures (e.g., peripheral pulmonary vessels) are affected proportionally much more than larger structures.

Intravenous Contrast Enhancement

Intravenous contrast enhancement only needs to be given in specific instances, because of the high contrast on CT between vessels and surrounding air in the lung and between vessels and surrounding fat within the mediastinum. One such instance is to aid the distinction between hilar vessels and a soft tissue mass. The exact timing of the injection of contrast media depends most on the time the CT scanner takes to scan the thorax. With multichannel CT scanners, the circulation time of the patient becomes an important factor.

Contrast medium rapidly diffuses out of the vascular space into the extravascular space, so that opacification of the vasculature after a bolus injection with a power injector quickly declines, and structures such as lymph nodes steadily increase in density over time. Such dynamics result in a point at which a solid structure may have exactly the same density as an adjacent vessel. The timing and duration of the contrast medium infusion must, therefore, be taken into account when interpreting a contrast-enhanced CT examination. Rapid scanning protocols with automated injectors tend to improve contrast enhancement of vascular structures at the expense of enhancement of solid lesions because of the rapidity of scanning.

With spiral CT, it is possible to achieve good opacification of all the thoracic vascular structures by use of small volumes of contrast media. Optimal contrast enhancement is a prerequisite for the diagnosis of pulmonary embolism (PE) or aortic and great vessel abnormalities. To achieve optimal contrast enhancement, many CT systems now use an automated triggering system. Thus, when examining the pulmonary arteries a low dose repeating scan will monitor the density in the pulmonary outflow tract once every second. When a predetermined density threshold is reached as a result of the arrival of intravenous contrast, the preplanned examination is triggered. The couch rapidly moves the patient from the monitoring position to the start position, a prerecorded breath hold instruction is given to the patient over a loudspeaker, and the data acquisition commences.

When examining inflammatory lesions, such as the reaction around an empyema, it may be necessary to delay scanning by 30 sec to allow contrast to diffuse into the extravascular space. When examining the liver and adrenals in the examination of a patient with suspected lung cancer, the optimal phase of contrast enhancement to maximize the conspicuity of hepatic metastases is during the portal venous phase of contrast enhancement, and this occurs 60–80 sec after contrast injection.

HIGH-RESOLUTION COMPUTED TOMOGRAPHY

Technical Considerations

In the past 10 years, the development of high-resolution computed tomography (HRCT) has had great impact on the approach to the imaging of diffuse interstitial lung disease and bronchiectasis. Images of the lung produced by HRCT correlate closely with the macroscopic appearances of pathologic specimens, so in the context of diffuse lung disease, HRCT represents a substantial improvement over chest radiography. Three factors significantly improve the spatial resolution of CT and so confer the description "high-resolution"

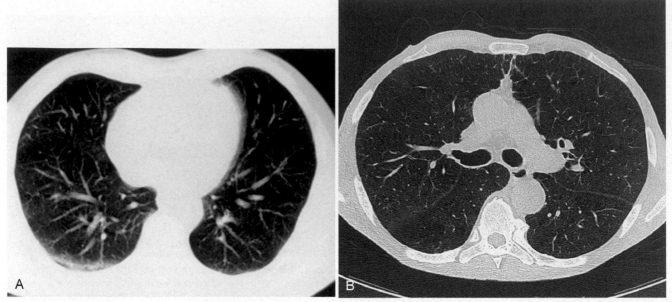

FIGURE 1-10 The effect of computed tomography section thickness and edge enhancement on image appearance. **A,** A 10-mm-thick section reconstructed without edge enhancement from a 64-channel CT data set. **B,** A 1.5-mm-thick section with high edge enhancement from the same data set and is typical of an HRCT lung image.

CT—narrow beam collimation, a high spatial reconstruction algorithm, and a small field of view.

Narrow collimation of the X-ray beam reduces volume averaging within the section and so increases spatial resolution compared with standard 10-mm collimation. For routine HRCT scanning, 1.50-mm beam collimation is generally regarded as optimal. Narrow collimation has a marked effect on the appearance of the lungs, notably the vessels and bronchi—the branching vascular pattern seen particularly in the mid zones on standard 10-mm sections has a more nodular appearance with narrow sections, because shorter segments of the obliquely running vessels are included in the section. In addition, parenchymal details become more clearly visualized (Figure 1-10).

In HRCT lung work, a high spatial-frequency algorithm is used to take advantage of the inherently high-contrast environment of the lung. The high spatial-frequency algorithm (also known as the edge-enhancing, sharp, or formerly "bone" algorithm) reduces image smoothing and makes structures visibly sharper, but at the same time makes image noise more obvious (see Figure 1-10).

Several artifacts are consistently identified on HRCT images, but they do not usually degrade the diagnostic content of the images. Nevertheless, it is useful to be able to recognize the more common ones. Probably the most frequently encountered is a streaking appearance that arises from patient motion. Cardiac motion sometimes causes movement of the adjacent lung and hence degradation of image quality. Some CT scanners are able to eliminate this artifact by triggering the acquisition of the slice from the ECG trace and so collect the data during diastole when cardiac motion is minimized. To optimize this technique the scanner must have a short rotation time and also be capable of acquiring a CT image from data from a partial rotation. This reduces the data acquisition time window to as little as 360 msec.

The size of the patient has a direct effect on the quality of the lung image—the larger the patient, the more conspicuous

the noise, which is seen as granular streaks because of increased X-ray absorption by the patient. This artifact is particularly evident in the posterior lung adjacent to the vertebral column. The phenomenon of aliasing results in a fine, streak-like pattern radiating from sharp, high-contrast interfaces. The severity of the aliasing artifact is related to the geometry of the CT scanner, and, unlike quantum mottle, aliasing is independent of the radiation dose. These artifacts are exaggerated by the nonsmoothing, high spatial resolution reconstruction algorithm but do not mimic normal anatomic structures and are rarely severe enough to obscure important detail in the lung parenchyma (Figure 1-11).

The degree to which HRCT samples the lung depends primarily on the spacing between the thin sections. An HRCT examination also may vary in terms of the number of sections, the position of the patient, the phase in which respiration is

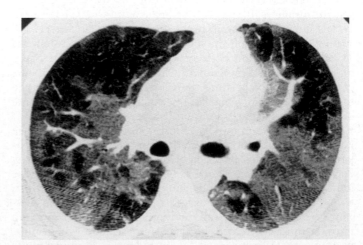

FIGURE 1-11 High-resolution computed tomography image demonstrating artifact caused by aliasing and quantum mottle. Detail is obscured in the posterior parts of the lungs. The patchy parenchymal opacification results from desquamative interstitial pneumonitis.

suspended, the window settings at which the images are displayed, and the manipulation of the image by postprocessing. No single protocol can be recommended to cover every eventuality. However, the simplest protocol entails 1.5-mm collimation sections at 20-mm intervals from apex to lung bases. Any given scanning protocol may need to be modified—a patient referred with unexplained hemoptysis ideally is scanned with contiguous standard sections through the major airways (to show a small endobronchial abnormality) and interspaced narrow sections through the remainder of the lungs (to identify bronchiectasis).

When early interstitial disease is suspected, for example, in asbestos-exposed individuals who have an apparently normal chest radiograph, HRCT scans are often performed in the prone position to prevent any confusion with the increased opacification seen in the dependent posterior-basal segments of many normal individuals scanned in the usual supine position. The increased density seen in the posterior dependent lung in the supine position disappears in normal individuals when the scan is repeated at the same level with the patient in the prone position. No advantage is gained by scanning a patient in the prone position if no obvious diffuse lung disease is found on a contemporary chest radiograph.

A limited number of scans taken at end expiration can reveal evidence of air trapping caused by small airways disease, which may not be detectable on routine inspiratory scans. Areas of air trapping range from a single secondary pulmonary lobule to a cluster of lobules that give a patchwork appearance of low attenuation areas adjacent to higher attenuation, normal lung parenchyma (Figure 1-12).

Alterations of the window settings of HRCT images sometimes make detection of parenchymal abnormalities impossible when there is a subtle increase or decrease in attenuation of the lung parenchyma. Uniformity of window settings from patient to patient aids consistent interpretation of the lung images. In general, a window level of −500 to −800 H and a width of between 900 and 1500 H are usually satisfactory. Modification of the window settings for particular tasks is often desirable; for example, in looking for pleuroparenchymal abnormalities in asbestos-exposed individuals, a wider window of up to 2000 H may be useful. Conversely, a narrower window of approximately 600 H may emphasize the subtle density differences that characterize emphysema and small airways disease.

The relatively high radiation dose to the patient inherent in all CT scanning needs to be appreciated. The radiation burden to the patient is considerably less with HRCT than with conventional CT scanning. It has been estimated that the mean radiation dose delivered to the skin with HRCT by use of 1.5-mm sections at 20-mm intervals is 6% that of conventional 10-mm contiguous-scanning protocols. A further method of reducing the radiation burden to the patient is to decrease the milliamperage; it is possible to reduce the milliamperage by up to 10-fold and still obtain comparably diagnostic images. Although future refinements in CT technology may reduce the radiation burden to patients, CT still represents a relatively high radiation dose to patients and, as such, must not be performed indiscriminately.

Clinical Applications of High-Resolution Computed Tomography

Increasingly, HRCT is used to confirm or refute the impression of an abnormality seen on a chest radiograph. It may also be used to achieve a histospecific diagnosis in some patients who have obvious, but nonspecific, radiographic abnormalities.

It is probably impossible to determine the frequency with which HRCT will show significant parenchymal abnormalities when the chest radiograph appears normal. Studies of individual diseases show that HRCT demonstrates abnormalities despite normal chest radiographs in 29% of patients who have systemic sclerosis and in up to 30% of asbestosis patients. For hypersensitivity pneumonitis, the proportion may be even higher. Taking the average sensitivity results of several studies, HRCT seems to have a sensitivity of approximately 94% compared with 80% for chest radiography; this increased sensitivity does not seem to be achieved at the expense of decreased specificity.

In patients with clinical, radiographic, and lung function evidence of diffuse lung disease, much evidence now indicates that HRCT correctly predicts more often, and with a greater degree of confidence than chest radiography allows, the correct histologic diagnosis. In the original study that compared

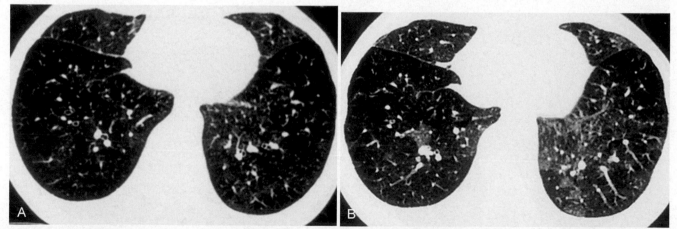

FIGURE 1-12 High-resolution computed tomography through the lower lobes of a patient who has severe dyspnea and rheumatoid arthritis. **A,** Minor inhomogeneity of the density of the lung parenchyma and some dilatation of the bronchus. **B,** A high-resolution computed tomogram taken at end expiration emphasizes the density differences. Appearances are consistent with obliterative bronchiolitis.

the diagnostic accuracy of chest radiography and CT in the prediction of specific histologic diagnoses in patients with diffuse lung disease, Mathieson *et al* showed that three observers could make a confident diagnosis in 23% of cases on the basis of chest radiographs and in 49% of cases by use of CT; the correct diagnoses were made in 77% and 93% of these readings, respectively (Figure 1-13).

In a later study, Grenier *et al* showed that for each of three observers, the high-confidence diagnoses that were correct from chest radiography findings alone were 29%, 34%, and 19%, respectively, whereas in HRCT the results were 57%, 55%, and 47%, respectively. Moreover, the intraobserver agreement for the proposed diagnosis was improved with HRCT compared with chest radiography. These studies show that HRCT is clearly useful in the assessment of patients suspected of having diffuse lung disease but for whom the clinical

features and chest radiograph do not allow a confident diagnosis to be made. Even without clinical information, a number of diffuse lung diseases can, in the hands of experienced chest radiologists, have a "diagnostic" appearance on HRCT; these include fibrosing alveolitis, sarcoidosis, Langerhans' cell histiocytosis, lymphangioleiomyomatosis, pneumoconiosis, and hypersensitivity pneumonitis (Figure 1-14). Intriguingly, the ability of HRCT to allow observers to provide correct histospecific diagnoses seems to be maintained in advanced "end-stage" disease.

However, HRCT is sometimes used indiscriminately for patients in whom the high certainty of diagnosis from clinical and radiographic findings does not justify the extra cost and radiation burden. No evidence shows that an HRCT examination adds anything of diagnostic value for a patient who has progressive shortness of breath, finger clubbing, crackles at

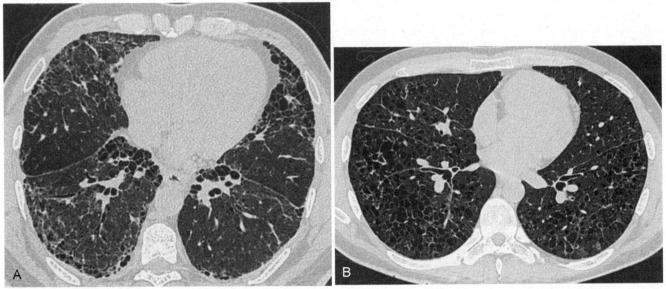

FIGURE 1-13 High-resolution computed tomography patterns. **A,** Subpleural reticular pattern typical of established fibrosing alveolitis. **B,** Multiple irregularly shaped cystic spaces within the lungs in a young patient with preserved lung volumes. Sections through the lung bases were normal. This high-resolution computed tomography pattern and distribution is virtually pathonomonic of Langerhans' cell histiocytosis.

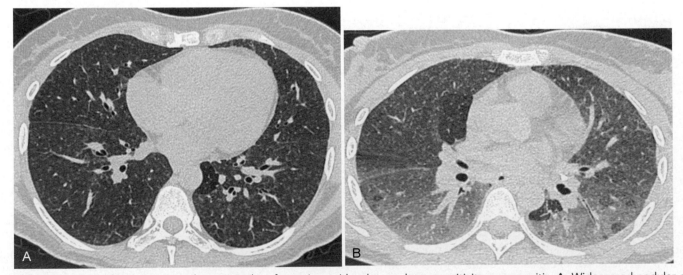

FIGURE 1-14 High-resolution computed tomography of a patient with subacute hypersensitivity pneumonitis. **A,** Widespread nodular and ground-glass patterns. **B,** Note the areas of decreased attenuation posteriorly, made more obvious on this scan obtained in expiration.

the lung bases, and the typical radiographic pattern and lung-function profile of fibrosing alveolitis. Nevertheless, the ability of HRCT to characterize disease, and often to deliver a definite and correct diagnosis in patients with nonspecific radiographic shadowing, is frequently helpful.

Much interest has been shown in defining the role of HRCT in staging disease activity, particularly for fibrosing alveolitis, in which cellular histology indicates disease activity and is used to predict both responses to treatment and prognosis. There is now evidence that a predominance of ground-glass opacification in fibrosing alveolitis predicts a good response to treatment and increased actuarial survival compared with patients with a more reticular pattern, which denotes established fibrosis. Similar observations about the potential reversibility of disease can be made by use of HRCT on patients who have sarcoidosis, in whom a ground-glass or a nodular pattern predominates. In other conditions, the identification of ground-glass opacification on HRCT, although nonspecific, almost invariably indicates a potentially reversible disease; for example, extrinsic allergic alveolitis, diffuse pulmonary hemorrhage, and *Pneumocystis jirovecii* pneumonia (Box 1-1). An important exception is bronchoalveolar cell carcinoma, in which there may be areas of ground-glass opacification that merge into areas of frank consolidation or a more nodular pattern. Another caveat is the situation in which fine, intralobular fibrosis is seen on HRCT as widespread ground-glass opacification; in this rare occurrence, evidence of traction bronchiectasis is usually present within the areas of ground-glass opacification.

The ability of CT to discriminate between various patterns of disease has clarified the reasons for the sometimes complex mixed obstructive and restrictive functional deficits found in some diffuse lung diseases. A good example is hypersensitivity pneumonitis, in which both interstitial and small airways disease coexist—patterns caused by these different pathologic processes can be readily appreciated on HRCT. The extent of the various HRCT patterns correlates with the expected functional indices of restriction and obstruction, respectively. Other conditions in which CT is able to tease out the morphologic abnormalities responsible for complex functional deficits include fibrosing alveolitis, when there is coexisting emphysema, and sarcoidosis, when there may be a combination of interstitial fibrosis and small airways obstruction by peribronchiolar granulomata.

In patients for whom lung biopsy is deemed necessary, HRCT may be invaluable to indicate which type of biopsy procedure is likely to be successful in obtaining diagnostic material. The broad distinction between peripheral disease

---

BOX 1-2 Indications for High-Resolution Computed Tomography of the Lungs

Narrow the differential diagnosis or make a histospecific diagnosis in patients with obvious but nonspecific radiographic abnormalities
Detect diffuse lung disease in patients with normal or equivocal radiographic abnormalities
Elucidate unexpected pulmonary function test results
Investigate patients presenting with hemoptysis
Evaluate disease reversibility, particularly in patients who have fibrosing alveolitis
Guide the type and site of lung biopsy

---

versus central and bronchocentric disease is easily made on HRCT. Thus, disease with a subpleural distribution, such as fibrosing alveolitis, is most unlikely to be sampled by transbronchial biopsy, whereas diseases with a bronchocentric distribution on HRCT, such as sarcoidosis and lymphangitis carcinomatosa, are consistently accessible to transbronchial biopsy. In patients for whom an open or thoracoscopic lung biopsy is contemplated, HRCT assists in determining the optimal biopsy site. Pathologic examination of a lung biopsy can still justifiably be regarded as the final arbiter for the presence or absence of subtle interstitial lung disease. Because HRCT images provide an "*in vivo* big picture," many lung pathologists now combine the imaging and pathologic information before assigning a final diagnosis, and in many centers, the benefits of a team approach to the diagnosis of diffuse lung disease are recognized. The indications for HRCT that have been developed over the past 10 years are summarized in Box 1-2.

MAGNETIC RESONANCE IMAGING (MRI) AND MAGNETIC RESONANCE ANGIOGRAPHY (MRA)

Plain radiographs, CT, ultrasound, contrast angiography, and isotope scanning form the mainstay of imaging thoracic diseases. Although MRI has developed a role complementary to these techniques, it generally remains a problem-solving tool rather than a technique of first choice.

Magnetic resonance imaging entails placing the subject in a very strong magnetic field (typically 0.2–1.5 Tesla) and then irradiating the area under examination with pulses of radiowaves. Anatomic MRI depends on the presence of water within tissue to produce the signal required for interpretation. Protons within this water exist within different local atomic environments and, consequently, they have different properties. These differences can be exploited by sequence manipulation to generate differences in contrast between tissues in the final MR image. Thus, the frequency of the radiofrequency (RF) pulse transmitted into the patient is carefully selected so that it causes hydrogen protons within water to be disturbed from the orientation that they have assumed as a result of being placed inside the powerful magnetic field within the bore of the magnet. After the transient disturbance caused by the RF pulse, these protons, which are acting akin to small bar magnets, relax back into their original resting position. As they do this, they release energy as a further pulse of radio waves, and these are detected by the receiver coils that

---

BOX 1-1 Causes of Ground-Glass Opacification

Pneumocystis jirovecii or cytomegalovirus pneumonia
Acute respiratory distress syndrome/acute interstitial pneumonia
Hypersensitivity pneumonitis—subacute
Desquamative interstitial pneumonitis
Pulmonary edema
Idiopathic pulmonary hemorrhage
Bronchioloalveolar cell carcinoma
Alveolar proteinosis
Lymphocytic interstitial pneumonia
Respiratory bronchiolitis-interstitial lung disease

are located in the wall of the bore of the magnetic or more commonly in a variety of receiver coils placed more directly around the area under investigation. These coils are frequently known by the body part they have been designed to examine, and thus a knee, head, neck, or body coil is placed appropriately at the start of the examination. In the case of thoracic imaging, the body coil usually comprises a pair of coil mats placed in front and behind the patient.

Historically, the main strengths of MRI are the high intrinsic soft tissue contrast generated, the lack of artifact from bone, the lack of ionizing radiation, and the ability to produce images in any chosen plane. The major weaknesses of MRI in the thorax has, until recently, been its susceptibility to image degradation because of respiratory and cardiac motion, as well as the relatively long times taken to perform an examination. In general, the quality of MR images is related to the field strength of the scanner and the peak power and speed of the amplifiers that generate the interrogating radiofrequency pulses.

For thoracic imaging, ECG-triggering facilities, whereby the acquisition of imaging data can be coordinated with the cardiac cycle to reduce flow artifact, are essential. Various methods of compensation for respiratory motion have been developed. Some use external devices such as respiratory bellows, which detect movement of the chest wall, with data collection occurring when motion is at its least. Other methods are essentially software developments, which compensate for respiratory disruption of magnetic spins. Most of these techniques have been superseded on modern scanners by the ability to acquire images of the thorax by use of breath-hold techniques.

Mediastinal and Chest Wall Imaging

The most common indications for the use of MRI in respiratory disease are for imaging of neoplastic disease, most commonly bronchogenic carcinoma. As well as the primary disease, secondary complications such as cerebral secondaries, spinal metastases, and retroperitoneal fibrosis all lend themselves to MRI. MRI also allows assessment of invasion of mediastinal structures such as the major airways, heart and great vessels, chest wall, and diaphragm and allows differentiation between different forms of soft tissue, fluid, hemorrhage, local hematoma formation, and aneurysms (Figures 1-15 and 1-16). With modern multichannel CT, there is now relatively little advantage of MRI over CT in assessing chest wall invasion

except for superior sulcus tumors. However, MRI does provide superb anatomic detail without the use of irradiation, an important consideration in the pediatric age group who may require a number of follow-up studies (Figure 1-17). The disadvantage of MRI in the very young child is the necessity for general anesthesia in many cases.

Lung Parenchymal Imaging

The lungs present an enormous challenge to MRI for a number of reasons. First, they are constantly moving because of respiratory and cardiac motion. Second, because they have a low water content relative to other biologic tissues, they have a low proton density and return relatively little signal.

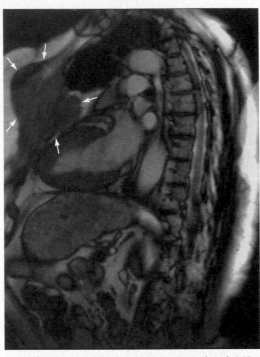

FIGURE 1-16 Chest wall invasion demonstrated with MRI. Oblique sagittal T2W image through the long axis of the left ventricle demonstrates an adjacent chest wall mass (*arrows*) extending through the interior chest wall into the overlying breast tissue. This was due to recurrent breast carcinoma.

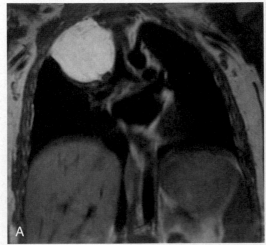
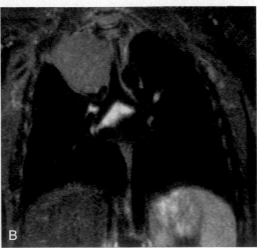

FIGURE 1-15 Right upper zone mass in an 11-year-old boy. **A,** A coronal T1W sequence demonstrates a high-signal-intensity apical mass. **B,** With the addition of fat saturation, reducing the signal returned from fat, the signal intensity in the mass falls significantly. This confirms the fatty nature of the mass, which was a large pleural lipoma.

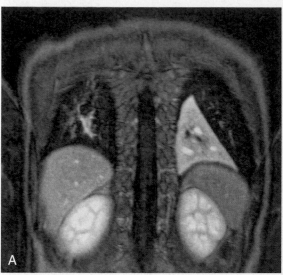
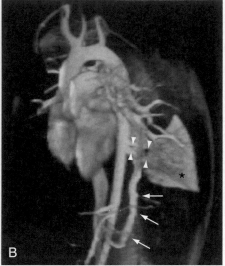

FIGURE 1-17 Extralobar pulmonary sequestration. **A,** A coronal contrast-enhanced breath-hold image demonstrates the avidly enhancing pulmonary sequestration at the left lung base. Note the clear plane between the triangular sequestrated segment and the diaphragm and underlying spleen. **B,** Volume-rendered angiographic image demonstrating the same triangular sequestrated segment (*asterisk*) with two supplying branches from the aorta (*arrowheads*) and complex venous drainage. The largest vein drains subdiaphragmatically (*arrows*) into the left renal vein.

Third, because of the multiple interfaces between air and soft tissue, there are innumerable small disturbances in the magnetic field. This loss of homogeneity at air–tissue interfaces results in a phenomenon known as magnetic susceptibility artefact, further reducing signal and increasing noise. Thus, on standard spin-echo sequences, normal lung exhibits little signal and is often obliterated by artefact. Various attempts to tackle these problems by designing particular pulse sequences have met with little success in the past 10–15 years. Paradoxically, the lack of signal from the lung may, in some situations, be an advantage because abnormalities that contain relatively greater amounts of tissue water may become more obvious.

Ventilation Studies

Another area of intense interest has been in the use of polarized gases (3-Helium and 129-Xenon) to show pulmonary ventilation. With this technique, a process of heating and irradiating with polarized light produces polarized gases. The gases (which have a short half-life) are inhaled and imaged by use of optimized sequences. The use of dual-frequency probes allows gas and proton images to be acquired and registered enabling function and anatomy to be correlated.

MAGNETIC RESONANCE ANGIOGRAPHY (MRA)

MR can also be used to demonstrate vascular anatomy by generation of contrast between flowing blood and stationary tissue, and this may be achieved with or without intravenous MR contrast agents. Generally, the use of contrast increases the signal returned from blood, increases the signal-to-noise ratio, and allows acquisition times to be shorter. MRA can be used to look at venous or arterial flow, together or separately (see Figure 1-17).

The contrast agents used in MR generally and MRA in particular are almost exclusively based on gadolinium chelates. Most are extracellular space agents, and they cause shortening of the T1 relaxation time and so increase the signal from the enhanced tissue on T1-weighted sequences. The distribution of these agents is very similar to the iodinated contrast agents used routinely in CT.

Pulmonary Emboli and Infarction

At present, MR is not routinely used in patients with suspected pulmonary embolism and infarction, but it has been the subject of much research, and a number of series have been published demonstrating that breath-hold pulmonary MRA can now show fifth-order pulmonary vessels and allow diagnosis of emboli to segmental level. Smaller pulmonary emboli can be inferred by lack of segmental and subsegmental perfusion. Three-dimensional MR angiographic data sets can be acquired and displayed on workstations as moving projections, and this can help show areas of deficient perfusion.

Vascular Malformations and Congenital Anomalies

There is increasing evidence that MR can clearly define a number of vascular and developmental anomalies of the lungs by combining anatomic and flow imaging. These include the scimitar syndrome, hypogenetic lung syndrome, pulmonary artery agenesis, bronchopulmonary sequestration, and vascular malformations (see Figure 1-17).

Cardiovascular Imaging

MR is now regarded as the definitive technique for imaging the aorta for dissection, aneurysms, and coarctation. MR is widely used for the assessment of congenital heart disease. It can also be used to assess cardiac anatomy and function, and software has been developed to allow rapid and accurate assessment of wall motion, ejection fraction, stress testing for reversible ischemia, hibernating myocardium, and valvular disease. The ultimate challenge, namely accurate imaging of the coronary arteries, is under intense investigation although has not yet reached routine practice. Nevertheless, MRI is now able to provide comprehensive noninvasive cardiac assessment that is likely to challenge more established techniques such as nuclear medicine and echocardiography.

PULMONARY ANGIOGRAPHY

Pulmonary angiography is used to investigate pulmonary circulation when other, less invasive, methods have failed to provide the requisite information. The most frequent indication is for suspected PE, usually following a nondiagnostic ventilation-perfusion scan (V/Q). Ideally, the angiogram is undertaken within 24 h of an acute presentation of suspected embolism. However, a delay of 48–72 h should not preclude the use of pulmonary angiography, although the diagnostic yield progressively declines because of fragmentation of thrombi over time, especially if anticoagulation has been instituted.

Pulmonary angiography is a technique that tends to be under used for a variety of reasons. Apart from the relative expense and invasive nature of angiography, it is perceived to have a high complication rate (although this is not supported by the published evidence). The imbalance between the rates of V/Q scan and angiography is striking, and it has been estimated that only one angiogram is requested for every 100 V/Q scans. This is a ratio that flatters the diagnostic abilities of V/Q scanning, which in most series yields an equivocal result in 30–60% of patients. The frequently quoted complications of angiography, namely respiratory compromise, arrhythmia, renal failure, and transient hypersensitivity reactions, are based on historical data that suggested a mortality rate of up to 0.5%, a major nonfatal complication rate of 1%, and a minor complication rate of 5%. More recent evaluation suggests pulmonary angiography is much safer. This improvement is attributed predominantly to the change from ionic contrast media to low, osmolar nonionic agents. Second, more flexible, small-gauge pigtail catheters have reduced the incidence of myocardial injury.

The technique of pulmonary angiography involves fluoroscopically directed insertion of a guidewire, followed by a modified pigtail catheter into the right and left main pulmonary arteries in turn, with injection of a nonionic contrast at an appropriate flow rate. At least two views per side are required, with additional oblique or magnification views as necessary. Catheter access is usually through the femoral vein, with the internal jugular and subclavian veins as possible alternatives. Despite the desirable high resolution of conventional film-screen angiography, most departments now undertake angiography with digital subtraction vascular equipment (Figure 1-18). Problems with misregistration artifact, inherent in digital subtraction systems and caused by respiratory or cardiac cycle-phase differences between the mask image and the contrast image, can usually be overcome by acquiring a series of mask views before contrast injection. Crossing the tricuspid valve may induce an arrhythmia that is usually transient. Therefore, electrocardiogram (ECG) monitoring is mandatory, and the use of prophylactic, antiarrhythmic agents or temporary pacing-wire insertion is common practice in some centers.

When a pulmonary embolus is present, it is most frequently situated in the posterior segments of the lower lobe. Thrombi beyond the segmental vessel level are detected less reliably than more central thrombi. However, the significance of thrombi confined to subsegmental vessels is unclear. The typical angiographic findings of PE are vascular cutoff or, when vascular occlusion is not complete, an intraluminal filling defect with contrast passing around and beyond the clot. Indirect signs of embolism include areas of relatively delayed or reduced perfusion, late filling of the venous circulation, and vessel tortuosity. When the angiogram is undertaken to investigate suspected chronic thromboembolic disease, the vascular changes include local stenosis or thin

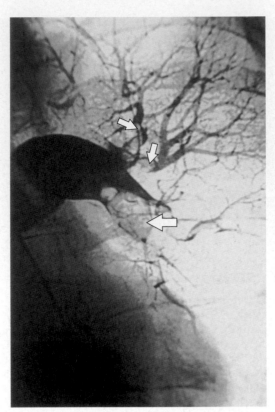

FIGURE 1-18 Digital subtraction pulmonary angiogram. A large thrombus causes a filling defect within the contrast in the artery of the left lower lobe (*large arrow*). Smaller thrombi are present within the proximal branches to the upper lobe (*small arrows*).

webs, luminal ectasia, and irregularities of the normal tapering pattern.

The high threshold for proceeding to pulmonary angiography when the diagnosis of PE remains in doubt has been central in the developing role of contrast-enhanced spiral CT scanning for the diagnosis of PE.

BRONCHIAL ARTERY EMBOLIZATION

Bronchial artery embolization is usually performed to stop massive hemoptysis in patients unsuitable for surgical management. The most common causes of bronchial artery hypertrophy and consequent hemorrhage are suppurative lung diseases (particularly bronchiectasis) and fibrocavitary disease that involves mycetomas. Less common causes of hemorrhage from the bronchial circulation include bronchial carcinoma, chronic pulmonary abscess, and congenital cyanotic heart disease. No absolute contraindications to bronchial artery embolization are known, although the patient should be hemodynamically stable and able to cooperate.

The most common anatomic arrangement on bronchial arteriography is one main right bronchial artery arising from a common intercostobronchial trunk, which comes off the thoracic aorta at approximately the level of T5, and two left bronchial arteries arising more inferiorly. However, bronchial arteries may arise from the thyrocervical trunk, internal mammary artery, costocervical trunk, subclavian artery, a lower intercostal artery, inferior phrenic artery, or even the abdominal aorta. The right intercostal bronchial trunk takes off from the aorta at an acute upward angle, whereas the left bronchial arteries leave the aorta more or less at right angles, and special catheters have been designed to facilitate selective catheterization. Superselective catheterization of the bronchial circulation allows precise delivery of embolic material and so prevents spillover into the aorta or inadvertent embolization of the spinal artery.

Fiberoptic bronchoscopy is often advocated before bronchial artery embolization to establish the site of hemorrhage. However, a large hemoptysis almost invariably results in vigorous coughing, and so blood is spread throughout the bronchial tree, which makes localization impossible. Few criteria exist to determine which angiographically demonstrated bronchial arteries should be embolized. Guidelines are particularly relevant when several bronchial arteries have been identified and the site of hemorrhage is not obvious from prior thoracic imaging. Embolization is directed at the vessels considered most likely to be the source of hemorrhage (Figure 1-19). Bronchial arteries of diameter >3 mm may be considered pathologically enlarged. In patients with diffuse, suppurative lung disease, most commonly cystic fibrosis, attempts are made to embolize all significantly enlarged bronchial arteries bilaterally. If no abnormal bronchial arteries are identified, a systematic search is made for aberrant bronchial arteries. When a patient continues to have hemoptysis after embolization of all suspicious systemic arteries, it may be necessary to investigate the pulmonary circulation for a source of hemorrhage.

A variety of embolic materials have been used for the embolization of bronchial arteries, ranging from spheres of polyvinyl alcohol in a variety of sizes to small pieces of Gelfoam. Although coils lodged proximally in the bronchial artery have been used, they can prevent subsequent catheterization.

After bronchial artery embolization, many patients experience transient fever and chest pain; after 2 days, some patients cough up a small amount of blood, which possibly arises from limited infarction of the bronchial mucosa. Serious complications after bronchial artery embolization are rare, the most serious being transverse myelitis, probably caused by contrast toxicity rather than inadvertent embolization. Inadvertent spillover of embolization material into the thoracic aorta may cause distant ischemia in the legs or abdominal organs.

The aim of bronchial artery embolization is the immediate control of life-threatening hemoptysis, which is achieved in more than 75% of patients. Failures usually result from nonidentification of significant bronchial arteries and an inability to maintain the catheter position and proceed to embolization. Up to 20% of patients re-bleed within 6 months of an initially successful bronchial artery embolization. The reasons cited for recurrent hemorrhage are recanalization of previously embolized vessels, incomplete initial embolization, and hypertrophy of small bronchial arteries not initially embolized. However, bronchial artery embolization usually can be satisfactorily repeated in patients who re-bleed.

SUPERIOR VENA CAVA STENTS

Superior vena cava obstruction (SVCO) is characterized by facial and upper limb swelling, headache, and shortness of breath, and is usually caused by advanced mediastinal malignancy. Conventional palliative treatment relies on radiotherapy, chemotherapy, and sometimes surgery. Radiotherapy usually produces an initial improvement, although subsequent recurrence of symptoms is frequent. Balloon angioplasty of both benign and malignant causes of SVCO has been reported, but not surprisingly symptoms are liable to recur soon after angioplasty alone.

The percutaneous placement of metallic stents for the treatment of SVCO has several attractions. With increasing

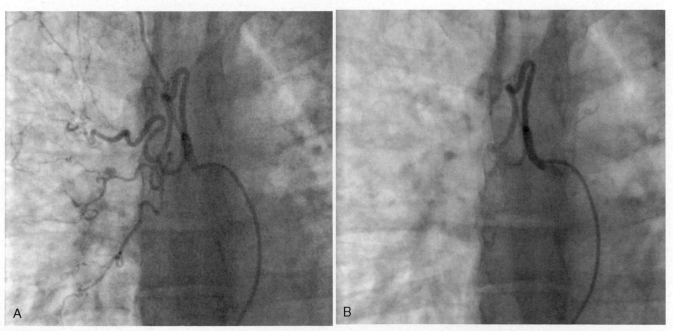

FIGURE 1-19 Bronchial arteriogram in a patient with hemoptysis. **A,** There is marked hypertrophy of the bronchial artery to the right upper zone. These changes were caused by cystic fibrosis. After embolization **B,** there is no further flow into these branches.

experience, reliable and successful palliation of SVCO has been reported by use of various stent designs. A superior venacavogram is necessary to identify the length of the stenosis and its site in relation to the confluence of the brachiocephalic veins and the right atrium. Identification of intraluminal thrombus or tumor is an absolute contraindication to the procedure. After balloon dilatation of the SVC stricture, the stent is positioned across the stricture, and a postplacement venacavogram is performed to confirm free flow of blood into the right atrium (Figure 1-20). After angioplasty and stent placement, relief of SVCO symptoms is usually rapid and dramatic. Recurrence of symptoms may be caused by venous thrombosis or tumor progression distal to the stent. Although rupture of the SVC at the time of angioplasty is a risk, this complication seems to be extremely rare, possibly because of the tamponade provided by surrounding tumor or postirradiation fibrosis.

The role of intravascular stents in nonmalignant SVCO has not yet been defined. Patients who have SVCO caused by benign fibrosing mediastinitis have been treated successfully, although occlusion of the stent by the progression of the mediastinal fibrosis or by endothelial proliferation may occur.

NORMAL RADIOGRAPHIC ANATOMY

The Mediastinum and Hilar Structures

The mediastinum is delineated by the lungs on either side, the thoracic inlet above, the diaphragm below, and the vertebral column posteriorly. Because the various structures that make up the mediastinum are superimposed on each other, they cannot be separately identified on a two-dimensional chest radiograph; for this reason, the normal anatomy of the individual components of the mediastinum is considered in more detail in the section on CT of the mediastinum. Nevertheless, because a chest radiograph is usually the first imaging investigation, it is necessary to appreciate the normal appearances of the mediastinum and the considerable possible variations, which result from the patient's body habitus and age.

The mediastinum is conventionally divided into superior, anterior, middle, and posterior compartments (Figure 1-21). Some texts add a superior compartment. The practical use of these arbitrary divisions is that specific mediastinal pathoses show a definite predilection for individual compartments (e.g., a superior mediastinal mass is most frequently caused by intrathoracic extension of the thyroid gland; a middle mediastinal mass usually results from enlarged lymph nodes). However, localization of a mass within one of these compartments does not normally allow a specific diagnosis to be made, and neither do the arbitrary boundaries preclude disease from involving more than one compartment.

Only the outline of the mediastinum and the air-containing trachea and bronchi (and sometimes esophagus) is clearly seen on a normal PA chest radiograph. On a chest radiograph, the right brachiocephalic vein and SCV form the right superior mediastinal border. This border is usually vertical and straight (in contrast to the situation in which there is right paratracheal lymphadenopathy, when the right superior mediastinal border tends to be undulate), and it becomes less distinct as it reaches the thoracic inlet. The right side of the superior mediastinum can appear to be considerably widened in patients who have an abundance of mediastinal fat (Figure 1-22); these

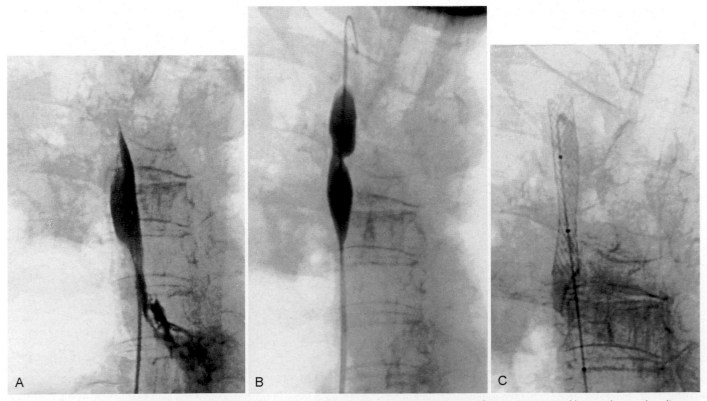

FIGURE 1-20 Stenting of superior vena cava obstruction. The patient had a superior vena cava obstruction caused by mediastinal malignancy. **A,** Superior venacavogram showing a tight stricture in the mid superior vena cava. **B,** Balloon dilation of the stricture. **C,** Placement of a meshed-wire stent in the patent superior vena cava.

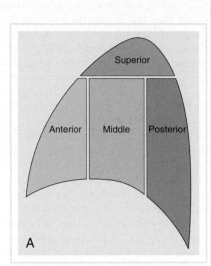 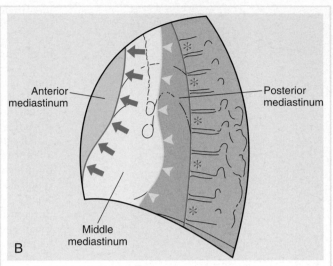

FIGURE 1-21 The mediastinal compartmental divisions. **A,** Arbitrary division of the mediastinum into superior, anterior, middle, and posterior compartments. **B,** An alternative scheme omits the superior mediastinal compartment. The area posterior to the sternum and anterior to the heart and great vessels (*blue arrows*) defines the anterior mediastinum in both cases. Likewise a line placed along the posterior aspect of the trachea and heart (*yellow arrowheads*) defines the middle from the posterior mediastinum, which is defined posteriorly by the vertebra (*red asterisks*).

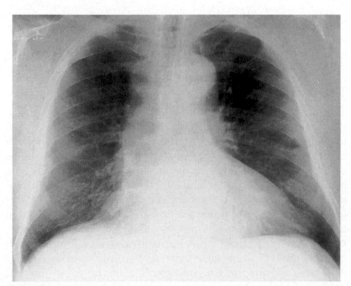

FIGURE 1-22 Widening of the superior mediastinum caused by abundance of mediastinal fat. In addition, bilateral cardiophrenic fat pads are present.

individuals often have prominent cardiophrenic fat pads. The mediastinal border to the left of the trachea above the aortic arch is the result of summation of the left carotid and left subclavian arteries, together with the left brachiocephalic and jugular veins. The left cardiac border comprises the left atrial appendage that merges inferiorly with the left ventricle. The silhouette of the heart should always be sharply outlined. Any blurring of the border results from loss of immediately adjacent aerated lung, usually by collapse or consolidation.

The density of the heart shadow to the left and right of the vertebral column should be identical—any difference indicates pathology (e.g., an area of consolidation or a mass in a lower lobe). On a well-penetrated film, a density with a convex lateral border is frequently seen through the right heart border—this apparent mass is caused by the confluence of the

right pulmonary veins as they enter the left atrium and is of no clinical significance.

The trachea and main bronchi should be visible through the upper and middle mediastinum. The trachea is rarely straight and is often to the right of the midline at its midpoint. In older individuals, the trachea may be markedly displaced by a dilated aortic arch below. In approximately 60% of normal subjects, the right wall of the trachea (the right paratracheal stripe) can be identified as a line of uniform thickness (<4 mm in width); when visible, it excludes the presence of any adjacent space-occupying lesion, most usually lymphadenopathy. The angle between the main bronchus, which forms the carina, is usually somewhat less than 80 degrees. Splaying of the carina is a relatively crude sign of subcarinal disease, either in the form of a massive subcarinal lymphadenopathy or a markedly enlarged left atrium. A more sensitive sign of subcarinal disease is obscuration of the upper part of the azygoesophageal line, which is usually visible in its entirety on a well-penetrated chest radiograph (Figure 1-23). The origins of the lobar bronchi, when they are projected over the mediastinal shadow, can usually be identified, but segmental bronchi within the lungs generally are not seen on plain radiography.

The normal hilar shadows on a chest radiograph represent the summation of the pulmonary arteries and veins, with little contribution from the overlying bronchial walls or lymph nodes of normal size. The hilar are approximately the same size, and the left hilum normally lies between 0.5 and 1.5 cm above the level of the right hilum. The size and shape of the hilar show remarkable variation in normal individuals, making subtle abnormalities difficult to identify.

Pulmonary Fissures, Vessels, and Bronchi

The two lungs are separated by the four layers of pleura behind and in front of the mediastinum. The resultant posterior and anterior junction lines are often visible on frontal chest radiographs as nearly vertical stripes, the posterior junction line lying higher than the anterior (Figure 1-24). Because these junction lines are not invariably seen (their visibility is largely

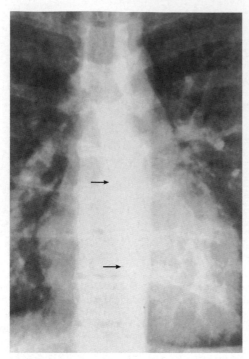

FIGURE 1-23 AMBER chest radiograph. The normal azygoesophageal line is demonstrated (*arrows*).

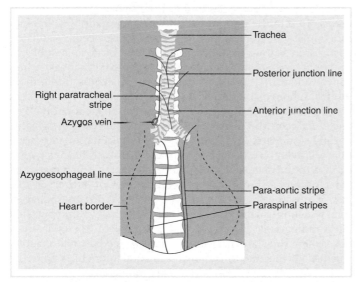

FIGURE 1-24 Some of the mediastinal lines and stripes frequently seen on a frontal chest radiograph.

dependent on whether the pleural reflections are tangential to the X-ray beam), their presence or absence is not usually of significance.

The lobes of lung are surrounded by visceral pleura—the major (or oblique) fissure separates the upper and lower lobes of the left lung. The major (or oblique) fissure and the minor (horizontal or transverse) fissure separate the upper, middle, and lower lobes of the right lung. The minor fissure is visible in more than half of normal PA chest radiographs. In normal individuals, the minor fissure is slightly bowed upward and runs horizontally; any deviation from this configuration is usually caused by loss of volume of a lobe. The major fissures are not visible on a frontal radiograph and are inconsistently

identifiable on lateral radiographs. Inability to detect a fissure usually reflects that the fissure is not exactly in the line of the X-ray beam. However, in a few individuals, fissures are incompletely developed, a point familiar to thoracic surgeons who sometimes encounter difficulty in performing a lobectomy because of incomplete cleavage between lobes. Accessory fissures are occasionally seen; for example, in the left lung a minor fissure can be present, which separates the lingula from the remainder of the upper lobe.

All of the branching structures seen within normal lungs on a chest radiograph represent pulmonary arteries or veins. The pulmonary veins may sometimes be differentiated from the pulmonary arteries—the superior pulmonary veins have a distinctly vertical course. However, it is often impossible to differentiate arteries from veins in the lung periphery. On a chest radiograph taken in the erect position, a gradual increase in the diameter of the vessels is seen, at equidistant points from the hilum, traveling from lung apex to base; this gravity-dependent effect disappears if the patient is supine or in cardiac failure.

The lobes of the lung are divided into segments, each of which are supplied by their own segmental pulmonary artery and accompanying bronchus. The walls of the segmental bronchi are rarely seen on the chest radiograph, except when lying parallel with the X-ray beam in which case they are seen end-on as ring shadows that measure up to 8 mm in diameter. The most frequently identified segmental airways are the anterior segmental bronchi of the upper lobes.

The Diaphragm and Thoracic Cage

The interface between aerated lung and the hemidiaphragms is sharp, and the highest point of each dome is normally medial to the midclavicular line. The right dome of the diaphragm is higher than the left by up to 2 cm in the erect position, unless the left dome is elevated by air in the stomach. Laterally, the hemidiaphragm forms an acute angle with the chest wall. Filling in or blunting of these costophrenic angles usually represents pleural disease, either pleural thickening or an effusion. In the elderly, localized humps on the dome of the diaphragm, particularly posteriorly (thus most obvious on a lateral radiograph), are common and represent minor weaknesses or defects of the diaphragm. Interposition of the colon in front of the right lobe of the liver is a frequently seen normal variant (so-called Chilaiditi syndrome).

Apparent pleural thickening along the lateral chest wall in the mid zones is a frequent observation in obese individuals; it is caused by subpleural fat bulging inward. Deformities of the thoracic cage may cause distortion of the normal mediastinum and so simulate disease. One of the most common deformities is pectus excavatum, which, by compressing the heart between the depressed sternum and vertebral column, causes displacement of the apparently enlarged heart to the left and blurring of the right heart border (Figure 1-25). A similar appearance may arise from an unusually straight thoracic spine, referred to as straight back syndrome.

Anatomy of the Lateral Chest Radiograph

Consistent viewing of lateral chest radiographs in the same orientation, whether a right or left lateral projection, improves the ability to detect deviations from normal. In the lateral view, the trachea is angled slightly posteriorly as it runs toward the carina, and its posterior wall is always visible as a fine

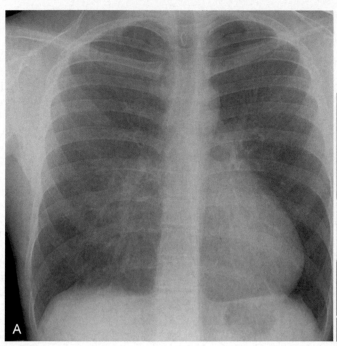

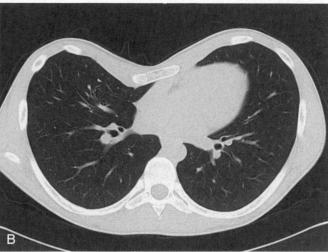

FIGURE 1-25 A, Frontal chest radiograph of a patient who has marked pectus excavatum. The blurring of the right heart border and apparent increase in heart size are a direct consequence of a depressed sternum. Note the "7" configuration of the ribs. **B,** CT scan shows the sternal depression.

stripe (Figure 1-26). The posterior walls of the right main bronchus and the right intermediate bronchus are outlined by air and are also seen as a continuous stripe on the lateral radiograph. The overlying scapulae are invariably seen running almost vertically in the upper part of the lateral radiograph (and may be misinterpreted as intrathoracic structures). Further confusing shadows are formed by the soft tissues of the outstretched arms, which project over the upper mediastinum. The carina is not visible as such on the lateral radiograph, and the two transradiancies projected over the lower trachea represent the right main bronchus (superiorly) and the left main bronchus (inferiorly).

Overlying structures on a lateral radiograph obscure most of the lung. In normal individuals, the unobscured lung in the retrosternal and retrocardiac regions should be of the same transradiancy. Furthermore, as the eye travels down the spine, a gradual increase in transradiancy should be apparent. The loss of this phenomenon suggests the presence of disease in the posterior-basal segments of the lower lobes (e.g., fibrosing alveolitis) (Figure 1-27).

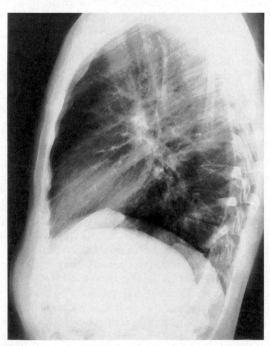

FIGURE 1-26 The lateral radiograph in a normal subject.

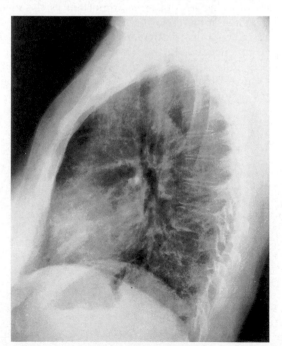

FIGURE 1-27 Loss of the normal increase in transradiancy toward the lower part of the dorsal spine in a patient with fibrosing alveolitis.

The two major fissures are seen as diagonal lines, of a hair's breadth, that run from the upper dorsal spine to the anterior surface of the diaphragm. Care must be taken not to confuse the obliquely running rib edges with fissures. The minor fissure extends horizontally from the mid right major fissure. It is often not possible to differentiate the right from the left major fissures with confidence. Similarly, although the two hemidiaphragms may be identified individually (especially if the gastric bubble is visible under the left dome of the diaphragm), differentiation between the right and the left hemidiaphragm is often impossible. A useful sign is the relative heights of the two domes—the dome furthest from the film is normally higher because of magnification.

The summation of both hilar on the lateral radiograph generates a complex shadow. However, one general point is useful in the interpretation of this difficult area—the right pulmonary artery lies anterior to the trachea and right main bronchus, whereas the left pulmonary artery arches over the left main bronchus so that a large part of it lies posterior to the major bronchi (Figure 1-28). A bandlike opacity is often seen along the lower third of the anterior chest wall behind the sternum. It represents a normal density and occurs because less aerated lung is in contact with the chest wall, because the space is occupied by the heart; it should not be confused with pleural disease.

POINTS IN THE INTERPRETATION OF A CHEST RADIOGRAPH

Even when an obvious radiographic abnormality is present, it is necessary to review a chest radiograph by use of a systematic method. With increasing experience, appreciation of deviation from normal appearances becomes rapid, which leads quickly to a directed search for related abnormalities. Before interpreting a chest radiograph, it is vital to establish whether any previous radiographs are available for comparison—the sequence and pattern of change is often as important as the identification of a radiographic abnormality. Information gained from preceding radiographs, particularly the lack of serial change, often prevents needless further investigation.

A check that the radiograph is of satisfactory quality includes an estimation of the adequacy of radiographic

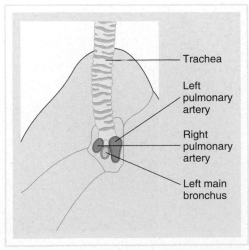

FIGURE 1-28 The proximal pulmonary arteries seen on a lateral chest radiograph.

exposure, depth of inspiration, and position of the patient. The intervertebral disk spaces of the entire dorsal spine should be visible on a correctly exposed chest radiograph, and the midpoint of the right hemidiaphragm lies at the level of the anterior end of the sixth rib if the (normal) subject has taken a satisfactory breath in. The medial ends of the clavicles should be equidistant from the spinous processes of the cervical vertebral bodies.

The order in which the various parts of a chest radiograph are examined is unimportant. A suggested sequence is to start with a check of the position of the trachea, mediastinal contour (which should be sharply outlined in its entirety), and then the position, outline, and density of the hilar shadows. The certain identification of a hilar abnormality often requires comparison with a previous radiograph; any suspicion of a hilar abnormality necessitates the retrieval of any previous chest radiographs. At least as important as an abnormal contour in detecting a mass at the hilum is a discrepancy in density between the two sides—both hilar shadows, at equivalent points, should be of equal density and a mass at the hilum (or an intrapulmonary mass projected over the hilum) is evident as an increased density of the affected hilum. For a questionably abnormal hilum, the lateral radiograph is sometimes helpful in clarifying the situation, providing the normal anatomy is remembered (i.e., most of the right pulmonary artery lies anterior to the trachea and the bulk of the left pulmonary artery lies behind the trachea). Thus, a suspected right hilar mass on a frontal radiograph that appears to be behind the trachea on a lateral view is unlikely to represent a prominent right pulmonary artery and is, therefore, most likely to be an abnormal mass (the converse rule applies to a suspicious left hilum).

The lungs may then be examined in terms of their size, the relative transradiancy of each zone, and the position of the horizontal fissure. Pulmonary vessels are seen as far out as the outer third of the lung, and the number of vessels should be roughly symmetric on the two sides. Next, the position and clarity of the hemidiaphragms should be noted, followed by an assessment of the ribs and soft tissues of the chest wall. Before regarding a chest radiograph as normal, it is useful to review areas that are poorly demonstrated or sometimes misinterpreted; these include the central mediastinum (where even a large mass may be invisible on the PA view), the lungs behind the diaphragm and heart, the lung apices (often obscured by the overlying clavicles and ribs), and the lung and pleura just inside the chest wall.

Radiographic Signs
Consolidation

Consolidation, or synonymously airspace shadowing, is caused by opacification of the air-containing spaces of the lung. The causes of consolidation are numerous (Table 1-1) and include almost any pathologic process that results in the filling of the normal alveolar spaces and small airways. The responsible material is almost invariably of fluid density, and usually the volume of the displacing fluid equals the volume of air displaced. This normally results in no net change in size of the lobar anatomy. Typically, it is not possible to tell from the radiologic appearances what has caused the airspace filling, especially in the absence of a clinical history. The possible exception to this generalization is airspace shadowing because of cardiogenic alveolar edema, when associated signs of congestive cardiac failure are found. When analyzing an area

TABLE 1-1 Causes of Consolidation

Common	Rare
Infection	Allergic lung diseases
Infarction	Connective tissue diseases
Cardiogenic pulmonary edema	Drug reactions
Noncardiogenic pulmonary edema	Hemorrhage
Adult respiratory distress syndrome	Lymphoma
Neurogenic edema	Radiation
Drug-induced edema	Amyloid
Miscellaneous	Eosinophilic lung disease
	Sarcoid
	Alveolar proteinosis

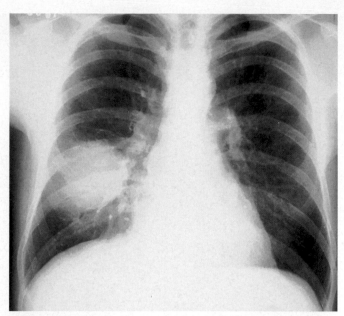

FIGURE 1-30 Well-defined, rounded opacity in the right mid zone, which fades out peripherally. Round pneumonia caused by pneumococcal infection.

of pulmonary opacification, the presence of a number of radiologic characteristics allows the confident characterization of airspace shadowing.

Typically, the shadowing is ill defined, except when it directly abuts a pleural surface (including the interlobar fissures), in which case it is sharply demarcated (Figure 1-29). Although consolidation respects lobar boundaries, there are no such barriers to spread into adjacent lung segments, which are frequently contiguously involved. Thus, an area of consolidation within a single lobe often enlarges in an irregular manner, and a discrete, well-defined opacity (so-called round pneumonia) is the exception and not the rule (Figure 1-30).

The vascular markings within an area of consolidation usually become obscured, because the contrast between the air-containing lung and the soft tissue density vascular markings is lost. By contrast, the bronchi, which are usually too thin walled to be differentiated from the surrounding lung parenchyma, become apparent in negative contrast to the airspace opacification, to produce the true hallmark of consolidation, the air bronchogram (Figure 1-31). A relatively uncommon, but very suggestive, radiologic sign of consolidation is the

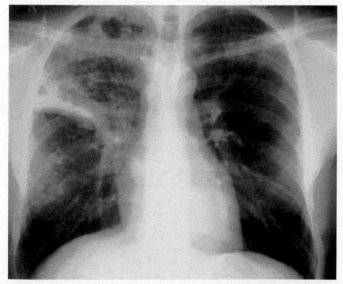

FIGURE 1-29 Patchy consolidation caused by tuberculosis. Where this abuts the horizontal fissure, the inferior surface of the consolidation is sharply defined.

acinar shadow, where an individual secondary pulmonary lobule becomes opacified but remains surrounded by normally aerated lung. The resultant soft tissue density nodule is usually on the periphery of a more confluent area of consolidation and normally measures 0.5–1 cm in diameter. These acinar opacities are most commonly seen in association with mycobacterial and varicella-zoster pneumonias but can occur in any other cause of consolidation (Figure 1-32). Occasionally, an acinus is left normally aerated but surrounded by opacified air spaces; this radiologic sign has been termed the air alveologram. When consolidation is not fully developed and has caused only partial filling of the air spaces, the resultant radiographic appearance is ground-glass opacification (Figure 1-33). Again, there is a wide range of possible causes, and in addition to causes of consolidation, this pattern may result from interstitial lung infiltration.

When an area of consolidation undergoes necrosis, because of either infection or infarction, liquefaction may result, and if either a gas-forming organism or communication with the bronchial tree is present, an air–fluid level may develop in addition to cavity formation (Figure 1-34). Consolidation frequently produces a silhouette sign, as described by Felson and Felson. Although this radiographic sign may be seen in association with a wide number of intrapulmonary pathologic processes, it is the relatively transitory nature of many forms of consolidation that best demonstrate the features of this finding. The original description stated that when an intrathoracic lesion touched a border of the heart, aorta, or diaphragm, it obliterated that border on the radiograph. Furthermore, a small area of consolidation may obliterate a normal air–soft tissue interface as effectively as a large area. This is demonstrated well by the obliteration of the right heart border by subtle middle-lobe consolidation that might otherwise be overlooked.

Understanding the significance of the silhouette sign allows the observer to localize an area of consolidation or other pulmonary opacity. Only if an area of consolidation lies in direct

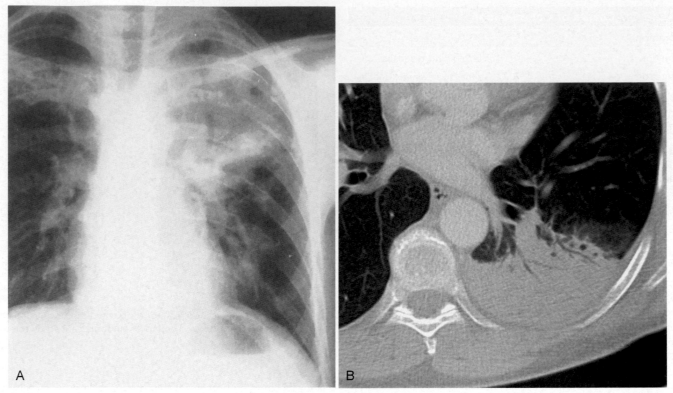

FIGURE 1-31 Air bronchogram in consolidation. **A,** Left, upper zone tuberculosis demonstrating an air bronchogram. **B,** Computed tomography scan through the left lower lobe in a different patient demonstrates an area of segmental pneumonia.

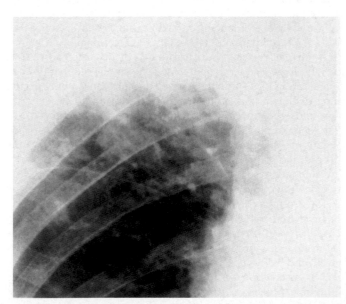

FIGURE 1-32 Acinar opacities seen at the periphery of confluent right upper lobe consolidation in a patient who has tuberculosis. Note the elevation of the horizontal fissure.

contact to a normal structure is the silhouette of that structure lost. If an area of consolidation and a normal structure–lung interface merely lie along the same X-ray path, they are superimposed on the radiograph but do not demonstrate the silhouette sign. Thus, lingular consolidation is likely to obscure the heart border, but left lower lobe consolidation usually does

not (Figures 1-35 through 1-37). There are several potential causes for a falsely positive silhouette sign. Some relatively common anatomic variants that result in a reduced AP diameter of the thorax, such as pectus excavatum or straight back syndrome, cause loss of the right heart border as the depressed sternum distorts the normal anatomy (see Figure 1-25). Occasionally, a scoliosis, usually concave to the left and which may be relatively trivial, causes the right heart border to be projected over the spine. It is only when the heart border is projected over the right lung that the silhouette sign can be elicited. Underexposed radiographs may appear to demonstrate the silhouette sign, so it is imperative that the technical quality of the radiograph is taken into account.

Collapse

When there is partial or complete volume loss in a lung or lobe, this is referred to as collapse or atelectasis. The terms are essentially interchangeable, and they imply a diminished volume of air in the lung with associated reduction of lung volume. Several different mechanisms result in lung or lobar collapse.

Relaxation or Passive Collapse. The lung retracts toward its hilum when air or an abnormal amount of fluid accumulates in the pleural space.

Cicatrization Collapse. The normal expansion of the lung, to contact the parietal pleura, depends on a balance between outward forces in the chest wall and opposite elastic forces in the lung. If the lung is abnormally stiff, this balance is disturbed, lung compliance is decreased, and the volume of the affected lung is reduced. Perhaps the best example of this phenomenon is volume loss associated with pulmonary fibrosis.

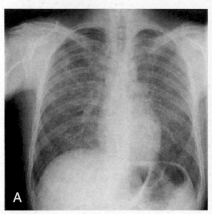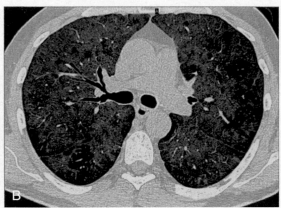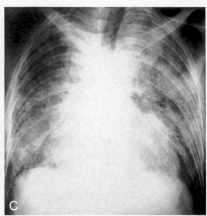

FIGURE 1-33 Ground-glass opacification in the mid and lower zones in a patient who has *Pneumocystis jiroveci* pneumonia. **A,** Chest radiograph of a young HIV-positive male patient presenting with *P. jiroveci* pneumonia. There is perihilar poorly defined increased (ground-glass) density. (Courtesy of Dr. M. Taylor.) **B,** HRCT image of the same patient demonstrating variation of lung attenuation with markedly black airways highlighted by the ground-glass patchy infiltrate. **C,** Diffuse and severe ground-glass and air space infiltrate in a different patient with *P. jiroveci* pneumonia.

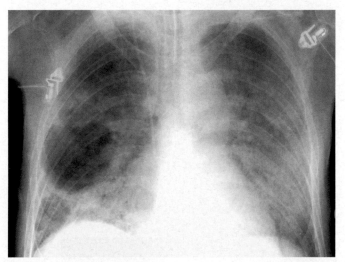

FIGURE 1-34 Large right lower lobe cavity in a patient with widespread pneumonic consolidation. In this supine patient, an air–fluid level is not evident.

Adhesive Collapse. In the normal lung, the forces that govern surface tension become more pronounced as the surface area of the airspace is reduced. Hence, the collapse of smaller airways and alveoli tends to occur at lower lung volumes, a tendency that is offset by surfactant, which reduces the surface tension of the fluid that lines the alveoli. This reduction is usually sufficient to overcome the tendency to collapse in the normal lung. However, if the mechanism is disturbed, as in respiratory distress syndrome, collapse of the alveoli occurs, and typically the larger airways remain patent.

Reabsorption Collapse. In acute bronchial obstruction, gases in the alveoli are steadily taken up by the blood in the pulmonary capillaries and are not replenished, which causes alveolar collapse. The degree of collapse may be counteracted by collateral air drift if the obstruction is distal to the main bronchus and also by infection and accumulation of secretions. If the obstruction becomes chronic, subsequent reabsorption of intraalveolar secretions and exudate may result in complete collapse, the usual mechanism of collapse seen in carcinoma of the bronchus. When the cause of collapse is a proximal obstructing mass, the S sign of Golden may be apparent. This sign refers to the S shape made by the relevant fissure as the distal part of a lobe collapses, but the proximal part of a lobe maintains its bulk because of the presence of a tumor.

Radiographic Signs of Lobar Collapse. The radiographic appearance in pulmonary collapse depends on a number of factors, which include the mechanism of collapse, the extent of collapse, the presence or absence of consolidation in the affected lung, and the preexisting state of the pleura. This last factor includes the presence of underlying pleural tethering or thickening and the presence of pleural fluid. Preexisting lung disease, such as fibrosis and pleural adhesions, may alter the expected displacement of anatomic landmarks in lung collapse. An air bronchogram is rare in reabsorption collapse but is usual in passive and adhesive collapse and may be seen in cicatrization collapse if fibrosis is particularly dense.

Signs of collapse may be direct or indirect. Indirect signs are the result of compensatory changes that occur as a consequence of the volume loss. The direct signs of collapse include displacement of interlobar fissures, loss of aeration, and vascular and bronchial signs. Indirect signs include elevation of the hemidiaphragm, mediastinal displacement, hilar displacement, compensatory hyperinflation, and crowding of the ribs. There tends to be a reciprocal relationship between the individual compensatory signs of collapse, so that if there is mediastinal shift to the side of collapse, there is unlikely to be significant diaphragmatic elevation. For example, in lower lobe collapse, if hemidiaphragmatic elevation is marked, hilar depression is less marked.

Displacement of Interlobar Fissures. Displacement of interlobar fissures is the most reliable sign, and the degree of displacement depends on the extent of collapse.

Loss of Aeration. The increased density of a collapsed area of lung may not become apparent until collapse is almost complete. However, if the collapsed lung is adjacent to the mediastinum or diaphragm, the presence of the silhouette sign may indicate loss of aeration.

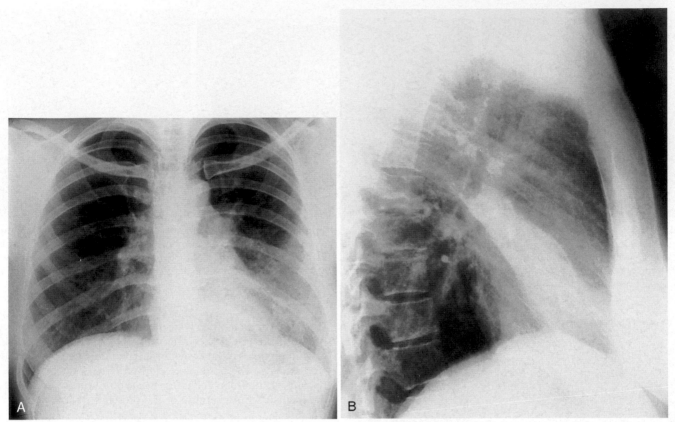

FIGURE 1-35 Lingular consolidation. **A,** Loss of the left heart border with a diffuse pulmonary infiltrate in the left mid and lower zone. The outer aspect of the left diaphragm is preserved. **B,** Lateral view of the same patient as in **(A),** showing consolidation within the lingula and delineated posteriorly by the major fissure.

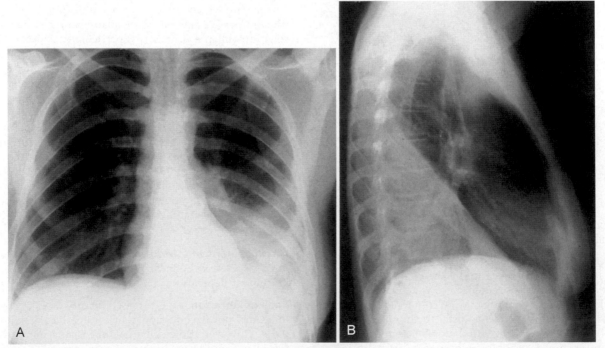

FIGURE 1-36 Mid and lower zone consolidation in the left lower lobe. **A,** There is preservation of the left heart border, but loss of the left hemidiaphragm. **B,** Lateral view showing the consolidation in the lower lobe delineated anteriorly by the major fissure.

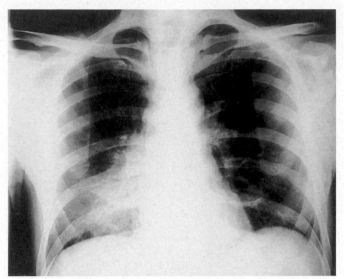

FIGURE 1-37 Right lower lobe consolidation. The right heart border is clearly defined. Because the consolidation is not complete, the hemidiaphragm has not been effaced.

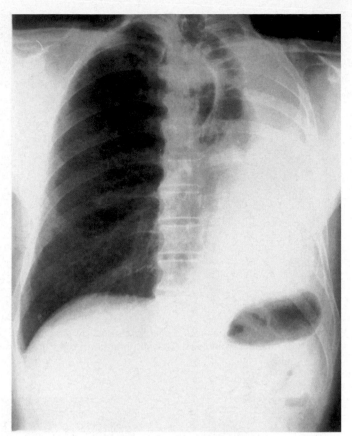

FIGURE 1-38 Collapse of the left lung. There is a proximal obstructing tumor within the left main bronchus, with complete collapse of the left lung and a mediastinal shift to the left.

Vascular and Bronchial Signs. If a lobe is partially collapsed, crowding of its vessels may be visible; also, if an air bronchogram is visible, the bronchi may appear crowded together.

Elevation of the Hemidiaphragm. Elevation of the hemidiaphragm may be seen in lower lobe collapse but is uncommon in collapse of the other lobes.

Mediastinal Displacement. In upper lobe collapse, the trachea is often displaced toward the affected side; in lower lobe collapse, the heart may be displaced to the same site.

Hilar Displacement. The hilum may be elevated in upper lobe collapse and depressed in lower lobe collapse.

Compensatory Hyperinflation. The remaining normal lung may become hyperinflated and thus may appear more transradiant, with the vessels more widely spaced than in the corresponding area of the contralateral lung. With considerable collapse of a lung, compensatory hyperinflation of the contralateral lung may occur, with herniation of lung across the midline.

Crowding of the Ribs. On the side of the collapse there is often narrowing of the intercostal spaces with crowding together of the ribs, which reflects the diminished overall volume of the affected hemithorax.

Complete Lung Collapse. When there is complete collapse of an entire lung (in the absence of an accompanying pneumothorax, large pleural effusion, or extensive consolidation), complete opacification of that hemithorax is seen, with displacement of the mediastinum to the affected side and elevation of the hemidiaphragm. Compensatory hyperinflation of the contralateral lung occurs, often with herniation across the midline. Herniation is most often in the retrosternal space, anterior to the ascending aorta, but may occur posterior to the heart (Figure 1-38).

Individual or Combined Lobar Collapse. The descriptions that follow apply to collapse of individual lobes, uncomplicated

by preexisting pulmonary or pleural disease. The alterations to the positions of the fissures, mediastinal structures, and diaphragms are shown in Figures 1-39 to 1-43.

Right Upper Lobe Collapse. As the right upper lobe collapses (see Figure 1-39), the horizontal fissure rotates around the hilum and the lateral end moves upward and medially toward the superior mediastinum. The anterior end moves upward, toward the apex. The upper half of the oblique fissure moves anteriorly. The two fissures become concave superiorly. In severe collapse, the lobe may be flattened against the superior mediastinum and may obscure the upper pole of the hilum. The hilum is elevated, and its lower pole may be prominent. Deviation of the trachea to the right is usual, and compensatory hyperinflation of the right middle and lower lobes may be apparent.

Middle Lobe Collapse. In right middle lobe collapse (see Figure 1-40), the horizontal fissure and lower half of the oblique fissure move toward each other, a feature best seen on the lateral projection. Because the horizontal fissure tends to be more mobile, it usually shows greater displacement. On the frontal radiograph, middle lobe collapse may be subtle because the horizontal fissure may not be visible, and increased opacity does not become apparent until collapse is almost complete. Critical analysis of the radiograph sometimes reveals obscuration of the right heart border as the only clue. The lordotic AP projection is rarely required but may be used to bring the displaced fissure into the line of the X-ray beam and occasionally may elegantly demonstrate middle lobe collapse. Because

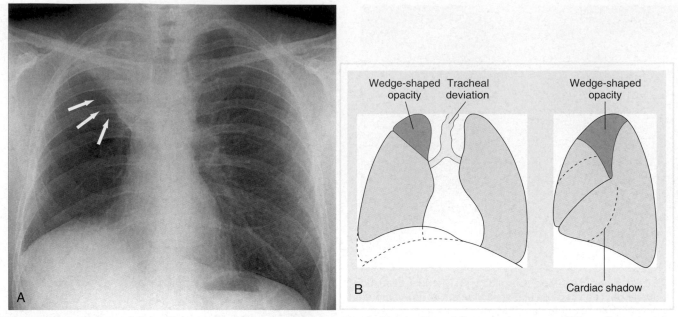

FIGURE 1-39 Right upper lobe collapse caused by a right hilar tumor. **A,** The horizontal fissure takes on an "S" configuration, known as the S sign of Golden (*arrows*). **B,** Line diagram of right upper lobe collapse.

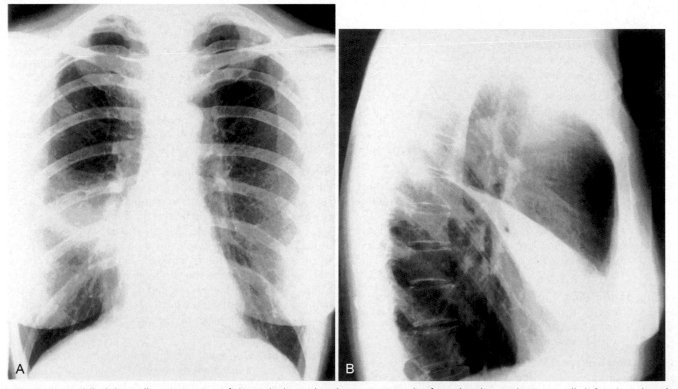

FIGURE 1-40 Middle lobe collapse. **A,** Loss of the right heart border is seen on the frontal radiograph. **B,** A well-defined wedge-shaped opacity on the lateral radiograph is delineated by the horizontal and oblique fissures (*arrows*).

the volume of this lobe is relatively small, indirect signs of volume loss are rarely obvious.

Left Lower Lobe Collapse. In left lower lobe collapse (Figure 1-41), the normal oblique fissures extend from the level of the fourth thoracic vertebra posteriorly to the diaphragm, close to the sternum anteriorly. The position of these fissures on the lateral projection is the best index of lower lobe volumes. When a lower lobe collapses, the oblique fissure moves posteriorly but maintains its normal slope. In addition to posterior movement, the collapsing lower lobe causes medial displacement of the oblique fissure, which may become visible in places on the frontal projection.

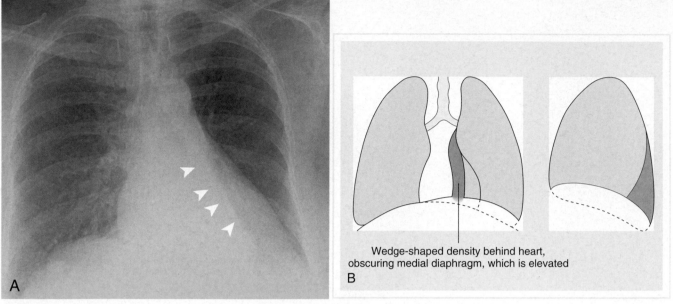

FIGURE 1-41 Left lower lobe collapse in a patient who has an occluding tumor. **A,** The left hemithorax is of reduced volume, and there is loss of the normal silhouette of the left lower lobe pulmonary artery. The left lower lobe has contracted behind the cardiac silhouette (*arrowheads*). **B,** Line diagram.

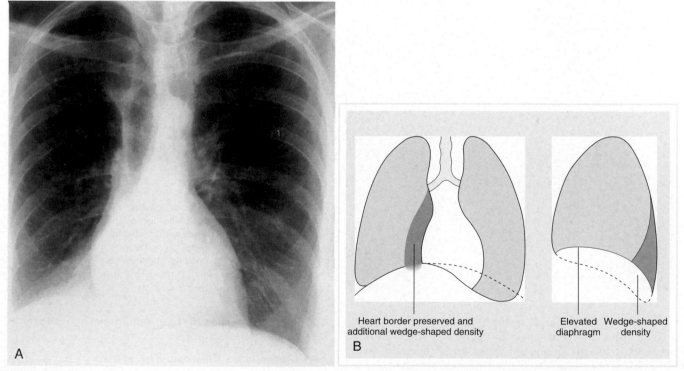

FIGURE 1-42 Right lower lobe collapse in a patient with asthma. **A,** There is preservation of the right heart border, but reduction in volume of the right hemithorax and shift of the trachea to the right side. **B,** Line diagram.

Right Lower Lobe Collapse. Right lower lobe collapse (see Figure 1-42) causes partial depression of the horizontal fissure, which may be apparent on the frontal projection. Increased opacity of a collapsed lower lobe is usually visible on the frontal projection also. A completely collapsed lower lobe may be so small that it flattens and merges with the mediastinum to produce a thin, wedge-shaped shadow. In left lower lobe collapse, the heart may obscure this opacity, and a penetrated view may be required to demonstrate it. Mediastinal structures and parts of the diaphragm adjacent to the nonaerated lobe are obscured. When significant lower lobe collapse occurs, especially when the collapsed lobe is so small

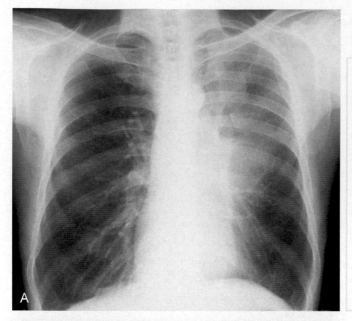

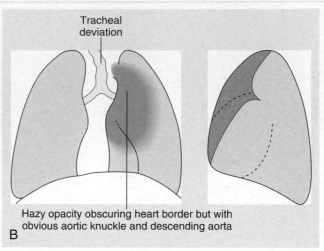

Tracheal
deviation

Hazy opacity obscuring heart border but with
obvious aortic knuckle and descending aorta

B

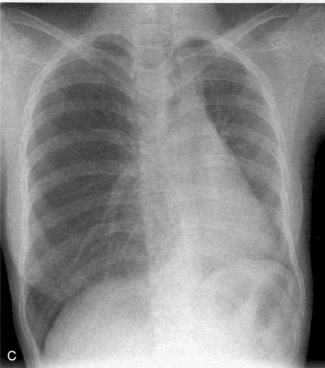

C

FIGURE 1-43 Left upper lobe collapse with shift of the mediastinum to the left and loss of definition of the mediastinal structures. **A,** In this patient, a large tumor is causing left upper lobe and lingula collapse. The opacification fades out more inferiorly. **B,** Line diagram. **C,** In another patient, there is very tight left upper lobe collapse because of a small tumor. The appearances are different, but there is still marked volume loss.

as to be invisible as a separate opacity, confirmatory evidence is usually apparent from close inspection of the relevant hilum. This is usually depressed and rotated medially, with loss of the normal hilar vascular structures, which is made all the more obvious if a previous film is available for comparison. In addition, indirect signs of collapse, such as upper lobe hyperinflation, are present. Diaphragmatic elevation is unusual.

Lingula Collapse. The lingula is often involved in collapse of the left upper lobe, but occasionally it may collapse individually, in which case the radiographic features are similar to those of middle lobe collapse. However, the absence of a horizontal fissure on the left makes anterior displacement of the lower half of the oblique fissure and increased opacity anterior

to it important signs. On the frontal projection, the left heart border becomes obscured.

Left Upper Lobe Collapse. The pattern of upper lobe collapse is different in the two lungs. Left upper lobe collapse (see Figure 1-43) is apparent on the lateral projection as anterior displacement of the entire oblique fissure, which becomes oriented almost parallel to the anterior chest wall. With increasing collapse, the upper lobe retracts posteriorly and loses contact with the anterior chest wall. With complete collapse, the left upper lobe may lose contact with the chest wall and diaphragm and retract medially against the mediastinum. On a lateral film, therefore, left upper lobe collapse appears as an elongated opacity that extends from the apex and reaches, or almost reaches, the diaphragm; it is anterior to the hilum and is bounded by the displaced oblique fissure posteriorly and by the hyperinflated lower lobe.

A collapsed left upper lobe does not produce a sharp outline on the frontal view. An ill-defined, hazy opacity is present in the upper, mid, and sometimes lower zones, the opacity being densest near the hilum. Pulmonary vessels in the hyperinflated lower lobe are usually visible through the haze. The aortic knuckle is usually obscured, unless the upper lobe has collapsed anterior to it, in which case hyperexpansion of the lower lobe apical segment may occur and separate the collapsed upper lobe from the mediastinal silhouette and aortic knuckle. This produces an unusual, but characteristic, medial crescent of lucency termed the Luftsichel sign. If the lingula is involved, the left heart border is obscured. The hilum is often elevated, and the trachea deviated to the left.

Combined Lobar Collapses
Right Lower and Middle Lobe Collapse. Because the right lower and middle lobes take their origin from the bronchus intermedius, an extensive lesion at that site may cause combined collapse. The appearances are similar to right lower lobe collapse (Figure 1-44), except that the horizontal fissure is not apparent, the opacification reaches the lateral chest wall on the frontal radiograph, and similarly extends to the anterior chest wall on the lateral view.

Right Upper and Middle Lobe Collapse. Combined collapse of the right upper and middle lobes is unusual because of the distance between the origins of their bronchi; it can generally be taken to imply the presence of more than one lesion. This combination produces appearances almost identical to those of left upper lobe collapse (Figure 1-45). On occasion, isolated

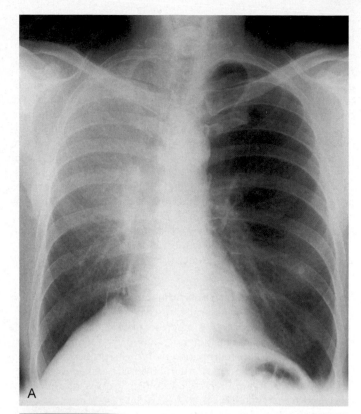

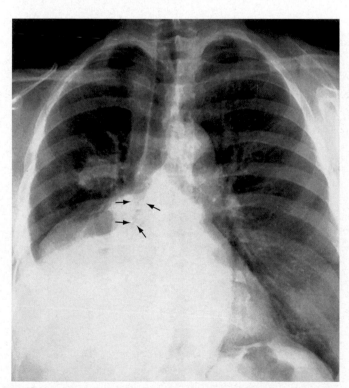

FIGURE 1-44 Right middle and lower lobe collapse caused by an obstructing lesion in the bronchus intermedius. A bronchial cut-off sign is visible (*arrows*). A separate pulmonary mass is present in the right upper lobe.

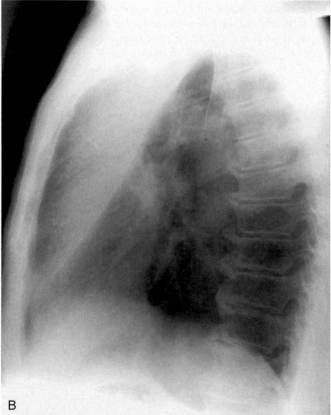

FIGURE 1-45 Right middle and upper lobe collapse. Occasionally, this combination mimics left upper lobe and lingular collapse. **A**, PA view and (**B**) lateral radiograph demonstrating changes similar to those seen on the opposite side. The major fissure shifts anteriorly and extends from the lung apex to the anterior costophrenic recess.

right upper lobe collapse also produces appearances that are identical to those of left upper lobe collapse.

Rounded Atelectasis. Rounded atelectasis is an unusual form of pulmonary collapse that may be misdiagnosed as a pulmonary tumor. On the plain film, there is an opacity that may be several centimeters in diameter, frequently with ill-defined edges. Rounded atelectasis is always pleura based and associated with pleural thickening. Vascular shadows may radiate from part of the opacity, said to resemble a comet's tail (Figure 1-46). The appearance is caused by peripheral lung tissue folding in on itself. Rounded atelectasis is usually related to previous asbestos exposure but may also occur secondary to any exudative pleural effusion. It is not of any other pathologic significance, although when present often raises the question of a malignancy. The CT appearance is usually sufficiently diagnostic to allow differentiation from other pulmonary masses.

Unilateral Increased Transradiancy. The most common causes of increased unilateral transradiancy are technical factors, such as patient rotation, poor beam centering, or an offset grid. Usually, hypertransradiancy caused by technical factors can be identified by comparison of the soft tissues around the shoulder girdle and particularly over the axillae. Nevertheless, there are a number of pathologic causes of unilateral increased transradiancy.

Chest Wall. A hemithorax may appear of increased transradiancy (blacker) if the X-rays are less attenuated because of a reduction in the amount of overlying soft tissue. The most common cause for this is a mastectomy. Rarely, the same phenomenon may be seen in patients who have congenital unilateral absence of pectoral muscles, known as Poland's syndrome (Figure 1-47). This may be accompanied by associated skeletal abnormalities in the ipsilateral ribs, but may be recognized by loss of the normal axillary skin fold.

Reduced Vascularity. Interruption or significant reduction in the blood supply to one lung, either congenital or acquired, has increased transradiancy (Figure 1-48).

Lung Hyperexpansion. If a lung is overexpanded because of either air trapping secondary to the presence of a foreign body or asymmetric emphysema, that hemithorax may demonstrate increased transradiancy. When the entire lung is affected, the hemithorax is usually relatively larger than the opposite side. However, the same phenomenon may occur with compensatory emphysema because of collapse or removal of an ipsilateral lobe. In this case, the transradiant hemithorax may be of normal volume, and the presence of the increased transradiancy should prompt a search for other evidence of collapse or prior surgery.

A relatively increased transradiancy of one hemithorax with no obvious cause suggests the possibility of a generalized increase in radiopacity of the opposite side (for example, the posterior layering of a pleural effusion in a supine patient) (Figure 1-49).

The Pulmonary Mass

The finding of a solitary pulmonary nodule on the chest radiograph requires careful analysis, because the diagnostic possibilities are numerous. Once a pulmonary mass has been identified, the observer must first decide if the lesion is genuine and second whether the lesion is truly intrapulmonary.

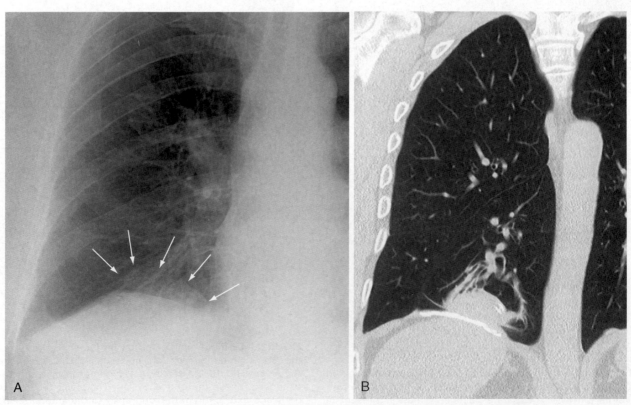

FIGURE 1-46 Rounded atelectasis. **A,** A poorly defined opacity is visible on the frontal radiograph (*arrows*). **B,** Coronal reformatted image from computed tomography scan reveals the characteristic pleurally based mass with radiating bronchovascular strands.

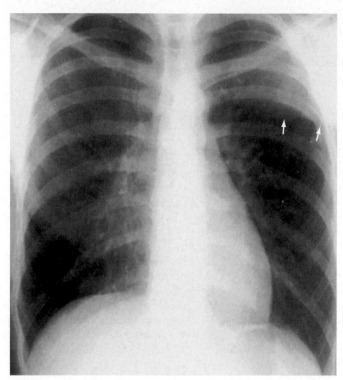

FIGURE 1-47 Poland's syndrome. Incidental finding on a chest radiograph of congenital absence of the left pectoralis major muscle. Note the alteration in the left axillary skin fold compared with the right (*arrows*).

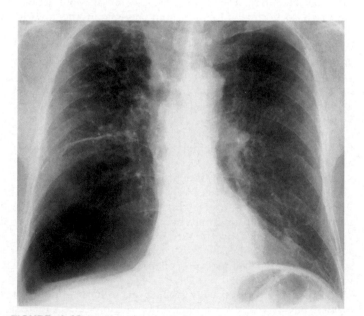

FIGURE 1-48 Increased transradiancy in the right lower zone. A large emphysematous bulla occupies the lower half of the right lung, and the apical changes are in keeping with previous tuberculosis.

The possibility of a cutaneous lesion should not be forgotten, especially if only a part of the nodule is well defined. If doubt remains, repeat radiographs are obtained, with a lateral view and, if relevant, nipple markers. What appears at first glance to represent a solitary pulmonary mass may, on closer

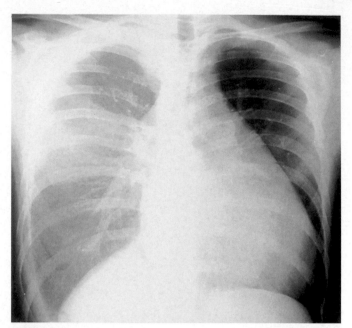

FIGURE 1-49 Supine radiograph of a patient who has a large right pleural effusion. The generalized increase in radiopacity of the right side is caused by posterior layering of a pleural effusion.

inspection, actually represent the most obvious of a number of pulmonary nodules. The radiology of multiple pulmonary nodules is discussed later.

When a pulmonary mass is clearly defined around its entire circumference and is projected over the lung on frontal and lateral projections, the mass is truly intrapulmonary (Figure 1-50). However, if a surface is in contact with another soft tissue structure, the possibility of an extrapulmonary mass projecting into the lung must be considered. Analysis of the breadth of the base of the lesion, the angle made with the adjacent structure, and the presence of bone destruction often allows the observer to differentiate between an extrapulmonary mass that extends into the adjacent lung from an intrapulmonary mass that has grown to contact the mediastinum, diaphragm, or chest wall.

The analysis of a solitary pulmonary mass relies on a number of radiologic and clinical factors. The latter include patient age, geographic and ethnic origins, smoking history, and medical history. The likelihood that a pulmonary nodule represents a malignancy in a young nonsmoker who comes from an area where histoplasmosis is endemic is clearly different from that for an elderly patient with a lifetime history of smoking.

Radiographic features of a pulmonary nodule that should be analyzed include size, density, margins, vascular markings, and growth rate.

Size

Generally, the likelihood of malignancy is greater with increasing size, although the opposite argument is not reliable.

Density

Most pulmonary masses are of soft tissue density. However, careful inspection must be made for the presence of calcification, because certain patterns of calcification are typical of benign lesions that may be safely observed rather than resected

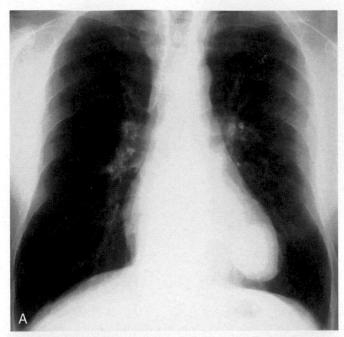

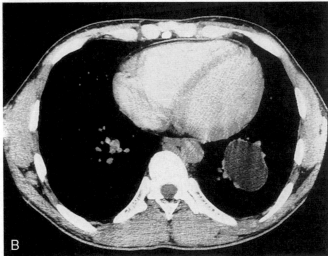

FIGURE 1-50 A rounded pulmonary mass. **A,** Posteroanterior radiograph of a patient who has a well-defined pulmonary mass. The entire circumference is visualized on the film, which indicates no surface of contact with the mediastinal structures. **B,** Computed tomography of this mass demonstrates it is of fluid density and was due to a hydatid cyst.

(Figure 1-51). A completely or centrally calcified nodule is diagnostic of a tuberculoma or histoplasmoma. Often, CT is required to confirm this pattern of calcification. Likewise, concentric rings of calcification are typical of healed histoplasmosis infection. Popcorn calcification, within the matrix of a pulmonary nodule, is highly suggestive of a hamartoma (Figure 1-52). Other forms of calcification do not reliably indicate whether a nodule is benign or malignant, and dystrophic calcification within a pulmonary malignancy is relatively common.

Margins

Perfectly smooth, round lesions are likely to be benign. However, this is not a completely reliable rule, because some primary lung malignancies and secondary deposits, particularly from soft tissue sarcomas, may be perfectly spherical. By contrast, lobulated or spiculated masses are much more likely to represent malignancy.

Vascular Markings

A rare, benign, but important cause of a pulmonary nodule is an arteriovenous malformation. The diagnosis may be suggested on the plain radiograph if a prominent feeding artery or draining vein is identified.

Growth Rate

Review of previous radiographs, when available, may establish whether a lesion is static or increasing in size. It is usual practice to express the growth of a pulmonary tumor in terms of the time taken for it to double in volume, which equates to an increase in diameter of 25%, assuming that the tumor is roughly spherical, as is usually the case. Tumors with a doubling time of <30 days or >2 years are very unlikely to result from malignancy. However, often no previous films are available, and thus the use of growth rate as a diagnostic aid is limited. Modern CT allows small pulmonary lesions to be followed over increasing intervals to confirm lack of growth. This is facilitated by the use of automated software that allows volumetric information to be derived form the CT data set (Figure 1-53).

Enhancement Characteristics

By the same token, it has been shown that failure of enhancement of a small lung mass, after a bolus of intravenous radiographic contrast, is also a strong indicator of a benign histology and may strengthen the case for an observational approach to a small (1–3 cm) lung nodule in the low-risk patient.

When a solitary lung mass is evident on the chest radiograph, and no features suggest whether it is of benign etiology or a malignant lesion, it should be assumed to be a primary lung carcinoma until proved otherwise. In the assessment of a potential lung primary tumor, certain guidelines may be helpful.

Approximately half of primary lung carcinomas arise centrally in a proximal or segmental bronchus and as a result present as a hilar mass.

Because carcinoma of the bronchus arises in the bronchial mucosa, the tumor is likely to grow into the bronchial lumen and around the bronchus. As the bronchial lumen narrows, the distal lung may become consolidated and lose volume. Depending on the site of the tumor, a malignant solitary lung mass may be associated with lobar or segmental collapse (Figure 1-54) or even collapse of an entire lung (see Figure 1-38).

Peripheral tumors usually appear as solitary nodules or masses, but no features on plain films reliably differentiate a benign from a malignant pulmonary nodule. As described previously, malignant tumors are often larger, poorly defined, spiculated, or lobulated. Satellite opacities around a mass are more commonly seen with benign lesions, notably granulomatous diseases (see Figure 1-32). At least 5% of bronchial carcinomas cavitate because of central necrosis or abscess formation; the resultant cavity is typically thick-walled with an irregular inner margin (Figure 1-55). Peripheral tumors may invade the ribs or spine directly. Bone destruction must be specifically looked for and, when present, almost invariably indicates malignancy (Figure 1-56).

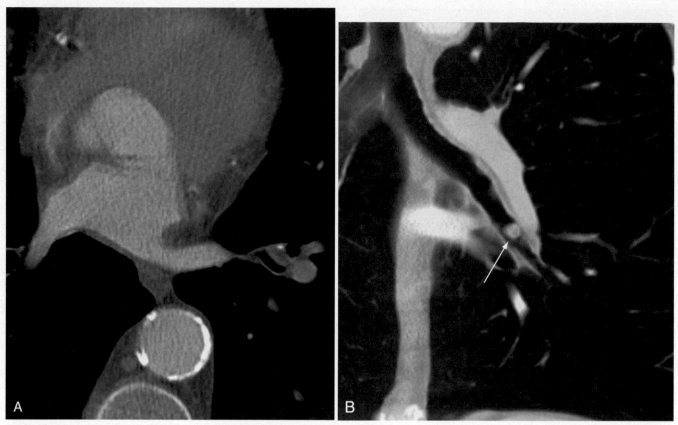

FIGURE 1-51 Fat and calcium density in a small endobronchial mass. CT of a small lesion in the left lower lobe bronchus on **(A)** axial and **(B)** coronal reformats. This density *(arrow)* confirms that the lesion is a hamartoma.

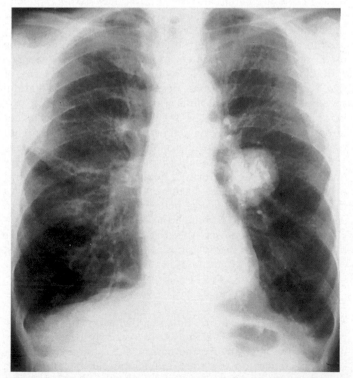

FIGURE 1-52 Pulmonary mass calcification. Posteroanterior chest radiograph of a mass that projects over the left hilum. This is smoothly marginated and contains central popcorn calcification; it is unusually large but otherwise a typical pulmonary hamartoma.

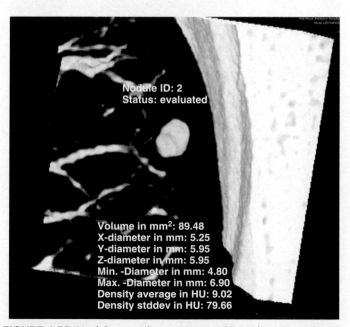

Nodule ID: 2
Status: evaluated

Volume in mm²: 89.48
X-diameter in mm: 5.25
Y-diameter in mm: 5.95
Z-diameter in mm: 5.95
Min. -Diameter in mm: 4.80
Max. -Diameter in mm: 6.90
Density average in HU: 9.02
Density stddev in HU: 79.66

FIGURE 1-53 Nodule growth assessment. CT workstation volumetric assessment allows accurate follow-up of small pulmonary nodules to determine whether there has been interval growth.

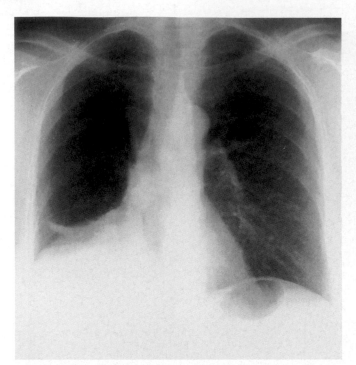

FIGURE 1-54 Right lower and partial middle lobe collapse secondary to a proximal bronchogenic carcinoma.

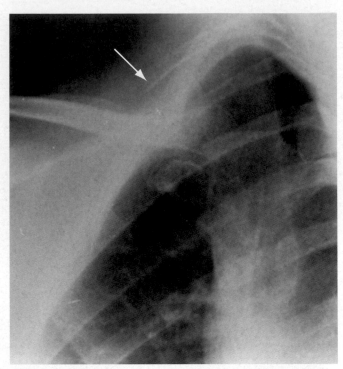

FIGURE 1-56 Oblique view of the right apex demonstrating bone destruction within the first rib (*arrow*). The patient has peripheral bronchogenic carcinoma.

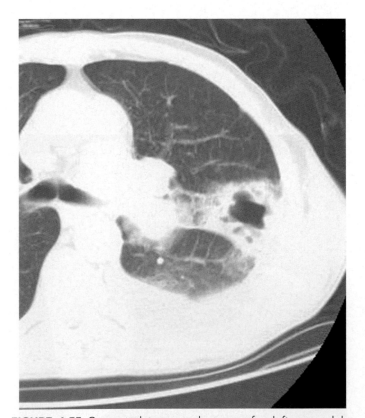

FIGURE 1-55 Computed tomography scan of a left upper lobe bronchogenic carcinoma with central necrosis and cavitation. The cavity wall is thick and irregular.

Multiple Pulmonary Nodules

The differential diagnosis of multiple pulmonary nodules is wide (Table 1-2), but analysis of the chest radiograph and a review of the clinical status of the patient rapidly narrow the number of possibilities. Many of the radiographic features used in the analysis of the solitary pulmonary nodule can be used usefully in the assessment of multiple lesions.

Radiographically, multiple nodules are described in terms of size, number, distribution, density, definition, cavitation, speed of growth (if serial films are available), and accompanying pleural, mediastinal, or skeletal abnormalities. Further important clinical clues may come from the clinical status of the patient. Specifically, evidence of infection, systemic illness, and prior malignancy is sought (Figures 1-57 to 1-60). Miliary nodules are a particular form of nodular shadowing. The term miliary derives from the likening of the size and shape of the nodules to millet seeds, being round, well defined, and 2–3 mm in diameter. Although the description is usually associated with tuberculosis, this pattern of nodular infiltrate may also be due to histoplasmosis, organic and inorganic dust diseases, sarcoid, or metastases.

Diffuse Shadowing

Many diseases cause diffuse lung shadowing on chest radiography. Careful analysis is required to correctly determine the nature of the abnormality and narrow the differential diagnosis. Appearances on the chest radiograph can be misleading, and the pattern of disease demonstrated at pathologic or HRCT examination may differ considerably from the pattern

TABLE 1-2 Causes of Acquired Pulmonary Nodules	
Acquired	
Neoplastic	Inflammatory

Benign
   Hamartomas
   Papillomatosis
   Bronchogenic cysts
 	
Malignant
   Metastases
   Lymphoma
   Multifocal tumor
   Kaposi's sarcoma
   Bronchoalveolar
      cell carcinoma
	Infectious
	   Granulomatous infections
	   Multiple embolic abscesses
	   Round pneumonias
	   Viral infections—chickenpox and
	      measles
	   Parasites—hydatid and
	      paragonimiasis
	Noninfectious
	   Caplan's syndrome and rheumatoid
	      nodules
	   Wegener's granulomatosis
	   Sarcoidosis
	Others
	   Progressive massive fibrosis
	   Amyloid
	   Infarcts
	   Bronchial impaction

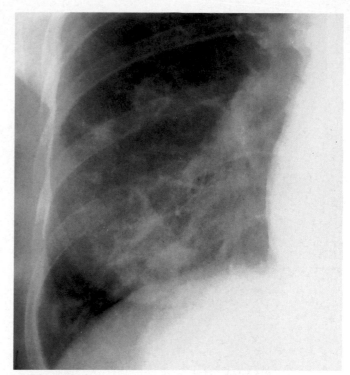

FIGURE 1-58 Magnified view of the right lower zone. The multiple pulmonary nodules are cavitating in this case of multiple staphylococcal abscesses in an intravenous drug abuser.

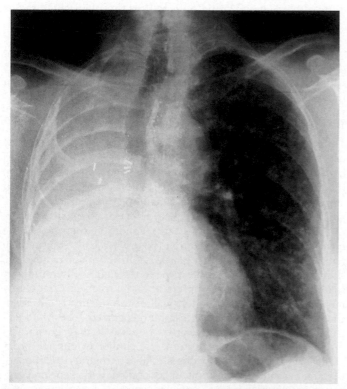

FIGURE 1-57 Chest radiograph of a patient who had a previous right pneumonectomy for adenocarcinoma. Multiple pulmonary nodules are now within the lung because of secondary deposits.

of abnormality suggested by the chest radiograph. The summation of multiple, small, linear opacities on the chest radiograph may produce the appearance of multiple small nodules. Likewise, the superimposition of multiple small nodules may produce a granular or ground-glass pattern. A variety of descriptive terms are used in the analysis of a chest radiograph in this context, and frequently appearances are classified as being either interstitial or airspace. However, a number of processes are capable of producing both patterns, so that the differential diagnosis may be erroneously narrowed at an early stage of analysis. Thus, it is preferable to analyze the pattern in purely descriptive terms, such as reticular or nodular shadowing, to avoid this pitfall.

Reticular Shadowing. Reticular or linear shadowing (Figure 1-61) is made up of multiple, short, irregular linear densities, usually randomly orientated, and often overlapping to produce a netlike pattern. When profuse, they may summate to form ring shadows or sometimes a nodular pattern. Occasionally, the linear shadows may be orientated at right angles to the pleural surface, so-called Kerley's B lines (Figure 1-62), which indicates thickening of the interlobular septa. When the linear opacities are extremely profuse or coarse, the impression of a ring or honeycomb pattern is given.

Nodular Opacities. Nodules may be well or poorly defined and of varying density, ranging from soft tissue to calcific (Figure 1-63). They may be discrete or coalescent, with areas of confluence producing consolidation. When the nodules are greater than a few millimeters in diameter, the differential

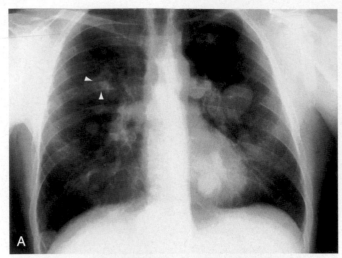

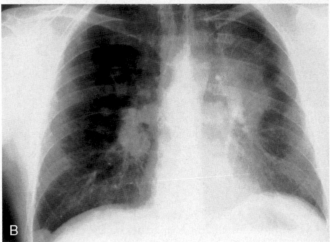

FIGURE 1-59 Multiple pulmonary nodules. **A,** The multiple pulmonary nodules are smoothly defined and vary in size; some are cavitating (*arrowheads*). **B,** Subsequent chest radiograph obtained shortly afterward. The left perihilar nodules are no longer visible because they lie within the now collapsed left upper lobe. The patient has multiple metastases from soft-tissue sarcoma.

diagnosis changes. Larger discrete nodules were discussed previously.

Reticulonodular Shadowing. Often, it is impossible to confidently assign a pattern of diffuse shadowing to one of the two previously described categories because they overlap. The reticulonodular pattern is probably the most common form of diffuse lung shadowing.

Ground-Glass Shadowing. Ground-glass shadowing (see Figure 1-33) refers to a generalized increase in density of the lung, which may be diffuse or patchy but is most commonly bilateral and mid and lower zonal or perihilar. The underlying vascular branching pattern is not totally obscured, as it is in consolidation, but the vessels become less distinct; likewise, the hilar and diaphragms may appear less sharp. This subtle abnormality is considerably easier to appreciate with the benefit of a previous normal film for comparison.

In addition to determining the radiographic pattern of diffuse abnormality, a number of other features must be sought, including whether the distribution of disease is central or peripheral, in the upper, mid, or lower zone, and whether

distortion of the lung architecture is associated. Additional important features include signs of cardiac failure or fluid overload, such as increased heart size, equalization of upper and lower lobe vein size, and pleural effusions. Hilar or mediastinal enlargement caused by lymph nodes or vascular enlargement should also be specifically sought. The bones and soft tissues of the chest wall may also provide important clues, such as evidence of previous breast surgery or an erosive arthritis. The accuracy of radiographic analysis is reduced in the absence of appropriate clinical information. For example, ascertaining whether the patient is well, acutely or chronically unwell, of normal immune status, or immunocompromised can dramatically narrow a wide radiologic differential diagnosis.

Airway Disease

Plain tomography has been replaced by CT as the investigation of choice for the examination of airway abnormalities.

Tracheal Narrowing

Tracheal narrowing may be caused by an extrinsic mass, mediastinal fibrosis, or an intrinsic abnormality of the tracheal wall. Chronic inflammatory causes include fibrosing mediastinitis, sarcoidosis, chronic relapsing polychondritis, infection (Figure 1-64), and Wegener's granulomatosis. Primary tumors of the trachea are rare. Benign tumors present as small, well-defined, intraluminal nodules that are difficult or impossible to visualize on the chest radiograph. Malignant tumors of the trachea tend to occur close to the carina (Figure 1-65), although they may be quite extensive and cause a long stricture. Tracheal wall thickening and tracheal luminal narrowing can be detected on the plain chest radiograph, especially when specifically sought, but is best appreciated on CT (Figure 1-66). The right lateral wall of the trachea (the right paratracheal stripe) above the level of the azygos vein, is typically a 2-mm thick soft tissue stripe, and tracheal wall thickening can be detected on the plain radiograph if this portion of the airway is involved.

Tracheal Widening

The normal dimensions of the trachea have been assessed by use of a variety of techniques, most recently CT. The trachea becomes slightly larger with increasing age. On CT scanning, the maximal coronal diameter of the trachea is 23 mm in a man and 20 mm in a woman. Dilatation of the trachea is rare and may result from a generalized defect of connective tissue.

Mounier–Kuhn syndrome is the condition that causes the most dramatic tracheal dilatation (Figure 1-67). It is extremely rare and was first described in 1932. On the plain radiograph, shift of the right paratracheal stripe to the right is often the only sign of tracheal widening, and because the trachea is frequently not central, it is only if the left wall of the trachea is also identified that tracheal widening can be recognized. The Mounier–Kuhn syndrome is underreported because it may go undiagnosed, because clinical symptoms are similar to chronic bronchitis, COPD, or bronchiectasis. There is marked dilation of the trachea and major bronchi associated with repeated respiratory infections and copious sputum production. CT scans demonstrate tracheobronchial dilatation; some will often reveal parenchymal scarring secondary to chronic infection. Bronchoscopy demonstrates dilated central airways with thickened walls. Dilatation results in ineffective mucociliary

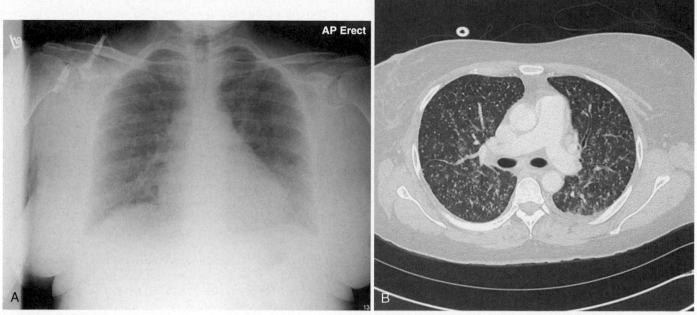

FIGURE 1-60 Miliary tuberculosis. **A,** Chest x-ray demonstrating innumerable 2-3–mm soft nodules. **B,** CT showing discrete miliary mottles or nodules. (Courtesy of Dr. M. Taylor.)

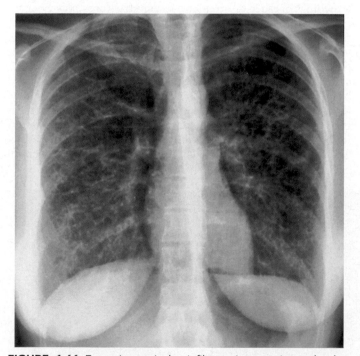

FIGURE 1-61 Extensive reticular infiltrate in a patient who has normal-volume lungs. The patient has Langerhans' cell histiocytosis.

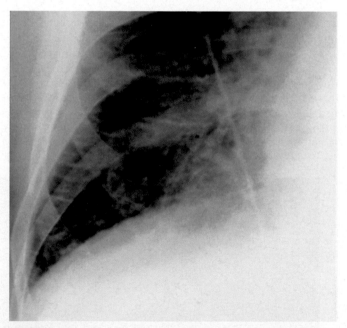

FIGURE 1-62 Kerley's B lines in a patient who has heart failure. Note how the reticular opacities are orientated at right angles to the pleural surface.

expectoration, and the subsequent chronic inflammation contributes to the cycle of infection and continued inflammation, leading to bronchiectasis and recurrent pneumonia and the development of emphysema.

At histologic inspection there is loss of cartilage and muscle within the airway walls associated with dilatation and saccular diverticulosis. There may be associated connective tissue diseases such as Ehlers–Danlos syndrome in adults and cutis laxa in children. Airways usually return to normal caliber at the fourth or fifth bronchial generation. In some cases, the disease may be acquired because there is a complete absence of symptoms until the third or fourth decades.

The chest radiograph is often reported to be normal even when there is extensive disease evident on CT. There are

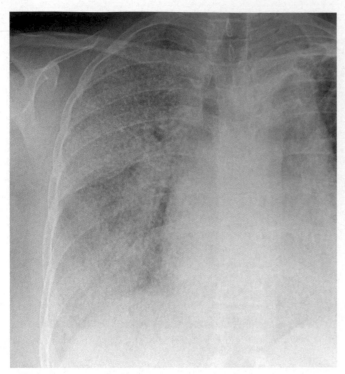

FIGURE 1-63 Very profuse nodular shadowing. The individual nodules are of high density. The patient has alveolar microlithiasis.

in early childhood with symptoms of cough, wheezing, and recurrent pulmonary infections. On examination, the chest was barrel-shaped, and there were inspiratory and expiratory wheezes and clubbing. In this original cohort, the plain radiograph and bronchography demonstrated thin-walled cystic bronchiectasis and ballooning of more peripheral airways on inspiration with collapse on expiration. Inspiratory and expiratory CT images have proven useful in the diagnosis of this syndrome in more recent reports.

Bronchiectasis

The chest radiograph is relatively insensitive for the detection of bronchiectasis, and in most series a significant portion of plain radiographs of patients who have bronchiectasis are judged to be normal (Figure 1-68). The use of HRCT is discussed later and is now the investigation of choice for bronchiectasis. Abnormalities present on the chest radiograph are as follows.

Bronchial wall thickening is evident as parallel, linear opacities radiating from the hilum, with lack of the normal convergence more peripherally. Ring shadows occur when the dilated airway is seen end on, may be thick or thin walled, and may contain secretions that produce an air–fluid level. Bronchiectatic airways that become plugged with secretions may produce tubular, soft tissue density opacities radiating from the hilum, more commonly in the lower lobes.

Distortion of the lobar anatomy with volume loss and crowding together of bronchovascular structures may be associated. However, patients who have cystic fibrosis, also characterized by bronchiectasis, may have significant air trapping, which results in overexpansion. Even severe bronchiectasis may be invisible within a completely collapsed lobe.

Cylindrical (or tubular) bronchiectasis produces a dilated bronchus with parallel walls, in varicose bronchiectasis the walls are irregular, and in saccular (or cystic) bronchiectasis the airways terminate as round cysts. In an individual patient, it is usual to see more than one pattern. Bronchiectasis usually involves the peripheral bronchi more severely than the central

limited management options, because the central airway involvement prevents extensive surgical intervention. Postural drainage and antibiotic therapy are necessary in parallel with other forms of bronchiectasis. There have been cases reported where bronchoscopy was used to clear secretions, tracheostomy has been necessary, and transplant has been attempted.

Another unusual form of airway dilatation was described by Williams and Campbell and colleagues. All patients presented

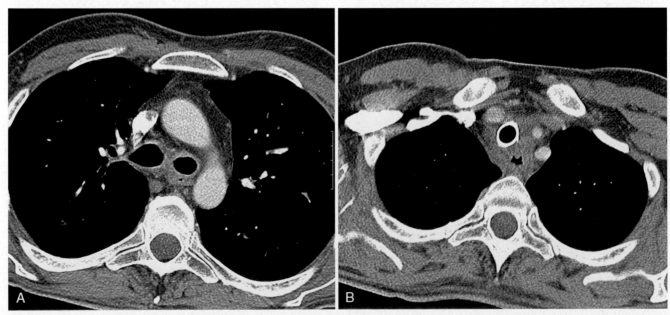

FIGURE 1-64 There is diffuse wall thickening in the left and right main bronchus, just below the level of the carina. Diffuse tracheal wall thickening is evident at the high level where there is a silicone stent *in-situ*.

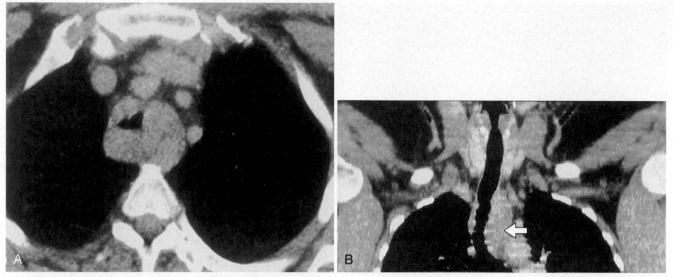

FIGURE 1-65 Adenoid cystic carcinoma. Extensive tracheal tumor. **A,** Circumferential soft tissue tumor of the trachea at the level of the great vessels. **B,** Coronal reformation showing extensive tracheal wall thickening measuring, on the left, almost 2 cm (*arrow*).

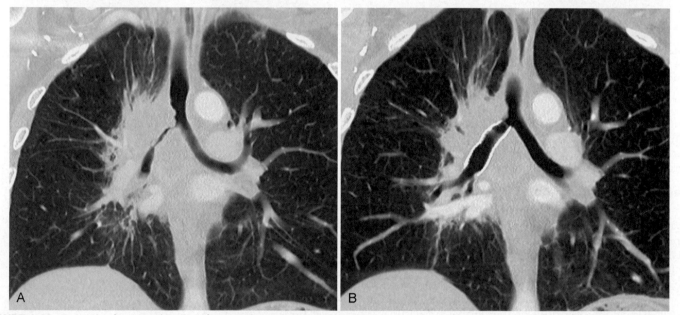

FIGURE 1-66 Coronal reformatted images from computed tomography **(A)** demonstrating an extensive mediastinal lymph node mass causing tracheal narrowing. **B,** After stent insertion, there is restoration of airway caliber.

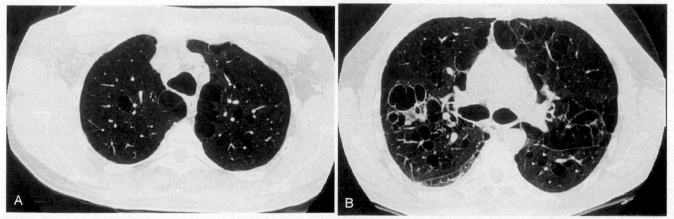

FIGURE 1-67 Tracheobronchomegaly. Computed tomography scans showing diffuse moderate dilatation of the trachea and main bronchi in association with cystic bronchiectasis. **A,** At the level of the trachea. **B,** At the level of the carina.

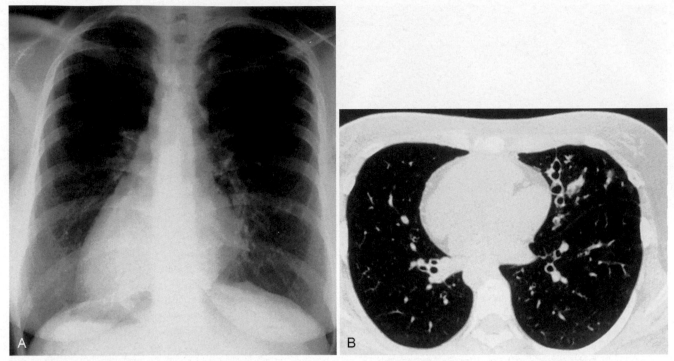

FIGURE 1-68 Bronchiectasis. **A,** The chest radiograph of a patient who has primary ciliary dyskinesia. There is dextrocardia. Some questionable bronchial wall thickening adjacent to the left heart border is obscured. **B,** The changes of bronchiectasis are much more convincingly demonstrated on high-resolution computed tomography.

bronchi. Although it has long been held that in allergic bronchopulmonary aspergillosis this pattern may be reversed, overall the distribution and morphology demonstrated by CT gives no more than a clue to the underlying etiology.

Mediastinal Abnormalities

The normal radiographic anatomy of the mediastinum was discussed earlier in this chapter. When a mediastinal abnormality is present on the PA radiograph, a lateral view should be obtained to aid anatomic localization. Today, the imaging of mediastinal masses depends heavily on CT scanning, which is discussed elsewhere. However, a familiarity with normal anatomy is required to detect mediastinal masses that at first appear as a subtle distortion of the normal mediastinal contours. A considerable volume of mediastinal tumor or lymph node enlargement may be present in the face of an apparently normal chest radiograph.

The most common cause of mediastinal enlargement visible on the chest radiograph in children is the normal thymus, which may enlarge and contract in certain disease states, but normally remains relatively prominent, especially on CT scans, until puberty (Figure 1-69). Lymphadenopathy, tumor, hiatus hernia, and vascular abnormalities account for most mediastinal masses seen in adults.

Mediastinal Lymphadenopathy

Lymph nodes are present in all compartments of the mediastinum but are visible on the chest radiograph only when they are calcified or enlarged. Causes of mediastinal nodal enlargement are discussed elsewhere. The chest radiograph is a relatively insensitive indicator of lymphadenopathy. Enlargement of right paratracheal nodes is identified more easily than that of left paratracheal nodes, aortic-pulmonary nodes, and

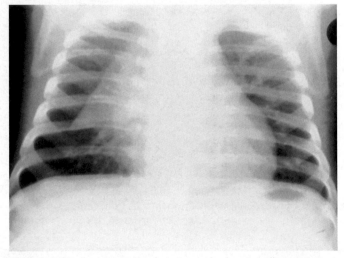

FIGURE 1-69 A prominent, but normal, thymic silhouette in an infant. Note the characteristic sail shape of the thymus as it projects over the right lung and the typically slightly lobulated contour as it conforms to the overlying ribs.

subcarinal lymphadenopathies (Figure 1-70). Barium swallow is a simple method of identifying some cases of subcarinal lymphadenopathy, but CT is the most comprehensive and accurate method of assessing mediastinal nodes.

Abnormalities of the Thoracic Aorta

The thoracic aorta arises in the middle mediastinum and then arches through the anterior, middle, and posterior mediastinal compartments. The greater vessels arise from the aortic arch in the superior mediastinum (Figure 1-71). Dilation or

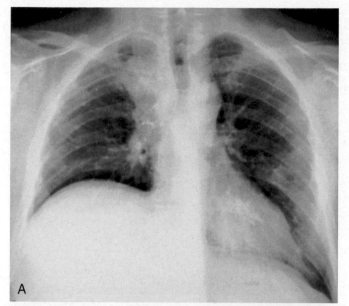

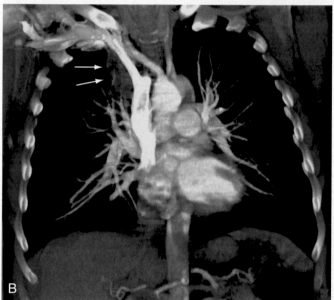

FIGURE 1-70 Right paratracheal lymph node enlargement caused by bronchogenic carcinoma. **A,** A right phrenic nerve palsy results in elevation of the right hemidiaphragm. **B,** Coronal volume rendered slab image from a multidetector CT from a different patient. There is again right paratracheal lymph node enlargement *(arrows)* that is abutting, but not distorting, the right brachiocephalic vein and superior vena cava.

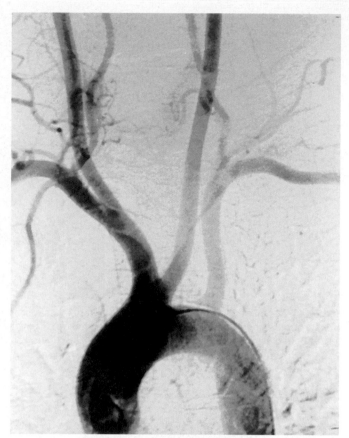

FIGURE 1-71 Digital subtraction arch aortogram. This patient has two vessels arising from the arch, a common variant of the normal three vessels. The image was obtained with the patient in a 30-degree left anterior oblique position.

tortuosity of the aortic arch or its branches may cause widening of the mediastinal shadow. So-called unfolding of the aorta is a common finding in the chest radiograph of elderly or hypertensive patients. Aneurysm of the aorta most often results from atherosclerosis (Figure 1-72). Cystic medial necrosis (Marfan's syndrome), infection (mycotic aneurysm), syphilitic aortitis, and a history of trauma are less common causes. Most aortic aneurysms are asymptomatic and present as mediastinal opacities on the radiograph, sometimes with curvilinear calcification visible in the wall. Aneurysms of the ascending aorta are best appreciated on the lateral radiograph

as a filling in of the retrosternal window. Aneurysms of the arch and descending aorta are frequently evident on the frontal radiograph, but a lateral view is often required for more accurate localization, and cross-sectional imaging is often required to confirm that the mediastinal abnormality in question is of vascular origin.

In the acutely injured patient, traumatic aortic rupture may be suspected from chest radiographic findings, and confirmation of injury usually requires angiography (Figure 1-73). However, when the chest radiograph is equivocal and the degree of trauma less than that usually associated with aortic injury, a spiral CT scan may be performed in the stable patient to exclude a mediastinal hematoma. If any doubt remains, the patient should proceed to angiography. If the aortic injury remains undetected and the patient survives, an aneurysm secondary to the trauma may develop subsequently. This is almost always confined to the junction of arch and descending aorta. Aortic abnormalities may produce pressure changes in adjacent skeletal structures.

Aneurysm of the ascending aorta may erode the posterior surface of the sternum, and descending aortic aneurysms may cause scalloping of the spine. Tortuosity of the innominate artery is a common cause of widening of the superior mediastinum in the elderly. Right-sided aortic arch (Figure 1-74) and pseudocoarctation of the aorta are two anomalies that may alter the appearance of the mediastinum and suggest a mass.

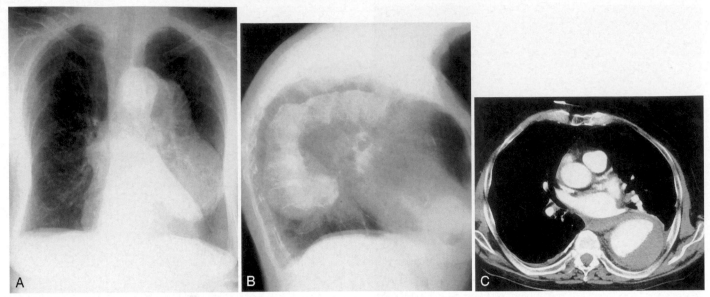

FIGURE 1-72 Thoracic aortic aneurysm. **A,** Marked dilatation and tortuosity of the descending thoracic aorta is present. Note how the left heart border is still evident, indicating the abnormality is likely to lie in the posterior thorax. **B,** Lateral view in the same patient demonstrates that the aneurysm involves the posterior arch and descending thoracic aorta. Note calcification within the ascending aorta. **C,** Computed tomography demonstrating extensive mural thrombus.

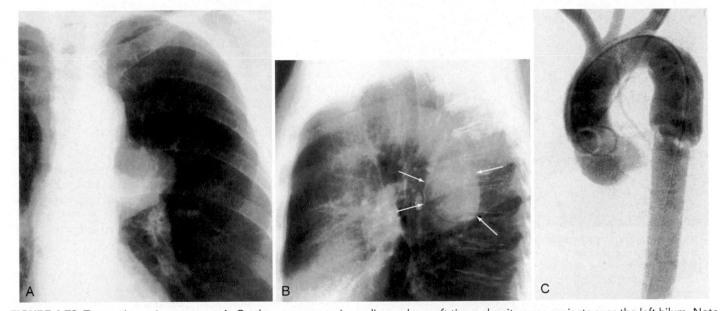

FIGURE 1-73 Traumatic aortic aneurysm. **A,** On the posteroanterior radiograph, a soft tissue density mass projects over the left hilum. Note how the left lower lobe artery is still visible through this mass, which indicates that it is separate from the hilum. The medial surface blends smoothly with the mediastinal structures, indicating it is likely to be extrapulmonary. **B,** The lateral view confirms an aneurysm secondary to previous trauma at the typical site, the junction of the posterior arch and descending thoracic aorta (*arrows*). **C,** The arch aortogram confirms the diagnosis of an acute aortic injury at the typical site.

Abnormalities of the Esophagus

Abnormalities of the esophagus are relatively common. They include infection and inflammation, trauma and perforation, and benign and malignant neoplastic processes. Esophageal abnormalities may be associated with diseases that also involve the lungs. This is best demonstrated by achalasia of the cardia (Figure 1-75) or systemic sclerosis (Figure 1-76), where esophageal motility disorders, resulting in significant dilatation and reflux, may be encountered in conjunction with pulmonary fibrosis and the results of recurrent aspiration.

Dilatation of Central Veins

The superior vena cava and azygos veins may dilate because of increased pressure, increased flow, obstruction, or congenital abnormality. Increased flow in the superior vena cava is seen in supracardiac, total, anomalous pulmonary venous drainage (Figure 1-77), and in the azygos vein in congenital absence of the inferior vena cava. Rarely, aneurysmal dilatation of the superior mediastinal veins produces an abnormal mediastinal silhouette. Likewise, obstruction of the superior vena cava may cause dilatation of the great veins in the

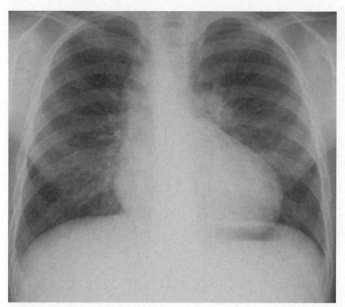

FIGURE 1-74 Tetralogy of Fallot. There is a right-sided aortic arch in addition to elevation of the ventricular apex because of developing ventricular hypertrophy. Note the relatively oligemic lungs.

superior mediastinum, which results in widening of the mediastinal contour. However, the clinical features are likely to be obvious by the time radiographic abnormalities become significant.

Other Mediastinal Abnormalities

Pneumomediastinum or mediastinal emphysema is the presence of air between the tissue planes of the mediastinum. This may occur secondary to interstitial pulmonary emphysema (most often caused by mechanical ventilation); to perforation of the esophagus, trachea, or a bronchus; or to a penetrating chest injury. Chest radiography may show vertical, translucent streaks in the mediastinum, which represent air separating the soft tissue planes (Figure 1-78). The air may extend up into the neck and over the chest wall (causing subcutaneous emphysema) and also over the diaphragm. The mediastinal pleura may be displaced laterally and then be visible as a thin stripe alongside the mediastinum.

Acute mediastinitis is usually caused by perforation of the esophagus, pharynx, or trachea, and a chest radiograph usually shows widening of the mediastinum. A pneumomediastinum is often apparent, and fluid levels may be visible in the mediastinum. Chronic or fibrosing mediastinitis usually presents as SVCO. Mediastinal hemorrhage may occur from venous or arterial bleeding. The mediastinum appears widened, and blood may be seen to track over the lung apices. It is obviously imperative to identify a life-threatening cause such as aortic rupture.

Hilar Abnormalities

Having identified a hilar abnormality, the observer must differentiate between a vascular and a nonvascular cause. Vascular prominence is often bilateral and accompanied by enlargement of the main pulmonary artery (Figure 1-79). Although the hila are large, they are of relatively normal density, and it is usually possible to trace the pulmonary artery branches in continuity from the adjacent lung to their point of convergence with

the interlobar arteries, known as the "hilar convergence" sign. By comparison, enlargement caused by lymph nodes or hilar tumor usually produces a lobulated hilar contour, with discernible lateral or inferior borders. Frequently, the normal hilar point is obliterated and, on the left, the aortopulmonary angle is filled in (Figure 1-80).

Occasionally, a pulmonary lesion is superimposed directly on the hilum on the frontal radiograph, which produces a spuriously large or dense hilum. The true position of the abnormality is revealed on the lateral radiograph (see Figure 1-72). A further pitfall is encountered when the vessels to the lingula or, more commonly, the right middle lobe are superimposed on the lower part of the hilar shadow, particularly when the film is taken anteroposteriorly, in a lordotic projection, or with a poor inspiratory effort. A lateral radiograph usually confirms the vascular nature of the shadowing.

Pleural Disease
Pleural Fluid

The most dependent recess of the pleural space is the posterior costophrenic angle, which is where a small effusion tends to collect. As little as 100–200 mL of fluid accumulated in this recess can be seen above the dome of the diaphragm on the frontal view. Even smaller effusions may be seen on a lateral radiograph, and it is possible to identify effusions of only a few milliliters by use of decubitus views with a horizontal beam, ultrasound, or CT. Eventually, the costophrenic angle on the frontal view fills in, and with increasing fluid a homogeneous opacity spreads upward, obscuring the lung base (Figure 1-81). The fluid usually demonstrates a concave upper edge, higher laterally than medially, and obscures the diaphragm. Fluid may track into the fissures. A massive effusion may cause complete opacification of a hemithorax with passive atelectasis. The space-occupying effect of the effusion may push the mediastinum toward the opposite side, especially when the lung does not collapse significantly (Figure 1-82).

Lamellar effusions are shallow collections between the lung surface and the visceral pleura, sometimes sparing the costophrenic angle. Subpulmonary effusions accumulate between the diaphragm and undersurface of a lung, mimicking elevation of the hemidiaphragm. Usually, the contour to the top of such an effusion differs from the normal diaphragmatic contour, the apparent apex being more lateral than usual. Also, some blunting of the costophrenic angle or tracking of fluid into fissures may be visible. On the left side, increased distance between the gastric air bubble and lung base may be apparent. A subpulmonary effusion may be confirmed by ultrasound. However, because the fluid is free to shift within the pleural cavity with changes in patient position, a decubitus film may be needed for confirmation.

Encapsulated or encysted fluid may be difficult to differentiate from an extrapleural opacity, parenchymal lung disease, or mediastinal mass. However, an encysted effusion is often associated with free pleural fluid or other pleural shadowing and may extend into a fissure (see Figure 1-81). Loculated effusions tend to have comparatively little depth, but considerable width, rather like a biconvex lens. Their appearance, therefore, depends on whether they are viewed face on, in profile, or obliquely. Extrapleural opacities tend to have a much sharper outline, with tapered, sometimes concave, edges where they meet the chest wall. Peripheral, pleurally based lung lesions may show an air bronchogram that differentiates

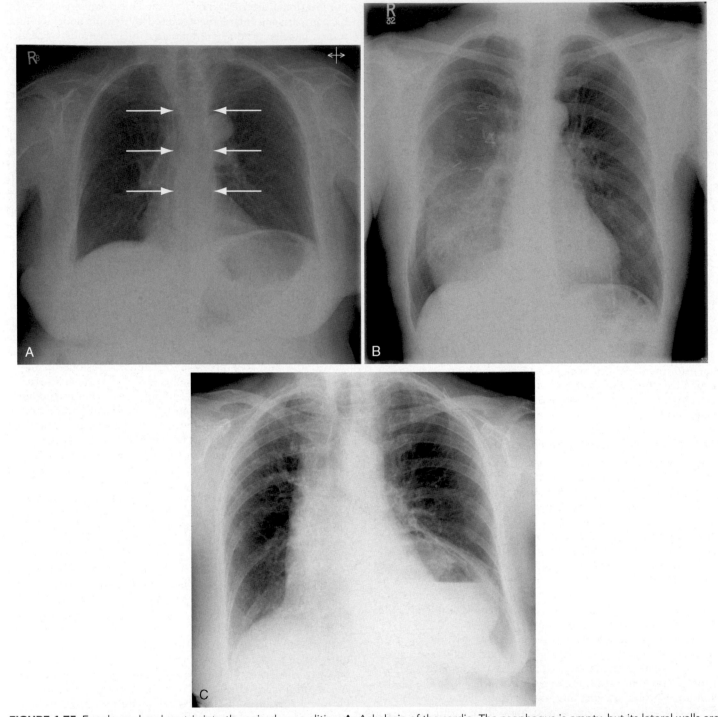

FIGURE 1-75 Esophageal and gastric intrathoracic abnormalities. **A,** Achalasia of the cardia. The esophagus is empty, but its lateral walls are seen running up the mediastinum (*arrows*). **B,** Chest x-ray of a patient who has had a gastric pull-up following esophagectomy. The wall of the stomach is seen near the right chest wall margin. The stomach contains solid matter in its lower part and mainly air in its upper part. Note rib resection for the necessary surgery. **C,** Large hiatus hernia with fluid level more or less overlying the heart. No stomach bubble is seen on the chest x-ray in the conventional site and the left diaphragm is poorly demarcated. (Courtesy of Dr. M. Taylor.)

them from true pleural disease. The differentiation between pleural thickening or mass and loculated pleural fluid may be difficult on plain films; CT and ultrasound are particularly useful in this context.

Fluid may become loculated in the interlobar fissures and is most frequently seen in heart failure. Fluid that collects in the horizontal fissure produces a lenticular, oval, or round shadow, with well-demarcated edges. Loculated fluid in an oblique fissure may be poorly defined on a frontal radiograph, but a lateral film is usually diagnostic because the fissure is seen tangentially, and the typical lenticular configuration of the effusion is demonstrated. Loculated interlobar effusions can

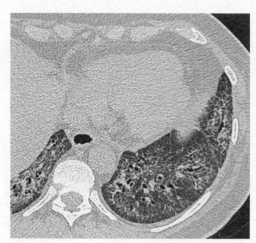

FIGURE 1-76 Systemic sclerosis with esophageal involvement. There is a coarse bibasal reticular infiltrate with marked traction bronchiectasis. In addition, the esophagus is moderately dilated and contains an air–fluid level.

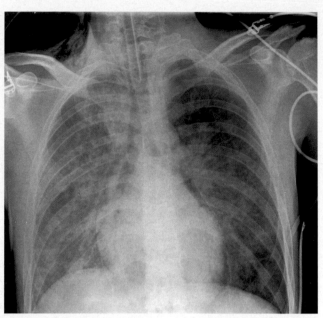

FIGURE 1-78 Pneumomediastinum. Air separates the tissue planes within the mediastinum and extends into the soft tissues of the neck and chest. A left-sided intercostal drain is *in situ.* (Courtesy of Dr. M. Taylor.)

Pneumothorax

A small pneumothorax is easily overlooked and, in an erect patient, usually collects at the apex. The lung retracts toward the hilum, and on a frontal chest film, the sharp white line of the visceral pleura is visible, separated from the chest wall by the radiolucent pleural space, which is devoid of lung markings. This should not be confused with a skinfold (Figure 1-84). The lung usually remains aerated, although perfusion is reduced in proportion to ventilation, and, therefore, the radiodensity of the partially collapsed lung remains relatively normal. A closed pneumothorax is easier to see on an expiratory film, although expiratory radiographs are not routinely required to detect clinically significant pneumothoraces. A lateral decubitus film with the affected side uppermost is occasionally helpful, because the pleural air can be seen along the lateral chest wall. This view is particularly useful in infants, because small pneumothoraces are difficult to see on supine AP films, because the air tends to collect anteriorly and medially.

A large pneumothorax may lead to complete relaxation and retraction of the lung, with some mediastinal shift toward the normal side (Figure 1-85). Because it is a medical emergency, tension pneumothorax is often treated before a chest radiograph is obtained. However, if a radiograph is taken in this situation, it shows marked displacement of the mediastinum (Figure 1-86). Radiographically, the lung may be squashed against the mediastinum or herniate across the midline, and the ipsilateral hemidiaphragm may be depressed.

Complications of Pneumothorax. Pleural adhesions may limit the distribution of a pneumothorax and result in a loculated or encysted pneumothorax. The usual appearance is an ovoid air collection adjacent to the chest wall, which may be radiographically indistinguishable from a thin-walled, subpleural pulmonary cyst or bulla. Pleural adhesions are occasionally seen as line shadows that stretch between the two pleural layers; they prevent relaxation of the underlying lung. Rupture of an adhesion may produce a hemopneumothorax.

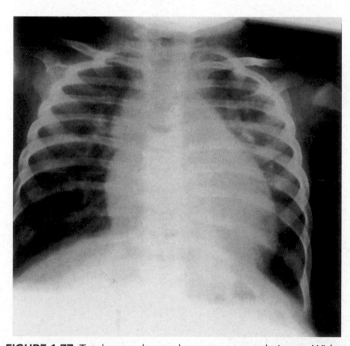

FIGURE 1-77 Total anomalous pulmonary venous drainage. Widening of the superior mediastinum caused by dilatation of the superior vena cava.

appear rounded on two views and may disappear rapidly. Hence, they are sometimes known as pulmonary pseudotumors (Figure 1-83). With subsequent episodes of heart failure, they may return at the same site.

Diagnosis of an empyema usually requires thoracentesis. Nevertheless, radiographically the diagnosis may be suspected on a plain film by the spontaneous appearance of an air–fluid level in a pleural effusion, because this usually equates with loculation and communication with the tracheobronchial tree or the presence of a gas-forming organism. Loculation is best demonstrated with ultrasound.

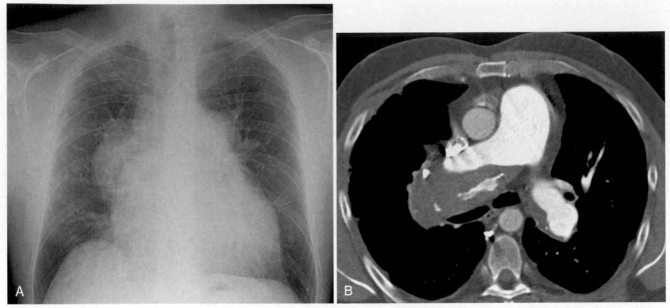

FIGURE 1-79 Recurrent pulmonary emboli resulting in marked dilatation of the proximal pulmonary arteries. **A,** The cardiac silhouette is enlarged. **B,** CT angiogram demonstrating contrast and clot in the pulmonary arteries.

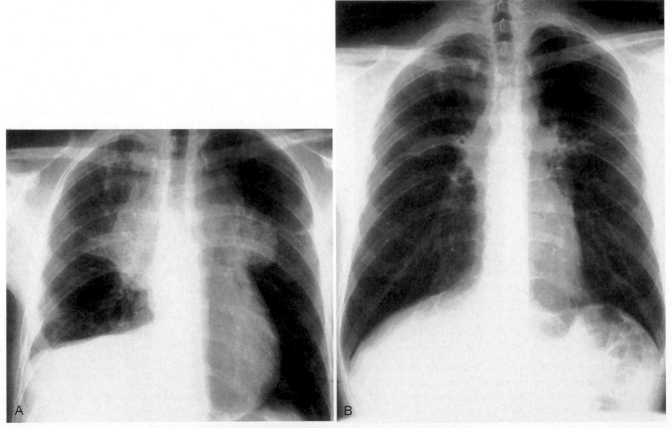

FIGURE 1-80 Non-Hodgkin's lymphoma. **A,** Bilateral hilar lymph node enlargement, with obliteration of the normal aortopulmonary angle and subcarinal nodes. A right-sided pleural effusion is present. **B,** The same patient showing residual abnormality after chemotherapy.

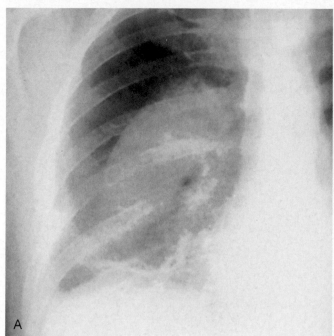
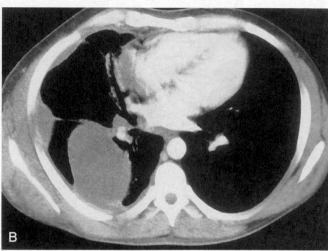

FIGURE 1-81 Small, right pleural effusion. **A,** The lentiform opacity in the right mid zone is caused by a loculated interlobar effusion. **B,** Computed tomography scan on mediastinal settings demonstrating the position of the loculated fluid within the oblique fissure.

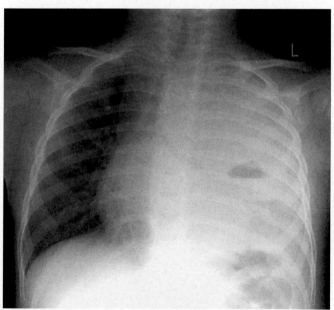

FIGURE 1-82 Large left pleural effusion. This patient presented with an acute empyema resulting from a lung abscess (note the air–fluid level). There is mediastinal shift to the right due to the space-occupying effects of the fluid.

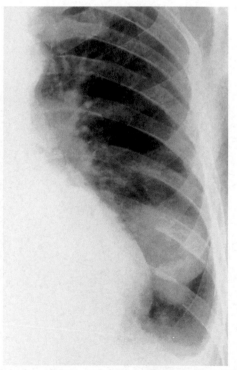

FIGURE 1-83 Small, left basal pleural effusion. The opacity in the left mid zone is caused by fluid loculated in the oblique fissure.

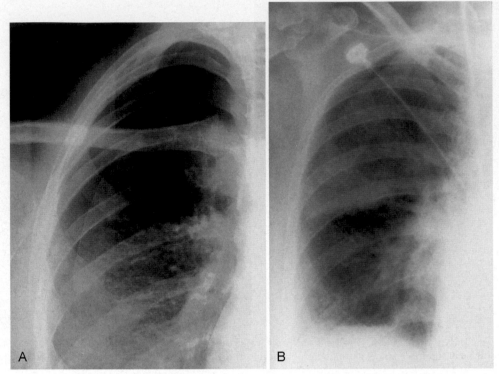

FIGURE 1-84 Shallow right pneumothorax. **A,** A discrete pleural white line is seen. Peripheral to this, there are no lung markings. **B,** In this skinfold, although a change in density parallels the chest wall, no discrete pleural line is present, and lung markings are seen to extend beyond the apparent lung edge. This appearance is caused by a superficial fold of skin produced by the X-ray cassette.

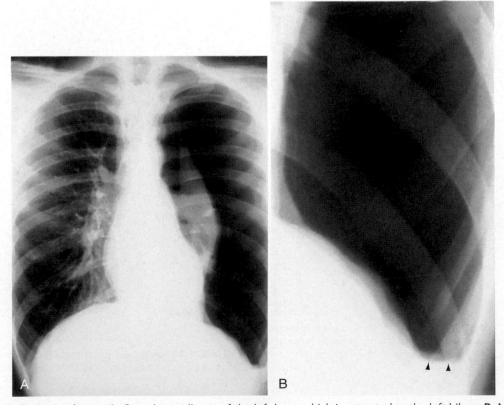

FIGURE 1-85 Left-sided pneumothorax. **A,** Complete collapse of the left lung, which is retracted to the left hilum. **B,** Magnified view of the left lower zone demonstrates the short air–fluid level commonly seen in a costophrenic angle when a pneumothorax is present (*arrowheads*).

Collapse or consolidation of a lobe or lung in association with a pneumothorax is important because it may delay re-expansion of the lung.

Because the normal pleural space contains a small volume of fluid, blunting of the costophrenic angle by a short fluid level is commonly seen in a pneumothorax (see Figure 1-85). In a small pneumothorax, this fluid level may be the most obvious radiologic sign. A larger fluid level usually signifies a complication and represents exudate, pus, or blood, depending on the etiology of the pneumothorax (Figure 1-87).

The usual radiographic appearance of a hydropneumothorax is that of a pneumothorax containing a horizontal fluid level that separates opaque fluid below from lucent air above. A hydrothorax or pyopneumothorax may arise as a result of a bronchopleural fistula (an abnormal communication between the bronchial tree and the pleural space). This may be a complication of surgery but may occur as a complication of a subpleural lung tumor (Figure 1-88).

Pleural Thickening

Blunting of a costophrenic angle is a common observation and usually is caused by localized pleural thickening secondary to previous pleuritis. In the asymptomatic patient and in the absence of other radiologic abnormalities, it is of no significance other than that it may simulate a pleural effusion. When relevant, the possibility of pleural fluid may have to be excluded by other techniques. Localized pleural thickening that extends into the inferior end of an oblique fissure may produce so-called tenting of the diaphragm and is of similar significance, although a similar appearance may result from scarring caused by previous pulmonary infection or infarction.

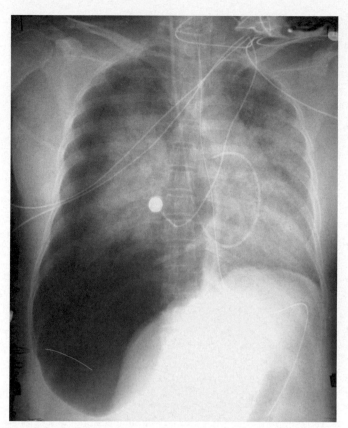

FIGURE 1-86 Tension pneumothorax after insertion of a Swan-Ganz catheter. Note the shift of the mediastinum toward the left and reversal of the normal contour of the right hemidiaphragm.

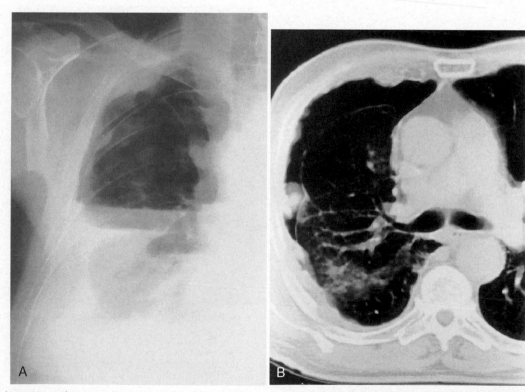

FIGURE 1-87 Hydropneumothorax in a patient with a mesothelioma. A, Note the normal thickness of the visceral pleura, but the lobulated soft tissue shadowing caused by tumor within the parietal pleura. B, Computed tomography scan in the same patient that demonstrates the lobulated pleural tumor.

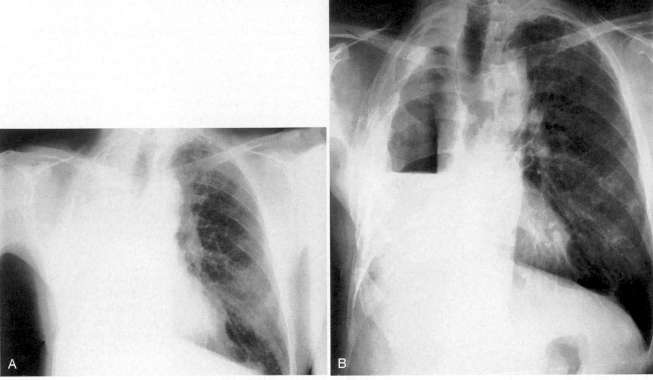

FIGURE 1-88 Pneumonectomy—appearances and complications. **A,** Chest radiograph showing the normal appearances after a right pneumonectomy. **B,** Spontaneous development of an air–fluid level caused by a bronchopleural fistula from local recurrence.

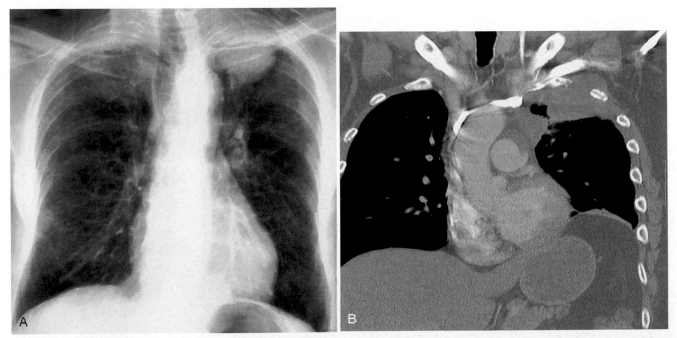

FIGURE 1-89 Apical abnormalities. **A,** Benign apical pleural thickening is visible on the right; on the left there is also a Pancoast's tumor. **B,** Coronal CT reformat from another patient who also has an apical tumor.

Bilateral apical pleural thickening is common, usually symmetric, more frequent in elderly patients, and does not necessarily indicate previous tuberculosis. The etiology is uncertain, but in some individuals the caps represent extrapleural fat that has descended because of scarring and consequent retraction of the upper lobes. In contrast, asymmetric or unilateral apical pleural thickening may be highly significant, especially if associated with pain. Asymmetric apical pleural shadowing may represent a Pancoast's tumor, and bone destruction should be specifically sought (Figure 1-89).

More extensive unilateral pleural thickening is usually the result of a previous thoracotomy or an exudative pleural effusion. A simple transudate usually resolves completely, but empyema and hemothorax are likely to resolve with pleural fibrosis. The thickened pleura may calcify (Figure 1-90), and the entire lung may become surrounded by fibrotic pleura, which may be as much as a few centimeters thick (Figure 1-91). Bilateral (parietal) pleural plaques are a common manifestation of asbestos exposure, and occasionally more diffuse, visceral pleural thickening is seen.

Pleural Calcification

In general, pleural calcification has the same causes as pleural thickening. Unilateral pleural calcification is, therefore, likely to be the result of previous empyema or hemothorax, and bilateral calcification occurs after asbestos exposure (Figure 1-92). Pleural calcification may be discovered in a patient who is not aware of previous chest disease.

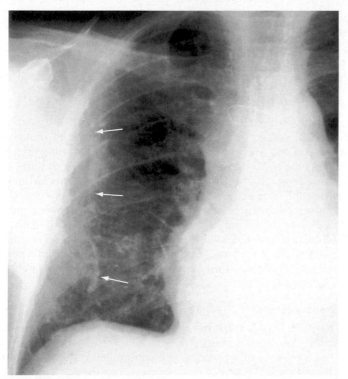

FIGURE 1-90 Previous thoracotomy (note sternotomy sutures) for mitral valve replacement. Pleural calcification is seen on the right side (*arrows*).

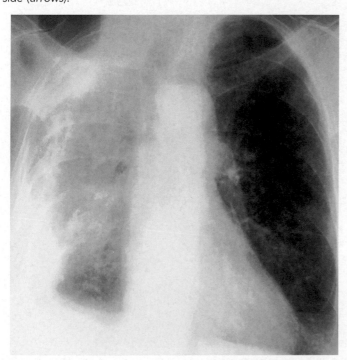

FIGURE 1-91 Previous tuberculosis. Extensive right-sided pleural thickening and calcification, with reduction in volume of the right hemithorax.

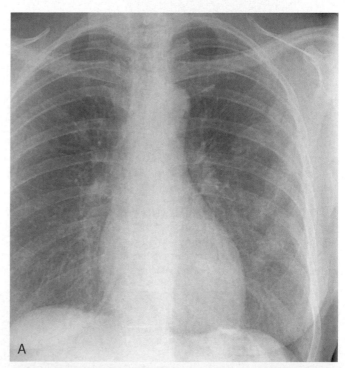

A

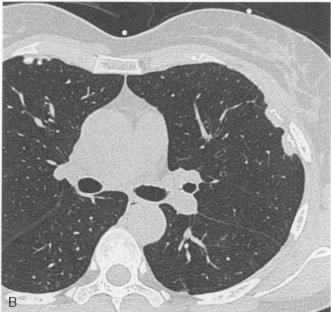

B

FIGURE 1-92 Calcified pleural thickening secondary to asbestos exposure. **A,** There are subtle plaques on the chest radiograph **(B)**, better demonstrated on CT.

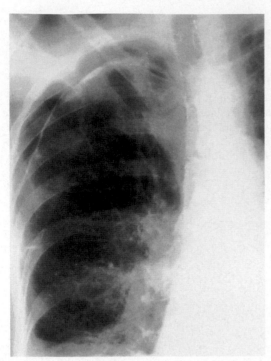

FIGURE 1-93 Previous sternotomy resulting in pleural thickening and calcification. A small pneumothorax is visible. Note how the pleural thickening is associated with the visceral pleura.

The calcification associated with previous pleurisy, empyema, or hemothorax occurs in the visceral pleura (Figure 1-93); associated pleural thickening is almost always present and separates the calcium from the ribs. The calcium may be in a continuous sheet or in discrete plaques, which usually produce dense, coarse, irregular shadows, often sharply demarcated laterally. When a plaque is viewed face on, it may be less well defined and mimic a pulmonary infiltrate.

Pleural Masses

Primary tumors of the pleura are rare. Benign tumors of the pleura include pleural fibroma and lipoma (Figure 1-94). The most common malignant disease of the pleura is metastatic, usually adenocarcinoma from the bronchus or breast (Figure 1-95). Malignant mesothelioma is usually associated with prior asbestos exposure.

COMPUTED TOMOGRAPHY

Anatomy of the Mediastinum

The soft tissue contrast provided by CT, as well as its cross-sectional nature, makes the diagnostic information available from CT far superior to that provided by two-dimensional radiography. Modern CT scanners can acquire a volume of information that includes the whole of the mediastinum within the time of a single breath hold. This three-dimensional data set can then be displayed as continuous or overlapping axial slices, free from breathing movement artifact. Usually, a collimation and slice width of between 5 and 10 mm is used, and it is usual, but not always essential, to give intravenous contrast. The normal mediastinal anatomy is demonstrated in Figures 1-96 to 1-101.

Great Vessels

The great vessels form the most familiar anatomic landmarks within the mediastinum. Knowledge of the relationship of these vessels to other mediastinal components allows accurate

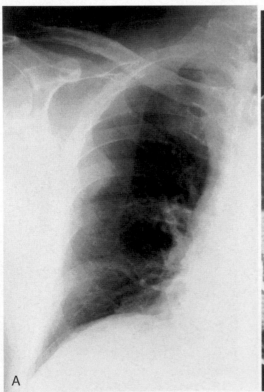
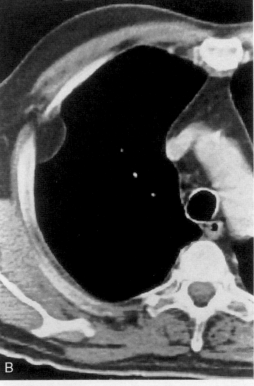

FIGURE 1-94 The appearances of a pleural lipoma. **A,** Localized view of the right lung from a posteroanterior chest radiograph. There is a pleurally based opacity in the right mid zone, well defined medially but fading out laterally. **B,** Computed tomography scan of the same. The opacity is caused by a pleural lipoma. Note the identical computed tomography attenuation of this mass compared with the subcutaneous fat.

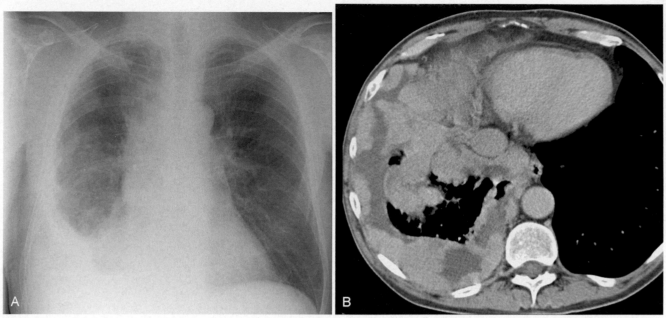

FIGURE 1-95 Malignant pleural involvement from metastatic adenocarcinoma. **A,** Chest radiograph and **(B)** CT after contrast enhancement. A lobulated rind of pleural thickening extends from the right apex down to the right diaphragm, which appears elevated. The overall volume of the right hemithorax is reduced.

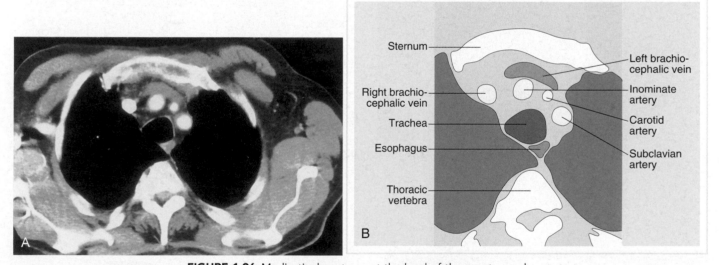

FIGURE 1-96 Mediastinal anatomy at the level of the great vessels.

description of the location of pathology and has important implications for planning the approach to either open operation or mediastinoscopy. The most common branching pattern of the aortic arch is for three arteries to arise from the upper arch—the right innominate, left common carotid, and left subclavian (see Figure 1-96). However, many variations to this basic anatomy exist (see Figures 1-71, 1-74, and 1-77). The transverse portion of the aortic arch is the most readily recognizable vascular structure within the mediastinum (see Figure 1-97). The great veins lie anterior to the arterial structures. The left brachiocephalic vein is situated above and anterior to the aortic arch and aortic branches, although its position is

variable. The right brachiocephalic vein descends more directly in the anterior right mediastinum to merge with its counterpart to form the superior vena cava. Because CT contrast is given from one arm, one brachiocephalic vein is heavily opacified, whereas the other remains of soft tissue density.

The pulmonary outflow tract ascends, usually outlined by fat within the pericardium, to divide adjacent and just posterior to the ascending aorta. Usually, the main pulmonary artery diameter is equal to or less than the ascending aorta as measured on CT. When the pulmonary artery diameter exceeds the aortic diameter, underlying pulmonary hypertension is likely. The right pulmonary artery swings dorsally and

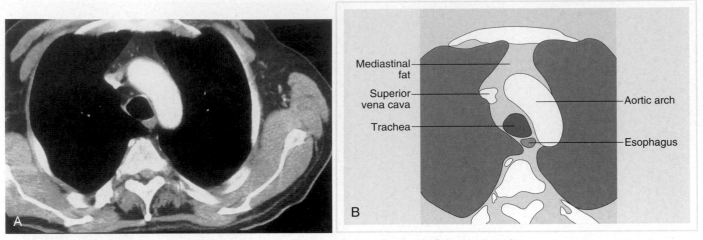

FIGURE 1-97 Mediastinal anatomy at the level of the aortic arch.

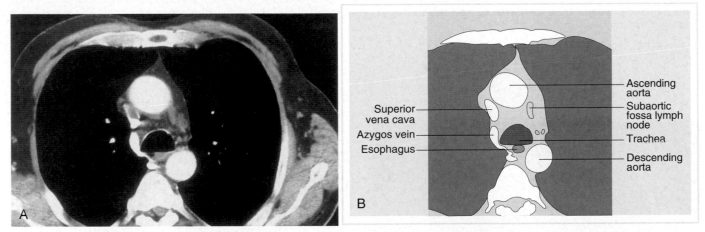

FIGURE 1-98 Mediastinal anatomy at the level of the subaortic fossa.

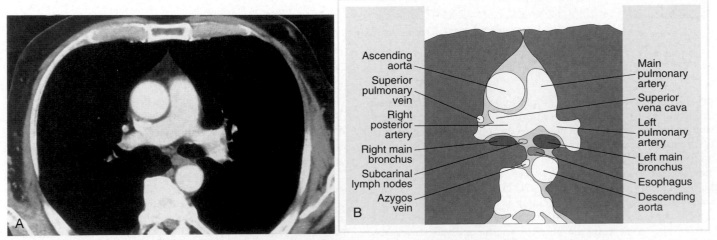

FIGURE 1-99 Mediastinal anatomy through the division of the main pulmonary artery.

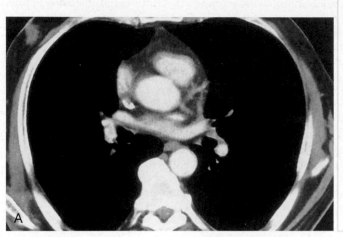
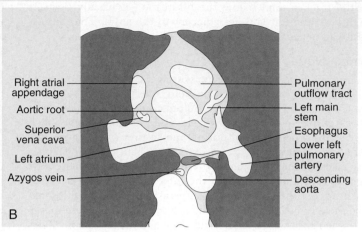

Right atrial appendage
Aortic root
Superior vena cava
Left atrium
Azygos vein

Pulmonary outflow tract
Left main stem
Esophagus
Lower left pulmonary artery
Descending aorta

FIGURE 1-100 Mediastinal anatomy through the aortic root.

to the right, behind the ascending aorta and SVC and anterior to the right main bronchus (see Figure 1-99). After giving a branch to the upper lobe, it descends posterolaterally to the bronchus intermedius. The left pulmonary artery follows a shorter course and arches up and over the left main bronchus.

Hilar anatomy is well demonstrated on contrast-enhanced CT, especially when vascular structures are traced sequentially over contiguous images. Knowledge of normal anatomy enables differentiation of vascular structures from normal or enlarged mediastinal lymph nodes, even on unenhanced scans; however, if there is any cause for doubt, intravenous contrast always clarifies the situation (Figure 1-101).

Airways

The trachea descends through the thoracic inlet, where reduction in caliber may occur, and usually appears rounded on scans obtained in full inspiration. If scans are obtained during expiration, the membranous posterior wall of the trachea is seen to bow forward into the tracheal lumen. The wall of the

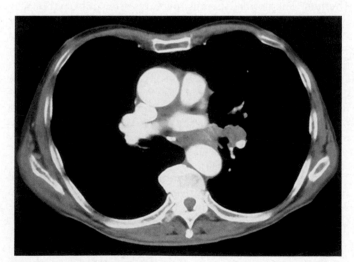

FIGURE 1-101 Contrast-enhanced computed tomography scan. Left hilar lymph node enlargement with extension of abnormal tissue anterior to the descending aorta.

trachea is only 2-mm thick, and any intramural thickening is well demonstrated on CT. Modern scanners also allow reformatting of the data in sagittal or coronal planes, thus providing more elegant demonstration of tracheal abnormalities. The anatomy of the bronchial tree can be traced from the tracheal carina out into the lungs, at least to segmental level, with excellent correlation between CT and bronchoscopic findings. Furthermore, the three-dimensional data set acquired on modern spiral scanners can be manipulated to provide a computer simulation of the bronchoscopic appearances (see Figure 1-7, *D*).

Thymus

The thymus, in the normal state, is not visible on the chest radiograph of the adult patient, but the thymic remnant is frequently evident on CT. The thymus reduces in size after puberty. It lies in the anterior mediastinum, just in front of the root of the aorta; it is bi-lobed, with the left lobe usually being the larger. Generally, the thymus is assessed by examining the contours of the gland, which should be concave, and the thickness of the individual lobes. In childhood, the thymus is of soft tissue density on CT scanning, but after puberty it starts to involute, and the gland undergoes atrophy and fatty replacement. Traces of thymic tissue within the anterior mediastinal fat are frequently identifiable on CT in young adults.

Thyroid

Usually, the thyroid is confined to the neck, but frequently mediastinal extension occurs with thyroid enlargement (see later). Typically, the thyroid lies on either side of the extrathoracic trachea and is bounded laterally by the carotid artery and internal jugular vein. On contrast enhancement, normal thyroid tissue enhances avidly and is usually of relatively high attenuation on unenhanced scans because of its relatively high iodine content.

Esophagus

Often the esophagus is completely collapsed on CT scanning and is thus inconspicuous but is easily identified if it contains air or contrast. Initially, the esophagus lies directly posterior to the trachea, and below the bifurcation it usually deviates slightly to the left and lies adjacent to the aorta. The esophageal wall is usually only 2–3 mm in thickness.

Lymph Nodes

Numerous lymph nodes occur within the mediastinum, usually <1 cm in long axis and discrete; they may not be visible on CT scanning. Previous granulomatous disease may result in extensive mediastinal lymph node calcification, which reveals the true extent of normal mediastinal lymph node distribution (Figure 1-102). An extensive chain of lymph nodes also accompanies the internal mammary vessels bilaterally. Further nodes are present in the intercostal chain adjacent to the heads of the ribs in a posterior, paraspinal position and alongside the esophagus and descending thoracic aorta. These merge with the retrocrural lymph node chain and the paraaortic nodes on the abdomen.

Pericardium

The pericardial membrane is composed of visceral and parietal layers and surrounds the heart. The visceral layer is separated from the myocardium by a variable amount of epicardial fat. The parietal layer is variably fused with the mediastinal pleura. Where they are separate, mediastinal fat may accumulate (such as in the epiphrenic fat pad). Fluid within the pericardial sac may be evident on the chest radiograph, CT, or ultrasound.

Computed Tomographic Evaluation of Mediastinal Masses

Most patients who have a mediastinal mass present with symptoms from the local compressive or invasive effects of the mediastinal mass, but in a surprising number, the mass is discovered on a chest radiograph taken for an unrelated cause. Generally, the PA and lateral chest radiographs enable localization of the mass to one of the compartments of the

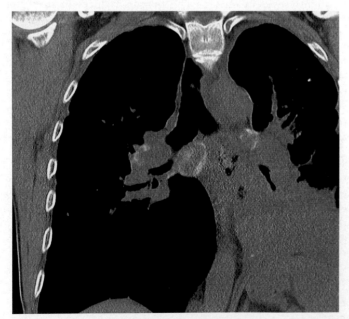

FIGURE 1-102 Unenhanced computed tomography scan through the thorax. There is faint eggshell calcification in mediastinal lymph nodes secondary to previous granulomatous disease.

mediastinum, which refines the differential diagnosis. However, current practice is for patients who present with a mediastinal mass to undergo a contrast-enhanced CT scan or sometimes MRI.

The differential diagnosis of a mediastinal mass is wide. Masses can arise from any of the normal structures in the mediastinum, as well as from metastatic disease from a distant primary tumor. In addition, mediastinal abscesses may also present as a mass. The diagnosis is considerably narrowed by CT, which enables the organ of origin of the mass to be assessed, defines the attenuation and enhancement characteristics, and detects evidence of invasion of adjacent structures. It is usual to classify mediastinal masses according to the anatomic portion of the mediastinum from which they appear to arise (Figure 1-103).

Superior Mediastinal Masses

Thyroid. An enlarged thyroid may extend inferiorly into the superior mediastinum and may be large enough to reach into the middle mediastinum. However, this rarely presents a diagnostic problem, because the mass is obviously continuous with the cervical thyroid tissue and enhances avidly after intravenous contrast. Frequently, the enlarged gland contains low-density cysts and areas of calcification, particularly within cyst walls. Large thyroid masses may cause tracheal deviation or narrowing and may enlarge acutely if there is hemorrhage into the gland (Figure 1-104). Although the thyroid originates anterior to the trachea, there may be extension to the right and even posterior to the trachea within the upper mediastinum.

Lymphatic Malformations. Lymphatic malformations are rare and may present in the superior mediastinum. The most common of these is the cystic hygroma, which usually presents in infants as a cervical mass with an extensive intrathoracic component. Although considered benign, these lesions are difficult to completely resect because of a tendency to spread around normal structures.

Anterior Mediastinal Masses

Most anterior mediastinal masses arise from the thymus, thyroid (see earlier), germ-cell tumors, and enlarged lymph nodes.

Thymus. The normal thymus involutes after puberty but may show reactive enlargement in certain disease states or after chemotherapy. However, intrinsic neoplasia of the thymus is a relatively common cause of an anterior mediastinal mass in adult life. Causes of thymic neoplasia include thymoma, thymic carcinoma, thymic cysts (Figure 1-105), thymic lipoma, thymic carcinoid, and thymic lymphoma. With CT, fat or fluid elements may be identified within a thymic mass, and invasion of adjacent structures can be shown. With the exception of thymolipoma and thymic cysts, histologic examination is usually required for definitive diagnosis.

Teratomas and Germ-Cell Tumors. Teratomas and germ-cell tumors originate from primitive stem cell rests. It is useful to separate these neoplasms into benign and malignant forms—the former is the benign cystic teratoma (synonymous with dermoid cysts). Benign cystic teratomas (Figure 1-106) may contain differentiated elements and so on CT may display a variety of densities, ranging from fat to calcified tissue and even that of teeth. The malignant teratomas comprise a variety of tumors that usually arise in the testes, namely seminomas,

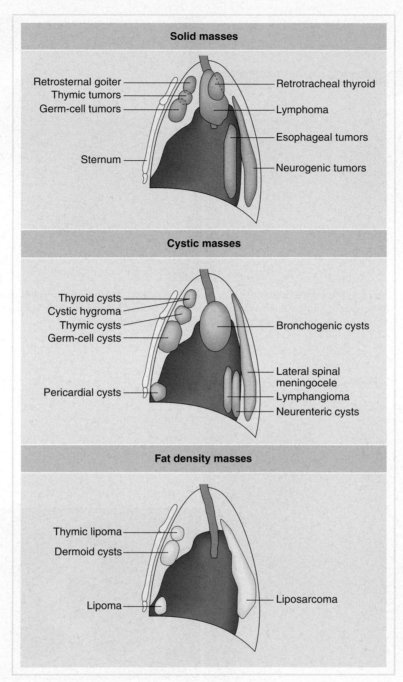

FIGURE 1-103 Distribution and classification of mediastinal masses depending on density derived from computed tomography.

teratocarcinoma, embryonal carcinoma, yolk sac tumors, and choriocarcinoma. Some mediastinal germ-cell tumors may be secondary to a primary tumor arising within the gonads. Malignant germ-cell tumors are usually found in young men, secrete tumor markers, and are chemosensitive.

Lymph Node Enlargement. Lymph node enlargement is a common cause of an anterior mediastinal mass, although many processes that involve lymph nodes cause generalized mediastinal nodal enlargement. These processes may be infective (such as tuberculosis or histoplasmosis), neoplastic, reactive, or of unknown etiology (such as sarcoidosis).

Lymphoma. Hodgkin's disease and, to a lesser extent, non-Hodgkin's lymphoma and lymphatic leukemia frequently involve the mediastinum, especially the paratracheal, tracheobronchial, and anterior mediastinal nodes. Typically, the lymph node enlargement is asymmetric.

Middle Mediastinal Masses

Middle mediastinal masses are most frequently malignant, usually from metastatic nodal enlargement. However, the presence of enlarged nodes is not an accurate predictor of malignancy, because reactive enlargement is also common.

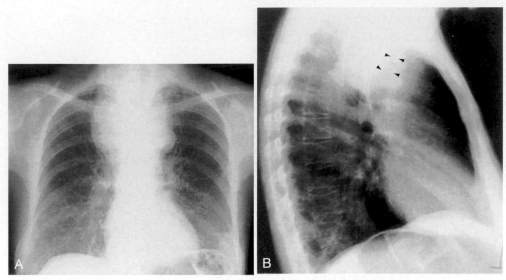

FIGURE 1-104 Retrosternal thyroid mass. **A,** Posteroanterior chest radiograph with a large superior mediastinal mass mainly to the right of the trachea. **B,** The lateral view demonstrates an extension behind the trachea, which is narrowed in its anteroposterior dimension (*arrowheads*). The thyroid frequently extends into a retrotracheal position in the upper mediastinum.

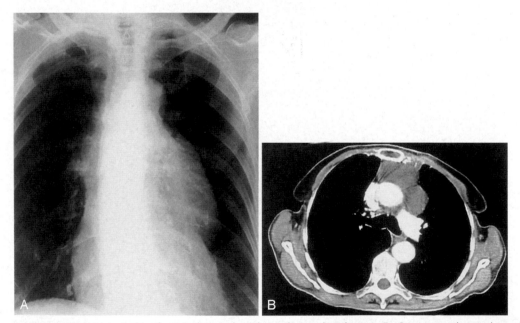

FIGURE 1-105 Thymic cyst. **A,** Anteroposterior chest radiograph with mediastinal widening. **B,** Contrast-enhanced computed tomography confirms an anterior mediastinal abnormality of fluid density.

The classification of mediastinal lymph node enlargement is discussed under staging of lung cancer.

There are some important developmental middle mediastinal masses. These lesions are frequently identified as an incidental abnormality in adult life, although they may present earlier if complications supervene. Bronchogenic cysts may arise anywhere along the course of the trachea, but are usually found close to a carina. On the chest radiograph they appear as well-defined, round masses that may, on rare occasions, calcify. On CT they may appear as either cystic or solid masses. Magnetic resonance imaging may be diagnostic.

Posterior Mediastinal Masses

The posterior mediastinum contains neural elements, which give rise to a range of benign and malignant neural tumors. These may become of considerable size before presentation, and modeling abnormalities may occur in the adjacent ribs and spine, which provide a clue to their chronicity. On CT scanning, they are typically paraspinal and of soft tissue density, with patchy calcification. Also, CT may show the typical dumbbell extension of a neurofibroma, from an extraspinal position through an intervertebral foramina. In the assessment of neurogenic tumors, MRI has distinct advantages over CT

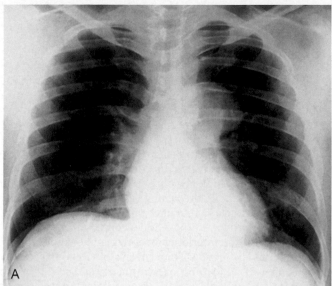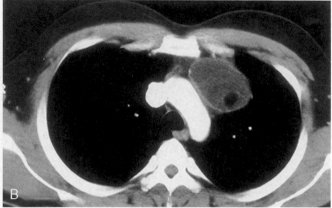

FIGURE 1-106 Cystic teratoma. **A,** Posteroanterior, erect chest radiograph showing a mass arising from the mediastinum. Note how the posterior aortic arch and descending aorta are still visualized, which indicates an anterior position. **B,** Computed tomography scan shows fluid and fat elements within an anterior mediastinal mass.

because of its ability to definitively confirm or exclude tumor extension into the spinal canal (Figure 1-107).

The esophagus lies in the posterior mediastinum. Esophageal carcinoma usually presents with dysphagia or weight loss without a mass being apparent on the chest radiograph. Usually, CT is reserved for the staging of esophageal malignancy, in addition to the assessment of local tumor bulk. Benign esophageal lesions may reach a considerable size before symptoms occur, and as a result, such large masses may be apparent on the plain radiograph. Such tumors include fibroma, leiomyoma, and lipomas.

Neuroenteric cysts are rare congenital masses that occur in the posterior mediastinum, usually inseparable from the esophagus, and sometimes within the esophageal wall. If a vertebral or neural canal abnormality is present, these are known as neuroenteric cysts, but if not, they are termed esophageal duplication cysts. Posterior mediastinal masses may arise directly from the spinal column and may represent primary or secondary tumors, infective processes, or the results of trauma or degeneration.

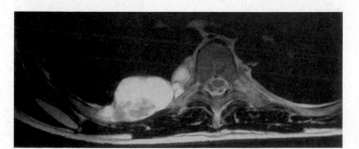

FIGURE 1-107 Paraganglionoma in an adult. A right paraspinal high T2W signal lobulated mass is present. There is no extension into the soft tissues of the chest wall or through the neural foramina into the spinal canal.

INTERPRETATION OF HIGH-RESOLUTION COMPUTED TOMOGRAPHY OF THE LUNGS

Appearance of Normal Lung Anatomy

Accurate interpretation of HRCT of the lung requires an understanding of the normal appearances of the bronchi, blood vessels, and the secondary pulmonary lobule. The close correspondence between the appearances of gross pathologic specimens and HRCT features enables the use of anatomic terms to describe the patterns of lung disease depicted by HRCT.

Throughout the lung, the bronchi and pulmonary arteries run together and taper slightly as they travel radially; this is easiest to appreciate in the bronchovascular bundles that run within and parallel to the plane of HRCT section. At any given point, the diameter of the bronchus is the same as its accompanying pulmonary artery. The bronchovascular bundle is surrounded by connective tissue from the hilum to the bronchioles in the lung periphery. The concept of connected components making up the lung interstitium is useful for the understanding of HRCT findings in interstitial lung disease—the peripheral interstitium around the surface of the lung beneath the visceral pleura extends into the lung to surround the secondary pulmonary lobules. Within the lobules, a finer network of septal, connective tissue fibers support the alveoli. The "axial" fibers form a sheath around the bronchovascular bundles. Thus, the connective tissue stroma of these three separate components is in continuity and so form a fibrous skeleton for the lungs.

In normal individuals, HRCT shows a clear and definite interface between the bronchovascular bundle and surrounding lung. Any thickening of the connective tissue interstitium results in apparent bronchial wall thickening and blurring of this interface. The size of the smallest subsegmental bronchi visible on HRCT is determined by the thickness of the bronchial wall rather than by the bronchial diameter. In general, bronchi with a diameter <3 mm and walls less than 300-mm thick are not consistently identifiable on HRCT. Airways reach this critical size at approximately 2–3 cm from the pleural surface. The secondary pulmonary lobule is the smallest anatomic unit of the lung that is surrounded by a connective tissue septum (Figure 1-108). Within the septa lie lymphatic vessels and venules. The lobule contains between 5 and 12 acini, which each measure approximately 6–10 mm in diameter. Each lobule is approximately 2 cm in diameter and polyhedral in shape and often resembles a truncated cone. In the lung periphery, the bases of the cone-shaped lobules lie on a visceral pleural surface. In the central parts of the lung, the interlobular septa, and thus the lobules, are less well developed. The centrilobular bronchiole and accompanying pulmonary artery enter through the apex of the lobule.

The interlobular septa measure approximately 100 μm in thickness. The lower limit of resolution of HRCT is approximately 200 μm, so normal septa are infrequently identified on HRCT. The few interlobular septa that are visible in normal individuals are seen as straight lines 1–2 cm in length that terminate at a visceral pleural surface. Sometimes several septa that join end to end are seen as a nonbranching, linear structure, which can measure up to 4 cm in length; these are most frequent at the lung bases, just above the diaphragmatic surface.

The secondary pulmonary lobule is supplied by a centrilobular artery and bronchiole that are approximately 1 mm in diameter as they enter the lobule. In the normal state, the core structures, effectively the 500-μm–diameter centrilobular artery, are visible as dots 1-cm deep to the pleural surface. On standard window settings, the lung parenchyma is of almost homogeneous low density, marginally greater than that of air.

Patterns of Parenchymal Disease

Vague terms traditionally used in the lexicon of plain chest radiography can be replaced by precise descriptions derived from an understanding of HRCT anatomy. Abnormal patterns on HRCT that represent pulmonary disease can usually be categorized into one of four patterns—reticular and linear opacities, nodular opacities, increased lung density, and cystic air spaces with areas of decreased lung density.

Although these HRCT patterns generally have a corresponding pattern on chest radiography, they are seen with much greater clarity on the cross-sectional images of HRCT and the precise distribution of disease can be more readily appreciated. There is increasing conformity in the terminology used to describe the HRCT abnormalities of diffuse infiltrative lung diseases.

Reticular Pattern

A reticular pattern on HRCT always indicates significant pathosis. A reticular pattern caused by thickening of interlobular septa is a cardinal sign of many interstitial lung diseases. Numerous interlobular septa that join up to form an obvious network indicate an extensive interstitial abnormality caused by infiltration with fibrosis, abnormal cells, or fluid (e.g., fibrosing alveolitis, lymphangitis carcinomatosa, and pulmonary edema, respectively). Interlobular septal thickening that results from fibrosing alveolitis is often associated with intralobular, interstitial thickening (beyond the resolution of HRCT) and a coarse reticular pattern that contains cystic air spaces and produces the "honeycomb" of destroyed lung. Thickening of the interlobular septa may be smooth or irregular, but this distinction is not always obvious. Irregular septal thickening is a feature of lymphangitic spread of tumor, whereas pulmonary edema and alveolar proteinosis cause smooth thickening. Sarcoidosis is typified by some nodular septal thickening, although widespread septal thickening is not characteristic of this condition.

Because the various parts of the lung interstitium are in continuity, widespread interstitial disease that causes interlobular septal thickening also results in bronchovascular interstitial thickening (e.g., by lymphangitis carcinomatosa). The bronchovascular thickening seen on HRCT is equivalent to the peribronchial "cuffing" seen around end-on bronchi on chest radiography. The HRCT finding of peribronchovascular thickening in isolation must be interpreted with caution, because it may be seen in reversible pure airways disease, for example, asthma. Thickening of the subsegmental and segmental bronchovascular bundles, for example, caused by lymphangitis carcinomatosa, sometimes gives the interface between the thickened bronchial wall and surrounding lung a "feathery" appearance (Figure 1-109).

The coarseness of the network that makes up the reticular pattern on HRCT is determined by the level at which the interstitial thickening is most severe. Thickening of the intralobular septa results in a very fine reticular pattern on HRCT,

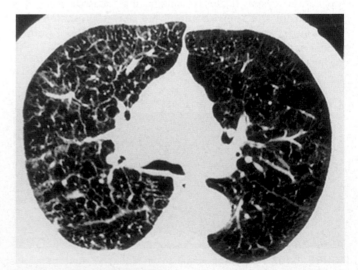

FIGURE 1-109 High-resolution computed tomography showing generalized, irregular thickening of the interlobular septa in the right lung. The patient has lymphangitis carcinomatosa.

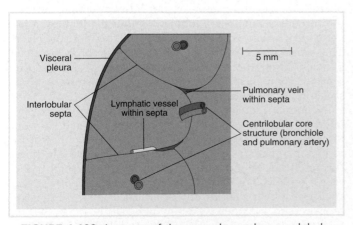

FIGURE 1-108 Anatomy of the secondary pulmonary lobule.

Visceral pleura

Interlobular septa

Lymphatic vessel within septa

5 mm

Pulmonary vein within septa

Centrilobular core structure (bronchiole and pulmonary artery)

only visible on an optimal HRCT scan. Some of the very delicate linear structures that make up such a fine reticular pattern are so small as to be below the resolution limits of HRCT, even with the narrowest collimation. The result is an amorphous increase in lung density ("ground-glass" opacification, see later) caused by volume averaging within the section.

Extensive pulmonary fibrosis causes complete destruction of the architecture of the secondary pulmonary lobules, which results in a coarse reticular pattern made up of irregular, linear opacities. The reticular pattern of end-stage fibrotic or honeycomb lung mirrors the appearances on chest radiography and is characterized by cystic spaces that measure a few millimeters to several centimeters across and are surrounded by discernible walls (Figure 1-110). Paradoxically, thickened interlobular septa are not an obvious feature of advanced fibrosing alveolitis, probably because of the severe disturbance of the normal lung architecture. The distortion that accompanies interstitial fibrosis may result in irregular dilatation of the segmental and subsegmental bronchi without honeycomb change, a phenomenon termed traction bronchiectasis (see Figure 1-110).

Nodular Pattern

A nodular pattern on HRCT comprises innumerable, small, discrete opacities that range in diameter from 1–10 mm and is a feature of both interstitial and airspace diseases. The location of nodules in relation to the lobules and bronchovascular bundles, as well as their density, clarity of outline, and uniformity of size, may indicate whether the nodules lie predominantly within the interstitium or airspaces. Because most

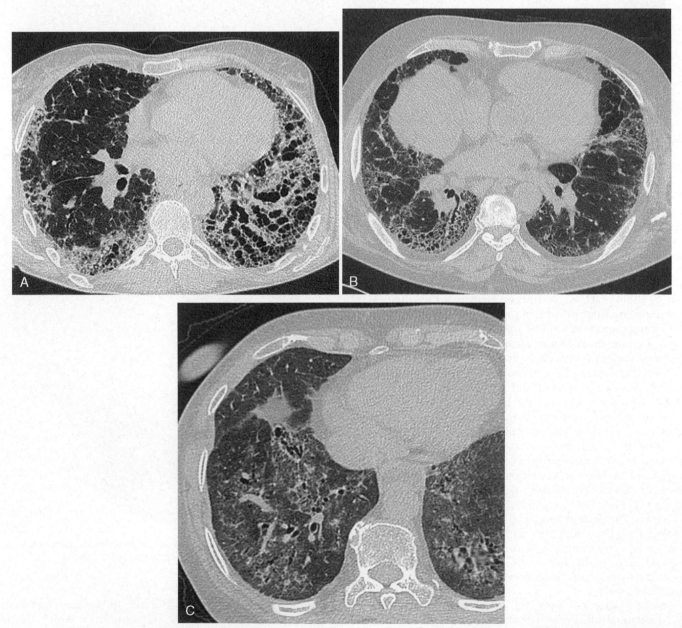

FIGURE 1-110 High-resolution computed tomography in fibrosing alveolitis. **A,** In the first patient, coarse cystic spaces are visible throughout the lung bases. **B,** In the second patient, there are finer fibrotic changes. Traction bronchiectasis is evident in both cases, which are typical of usual interstitial pneumonitis pattern. **C,** In another patient, there is much more marked ground-glass change characteristic of nonspecific interstitial pneumonia (NSIP) pattern.

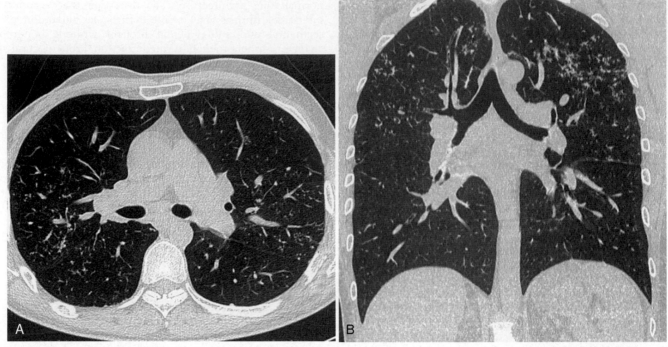

FIGURE 1-111 High-resolution computed tomography of sarcoidosis. **A,** Parenchymal nodularity together with thickening and beading of the bronchovascular bundles typical of sarcoidosis. **B,** Coronal reformat through the lungs of the same patient demonstrating the mid and upper zone predominance of disease.

diffuse lung pathoses have both interstitial and airspace components, this distinction does not always aid in the diagnosis. Whether pulmonary nodules can be detected on CT depends on their size, profusion, density, and the scanning technique. Narrow collimation HRCT is clearly superior to conventional CT for the detection of micronodular disease, because there is less partial volume effect, which can average out the attenuation of tiny nodules. A further refinement is the use of maximum-intensity projection images obtained with spiral CT to detect extremely subtle micronodular disease. Nodules within the lung interstitium are seen in the interlobular septa, subpleural regions (particularly in relation to the fissures), and in a peribronchovascular distribution. Nodular thickening of the bronchovascular interstitium results in an irregular interface between the margins of the bronchovascular bundles and the surrounding lung parenchyma. These features are most pronounced in cases of sarcoidosis, in which coalescent, perilymphatic granulomas cause a beaded appearance of the thickened bronchovascular bundles. The bronchovascular distribution of nodules, in conjunction with a perihilar concentration of disease, is virtually pathognomonic of sarcoidosis (Figure 1-111).

The nodular pattern seen in coal-worker's pneumoconiosis and silicosis is generally more uniform in distribution; the distribution of centrilobular nodules may be more in the upper zone and subpleurally, but overall they tend to be more evenly spread throughout the lung parenchyma than those seen in sarcoidosis.

When the airspaces are filled, or partially filled, with exudate, individual acini may become visible as poorly defined nodules approximately 8 mm in diameter. Acinar nodules may merge with areas of ground-glass opacification and are sometimes seen around the periphery of areas of dense parenchymal consolidation (Figure 1-112). Such nodules are usually

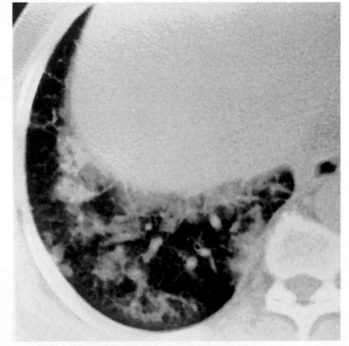

FIGURE 1-112 Poorly defined acinar nodules and patchy consolidation. The patient has cardiogenic pulmonary edema.

centrilobular, although this may be difficult to appreciate if the nodules are very profuse. Conditions in which this nonspecific pattern is seen include organizing pneumonia, hypersensitivity pneumonitis (Figure 1-113), endobronchial spread of tuberculosis, idiopathic pulmonary hemorrhage, and some cases of bronchoalveolar cell carcinoma.

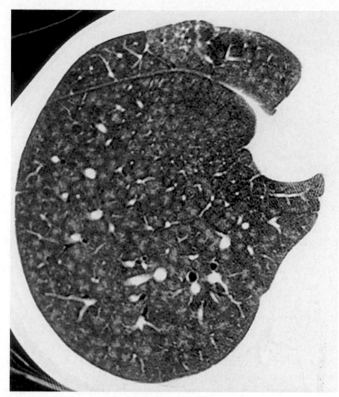

FIGURE 1-113 High-resolution computed tomography showing poorly defined nodular opacities merging with ground-glass opacification. The patient has subacute hypersensitivity pneumonitis.

Increased Lung Density

An amorphous increase in lung density on HRCT is often described as a ground-glass opacification appearance (Figure 1-114). Unlike the equivalent abnormality on chest radiography, in which the pulmonary vessels are often indistinct, a ground-glass pattern on HRCT does not obscure the pulmonary

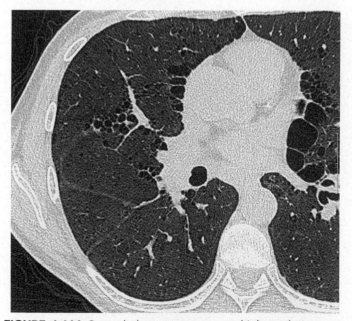

FIGURE 1-114 Ground-glass appearance on high-resolution computed tomography. Extensive ground-glass opacification in a patient who has desquamative interstitial pneumonitis. Note that the vessels are visible within the areas of ground-glass opacification.

vasculature. In cases in which the presence of a ground-glass pattern is equivocal, HRCT is often useful to compare the density of the lung parenchyma with air in the bronchi—in the normal state, the difference in density is marginal. Although this HRCT abnormality is usually easily recognizable, particularly when it is interspersed with areas of normal lung parenchyma, subtle degrees of increased parenchymal opacification may not be obvious. It is important to recognize that a normal increase in parenchymal density, indistinguishable from a generalized opacification caused by infiltrative lung disease, results in a ground-glass pattern in patients who breath-hold at end expiration.

On a pathologic level, the changes responsible for ground-glass opacification are complex and include partial filling of the airspaces and thickening of the interstitium or a combination of the two (Figure 1-115). Conditions that are characterized by these pathologic changes and result in the nonspecific pattern of ground-glass opacification include fibrosing alveolitis in the active cellular phase, *Pneumocystis carinii* pneumonia, subacute hypersensitivity pneumonitis, sarcoidosis, drug-induced lung damage, diffuse pulmonary hemorrhage, and acute lung injury. The amorphous ground-glass density seen on HRCT in these conditions usually represents a potentially reversible process. However, mild thickening of the intralobular interstitium by irreversible fibrosis may rarely produce a ground-glass appearance in fibrosing alveolitis. Furthermore, ground-glass opacification may be seen in areas of bronchoalveolar cell carcinoma, usually in conjunction with patches of denser, consolidated lung (Figure 1-116).

A pitfall in identifying a ground-glass pattern on HRCT occurs when regional differences in pulmonary perfusion are present—regional alterations in pulmonary blood flow, caused by thromboembolism, for example, may result in striking differences in lung density (Figure 1-117). The density difference between the underperfused lung and normal lung may give the appearance of a ground-glass density in normal (but relatively overperfused) lung parenchyma. These areas of different density have often been termed mosaic oligemia. A similar appearance is seen in patients who have patchy air-trapping caused by small airways disease, for example, an obliterative bronchiolitis; the relatively transradiant areas of underventilated and thus underperfused lung make the normal lung parenchyma appear more than usually dense and thus simulate a ground-glass infiltrate. This potential pitfall can often be recognized for what it is by the relative paucity of vessels in the underventilated parts of the lungs caused by hypoxic vasoconstriction. The vessels in the relatively normal lung of higher density are engorged because of shunting of blood to these regions (see Figure 1-117).

Cystic Airspaces

The term *cystic airspace* describes a clearly defined, air-containing space that has a definable wall 1–3-mm thick. Many conditions are characterized by a profusion of cystic airspaces, which may not be recognizable as such on chest radiography (Figure 1-118), whereas the size and distribution of these cysts on HRCT may suggest the diagnosis.

The destruction of alveolar walls that characterizes emphysema produces areas of low attenuation on HRCT, which often merge imperceptibly with normal lung (Figure 1-119). In patients who have predominantly centrilobular emphysema, circular areas of lung destruction may resemble cysts; however, the centrilobular core is usually visible as a dotlike structure in

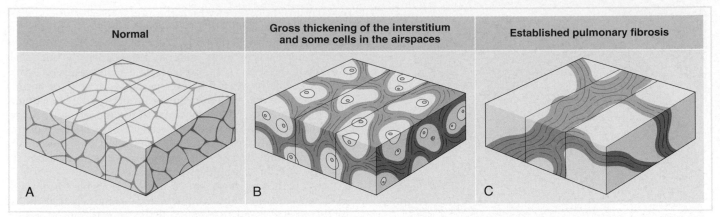

Normal	Gross thickening of the interstitium and some cells in the airspaces	Established pulmonary fibrosis
A	B	C

FIGURE 1-115 Normal and diseased lung voxels. **A,** In the normal state, most of the volume of these voxels is made up of air. **B,** Gross thickening of the interstitium and some cells within the air spaces causes displacement of air and thus an increase in density within the voxels—this produces ground-glass opacification on a high-resolution computed tomography image. **C,** In established pulmonary fibrosis, the strands of fibrotic lung occupy much of the volume of individual voxels, which is reflected in their density; pulmonary fibrosis thus has a reticular pattern on high-resolution computed tomography.

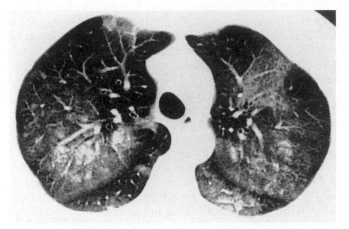

FIGURE 1-116 Patchy areas of ground-glass opacification in a patient who has biopsy-proven bronchoalveolar cell carcinoma.

the center of the apparent cyst. Although bullae of varying sizes are clearly seen on HRCT in patients who have emphysema, usually a background permeative, destructive parenchyma prevents confusion with other conditions in which cystic airspaces are a prominent feature.

Cystic airspaces as the dominant abnormality are seen in only a few conditions, which include lymphangioleiomyomatosis, Langerhans' cell histiocytosis, end-stage fibrosing alveolitis, and postinfective pneumatoceles. In lymphangioleiomyomatosis, the cysts are usually uniformly scattered throughout the lungs, with normal lung parenchyma intervening; the individual cysts are rarely larger than 4 cm in diameter (Figure 1-120). As the disease progresses, the larger cystic airspaces coalesce; the circumferential, well-defined walls of the cysts become disrupted; and the HRCT pattern of advanced lymphangioleiomyomatosis, and indeed of Langerhans' cell histiocytosis,

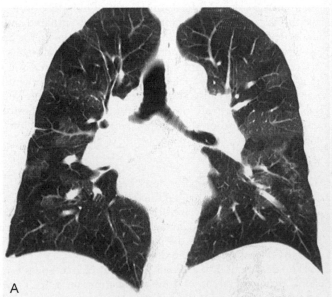
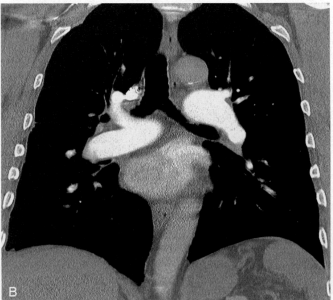

FIGURE 1-117 Uneven density of the lung parenchyma caused by perfusion inhomogeneity. The patient has chronic thromboembolism. **A,** Coronal reformat on lung window settings demonstrates the mosaic attenuation pattern. **B,** On mediastinal window settings, the large central pulmonary arteries are evident.

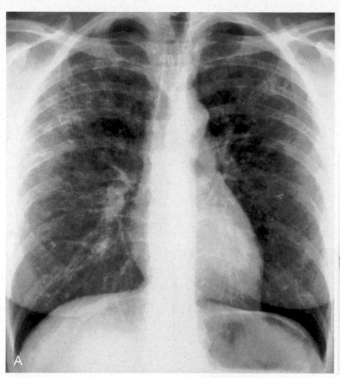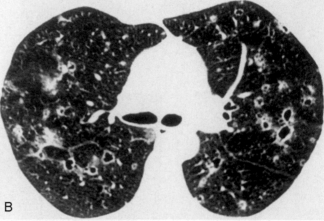

FIGURE 1-118 Cystic airspaces. **A,** Nonspecific shadowing on a chest radiograph, with the suggestion of a cavitating nodule in the right upper zone. **B,** High-resolution computed tomography through the upper lobes reveals multiple, curious-shaped, cavitating lesions, typical of Langerhans' cell histiocytosis.

may be practically indistinguishable from severe centrilobular emphysema. Distinction of the delicate, "lacelike" reticular pattern of lymphangioleiomyomatosis on HRCT from that of end-stage fibrosing alveolitis is usually possible because the cystic airspaces in a fibrotic honeycomb lung are smaller and have thicker walls. Furthermore, the tendency for fibrosing alveolitis to have a peripheral distribution, even in its end stage, is usually still obvious in the upper zones.

Similar, confluent cystic airspaces that give a delicate pattern on HRCT are seen in patients who have advanced Langerhans' cell histiocytosis. However, earlier in the disease, a nodular component is present and some of the nodules cavitate. The combination of cavitating nodules, some of which have curious shapes (e.g., clover-leaf shape), and cystic airspaces with a predominantly upper-zone distribution is virtually pathognomonic for the diagnosis (see Figure 1-118). Serial HRCT scans show the natural history of nodules, which cavitate, become cystic airspaces, and, in the end stages, coalesce. In a few cases, the cavitating nodules and cystic airspaces may resolve, with the lung parenchyma reverting to a normal appearance. Some of the cavitating nodules in Langerhans' cell histiocytosis superficially resemble bronchiectatic airways, but there is a lack of continuity between these lesions on adjacent sections, and the segmental bronchi, where they can be identified, do not have any of the HRCT features of bronchiectasis.

Diseases of the Airways

The imaging test of choice for the detection of bronchiectasis is now HRCT. The diagnosis of bronchiectasis on chest radiography can rarely be made with certainty unless the disease is severe. The opportunity for prospective studies to compare the accuracy of HRCT with what used to be the "gold standard," bronchography, has passed. Most of the evidence

that suggests HRCT is at least as good as bronchography is based on small, retrospective studies with different bronchographic and CT techniques. However, now that bronchography is rarely performed, no other imaging technique begins to compare with the sensitivity and specificity of an optimal HRCT examination.

Bronchiectasis is defined as damage to the bronchial wall that results in irreversible dilatation of the bronchi, whatever the cause. Thus, the main feature of bronchiectasis on HRCT is dilatation of the bronchi with or without bronchial wall thickening. Criteria for the HRCT identification of abnormally dilated bronchi depend on the orientation of the bronchi in relation to the plane of the HRCT section (Figure 1-121).

Vertically orientated bronchi are seen in the transverse section, so reference can be made to the accompanying pulmonary artery, which in normal individuals is of approximately the same caliber; any dilatation of the bronchus results in the so-called signet ring sign (Figure 1-122). Although this is generally a reliable sign of abnormal bronchial dilatation, care must be taken when comparing the diameter of the bronchi and adjacent pulmonary arteries just below the division of the lower lobe bronchus. At this level, pairs of segmental and sometimes subsegmental bronchi converge, and the resulting fusion of the two bronchi may give the spurious impression of an abnormally dilated bronchus. Bronchi that have a more horizontal course on CT, particularly the anterior segmental bronchi of the upper lobes and the segmental bronchi of the lingula and right middle lobe, are demonstrated along their length, and abnormal dilatation is seen as nontapering parallel walls or even flaring of the bronchi as they course distally (Figure 1-123). In more severe cases of bronchiectasis, the bronchi are obviously dilated and have a varicose or cystic appearance.

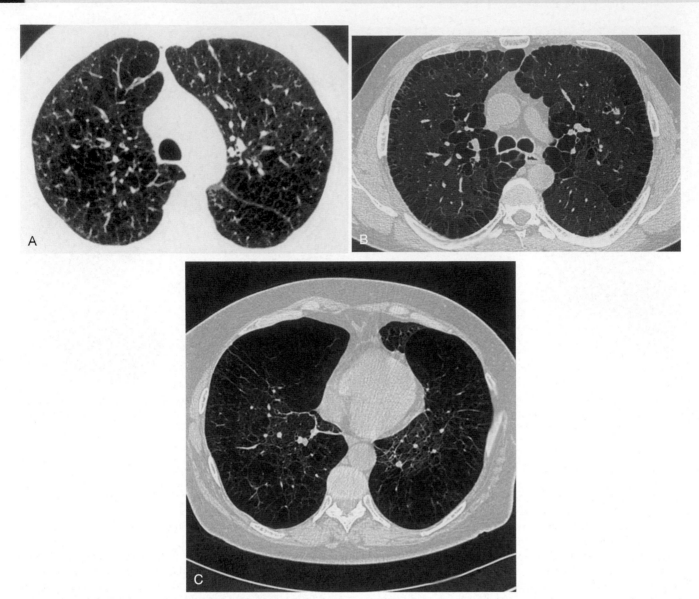

FIGURE 1-119 High-resolution computed tomography of centrilobular emphysema. **A,** Centrilobular emphysema. Note the permeative destruction of the lung parenchyma with scattered centrilobular lucent areas. **B,** Paraseptal emphysema. Note, however, the disease is concentrated in the subpleural lung. **C,** Panacinar emphysema. Large swathes of completely destroyed lung are evident, with almost no vascular or soft tissue structures demonstrated within.

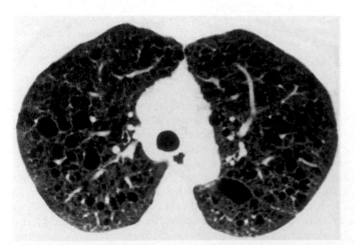

FIGURE 1-120 High-resolution computed tomography of advanced lymphangioleiomyomatosis. Note the coalescence of cystic air spaces, which resembles severe centrilobular emphysema.

Bronchial wall thickening is a frequent, but not invariable, feature of bronchiectasis. The definition of what constitutes abnormal bronchial wall thickening remains contentious, particularly because mild degrees of wall thickening are seen in normal subjects, asymptomatic smokers, asthmatic individuals, and patients affected by an acute, lower respiratory tract, viral infection. In brief, no robust and reproducible criterion for the identification of abnormal bronchial wall thickening exists, so bronchial wall thickening remains a subjective sign with an attendant high variation in observer interpretation. However, it is the presence of peribronchial thickening that renders the smaller peripheral airways visible on HRCT. Although there is no exact level beyond which visualization of the bronchi can be regarded as abnormal on HRCT, normal bronchi should not be visible within 2–3 cm of the pleural surface. The appearance of large elliptical and circular opacities, which represent secretion-filled, dilated bronchi, is a sign of gross bronchiectasis and is almost invariably seen in the presence of other obviously dilated bronchi,

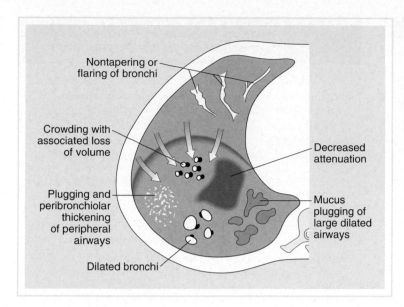

FIGURE 1-121 High-resolution computed tomography features of bronchiectasis. Nontapering or flaring of bronchi lying within the plane of section. "Signet ring" sign of dilated bronchi running perpendicular to the plane of computed tomography section. Mucus plugging of large, dilated airways. Plugging and peribronchiolar thickening of small peripheral airways. Crowding with associated loss of volume (see position of oblique fissure). Areas of decreased attenuation, which reflect associated small airways disease.

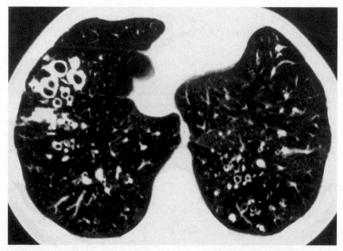

FIGURE 1-122 Severe bronchiectasis in the right lower lobe with plugging of the dilated bronchi. Mild, cylindric bronchiectasis in the left lower lobe showing the signet ring sign.

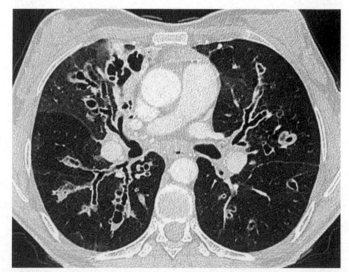

FIGURE 1-123 High-resolution computed tomography of a patient who has cystic fibrosis. Nontapering and flaring of the bronchiectatic airways is visible in the apical segment of the right lower lobe. In addition, mosaic perfusion is present, reflecting associated small airways disease.

some of which may contain air–fluid levels (Figure 1-124). When mucus plugging of the smaller airways occurs, minute branching structures or dots in the lung periphery may be identifiable. In some cases, plugging of the numerous centrilobular bronchioles gives a curious nodular appearance to the lungs (Figure 1-125).

Supplementary HRCT signs of bronchiectasis are crowding of the affected bronchi, with obvious volume loss of the lobe as shown by the position of the major fissures. In many lobes affected by bronchiectasis, areas of decreased attenuation of the lung parenchyma adjacent to the abnormal airways can be identified; this pattern of mosaic attenuation is

thought to reflect accompanying small airways disease, and the extent of the pattern correlates well with functional evidence of airflow obstruction, particularly indices of small airways dysfunction.

A positive diagnosis of bronchiectasis on HRCT is straightforward in patients who have moderate and severe disease. However, in some situations subtle signs of bronchiectasis may be obscured by technical artifacts. Conversely, the HRCT appearances of bronchiectasis may be mimicked by other lung pathoses. Some of the causes of false-negative and false-positive diagnoses of bronchiectasis are listed in Table 1-3.

Interest in the ability of HRCT to detect small airways disease is increasing. In the exudative form of bronchiolar disease

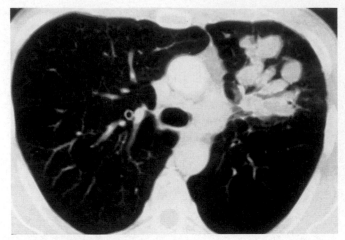

FIGURE 1-124 Severe bronchiectasis in the left upper lobe. The bronchi are completely filled with fluid, which results in multiple round and elliptical opacities. The patient has allergic bronchopulmonary aspergillosis.

TABLE 1-3	Causes of False-Positive and False-Negative Diagnoses of Bronchiectasis on High-Resolution Computed Tomography	
False Negatives		**False Positives**
Inappropriately thick computed tomography section		Cardiac pulsation causing "double vessels"
Movement artifact obscures lung detail		Confluence of subsegmental bronchi may give spurious impression of bronchiectasis, at a single level (particularly in the lower lobes)
Focal, inconspicuous, thin-walled bronchiectasis		Cavitating nodules mimicking bronchiectasis (e.g. Langerhans cell histiocytosis)
Bronchiectatic airways masked by surrounding fibrosis		Reversible dilatation of bronchi with acute pneumonic consolidation

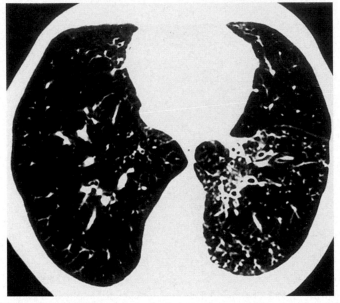

FIGURE 1-125 Numerous small irregular opacities in the left lower lobe representing plugged bronchioles. This is a case of panbronchiolitis.

(typified by Japanese panbronchiolitis), HRCT directly shows the plugged small airways as small irregular branching opacities. The HRCT signs of constrictive obliterative bronchiolitis (e.g., in patients who have rheumatoid arthritis or postviral obliterative bronchiolitis) are indirect—areas of decreased attenuation occur within which the vessels are of reduced caliber (but not distorted, in contrast to emphysema). The areas of decreased attenuation may merge with those of more normal lung or may have sharply demarcated, "geographic" boundaries (mosaic attenuation pattern). The density differences that characterize constrictive obliterative bronchiolitis may be extremely subtle, but because they represent areas of reduced ventilation, and thus air trapping, they may be dramatically emphasized on scans performed at end expiration. Most patients affected by small airways disease have some bronchiectatic changes on HRCT, which tend to be more severe in those who have immunologically mediated obliterative bronchiolitis (e.g., after lung transplantation).

SUGGESTED READINGS

Felson B, Felson H: Localization of intrathoracic lesions by means of the postero-anterior roentgenogram: The silhouette sign. Radiology 1950; 55:363–374.

Fraser RS, Muller N, Colman N, et al: Diagnosis of Diseases of the Chest. London: Saunders; 1999.

Golden R: The effect of bronchostenosis upon the roentgen-ray shadows in carcinoma of the bronchus. AJR 1925; 13:21–30.

Hansell D, Armstrong P, Lynch D, et al: Imaging Diseases of the Chest, 4th ed. London: Mosby; 2005.

Naidich D, et al: Computed Tomography and Magnetic Resonance of the Thorax, 4th ed. London: Lippincott Williams and Wilkins; 2007.

Webb WR, Muller N, Naidich D: High Resolution CT of the Lung. London: Lippincott Williams and Wilkins; 2000.

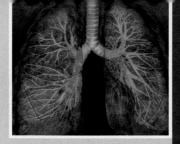

2 PET Imaging

JOHAN VANSTEENKISTE • CHRISTOPHE DOOMS • JOKKE WYNANTS

Conventional imaging is based on differences in the *structure* of tissues, measured by differences in density (chest X-ray and CT), surface reflectivity (ultrasound), or chemical environment (magnetic resonance imaging). They allow exquisite anatomic detail and interpretation, and they help in the assessment of many respiratory problems. Nonetheless, structural differences often do not allow a definitive diagnosis, and invasive tests with tissue sampling are needed.

Positron emission tomography (PET) has brought a revolutionary novelty in imaging, because it allowed accurate noninvasive measurement of regional metabolic tissue functions. Because PET relies on the detection of metabolic alterations observed in cells, this examination yields data other than the associated structural characteristics. It also allows detection or monitoring of specific metabolic alterations, which are not always associated with, or even precede, the anatomic changes.

USE OF PET IN RESPIRATORY MEDICINE

Because of its power to study metabolic processes, PET was originally developed as a research tool for brain function and cardiac metabolism studies. In the past decade, rapidly growing data on its use in patients with cancer came in place, and now PET cameras are primarily used for oncologic indications.

In respiratory medicine (Box 2-1), PET has its main indication in the assessment of non-small-cell lung cancer (NSCLC), with more limited experience in small-cell lung cancer (SCLC) and pleural mesothelioma (see Chapter 70 for the latter).

Because uptake of several tracers used in PET imaging is also enhanced in inflammatory tissues, PET has been studied in a variety of infectious or inflammatory respiratory disorders, such as environmental lung diseases (pneumoconiosis), sarcoidosis, chronic granulomatous disease, or even asthma. This use of PET generally belongs in a research context because easier and less expensive tests to measure activity of these inflammatory conditions are available. Therefore, PET outside of the neoplastic indications will not be commented on further in this chapter.

PRINCIPLES OF PET IMAGING

PET Cameras

The detection limit of a PET camera is about twice its spatial resolution (4–6 mm for current cameras). PET thus has good sensitivity for lesions of 10 mm or larger. Imaging of smaller lesions is less reliable, except for strongly FDG-avid lesions.

At present, three different types of PET scanners exist: dedicated PET, gamma coincidence PET (dual-head gamma camera coincidence imaging, GCI), and integrated PET-CT.

The main difference between standard radionuclide imaging with gamma cameras and dedicated PET is that the latter has a full ring of several thousands of scintillation detectors and does not need lead collimators, which may absorb up to 90% of the emitted photons, to generate the image. GCI has been developed as a cheap alternative to dedicated PET and is based on adding coincidence imaging to a simple dual-head gamma camera. The detectors used in GCI have less stopping power for high-energy photons, which results in a much worse sensitivity and resolution than dedicated PET (e.g., in the detection of small metastatic deposits in mediastinal nodes or distant sites). It should be emphasized, therefore, that the body of evidence for PET in respiratory oncology described in this chapter rests on dedicated scanners and may not be extrapolated to GCI.

The relative lack of anatomic detail of PET images limits the ability to properly localize hypermetabolic lesions. Therefore, visual correlation with CT images is the current minimum standard in the interpretation of PET images. From 2001 onward, integrated PET-CT scanners have made their entrance in clinical practice. PET-CT allows adequate fusion of metabolic and anatomic information and reduces the scanning time (see later). Many studies on lung cancer listed in this chapter have been performed with PET-alone cameras, but integrated PET-CT is rapidly gaining widespread use, because nearly all newly installed systems offer the fusion modality. The drawback of PET-CT is an increase in radiation dose, because the CT adds approximately 10 mSv to the 8 mSv generated by PET scanning.

Metabolic Tracers

The glucose analog ^{18}F-fluoro-2-deoxy-D-glucose (FDG), by far the most popular tracer for cancer imaging, was described in 1978. Its use is based on the increased cellular uptake of glucose, because of an increased expression of glucose transporter proteins and a much higher rate of glycolysis of cancer cells. FDG, a glucose analog in which the oxygen molecule is in position 2, is replaced by a positron-emitting ^{18}fluorine, undergoes the same uptake as glucose but is metabolically trapped and accumulated in the neoplastic cell after phosphorylation by hexokinase.

Acquisition Protocols

The behavior of FDG in normal and neoplastic tissues can be studied with different PET acquisition protocols.

Absolute quantification protocols allow for expression of the FDG uptake milligram per gram tissue, on the basis of kinetic models that describe the behavior of FDG in a tumor cell. This requires a dynamic acquisition over the target lesion (at least 1 h) and arterial blood sampling to measure the FDG input function. The use is mainly limited to more fundamental research studies (e.g., functional brain research).

Nonattenuation corrected whole-body images were common in the 1990s (Figure 2-1). FDG is injected outside the PET camera. After an uptake period of at least 60 min, different bed positions are scanned to obtain a whole-body survey, usually from the base of the skull to the pelvis. This took approximately 45 min, but the disadvantage was that no measure of FDG uptake was available.

Attenuation-corrected images correct for absorption of the emitted photons in the patient's body and are a better reflection of the actual FDG uptake. A so-called transmission scan estimates the attenuating characteristics of the patient, and semiquantification of the FDG metabolism becomes possible, expressed as standardized uptake value (SUV). The SUV of a lesion is obtained by normalizing its accumulation of FDG to the injected dose and the patient's body weight or surface area. In the early days of clinical PET, the transmission scan to correct for photon attenuation could only be performed before FDG injection and emission scanning ("cold transmission," total camera time nearly 3 h, see Figure 2-1). This has become much faster (45–60 min) with "hot transmission" (i.e., acquisition of transmission images after injection, alternating with emission images). The examination time was further reduced by approximately 30% in integrated PET-CT machines, where CT can be used for attenuation correction. By this, the latest generation of PET scans combined with multislice CT generate whole-body PET/CT fusion images in 25–30 min (see Figure 2-1).

INTERPRETATION OF PET IMAGES

General Principles

If the aim of the PET study is just to stage the patient, visual analysis of nonattenuation corrected images (i.e., hot spots higher than background activity being regarded positive for tumor) is probably just as good as SUV images, as has been pointed out by different prospective studies, both for the discrimination of nodules and for the evaluation of mediastinal involvement.

The Normal PET Image

A low degree of physiologic uptake of FDG exists in thoracic structures, including the lung, the heart, the aorta and large arteries, esophagus, thymus, trachea, thoracic muscles, bone marrow, joints, and soft tissues. This low background tracer activity builds the image contour. The high degree of FDG uptake in the brain and the excretory system impedes sensitive detection in these organs.

False-Positive Findings

FDG uptake is not tumor specific and can be found in all active tissues with high glucose metabolism, particularly inflammation. Therefore, clinically relevant FDG-positive findings, especially if isolated and decisive for patient management, require confirmation. The differentiation between metastasis, a benign or inflammatory lesion, or even an unrelated second malignancy should be made by other tests or tissue diagnosis.

The major causes of false-positive results (Box 2-2) in chest disease are infectious, inflammatory, and granulomatous disorders (Figure 2-2). Iatrogenic procedures may also give false-positive results: thoracocentesis, placement of a chest tube, percutaneous needle biopsy, mediastinoscopy, and talc pleurodesis.

False-Negative Findings

False-negative results are less common and may be due to lesion-dependent or technical factors (see Box 2-2).

A critical mass of metabolically active malignant cells is required for PET detection. Interpretation thus should be careful in tumors with decreased FDG uptake such as very well-differentiated adenocarcinoma (Figure 2-3), bronchioloalveolarcarcinoma, or carcinoid tumors. FDG-avid lesions

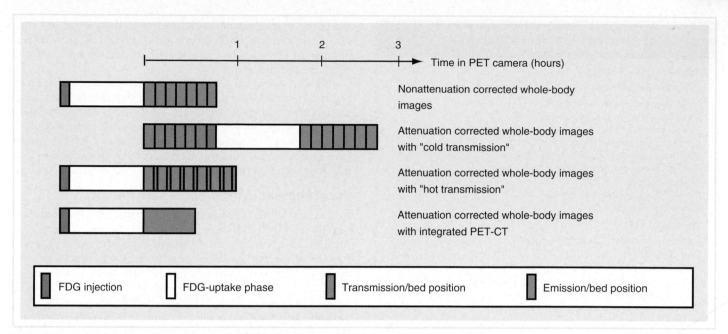

FIGURE 2-1 Different PET acquisition protocols. Nonattenuation corrected whole-body images, "cold transmission" attenuation correction, "hot transmission" attenuation correction, and CT-based attenuation correction in integrated PET-CT.

smaller than 5 mm may be false negative because of the limitations in spatial resolution and partial volume effects. In the lower lung fields, the detection limit may even go down to 10 mm because of additional respiratory motion.

Factors inherent in the technique are paravenous FDG injection or high baseline glucose serum levels. Blood glucose levels should be checked, and it is advised to proceed only if the glucose level is within a normal range before tracer injection. Although diabetic patients were often excluded in the prospective studies, FDG uptake is probably not significantly influenced in these patients if the blood glucose levels are reasonably controlled.

PET IN DIAGNOSIS

The Solitary Pulmonary Nodule

The value of PET in differentiating benign from malignant lesions (see Figure 2-3) has been studied in many prospective studies and documented in different meta-analyses. In these different series—in which a cutoff SUV of >2.5 was often used to suggest malignancy—a sensitivity of approximately 90–95% (range, 83–100%), a specificity of approximately 80% (range, 52–100%), and an accuracy of approximately 90% (range, 86–100%) can be expected. Differences in the results can be explained by the prevalence of malignancy in the study population, which is the result of the varying epidemiology of solitary pulmonary lesions in different areas of the world (e.g., regions with more tuberculosis or histoplasmosis). Other factors are the inclusion criteria of the different series (e.g., a lower sensitivity can be expected in series with smaller nodules). The causes for false-negative and false-positive findings in SPNs are listed in Box 2-2.

On the basis of recent experience, the use of a threshold SUV of >2.5 for the diagnosis of malignancy in a pulmonary nodule is questionable, because some lesions <2.5 are malignant. A Japanese series documented that the use of the SUV cutoff 2.5 may lead to false-negative results in smaller or faint

lesions. In these patients with SPNs between 1 and 3 cm—including many ground-glass opacity lesions—the use of SUV >2.5 missed malignancy in a quarter of the cancerous lesions. Many of these could be diagnosed on the basis of weak FDG uptake on visual analysis (corresponding to an SUV of approximately 1.5). Likewise, large prospective experience with integrated PET-CT documented a 24% chance of malignancy if maximal SUV was between 0 and 2.5, an 80% chance if between 2.6 and 4.0, and 96% if 4.1 or greater.

The use of PET has been shown to reduce the number of patients with an indeterminate SPN undergoing unnecessary resection of a benign lesion by about 15% and to reduce the cost per patient.

In the interpretation of the PET results, one should be aware of possibilities and limitations (see Box 2-1). Data are strong for the use of PET for characterization of solid pulmonary nodules >2 cm. Sensitivity is approximately 95%, negative predictive value (NPV) is very high, and malignancy can be excluded correctly in most cases. In these patients, a thoracotomy can be avoided, and repeat chest X-ray or CT can be used to confirm the absence of growth.

To minimize the chance of missing a malignancy in smaller or faint pulmonary nodules, however, any lesion with FDG uptake higher than background should be considered suspect, and the "magic" SUV threshold of 2.5 should be abandoned in this setting. Other clinical (age, smoking history) and radiologic (spiculation) factors determining the likelihood of malignancy should be considered. Specific CT study, close follow-up, or more invasive tests can be appropriate.

Finally, specificity and good positive predictive value are lower, and one should be aware that a positive scan is possible in the conditions listed in Box 2-2, which should be evaluated by appropriate tests. In case of doubt, lesions with increased FDG uptake should be considered malignant until proven otherwise and managed accordingly.

PET has also been studied in the assessment of nodules detected in lung cancer screening protocols (see Chapter 47).

BOX 2-2   Causes of False-Positive and False-Negative PET Findings

False-Positive Findings

Infection/Inflammation

(Postobstructive) pneumonia/abscess
Mycobacterial or fungal infection
Granulomatous disorders (sarcoidosis, Wegener)
Chronic nonspecific lymphadenitis
(Rheumatoid) arthritis
Occupational exposure (anthracosilicosis)
Bronchiectasis
Organizing pneumonia
Reflux esophagitis

Iatrogenic Causes

Invasive procedure (puncture, biopsy)
Talc pleurodesis
Radiation esophagitis and pneumonitis
Bone marrow expansion after chemotherapy
Colony-stimulating factors
Thymic hyperplasia after chemotherapy

Benign Mass Lesions

Salivary gland adenoma (Wharton)
Thyroid adenoma
Adrenal adenoma
Colorectal dysplastic polyps

Focal Physiologic FDG Uptake

Gastrointestinal tract
Muscle activity
Brown fat
Unilateral vocal cord activity
Atherosclerotic plaques

False-Negative Findings

Lesion Dependent

Small-sized lesion
Bronchioloalveolar carcinoma
Carcinoid tumors
Ground-glass opacity neoplasms

Technique Dependent

Hyperglycemia
Paravenous FDG injection
Increased time between injection and scanning

PET IN STAGING

Local or distant relapse after curative treatment such as surgery or radical chemoradiotherapy remains frequent. Therefore, reliable noninvasive methods for accurate staging are highly warranted. CT scan, endoscopic techniques, and surgical procedures are key players, but the addition of PET to these conventional methods has been shown to improve the staging process substantially in the past decade by distinguishing patients who are candidates for radical approaches such as surgical resection or intense multimodality treatments from those who are not.

The Primary Tumor (T Factor)

In general, CT has gained a central role in lung cancer staging and is now available for every treatable patient. Current multislice CT, with its exquisite anatomic detail, remains the preferred test to evaluate the T factor (e.g., relationship of the tumor to the fissures), which may determine the type of resection, to mediastinal structures or to the pleura and chest wall. Stand-alone PET offers little extras in this respect because of its limitations in spatial resolution and anatomic detail within the image.

PET has been used to assess pleural disease with varying results. If pleural staging determines the chance for radical treatment, often pathologic verification with cytologic studies or thoracoscopic biopsy should be sought, because small pleural deposits can be missed on PET because of their low tumor load and/or partial volume effects, whereas false-positive findings may occur in patients with inflammatory pleural lesions.

Locoregional Lymph Nodes (N Factor)

In the late 1990s, several prospective studies from dedicated centers demonstrated that PET is more accurate than CT for mediastinal LN staging, and this has been confirmed in several meta-analyses. An overall sensitivity of 80–90% and a specificity of 85–95% was reported, significantly better than the performance of CT in the same cohorts. From the beginning onward, it became clear that results of PET images interpreted with the aid of visual correlation with CT images was superior because of the complementary nature of anatomic and metabolic information, allowing better distinction between, for example, central tumors and adjacent LNs (Figure 2-4).

A prospective randomized study compared staging with upfront PET (i.e., directly after first presentation) versus routine clinical staging in 465 patients. Patients with FDG-avid, noncentrally located tumors without signs of mediastinal or distant spread on PET proceeded directly to surgical resection. Quality of staging was measured by comparison of the clinical stage to the final stage and was similarly good in both arms. Noninvasive tests to reach a clinical TNM were similar in both arms, but invasive tests (i.e., mainly mediastinoscopy) were significantly reduced with PET, again a consequence of the successful implementation of the NPV of PET for mediastinal node metastases.

In addition, PET can document suspect LNs in stations not amenable to mediastinoscopy, such as lower mediastinal nodes, and PET can be of help to guide and improve the yield of invasive procedures. In a recent prospective study, endobronchial ultrasound-guided transbronchial needle aspiration (EBUS-TBNA) for detection of mediastinal and hilar LN metastases was guided by the information on thoracic PET and CT images, and the sensitivity of the aspiration was up to 92% in this setting.

The high NPV of PET correlated with CT allows us to proceed to straightforward surgical resection in operable patients without signs of mediastinal lymph node (LN) involvement, thereby sparing invasive staging tests in a substantial number of patients. In North American data, a strategy with PET and CT also was more cost-effective than a strategy with CT alone in the staging of NSCLC.

To minimize the chance of missing clinically important LN metastasis, some important side conditions in the interpretation should be taken into account (see Box 2-1): sufficient FDG uptake in the primary tumor and no centrally located tumor or important hilarnodal disease that may obscure coexisting N2 disease on PET. If this approach is used, an occasional patient with a false-negative mediastinal PET will proceed to straightforward thoracotomy, but then minimal N2 will be in place, a situation where surgery followed by adjuvant chemotherapy is appropriate (the size of the LN tumor deposits that may escape detection by PET is approximately 4–6 mm).

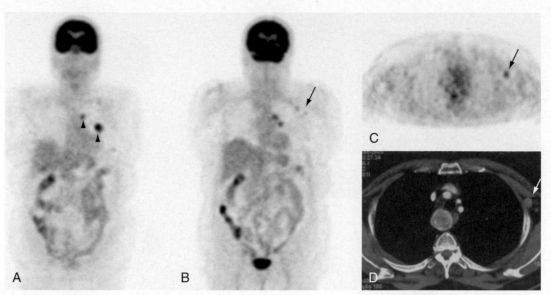

FIGURE 2-2 A, Left lung tumor with accompanying left paraaortic lymph nodes *(arrowheads).* **B** and **C,** PET also suggested left axillary lymph node metastases *(arrow).* **D,** Corresponding picture on CT. Biopsy revealed inflammatory hydradenitis. Final stage cT2N2, candidate for radical multimodality treatment.

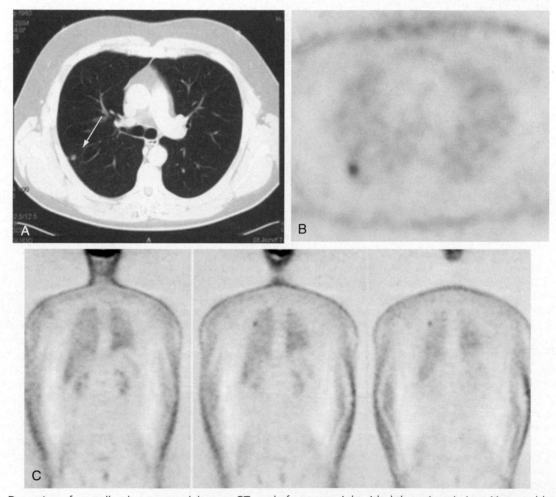

FIGURE 2-3 A, Detection of a small pulmonary nodule on a CT made for vague right-sided thoracic pain in a 41-year-old patient. **B** and **C,** The lesion is moderately FDG avid with no signs of lymph node or pleural disease, but no explanation for thoracic pain. At thoracoscopy, diffuse superficial pleural metastases from a well-differentiated lung adenocarcinoma were present.

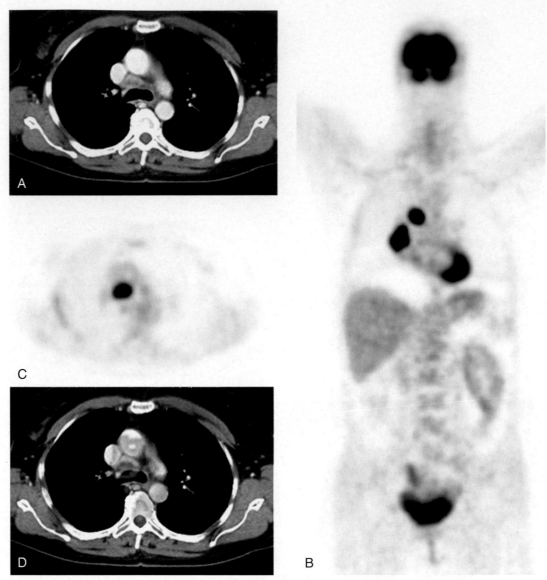

FIGURE 2-4 A, CT of a patient with centrally located right lung tumor (not shown) and adenopathy. **B** and **C,** Tumor on the PET images, visual correlation strongly suggestive of right paratracheal adenopathy. **D,** Integrated image confirmation.

False-positive images are possible in LNs on the basis of the conditions listed in Box 2-2. Therefore, tissue proof of LN involvement should be sought in most patients with positive mediastinal nodes on PET, except those with obvious bulky LN metastases.

Extrathoracic Spread (M Factor)

In the evaluation of metastases by site, PET is almost uniformly superior to conventional imaging, except for brain imaging, where sensitivity is unacceptably low because of the high glucose uptake of normal surrounding brain tissue. CT and/or MRI remain the method of choice there.

For bone metastases, several prospective studies and retrospective surveys have shown that PET is more accurate than a 99mTcMDP bone scan: sensitivity is at least as good (90–95%) and specificity is far better (95% vs 60% for bone scan). Limitations are that standard PET images are from the head to just below the pelvis, and thus could miss metastases in the lower extremities, and that some breast cancer studies

reported false-negative findings in osteoblastic lesions, a rare event in lung cancer.

The adrenal glands are a challenge in lung cancer staging because adrenal metastases originating from NSCLC are quite frequent (up to 20% of patients at presentation), but adrenal enlargement is quite often caused by asymptomatic adrenal adenoma as well (up to 60%). Smaller prospective series and larger retrospective evidence point at a high sensitivity of PET in detecting adrenal metastasis, so that an equivocal lesion on CT without FDG uptake will usually not be metastatic. One should be careful with the interpretation of small lesions (<1 cm), but, on the other hand, smaller size often suggests adenoma as well. Specificity is high, but not perfect, because some adenomas are quite FDG avid. For this reason, pathologic proof is warranted in case the decision on curative treatment intent relies on the adrenal gland interpretation.

Liver staging is, in general, less problematic, because both ultrasound (US) and CT are reliable tools. No specific series exist on the use of PET in liver assessment, but general staging

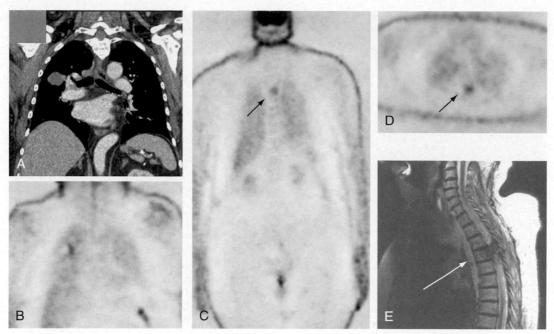

FIGURE 2-5 **A** and **B,** Patient with large-cell lung cancer in the right upper lobe. **C** and **D,** Suspicion of bone lesion in the thoracic spine on PET *(arrow).* **E,** Bone CT was equivocal, but MRI of the spine confirmed bone and soft tissue metastasis *(arrow).*

series in NSCLC suggest a superiority of PET by being more accurate than CT, mainly by differentiating hepatic lesions that remain indeterminate by conventional studies.

Obviously, PET may also reveal metastases in sites that escape our attention in conventional staging (e.g., soft tissue lesions, retroperitoneal LNs, hardly palpable supraclavicular nodes, and painless bone lesions).

It is clear that PET is a significant complement to conventional imaging for two reasons: (1) detection of unexpected metastatic spread (Figure 2-5). After a negative conventional staging, unknown metastases were found on PET in 5% to as high as 29% of the patients, in increasing numbers from pre-PET stage I–III. Variation in this number is also due to differences in the definition of conventional staging (consisting of thoracic/upper abdomen CT alone, or with systematic brain CT and/or bone scintigraphy), in the definition of unexpected lesions (taking into account only negative conventional staging findings or equivocal readings as well), or to the quality of the conventional staging. (2) PET is able to determine the nature of equivocal lesions on conventional imaging, present in 7–19% of the patients.

Despite the overall better accuracy, it is not fully understood whether PET is ready to replace conventional imaging. This is unlikely, however, because most PET studies were performed in an additional setting, and it is difficult to estimate how solid the exclusion of very small lesions is by PET. With the rapid transition toward integrated PET-CT, this question may soon become an academic one.

Exclusion of malignancy by PET in equivocal conventional findings requires caution in case of smaller lesions (<1 cm) (see Box 2-1). In this regard, we mention the problem of small pulmonary nodule(s) in a different lobe or lung, a common finding in patients with lung cancer in the era of spiral multislice CT. Because of the low volume of these lesions, PET or even integrated PET-CT often does not solve this problem, and invasive sampling by, for example, thoracoscopy is still needed.

Interpretation is not a problem when whole-body PET shows multisite metastases, but it is imperative to seek verification by other tests or tissue sampling of an isolated positive finding that determines the radical treatment intent. In large retrospective survey findings on whole-body PET, solitary extrathoracic lesions were documented in approximately 20% of the patients. Approximately half of these, indeed, were metastatic, whereas the other half were not related to lung cancer, mostly inflammatory or other benign lesions (see Figure 2-2) and some second primary tumors. The drawback of this "seek for verification" strategy is that many indeterminate findings on PET may lead to additional studies or interventions. However, after the initial learning curve in interpretation, it is usually possible to distinguish well-known areas of physiologic FDG uptake from suspect findings (see "Interpretation of PET Images").

IMPACT ON OVERALL STAGING AND TREATMENT

The unique aspect of PET is that it gives reasonably reliable information on locoregional and extrathoracic spread in one single test. PET induces a change of stage in 27–62% of NSCLC patients, in general more upstaging than downstaging, related mainly to the detection of unexpected distant lesions (Table 2-1). This leads to a change in patient management in 25% to even 52% of the patients. Changes were both in treatment intent (curative vs palliative) and in alterations in treatment modalities (chemotherapy vs radiotherapy, radical radiotherapy vs surgery).

The additive value of PET was investigated in two randomized controlled trials comparing implementation of PET added to conventional staging versus conventional staging alone. The outcome measure was reduction in the number of futile surgical procedures. A clear reduction was found in a Dutch trial, with approximately 20% absolute reduction of futile

TABLE 2-1 Impact of PET on Stage Designation and Patient Management in NSCLC

Study	Year	N	Change of Stage	Change in Management
Lewis et al.	1994	34	NR	41%
Bury et al.	1997	109	34%	25%
Saunders et al.	1999	97	27%	37%
Pieterman et al.	2000	102	62%	NR
Hicks et al.	2001	153	43%	35%
Schmucking et al.	2003	63	NR	52%
Hoekstra et al.	2003	57	30%	19%

NR, Not reported.

surgery, thus five patients needing a PET to avoid one futile surgery. A similar trial in clinical stage I–II patients in Australia did not reveal this difference. Further trials are needed to estimate the additional value of PET in NSCLC staging.

Integrated PET-CT

Sometimes confusion exists about the term *fusion PET-CT*. Visual correlative reading is always the minimum requirement. Before the advent of integrated PET-CT machines, there was software fusion—where images from a patient lying in the same position during consecutive PET and CT acquisition in different scanners—were fused by a computer algorithm. This fusion was far from perfect because patient position and respiratory status were difficult to control. In truly integrated PET-CT, a combined scanner creates both data sets that are subsequently merged into a single image.

The most significant improvement by integrated PET-CT relates to the accuracy of T staging rather than N staging (see Figure 2-4). For the T factor, more precise evaluation of chest wall and mediastinal infiltration or correct differentiation between tumor and peritumoral inflammation or atelectasis has been described. In a large retrospective survey on patients with different tumors, a significant advantage of integrated PET-CT versus PET or CT alone was found, but not versus side-to-side correlated images. As a whole, it seems that visual side-by-side comparison of images is a reasonable approach at present, even if technological evolution will lead to integrated scanning as the standard approach in the near future.

Small-Cell Lung Cancer

It can be assumed that the principles of PET for NSCLC are applicable to SCLC, but there are far less data on PET for the latter patients. Several things may account for this. First, SCLC today represents only 15–20% of all lung cancers. Second, it is a tumor with early spread into distant sites, thereby obviating the need for PET in many patients. For that reason, patients with SCLC are often grouped in "limited disease" (LD), treated with radical concurrent chemoradiotherapy, and "extensive disease" (ED), treated with palliative chemotherapy only.

The main merit of PET is that it may change the LD or ED status on the basis of conventional staging, thereby changing the treatment intent. In several small prospective series, PET, indeed, caused a stage migration, more often upstaging of LD patients to ED than downstaging ED patients to LD.

PET in Follow-Up

After radical locoregional therapy for lung cancer, early detection of recurrence is important because salvage therapies can

be rewarding. It can be difficult to differentiate therapy-induced fibrosis from tumor recurrence on conventional imaging. Moreover, tissue sampling can be technically impossible or yield a false-negative result.

Several—mostly prospective—studies have brought convincing evidence that PET is a valid tool to differentiate local recurrence from posttreatment changes. Specificity is more critical because false-positive findings may occur if PET is performed shortly after radiotherapy or surgery. To minimize the postradiotherapy changes interfering with correct staging, an interval of 3–6 months is recommended between the initial treatment and reassessment by PET. PET cannot be recommended for general follow-up of patients treated for lung cancer, but selective use in case of suspicion of local recurrence on conventional imaging can be appropriate.

PET in Prognosis and Assessment of Therapy

FDG uptake in tumors is related to the number of viable cancer cells and their proliferation capacity. Therefore, PET has been proven to be useful to measure the biological properties of lung cancer and to be of help in the prognostic and therapeutic assessment of lung cancer. For a more extensive overview, we refer to our review listed at the end of this chapter.

One aspect, the restaging of patients after induction therapy for locally advanced NSCLC, is of particular interest for the pulmonologist. In the late 1990s, different prospective studies looked at the value of PET—in visual correlation with CT—to assess the effect of induction chemo(radio)therapy for locally advanced NSCLC (Table 2-2). In the restaging of mediastinal LNs, PET was more accurate than CT alone (Figure 2-6), but with more moderate results than when used for baseline LN staging (sensitivity 50–70%, specificity 60–90%).

More important were the findings on outcome prediction in these studies. One of the difficult issues in combined modality treatment is the decision concerning which patient is a candidate for surgical resection after induction. This is difficult, because factors associated with better outcome are the downstaging of mediastinal LNs and the pathologic response in the primary tumors, both of which are poorly predicted by CT. In these prospective studies, both the residual FDG uptake in the primary tumor after induction as well as the change in FDG uptake when comparing preinduction and postinduction values had strong power to predict outcome after combined modality treatment.

Three recent studies looked at the value of integrated PET-CT (see Table 2-2). The integrated scan performed better in this setting, with a sensitivity to detect persistent mediastinal LN disease after induction of approximately 60–80%

TABLE 2-2   Result of PET and Integrated PET-CT in Restaging after Induction Treatment for Locally Advanced NSCLC

Study	Year	N	Stage	CTRT	Imaging	Sensitivity	Specificity
Vansteenkiste et al.	2001	31	IIIA-N2	0%	PET + CT (visual corr.)	71%	88%
Akhurst et al.	2002	56	I-IV	29%	PET + CT (visual corr.)	67%	61%
Ryu et al.	2002	26	III	100%	PET + CT (visual corr.)	58%	93%
Cerfolio et al.	2003	34	IB-IIIA	21%	PET + CT (visual corr.)	50%	99%
Hellwig et al.	2004	37	III	70%	PET + CT (visual corr.)	50%	88%
Port et al.	2004	25	I-IIIA	0%	PET + CT (visual corr.)	20%	71%
Hoekstra et al.	2005	25	IIIA-N2	0%	PET + CT (visual corr.)	50%	71%
Cerfolio et al.	2006	93	IIIA-N2	100%	Integrated PET-CT	62%	88%
Pottgen et al.	2006	37	IIIA/B	100%	Integrated PET-CT	73%	89%
De Leyn et al.	2006	30	IIIA-N2	0%	Integrated PET-CT	77%	92%

CTRT, Percent of patients with chemoradiotherapy.

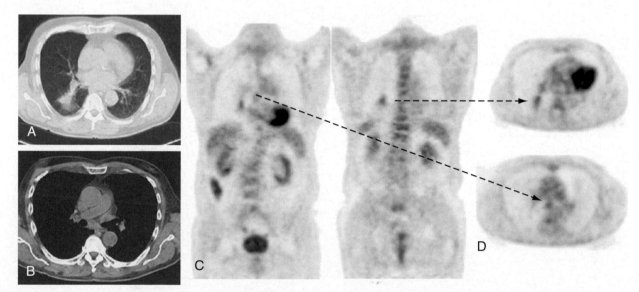

FIGURE 2-6 Patient with stage IIIA-N2 after induction chemotherapy. Both the primary tumor in the right lung (**A**) as well as the subcarinal adenopathy (**B**) have decreased in size. On coronal (**C**) and transaxial (**D**) PET images, moderate FDG uptake is still present in the primary tumor and in the subcarinal space. Endoscopic needle aspiration confirmed persistent N2 disease.

and preserved specificities of approximately 80–90%. One of these studies prospectively compared integrated PET-CT and redo mediastinoscopy in the assessment of residual mediastinal LN involvement after chemotherapy induction and described significant superiority of PET-CT for sensitivity and accuracy. SUV on PET-CT after induction again correlated with the degree of pathologic response in the primary tumor.

PET in Planning of Radiotherapy

Modern radiotherapy tries to minimize healthy tissue irradiation by reducing treatment fields, thereby seeking to increase the dose to the involved sites to improve outcome. Several studies have consistently demonstrated that delineation of radiation fields is improved by use of PET-CT information. A substantial reduction in radiation fields can occur, especially in case of centrally located tumors with postobstructive

atelectasis. Adding PET information to standard radiotherapy planning results in changes in treatment volume in approximately 30–60% of the patients (see Suggested Readings for more detail).

FUTURE DEVELOPMENTS

FDG allows excellent discrimination between normal tissues and tissues with enhanced glucose metabolism, but false-positive uptake of FDG in inflammatory tissues is one of the major limitations of this tracer. Therefore, tracers with an equally high sensitivity but a better specificity are the focus of ongoing research, but none has shown a clear improvement over FDG at this time in clinical lung cancer imaging.

An entire new field that uses PET is molecular imaging to study cellular functions such as receptors, transport proteins, or intracellular enzymes. These results are eagerly awaited because targeted agents are the emerging new treatments for lung cancer, and targeting these expensive drugs by proper selection of patients by predictive markers is a key question.

With the advent of integrated PET and multislice spiral CT, the hardware for lung cancer imaging has come to a high technical standard. Future expectations are a further decrease of the spatial resolution of PET cameras to as low as 2 mm, which will probably be the limit of this technique, because the emitted photons are emitted with some scatter and with a slight deviation from the 180-degree angle of the detectors.

Another feature that could improve the quality of the images, especially in respiratory medicine, is respiratory gating of PET acquisition. Because of respiratory motion, the volume of a lung lesion is smeared out and thus overestimated, whereas the FDG intensity is underestimated, especially in the lower lung fields. Synchronization of the acquisition of the PET emission images with respiratory motion may overcome this problem.

SUGGESTED READINGS

Juweid ME, et al: Positron-emission tomography and assessment of cancer therapy, N Engl J Med 2006; 354:496–507.

Mavi A, et al: Fluorodeoxyglucose-PET in characterizing solitary pulmonary nodules, assessing pleural diseases, and the initial staging, restaging, therapy planning, and monitoring response of lung cancer, Radiol Clin North Am 2005; 43:1–21.

Oehr P, et al: PET and CT-PET in Oncology, Berlin, 2003, Springer.

Van Baardwijk A, et al: The current status of FDG-PET in tumour volume definition in radiotherapy treatment planning, Cancer Treat Rev 2006; 32:245–260.

Vansteenkiste J, et al: Positron emission tomography in non-small cell lung cancer, Curr Opin Oncol 2007; 19:78–83.

Vansteenkiste J, et al: Positron-emission tomography in prognostic and therapeutic assessment of lung cancer: systematic review, Lancet Oncol 2004; 5:531–540.

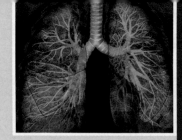

3 Basic Science of Genetics Applied to Lung Diseases

CHRISTOPHER D. COLDREN • SARAH MCKINLEY • MARK W. GERACI

INTRODUCTION

Genetics and the biochemistry and molecular biology associated with genes are some of the most highly developed areas of modern science, and our understanding of the role of individual genes in the pathophysiology of pulmonary disease has grown exponentially in recent years. Despite this explosion in genetic information, genetic testing is used most frequently in the context of only three clinical conditions in pulmonary medicine: cystic fibrosis, α_1-antitrypsin deficiency, and pulmonary hypertension. Although gene therapies for these diseases remain elusive, the effect of genetic testing on the lives of patients and families can be profound. This chapter provides a review of the foundations of human genetics, the state of genetics in current medical research, and the use of genetic evaluation in the diagnosis of lung diseases.

BASIC GENETIC CONCEPTS:

The Human Genome

The Human Genome Project has changed the face of medical genetics. The goal of this project has been to provide a detailed map of the human chromosomes, including the base sequences of all human genes. This map provides information that has proven essential in identifying the genetic elements of many diseases and has resulted in an explosion of knowledge about the contribution of individual genes to the pathophysiology of disease, including selected pulmonary conditions. Despite this rapidly expanding knowledge, few disorders in pulmonary medicine currently mandate specific DNA tests for definitive diagnosis. The role of genetic evaluation in pulmonary disease before the Human Genome Project was primarily limited to single-gene (also known as Mendelian) disorders, such as cystic fibrosis and α_1-antitrypsin deficiency. The project has provided insight into genes that, although not directly causative, alter disease susceptibility and contribute to pathogenesis. Genes are now known to play a role in many diseases that were once believed to be caused solely by environment. For example, observations of higher rates of asthma within families and a greater concordance of asthma between monozygotic than dizygotic twins have suggested that a genetic component exists for this disease. However, pedigree analysis does not reveal a pattern consistent with mutations in a single gene. This has led to the hypothesis that asthma is caused by interactions of multiple genes (polygenic) that increase susceptibility. The map created by the Human Genome Project is providing tools necessary to help identify these susceptibility genes.

As our understanding of complicated genetic conditions grows, genetic testing will become more important in explaining the pathogenesis of non-Mendelian diseases and guiding their treatment.

A popular and apt analogy casts the human genome as an encyclopedia of instructions for the construction of the human organism. Each volume of this encyclopedia represents one of the 23 pairs of chromosomes. Each subject entry in a volume represents 1 of approximately 25,000 genes, and each letter in the text stands for an individual base pair of DNA in the 3.2 billion base pair human genome sequence. However, the science of genetics predates our understanding of genes as chemical and physical entities. Whereas the molecular basis of genetic phenomenon is a major focus of modern research, classical geneticists made enormous strides by considering genes as conceptual "units of inheritance" by charting their passage through generations and by correlating this transmission to the resulting variation between organisms.

Three concepts form the foundation for our understanding of the transmission of inherited characteristics from parent to child: the two laws of Mendelian inheritance and the chromosome theory of inheritance.

Mendel's first law, the law of segregation, has four parts:

1. Alternative versions of genes (alleles) account for variations in phenotype.
2. Humans inherit two alleles of each gene, one from each parent.
3. When two different alleles are inherited, one allele is dominant and determines the phenotype.
4. The two alleles of each gene segregate in the process of gamete production.

Mendel's second law states that genes are inherited independently of one another and that the allele state of any given gene is not statistically associated with the allelic state of any other gene. The association of inheritable traits with specific cellular material is embodied in the chromosome theory of inheritance, which postulates that chromosomes are linear sequences of genes and that inheritance patterns may be explained by the location of individual genes at a specific location on a specific chromosome (the genetic locus).

Gene Structure

Each of the approximately 25,000 human genes exists physically as a linear region of double-stranded DNA embedded in the linear sequence of 1 of the 25 unique genetic structures. These genes are distributed across each of the 22 pairs of distinct autosomal chromosomes, the two sex chromosomes, and the mitochondrial DNA. Human autosomes vary widely—the smallest contains fewer than 400 individual genes (chromosome 21), whereas the largest contains more than 3000 (chromosome 1). Approximately 1100 and 200 exist on chromosomes X and Y, respectively, and 37 are encoded in mitochondrial DNA. The linear region of DNA representing a typical gene is approximately 3000 base pairs (3 kb) long, although extremely long (2.4 mb) and short (200 bp) human genes exist.

Genes contain regions of sequence with distinct features (Figure 3-1): these include sequences that are transcribed into the final messenger RNA (mRNA) molecule (exons) and the intervening regions that separate exons (introns). Exons consist of a sequence that directly encodes the protein product and regulatory regions that control the rate of translation of mRNA into protein and the half-life of the mRNA. Introns encode the regions that dictate the assembly of exons and the removal of introns from the mature mRNA (splice sites).

Alleles of a given gene typically differ from one another at only one or a few base positions, but the resulting difference in the gene product can affect the phenotype. For example, many genes encode enzymes. Intronic allelic variation can alter or destroy the activity of an enzyme through changes in the sequence of the expressed protein. Splice site variant alleles can also exhibit diminished enzyme activity; by modifying the way in which introns are assembled, the resulting transcript is radically changed, as is the expressed protein. Allelic variation in the regulatory region of a gene can change the transcription level of that allele, resulting in a change in the abundance of the enzyme and its activity.

Dominance Relationship

Almost all human cells are diploid; each cell contains two copies of each autosomal chromosome and, therefore, two copies of most genes. When the two alleles of a given gene are identical (homozygous), the phenotype associated with the allele is expressed. When different alleles for a gene are present (heterozygous), one allele is dominant and determines the phenotype. This dominance relationship is represented in the designation of alleles as recessive or dominant.

Simple Dominance

The condition of simple dominance exists when one allele (the dominant allele) effectively masks the phenotype associated with other recessive alleles. Because inheriting only a single copy of a dominant allele results in expression of the associated phenotype, offspring of a heterozygous individual are 50% likely to express the phenotype. This results in a characteristic inheritance pattern (Figure 3-2). Clinical conditions with

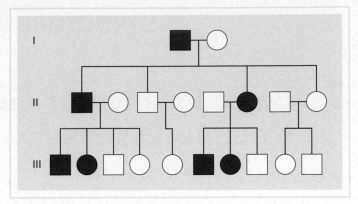

FIGURE 3-2 Pedigree chart showing the autosomal-dominant inheritance of a trait. Symbols indicate male (*squares*) and female (*circles*) individuals over three generations (horizontal rows I–III). Symbols representing affected individuals are filled.

autosomal-dominant inheritance patterns and significant pulmonary involvement include hereditary hemorrhagic telangiectasia type 1 (HHT1), familial idiopathic pulmonary fibrosis, and familial pulmonary arterial hypertension (FPAH).

Codominance

In contrast to simple dominance, codominant alleles do not mask one another, and heterozygous individuals express phenotypes associated with both codominant alleles. An important clinical condition with pulmonary involvement and elements of codominance is α_1-antitrypsin deficiency (A1AD), reviewed in the following text.

Autosomal Recessive

An allele is recessive when the phenotype associated with it is only expressed in homozygous individuals. Because recessive alleles are masked by dominant alleles, the traits associated with recessive alleles can skip generations, and the frequency of the carrier state is governed by the Hardy–Weinberg formula: $p^2 + 2pq + q^2 = 1$, where p and q are the frequencies of the two alleles (Figure 3-3). Cystic fibrosis, the most common

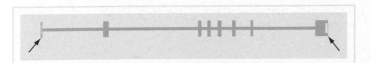

FIGURE 3-1 Structure of the human gene encoding pulmonary-associated surfactant protein D (SFTPD). This 11.3-mbp region of chromosome 10 encodes eight exons (*blue boxes*), including the 5′ and 3′ regulatory regions (*red arrows*), and seven intervening introns (*blue line*).

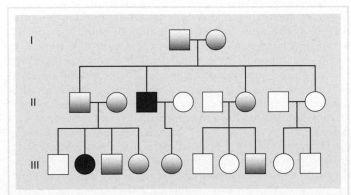

FIGURE 3-3 Pedigree chart showing the autosomal-recessive inheritance of a trait. Symbols indicate male (*squares*) and female (*circle*) individuals over three generations (horizontal rows I–III). Symbols representing affected individuals are filled, and unaffected carriers are shaded.

Genetic Penetrance

The penetrance of a trait is the degree to which the genetically determined phenotype is expressed in an individual. Complete penetrance indicates that all individuals possessing the associated genotype will exhibit the phenotype, whereas traits with incomplete or low penetrance will only be expressed in some fraction of individuals inheriting the genotype. The expression of a trait with incomplete penetrance may depend on other factors such as age, environment, or other inherited factors. Most genetic disorders exhibit incomplete penetrance.

Complex Genetic Disorders

In contrast to the single gene disorders discussed previously, complex genetic disorders are the result of interactions between multiple genes and environmental factors. As a result, complex genetic disorders cluster within a family but do not show a clear pattern of inheritance. This is manifest as a genetic predisposition to a lung disease, differentially expressed through lifestyle, occupational, and environmental factors. For example, not all persons exposed to significant levels of cigarette smoke have lung disease develop, and, indeed, most remain free of lung diseases as assessed by conventional pulmonary function testing. However, continuous smokers have a 25% absolute risk of chronic obstructive pulmonary disease (COPD) developing. Familial aggregation of COPD cases, as well as studies of adult monozygotic and dizygotic twins, establishes COPD as a prototypical gene by environment interaction.

One approach to discovering genes contributing to complex genetic disorders involves the analysis of genetic differences between cases (subjects who have been determined to have the disease) and controls (subjects matched for various factors who do not have nor are likely to develop the same disease). By carefully matching cases and controls, investigators have begun to uncover differences in genetic composition that predispose individuals to particular lung diseases. The most common studies used in this manner are genetic association studies that compare the distribution of genetic variation between cases and controls. Implicit within these studies is a strict rule that important genetic factors are carefully controlled. One of the most important factors is race, because genetic variation between races can overshadow genetic predisposition to diseases. Therefore, most complex genetic disorders are described in terms of "monoethnic" populations. Generalizing these discoveries to all individuals will require much larger studies.

One of the most common forms of DNA sequence variation in humans is single nucleotide polymorphisms (SNPs) (Figure 3-4). Although more than 99% of human DNA sequences are the same across the population, polymorphic loci are found approximately every 300 base pairs. For example, within the fifth exon of the human gene encoding glutathione S-transferase pi (GSTP1), approximately 80% of alleles bear the sequence ...AAATAC A TCTCCC... (the major allele), whereas 20% of alleles are ...AAATAC G TCTCCC... (the minor allele). Furthermore, a haplotype is a series of genetic variants on one chromosome that seem to be inherited from one parent with high frequency. In point of fact, SNPs that are located in close proximity are more likely to be inherited together, and thus seem to be linked. This

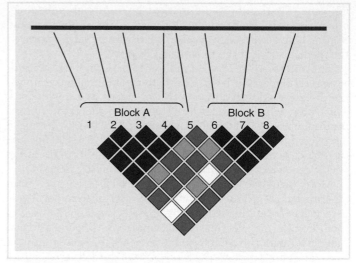

FIGURE 3-4 Linkage disequilibrium between SNP loci in close physical proximity. Eight consecutive loci are represented in this diagram, and the shade of the cell at the intersection of two columns indicates the degree of association between the two corresponding SNPs. Cells connecting loci within the two indicated blocks are darkly shaded, indicating that the inheritance of alleles at these loci is linked.

phenomenon is known as linkage disequilibrium (LD). Beyond the sequencing of the human genome, investigators have been working to resequence many genomes and characterize the genetic variation in populations. This project has been termed the HapMap Project. This project uses the blocklike structure of the genome to create a roadmap of genetic variations between individuals. Most of the common pulmonary diseases with genetic aspects are complex disorders, including asthma, COPD, lung cancer, and several forms of pulmonary fibrosis.

SUSPECTING GENETIC LUNG DISEASE

Diagnosis of genetic lung disease requires high clinical suspicion. Careful history taking, including a review of childhood illness and family history of disease, can provide clues to a genetic origin of disease. For example, key historical elements that should raise concern for cystic fibrosis include symptoms of recurrent cough, sputum production or respiratory tract infections (including otitis and sinusitis), symptoms present since childhood, disease presenting at age younger than expected, history of sterility in patient or family members, history of pancreatic insufficiency in patient or family members, or a history of idiopathic cirrhosis in the patient or in family members. Characteristics of disease presentation, such as distribution of disease, can also suggest genetic disease (e.g., basal rather than apical-predominant bullous emphysema should prompt consideration of α_1-antitrypsin deficiency).

Cystic Fibrosis

Cystic fibrosis (CF) is an autosomal-recessive chronic disease that affects the lungs and digestive system. Worldwide, approximately 70,000 individuals are affected with CF, making it the most common inherited pulmonary disease. Given a carrier rate in Caucasian populations of 1 in 20 persons, it is estimated that the United States has 7 million heterozygous carriers of the

CF gene. Cystic fibrosis is marked by recurrent pulmonary infections with eventual development of bronchiectasis and fibrotic lung disease. Advances in CF treatment have improved the median survival age to almost 37 years.

The autosomal-recessive inheritance pattern of cystic fibrosis was recognized in 1946. This pattern of inheritance implied the disease was caused by a defect of a gene at a single locus. This locus, which encodes a protein called the cystic fibrosis transmembrane conductance regulator (CFTR), was finally discovered on the long arm of chromosome 7 in 1989. Because the defect is autosomal recessive, defects in both copies of the CFTR gene are required to produce classic cystic fibrosis.

More than 800 mutations of the CFTR gene have been described that produce the cystic fibrosis phenotype. These defects have been divided into five broad classes on the basis of their impact on the final CFTR molecule (Figure 3-5 and Table 3-1) with the $\Delta F508$ mutation being the most common. The name of this mutation is descriptive of the defect: Δ signifies deletion, F signifies the amino acid phenylalanine, and 508 signifies the position of this amino acid in the normal CFTR protein product. The $\Delta F508$ mutation is responsible for two thirds of all CFTR mutations worldwide, but causes up to 90% of cystic fibrosis in persons of Northern European descent.

Although sweat testing remains the "gold standard," genetic testing can also be used to confirm the diagnosis of CF in suspected cases. The Cystic Fibrosis Foundation Consensus Statement published in 1998 included a new diagnostic criterion for cystic fibrosis: the identification of mutations known to cause CF in *both* CFTR genes in patients with a characteristic phenotype.

Testing is most commonly performed at central specialized laboratories. Blood samples or buccal swabs are collected and sent to the laboratory for DNA analysis and comparison with known mutations. Currently, testing can identify approximately 80 of the more than 700 known mutations that can cause CF, including the $\Delta F508$ mutation.

Identification of only one defective CFTR gene, although insufficient for diagnosis of CF, can prompt further testing. The allele that is "normal" by genetic testing may represent a mutation not included in the limited test panel. Further testing for cystic fibrosis, such as by nasal epithelial ion transport or further sweat testing, may be pursued.

Single allele defects in CFTR may predispose patients to diseases other than classic cystic fibrosis. These conditions, termed "CFTR-related diseases," include pulmonary conditions, such as asthma, allergic bronchopulmonary aspergillosis in asthmatics, and disseminated bronchiectasis. Other organ systems are affected by conditions associated with one CFTR mutation, including infertility caused by congenital bilateral absence of the vas deferens and chronic pancreatitis.

Alpha₁-Antitrypsin Deficiency

A small minority of cases of emphysema in the United States results from α_1-antitrypsin deficiency. This disorder is caused by an insufficient amount of the serpin peptidase inhibitor SERPINA1, commonly known as α_1-antitrypsin. Alpha₁-antitrypsin is critical in preserving lung structure because it inhibits many proteinases that can be released during inflammation and with exposure to cigarette smoke. The production of this protein is controlled by the Pi gene locus on the long arm of chromosome 14. The two alleles of Pi are expressed in a codominant fashion, each allele in a normal person contributing 50% of the total α_1-antitrypsin level. The normal allele is called the M allele based the electrophoretic mobility of its protein product. Most people are homozygous for the M allele (symbolized *PiMM*). Two other alleles have been described, the S allele and the Z allele. The S allele produces α_1-antitrypsin levels that are 60% of the normal M allele. Because of these relatively preserved proteinase levels, patients with one or both S alleles have adequate α_1-antitrypsin levels and do not have increased rates of pulmonary disease. The Z allele, however, results in abnormal α_1-antitrypsin with a single amino acid substitution that causes the protein to fold abnormally. The protein becomes trapped within hepatocytes where it is made. Persons homozygous for the Z allele (*PiZZ*) produce serum α_1-antitrypsin levels only 20% of those produced by those homozygous for the M allele. These patients have an accelerated rate of decline in lung function even in the absence of smoking.

The *PiZZ* phenotype is found in 1 in 1500 to 1 in 5000 births and is responsible for 1–10% of emphysema diagnosed in the United States. It is estimated that patients who have homozygous *PiZZ* α_1-antitrypsin deficiency have a 50–80% chance of clinically significant emphysema developing. Cigarette smoking produces emphysema in these patients at a younger age, typically in the third or fourth decade of life. Heterozygotes with one Z allele and one M allele (*PiMZ*) may show low or low-normal α_1-antitrypsin levels, but rarely have clinical disease. Patients with the *PiSZ* genotype may have emphysema, but it is generally milder than in *PiZZ* patients and only in those who smoke.

Alpha₁-antitrypsin deficiency is usually diagnosed by phenotypic analysis of the protein products themselves rather than by genetic testing. However, gene analysis by polymerase chain reaction (PCR) can be performed on dried blood spot specimens. The World Health Organization in 1997 advocated the use of protein-based screening for patients who have COPD and asthma, followed by genetic testing in those with abnormal screening results. Testing may also be considered in patients with a personal or family history of α_1-antitrypsin deficiency considering having children. Neonatal testing with heel stick blood sample analysis can also be considered in this context.

Infrequently, patients are seen with decreased levels of α_1-antitrypsin but lack the abnormal protein electrophoresis pattern seen with the Z or S alleles. Two classes of the alleles are responsible for this: M_{Duarte} and the "null allele" for α_1-antitrypsin. The protein product of the M_{Duarte} allele is electrophoretically indistinguishable from the M allele product; however, it is rapidly degraded within hepatocytes and, therefore, does not contribute to serum α_1-antitrypsin levels. A number of distinct null alleles exist. In each of these, a

TABLE 3-1	Classification of Genetic Mutations Causing Cystic Fibrosis	
Class	**Nature of defect**	**Effect on CFTR protein**
I	Defective protein synthesis	Absence of CFTR
II	Production of abnormal protein (includes $\Delta F508$)	CFTR unable to reach cell membrane
III	Disrupted activation and regulation	Decreased CFTR activity
IV	Altered chloride conductance	Decreased CFTR activity (mild disease)
V	Defective splicing	Decreased amount of protein (mild disease)

premature stop codon is present in a Pi exon. As a result, this allele contributes no α_1-antitrypsin at all. These diagnoses may be considered in patients with typical disease who have low α_1-AT level but a normal electrophoresis pattern. The diagnosis of α_1-antitrypsin deficiency caused by these genetic defects can be confirmed by genotyping by PCR.

Primary Pulmonary Hypertension

Idiopathic pulmonary arterial hypertension (IPAH, formerly known as primary pulmonary hypertension) is a rare, severe disease marked by a progressive increase in pulmonary vascular pressures without apparent cause. IPAH ultimately results in right heart failure if it is untreated and predominantly affects women of childbearing age. One to two persons per million are affected each year in the United States. IPAH progresses rapidly without therapy, with a mean survival of less than 3 years. Early therapy improves survival and quality of life, although treatment must be life long. IPAH usually occurs sporadically, but 6% of patients with IPAH have a family history of pulmonary hypertension. Familial pulmonary arterial hypertension (FPAH) is clinically indistinguishable from sporadic IPAH; however, genetic anticipation seems to occur in affected families, meaning that the disease occurs at a younger age in subsequent generations of affected family members.

Review of familial cases suggests that FPAH follows an autosomal-dominant transmission pattern with incomplete penetrance. More females seem to have the disease-associated allele, and more females than males have FPAH develop, but examples of direct father-to-son transmission rule out X-linkage. Affected members and carriers are more likely to have female children, suggesting the genetic defect of FPAH may play a role in fetal development and cause increased intrauterine loss of male offspring.

Linkage analysis has been performed to identify a responsible gene. This technique involves a review of known polymorphisms, or normal highly variable genes, in individuals and families affected by FPAH to detect patterns in genes that correlate with the presence of disease. This technique localized a potential gene to chromosome 2q. The specific gene was identified when mutations of the bone morphogenetic protein receptor type II (BMPR2) on chromosome 2q were shown to produce FPAH. Of patients with FPAH, newer investigation demonstrates that approximately 70% of patients demonstrate mutations, including exonic deletions or duplications. Studies of patients with sporadic IPAH suggest that *de novo* BMPR2 mutations may contribute to that condition. At least 26% of patients with IPAH had BMPR2 mutations, and none of more than 350 normal persons had a similar mutation. In some cases, when parental DNA is examined, these IPAH cases with mutations represent *de novo* mutations in the affected individual. Approximately 144 distinct mutations have been identified in 210 independent patients with FPAH. BMPR2 mutations are not detectable in 30% of patients with FPAH.

Despite the identification of a genetic defect responsible for many cases of FPAH and IPAH, the way in which this defect produces disease is not yet understood. BMPR2 is a receptor in the transforming growth factor (TGF)–ß family and is expressed in many human tissues. It acts as a receptor for growth factors known as bone morphogenetic proteins. These proteins are key growth factors in embryonic development (homozygous mutation of BMPR2 results in fetal loss), although their role in adults is poorly understood. Why mutation of such a ubiquitous receptor produces disease isolated to the pulmonary vasculature is unknown. Description of the functional effects of BMPR2 receptor mutations, such as effects of mutations on the amount or function of receptor produced, is vital to understanding this disease. The low penetrance of FPAH suggests that other genetic or environmental factors must be present in addition to the BMPR2 mutation to produce clinical disease.

The role for genetic testing in IPAH is uncertain. Although testing can identify some individuals who are at risk, heterozygous mutation does not predict disease development, because the disorder exhibits incomplete penetrance. In addition, most patients with IPAH and up to 50% with FPAH do not demonstrate BMPR2 mutations.

Hereditary Hemorrhagic Telangiectasia

Hereditary hemorrhagic telangiectasia, also known as Osler–Weber–Rendu, is a heritable systematic disorder marked by mucocutaneous telangiectasias with a predilection to develop arteriovenous malformations in many organs, including the lung, liver, and brain. The incidence of this disorder is as high as 1 per 10,000 persons. It follows an autosomal-dominant inheritance pattern with age-related penetrance (increase in clinical disease develops with advancing age). Mutations in two genes have been identified in families with hereditary hemorrhagic telangiectasia, activin receptor-like kinase (ALK)–1 on chromosome 12 and endoglin on chromosome 9. Both are proteins involved in TGF-ß superfamily receptor complexes, similar to the BMPR2 protein associated with primary pulmonary hypertension. Most cases involve a heterozygous mutation in one of these proteins, although a few reports of homozygous defects exist. This disease is believed to arise from these mutations because of TGF-ß effects on vasculogenesis, although the mechanisms by which this occurs are only speculative. Identification of the genes responsible for this disease is providing insight into pathogenesis and possibly future treatments. The disease is usually diagnosed by radiographic and physiologic testing, but genetic testing can provide information for families at risk. Because this disease can vary from asymptomatic minor telangiectasias to life-threatening arteriovenous malformations, genetic testing provides information only regarding relative risk, not severity of disease.

PHARMACOGENETICS

Pharmacogenetics is the study of how gene expression influences responses to medications. One of the best-studied examples of this phenomenon is response to ß$_2$-receptor agonist medications. These medications have therapeutic effects by means of cell surface receptors called ADRB2. Some individuals experience significant downregulation of these receptors after exposure to ß$_2$-receptor agonist therapy, leading to decreasing effect of subsequent doses of medication. The process of receptor downregulation resulting in decreased therapeutic effect is called desensitization or tachyphylaxis. Different genes that produce the ADRB2 receptor (polymorphisms) are associated with different degrees of receptor downregulation. Some polymorphisms show little downregulation; these patients experience very little desensitization in response to ß₂-receptor agonist therapy. Patients with higher degrees of desensitization may require less frequent dosing of medication to maintain adequate response. More studies are under way to better delineate which polymorphisms are present in populations and what effects they have on medication response. Pharmacogenetics may eventually play an important role in the management of many diseases, such as predicting response to therapy in lung cancer or interstitial lung disease guiding choices of medications or administration regiments.

TYPES OF GENETIC TESTS

Genetic testing is not synonymous with DNA testing. Many tests provide information about a patient's genotype, such as protein electrophoresis in patients with α_1-AT deficiency, without involving DNA analysis. DNA testing is also available and provides specific information regarding an individual's genetic code. DNA tests can be performed on many different samples, including buccal swabs or small samples of blood, such as from heel stick specimens in neonates.

The type of genetic test performed depends on the suspected diagnosis. DNA analysis by PCR is most commonly used for diseases in which the responsible gene and mutation are known. The PCR technique involves accurate amplification of small quantities of DNA, such as from a buccal swab. The DNA can then be compared with known mutations. One example of this type of testing is in CF, where DNA collected from a patient is compared with known mutations, such as ΔF508. The number of mutations that can be tested for is rapidly growing. Internet-based databases, such as Genetest (www.genetest.org), provide clinicians with searchable databases of available tests and laboratories that perform them.

Specialists in medical genetics can also test for suspected genetic diseases when neither the specific mutation nor the causative gene is known. This is done through linkage analysis. A thorough family history is performed to identify affected family members. Markers present on all genes are then used to determine which markers seem to travel with the disease in the affected family. DNA must be obtained from multiple family members to perform this testing. Linkage analysis allows medical geneticists to localize unknown genes to a specific region of one chromosome and identify other family members who may be affected.

Neonatal Screening of Cystic Fibrosis

Population-based genetic screening for CF is feasible because many of the mutations responsible for it have been identified. DNA microarray technology facilitates rapid screening for multiple mutations. Studies are ongoing to determine the long-term clinical benefits and social effects of such screening on patients and their families. Short-term analysis suggests that neonatal screening for CF may result in better nutrition and lung function. Despite this short-term evidence, the National Institutes of Health does not currently recommend routine neonatal screening of the general population for CF.

Neonatal screening in families with an increased likelihood of having children with CF is common. Between 50% and 90% of families at risk are considering or have had genetic testing. Of these families, 17–84% report they would terminate a pregnancy for a finding of CF.

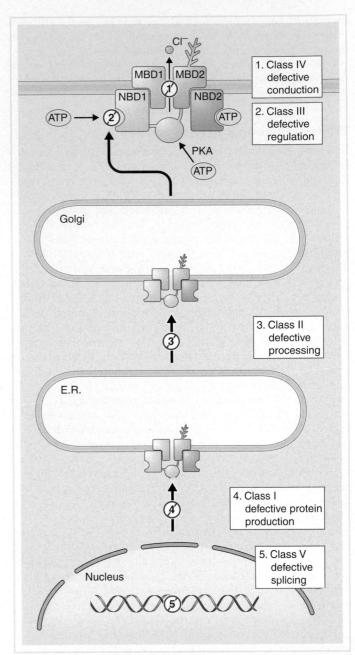

FIGURE 3-5 Functional consequences of the five different classes of CFTR mutant alleles in the airway epithelial cell. Adapted from Welsh MJ, Smith AE: Molecular mechanisms of CFTR chloride channel dysfunction in cystic fibrosis. Cell 1993; 73:1251–1254.

Genetic Testing in Other Pulmonary Diseases

Genetic testing in other pulmonary diseases generally relies on advanced technologies for genomic study. Because most of the common pulmonary genetic diseases are complex disorders, examination of SNPs and haplotypes has moved to the forefront in terms of defining genes that may have an association with particular diseases. The diseases included in this category include asthma, COPD, lung cancer, the acute respiratory distress syndrome/acute lung injury, and pulmonary fibrosis, to name but a few. Testing involves the analysis of, in general, very well-defined cases and controls. As previously mentioned, the phenotype (i.e., disease presence or absence and degree of discase severity) should be exquisitely well defined for these studies to have optimum power. Moreover, family-based association studies have the added benefit of examining common genetic elements within families and determining which distinct genetic elements are different between patients with disease and control patients. New technologies to assay up to 1 million simultaneous SNPs have been made commercially available. These technologies, based on microarrays, enable investigators to accurately access SNPs at nearly 1 million different loci within the human genome. With this great power has come complex and, as yet, unanswered questions on how to interpret the data. As with many high-throughput technologies, interpreting data with multiple testing is difficult. Several strategies, including the use of training and testing paradigms and independent validation cohorts are more generally accepted. Statistical analysis that uses correction for false discovery rates (FDR) is an agreed-on method to diminish the potential for false discovery occurring as a result of multiple testing. In more complex terms, analysis of individual SNPs, or haplotype blocks along chromosomes, have both been used in genetic determination of disease. There are inherent complexities with this approach, however, because SNPs that may be very close in physical distance to one another may reside in different haplotype blocks. Until computational analysis of high-throughput SNP arrays can be matched with the complexity of the HapMap Project, analysis will remain a difficult issue. Nonetheless, the promise of more rapidly unraveling genetic contributions to complex lung diseases will certainly be expedited through the use of these extraordinary technologies.

ETHICAL CONSIDERATIONS

Because genetic testing has many implications to patients and their family members, genetic counseling should precede most testing. Positive tests can affect reproductive decisions, patients' ability to get insurance or employment, and patient confidentiality, because family members may require testing as well. Consultation of a medical geneticist may be appropriate to assist with informed consent, interpretation of test results, and family and reproductive counseling. Genetic testing usually requires specialized laboratories. Because current understanding of the role of specific genes in disease is expanding, practitioners should stay informed of new testing available.

SUGGESTED READINGS

Cookson WO: State of the art. Genetics and genomics of chronic obstructive pulmonary disease. Proc Am Thorac Soc 2006; 3:473–475.

Cutting GR: Modifier genetics: cystic fibrosis. Annu Rev Genomics Hum Genet 2005; 6:237–260.

Garcia JG, ed: Virtual symposium: Making genomics functional in lung disease. Proc Am Thorac Soc 2007; 4:3–132.

Jorde LB, Carey JC, Bamshad MJ, White RL: Medical Genetics, 3rd ed, St. Louis: Mosby/Elsevier; 2005.

Knowles MR: Gene modifiers of lung disease. Curr Opin Pulm Med 2006; 12:416–421.

Manolio TA, Bailey-Wilson JE, Collins FS: Genes, environment and the value of prospective cohort studies. Nat Rev Genet 2006; 7:812–820.

Newman JH, Trembath RC, Morse JA, et al: Genetic basis of pulmonary arterial hypertension: current understanding and future directions. J Am Coll Cardiol 2004; 43:33S–39S.

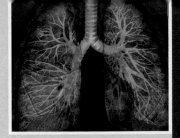

4 Respiratory Mechanics

BRUCE H. CULVER

INTRODUCTION

This chapter describes the physical properties of the lungs and chest wall involved in the cyclical processes of ventilation supporting the metabolic needs of the body. The respiratory muscles are introduced, but their function is more fully described in Chapter 8. Clinical measurements of some of these mechanical properties are an important part of pulmonary function testing at rest and with exercise as discussed in Chapter 10.

STRUCTURE OF THE THORAX AND LUNGS

Thorax

The bony thorax protects the lungs, heart, and great vessels but also allows the lungs to change volume from a minimum of 1.5–2.0 L to a maximum of 6–8 L. This large expansion is made possible by the articulation of the ribs with the spine and the sternum, the arrangement of the muscles, and the motion of the diaphragm. The ribs articulate with the transverse processes of the thoracic vertebrae and have flexible cartilaginous connections with the sternum. The ribs angle down, both from back to front and from midline to side, so that as they elevate, both the anteroposterior and the transverse dimensions of the thorax increase (Figure 4-1). The external intercostal muscles that angle down from posterior to anterior (Figure 4-2) are well situated to elevate the ribs. With deep inspiratory efforts, the first and second ribs are elevated and stabilized by the accessory muscles of respiration in the neck. If the upper extremities are fixed, the pectoralis muscles can also act to raise the ribs (e.g., holding onto a chair back or leaning against a wall when out of breath). Expiration is normally passive, driven by the elastic recoil of the lung, but can be assisted by the internal intercostal muscles. Forced expiration (or coughing) requires the abdominal muscles to force the diaphragm upward.

The diaphragm is dome shaped in its relaxed position and can be pulled flatter by muscle contraction. The diaphragm is most often described as fixed at the periphery so that its action pulls down the center of the dome, lengthening the lungs. However, if it is fixed centrally by the pressure of the abdominal contents, the peripheral attachments will lift the ribs, which swing outward when elevated, increasing the transverse diameter of the chest. In addition, the increase in abdominal pressure associated with descent of the diaphragm acts on the lower ribs in the "zone of apposition" to impart an outward force. The actual action of the diaphragm is a combination of these mechanisms in a proportion that varies with position and abdominal wall tension.

The intercostal muscles are innervated from the thoracic spine at their own level, and the abdominal muscles are innervated from lower thoracic and lumbar level, but the diaphragm is served by the phrenic nerves that originate at the cervical level (C3–C5). Thus, the diaphragm remains functional in patients who have spinal injuries below the midcervical level. The long course of each phrenic nerve along the mediastinum, however, makes it vulnerable to both transient and permanent interruptions by disease, injury, or surgery. Occasionally, local irritation of a phrenic nerve leads to intractable singultus (i.e., hiccups.) The respiratory muscles are more fully discussed in Chapter 8.

Pleural Space

The lungs are covered by a thin visceral pleura, which is invaginated into the lobar fissures. The inner aspect of each hemithorax, including the top of the diaphragm and the mediastinal surface, is lined with the parietal pleura, which joins the visceral pleura on each side at the lung hilum. The pleural space extends deeply into the posterior and lateral costophrenic recesses and is a potential space, normally containing only a few milliliters of fluid to serve a lubricating function.

The inspiratory force of the chest wall and diaphragm is transmitted to the lung by creation of a more negative pressure in this potential space. In pathologic states, pleural effusions may form and necessarily make the lung volume smaller by occupying part of the intrathoracic space. Penetration of the chest wall or rupture of the lung surface can allow air to enter the pleural space and create a pneumothorax.

The Airways

The upper respiratory passages (nasal cavities and pharynx) conduct, warm, and moisten air as it moves into the lungs. The respiratory system develops as an offshoot from the digestive system and, like the digestive system, has an absorptive function. The entire system is continuously exposed to particulate and infective agents and, accordingly, is protected by a well-developed lymphoid barrier and, more superficially, a mucous barrier. The upper respiratory passages contain the olfactory areas and also conduct and help shape the sounds that produce speech.

The larynx opens off the lowest part of the pharynx. During swallowing, the larynx is closed off from both the pharynx above and the esophagus posteriorly by the epiglottis. The trachea begins at the lower border of the cricoid cartilage of the larynx, at the level of the sixth cervical vertebra. The lumen of the trachea is held open by incomplete, C-shaped cartilaginous rings. The posterior membranous portion contains smooth muscle. When the intrathoracic pressure exceeds the intraluminal pressure, the membranous portion becomes invaginated, the ends of the rings may overlap, and the lumen is greatly narrowed. Smooth muscle contraction narrows the lumen, but

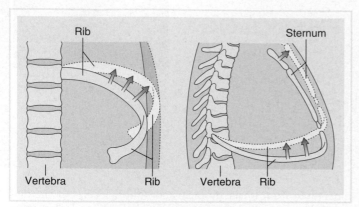

FIGURE 4-1 Frontal and lateral views of thorax movement. With rib elevation, both the transverse and anteroposterior dimensions increase.

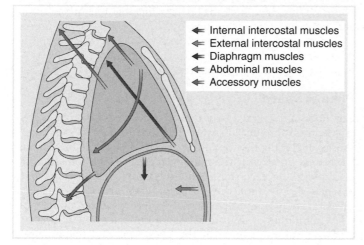

← Internal intercostal muscles
← External intercostal muscles
► Diaphragm muscles
◄ Abdominal muscles
← Accessory muscles

FIGURE 4-2 Action of the major respiratory muscle groups (intercostals, accessories, diaphragm, and abdominal).

increases its rigidity. With deep inspiration, the trachea enlarges and lengthens. The trachea bifurcates into the main bronchi, which in turn become lobar, segmental, then subsegmental bronchi, and end in bronchioles that lack cartilage and are approximately 1 mm in diameter. Beyond these are the respiratory bronchioles, alveolar ducts, sacs, and alveoli that make up the respiratory zone in which gas exchange and other functions take place.

The intraparenchymal bronchi are invested with overlapping helical bands of smooth muscle wound in clockwise and counterclockwise fashion. The amount of smooth muscle increases proportionately in the smaller bronchioles to occupy approximately 20% of the wall thickness. Elastic fibers are present at every level of the respiratory system and become a rich component of the connective tissue in the smaller bronchi and bronchioles. They stretch when the lungs are expanded in inspiration, and their recoil helps to return the lungs to their end-exhalation volume. Although the smooth muscle stops at the portals of the respiratory zone, elastic and collagen fibers contribute to the alveolar wall and form an irregular, wide-meshed net of delicate interlacing fibers.

The number of airway generations required to reach the respiratory zone varies with pathway length, so that areas near the hilum may be reached in 15 generations, whereas those in the periphery may require 25 generations. Although the size of individual airways becomes smaller, the number of airways

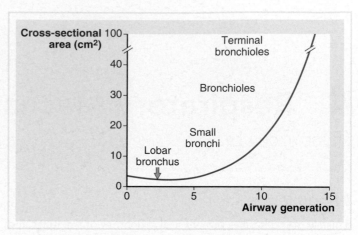

FIGURE 4-3 Total cross-sectional area of the airways. The aggregate luminal area increases greatly from approximately 2.5 cm² in the trachea and major airways to more than 100 cm² at the level of the terminal bronchioles. (Modified with permission from Culver BH, ed: The respiratory system. Seattle: University of Washington Publication Services; 2006, data from Weibel ER. Morphometry of the human lung. Berlin and New York: Springer-Verlag; 1963.)

approximately doubles with each new generation, so that the total cross-sectional area of the combined air path increases. This is especially so in the smaller bronchi and bronchioles, where the "daughters" of each division are only slightly smaller than the "parent." The rapidly increasing total cross-sectional area of small airways, shown diagrammatically in Figure 4-3, means that their contribution to airflow resistance in the lungs is small. Thus, diseases that affect these peripheral airways may be functionally "silent" until an advanced state.

Interdependence in the Lung

Because the lung parenchyma is made up of interconnected alveolar walls, interstitial tissues, and fibers, any local distortion is opposed by the surrounding tissue. That is, if a small zone of alveoli within a lobe begins to collapse, the surrounding tissue is stretched and thus tends to pull the alveoli back open. This property is termed structural interdependence. It, along with surfactant and the presence of collateral air pathways, helps to prevent alveolar collapse even when small bronchioles become plugged. When collapsed areas of lung cannot expand despite distention of the surrounding alveoli, lung injury may develop as a result of extremely large stretching forces that are generated at the interface. Because the bronchi and blood vessels travel through, and have attachments to, the lung parenchyma, they too are affected by the surrounding tissue. As the lung expands, the caliber of these channels also increases, and at low lung volume airway closure may occur.

RESPIRATORY MECHANICS

The properties of the lung and chest that affect and effect the movement of air in and out of the lungs are central to understanding both normal and abnormal lung function.

Lung Volumes

The total gas-containing capacity of the lungs can be divided into a series of volumes, as shown in Figure 4-4, which, in combination, give lung capacities. The largest amount of air that can be held in the lungs at full inspiration is the total lung capacity (TLC). After a complete forced exhalation, the lungs

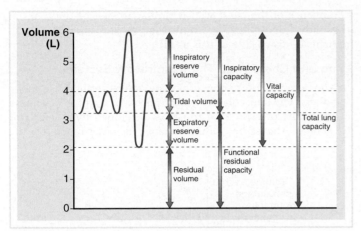

FIGURE 4-4 The normal spirogram and subdivisions of lung volume. By convention, "volume" is used to describe the smallest subdivisions that do not overlap (residual volume, expiratory reserve volume, tidal volume, and inspiratory reserve volume), and "capacity" is used to describe combinations of these volumes (functional residual capacity, inspiratory capacity, vital capacity, and total lung capacity). (From Pulmonary terms and symbols: A report of the ACCP-ATS Joint Committee on Pulmonary Nomenclature. Chest 1975;67:583–593.)

are not empty but contain a residual volume (RV). The difference between TLC and RV, that is, the greatest volume of air that can be inhaled or exhaled, is the vital capacity (VC). The vital capacity can be affected by factors that either limit expansion of the lung (restrictive processes) or limit lung emptying (airflow obstruction).

A normal breath has a tidal volume (V_T) that is only a small portion of the vital capacity (approximately 10%), and even during strenuous exercise, V_T increases to only 50–60% of VC. Increases in V_T occur by the use of parts of the inspiratory

reserve and expiratory reserve volumes as shown in Figure 4-4. At the end of a relaxed tidal exhalation, the lungs return to a resting volume, which is normally approximately 50% of TLC. The volume contained in the lungs at this end-tidal position is the functional residual capacity (FRC), and the volume that can be inhaled from this point is the inspiratory capacity (IC).

The Lung–Chest Wall System

To understand the process of normal breathing, special maneuvers such as coughing and the effects of positive pressure ventilators requires knowledge of the mechanical properties of the thorax. Three primary forces are involved:

1. Elastic recoil properties of the lung
2. Elastic recoil properties of the chest wall
3. Muscular efforts of chest wall, diaphragm, and abdomen

In combination, these result in changes in lung (and thorax) volume, in alveolar pressure, and in intrapleural pressure.

Volumes of Elastic Structures

The recoil tendency of a spring can be expressed in terms of its unstressed or resting length and its length–tension relationship. Similarly, for expandable volumetric structures, the relevant properties are the unstressed volume and the relationship between volume and the transmural pressure required to achieve that volume (Figure 4-5). By convention, transmural pressures are expressed as the difference between the pressure inside and the pressure outside the structure (P_{IN}–P_{OUT}). It is convenient to think of this as the "distending pressure" required to achieve a certain volume. In addition, this distending pressure also represents the "recoil pressure," or the tendency of the structure to return to its unstressed volume (where transmural pressure is zero). A positive recoil pressure indicates a tendency to become smaller. A structure distorted to a volume below its unstressed volume has a negative recoil pressure, which indicates its tendency to become larger.

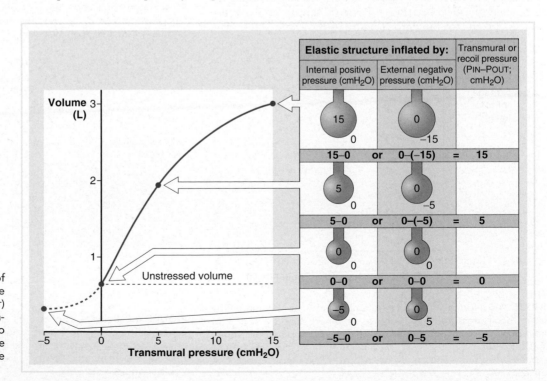

FIGURE 4-5 Elastic recoil of an expandable structure. The transmural pressure (P_{IN}–P_{OUT}) associated with each volume indicates the tendency to return to the unstressed volume. Positive pressure and negative pressure inflation are equivalent.

Elastic Properties of the Lung

The lungs are elastic structures with a tendency to recoil to a small "unstressed volume" (usually slightly less than RV). To maintain any lung volume larger than this unstressed volume requires a force that distends the lungs; this force is the difference between the alveolar pressure (PA) and the pressure surrounding the lungs, the intrapleural pressure (PPL). The elastic properties of the lungs and their tendency to recoil are represented by a plot of the relationship between lung volume and transmural pressure (Figure 4-6). Such graphs apply to an excised lung being inflated by a pump, an *in vivo* lung inflated by a ventilator, or the more physiologic normal lung inflated by expanding the chest (to create a more negative pleural pressure). In each case, the curve of volume versus the transpulmonary pressure difference (PA – PPL) is the same.

The slope of this pressure–volume curve represents the compliance of the lungs (CL), as represented by Equation 4.1.

$$C_L = \Delta V / \Delta P \qquad (4.1)$$

The CL decreases as the lungs near the limit of their distensibility at TLC. Usually, CL is measured just above FRC in the tidal breathing range. Because it is normally expressed in absolute volume units (e.g., L/cmH$_2$O), CL is strongly dependent on the lung size. A single lung, for example, only has 50% of the volume change for the same pressure change as two lungs. A small child's normal CL is considerably lower than that of an adult's. For this reason, CL is often divided by lung volume to give the volume-independent "specific compliance."

Elastic Properties of the Chest Wall

The chest wall has elastic properties that can be expressed in the same way as those of the lung (Figure 4-7). The chest wall differs from many common elastic structures in that its unstressed volume (where recoil pressure = 0) is normally quite high. When expanded above its unstressed volume, it recoils inward, but if the chest wall is "distorted" to a smaller volume, its tendency is to recoil outward. Recoil pressure for the relaxed chest wall is PPL – PATM or simply PPL, because PATM is taken to be zero (Figure 4-8; Table 4-1). The

compliance of the chest wall is similar to that of the lungs in the midvolume range, but note that at TLC, the chest wall remains as distensible as it is at FRC.

Lung and Chest Wall: The Respiratory System

In the intact thorax, the lungs and chest wall must move together. The muscular effort required to inspire a volume of air or the pressure that must be developed by a ventilator to achieve the same volume change is determined by the

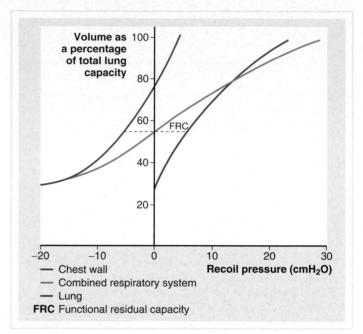

FIGURE 4-7 Pressure–volume curves of the combined thoracic system. The relaxed chest wall has a relatively high unstressed volume. The recoil of the combined respiratory system is the sum of the recoil of the chest wall plus lung. (Modified with permission from Culver BH, ed: The respiratory system. Seattle: University of Washington Publication Services; 2006. Data from Rahn H, Otis AB, Chadwich LE, Fenn WO: The pressure–volume diagram of the thorax and lung. Am J Physiol. 1946;146:161–178.)

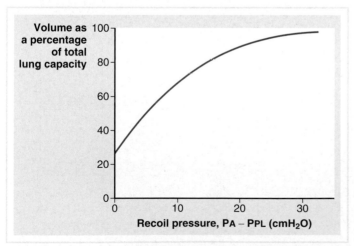

FIGURE 4-6 Normal "pressure–volume" curve of the lung. The elastic recoil pressure of the lung as obtained during a very slow expiration from total lung capacity (the curve on inspiration is somewhat different). (Modified with permission from Culver BH, ed: The respiratory system. Seattle: University of Washington Publication Services; 2006.)

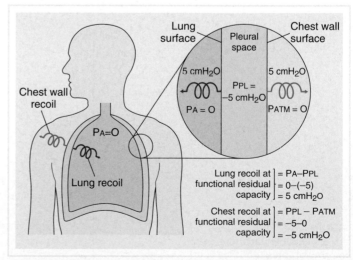

FIGURE 4-8 Balance of pressures and forces at functional residual capacity. The opposing recoils of lung and chest wall create a negative intrapleural pressure. (Modified with permission from Culver BH, ed: The respiratory system. Seattle: University of Washington Publication Services; 2006.)

TABLE 4-1	Recoil Pressures of the Lungs, Chest Wall, and Respiratory System, Measured as the Transmural Pressure Difference (Inside – Outside)	
Transmural Pressure	**Pressure Inside – Pressure Outside**
Lungs	Alveolar pressure (P_A) – pleural pressure (P_{PL})
Chest wall	P_{PL} – atmospheric pressure (P_{ATM}), or simply P_{PL}
Respiratory system	$(P_A - P_{PL}) + (P_{PL} - P_{ATM}) = P_A - P_{ATM}$

pressure–volume curve of the combined respiratory system, shown by the red line in Figure 4-7. The lungs and chest wall normally contain the same volume of air, so that only points at the same horizontal level in Figure 4-7 can coexist. Because both the lungs and the chest wall are expanded together, the distending pressure for the respiratory system is the sum of the distending pressures required by the lungs and chest wall. The transmural pressure for the respiratory system is $P_A - P_{ATM}$ (see Table 4-1). Figure 4-7 shows that a greater pressure change is required to add volume to the respiratory system than to either of its components alone, and thus the compliance of the respiratory system is lower than that of either lungs or chest wall at the same volume. This may at first seem paradoxical, because the tendency of the chest wall to expand might be thought to help lung expansion; however, as the system volume is increased, the outward recoil of the chest wall decreases, and this force must be replaced by additional work.

The third mechanical factor, muscle force, is not considered in Figure 4-7. Thus, the pressure difference across the lung, which has no muscle, can always be taken from its curve, but the pressure across the chest wall (and diaphragm) may reflect muscle tension and is only described by this curve during complete relaxation. Similarly, the curve for the respiratory system shows the pressure that would be measured by a manometer held tightly in the mouth after a subject has inhaled or exhaled to a particular volume and then relaxed all muscle effort.

At the resting end-tidal position of the respiratory system (FRC), no active muscular forces are applied and $P_A = P_{ATM}$ (distending pressure = 0). The lung is distended above its low unstressed volume, and the chest wall is held below its relatively high unstressed volume. The relaxed FRC is the volume at which the opposing tendencies of the lungs to recoil inward and the chest wall to recoil outward are evenly balanced. Any change in the unstressed volume or the compliance of either lungs or chest wall results in a new FRC. For example, obesity reduces the unstressed volume of the chest wall and thus reduces the FRC (and expiratory reserve volume; see Chapter 74). Emphysema increases both compliance and unstressed volume of the lung, which results in a higher FRC and a "shift to the left" of the respiratory system pressure–volume curve.

The opposing forces of lung and chest wall create a subatmospheric (negative) pressure in the intrapleural space at the FRC (see Figure 4-8). Because the lungs and chest wall are not directly linked, it is actually the intrapleural pressure that opposes lung recoil and chest wall recoil. Thus, at a relaxed FRC, it must have the same magnitude as each of these recoil forces. The average pleural pressure is normally approximately $-5\ cmH_2O$ at FRC.

Events of the Respiratory Cycle

Inspiration is an active process. Contraction of the inspiratory muscles (primarily the intercostals and the diaphragm) tends to expand the thorax, which creates a more negative intrapleural pressure. This increases the distending pressure applied to the lung, and the subsequent expansion causes the alveolar pressure to become negative with respect to the atmosphere, drawing air into the lungs. This process continues until the lung volume increases to a point where its recoil pressure is increased to balance the combined muscular and elastic forces of the chest wall. At this point, alveolar pressure becomes zero, and the inspiratory flow stops, because a pressure gradient no longer exists along the airways.

During normal breathing, expiration is a passive process. The inspiratory muscles relax, and the balance of forces shifts so that lung recoil predominates. The alveolar pressure becomes positive, and the air moves from alveoli through the airways to the outside atmosphere until FRC conditions are reached, with the forces again balanced and the alveolar pressure zero. Note that with a typical small V_T, the chest wall remains below its unstressed volume, with a small outward recoil force, and pleural pressure can be negative throughout the cycle. During active expiration, this process can be assisted by contraction of the expiratory muscles (intercostal and abdominal wall muscles), which makes pleural pressure positive.

Respiratory Muscle Effort

The maximum inspiratory and expiratory pressures measure the maximal efforts of the respiratory muscles (Figure 4-9). That is, if one were to try to inhale against a closed pressure manometer, the negative pressure that can be generated at the mouth is approximately $100\ cmH_2O$ at a low lung volume. At TLC, no negative pressure can be generated, and thus no more air can be drawn into the chest. Maximum expiratory pressures are somewhat greater, $150–200\ cmH_2O$ at high lung volume, and fall to 0 at RV.

Surface Tension

At the surface of a liquid, the intramolecular forces are not balanced by the more widely spaced molecules of the gas phase, which creates a surface tension. The surface tension of the air–liquid interface that lines the alveoli contributes an important part of the elastic properties of the lung shown by the pressure–volume curve. If a lung is filled with liquid,

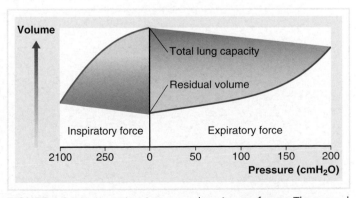

FIGURE 4-9 Maximum inspiratory and expiratory forces. The normal maximum force generated by inspiratory muscles is greatest at low lung volume, and the expiratory force is greatest at high lung volume. (Modified with permission from Culver BH, ed: The respiratory system. Seattle: University of Washington Publication Services; 2006.)

surface forces are abolished, and the resultant pressure–volume curve (Figure 4-10) reflects only the tissue properties of the lung. This liquid-filled curve is shifted to the left, indicating that the lung can be distended with much less pressure. The air-filled lung, in addition to requiring greater pressures, demonstrates marked hysteresis; that is, the pressure–volume curve during inflation is different from that during deflation.

The air-filled deflation curve approaches the liquid-filled curve at low lung volume, indicating that the pressure from surface tension becomes small at this volume. Given no other parameters, however, the prediction would be that pressure from surface forces should *increase* as alveoli become smaller. Laplace's law relates the pressure within a sphere to wall tension (T) and radius (r), P = 2T/r, whereas for a cylinder P = T/r.

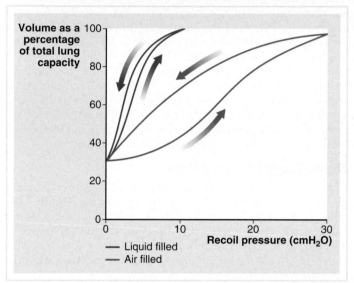

FIGURE 4-10 Effect of surface tension on recoil force. Pressure–volume curves obtained on inflation and deflation of a normal air-filled lung and the same lung when filled with saline. The horizontal difference between the curves reflects the effect of surface tension, which is greater on inspiration than expiration and abolished when the lung is liquid filled. (Modified with permission from Culver BH, ed: The respiratory system. Seattle: University of Washington Publication Services; 2006. Data from Bachofen H, Hildebrandt J, Bachofen M: Pressure–volume curves of air- and liquid-filled excised lungs—Surface tension in situ. J Appl Physiol. 1970; 29:422–431.)

If the surface tension remains constant as "r" decreases (smaller alveoli or airway), the pressure from the surface tension should rise. This situation is avoided in the lung by the presence of a unique surface-lining material, surfactant, that not only reduces surface tension but does so in a volume-dependent manner. As lung volume and surface area decrease, the lining layer compresses, and surface tension decreases until it is nearly abolished at RV. This property has important consequences in the lung including the following:

- The work needed to expand the lungs is greatly reduced.
- Stability of alveoli and terminal airways is maintained. (If pressure increased within an alveolus as it became smaller, the alveolus would tend to empty into interconnected, larger alveoli with lower pressure.)
- Inwardly directed forces of surface tension in the "corners" of alveoli act to draw fluid from the capillaries and interstitium into the alveoli, so lowering surface tension helps prevent alveolar edema (discussed in Chapter 6).

Pulmonary surfactant is produced in alveolar type II cells in the form of lamellar bodies, appears in the alveolar lining liquid as tubular myelin, then spreads as a monolayer at the air–liquid interface. The major component, and the component that is primarily responsible for the surface tension–lowering effects, is dipalmitoyl phosphatidylcholine (DPPC). DPPC has a nonpolar end made up of two saturated fatty acid chains and a polar end that tends to have a positive charge. At the air–liquid interface, the molecules orient with the hydrophilic polar end in the liquid and the fatty acid chains project into the air (Figure 4-11). Both ends have similar cross-sectional area allowing them to pack closely together. The molecules may also adsorb directly to the epithelial surface, which tends to have a negative charge, in areas where a liquid subphase is absent.

Flow Resistance

Airflow between the atmosphere and alveolar gas depends on the driving pressure (i.e., alveolar–atmospheric) and the airway resistance, as shown in Equation 4.2.

$$\text{Flow} = \dot{V} = \Delta P/R = (P_A - P_{ATM})/R_{AW} \qquad (4.2)$$

The normal airway resistance (R_{AW}) during quiet breathing (or a panting maneuver, as it is usually clinically measured) is less than 2 cmH$_2$O/L/sec. Airflow resistance is affected by:

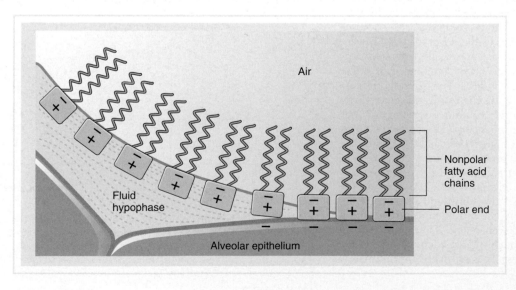

FIGURE 4-11 Pulmonary surfactant at the air–liquid interface in an alveolus. The nonpolar fatty acid chains project into the alveolar gas phase, whereas the hydrophilic polar end lies within the surface of the liquid phase or may be able to bond directly to the epithelium. The close arrangement of the molecules facilitates their surface tension–lowering properties. The fluid hypophase tends to fill alveolar corners and surface irregularities.

- Viscosity of air
- Length of airways (R_{AW} is directly proportional to length)
- Caliber of airways (R_{AW} is proportional to $1/r^4$)

Thus, a doubling of length doubles resistance, but a halving of caliber causes a 16-fold increase in resistance. Factors affecting airway caliber include:

- Position of the airway in the bronchial tree
- Lung volume
- Bronchial muscle tone
- Mucous secretion
- Pressure across the airway wall

All these factors are similar during both inspiration and expiration, except the last. During inspiration, the intrathoracic pressure that surrounds the airways is more negative than the intraairway pressure, so airways tend to be distended (Figure 4-12). During passive exhalation, the magnitude of the airway distending force is lower, and thus airflow resistance is somewhat higher. With active expiratory efforts, the pleural pressure becomes positive and, with the addition of lung recoil, the pressure in the alveoli is even higher. However, the intraluminal pressure decreases progressively in airways mouthward of the alveoli, reflecting both frictional losses and a decrease in lateral pressure through the Bernoulli effect as the decreasing cross-sectional area of the composite airway requires a marked increase in velocity of air movement (convective acceleration). Because their cartilaginous structure is incomplete, airways are compressed under such forces, and calculated resistance is much higher.

Maximum airflow rates are evaluated by having the subject take a full inspiration to TLC and blow the air out as forcefully and completely (to RV) as possible. By use of a spirometer, this forced vital capacity (FVC) is recorded as an expiratory spirogram (volume vs time) or, if the flow rate is directly measured, the same information can be recorded as a maximum expiratory flow versus volume curve (Figure 4-13). A remarkable feature of this maneuver is that the maximum flow rate for any volume, except the higher lung volumes near the beginning of the exhalation, is achieved with submaximal effort and cannot be exceeded with further effort. This flow limitation or "effort independence" is demonstrated in Figure 4-14 and is a consequence of the dynamic compression noted previously. The mechanism of this flow limitation is related to the rate of propagation of a pressure wave through a compliant tube, but the result can be understood with a simpler conceptual model of dynamic compression. Because this compression begins just beyond the point where intraairway pressure falls to equal pleural pressure, the effective pressure driving flow from the alveoli to this point becomes P_A–P_{PL} [(30 – 20) = 10 cmH$_2$O in Figure 4-13, forced expiration]. This is the same as the elastic recoil pressure of the lung and is a function of lung volume, not effort. If, in the example of Figure 4-13, a greater expiratory effort is made and the pleural pressure is raised to 40 cmH$_2$O at the same lung volume, the alveolar pressure becomes 50 cmH$_2$O and the effective driving pressure = (50 – 40) = 10 cmH$_2$O, so the resultant flow rate remains unchanged.

This mechanism may have its major physiologic significance in normal individuals during a cough. Although overall airflow rate (L/sec) out of the lungs is not increased by the high pleural pressure generated, the airflow velocity (m/sec) through the narrowed major airways is greatly increased, which aids the removal of secretions and foreign material.

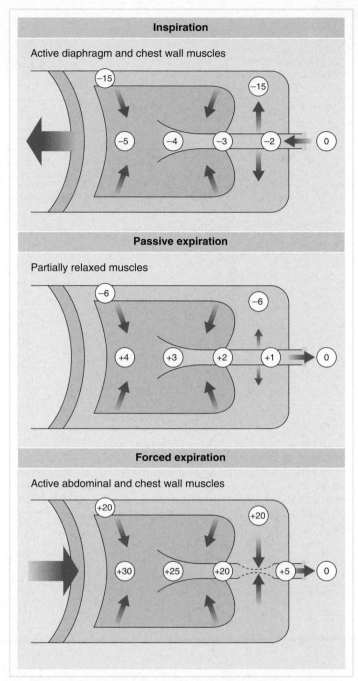

FIGURE 4-12 Dynamic compression. Comparison of intrathoracic and intraluminal pressures during inspiration, passive expiration, and forced expiration. In each case, the lung volume is the same, with a recoil pressure of 10 cmH$_2$O. During inspiration, the intrathoracic airways tend to be distended, which lowers airway resistance. In passive expiration, although intrapleural pressure may remain slightly negative, a positive alveolar pressure is generated by lung elastic recoil. Central airways are less distended than during inspiration. In forced expiration, high intrapleural pressure, plus lung recoil, creates a large, positive alveolar pressure to drive flow but also compresses central airways. Flow is limited once dynamic compression begins downstream from the point where intraluminal pressure falls below pleural pressure (equal pressure point). Further effort increases alveolar driving pressure but also increases compression. Airway resistance becomes high and varies with the degree of effort.

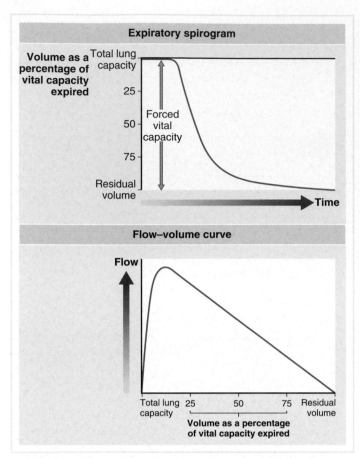

FIGURE 4-13 Forced vital capacity maneuver. This common breathing test can be displayed as an expiratory spirogram or as a flow–volume curve. Volume axes show percentage of vital capacity expired. (Modified with permission from Culver BH, ed: The respiratory system. Seattle: University of Washington Publication Services; 2006.)

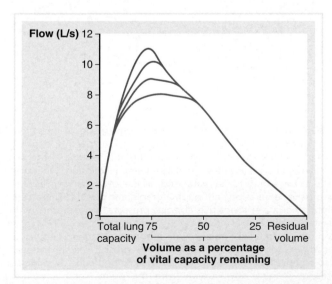

FIGURE 4-14 Effort-independent flow. The top curve represents a maximum expiratory effort, and the lower curves show the flow that results from progressively less effort. At lower lung volumes, the maximum flow rate is relatively independent of effort. (Modified with permission from Bates DV, Macklem PT, Christie RV: Respiratory function in disease, 2nd ed. Philadelphia: WB Saunders; 1971:10–95.)

Work of Breathing

The muscle effort required to raise lung volume above the FRC during inspiration is a form of work. Part of this is the elastic work used to stretch the tissues and the surface lining of the lung, whereas another part is the frictional work required to overcome airflow resistance in the airways. The elastic work stored in stretched fibers on inspiration then provides the energy needed to push air out on the subsequent passive exhalation. With active expiratory efforts, additional muscle work is done on expiration as well.

The elastic and frictional components of respiratory work are affected differently by lung volume. At low lung volume, airways are narrower, and resistance (and thus frictional work) increases rapidly (R is proportional to $1/r^4$). At higher lung volumes, the airways are larger, but muscles must do more elastic work to keep the lungs stretched. The relaxed FRC is the volume at which the static recoil forces of the lung and chest wall are balanced, but Figure 4-15 shows that FRC is also the volume at which work of breathing is least. If either the elastic or frictional contributions to work of breathing change, FRC may change rapidly or chronically.

The narrowed airways in obstructive disease increase frictional work and the volume at which work is the least increases. The accompanying shift of the tidal breathing range to a higher volume may occur quite suddenly in an asthma attack or may develop slowly with chronic obstructive disease. When airflow rates increase, frictional work becomes relatively more important, so that patients who have obstructive disease may shift to a higher end-expiratory volume during exercise or voluntary hyperventilation.

Restrictive disease processes reduce lung compliance (C_L). Accordingly, the force the muscles must generate to stretch the lung increases. The elastic work required to breathe at any lung volume is higher, and this shifts the volume for least work lower. Increased C_L, as with emphysema, has the opposite effect. Figure 4-7 shows that the static forces predict the same changes in FRC (greater lung recoil results in lower FRC volume and vice versa).

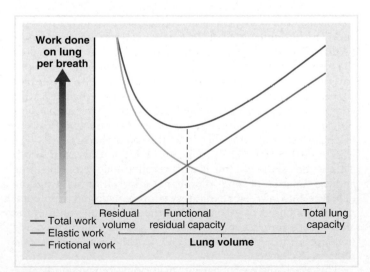

FIGURE 4-15 Work of breathing. The combined work of lung and chest wall expansion (elastic) and airflow resistance (frictional) is normally lowest near functional residual capacity. (Modified with permission from Culver BH, ed: The respiratory system. Seattle: University of Washington Publication Services; 2006.)

Normally, the energy consumed by breathing is very small. In metabolic terms it requires less than 1 mL/min of oxygen consumption for each liter per minute of ventilation, or only a few percent of a person's total body oxygen consumption at rest. With severe airway obstruction, the energy cost of breathing becomes much higher (as much as 30% during an acute exacerbation).

Distribution of Ventilation

The incoming air of each tidal breath is not distributed evenly to all alveoli in the lung. Pleural pressure is not the same throughout the chest but has a vertical gradient of several centimeters of water because of the effects of gravity, the configuration of the chest and diaphragm, the presence of the heart and mediastinal structures, and the need for the lung to fit within the thorax irrespective of the shape of either the lung or the thorax. At FRC in upright humans, $-5\,cmH_2O$ is an average value at chest midlevel, but near the apices the pressure outside the lung might be $-8\,cmH_2O$, whereas near the bases only $-2\,cmH_2O$. Because alveoli throughout the lung seem to have similar maximum volume and pressure–volume relationships, and because alveolar pressure is everywhere the same, those alveoli near the top of the lung are held at larger volume (distending pressure of $8\,cmH_2O$) than those near the bottom (distending pressure of $2\,cmH_2O$). This places the lower alveoli on a steeper (more compliant) portion of their pressure–volume curve. In addition, the proximity of the basal alveoli to the motion of the diaphragm exposes them to a greater increase in distending pressure with inspiration.

These two factors combine to give the lower portion of the normal lung a relatively greater proportion of the tidal ventilation than the apices.

A second consequence of the higher (i.e., less negative) pleural pressure in the basal portions of the lung is that the distending pressure of the small airways is also less. At low lung volume, airways may close, and the dependent portions of the lung reach this "closing volume" first, whereas higher portions of the lung are still partially distended. Thus, a patient who breathes at very low lung volumes, near residual volume (e.g., obese patients), may have basal airway closure and consequently little ventilation to the lung bases.

In summary, respiratory units in the basal portion of the lung contain less gas but receive more ventilation as long as they remain open. However, they are more susceptible to airway closure and loss of ventilation at low lung volume.

SUGGESTED READINGS

Gibson GJ: Lung volumes and elasticity. In Hughes JMB, Pride NB, eds. Lung Function Tests: Physiologic Principles and Clinical Applications. London: WB Saunders; 1999:45–56.

Hills BA: Surface-active phospholipids: A Pandora's box of clinical applications. Part I: The lung and air spaces. Int Med J 2002; 32:170–178.

Pride NB: Airflow resistance. In Hughes JMB, Pride NB, eds. Lung Function Tests: Physiologic Principles and Clinical Applications. London: WB Saunders; 1999:27–44.

Schurch S, Bachofen H, Possmeyer F: Alveolar lining layer. Functions, composition, structures, In Hlastala MP, Robertson HT, eds. Lung Biology in Health and Disease, vol 121: Complexity in Structure and Function of the Lung. New York. Marcel Dekker; 1998:35–98.

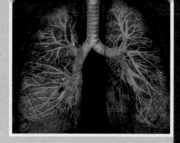

5   Gas Exchange in the Lung*

BRUCE H. CULVER

INTRODUCTION

The primary function of the lung is to provide adequate oxygenation of the blood and to remove carbon dioxide, as first described by Lavoisier in 1777:

> Eminently respirable air that enters the lung, leaves it in the form of chalky aeriform acids [carbon dioxide] . . . in almost equal volume. . . . Respiration acts only on the portion of pure air that is eminently respirable [which he later named 'oxygine']. . ., the excess [nitrogen], is a purely passive medium which enters and leaves the lung . . . without change or alteration. The respirable portion of air has the property to combine with blood and its combination results in its red color.
> Quoted in West JB, ed: Pulmonary gas exchange, Vol. 1. Ventilation, Blood Flow, and Diffusion. New York: Academic Press; 1980.

This gas exchange process can be considered in three parts:

1. Ventilation of the lungs, which determines the alveolar levels of oxygen and carbon dioxide
2. Storage and transport of these gases in the blood
3. Process of equilibration between alveolar gas and arterial blood

The terminology and abbreviations particular to gas exchange are introduced in Table 5-1.

FUNCTIONAL ANATOMY OF GAS EXCHANGE

The lung can be functionally divided into a conducting zone of air passages and a respiratory zone that consists of the last few branches of airways and alveoli, in which gas exchange with blood takes place. In the conducting zone, from the upper respiratory tract to the terminal bronchioles, essentially no exchange of respiratory gases with the atmosphere occurs. These airways warm and humidify the incoming air and can remove some gaseous and particulate pollutants.

The terminal bronchioles are succeeded by two to five generations of respiratory bronchioles (Figure 5-1), which have increasing numbers of alveoli in their walls. The next branches are alveolar ducts, which are completely alveolated, with no ciliated epithelium remaining, and terminate in alveolar sacs and individual alveoli. Helical bands of smooth muscle extend

to the alveolar ducts and may aid control of the distribution of ventilation. The entire respiratory unit served by one terminal bronchiole is an acinus. Several adjacent acini make up a pulmonary lobule, which has incomplete connective tissue septae that separate it from adjacent lobules. The collateral communication of both airflow and blood flow is better within a lobule than between lobules, although canals of Lambert apparently connect bronchioles of adjacent lobules.

Alveoli are irregular polyhedrons approximately 250 μm in diameter. They increase in number in early childhood to the average adult number of 300 million (varying with body size). The total alveolar surface area is 85–90% covered with capillaries, which provides an impressive surface area of 70 m^2 for gas exchange. Adjacent alveoli are connected by pores of Kohn that provide routes for collateral airflow, fluid movement, phagocyte mobility, and bacterial spread.

Most of the alveolar surface is covered by epithelial cells that have very attenuated cytoplasm sitting directly on a basement membrane. The capillary endothelial cells are also very thin (except where their nuclei bulge) and again sit directly on a basement membrane. Over much of the area where gas exchange takes place, these basement membranes are fused into one with no intervening interstitial space (Figure 5-2). Thus, the diffusion distance from alveolar gas to plasma may be less than 0.5 μm. The distance to a red cell or even within a red cell (approximately 8 μm) may be much greater than that across the alveolar and capillary membrane itself.

Despite the anatomic complexity of the lung, its gas exchange function can be well described by simple models that consist of a conducting zone (branched tube) and a respiratory zone (usually depicted as one or more giant alveoli) with blood flow.

Ambient Gas Partial Pressures (Tensions)

Atmospheric or barometric pressure (PB) is the total pressure exerted by the kinetic energy of all the molecules in the atmospheric mixture. It varies with altitude, but at sea level it raises a column of mercury in an evacuated tube to a height of 760 mm (equivalent to 29.9 inches of mercury or 100 kPa) and varies slightly from day to day.

In discussing lung mechanics, the pressure in the chest or lungs is measured relative to atmospheric pressure, so PATM is set at zero. This is termed *gauge pressure* and is commonly used, for example, to measure blood pressure or tire pressure. However, gas pressures in the atmosphere, alveoli, and blood are reported in absolute pressure terms, expressed as millimeters of mercury (mmHg) or Torr. An alveolar pressure of 13 cmH$_2$O, or 10 mmHg (gauge), is equivalent to 770 mmHg in absolute pressure.

Atmospheric air is a mixture that consists of oxygen (20.95%), nitrogen (78.09%), argon (0.93%), and carbon dioxide (0.03%),

---

*Author note: Units in this chapter are expressed in cmH$_2$O, mmHg, or Torr. Should the reader need SI units at any point, the conversion factors are:
1cmH$_2$O = 0.1 kPa
1 mmHg=1 Torr = 0.132 kPa
1 kPa=7.6 mmHg or Torr = 10 cmH$_2$O

TABLE 5-1 Gas Exchange Terminology and Abbreviations

Symbol	Definition	Units
P	Pressure or partial pressure; e.g., P_{O_2} = partial pressure of oxygen	mmHg (millimeters of mercury) or torr (1 torr = 1 mmHg under standard gravitational conditions, i.e., sea level) kPa (kiloPascal; 1 kPa = 7.6 mmHg or torr) cmH_2O (centimeters of water; 1 mmHg = 1.3 cmH_2O)
F	Fraction of a given gas present in a mixture (F × 100 = percentage concentration)	–
V	Volume of gas	L (liters) or mL (milliliters)
$\dot{V}$	Flow (volume per time)	mL/min (milliliters per minute; e.g., oxygen consumption, $\dot{V}_{O_2}$) L/min (e.g., ventilation, $\dot{V}_E$) L/s (e.g., airflow rates)

The symbols and modifiers used in this chapter are based on those recommended in the *American Medical Association Manual of Style* and the ATS-ACCP Joint Committee on Nomenclature. Main symbols indicating the type of measurement are in capital letters followed by one or more modifiers to indicate location or the gas measured. By convention, locations related to ventilation are given in small capital letters (e.g., I, inspired; E, expired; A, alveolar), and vascular locations are given in lower-case letters (e.g., a, arterial; v, venous; c, capillary).

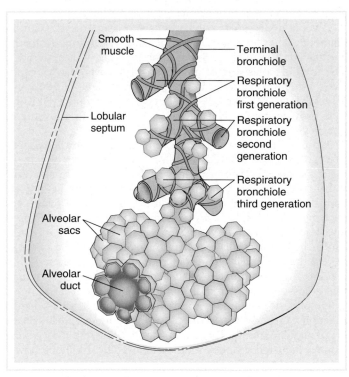

FIGURE 5-1 Gas exchange portion of the lung.

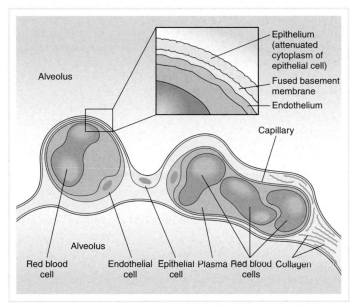

FIGURE 5-2 Structure of the interalveolar septum facilitates gas exchange. Capillaries tend to lay asymmetrically within the septum, with most of the interstitial space, structural elements, and cell nuclei on a "thick side," whereas the "thin side" presents a very short path for gas diffusion. Based on information from Siegwart B, Gehr P, Gil J, Weibel E: Morphometric estimation of pulmonary diffusing capacity. IV. The normal dog lung. Respir Physiol 1971; 13:141–159.

with water vapor that varies from 0–2% and dilutes the other gases accordingly. For practical purposes, oxygen is taken to be 21%, nitrogen 79%, and carbon dioxide and other trace gases are ignored. Water vapor requires special consideration (see later).

Concept of Partial Pressure

In a mixture of gases, the pressure exerted by the kinetic energy of each separate gas is referred to as its partial pressure. If the mixture is enclosed in a sealed container, it develops a pressure on the walls of the container by the mechanism of collisions between the gas molecules and the container walls. The force or pressure developed by all the molecules of the mixture as they bounce off the container walls is the total pressure developed by the gas. The partial pressure of any component is the pressure developed by the molecules of that component acting alone. Because the random motion that causes collisions is the same motion that allows diffusion to take place, the partial pressure of a gas is a measure of its tendency to diffuse through either gas or fluid media.

The total pressure of a mixture of gases is equal to the sum of the partial pressures of each gas in the mixture (Dalton's law). Because the alveoli and airways are open to the atmosphere, the sum of the partial pressures in the lung must add up to the barometric pressure (Eq. 5-1). The small variations in alveolar pressure during the respiratory cycle are ignored.

$$P_{ATM} = P_{CO_2} + P_{O_2} + P_{N_2} = P_{H_2O} \qquad \text{(Dalton's law)}$$

In the gas phase, partial pressure is proportional to concentration. By convention, gas fractions are measured after water vapor has been removed ("dry" gas). Thus, the partial pressure of a gas is found by multiplying the concentration or fraction of the gas by the total pressure of dry (i.e., no water vapor) gases.

The concept of partial pressure also applies to gases in a liquid, including plasma or blood. When a gas-free liquid is in contact with air, gas molecules move into the liquid by diffusion until the partial pressure in the liquid and air are the same. The relationship of partial pressure of a gas in a liquid to the content of that gas depends on solubility and any chemical binding that takes place. For example, nitrogen and oxygen are both poorly soluble, but large amounts of oxygen can be bound to hemoglobin (Hb).

Water Vapor

Water vapor requires special consideration, because water is present as both a gas and a liquid in the body. When a gas mixture is in contact with liquid and is saturated with the vapor of that liquid, the partial pressure of that vapor is a function of temperature (Table 5-2).

Atmospheric gas is cooler than body temperature and, although it contains some water, it is rarely 100% saturated. Inspired gas that enters the upper portion of the respiratory system is rapidly warmed to body temperature and becomes fully saturated with water vapor. The small volume change associated with warming and added water vapor can be calculated from gas laws if necessary (Table 5-3). At 37°C, water vapor has a partial pressure of 47 mmHg. This pressure does not vary with changes in barometric pressure or changes in the other components in the gas mixture. Thus, if P_B is 760 mmHg,

and P_{H_2O} is 47 mmHg, the difference, 713 mmHg, is the partial pressure of the remaining dry, inspired gases. Of this total, 21% is oxygen and 79% is nitrogen, so $P_{IO_2}=0.21\times713=150$ mmHg and $P_{IN_2}=0.79\times713=563$ mmHg.

Air has the same relative concentration of gases, even when P_B is lowered. For example, at the top of Mt. Everest (altitude approximately 29,000 feet), $P_B=253$ mmHg, and the atmospheric $P_{O_2}=0.21\times253=53$ mmHg.

VENTILATION

The total ventilation per minute ($\dot{V}_E$=volume exhaled per minute) can be determined by collecting exhaled gas for a measured time. The volume of gas exhaled during one normal respiratory cycle is the tidal volume (V_T). The total ventilation is equal to V_T multiplied by the breathing frequency, f or ($\dot{V}_E=V_T\times f$).

Alveolar Ventilation and Dead Space

Gas exchange occurs in alveoli when freshly inspired air comes in contact with capillary blood. However, not all of each inspired breath reaches the alveoli to participate in gas exchange. Inspired air must first pass through the conducting airways, from the nose to the distal bronchioles, which contain no alveoli and do not participate in gas exchange. At the end of inspiration, the volume of air that remains in the conducting airways, and therefore does not participate in gas exchange, is the anatomic dead space. The effect of the conducting airways on ventilation and gas exchange can be considered in two ways. After inspiration, atmospheric air (plus a little water vapor) remains in these airways and leaves as the first gas out on the subsequent exhalation. After expiration, alveolar gas (with carbon dioxide added and oxygen partially removed) fills the anatomic dead space and reenters the alveoli with the next breath. Thus, a tidal breath may inspire 500 mL of air and result in a 500-mL expansion of the alveolar volume followed by the expiration of 500 mL, but the volume of *fresh* air delivered to the alveoli and the volume of alveolar air exhaled to the atmosphere are each less than 500 mL by an amount equal to the volume of the anatomic dead space.

In addition to the conducting airways, any alveoli that are ventilated with air but not perfused with blood cannot participate in gas exchange. The volume of ventilation that goes to these alveoli is also wasted and is called alveolar dead space. Ventilation to areas of lung that have reduced, but not absent, perfusion can be treated as if a portion were going to alveoli with normal perfusion and a portion to alveoli with no perfusion. This latter portion is also part of the alveolar dead space (Figure 5-3). The sum of anatomic and alveolar dead space makes up the physiologic dead space.

The volume of the anatomic dead space ($V_{D_{an}}$) in a normal adult male is 150–180 mL (approximately equal to the lean body weight in pounds). In a young normal individual, the volume of the physiologic dead space (V_D) is only slightly greater than this or approximately 25–35% of an average V_T (referred to as the V_D/V_T ratio). The anatomic dead space is not fixed but increases at higher lung volumes, because the intrapulmonary airways increase in size along with the surrounding lung tissue through interdependence. Thus, breathing with a large V_T, and the accompanying larger end-inspiratory lung volume, is associated with a modest decrease in V_D/V_T ratio. With exercise, V_T may increase to 2.5–3.0 L, and V_D/V_T normally falls to 15% or less, but an important additional factor is

TABLE 5-2 Water Vapor Pressure

Temperature (°C)	Water Vapor Pressure	
	mmHg	kPa
0	4.6	0.6
20	17.5	2.3
37	47.0	6.2
100	760.0	100

The partial pressure due to water vapor at full saturation varies with temperature.

TABLE 5-3 Gas Conditions and Corrections

The volume occupied by an amount of gas is directly proportional to its absolute temperature (°Kelvin), is inversely proportional to its total pressure, and is further affected by the volume of water vapor present.

Exhaled gas collected in a spirometer or bag is saturated at ambient temperature and pressure (ATPS).

Lung and ventilatory volumes are conventionally converted into body temperature and pressure, saturated (BTPS) conditions, a volume expansion of 9–10%.

Gas transfer quantities ($\dot{V}_{O_2}$, $\dot{V}_{CO_2}$, and diffusing capacity) are conventionally expressed at standard temperature (273°K), pressure (760 mmHg), and dry (STPD) conditions.

For quantitative calculations, gas volumes must be corrected for changes in temperature, pressure, and water vapor, but these corrections or conversions can be largely ignored for conceptual understanding.

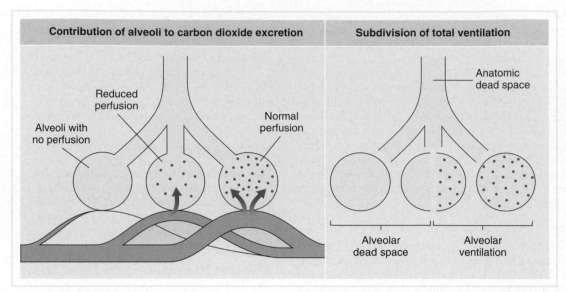

FIGURE 5-3 Physiologic dead space. Alveoli with no perfusion, reduced perfusion, and normal perfusion and their contribution to carbon dioxide excretion. Subdivision of the total ventilation into anatomic dead space, alveolar dead space with no perfusion, and alveolar ventilation with ideal perfusion. (Modified with permission from Culver BH, ed: Seattle: University of Washington Publication Services; 2006.)

the increase in pulmonary blood flow, which tends to eliminate any poorly perfused alveolar dead space. At the other extreme, it would seem that as V_T became small, approaching the anatomic dead space, alveolar ventilation should fall to zero and gas exchange become impossible. However, with high-frequency ventilation, it has been demonstrated that gas exchange can be maintained even with V_T equal to or smaller than the measured anatomic dead space. Some fresh gas reaches alveoli, because some path lengths are shorter than others and because airway gas will exchange with alveolar gas by diffusion and by physical mixing induced by the heartbeat.

The physiologic dead space and wasted ventilation may be considerably increased with diseases of the air spaces and vasculature, primarily because of an increase in the alveolar component. (Importantly, increases in the "physiologic" dead space are almost always abnormal, i.e., pathologic.) The fraction of ventilation "wasted" by going to physiologic dead space can be calculated from arterial and expired gas values (see Table 5-4). Dead space has the effect of diluting the carbon dioxide content of expired gas below the alveolar level, and the equation derived in Table 5-4 is simply a calculation of this dilution. Because the body needs to eliminate a certain volume of carbon dioxide per minute, the effect of a low expired CO_2 level is to require more total ventilation to maintain homeostasis.

The volume of air that does participate in gas exchange, because it is in contact with perfused alveoli, is termed the *alveolar ventilation* ($\dot{V}_A = \dot{V}_E - \dot{V}_D$). The volume per minute of alveolar ventilation is critical, because it determines the amount of air presented to alveoli into which carbon dioxide can be excreted and from which oxygen can be removed. Note that "alveolar ventilation," as defined here and widely used in respiratory physiology, is a conceptual term and might better be called "gas exchange ventilation." It is not the same as the volume of gas that enters or leaves the alveoli each minute.

Carbon Dioxide Elimination

Because the body's carbon dioxide production ($\dot{V}_{CO_2}$) is only eliminated by ventilation, it must equal the volume of carbon

TABLE 5-4 Physiologic Dead Space Calculations

The physiologic dead space, made up of ventilation to anatomic dead space plus that to unperfused alveoli and a portion of that to poorly perfused alveoli, is not an anatomically identifiable volume, but an "as if" volume may be obtained by calculation from a collection of exhaled gas over 1–3 minutes.

Using a "conservation of mass" concept, the total expired volume of gas per minute is considered to have two sources:

ideal alveoli with equal alveolar and arterial partial pressures of carbon dioxide ($P_{ACO_2} = P_{aCO_2}$); and

unperfused areas (conducting airways or alveolar dead space) with $P_{ACO_2} = $ inspired $P_{CO_2} = 0$.

The total expired volume of carbon dioxide comes entirely from the effective (nondead space) alveolar ventilation ($\dot{V}_E - \dot{V}_D$).

$$\dot{V}_{CO_2} = \dot{V}_E \times F_{ECO_2} = (\dot{V}_E - \dot{V}_D) \times F_{ACO_2}$$

Algebraic manipulation yields:

$$\dot{V}_D \times F_{ACO_2} = \dot{V}_E \times F_{ACO_2} - \dot{V}_E \times F_{ECO_2}$$

$$\dot{V}_D/\dot{V}_E = (F_{ACO_2} - F_{ECO_2})/F_{ACO_2}$$

Multiplying top and bottom by ($P_{ATM} - 47$) converts fractions to partial pressure:

$$\dot{V}_D/\dot{V}_E = (P_{ACO_2} - P_{ECO_2})/P_{ACO_2}$$

P_{ACO_2} cannot be readily measured, but in these assumed ideal alveoli $P_{ACO_2} = P_{aCO_2}$, so the measured arterial blood gas value can be substituted to create the final equation below. P_{ECO_2} is obtained from a collection of expired gas.

By convention, the results are reported as the $\dot{V}_D/\dot{V}_T$ or wasted fraction of each tidal breath, but actually they are measured as the average wasted ventilation over 1–3 minutes.

$$V_D/V_T = \dot{V}_D/\dot{V}_E = (P_{aCO_2} - P_{ECO_2})/P_{aCO_2}$$

Multiplying this fraction by the tidal volume or minute ventilation gives the volume of physiologic dead space or wasted ventilation. (In carrying out this measurement, it must be remembered that the volume of air in mouthpiece, connections, and valve [mechanical dead space] also contribute air free of carbon dioxide to the expired collection.)

dioxide exhaled per minute minus the volume of carbon dioxide inhaled, which is negligible and can be disregarded. All of the carbon dioxide expired must come from alveolar ventilation and is equal to the volume of this ventilation times the concentration of carbon dioxide in the effective gas-exchanging space (F_{ACO_2}) (Eq. 5-2).

$$\dot{V}_{CO_2} = \dot{V}_A \times F_{ACO_2} \qquad (5\text{-}2)$$

Rearranging this equation demonstrates that for a given level of metabolic carbon dioxide production, a reciprocal relationship exists between alveolar ventilation and the level of alveolar carbon dioxide (Eq. 5-3).

$$F_{ACO_2} = \dot{V}_{CO_2}/\dot{V}_A \qquad (5\text{-}3)$$

Multiplying both sides of Eq. 5-3 by the total pressure of dry gases in the alveoli ($P_B - 47$) converts the fraction into the partial pressure units in which carbon dioxide is commonly measured and yields the useful relationship in Eq. 5-4, which states that alveolar P_{CO_2} is directly related to the production of carbon dioxide and inversely related to alveolar ventilation ($\dot{V}_A$).

$$P_{ACO_2} = (\dot{V}_{CO_2}/\dot{V}_A) \times (P_B - 47) \qquad (5\text{-}4)$$

The body maintains a normal alveolar (and arterial) P_{CO_2} of 40 mmHg by adjusting ventilation appropriately for the $\dot{V}_{CO_2}$ dictated by metabolic demand.

Hyperventilation is defined as ventilation in excess of metabolic needs. Therefore, a P_{ACO_2} below normal indicates alveolar hyperventilation. Conversely, a P_{ACO_2} greater than normal indicates alveolar hypoventilation.

Any depression in central nervous system function can change $\dot{V}_E$ and, therefore, $\dot{V}_A$; for example, many drugs such as narcotics and sedatives can reduce $\dot{V}_E$. Any increase in V_D will also reduce $\dot{V}_A$ unless $\dot{V}_E$ increases proportionally. Many disease processes increase physiologic dead space, which is a contributory cause of ventilatory failure when the patient can no longer increase total ventilation.

The alveolar P_{CO_2} level reflects a balance between carbon dioxide that enters the alveoli as it escapes from the blood and that which leaves with exhaled gas. In a steady state, production and excretion must be the same. Under resting conditions, $\dot{V}_{CO_2}$ is relatively constant at approximately 200 mL/min for an individual of normal size. If a person hyperventilates, initially carbon dioxide is exhaled at a greater rate than carbon dioxide production; P_{ACO_2} falls (and with it arterial P_{CO_2}). As P_{ACO_2} falls, the carbon dioxide exhaled per minute decreases, because less is loaded into exhaled air, until carbon dioxide elimination is again equal to carbon dioxide production and a new steady state is established. In hypoventilation, the rate of carbon dioxide exhalation initially falls, so P_{ACO_2} and P_{aCO_2} rise until a new steady state is reached at which excretion again equals production, with less ventilation but with each liter of gas leaving the alveoli carrying more carbon dioxide. This mechanism allows patients who have severe lung disease and high work of breathing to excrete their carbon dioxide production at less energy cost.

Alveolar Oxygen

The level of alveolar oxygen also reflects a balance of two processes:

- Oxygen delivery to the alveoli by ventilation
- Oxygen removal from the alveoli by capillary blood

Oxygen delivery to alveoli is determined by their ventilation ($\dot{V}_A$) and the fraction of inspired oxygen (F_{IO_2}), but oxygen is also carried away in exhaled air. The gas that leaves alveoli has the alveolar oxygen concentration (F_{AO_2}), so the net oxygen taken up from alveoli is given by $\dot{V}_A \times (F_{IO_2} - F_{AO_2})$. This relationship can be written as a conservation of mass equation that states that the oxygen consumed to meet metabolic demand ($\dot{V}_{O_2}$) equals that removed from the alveolar ventilation (none is removed from dead space ventilation) (Eq. 5-5).

$$\dot{V}_{O_2} = \dot{V}_A(F_{IO_2} - F_{AO_2}) \qquad (5\text{-}5)$$

Rearranging this equation demonstrates that for a given level of metabolic oxygen consumption, a reciprocal relationship exists between alveolar ventilation and the fraction of oxygen removed from the incoming air. That is, when alveolar ventilation is decreased, more oxygen must be extracted from each unit of that incoming ventilation, which results in a lower residual level of alveolar oxygen (Eq. 5-6).

$$F_{IO_2} - F_{AO_2} = \dot{V}_{O_2}/\dot{V}_A \qquad (5\text{-}6)$$

Conversion of equation (5-6) into partial pressure by multiplying both sides by ($P_B - 47$) gives Eq. 5-7.

$$P_{IO_2} - P_{AO_2} = (\dot{V}_{O_2}/\dot{V}_A) \times (P_B - 47) \qquad (5\text{-}7)$$

Eq. 5-7 shows that for a given inspired oxygen level, P_{AO_2} is determined by $\dot{V}_A$ and $\dot{V}_{O_2}$. If P_{IO_2} and $\dot{V}_{O_2}$ are constant and $\dot{V}_A$ increases, P_{AO_2} must also increase; if $\dot{V}_A$ decreases, P_{AO_2} must also decrease. The amount of oxygen taken from inspired air is governed by tissue oxygen consumption and varies with activity, but under resting conditions it is approximately 250 mL/min for a person of average size. In a steady state, P_{AO_2} does not change, so the extraction of oxygen from inspired air just matches the transfer of oxygen to the blood. In hyperventilation, initially alveolar oxygen is added at a greater rate than it is consumed and P_{AO_2} rises. As P_{AO_2} rises, the amount of oxygen exhaled increases and that unloaded to the alveoli decreases, until a new steady state is established at a higher P_{AO_2}. In hypoventilation, the rate of oxygen delivery to the alveoli initially falls, and P_{AO_2} falls until a new steady state is reached with less ventilation, but each liter of gas that enters and leaves the alveoli has given up more oxygen.

Estimating the Alveolar Partial Pressure of Oxygen

Abnormalities in oxygenation often cause a wide disparity between the level of alveolar oxygen and that measured in the arterial blood. To understand fully the clinical arterial blood gas values, it is necessary to estimate quantitatively the P_{AO_2}, but this cannot be readily obtained from equation (5-7), because neither $\dot{V}_{O_2}$ nor $\dot{V}_A$ are easily measured. However, because carbon dioxide production is the metabolic product of oxygen consumption, the quantities $\dot{V}_{CO_2}$ and $\dot{V}_{O_2}$ are tightly linked and their ratio, $\dot{V}_{CO_2}/\dot{V}_{O_2}$, is the respiratory exchange ratio (R). If these values are identical (R=1), the solutions to Eqs. 5-4 and 5-7 are identical and show that the fall in P_{O_2} from inspired to alveolar air is exactly the same as the rise in P_{CO_2} from zero to the alveolar level. With a more typical R of 0.8, the consumption of five molecules of oxygen results in the production of four molecules of carbon dioxide, and it follows that in the lung the addition of carbon dioxide to a level of 40 mmHg in alveolar air would be associated with a $P_{A}O_2$ that showed a 50 mmHg extraction from the inspired air (Eq. 5-8).

$$P_{A}O_2 = P_{I}O_2 - (P_{A}CO_2/R) \quad (5\text{-}8)$$

Because the measured $P_{a}CO_2$ is very close to $P_{A}CO_2$, this can be substituted and rewritten as Eq. 5-9.

$$P_{A}O_2 = P_{I}O_2 - (P_{a}CO_2/R)$$

(5-9: The alveolar gas equation [simplified])

For typical normal values, $R = 0.8$, $P_{I}O_2 = 0.21(760 - 47)$, and $P_{a}CO_2 = 40$ (Eq. 5-10).

$$P_{A}O_2 = 150 - (40/0.8) = 100 \text{ mmHg} \quad (5\text{-}10)$$

The alveolar gas equation is often misinterpreted as indicating that inspired oxygen is displaced by carbon dioxide in the alveoli. This is incorrect, because the removal of oxygen from inspired air and the addition of carbon dioxide proceed as independent processes in the lung, but because the normal respiratory quotient (RQ; see later) in the tissues is typically 0.8–1.0, extraction of oxygen from the inspired air to the blood is approximately equal to the increase in carbon dioxide.

Appropriate interpretation of arterial blood gas values always requires thinking through the alveolar gas equation. This helps, for example, to establish whether a low $P_{a}O_2$ is explained by hypoventilation or whether the $P_{a}O_2$ is appropriate for the $F_{I}O_2$. Table 5-5 gives examples of the use of the alveolar gas equation. The amount of ventilation relative to metabolic need markedly affects the $P_{A}O_2$ available to equilibrate with capillary blood. The $P_{A}O_2$ calculated from the alveolar gas equation, which ranges from 70–125 mmHg in these examples, is a somewhat theoretical value for average alveoli; some areas of the lung may have higher or lower values.

Metabolism and the Respiratory Exchange Ratio

Energy necessary for life processes is produced by oxidation of carbohydrates, protein, and fats, which produce principally carbon dioxide and water as breakdown products. The RQ is the ratio of metabolic carbon dioxide production to the oxygen consumption of the tissues ($\dot{V}CO_2/\dot{V}O_2$). When carbohydrate is

metabolized, RQ = 1.0; when fat is metabolized, RQ = 0.7; and when protein is metabolized, RQ averages 0.8. Thus, the RQ for the entire body varies with the percentages of carbohydrate, fat, and protein being oxidized at any given time. The respiratory exchange ratio (R) relates the volume of carbon dioxide eliminated and the net volume of oxygen taken up in the lungs. In a steady state or over a long period of time, R must equal RQ, but R may vary transiently with factors other than metabolism. For example, if an individual suddenly increases ventilation, R rises because carbon dioxide is "blown off" from blood and tissue stores (but little oxygen can be added). During exercise, R may reach 1.4 because of hyperventilation and continued excretion of carbon dioxide while an oxygen debt is contracted.

TRANSPORT OF GASES IN THE BLOOD

Oxygen Transport

Respiratory gases are carried in blood in physical solution, by binding proteins, and (for carbon dioxide) through chemical conversion. The small quantities carried in physical solution are calculated in Table 5-6. For oxygen, with only 3 mL of oxygen per liter in physical solution at a normal arterial P_{O_2}, it would be impossible to pump enough blood to meet tissue demand without the large additional transport provided by hemoglobin.

Hemoglobin

Hemoglobin (Hb) is a complex protein consisting of four polypeptide chains (two α-chains and two β-chains), with four heme groups to bind oxygen. One mole of Hb can carry four moles of oxygen, so the theoretical maximum oxygen carrying capacity is calculated as 1.39 mL/g of Hb (but the actual maximum seems to be slightly less, because some sites are not available). Normal blood has an Hb concentration of 15 g/100 mL blood and thus can potentially carry approximately 20 mL oxygen per 100 mL of blood as oxyhemoglobin.

TABLE 5-5 **Application of the Alveolar Gas Equation**			
	Normal Ventilation	Hyper-ventilation	Hypo-ventilation
$P_{I}O_2 =$ (0.21 × 713) (mmHg)	150	150	150
$P_{a}CO_2$ (mmHg)	40	20	64
R	0.8	0.8	0.8
$P_{A}O_2 = P_{I}O_2 - (P_{a}CO_2/R)$ (mmHg)	150−50=100	150−25=125	150−80=70

The amount of ventilation relative to metabolic need markedly affects the $P_{A}O_2$ available to equilibrate with capillary blood; this can be estimated using the alveolar gas equation. The $P_{A}O_2$ calculated, which ranges from 70 to 125 mmHg in these examples, is a somewhat theoretical value for average alveoli; some areas of the lung may have higher or lower values.

TABLE 5-6 **Gases in Physical Solution**
The content of a gas (oxygen, carbon dioxide, or nitrogen) carried in physical solution in the blood is proportional to its partial pressure and solubility (Henry's law), where C is the concentration (mL/100 mL blood), P is the partial pressure (mmHg), and α is the solubility (mL/100 mL blood per mmHg).
Henry's Law $$C = \alpha P$$
The solubility of gases in liquid decreases as temperature increases. For blood at 37°C, the solubility of oxygen (α_{O_2}) is 0.003 mL/100 mL blood per mmHg, and α_{CO_2} is 0.072 mL/100 mL blood per mmHg.
The amount of oxygen stored in blood in physical solution at a normal arterial P_{O_2} of 13.3 kPa (100 mmHg) is given by the following equation: $$C_{O_2} = \alpha_{O_2} \times P_{O_2} = 0.003 \times 100 = 0.3 \text{ mL/100 mL blood}$$
The amount of carbon dioxide stored in blood in physical solution at a normal arterial P_{CO_2} of 5.3 kPa (40 mmHg) is given by the following equation: $$C_{CO_2} = \alpha_{CO_2} \times P_{CO_2} = 0.072 \times 100 = 2.9 \text{ mL/100 mL blood}$$

The Hb sites fill with oxygen in relation to its partial pressure in solution; the percentage of saturation of Hb indicates the portion of the total oxygen-binding sites actually occupied. The relation between P_{O_2} and Hb oxygen content or percentage saturation is nonlinear (Figure 5-4). The curve is S-shaped, which has particular physiologic advantages. In the normal arterial range, the curve is fairly flat, so that moderate decreases in arterial P_{O_2} cause only small decrements in arterial oxygen saturation (Sa_{O_2}) and content. A normal saturation of 97.5% occurs at a P_{O_2} of 100 mmHg. A decrease in P_{O_2} to 60 mmHg still allows the Hb to be 90% saturated. The curve is fairly steep in the normal range of systemic venous P_{O_2} (Pv_{O_2}), which allows further unloading of oxygen to active tissues, with only a small reduction in the partial pressure that drives oxygen diffusion to the cells. The oxygen unloaded under normal resting conditions leaves a Pv_{O_2} of 40 mmHg and a saturation of 75%.

The relative affinity of Hb for oxygen is described by the parameter P_{50} (the P_{O_2} at 50% saturation). Decreased P_{50} or a curve shift to the left means increased affinity or more oxygen bound for any P_{O_2}; increased P_{50} or a curve shift to the right means decreased affinity (Figure 5-5). Physiologic factors that affect the affinity of Hb for oxygen include H^+ concentration, P_{CO_2}, and temperature. Increases in all of these, as seen in an exercising muscle, shift the curve to the right, which decreases affinity and helps to unload oxygen at the tissues.

The effect of P_{CO_2} is particularly important because the loading of carbon dioxide in tissues produces a right shift of the dissociation curve and enhances the simultaneous unloading of oxygen. Part of this shift is caused by the associated pH change, and part results from the binding of carbon dioxide with Hb to form carbamino compounds, which have lower affinity for oxygen. The reverse occurs in the lungs as the unloading of carbon dioxide shifts the dissociation curve to the left, which enables the blood to load more oxygen at a given Pa_{O_2}. This bidirectional shift is called the Bohr effect.

Additional regulation of Hb-O_2 affinity over a time frame of hours to days occurs by means of 2,3-diphosphoglycerate (2,3-DPG), an intermediate metabolite in the red-cell metabolic pathway. When upregulated by a stimulus like chronic hypoxia (e.g., altitude), increased 2,3-DPG concentration decreases oxygen affinity by binding to the Hb molecule. Changes in the 2,3-DPG level also play an adaptive role during acid–base abnormalities and with anemia.

Affinity for oxygen can also be affected by variation in the Hb polypeptides. At 37°C and pH 7.4, normal adult Hb A has a P_{50} of 27 mmHg, whereas human fetal Hb has a P_{50} of 20 mmHg. Several abnormal hemoglobin types have been identified that have either high or low oxygen affinity.

The physiologic advantage of a curve shift for oxygen delivery depends on the conditions of loading and unloading. An increased affinity means the blood that leaves the alveoli, equilibrated with the alveolar P_{O_2}, has a slightly higher oxygen content, but when required to give up 5 mL/100 mL or more

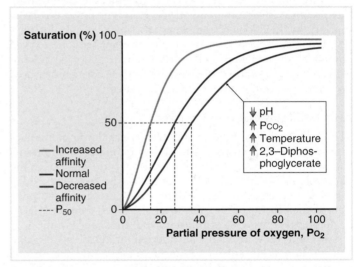

FIGURE 5-5 Normal, increased affinity (*left shift*) and decreased affinity (*right shift*) Hb-O_2 curves. Note that decreased affinity means a higher P_{O_2} at a given saturation (e.g., 50%) or a lower saturation at a given P_{O_2} (e.g., P_{O_2} of 40). (Modified with permission from Hlastala MP: Blood gas transport. In Culver BH, ed: The respiratory system. Seattle: University of Washington Publication Services; 2006.)

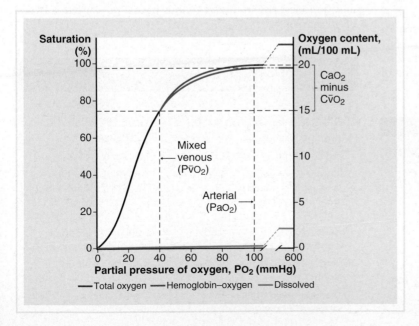

FIGURE 5-4 Hemoglobin-oxygen (Hb-O_2) dissociation curve shows the percentage saturation of hemoglobin at each P_{O_2}. When the hemoglobin concentration is known, the content of oxygen can be calculated. The total content includes the small additional content of oxygen in solution, which becomes significant at high levels of P_{O_2}. The saturation scale on the left applies only to the Hb-O_2 line. The scale on the right shows content values for a normal hemoglobin level of 15 g/100 mL blood. (Modified with permission from Hlastala MP: Blood gas transport. In Culver BH, ed: The respiratory system. Seattle: University of Washington Publication Services; 2006.)

of its content to metabolically active tissue, the P_{O_2} at the delivery point has to fall to a lower-than-normal value (see Figure 5-5). A decreased affinity means that the blood leaving alveoli has a slightly lower content, but not very much lower because of the nearly flat top of the Hb-O_2 curve. This blood can give up the same amount (5 mL/100 mL) to the tissues and still maintain a higher P_{O_2} at the delivery point. Thus, at near-normal levels of alveolar P_{O_2}, a right shift is usually advantageous, but when loading at a markedly reduced P_{O_2} (e.g., from placental exchange or at extreme altitude), a left shift is more helpful.

Carbon Monoxide

Carbon monoxide is a particularly dangerous gas because its affinity for Hb is 200–250 times that of oxygen, and thus it can fully saturate Hb at a very low ambient concentration. The presence of carbon monoxide decreases the oxygen-carrying capacity by functionally removing Hb sites available for oxygen binding. It also causes an effective increase in oxygen affinity of the remaining Hb sites. Carbon monoxide poisoning can create a marked disparity between a normal measured Pa_{O_2} and a severely reduced oxygen content.

Arterial Blood Oxygen Content

The equilibration of blood with alveolar gas in the pulmonary capillaries determines the partial pressure of oxygen in plasma and would do so even if Hb were totally absent. The P_{O_2} in the plasma is in equilibrium with the Hb in the red cells, which yields an oxygen saturation determined by the shape and position of the Hb-O_2 curve. The arterial oxygen content (Ca_{O_2}) is determined by this saturation and the concentration of Hb present plus a small contribution of dissolved oxygen. With a normal Hb concentration of 15 g/100 mL, the normal arterial oxygen content is approximately 20.5 mL/100 mL (Table 5-7). Blood with decreased Hb concentration (anemia) holds less oxygen, whereas that with an increased Hb concentration (polycythemia) holds an increased amount of oxygen.

Venous Blood Oxygen Content

A portion of the oxygen carried in arterial blood is given up to the tissues to meet metabolic needs, which leaves a lower oxygen content in the venous blood that returns to the right heart and lungs. This mixed venous oxygen content ($C\bar{v}_{O_2}$) depends on arterial oxygen content and the balance between tissue oxygen consumption ($\dot{V}_{O_2}$) and blood flow ($\dot{Q}$). It is described by the Fick equation (Eq. 5-11), which states that the volume of

oxygen consumed per minute is equal to the cardiac output times the content of oxygen removed from each unit volume of blood (Table 5-8).

$$\dot{V}_{O_2} = \dot{Q} \times (Ca_{O_2} - C\bar{v}_{O_2}) \qquad \text{(5-11; Fick equation)}$$

An increased oxygen demand in the face of a constant blood flow requires more oxygen be extracted from each portion of that blood, leaving a lower venous content and an increased arterial-venous (a-$\bar{v}$) oxygen content difference. Alternately, an increased blood flow in the face of a constant metabolic demand yields a decreased (a-$\bar{v}$) oxygen difference.

The mixed venous partial pressure of oxygen ($P\bar{v}_{O_2}$) is determined by the venous oxygen content and the oxygen dissociation curve. The venous oxygen content and P_{O_2} vary in the blood that returns from different capillary beds, depending on the matching of blood flow to metabolic demand. For example, blood that leaves exercising muscle may have a very low venous oxygen content, whereas the kidneys have high blood flow and relatively little oxygen extraction. After these flows combine in the right heart, the mixed venous (designated by the symbol $\bar{v}$) content reflects total body oxygen extraction.

Carbon Dioxide Transport

As the blood passes through the lung, carbon dioxide equilibrates with the alveolar gas, so the arterial P_{CO_2} is very close to alveolar P_{CO_2}. The alveolar P_{CO_2}, and hence arterial P_{CO_2}, is determined by the balance between alveolar ventilation and carbon dioxide production. Under normal conditions, arterial P_{CO_2} is regulated near 40 mmHg with an arterial carbon dioxide content related to partial pressure in a nonlinear fashion, normally 47 mL/100 mL.

The venous carbon dioxide is determined by the arterial carbon dioxide content and the relationship between blood flow and carbon dioxide production, again described by the Fick principle. With a typical RQ of 0.8, a resting oxygen consumption of 250 mL/min is associated with a carbon dioxide production of 200 mL/min, and a cardiac output of 5 L/min requires the loading of an additional 4 mL/100 mL of carbon dioxide into the systemic venous blood. This increase to a venous carbon dioxide content of 51 mL/100 mL occurs with only a modest rise in mixed venous partial pressure to a $P\bar{v}_{CO_2}$ of 46 mmHg.

TABLE 5-7 Normal Arterial Oxygen Content

Parameter	Value
Arterial partial pressure of O_2	90–100 mmHg
Arterial saturation of O_2	97%
Hemoglobin (Hb) content	15 g/100 mL
O_2 carrying capacity of Hb	1.39 mL/g Hb
Arterial O_2 content	O_2 bound to Hb plus dissolved O_2 = $(15 \times 1.39 \times 0.97) + (0.003 \times 100)$ = 20.2 + 0.3 mL/100 mL = 20.5 mL/100 mL

TABLE 5-8 The Fick Equation, $\dot{V}_{O_2} = \dot{Q} \times (Ca_{O_2} - C\bar{v}_{O_2})$

Parameter	Symbol	Typical Normal Values at Rest
Oxygen consumption	$\dot{V}_{O_2}$	250 mL/min
Cardiac output	$\dot{Q}$	5 L/min
Difference between arterial and mixed venous oxygen content	$Ca_{O_2} - C\bar{v}_{O_2}$	50 mL/L blood (or 5 mL/100 mL blood)
Arterial oxygen content	Ca_{O_2}	200 mL/L blood (or 20 mL/100 mL blood)
Mixed venous oxygen content	$C\bar{v}_{O_2}$	150 mL/L blood (or 15 mL/100 L blood)
Mixed venous partial pressure of oxygen	$P\bar{v}_{O_2}$	~40 mmHg

Carbon Dioxide Dissociation Curve

The overall relationship between carbon dioxide content (Cco_2) and Pco_2 is curvilinear, as indicated in Figure 5-6, but the curve is essentially linear over the limited range between arterial and venous Pco_2 (40–46 mmHg). Although the quantity of carbon dioxide exchanged is similar to that of oxygen (as governed by the RQ), this narrow range of arterial-to-venous Pco_2 is made possible by the steepness of the carbon dioxide dissociation curve. Oxygenation of Hb decreases its ability to carry carbon dioxide (the Haldane effect), which facilitates the unloading of carbon dioxide at the lung, whereas the opposite effect occurs at tissues. This shift between the dissociation curves of venous and oxygenated blood increases the effective slope of the carbon dioxide curve (as shown in the inset in Figure 5-6). The ability to load or unload carbon dioxide with minimal change in Pco_2 helps to minimize the change in pH between arterial and venous blood.

Carbon Dioxide Storage in Blood

Carbon dioxide is stored in physical solution and in chemical combination with Hb, but, in addition, a major portion of the carbon dioxide is stored in the blood as bicarbonate (HCO_3^-). The blood stores of carbon dioxide are greater than those of oxygen, and, because bicarbonate is also present in the extravascular interstitial fluid, the body stores of carbon dioxide are much greater than those of oxygen. Thus, with a change in ventilation or if breathing ceases (apnea or asphyxia), the carbon dioxide level changes much more slowly than does that of oxygen.

Because the solubility of carbon dioxide is more than 20 times that of oxygen, a greater content of carbon dioxide is carried in physical solution at physiologic partial pressures (see Table 5-6), normally 2.9 mL/100 mL, representing approximately 6% of the total amount of carbon dioxide carried in arterial blood.

Carbon dioxide binds with Hb to form carbamino compounds and also, to a small extent, it binds with other proteins. At a normal arterial Pco_2, carbamino binding of carbon dioxide amounts to approximately 2.1 mL/100 mL blood, or 4% of the total carbon dioxide content. Formation of carbamino compounds tends to weaken the Hb-oxygen affinity (the Bohr effect). Conversely, as Hb binds oxygen, there is a decrease in carbamino compound formation (the Haldane effect). These interactions assist in the appropriate loading and unloading of oxygen and carbon dioxide in the lungs and tissues. Even though carbamino binding makes up a small part of the blood carbon dioxide storage, it undergoes a relatively large change between venous and arterial blood, so that it accounts for more than 25% of the carbon dioxide loaded in tissue and unloaded at the lung.

By far the major storage of carbon dioxide in blood is in the form of bicarbonate ion. In blood, carbon dioxide combines with water to form carbonic acid, which then dissociates to form hydrogen ion and bicarbonate ion. The first reaction is slow unless catalyzed by carbonic anhydrase (CA), present in the red cell and other tissues

$$CO_2 + H_2O \overset{CA}{\Longleftrightarrow} H_2CO_3 \Longleftrightarrow H^+ + HCO_3^- \qquad \text{(5-12)}$$

The whole-blood bicarbonate concentration of carbon dioxide is equivalent to approximately 42 mL/100 mL at a normal arterial Pco_2, with most of that in the plasma. This is approximately 90% of the total amount of carbon dioxide stored in the arterial blood.

As shown in Figure 5-7, carbon dioxide is carried in plasma as dissolved carbon dioxide or as bicarbonate and is carried inside red cells as dissolved carbon dioxide, bicarbonate, or carbamino compounds. The formation of bicarbonate in the red cell is extremely rapid because of the presence of carbonic anhydrase. Hydrogen ions formed are buffered by Hb, which shifts the Hb-O_2 curve to the right and thus enhances oxygen release. As a result of the high concentration of bicarbonate formed, some bicarbonate diffuses out into the plasma and, to maintain charge neutrality, chloride diffuses into the cell. The uncatalyzed formation of bicarbonate extracellularly is extremely slow. Thus, even though most blood carbon dioxide content is carried as plasma HCO_3^-, the red cell plays a very important role in facilitating its interconversion to and from diffusible gas and in buffering the associated hydrogen ions.

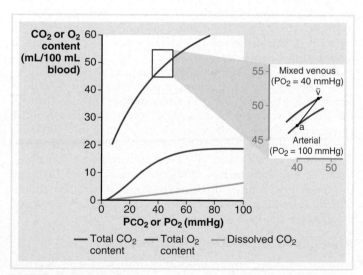

FIGURE 5-6 Curve of carbon dioxide content versus Pco_2 is steeper than the hemoglobin-oxygen curve, shown for comparison. It includes carbon dioxide bound to hemoglobin plus bicarbonate (the largest fraction) and dissolved carbon dioxide. *Inset,* Increasing the Po_2 decreases the carbon dioxide content for any Pco_2 (Haldane effect). As the blood shifts between the oxygenated and the deoxygenated curves, the functional steepness (i.e., $\Delta Cco_2/\Delta Pco_2$) between the arterial point and mixed venous point is increased. (Modified with permission from Hlastala MP: Blood gas transport. In Culver BH, ed: The respiratory system. Seattle: University of Washington Publication Services; 2006.)

ALVEOLAR-ARTERIAL OXYGEN EQUILIBRATION

In the discussion of alveolar ventilation, the factors that determine the average alveolar Po_2 of the lung were shown to be the inspired Po_2 and the relationship of alveolar ventilation to oxygen consumption. In an ideal cardiorespiratory system, the arterial blood would be perfectly equilibrated with the alveolar Po_2, but even normal individuals fall somewhat short of this; thus, an alveolar-arterial difference in Po_2 [$P(A-a)O_2$] occurs. With lung disease or circulatory abnormalities, $P(A-a)O_2$ may become quite wide. The three factors involved in

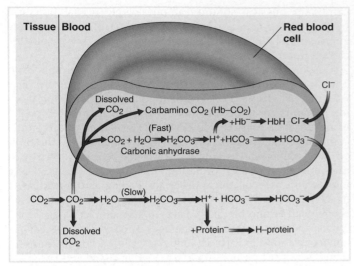

FIGURE 5-7 Uptake and storage of carbon dioxide. In the pulmonary capillaries, all the reactions and diffusions are reversed. Modified with permission from Hlastala MP: Blood gas transport. In Culver BH, ed: The respiratory system. Seattle: University of Washington Publication Services; 2006.

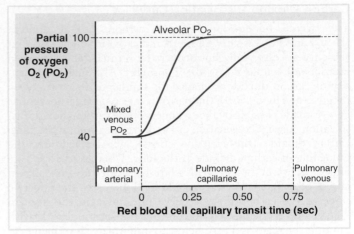

FIGURE 5-8 Mixed venous blood equilibrates to the alveolar Po_2 level by diffusion during transit through the pulmonary capillaries. Even when the diffusion rate is abnormally slow (*blue line*), the blood may be fully oxygenated within the normal transit time. Based on data from Wagner PD, West JB: Effects of diffusion impairment on O_2 and CO_2 time courses in pulmonary capillaries. J Appl Physiol 1972; 33:62–71.

alveolar-arterial equilibration are diffusion, shunt, and ventilation-perfusion matching.

Diffusion

Oxygen moves from alveolar gas to arterial blood by a passive process of diffusion from higher to lower partial pressure. The flux of a gas across a membrane is equal to a coefficient called the diffusion capacity (D_L) times the partial pressure gradient, which in the case of the lung is between alveolar gas and capillary blood. In the gas phase, diffusion is proportional to the inverse of the square root of the molecular weight (i.e., smaller molecules move faster). In a liquid, diffusion is proportional to solubility divided by the square root of the molecular weight. In the lung, diffusion also depends on the nature and length of the diffusion pathway and the total surface area available for diffusion, which reflects the effective alveolar capillary bed. The total diffusion capacity of the lung is made up of two components:

- Diffusion through the alveolar membrane itself
- Effective resistance of the red cell plus the process of chemical combination with Hb

The average red blood cell spends approximately 0.75 sec in the alveolar capillaries (i.e., the capillary transit time). With a normal diffusion capacity, enough oxygen crosses the membrane to bring the red cell Hb to equilibrium with the alveolar Po_2 in 0.25 sec or less. A diffusion abnormality slows the rate at which oxygen crosses, but usually sufficient time reserve is available for the red cell to be fully oxygenated by the time it leaves the capillary (Figure 5-8). Only when the diffusion capacity is severely limited (e.g., < 25% of normal) or the transit time is markedly shortened is it likely that blood leaving the alveolar capillaries will have a Po_2 lower than that of the alveolar gas. Thus, a diffusion abnormality, although present in many diseases, is very rarely the physiologic cause of a low Pao_2 at rest. If diffusion limitation for oxygen exists when breathing air, it may be virtually eliminated by breathing

oxygen, because the very high driving pressure of oxygen in alveolar gas increases the rate of equilibration. Thus, on 100% oxygen ($Pao_2 \approx 670$ mmHg) it can be arbitrarily stated that diffusion limitation makes no contribution to any $P(A-a)o_2$.

Although it may not indicate the physiologic reason for hypoxemia, it is often useful to measure the diffusion capacity of the lung to help establish the condition of the alveolar-capillary membrane (i.e., the alveolar surface area and capillary blood volume). Because it is technically difficult to estimate the back pressure of capillary Po_2 (it is changing, of course, from Po_2 to Pao_2), the clinical measurement of diffusion capacity is established with carbon monoxide. The test is described in Chapter 9.

Carbon dioxide also moves from blood to alveolus by diffusion. Although it is a larger molecule, diffusion in a liquid is proportional to solubility, so carbon dioxide diffuses through the alveolar wall more readily than oxygen by a factor of 20. However, the transfer of carbon dioxide out of the blood also depends on chemical reaction rates (remember that much carbon dioxide is carried as HCO_3^-, which must be converted, again by CA, into carbon dioxide). As a result of this, and the much lower initial driving pressure difference for carbon dioxide unloading, the equilibration rates between blood and alveolus are similar for carbon dioxide and oxygen.

Alveolar-Arterial Oxygen Difference

Because the lung is not a single unit, but consists of approximately 300 million alveoli, one might expect variation from one region to the next. All alveoli do not receive the same amount of ventilation ($\dot{V}_A$) or perfusion ($\dot{Q}$), and neither is the matching of ventilation to blood flow ($\dot{V}_A/\dot{Q}$) the same for each alveolus; because of this, gas partial pressures vary from one alveolus to the next. A diffusion limitation, if it exists, would create a difference between the alveolar gas partial pressure and that in the capillary blood leaving it, which would lead directly to a measured alveolar-arterial oxygen difference. In considering ventilation-perfusion abnormalities and shunt, it is assumed that each capillary is in complete equilibrium with the alveolus that it passes, but the subsequent mixture of blood from different areas of the lung results in an arterial P_{O_2} less than the value calculated for alveolar P_{O_2}, that is, a positive $PA_{O_2} - Pa_{O_2}$, or a $P(A-a)_{O_2}$ difference.

Shunt

Shunt refers to blood that passes from the systemic venous to arterial system (i.e., right to left) without going through gas-exchange areas of the lung. Some normal shunting of blood always occurs as a result of the bronchial arterial blood that drains to the pulmonary veins after having perfused and given up oxygen to the bronchial tissues and a small amount of coronary venous blood, which drains directly into the cavity of the left ventricle through the thebesian veins. An abnormal shunt may occur through congenital defects in the heart or blood vessels, or more commonly through areas of atelectasis or consolidation in the lung. For example, if one lung collapses but continues to receive half the cardiac output, deoxygenated blood mixes with oxygenated blood (Figure 5-9) to cause a marked reduction in the oxygenation of the arterial blood. Note that because of the shape of the Hb-O_2 dissociation curve, the final P_{O_2} is much closer to that of the shunted blood than to that leaving well-ventilated units.

If a patient who has a 50% shunt breathes 100% oxygen, the alveolar gas equation shows that the PA_{O_2} in well-ventilated units increase to approximately 670 mmHg, but this causes only a small increase in the content of oxygen in the blood that leaves them. The shunt blood continues to have the mixed venous content (which will be slightly higher if tissue oxygen extraction, $C[a-\bar{v}]_{O_2}$, remains constant). The mixed arterial blood remains somewhat hypoxemic, with a very large $P(A-a)_{O_2}$ difference.

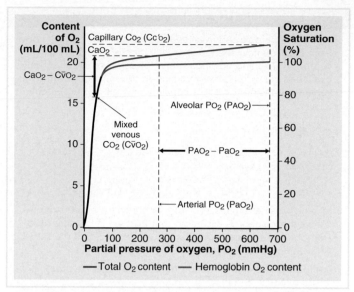

FIGURE 5-10 Analysis of right-to-left shunt in a patient who is breathing 100% oxygen. In this example, shunt fraction is 20% of cardiac output, so the arterial oxygen content (Ca_{O_2}) represents the mixture of one part venous blood and four parts fully oxygenated blood from alveolar capillaries. Breathing 100% oxygen, the P_{O_2} of well-ventilated alveoli is approximately 670 mmHg; the content in capillary blood leaving them is shown as Cc'_{O_2}. A normal $Ca_{O_2}-C\bar{v}_{O_2}$ difference gives the mixed venous content shown. With a 20% shunt, the arterial blood content (Ca_{O_2}) is one fifth of the distance from Cc'_{O_2} to $C\bar{v}_{O_2}$ on the vertical axis. Projecting horizontally gives the Pa_{O_2} associated with this content. Modified with permission from Culver BH, ed: The respiratory system. Seattle: University of Washington Publication Services; 2006.

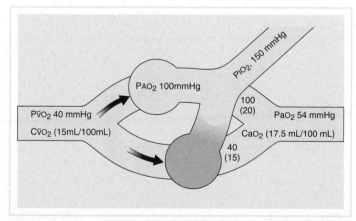

FIGURE 5-9 Shunt is blood flow not exposed to alveolar gas. To find the P_{O_2} of the mixed arterial blood (Pa_{O_2}), the relative blood flow (50:50 in this example) and oxygen *content* (shown in parentheses) contributed by each side must be considered; that is, Ca_{O_2} = (shunt fraction × mixed venous content) + (nonshunt fraction × ventilated capillary content). After determining the content (or percentage saturation) of the mixture, the resultant Pa_{O_2} can be found from the hemoglobin-oxygen dissociation curve. (In this example, $Ca_{O_2}-C\bar{v}_{O_2}$ has narrowed to 2.5 mL/100 mL, which implies an increase in cardiac output. If this does not occur, $C\bar{v}_{O_2}$ must drop below 15 and the final Pa_{O_2} will be lower than shown.) Modified with permission from Culver BH, ed: The respiratory system. Seattle: University of Washington Publication Services; 2006.

The effect of shunt can also be visualized graphically from the Hb-O_2 dissociation curve (Figure 5-10). Because Hb is fully saturated above a Pa_{O_2} of 150 mmHg, the additional content results from dissolved oxygen and is linearly related to P_{O_2}. Thus, a fixed relationship exists in this range between an increasing shunt fraction (movement of Ca toward C$\bar{v}$ on the vertical axis) and a decreasing Pa_{O_2}. For a normal $C(a-\bar{v})_{O_2}$ value of 5 mL/100 mL, this calculates as a fall in P_{O_2} of approximately 20 mmHg below the alveolar value for each 1% shunt. This rule of thumb is useful to estimate shunt fraction from arterial blood gas values obtained while breathing 100% oxygen. Plotting the appropriate points on Figure 5-10 also shows why the same normal shunt of approximately 5% causes a $P(A-a)_{O_2}$ of 10–15 mmHg while breathing air, but one of approximately 100 mmHg on 100% oxygen.

If $C\bar{v}_{O_2}$ is measured directly, the shunt fraction can be more accurately calculated from the shunt equation (Table 5-9). The impact of any given shunt fraction on arterial oxygenation is greater if $C\bar{v}_{O_2}$ is abnormally low, as in a low cardiac output state.

Shunt also has an impact on carbon dioxide elimination. Blood flowing through a R-L shunt does not unload CO_2, so in the 50% example shown in Figure 5-9, the expected mixed venous P_{CO_2} of approximately 46 in the shunted blood would increase the arterial level, unless ventilatory adjustments were made. However, this is easily corrected. If the ventilation in the normal alveoli increases enough for their P_{CO_2} to decrease

TABLE 5-9 Shunt Calculation

The oxygen transported in arterial blood is considered to come from two sources: shunt flow ($\dot{Q}s$) with mixed venous oxygen content ($C\bar{v}o_2$) and nonshunt flow (total flow minus shunt flow, or $\dot{Q}_T - \dot{Q}s$), with an oxygen content in equilibrium with well-ventilated alveoli ($Cc'o_2$ for capillary oxygen content), hence:

$$\dot{Q}_TCao_2 = \dot{Q}sC\bar{v}o_2 + (\dot{Q}_T - \dot{Q}s)Cc'o_2$$

Algebraic manipulations yield:

$$\dot{Q}_TCao_2 = \dot{Q}sCvo_2 + \dot{Q}_TCc'o_2 - \dot{Q}sCc'o_2$$
$$\dot{Q}sCc'o_2 - \dot{Q}sCvo_2 = \dot{Q}_TCc'o_2 - \dot{Q}_TCao_2$$
$$\dot{Q}s\,(Cc'o_2 - Cvo_2) = \dot{Q}_T(Cc'o_2 - Cao_2)$$
$$\dot{Q}s/\dot{Q}_T = (Cc'o_2 - Cao_2)/(Cc'o_2 - Cvo_2)$$

Cao_2 and $C\bar{v}o_2$ are measured from appropriate blood samples; $Cc'o_2$ is obtained by assuming that $Pc'o_2 = Pao_2$ calculated from the alveolar gas equation ($Pio_2 - Pco_2/R$) or, if the subject is breathing 100% oxygen, only ($Pio_2 - Pco_2$).

To truly calculate shunt fraction the subject must be breathing 100% oxygen. If the measurements are made breathing air or any fraction of inspired oxygen other than 1.0, the "shunt" calculated is termed venous admixture (or "physiologic shunt") because it includes any contribution of low V/Q areas as well as diffusion limitation. The calculation answers the question: if the observed reduction in Pao_2 were entirely caused by shunt, how large would that shunt have to be? Thus, for example, a calculation of 10% venous admixture in a patient breathing air might be caused by a 10% true shunt, or by a larger volume of blood flowing through low V/Q areas, or to some combination of true shunt, low, and high V/Q areas.

---

to 34, the final arterial mixture would have a normal Pco_2 of 40. (Unlike oxygen, the relationship of CO_2 content and partial pressure is nearly linear in this range.) To some extent this adjustment may occur automatically, because ventilation unable to reach closed or filled alveoli is diverted to the open units. Any tendency for arterial Pco_2 to rise would stimulate respiratory centers to increase ventilation further. Where this problem manifests clinically is in patients who are unable to increase their minute ventilations because of disease or because their ventilation is determined by a fixed mechanical ventilator rate.

Ventilation-Perfusion Abnormalities

The average ratio of ventilation to perfusion ($\dot{V}A/\dot{Q}$) in the lung is approximately (4.0 L/min)/(5.0 L/min), that is 0.8, but this average derives from alveoli with $\dot{V}A/\dot{Q}$ ratios ranging from near zero (unventilated) to near infinity (unperfused). In the normal lung the regional distribution of blood flow is influenced by the vascular branching pattern, gravity, and other factors resulting in more perfusion being directed to the dorsal, caudal lung regions and less to the cephalad regions. A number of mechanical factors cause ventilation to be greater in the dorsal, caudal region as well. However, the difference in perfusion from the bottom to the top of the lung is greater than the difference in ventilation. Accordingly, the ratio of ventilation to perfusion is low in the bottom of the lung and high at the top of the lung. Because the matching of ventilation and perfusion varies, the Pao_2 and $Paco_2$ also vary in different areas of the lung. In lung diseases, the scatter of $\dot{V}A/\dot{Q}$ around the mean ratio may be much greater than normal.

For alveolar gas in individual alveoli, groups of alveoli, or regions of lung, the partial pressures of O_2 and CO_2 are determined by the balance of influx and efflux of each gas, respectively. Thus, with a decrease in ventilation (or an increase in perfusion), the $\dot{V}A/\dot{Q}$ ratio of an alveolus is decreased, which causes Pao_2 to fall. That is, when ventilation is low relative to the amount of blood flow that carries oxygen away, more oxygen molecules must be extracted from each unit of incoming air, the local Pao_2 falls, and as it does, progressively less oxygen is loaded onto the perfusing blood until a new local steady state is reached.

The normal balance of ventilation and oxygen uptake causes the Po_2 to fall from 150 mmHg in inspired air to 100 mmHg in ideally ventilated and perfused alveoli. As the $\dot{V}A/\dot{Q}$ ratio falls toward zero (near shunt), the Pao_2 falls toward the mixed venous value (approximately 40 mmHg), and $Paco_2$ rises toward its mixed venous value (approximately 46 mmHg). Accordingly, with $\dot{V}A/\dot{Q}$ ratios below normal, any Pao_2 from 100 down to 40 mmHg is possible (whereas $Paco_2$ values are in the range of 40-46 mmHg). This range of possible values can be displayed on a Po_2–Pco_2 graph (Figure 5-11). The specific $\dot{V}A/\dot{Q}$ ratio in a given lung unit and the rise in oxygen content in the capillaries leaving that unit determine the extraction of oxygen from inspired air, which, in turn, determines the magnitude of the drop in Po_2 from inspired air to alveolar air. The blood perfusing low $\dot{V}A/\dot{Q}$ alveoli equilibrates with these lower levels of Pao_2 and leaves with lower-than-normal oxygen content. When this blood mixes downstream with blood coming from normal alveoli, the resulting mixture of contents causes arterial hypoxemia (Figure 5-12).

Figure 5-13 shows that, unlike shunt, if the inspired Po_2 is raised even moderately, the Pao_2 in these poorly ventilated alveoli rises sufficiently that the hypoxemia is eliminated (although $P[A-a]O_2$ is still large). If a patient with a low ratio of $\dot{V}A/\dot{Q}$ is placed on 100% oxygen, the inert gas nitrogen is washed out of the alveoli and blood. (Even if alveoli are very poorly ventilated, the nitrogen is washed out by means of the blood perfusing them and subsequently eliminated by more functional units.) Once this occurs, oxygen, carbon dioxide, and water are the only gases left in the lung, and their partial pressure must add up to P_B (if not, more gas is drawn in from the airways,

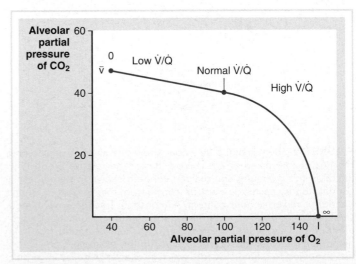

FIGURE 5-11 Spectrum of alveolar Po_2 and Pco_2 values possible as ventilation/perfusion ratio ($\dot{V}/\dot{Q}$) ranges from zero to infinity. The values follow a line from the mixed venous point ($\bar{v}$) to that representing inspired gas (I).

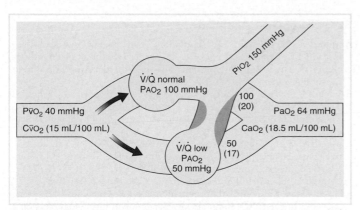

FIGURE 5-12 In alveoli with a low ventilation/perfusion ratio ($\dot{V}/\dot{Q}$), the alveolar P_{O_2} (PA_{O_2}) is low as more oxygen is removed from the incoming air. In this example, the $\dot{V}/\dot{Q}$ ratio has been arbitrarily chosen to result in a PA_{O_2} of 50 mmHg, and blood flow is equally divided. The mixture of contents (shown in parentheses) yields a PA_{O_2} well below normal.

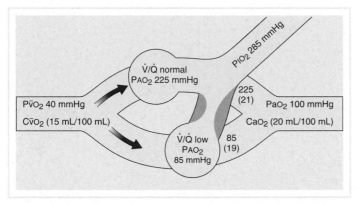

FIGURE 5-13 Effect of increased fraction of inspired oxygen (FI_{O_2}) when low ventilation/perfusion ($\dot{V}/\dot{Q}$) alveoli are present. Ventilation and perfusion are identical to the example in Figure 5-12, but the FI_{O_2} has been increased to 0.4, which results in a normal arterial P_{O_2}. Unlike the case with the shunt, the added oxygen increases the P_{O_2} in both low and normal $\dot{V}/\dot{Q}$ areas. (The drop in P_{O_2} from inspired to alveolar air on the obstructed side [285 − 85 = 200 mmHg] is now twice as large as it was breathing air, because it takes twice as much oxygen to raise the blood content from 15 to 19 versus 15 to 17 mL/100 mL; this is also seen to a smaller extent on the normal side.)

or the alveolus shrinks). If the uptake of oxygen by blood is faster than the inflow of oxygen through a severely obstructed bronchiole (e.g., $\dot{V}_A/\dot{Q}$ <0.1), the alveoli do shrink and eventually collapse in a process known as "absorption atelectasis" after which they behave as shunt—one reason to avoid the use of 100% oxygen. Because PA_{H_2O} is fixed at 47 mmHg and PA_{CO_2} cannot exceed $P\bar{v}_{CO_2}$, the Pa_{O_2} of any open alveolus is more than 650 mmHg no matter how low its $\dot{V}_A/\dot{Q}$ ratio falls. Thus, on 100% oxygen the effect of abnormal $\dot{V}_A/\dot{Q}$ ratios on the equilibration of mixed arterial blood with alveolar P_{O_2} is completely eliminated; that is $\dot{V}_A/\dot{Q}$ mismatching no longer, contributes to the observed $P(A-a)_{O_2}$ difference.

If an alveolus is unperfused (e.g., vessels blocked by an embolus), no oxygen can be removed or carbon dioxide added to it. With less severe underperfusion (or overventilation), the $\dot{V}_A/\dot{Q}$ ratio rises toward infinity and the alveolar gas values approach that of inspired gas (P_{O_2} = 150, P_{CO_2} = 0 mmHg; see Figure 5-11). Note that a high $\dot{V}_A/\dot{Q}$ abnormality (Figure 5-14)

does not cause hypoxemia; in fact, it would tend to increase Pa_{O_2} (but not very much, because the oxygen content is only slightly increased and the reduced blood flow from these alveoli is greatly outweighed by that from an equal number of normal alveoli). Carbon dioxide excretion from the high $\dot{V}/\dot{Q}$ portion of the blood flow is increased, which gives a lower end-capillary Pc_{CO_2} (and a proportionately lower content), but again, because blood flow is small, this has only a modest effect on the overall Pa_{CO_2}. In terms of the ventilation, this is inefficient gas exchange, because the ventilation going to the high $\dot{V}/\dot{Q}$ units carries away less carbon dioxide per liter, and thus the overall ventilation must increase to maintain homeostasis. These alveoli then contribute to physiologic dead space or "wasted ventilation."

Disease processes may cause both low and high $\dot{V}_A/\dot{Q}$ areas simultaneously, possibly with a normal overall mean $\dot{V}_A/\dot{Q}$. However, the shape of the Hb-O_2 curve shows that little oxygen content is added as the P_{O_2} increases above 100, so the blood from these high $\dot{V}_A/\dot{Q}$ units is unable to compensate for the drop in oxygen content contributed by the low $\dot{V}_A/\dot{Q}$ areas. In addition, by definition, less blood comes from high $\dot{V}_A/\dot{Q}$ units than from an equal volume of low $\dot{V}_A/\dot{Q}$ units. Thus, even a process that results in both high and low $\dot{V}_A/\dot{Q}$ areas results in arterial hypoxemia.

Abnormal $\dot{V}_A/\dot{Q}$ relationships also interfere with the elimination of carbon dioxide, but an elevation of Pa_{CO_2} is not commonly seen in such patients, because the normal response to a rising Pa_{CO_2} is to increase overall ventilation. This increases the carbon dioxide excretion in both high and low $\dot{V}/\dot{Q}$ areas, which brings Pa_{CO_2} back to normal. The increase in ventilation also increases Pa_{O_2} somewhat, which improves the oxygen content of blood that leaves low $\dot{V}/\dot{Q}$ alveoli, but does little for that of high $\dot{V}/\dot{Q}$ areas. The net result of this ventilatory response is to normalize Pa_{CO_2} and improve, but not fully correct, Pa_{O_2}.

Arterial Hypoxemia

Arterial hypoxemia (i.e., a low Pa_{O_2}) can result from one or more of five physiologic mechanisms summarized in Table 5-10. Two of these lower Pa_{O_2}, but do not contribute to the calculated $P(A-a)_{O_2}$ difference. The remaining three mechanisms all act to lower Pa_{O_2} below PA_{O_2} and therefore widen $P(A-a)_{O_2}$.

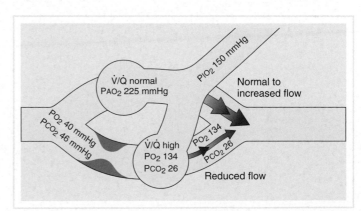

FIGURE 5-14 Gas exchange in high ventilation/perfusion ($\dot{V}/\dot{Q}$) alveoli. In this example, blood flow is reduced to approximately one fourth normal. (The missing blood flow must be shifted elsewhere, which affects the ratio of "normal" alveoli.) In the high $\dot{V}/\dot{Q}$ alveoli, P_{O_2} is increased and arterial P_{CO_2} decreased. (The specific values are for illustration only; as a result of the interaction of $\dot{V}/\dot{Q}$ and blood gas contents, these values are most easily obtained from tables or nomograms.)

TABLE 5-10 Physiologic Mechanisms of Hypoxemia

Decreased alveolar partial pressure of oxygen (P_{AO_2}); normal alveolar minus arterial difference ($P_{AO_2} - Pa_{O_2}$)

Decreased P_{IO_2}:
  Lower atmospheric pressure (P_{ATM}) with normal fraction of inspired oxygen (F_{IO_2}) (e.g., high altitude)
  Lower F_{IO_2} with normal P_{ATM} (e.g., iatrogenic)

Alveolar hypoventilation:
  $P_{AO_2} = P_{IO_2} - Pa_{CO_2}/R$ (e.g., depressed respiratory drive)

Increased $P_{AO_2} - Pa_{O_2}$

Diffusion limitation—blood leaving an alveolus fails to reach equilibration with alveolar gas; rarely significant as a cause of clinical hypoxemia

Ventilation/perfusion ($\dot{V}/\dot{Q}$) mismatching—specifically, the low $\dot{V}_A/\dot{Q}$ areas cause hypoxemia by contributing blood with reduced content to the arterial mixture

Shunt—the extreme of low $\dot{V}/\dot{Q}$; shunt flow of deoxygenated blood has no contact with alveolar gas

On 100% oxygen ($F_{IO_2} = 1.0$), only the shunt mechanism contributes to the $P_{AO_2} - Pa_{O_2}$ difference. Breathing air or on any $F_{IO_2} < 1.0$, both shunt and low $\dot{V}/\dot{Q}$ areas (plus any diffusion limitation) contribute to the $P_{AO_2} - Pa_{O_2}$ difference. This combined effect is termed *venous admixture* and has also been called *physiologic shunt*.

SUGGESTED READINGS

Anthonisen NR, Fleetham JA: Ventilation: Total, alveolar and dead space. In Fahri LE, Tenney SM, eds. Gas Exchange, Handbook of Physiology, section 3. The Respiratory System, Vol. 4. Bethesda: American Physiological Society; 1987:113–130.

Baumann R, Bartels H, Bauer C: Blood oxygen transport. In Fahri LE, Tenney SM, eds. Gas Exchange, Handbook of Physiology, section 3. The Respiratory System, Vol. 4. Bethesda: American Physiological Society; 1987:147–172.

Klocke RA: Carbon dioxide transport. In Fahri LE, Tenney SM, eds. Gas Exchange, Handbook of Physiology, section 3. The Respiratory System, Vol. 4, Bethesda: American Physiological Society; 1987:173–197.

Lucangelo U, Blanch L: Dead space. Intens Care Med 2004; 30:576–579.

Rahn H, Fahri LE: Ventilation, perfusion and gas exchange—The $\dot{V}_A/\dot{Q}$ concept. In Fenn WO, Rahn H, eds. Handbook of Physiology, section 3. Respiration, Vol. 1. Washington: American Physiological Society; 1964.

Wagner PD, Laravuso RB, Uhl RR, West JB: Continuous distribution of ventilation-perfusion ratios in normal subjects breathing air and 100% O_2. J Clin Invest. 1974; 54:54–68.

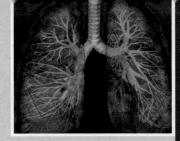

6 Pulmonary Circulation

BRUCE H. CULVER • JONATHAN E. SEVRANSKY • ROY G. BROWER

The lungs are served by two circulations—the pulmonary circulation, which accommodates the entire cardiac output from the right heart through a low-pressure circulation, and the bronchial circulation, which arises from branches off the aorta with systemic pressures and usually carries less than 1% of the cardiac output.

CIRCULATORY STRUCTURE

Pulmonary Circulation

The pulmonary arteries lie near and branch with the airways in the bronchovascular bundle. They are much thinner than systemic arteries and have, proportionately, more elastic tissue in their walls. The walls of the arterioles (diameter < 100 μm) are so thin, relative to their systemic counterparts, that fluid and gas can move across them. Within the gas-exchanging zone, the arterioles give rise to a network of pulmonary capillaries in the alveolar walls that is continuous throughout the lungs. They are so numerous that, when distended, blood flows almost as an unbroken sheet between the air spaces (Figure 6-1). "Sheet flow" reduces vascular resistance and optimizes gas exchange. When the transmural pressure difference between the inside and outside of the vessels is low, many of the capillary segments are closed, but flow switches frequently as some open and others close. Nonflowing segments are rapidly recruited into the pulmonary vascular bed as needed to accommodate increased flow and may be further distended by an increase in transmural pressure. A red cell that follows a capillary path from the pulmonary artery to a vein may cross several alveoli, with the average transit time through the vessels engaged in gas exchange calculated to be approximately 0.75 sec. The capillaries unite to form larger alveolar microvessels, which become venules and then veins that run between the lobules toward the hila, where upper and lower pulmonary veins from each lung empty into the left atrium.

Bronchial Circulation

The bronchial arteries arise directly from the aorta or from intercostal arteries to supply the walls of the trachea and bronchi and also to nourish the major pulmonary vessels, nerves, interstitium, and pleura. Extensive small-vessel anastomoses occur between these (systemic) vessels and both the precapillary and postcapillary pulmonary vasculatures. The bronchial veins from the larger airways and hilar region drain through the systemic veins (particularly the azygos system) into the right atrium. However, bronchial flow to the intrapulmonary structures connects to the pulmonary circulation and drains through the pulmonary veins into the left atrium. This small contribution of desaturated blood contributes to the normal (2–5%) anatomic shunt, which may become increased when the bronchial circulation hypertrophies to supply inflammatory and neoplastic lesions. The bronchial circulation has a role in the regulation of temperature and humidity in the airways and supplies the fluid for secretion through the airway mucosa.

Lymphatic Circulation

Pulmonary lymphatics are not found in alveolar walls but originate in interstitial spaces at the level of the respiratory bronchioles and at the pleural surface, then follow the bronchovascular bundles to the hila. The lymph flows through the right lymphatic duct and the thoracic duct into the right and left brachiocephalic veins. The total flow from the lungs is quite low under normal conditions (< 0.5 mL/min in experimental animals) but can increase many fold with pulmonary edema. The lymphatics have valves to prevent backflow and can generate sufficient pressures to maintain flow when systemic venous pressure is as high as 20 cmH$_2$O.

CIRCULATORY PHYSIOLOGY

The pulmonary circulation conducts the entire cardiac output with a remarkably low driving pressure between the pulmonary artery (mean Ppa = 15–20 mmHg) and the left atrium (Pla = 7–12 mmHg). Like the airways, the branching pattern of vessels leads to an increase in total cross-sectional area as the alveolar vessels are approached, but (unlike the airways) this increase is not associated with a decrease in resistance. Total cross-sectional area increases at a branching point if the number of daughter branches (n) is greater than the ratio of the parent-to-daughter radii squared, $(a/b)^2$, but resistance decreases only if n is greater than $(a/b)^4$. The latter case occurs in the peripheral airways but not in the vessels, so although small peripheral airways contribute little to normal airflow resistance, pulmonary microvessels make up a substantial portion of vascular resistance. Efforts to partition the pressure drop longitudinally suggest that approximately 20–30% is in the arterial portion (including arterioles), 40–60% in the microvascular portion, and the remainder in the veins. With increases in flow, recruitment occurs mainly at the microvascular level, so their relative contribution to resistance becomes less.

Pulmonary vascular resistance, R, is calculated as transvascular driving pressure, ΔP (mean upstream Ppa minus mean downstream Pla), divided by the flow, $R = \Delta P / \dot{Q}$. The calculated resistance must be interpreted in the context of flow because the relationship of driving pressure to flow is usually not linear and does not pass through zero. As shown in Figure 6-2, pulmonary vascular resistance decreases as flow and pressure increase with the attendant recruitment and distention of vessels.

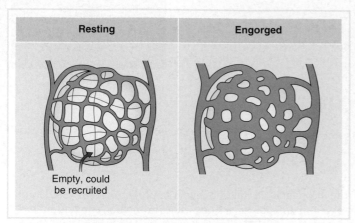

FIGURE 6-1 Alveolar capillaries. The normal cardiac output requires only a portion of the sheet of capillaries; any remaining vessels can be recruited when cardiac output rises during exercise. (Modified with permission from Butler J: The circulation of the lung. In Culver BH, ed: The respiratory system. Seattle: University of Washington Publication Services; 2006: 8.2.)

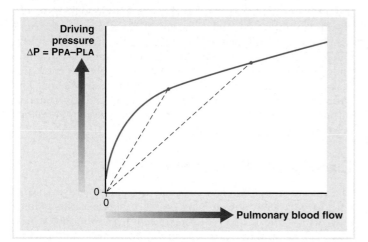

FIGURE 6-2 Driving pressure across the pulmonary circulation (mean pulmonary artery pressure [P_{PA}] minus mean left atrial pressure [P_{LA}]) increases nonlinearly with cardiac output. Resistance, represented by the slope from the origin to any point on the line, decreases with increased pulmonary blood flow, which reflects recruitment and distention of vessels.

The resistance to flow through a vessel increases with its length, with the viscosity of the fluid, and, most importantly, with the inverse of the radius to the fourth power. In addition to muscle activity in the wall, the caliber of a distensible vessel depends passively on the transmural pressure difference between intravascular and extravascular pressure. This is particularly important in the lungs, where the vessels are embedded in expandable parenchyma. It is convenient to consider separately the effect of lung expansion on the extraalveolar arterial and venous vessels, which differs from the effect on the microvessels of the alveolar zone. With lung volume increase, extraalveolar vessels are distended as the pressure is lowered in the expanding perivascular space around them (Figure 6-3), and they are elongated as the lung expands.

By contrast, the alveolar microvessels in the alveolar walls are elongated but partially collapsed by lung inflation, because the alveolar pressure that surrounds them tends to increase relative to the intravascular pressure. This is easy to recognize

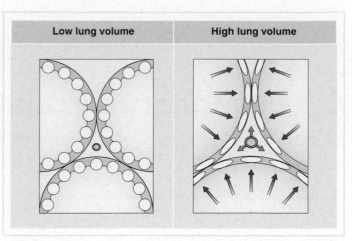

FIGURE 6-3 Lung volume affects alveolar and extraalveolar vessels differently. At high lung volume, alveolar microvessels are stretched and compressed as vascular pressures fall relative to alveolar pressure. Extraalveolar vessels, however, tend to be expanded as the pressure surrounding them decreases. (Modified with permission from Butler J: The circulation of the lung. In Culver BH, ed: The respiratory system. Seattle: University of Washington Publication Services; 2006: 8.4.)

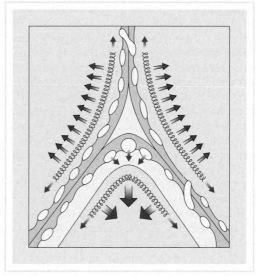

FIGURE 6-4 Alveolar "corner" at the junction of three alveolar walls. Surface tension (depicted by springs) holds vessels open, particularly in corners, and promotes fluid transudation by lowering the pressure around vessels. (Modified with permission from Butler J: The circulation of the lung. In Culver BH, ed: The respiratory system. Seattle: University of Washington Publication Services; 2006: 8.5.)

with positive-pressure ventilation, but it also occurs with spontaneous inspiration, because intravascular pressures fall relative to atmospheric and alveolar pressure. The sheets of capillaries in the alveolar walls are protected from the full compressive force of the alveolar pressure by the surface tension of the fluid that lines curved portions of the alveolar surface. Microvessels in the corners, where alveolar walls meet, are more fully protected from compression by the sharper curvature of the surface film and perhaps by local distending forces, analogous to the extraalveolar vessels (Figure 6-4). The pulmonary vascular resistance is the sum of that through alveolar and extraalveolar vessels and thus has a complex relationship with lung volume. It is lowest at approximately the normal resting lung volume (functional residual capacity) but increases at higher and lower volumes.

BLOOD FLOW DISTRIBUTION

Anatomy and gravity influence the distribution of blood flow within the lung. If the upright lung is viewed as a stacked series of slices, a vertical gradient occurs in which the average flow of the slice rises progressively down the lung, largely influenced by gravity. However, within each slice, a marked variability of blood flow is found among regions, with high-flow areas distributed dorsally. The tendency of blood flow to be higher in dorsal and basal regions is largely preserved even when the gravitational direction is opposite, which indicates that anatomic branching patterns are a major determinant of flow distribution.

The gravitational effect has been conceptualized by dividing the lung into four zones, one above another, on the basis of the relationship of vascular and alveolar pressures (Figure 6-5). Intravascular pressures are higher at the bottom of the lung than at the top by an amount equal to a vertical hydrostatic column as high as the lung. Near the lung apex, zone I, the pressure in the alveoli (PA) exceeds that in both the pulmonary arteries (Ppa) and pulmonary vein (Ppv) and collapses the alveolar vessels, except those in the alveolar corners, which remain patent and allow flow to continue. Below this, in zone II, Ppa exceeds PA, but PA is greater than Ppv, so flow depends on the pressure difference between Ppa and PA. The vessels remain open but are critically narrowed at the downstream end, where venous pressure is lower than alveolar pressure. This creates independence of flow from the downstream venous pressure, analogous to a waterfall in which a stream that flows over a precipice is unaffected by a rising level in the pool below until it rises above the level of the lip. In the mid to lower portion of the lung, zone III, both Ppa and Ppv exceed PA, the vessels are distended, and blood flow is the

highest. Zone IV is restricted to a small area in the most dependent region where flow diminishes. It has been postulated that this reduction is the result of increased vascular resistance because of low lung volume or perivascular edema in this area.

Although the gravitational effect expressed in the vertical zone concept contributes to the average increase in flow down the lung, it does not explain the observed large variability in flow within an isogravitational slice, which implies that other anatomic or vasoregulatory factors are important at this level. Rather than defined levels, these "zone" conditions may be dispersed within the lung on the basis of local microvascular pressure.

REGULATION OF PULMONARY BLOOD FLOW

Besides their responses to passive mechanisms (anatomy, gravity, lung volume, alveolar pressure), the pulmonary vessels show vasomotor activity as a result of both neural and nonneural factors. Motor efferents from three autonomic networks are in anatomic proximity to the vasculature—sympathetic, parasympathetic, and nonadrenergic noncholinergic fibers. The sympathetic efferents probably have little effect, whereas parasympathetic stimulation dilates constricted vessels. Although acetylcholine is a potent pulmonary vasodilator, there is little cholinergic innervation of the pulmonary resistance vessels. The nonadrenergic noncholinergic system is inhibitory, constantly releasing small vasodilatory peptides at the ganglia and postganglionic ends of its unique network. This vasodilator function is augmented with exercise.

Pulmonary arteries demonstrate an intrinsically low tone as they remain relaxed when isolated from the lung. This represents a balance of endothelium-derived vasoconstrictor and vasodilator substances. Although their relative roles are yet to be clarified, many vasoactive peptides are found in the lung. Those having vasoconstrictor activity on the pulmonary circulation include angiotensin II, arginine vasopressin, endothelin 1, peptide tyrosine Y, and substance P. Vasodilatory peptides include adrenomedullin, atrial natriuretic peptide, calcitonin gene–related peptide, endothelin 3, somatostatin, and vasoactive intestinal peptide.

Nitric oxide is produced in endothelial cells in the pulmonary circulation and elsewhere and is now recognized as an important mediator of vasodilatation. The oxidation of a nitrogen from L-arginine is catalyzed by nitric oxide synthase, present in both a constitutive form and a form that is inducible by products of inflammation. Nitric oxide activates guanylate cyclase, which increases cyclic guanosine monophosphate within vascular smooth muscle cells. This, in turn, reduces intracellular Ca^{++} by several mechanisms, leading to vascular relaxation. Nitric oxide is also abundantly produced in the nasal sinuses, providing an intriguing mechanism whereby inhaled nitric oxide may enhance blood flow to the best-ventilated areas of lung.

Although the role of nasal nitric oxide in ventilation-perfusion matching is still speculative, the role of alveolar hypoxia in vasoregulation has been recognized for more than 50 years, but the mechanisms involved are still uncertain. The arterioles constrict when the P_{O_2} in the alveoli they serve falls, and additional vasoconstriction results if alveolar P_{CO_2} rises (Figure 6-6). This hypoxic vasoconstriction seems to be a response to a low P_{O_2} in the air spaces rather than in the intraluminal blood, which is

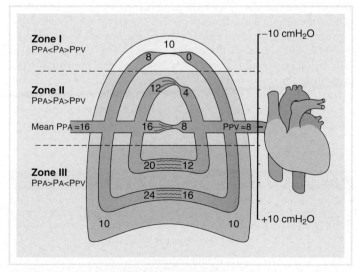

FIGURE 6-5 Perfusion in the lungs is influenced by the relationship of arterial and venous pressures to alveolar pressure. In this example, the alveolar pressure is 10 cmH_2O, as might be found in a patient who receives positive pressure ventilation. (Modified with permission from Culver BH: Hemodynamic monitoring: physiologic problems in interpretation. In Fallat RJ, Luce JM, eds: Cardiopulmonary critical care. Edinburgh: Churchill Livingstone, 1988.)

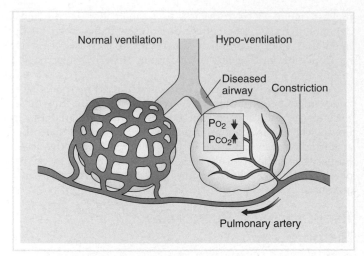

FIGURE 6-6 Hypoxic vasoconstriction reduces blood flow to poorly ventilated areas. This improves V̇/Q̇ matching and oxygenation but, if generalized, contributes to pulmonary hypertension. (Modified with permission from Butler J: The circulation of the lung. In Culver BH, ed: The respiratory system. Seattle: University of Washington Publication Services; 2006: 8.7.)

normally desaturated in these prealveolar vessels. The site and mechanism of this local signal pathway are unclear, but the microvascular endothelium seems to be necessary to signal the constriction of the more proximal arteriolar smooth muscle. Current interest is focused on potassium channels and their role in regulation of membrane potential. When ventilation is decreased by an obstructed airway or other injury, local hypoxic pulmonary vasoregulation decreases blood flow to the affected region, which tends to restore the local ventilation-perfusion (V̇/Q̇) ratio toward normal and thereby improve the P_{O_2} of the blood flowing through that area. The diverted blood flow can be directed to better-ventilated regions, which further contributes to an improvement in overall matching.

Considerable individual variability is found in the hypoxic vasoconstrictor response, and it may be diminished by vasodilating drugs. Diversion of blood flow is most effective in atelectatic areas of lung, in which hypoxic vasoconstriction is unopposed by the radial traction of surrounding expanded lung tissue. A reciprocal reflex in the airways also contributes to better matching, as small airways constrict when intraluminal P_{CO_2} falls and dilate when it rises. Hypoxic vasoconstriction is a helpful, adaptive response to local or regional lung abnormalities, but when alveolar hypoxia is generalized (e.g., hypoventilation or altitude), the increased resistance can lead to pulmonary hypertension.

NONRESPIRATORY FUNCTIONS OF THE PULMONARY CIRCULATION

Filtering

Aggregates of blood elements and emboli of various types (e.g., fat, air, particulate matter) carried in the systemic venous return are continually filtered out, dissolved, or engulfed by the cells of the pulmonary capillary bed. This is vital protection for the cerebral, coronary, and other systemic vascular beds. The small, potentially ischemic regions that may occur with larger emboli may receive limited perfusion by the bronchial circulation by means of bronchopulmonary anastomoses and may be exposed to oxygenated pulmonary venous blood that backflows into

the occluded region during tidal lung volume changes. Thus, ischemic damage to the alveoli is prevented while a thrombus is lysed and the pulmonary flow restored.

Large numbers of white cells (mainly polymorphonuclear leukocytes) are sequestered in the small vessels of the pulmonary bed. Many reticuloendothelial cells occur in the lung, and some evidence suggests that the vascular endothelial cell itself can be phagocytic when stimulated.

Modification of Mediators

Some mediators in the blood, which have regulatory functions throughout the body, are secreted, taken up, or inactivated through specific receptors and enzyme systems in the pulmonary endothelial cells. Best known is angiotensin-converting enzyme, which converts inactive angiotensin 1 into the systemic vasoconstrictor angiotensin 2. Histamine, bradykinin, serotonin, and acetylcholine are largely inactivated by the pulmonary endothelium in one passage through the lungs.

Coagulation

When local injury is present, pulmonary endothelial cells can be a source of thromboplastin and tissue plasminogen activator. Despite vascular stasis and closure of vessels when flow decreases, clots do not form in pulmonary vessels because of the structure of the endothelial surface and because the secretion of anticlotting substances bathes the surface and prevents the adherence of platelets and cells. Embolic thrombi are dissolved remarkably quickly by local thrombolytic secretions.

FLUID EXCHANGE IN THE PULMONARY CIRCULATION

The fluid flux across the pulmonary vascular endothelium is influenced by the same pressure relationship as in the systemic capillaries, summarized in the modified Starling equation (Table 6-1). The hydrostatic pressure in the pulmonary microvessels (Pmv) exceeds the interstitial hydrostatic pressure (Ppmv) outside the microvessels. This effect favors filtration. The interstitial tissue fluid protein osmotic pressure is probably approximately two thirds that in the vessel; thus, the net osmotic force is absorptive and inward. The components of this equation make it convenient to categorize abnormal fluid flux into the lung into two broad types: hydrostatic edema, when the primary abnormality is an increase in Pmv minus Ppmv, and permeability edema, when endothelial injury increases fluid conductivity across the membrane (incorporated

TABLE 6-1 The Starling Equation	
$F = Kf[(Pmv - Ppmv) - \sigma(pv - pt)]$	
Symbol	**Description**
F	Net fluid flux out of vessels
Kf	Permeability factor
σ	Reflection coefficient to oncotic agents
Pmv	Pressure in microvessels
Ppmv	Perimicrovascular pressure
pv	Osmotic pressure in vessels
pt	Osmotic pressure of tissues

into the permeability factor) and decreases the osmotic reflection coefficient and osmotic gradient. The terms *cardiogenic* and *noncardiogenic* are also commonly used for these two mechanisms of edema formation.

Fluid flux is sensitive to small intravascular or perivascular pressure changes. Intravascular pressure rises may originate downstream (left heart failure) or may follow overall vascular volume increments (overhydration) or displacement of blood from the systemic to the pulmonary vessels. Fluid is exchanged across the capillary walls, but the interstitial space around alveolar microvessels is tightly restricted by the collagen network between the alveolar walls. The two alveolar epithelial layers and the contained capillary bed form an inexpansible sandwich, so leakage is limited. The extraalveolar arterioles and venules, which are not so confined and are also very thin walled, may be an additional important site of fluid leakage.

Surface tension in the fluid film that lines the alveoli opposes alveolar pressure and tends to lower the interstitial pressure around pulmonary microvessels, particularly in corner areas (see Figure 6-4). An increase in surface tension may contribute to edema when surfactant is lost in an injured lung. Interstitial pressure around the extraalveolar vessels is close to intrathoracic (pleural) pressure and falls as the lungs are distended, which favors relatively more leakage from them at high rather than low lung volumes (see Figure 6-3).

Interstitial Edema

Normally, a net outflow of fluid from the upstream capillaries is reabsorbed into the downstream capillaries, where the intravascular pressure is lower.

Several factors tend to keep the lung from becoming edematous. Fluid leakage causes local perivascular pressures to rise, particularly in the "sandwich" between the alveolar walls, which reduces the outward fluid flux. It may also compress the vessels, which reduces the total surface available for leakage. Because the fluid that leaks through intact endothelium is largely protein free, it dilutes and washes out the interstitial protein. This reduces the perivascular osmotic pressure of tissues and thus increases the inward osmotic pressure difference and reduces the local fluid leak. If excess leakage does occur, the fluid moves from the alveolar walls, where it could interfere with gas exchange, into the low-pressure interstitial zones around the bronchovascular bundles, where it forms relatively innocuous venous, arterial, and peribronchial cuffs. This fluid may be absorbed in part by the rich bronchial vascular network and by the many lymphatics in the adventitia of the airways and vessels. Edema fluid may also reach the pleural space, where it is absorbed by the pleural lymphatic and blood vessels. Finally, experimental data suggest that all the blood perfusing the capillaries in alveolar walls must first pass through capillaries located in alveolar corners and that the negative interstitial pressure surrounding these corner capillaries (and, accordingly, the transmural pressure) is critically dependent on alveolar surface tension. When surface tension is eliminated by alveolar flooding, interstitial pressure around these vessels increases, thus serving to compress the corner vessels and diminish flow through the capillaries in the alveolar wall of these flooded alveoli. This mechanism provides for much more precise control of perfusion, virtually on an alveolus-to-alveolus basis, compared with the effects of alveolar hypoxia, which are directed to much more proximal vessels.

When the capillary endothelium is injured, locally or through the effect of circulating mediators, the vascular permeability to fluids and solutes is increased so that even a modest outward pressure gradient causes a large fluid leak. The ability to retain large molecules is lost, protein-rich plasma leaks out, and the osmotic pressure in tissues approaches that in vessels, so that the osmotic force opposing intravascular hydrostatic pressure is lost. This high-permeability or "leaky capillary" edema can be a fulminant process and lead to severe abnormalities of gas exchange.

Alveolar Edema

The epithelial cells that line the air spaces have tight junctions along their apical surface, so this membrane is normally much less permeable than the endothelial membrane, protecting alveolar spaces as interstitial edema increases. After total lung water has increased by approximately 50%, the edema fluid appears in the alveoli. A structural failure, at the epithelial cell junctions or elsewhere, is suspected, because there is no protein gradient between interstitial and alveolar edema fluid. Fluid is initially seen only in the corners of the alveoli, where the pressure below the curved fluid film is lowest. As more fluid accumulates, the alveoli rapidly become completely filled, again because of surface tension effects. As alveoli fill, the radius of the curvature of the meniscus of the fluid becomes shorter, and the effect of surface tension becomes greater (Laplace's law), which pulls fluid in more strongly (Figure 6-7). Thus, the sequence of edema development progresses from the perimicrovascular interstitium to peribronchovascular "sump" to patchy alveolar flooding.

Fluid and ions normally exchange across the bronchial and alveolar epithelial surfaces to regulate the character of the mucous blanket and maintain the subphase film beneath the surfactant that lines the alveoli. Alveolar edema can be cleared by an active process of sodium reabsorption with water after osmotic transport. The type II epithelial cells take in sodium through channels on their apical surface and move it by active Na^+,K^+-ATPase pumping on the basolateral surfaces into the interstitium. The type I cells seem to have similar, though less prominent, apparatus and, because they make up 95% of the surface, might have a significant role. This has not been demonstrated, however, because type I cell culture models are lacking. Fluid removal may also occur in distal airways where epithelial and Clara cells actively transport sodium.

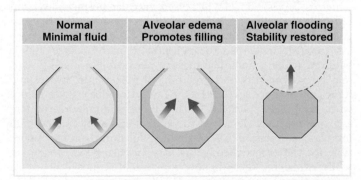

Normal Minimal fluid	Alveolar edema Promotes filling	Alveolar flooding Stability restored

FIGURE 6-7 Alveoli tend to fill with fluid in an "all-or-none" fashion. In the normal alveolus, a small amount of fluid rounds off the corners. Alveolar edema decreases the radius, which increases the inward force of surface tension and pulls in more fluid. When the alveolus is filled, the radius of the surface increases, so stability is regained. (Modified with permission from Butler J: The circulation of the lung. In Culver BH, ed: The respiratory system. Seattle: University of Washington Publication Services; 2006: 8.11.)

These active mechanisms are also crucial in the initial clearance of fetal lung fluid at birth. In experimental models, fluid clearance from air spaces is enhanced by β_2-agonists and blocked by the antagonist propranolol.

High-Altitude Pulmonary Edema

Some individuals traveling or climbing to high altitudes have pulmonary edema develop that may be severe and life threatening. The mechanisms are becoming better understood and seem to involve both hydrostatic and permeability factors. The underlying abnormality in individuals who are susceptible to high-altitude pulmonary edema (HAPE) and who are subject to repeated episodes with repeated exposures is an exaggerated elevation of pulmonary artery pressure in response to hypoxia that is further increased by exertion. Susceptible individuals may have only slight elevations of Ppa at rest or during routine activities when breathing air at sea level but have a greater increase in response to exercise than control subjects do. In response to a hypoxic challenge, HAPE-susceptible subjects have a rise in Ppa that is threefold to fourfold higher than that of controls. At altitude, typically greater than 3000 m, Ppa in these individuals would be expected to rise rapidly in response to alveolar hypoxia and to increase further with the exertion that is common to mountaineering activities. Symptomatic edema develops more than 24 hours to a few days but rarely occurs after 5 days at altitude. The few hemodynamic measurements made under these circumstances have shown marked elevation of pulmonary artery systolic pressure, as high as 80–100 mmHg, but usually normal pulmonary arterial occlusion pressure. Thus, although high hydrostatic forces are involved, this is not a typical cardiogenic mechanism with elevation of left atrial pressure reflected into the pulmonary microvasculature. The site of hypoxic vasoconstriction is in small pulmonary arteries and arterioles, although there is some venoconstriction that could contribute to a pressure increase at the capillary level. It has been hypothesized that a heterogeneous distribution of the increased pulmonary vascular resistance might divert relatively high blood flow to low-resistance arterioles, increasing local microvascular pressure sufficient to cause the patchy edema pattern typically seen in radiographs of those with HAPE. Interestingly, bronchoalveolar lavage fluid obtained from climbers on Mt. McKinley and elsewhere with symptomatic HAPE has shown high levels of protein, which is consistent with increased vascular permeability, and red cells, suggesting further loss of barrier function. Because granulocytes and inflammatory markers are seen in only modest quantities and tend to appear later in the course, this is believed to be a noninflammatory permeability change. This may be explained by the stretching of pores under hydrostatic forces or, in more severe cases, by overt capillary stress failure with endothelial, epithelial, and basement membrane disruption, as experimentally described in rabbit lungs subjected to high intravascular pressure. Although the cellular mechanisms responsible for the exaggerated pulmonary vascular response are yet to be explained, there is now a plausible sequence of events leading to pulmonary edema in HAPE-susceptible individuals.

RESPIRATORY-CIRCULATORY INTERACTIONS

Spontaneous Breathing

The phasic changes of intrathoracic pressure and lung volume of the respiratory cycle alter the preload and afterload of the right and left heart, which interact to vary cardiac output and blood pressure with the respiratory cycle. The changes are modest during normal tidal breathing but can be more notable in pathologic states. During inhalation, the decrease in intrathoracic pressure enhances systemic venous return to the chest. The right atrium and ventricle fill, and right heart output to the pulmonary vessels increases as the alveoli fill with air. Lung expansion dilates the extraalveolar pulmonary arterial vessels, which reduces their resistance and helps to accommodate the increased flow. Ppa stays almost constant relative to PA. The increase in right ventricular volume tends to stiffen or compress the left ventricle within the common pericardium, but the surge of pulmonary flow reaches the left heart after two to three beats, so that systemic output and blood pressure begin to rise in late inspiration or early expiration. This preload effect is normally dominant, but the inspiratory drop in intrathoracic pressure can also add effective afterload to the left ventricle. When the pressure surrounding the heart is lower, the myocardium would have to generate a greater transmural pressure difference to maintain the same stroke volume and systemic arterial pressure. Accordingly, systemic blood pressure falls a few millimeters of mercury coincident with inspiration and rises a few millimeters of mercury during exhalation. Depending on the respiratory rate, this direct pressure effect may be enhanced or countered by the arrival at the left ventricle of the inspiratory surge of pulmonary flow.

When intrathoracic pressure swings are exaggerated, as occurs during an asthma attack or an exacerbation of chronic obstructive pulmonary disease, the inspiratory drop in blood pressure can be 20–30 mmHg, creating the clinical finding of pulsus paradoxus. Interestingly, such markedly negative inspiratory pressures do not generate a proportionate increase in systemic venous return because of a flow-limiting, or waterfall, mechanism in the central veins. When the intraluminal pressure falls in these intrathoracic veins, the vessels collapse at the point where they are first exposed to atmospheric pressure, in the neck, axilla, and abdomen, and their flow becomes independent of the increasingly negative downstream right atrial pressure.

When the pericardial space is limited (e.g., pericardial effusion, constrictive pericarditis, enlarged heart), the interaction between the two ventricles is more prominent. Inspiratory filling of the right heart limits the diastolic expansion of the left heart. This ventricular interaction contributes to an inspiratory decrease in systemic outflow and blood pressure and allows them to increase when the right heart is less full during expiration.

Positive-Pressure Ventilation

When patients are mechanically ventilated with positive inspiratory pressure, the same mechanisms seen in spontaneous breathing are involved, but the pressure effects shift phase in the tidal cycle. For example, the pressure outside the left ventricle rises during inspiration, so the same contraction yields a higher blood pressure early in the inspiratory phase. This may be augmented by blood pushed out of the capillaries by the positive alveolar pressure (see Figure 6-3). During late inspiration or early expiration, the blood pressure decreases as the effect of an inspiratory decrease in venous return to the right heart reaches the left side. If the expiratory phase is long enough, the blood pressure will begin to rise, reflecting enhanced venous return to the right heart earlier in expiration.

In addition to the cyclic changes, there are overall effects on cardiac output when spontaneous breathing is replaced by positive-pressure ventilation, particularly when positive end-expiratory pressure (PEEP) is added. The mean airway pressure and mean intrathoracic pressure are both high and the latter is reflected in the pressure outside the right heart. This, in turn, causes the right atrial pressure to be higher, which may decrease the pressure difference drives venous flow from the systemic capacitance vessels. In addition, the increase in lung volume may partially compress the inferior vena cava as it runs through the lung just above the diaphragm, thereby increasing resistance to venous return. A resultant decrease in cardiac output is typically seen, accompanied by a decrease in right atrial transmural pressure and a decrease in right ventricular end-diastolic volume, particularly if intravascular volume is low. This may be opposed by a rise in abdominal pressure as thoracic volume increases and by increased venous tone to help restore the driving pressure for venous return.

When an increase in end-expiratory lung volume is recruited by PEEP, the chest wall must also be passively expanded, and its pressure-volume relationship (see Figure 4-7) would predict at least a modest increase in pleural pressure. However, direct measurements with suitable flat devices show that when the lungs are distended with PEEP, the pressure in the cardiac fossa may rise more than that measured by an esophageal balloon, and the pressure in the pericardium may be still higher. Bedside measurements of a decreased cardiac output accompanied by a higher pulmonary arterial occlusion pressure may suggest a decrease in cardiac function or contractility, but when accurate measurements of juxtacardiac pressure or left ventricular end-diastolic volume are made, the ventricle is seen to be operating at a lower preload on the same function curve. The same phenomenon may be seen when patients with severe airflow obstruction develop dynamic hyperinflation with an associated increase in cardiac fossa pressure.

High levels of PEEP and of end-inspiratory alveolar pressure compress alveolar septal capillaries, outweighing any distention of extraalveolar vessels with the lung volume increase, and thus increase pulmonary vascular resistance and right ventricular afterload. If this effect becomes dominant, a decrease in cardiac output may be associated with an increase in right ventricular end-diastolic volume.

The increase in juxtacardiac pressure with PEEP decreases the stroke work the left ventricle must do to maintain any given systemic blood pressure, thus effectively decreasing left ventricular afterload. In most circumstances, the preload effect previously described dominates, but a failing ventricle is quite sensitive to afterload, and this effect becomes more important in patients with severe heart disease.

HEMODYNAMIC MONITORING IN CRITICAL ILLNESS

Many critically ill patients require frequent or continuous assessments to identify potentially life-threatening conditions and to guide the use of life-sustaining treatments. Hemodynamic monitoring devices aid clinicians in assessing circulatory function, arterial blood oxygenation, and oxygen delivery to systemic tissues. Devices used frequently in intensive care units include central venous catheters, pulmonary artery catheters, pulse oximeters, and systemic arterial catheters. The rationale for the use of each of these monitoring devices is reviewed in this section. Fine points and caveats for data interpretation are discussed.

Central Venous Catheters

A catheter placed in the superior vena cava allows measurement of central venous pressure (CVP), which is usually similar to right ventricular end-diastolic pressure. It may, accordingly, reflect right ventricular preload and, therefore, be used to estimate right ventricular end-diastolic volume (preload). Because both right and left ventricular end-diastolic volumes are primary determinants of stroke volume and cardiac output, CVP is sometimes useful in the assessment of patients with circulatory dysfunction. For example, a low CVP in a patient with hypotension suggests that vascular volume is inadequate and that administration of intravenous fluids or blood products may be appropriate. A high CVP in a patient with diffuse pulmonary infiltrates and hypoxemia may suggest volume overload or congestive heart failure and the need for diuretics and fluid restriction. Central venous catheters are also frequently necessary for the intravenous administration of vasoactive drugs and caustic infusates.

The reader is referred elsewhere for detailed instructions on the placement of central venous catheters. New evidence suggests that complications of placement can be minimized by use of maximal barrier precautions and chlorhexidine antisepsis and avoiding the femoral site. The most common sites of insertion of central venous catheters are the internal jugular vein and the subclavian vein. Under some circumstances, the external jugular, brachial, cephalic, and femoral sites are used.

Sites of Central Venous Catheterization

The decision of which vessel to cannulate should take into consideration the patient's clinical status, risk of infectious and mechanical complications, anatomy, and operator experience. The subclavian vein may be the preferred approach in a patient who is hypovolemic and has normal coagulation parameters. It is also the preferred site to minimize infectious complications. During cardiopulmonary resuscitation, the femoral site might be preferred while the airway is being secured. In patients with uncorrected coagulopathies, the cephalic, brachial, and femoral sites may be preferred, because they can be more easily compressed to reduce bleeding. If possible, the subclavian vein should be avoided in patients with hyperinflated lungs or bullae, which predispose to pneumothorax. In patients with ascites or elevated pleural pressures, a femoral CVP may not accurately reflect right atrial pressure. The risks and benefits of the different approaches to central venous access are compared in Table 6-2.

Complications of Central Venous Catheterization

All catheters represent potential sources of infection. To prevent catheter-related bloodstream infections, sterile procedure and maintenance techniques should be strictly followed. The femoral site is more prone to infectious complications and venous thrombosis than the subclavian site. Other complications of central catheters are often related to the site of insertion. The most frequent mechanical complications from internal jugular cannulation are carotid artery puncture, hematoma, and pneumothorax. With subclavian vein catheterization, patients are at risk for pneumothorax, subclavian artery puncture, hemothorax, and hematoma. Risks of femoral vein catheterization include femoral artery puncture, which may cause a retroperitoneal hematoma; an increased incidence of

TABLE 6-2 Advantages and Disadvantages of Major Routes of Access for Central Line Insertion

Site	Advantages	Disadvantages
Internal jugular	↓ Risk of pneumothorax Easily compressible Higher rate success with inexperienced operators	Landmarks may be obscured with intubated patient or patients who have a tracheostomy More difficult in hypovolemic patient ? ↑ Risk of infection
Subclavian	Consistent landmarks Patient comfort Most reliable access in hypovolemic patient	Noncompressible site May be higher risk of complications with inexperienced operators ↑ Risk of pneumothorax
Femoral	Easily accessed during cardiopulmonary resuscitation Compressible site No need for Trendelenburg	Difficult access in hypovolemic patient ? ↑ Risk of infection ? ↑ Risk of thromboembolism May be less effective for monitoring central venous pressure in some patients

catheter-related bacteremia; and venous thrombosis. All central venous catheters can cause venous thrombosis, but the clinical significance of these clots is not clear. Mechanical complications of central venous catheterization are included in Table 6-2.

The risk of complications, both mechanical and infectious, is directly proportional to the number of attempts at catheterization. In some studies, the incidence of complications was substantially higher when the procedures were performed by less experienced operators. As a general rule, operators who are unsuccessful at gaining access at a single site with two to three passes should attempt to obtain access from another site or seek assistance from a more experienced operator. Recent studies suggest that the use of real-time sonographic devices may minimize complications, especially for inexperienced operators, but the value of such devices for experienced operators is unclear. When attempts to obtain access by means of the subclavian or internal jugular route are unsuccessful, a chest radiograph should be obtained to rule out pneumothorax before attempting insertion on the contralateral site.

Limitations of Central Venous Pressure Monitoring

In many clinical situations, CVP does not accurately reflect left ventricular end-diastolic pressure and, therefore, cannot be used to estimate left ventricular preload. For example, a patient with pulmonary hypertension might have elevated CVP but normal or low left ventricular end-diastolic pressure and volume. In patients with acute left ventricular myocardial infarction, CVP may be modestly elevated, whereas left atrial and left ventricular end-diastolic pressures are severely increased, with radiographic and clinical evidence of pulmonary edema. In patients with ascites or elevated pleural pressures, the pressures measured in the femoral vein may not accurately reflect right atrial pressure. Moreover, changes in CVP frequently do not predict the changes in left heart pressures.

In more than 25% of patients with mitral valve disease, right atrial pressure is discordant with left atrial pressure. In some of these patients, fluid loading causes right and left atrial

pressures to diverge, and responses of right atrial pressure and left ventricular end-diastolic volume to pressor agents are inconsistent. Thus, in many critically ill patients, CVP may provide misleading information about left heart pressure and preload or response to therapy. Additional methods for evaluating cardiac filling pressures and function are frequently required.

Pulmonary Artery Catheters

In 1970, Swan and colleagues reported the development of a balloon-tipped flow-directed catheter to measure pulmonary artery pressure and estimate left ventricular end-diastolic pressure (Figure 6-8). The catheter was introduced through a central vein, such as the subclavian or internal jugular, and advanced through the chambers of the right heart into a medium-sized pulmonary artery. When positioned in a pulmonary artery and inflated, the small balloon at the catheter tip caused cessation of blood flow distal to the catheter, resulting in a stagnant column of blood from the pulmonary capillary bed to a confluence of medium-sized veins where flow was continuing. Thus, the pressure measured at the catheter tip immediately distal to the balloon-pulmonary arterial occlusion pressure (Ppao) reflected a pressure close to the left atrium and therefore could, under most circumstances, be used to estimate left ventricular end-diastolic pressure. Use of Ppao avoids some of the previously described limitations of CVP for assessing vascular filling and ventricular preload.

Several years after the introduction of the balloon-tipped flow-directed catheter, techniques were developed by which cardiac output could also be measured by means of a pulmonary artery catheter (PAC) by use of a modification of the catheter developed by Swan. Cooled fluid is injected through a separate channel of the catheter, exiting the channel through a side hole in the right heart. Blood temperature is monitored with a thermistor at the catheter tip. When the change in blood temperature is graphed against time, analysis of the area and shape of the curve allows a calculation of flow (cardiac output) between the sites of cool fluid injection and the thermistor at the distal catheter tip. With concomitant

FIGURE 6-8 Pulmonary artery catheter. **A,** Red channel for balloon inflation; blue channel to proximal port (for right atrial pressure and injectate); yellow channel to distal port (for measurement of pulmonary artery pressure and pulmonary capillary wedge pressure); bright yellow thermistor connection. **B,** Cross section of pulmonary artery catheter. Clockwise from left, thermistor wire, distal port channel, balloon channel, proximal port channel.

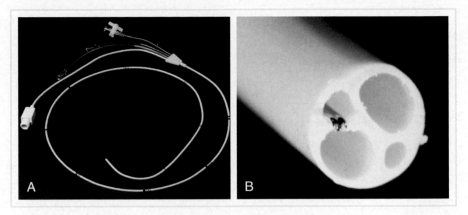

measurements of blood pressure, right and left atrial pressures, and arterial and mixed venous blood gases, the PAC allows the determination of systemic and pulmonary vascular resistance, systemic oxygen delivery, and oxygen extraction by systemic tissue. Since its development and introduction to clinical practice, the PAC has become an important part of the hemodynamic monitoring armamentarium of many intensivists.

Interpretation of Data

Several assumptions are required to use Ppao to estimate left ventricular end-diastolic volume (Figure 6-9). These assumptions pertain to two key questions: (1) How well does Ppao represent left ventricular end-diastolic pressure (see Figure 6-9, assumptions a, b, c, and d)? (2) How well does left ventricular end-diastolic pressure represent left ventricular end-diastolic volume (see Figure 6-9, assumptions e and f)? Intensivists must

consider these assumptions to avoid errors when reading Pcw tracings and interpreting their significance.

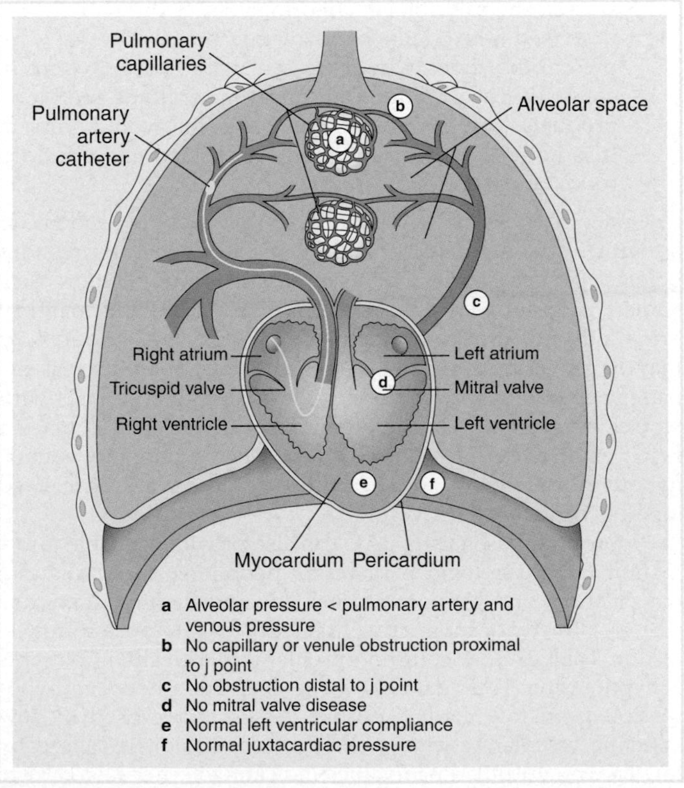

Some mechanically ventilated patients require high levels of PEEP or continuous positive airway pressure (CPAP) to improve oxygenation. This raises juxtacardiac pressure and tends to cause a misleading elevation in Ppao (see Figure 6-9, assumption f). To correct for this effect, some workers have advocated measuring Ppao approximately 1 sec after briefly disconnecting the ventilator from the endotracheal tube. However, this could cause hypoxemia from abrupt decreased alveolar derecruitment or could contribute to lung injury from repeated closing and reopening of small airways. Another approach is to assume that approximately 25% of the PEEP or CPAP is transmitted to the juxtacardiac pressure space and subtract this amount from the measured Ppao (after correcting for the difference in units, because PEEP and CPAP are reported in cmH_2O and Ppao is measured in mmHg). As a rule of thumb, this adjustment can be made by subtracting 25% of the PEEP or CPAP value from Pcw.

It is important to read the Ppao at end-expiration. This is the point in the respiratory cycle when the juxtacardiac pressure is closest to atmospheric pressure (regardless of the level of PEEP or CPAP; see Figure 6-9, assumption f). Identifying the point of end-expiration on the Ppao tracing is straightforward in patients breathing spontaneously, without positive pressure ventilatory assistance: the Ppao should be read immediately before the dip in pressure that signifies the beginning of inspiration (Figure 6-10, *A*). In patients receiving positive-pressure ventilation and who are making no inspiratory efforts of their own, end-expiration is easily identified on the Ppao tracing as the point immediately before the increase in pressure that accompanies the effects of positive pressure inspiration (see Figure 6-10, *B*). In patients who continue to make inspiratory efforts while receiving positive-pressure ventilation, the appearance of Ppao tracings is highly variable and often ambiguous. The patient's inspiratory effort usually causes a dip in Ppao, which may or may not be followed by a rise in Ppao from the effects of positive-pressure inspiration (see Figure 6-10, *C*). The size of the dip in Ppao in early inspiration and the subsequent rise in Ppao from ventilator pressure depend on the magnitude of the patient's effort in relation to the ventilator flow rate. In patients with vigorous inspiratory efforts, Ppao tracings resemble those of patients breathing spontaneously without positive-pressure assistance: the rise in Ppao because of ventilator assistance may not occur at all. Regardless of the magnitudes of these dips and rises in Ppao, it is critical to read Ppao at end-expiration. Reading Ppao at the wrong point in the cycle can lead to wrong treatment decisions.

a Alveolar pressure < pulmonary artery and venous pressure
b No capillary or venule obstruction proximal to j point
c No obstruction distal to j point
d No mitral valve disease
e Normal left ventricular compliance
f Normal juxtacardiac pressure

FIGURE 6-9 Assumptions required the use of capillary wedge pressure to estimate left ventricular preload.

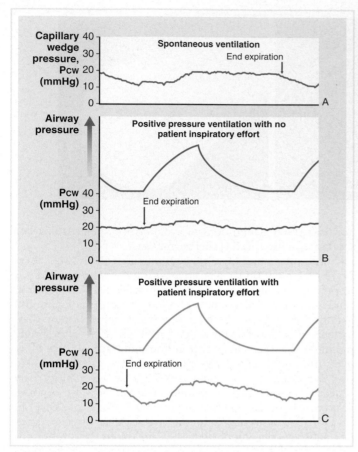

FIGURE 6-10 Representative capillary wedge pressure traces. **A,** Spontaneous ventilation; **B,** positive pressure ventilation with no patient inspiratory effort; and **C,** positive pressure ventilation with patient inspiratory effort.

The effect of left ventricular end-diastolic compliance must also be considered when interpreting a Ppao value (see Figure 6-9, assumption e). In a patient with normal left ventricular end-diastolic compliance, a Ppao of 12 mmHg may reflect ample diastolic filling. In contrast, in a patient with reduced diastolic compliance, as in hypertrophic cardiomyopathy, a Ppao of 12 mmHg may reflect inadequate end-diastolic volume.

When there is increased atrial filling during ventricular systole, as in mitral regurgitation, the Ppao tracing may show enlarged v waves (Figure 6-11). These may also appear in other conditions, such as mitral stenosis and hypervolemia. If the mean Ppao is read in the presence of large v waves, left ventricular end-diastolic pressure and diastolic filling may be overestimated. To avoid this error, the Ppao tracing should be read immediately before the start of the v wave, as close as possible to end-expiration. This usually appears around the time of the T wave during simultaneous electrocardiogram recordings.

Role of the Pulmonary Artery Catheter

Experienced physicians frequently have difficulty using common clinical and laboratory data to assess circulation in critically ill patients. This is especially true in patients requiring mechanical ventilation. Noninvasive techniques such as echocardiography are often not helpful in distinguishing among the different forms of shock.

In a study of patients in whom PACs were placed, attending intensivists and critical care fellows were correct in slightly

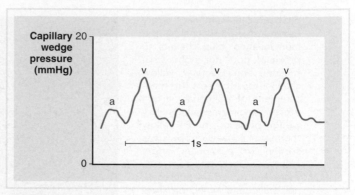

FIGURE 6-11 Proximal v waves in a capillary wedge pressure tracing.

more than 50% of their estimations of cardiac index, Ppao, and mean pulmonary artery pressure on the basis of their clinical assessments. Changes in therapy were made in almost half of the patients on the basis of information subsequently obtained from PACs.

In general, PACs should be considered when two conditions occur together:

1. Usual clinical observations and laboratory data are ambiguous with respect to the assessment of circulation, particularly in the presence of hypotension. For example, a patient may have hypotension and low urine output, suggesting low cardiac output from inadequate vascular volume. However, the same patient may also have clinical or radiographic findings consistent with pulmonary edema and diffuse pulmonary infiltrates, suggesting volume overload or cardiac dysfunction.

2. Consequences of the wrong treatment decision may worsen the physiologic abnormalities. If the patient just described were truly hypovolemic but a diuretic were prescribed, shock would worsen. If the patient were in congestive heart failure but intravenous fluids and blood products were given, pulmonary edema would worsen. It is necessary to carefully adjust preload and afterload to maximize cardiac output.

Under most other circumstances, it may be prudent to attempt a trial of therapy on the basis of clinical impressions before PAC placement. For example, in a young hypotensive patient with apparent sepsis, warm extremities, and marginal urine output, intravenous fluids followed by vasopressors may be prescribed. If improvement is not apparent or if the patient deteriorates over the next several hours, perhaps with worsening azotemia and hypotension, the decision to place a PAC can be reconsidered. In the absence of pulmonary edema, hypotension and low urine output should always be treated rapidly with additional volume.

Appropriate use of the PAC can also provide valuable information on physiologic parameters pertaining to circulation, oxygenation, and organ perfusion. Hemodynamic parameters that are directly or indirectly obtained with PACs are summarized in Table 6-3. A common problem in critically ill patients is hypotension. PAC data allow the distinction between hypotension from low cardiac output versus that caused by low systemic vascular resistance. When hypotension is caused by low cardiac output, Ppao values indicate whether low cardiac output is the result of inadequate preload or poor cardiac performance. Typical hemodynamic profiles in various shock

TABLE 6-3 Hemodynamic Equations and Normal Values

Parameter	Formula	Normal Values
Mean arterial pressure (MAP)	[(Diastolic pressure $\times$ 2) + systolic pressure]/3	10.6–13.3 kPa (80–100 mmHg)
Cardiac index (CI)	Cardiac output/body surface area	2.5–4.0 L/min/m^2
Stroke index (SI)	CI/heart rate	30–65 mL/beat/m^2
Systemic vascular resistance	[(MAP – Right atrial pressure) $\times$ 80]/Cardiac output	1200–1600 dyn . sec . cm^{25}
Pulmonary vascular resistance	{[Mean pulmonary arterial pressure (MPAP) – pulmonary capillary wedge pressure (Pcw)] $\times$ 80}/cardiac output	200–400 dyn . sec . cm^{25}
Left ventricular stroke work index	(MAP – Pcw) $\times$ SI $\times$ 0.0136	45–60 g/beat/m^2
Right ventricular stroke work index	(MPAP – central venous pressure) $\times$ SI $\times$ 0.0136	5–10 g/beat/m^2
Oxygen delivery	CI $\times$ 10 $\times$ Cao$_2$	500–750 mL/min/m^2
Arterial oxygen content (Cao$_2$)	1.34 $\times$ Hemoglobin $\times$ Sao$_2$ + [0.0031 $\times$ arterial partial pressure of oxygen (Pao$_2$)]	16–20 mL/dL
Mixed venous oxygen content (Cvo$_2$)	1.34 $\times$ Hemoglobin $\times$ Svo$_2$ + (0.0031 $\times$ Pao$_2$)	13–15 mL/dL
Difference between Cao$_2$ and Cvo$_2$	Cao$_2$ – Cvo$_2$	3.5–5.0 mL/dL
Oxygen consumption	(Cao$_2$ – Cvo$_2$) $\times$ CI $\times$ 10	100–175 mL/min/m^2

TABLE 6-4 Typical Hemodynamic Parameters of Shock

Cardiac Index	Pulmonary Capillary Wedge Pressure	Central Venous Pressure	Systemic Vascular Resistance	Diagnosis
↑	↓⇔	↓	↓	Distributive shock (e.g., septic shock, anaphylactic shock)
↓	↑	↑	↑	Cardiogenic shock
↓	↓⇔	↑	↑	Left ventricular myocardial infarction / Right ventricular myocardial infarction
↓	↓	↓	↑	Hypovolemic shock (e.g., massive gastrointestinal hemorrhage)
↓	↑	↑	↑	Extracardiac obstructive
↓	↓	↑⇔	↑	Tension pneumothorax
↓	↑	↑	↑	Massive pulmonary embolism / Pericardial tamponade

conditions are shown in Table 6-4. The PAC is frequently useful for guiding therapy with intravenous fluids and blood products, vasopressors, and inotropic drugs in patients with circulatory failure. The PAC can also be diagnostic of cardiac tamponade.

Complications of Pulmonary Artery Catheterization

As with any invasive procedure, PAC insertion can cause complications. These can be grouped into several categories. First, there are mechanical complications of vascular access, as outlined in Table 6-2. Second, there are mechanical complications of PAC placement, as outlined in Table 6-5. The third group of complications includes infections involving the insertion site, the catheter itself, and the tricuspid and pulmonic valves.

Finally, there are complications caused by the incorrect interpretation and use of PAC data.

Arterial Pressure Monitoring

Arterial pressure must be assessed frequently to identify life-threatening changes in circulatory status and to monitor the effectiveness of life-sustaining treatments, such as blood products and vasopressors. Traditional blood pressure assessment by sphygmomanometry is impractical in critically ill patients because of the time required for each measurement. Invasive blood pressure monitoring allows continuous measurement through an indwelling vascular catheter. Automated noninvasive techniques allow frequent blood pressure measurements with an inflatable pneumatic cuff wrapped around the upper or lower extremity.

TABLE 6-5 Complications of Pulmonary Artery Catheterization

Complication	Risk Factor for Complication	Measures to Avoid Complication
Arrhythmia	Catheter coiled in right ventricle Balloon not inflated while advancing	Familiarity with usual distance to wedged position Check balloon
Complete heart block	Left bundle branch block	Have transvenous or external pacer available
Balloon rupture	Overinflation	Check balloon prior to insertion Use only 1.5 mL air to inflate balloon
Pulmonary artery rupture	Inflation of balloon too distal Use of more than 1.5 mL air for inflation Catheter use during coronary artery bypass surgery during cold cardioplegia	Do not overwedge Use only 1.5 mL air to inflate balloon Remove pulmonary artery catheter to right atrium during coronary artery bypass surgery
Pulmonary infarction	Catheter tip too distal Prolonged balloon inflation	Check chest radiograph Always deflate balloon
Catheter-associated thrombosis and embolism	Prolonged catheterization	Remove catheter as soon as feasible
Infection	Prolonged catheterization	Remove catheter as soon as feasible Maximal barrier precautions during insertion
Valvular or papillary muscle damage	Knotting of catheter around papillary muscle Withdrawal of catheter with balloon inflated	Familiarity with usual distance to wedge position Deflate balloon prior to catheter withdrawal
Cardiac rupture	Myocardial infarction Stiff catheter Small ventricular chamber	Keep catheter tip out of right ventricle Remove catheter to right atrium during coronary artery bypass surgery

Invasive Arterial Pressure Monitoring

Measurement of arterial blood pressure by an indwelling vascular catheter is more accurate than other methods of measurement. Moreover, a graphic display of arterial pressure can be viewed in "real time" to provide diagnostic and therapeutic information that is not available with other techniques (Figure 6-12). Invasive pressure monitoring is of greatest value in conditions in which large changes in arterial pressure occur quickly, such as shock, or when intravenous vasodilators are used for hypertensive emergencies. Another advantage of invasive arterial pressure monitoring is that arterial blood gases can be drawn frequently through the catheter. This is especially important in patients with severe acid–base disorders or acute respiratory failure requiring mechanical ventilation.

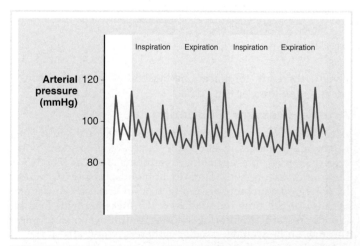

FIGURE 6-12 Arterial pressure tracing showing pulsus paradoxus. Systolic pressure falls by greater than 1.3 kPa (>10 mmHg) during inspiration.

Automated Noninvasive Blood Pressure Monitoring

This technique provides intermittent measurements of arterial blood pressure. An inflatable pneumatic cuff is wrapped around the upper arm and inflated to a pressure that exceeds arterial systolic pressure. The cuff pressure is then slowly deflated while pressure in the cuff is continuously monitored by the automated system. When cuff pressure decreases below arterial systolic pressure, oscillations in cuff pressure are created by the pulsations of arterial blood. Analysis of the pressures at which these oscillations begin, become maximal, and cease provides estimations of systolic, mean, and diastolic pressures.

Automated noninvasive blood pressure measurements can be obtained at frequent intervals, such as every 5 min. However, these pressure measurements are not as accurate as those obtained by an indwelling vascular catheter, especially when there is systemic vasodilatation, as in septic shock. Moreover, intermittent measurements of arterial pressure with noninvasive techniques do not provide graphic displays (see Figure 6-12).

Pulse Oximetry

Pulse oximetry provides a virtually continuous assessment and digital display of oxyhemoglobin saturation, which is one of the key determinants of oxygen delivery to systemic tissues. Light-emitting diodes are applied comfortably to the skin or fingernail. Light absorbance by oxyhemoglobin and reduced hemoglobin during arterial pulsations is compared with light absorbance between pulsations. This allows adjustments for absorbance by tissue, skin pigmentation, and capillary and venous blood. Because pulse oximeters are relatively inexpensive, noninvasive, and easily applied and usually provide useful data, they are widely used in the care of critically ill patients.

Several limitations of pulse oximetry are listed in Table 6-6. Pulse oximetry provides fairly accurate estimations of oxygen

TABLE 6-6 Factors that Affect Accuracy of Pulse Oximetry

Poor circulation (low cardiac output, vasoconstriction)
Low true oxygen saturation (< 90%)
Ambient light
Effects of nail polish, skin pigmentation
Carboxyhemoglobin and methemoglobin
Motion artifact

saturation when true oxygen saturation exceeds 90%. Some studies suggest 90% confidence limits of approximately ±4% for pulse oximetry values greater than 90%. However, the confidence limits increase substantially when pulse oximetry values fall below 90%. Thus, pulse oximetry values greater than 92% can usually be interpreted as "safe." Values below 92% should trigger additional investigations to confirm the accuracy of the pulse oximetry value.

CONTROVERSIES IN HEMODYNAMIC MONITORING

Health care workers are frequently tempted to adopt new methods of hemodynamic monitoring. The rationale for rapid and more accurate assessment of the circulatory status is compelling, and the aura of new technology is seductive. However, many new "advances" in monitoring entail risks to patients, and complications may outweigh any beneficial effects.

Although PACs have been used in critically ill patients for more than 25 years, it is not yet clear that patient outcomes improve with this monitoring technique; nor is it clear in which patients such monitoring is likely to be beneficial. Although some studies suggest that physicians' clinical assessments of circulatory status are frequently inaccurate and that information from PACs allows a beneficial redirection of treatment, other studies suggest that the use of PACs is associated with worse outcomes. Complications from PACs (see Table 6-5) may substantially reduce a patient's chance of recovery.

In a recent retrospective analysis of outcomes among critically ill patients, survival was significantly worse in patients in whom PACs were used on the first day in the intensive care unit than in those in whom PACs were not used. This study was notable in that the patient groups were carefully matched to avoid the confounding effects of uncontrolled variables such as age and severity of illness. This study strongly suggests that health care workers should reconsider the use of PACs. However, although this study demonstrated a clear association between PAC use and increased mortality, it did not prove a causal relationship. Although the risks of PAC insertion and use may outweigh the beneficial effects, other factors could have influenced the results of this study. For example, it is likely that some clinical information that triggered PAC insertion was not available to the investigators. If so, then the two groups would not have been matched for risk of death, tilting the table in favor of patients who did not receive PACs. Another explanation is that physicians with less critical care experience may be more likely to rely on information from PACs. PAC data may improve the outcomes in patients under the care of less experienced physicians. However, the same patients might fare better if cared for by more experienced physicians who are less reliant on technology.

Measurements from both pulmonary artery and central venous catheters have been used to optimize oxygen delivery in select patient subgroups. However, the use of PACs to reach supranormal physiologic goals has not led to improved outcomes in either critically ill patients in the medical intensive care unit or high-risk surgical patients. One study suggested that patients with severe sepsis and renal failure might benefit from early goal-directed therapy on the basis of central venous oxygen saturation on presentation to the emergency room.

Another controversial issue in hemodynamic monitoring is the optimal period to leave a vascular catheter in place before removing it. The risk of catheter-related infection increases substantially with the length of time a catheter remains in place, and each infection contributes substantially to intensive care unit length of stay, hospital cost, and mortality. Some policies require the removal of catheters after 3 days, replacing them in new sites if necessary. However, each new catheter placement involves risks, and the costs of catheter replacement are not trivial. In a recent study, the incidence of bloodstream infections and mechanical complications was compared in groups of patients randomly assigned to receive catheter replacements either every 3 days or when clinically indicated. As expected, frequent catheter reinsertion was associated with more mechanical complications such as pneumothorax. However, the incidence of bloodstream infection was not higher in patients whose catheters were changed only when clinical signs suggested infection. This study strongly suggests that the risks of new catheter placement outweigh the benefits of reduced infectious complications. However, the risks associated with catheter placement vary with the experience of the operator, and the likelihood of infectious complications may also vary with insertion and maintenance techniques. It is possible that different results would occur under different conditions.

SUGGESTED READINGS

Bartsch P, Mairbaurl H, Maggiorini M, Swenson ER: Physiological aspects of high-altitude pulmonary edema. J Appl Physiol 2005; 98: 1101–1110.

Baumgartner WA Jr, Jaryszak EM, Peterson AJ, et al: Heterogeneous capillary recruitment among adjoining alveoli. J Appl Physiol 2003; 95:469–476.

Bhattacharya J: Physiological basis of pulmonary edema. In Matthay M, Ingbar D, eds: Pulmonary edema. Vol 116 of Lenfant C, ed: Lung biology in health and disease. New York: Marcel Dekker; 1998.

Butler J, ed: The bronchial circulation. Vol 57 of Lenfant C, ed: Lung biology in health and disease. New York: Marcel Dekker; 1992.

Culver BH, Butler J: Mechanical influences on the pulmonary circulation. Ann Rev Physiol 1980; 42:187–198.

Glenny RW: State of the art: blood flow distribution in the lung. Chest 1998; 114:8S–16S.

Glenny RW, Bernard S, Robertson HT, Hlastala MP: Gravity is an important but secondary determinant of regional pulmonary blood flow in upright primates. J Appl Physiol 1999; 86:623–632.

Matthay M, Folkesson HG, Clerici C: Lung epithelial fluid transport and the resolution of pulmonary edema. Physiol Rev 2002; 82:569–600.

Tyberg JV, Grant DA, Kingma I, et al: Effects of positive intrathoracic pressure on pulmonary and systemic hemodynamics. Respir Physiol 2000; 119:163–171.

Ware LB, Matthay MA: Clinical practice. Acute pulmonary edema. N Engl J Med 2005; 353:2788–2796.

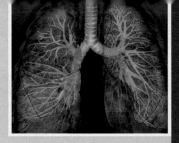

7 Acid–Base Balance and Control of Ventilation

BRUCE H. CULVER

ACID–BASE BALANCE

The respiratory system is closely interrelated to the acid–base status of the body because the carbon dioxide produced by tissue metabolism dissolves in water in the tissues or blood and becomes hydrated to form carbonic acid. In red blood cells, as well as some other cells of the body, the hydration reaction is greatly accelerated by carbonic anhydrase (CA) (Eq. 7-1).

$$\overset{CA}{CO_2 + H_2O \leftrightarrow H_2CO_3 \leftrightarrow H^+ + HCO_3^-} \tag{7-1}$$

Normal values for the components of the carbonic acid system are given in Table 7-1, and the quantitative relationship among them is expressed by the Henderson–Hasselbalch equation.

It is convenient to consider acids produced by the body to be of two types—carbonic acid from the preceding reaction and noncarbonic or metabolic acids such as phosphoric, sulfuric, and a variety of organic acids. Carbonic acid can be effectively removed or regulated through the lung as carbon dioxide, whereas the metabolic acids must be either excreted, primarily through the kidney, or metabolized. Changes in the carbonic acid component, which present as changes in Pa_{CO_2}, are termed respiratory acid–base abnormalities, and changes in the handling of metabolic acid or alkali result in metabolic acid–base derangements. On the basis of measurements of arterial pH, P_{CO_2}, and $[HCO_3^-]$, it is possible to quantify the clinical acid–base status of a patient in terms of a respiratory component, indicated by Pa_{CO_2}, and a metabolic component, reflected by changes in $[HCO_3^-]$.

From inspection of the reaction (see Eq. 7-1), it is apparent that an increase in P_{CO_2}, and thus in $[CO_2]$, drives the reaction to the right, which increases $[H^+]$ and leads to a respiratory acidosis, whereas a decrease in P_{CO_2} has the opposite effect, leading to a respiratory alkalosis. Similarly, the addition of H^+ from a metabolic source drives the reaction to the left, consuming HCO_3^- and creating additional carbon dioxide, which can be removed by ventilation. The magnitude of metabolic acidosis is reflected by the decrement in $[HCO_3^-]$. With an excess of a metabolic base, H^+ ions are removed from the right side of the equation, and the resultant shift of equilibrium causes $[HCO_3^-]$ to rise in relationship to the magnitude of the metabolic alkalosis. Understanding these relationships quantitatively requires a more detailed analysis and is further complicated in the body by the concurrent activity of other buffer systems.

Note that the concentration of hydrogen ions $[H^+]$ in body fluids is approximately a million times less than the concentration of other ions. Small changes in absolute $[H^+]$ can produce significant physiologic alterations, yet the body tolerates a wide range of relative activity. The range of viable arterial pH, from approximately 7.7–6.8, represents an eightfold change in $[H^+]$, from 20–160 nmol/L (and gastric $[H^+]$ is a million times higher).

Handling of Metabolic Acids

Metabolic (noncarbonic) acid or alkali is buffered by carbonic acid plus its salt, primarily sodium bicarbonate in extracellular fluid (ECF), as in Equation 7-2.

$$HCl + NaHCO_3$$
$$\Updownarrow$$
$$H^+ + HCO_3^- \leftrightarrow H_2CO_3 \leftrightarrow CO_2 + H_2O \tag{7-2}$$
$$+$$
$$NaCl$$

Some true chemical buffering occurs because the resultant carbonic acid is a weaker acid than the HCl added, but the major buffering in the body is physiologic, because virtually all the carbonic acid formed is excreted by the lungs under conditions of constant Pa_{CO_2}.

The effects of adding metabolic acid to water, to a bicarbonate solution, and to physiologic ECF are shown in Table 7-2. Quantitatively, if 12 mmol HCl is added to 1 L of water, it dissociates, and the resultant $[H^+]$ is 12 mmol/L, a pH of 1.9. However, if 12 mmol HCl is added to 1 L of a solution that contains 24 mmol $NaHCO_3^-$, the added H^+ ions combine with HCO_3^-, ultimately to form carbon dioxide. If the solution is equilibrated to a constant P_{CO_2} of 40 mmHg, all the carbon dioxide formed is removed, and the reaction continues until the 12 mmol of H^+ added has reacted with 12 mmol of HCO_3^-, which reduces its concentration from 24 to 12 mmol/L. Solving the Henderson–Hasselbalch equation (see Table 7-1) for $P_{CO_2} = 40$ mmHg and $[HCO_3^-] = 12$ mmol/L yields a pH of 7.1 and an $[H^+]$ of 80 nmol/L. Thus, in this example, 12 million nanomoles of H^+ are added as HCl, but $[H^+]$ increases by only 40 nmol/L. Virtually all the carbonic acid formed is eliminated as carbon dioxide, as long as P_{CO_2} is kept constant, and the change in $[HCO_3^-]$ is equal to the amount of acid added.

In the body, however, the ECF contains additional buffers and, to the extent that these take up some of the added H^+, the change in HCO_3^- is less than the added metabolic acid. To mitigate a pH change from either carbonic or metabolic aberrations, H^+ can be taken up by, or donated from, hemoglobin (Hb), plasma proteins, and inorganic chemical buffers. If the same experiment is carried out with 12 mmol of HCl added to 1 L of ECF, again equilibrated to a P_{CO_2} of

TABLE 7-1   Carbonic Acid System

$$CO_2 + H_2O \rightleftharpoons H_2CO_3 \rightleftharpoons H^+ + HCO_3^-$$

Component	Value
$[HCO_3^-]$	~ 24 mmol/L, as sodium bicarbonate
$[H^+]$	~ 40×10^{-9} mol/L at a normal arterial pH = 7.40 By convention $[H^+]$ is expressed as its negative logarithm: pH = $-$ log $[H^+]$
$[CO_2]$	~ 1.2 mmol/L at a normal arterial P_{CO_2} $[CO_2]$ includes the CO_2 in physical solution in plasma plus the very small amount of undissociated carbonic acid (H_2CO_3)

The Henderson–Hasselbalch equation for the carbonic acid system is:

$$pH = 6.1 + \log\,([HCO_3^-]/0.03\; P_{CO_2})$$

If any two of the components are measured, the third can be calculated

TABLE 7-3   Handling of Respiratory Acid

$$CO_2 + H_2O \rightleftharpoons H_2CO_3 \rightleftharpoons H^+ + HCO_3^-$$

Effect of doubling P_{CO_2} in a bicarbonate solution

	P_{CO_2} (mmHg)	pH	$[H^+]$ (nmol/L)	$[HCO_3^-]$ (mmol/L)
Initial	40	7.40	40	24
Final	80	7.10	80	24.000040

Effect of doubling P_{CO_2} in physiologic extracellular fluid

$$CO_2 + H_2O \rightleftharpoons H_2CO_3 \rightleftharpoons \underset{\displaystyle \Updownarrow}{H^+} + HCO_3^-$$

$$\overset{\displaystyle KHb}{+}$$

$$HHb + K^+ + HCO_3^-$$

	P_{CO_2} (mmHg)	pH	$[H^+]$ (nmol/L)	$[HCO_3^-]$ (mmol/L)
Initial	40	7.40	40	24
Final	80	7.15	71	26.5

40 mmHg, the result is a decrease in $[HCO_3^-]$ to 14, with a pH of 7.2 and an $[H^+]$ of 68 nmol/L. The pH change is less, because more total buffering has occurred, but the decrement in $[HCO_3^-]$ is only 10, which indicates that 2 mmol of H^+ has been buffered by the noncarbonic buffers. Empirical evidence such as this shows that the buffering capacity of the noncarbonic system in normal ECF is approximately 1 mmol/L per 0.1 change in pH. That is, with an increase in $[H^+]$ sufficient to lower the pH by 0.1 unit, the buffers take up 1 mmol/L of H^+ or release the same amount for a change in the opposite direction.

Handling of Respiratory Acid

The effect of adding carbonic acid to a bicarbonate solution is shown in Table 7-3. In this example, when P_{CO_2} is increased from 40–80 mmHg, the increase in $[CO_2]$ drives the reaction to the right, and because the P_{CO_2} is doubled, the final product of reactants on the right must also be doubled. This occurs when 40 nmol of H^+ have been formed, increasing $[H^+]$ to 80 nmol/L (pH falls from 7.4 to 7.1). Each new H^+ formed is associated with one new HCO_3^-, and thus $[HCO_3^-]$ also increases by 40 nmol/L, but this is negligible compared with the 24 mmol/L of HCO_3^- originally present. Thus, $[HCO_3^-]$ does not change measurably when carbon dioxide is added to an HCO_3^- solution with no other buffers present.

In the ECF of the body, however, the presence of noncarbonic buffers alters this relationship as well. Quantitatively, the most important of these is Hb, which is used, with its potassium salt, to represent all the noncarbonic buffers in the example shown (see Table 7-3). Again, the P_{CO_2} is increased from 40–80 mmHg, this time in the presence of Hb equivalent to

the amount distributed in normal ECF. In the simple bicarbonate solution, the reaction reaches equilibrium after only 40 nmol/L of H^+ have been formed, but in ECF, some of the newly formed H^+ can be taken up by Hb, so the reaction continues to the right and HCO_3^- ions accumulate. The plasma $[HCO_3^-]$ rises by an amount that reflects the number of H^+ ions buffered by Hb. As the pH decreases by 2.5 units to 7.15, the Hb and other noncarbonic buffers accept approximately 2.5 mmol of H^+, and the $[HCO_3^-]$ increases by 2.5 mmol/L. Again, the participation of noncarbonic buffers allows a smaller pH change than that observed in the bicarbonate solution.

A decrease in P_{CO_2} and the associated increase in pH of a respiratory alkalosis results in a fall in plasma $[HCO_3^-]$. When P_{CO_2} goes up or down, the buffering effect of noncarbonic buffers can be measured as the change in $[HCO_3^-]$ for a given change in pH and expressed as a buffer value, $b = -\Delta[HCO_3^-]/\Delta pH$, with the negative sign indicating that the $[HCO_3^-]$ change is opposite to the change in pH. The units of this ratio (mmol/L per pH unit) are more simply referred to as slykes (sl).

The greater the concentration of Hb and other noncarbonic buffers present, the greater the buffering of H^+ for a given change of pH. For blood with 15 g/100 mL Hb, $b = 30$ sl. In the body, however, the blood and its plasma are in equilibrium for these ions with the extravascular interstitial fluid (but not readily with the intracellular fluid). Interstitial fluid contains no Hb and very little protein, so it contributes little to noncarbonic buffering, but as H^+ ions are buffered in the blood and HCO_3^- levels are altered, these ions come into diffusional equilibrium with the interstitial fluid over 10–30 min. In effect, the buffering capacity of the blood is diluted by the interstitial fluid, and because blood volume is approximately one third the total ECF volume, the buffering capacity of

TABLE 7-2   Handling of Metabolic Acid

	Effect of Adding 12 mmol/L of a Metabolic Acid to		
	Water	Bicarbonate Solution	Extracellular Fluid
Initial $[HCO_3^-]$ (mmol/L)	0	24	24
Final $[HCO_3^-]$ (mmol/L)	0	12	14
Final $[H^+]$	12 mmol/L	80 nmol/L	68 nmol/L
Final pH	1.9	7.1	7.2

ECF is approximately one third that of blood. For total ECF, $b \cong {}^{1}/_{3} \times 30 \cong 10$ sl.

Primary Acid–Base Disorders

Before acid–base abnormalities can be understood, the presence and extent of the four primary disorders must be recognized.

- Respiratory acidosis results from a high P_{CO_2}, which reflects hypoventilation and is present, by definition, whenever P_{CO_2} is greater than 43. It is associated with a small increase in HCO_3^-, predictable as $\Delta[HCO_3^-] \cong -10 \times \Delta pH$, or 1 mEq/L per 0.1 pH unit fall.
- Respiratory alkalosis results from a low P_{CO_2}, which reflects hyperventilation and is present, by definition, whenever P_{CO_2} is less than 37. It is associated with a small decrease in HCO_3^-, predictable as $\Delta[HCO_3^-] \cong -10 \times \Delta pH$, or 1 mEq/L per 0.1 pH unit rise.
- Metabolic acidosis is recognized by a decrement in HCO_3^- greater than that expected for the pH effect alone and can be quantitated as a decrease in base excess (defined later and in Box 7-1).
- Metabolic alkalosis is recognized by a rise in HCO_3^- greater than that expected for the pH effect alone and can be quantitated as an increase in base excess.

Note that the terms *acidosis* and *alkalosis* are applied to the pathophysiologic processes that tend to cause an excess or deficit of H^+. It is possible—indeed, common—to have processes of both acidosis and alkalosis present simultaneously (e.g., respiratory acidosis plus metabolic alkalosis) with a pH that is low, high, or normal, depending on their relative magnitude. *Acidemia* and *alkalemia* are more precise terms when referring to blood pH.

As a first approximation, metabolic abnormalities are recognized by a deviation of $[HCO_3^-]$ from the normal value of 24, but it must be remembered that because of the action of the noncarbonic buffers, even a pure respiratory abnormality is associated with changes in $[HCO_3^-]$ of ± 3 mmol/L over the pH range 7.1–7.7. The base excess (BE) or base deficit (usually expressed as a negative BE) of the ECF is a better quantification of any metabolic component present. At a pH of 7.4, the noncarbonic buffers hold only their normal complement of H^+ ions and thus do not contribute to buffering. The BE calculates any deviation of $[HCO_3^-]$ from 24 that would exist at a pH of 7.4 and thus is equal in magnitude to the amount of excess metabolic acid or base added to the system, just as in a simple HCO_3^- solution. Many laboratories report this value along with blood gas measurements, but it can be estimated with a simple mental calculation (see Box 7-1) or obtained from a graphic display, as described later.

Compensation for Acid–Base Disorders

If the underlying pathology prevents the body from correcting a primary acid–base disorder (e.g., by restoring hypoventilation to normal), mechanisms come into play to minimize the deviation of pH from normal. The immediate effects of buffering are aided by a second type of homeostatic mechanism, termed *physiologic compensation*. The Henderson–Hasselbalch equation shows that pH is a function of the ratio of $[HCO_3^-]$ to P_{CO_2}, so pH is improved if this ratio is restored toward normal. If, for example, the primary disorder is a metabolic acidosis, $[HCO_3^-]$ is low and the physiologic compensation is to lower P_{CO_2} by increasing ventilation. This restores the $[HCO_3^-]/$

BOX 7-1 Base Excess Calculation

Base excess (BE) is defined as the difference between the patient's $[HCO_3^-]$ after correction to pH 7.40 by change of P_{CO_2} and the normal $[HCO_3^-]$ at pH 7.40 of 24.0 mmol/L.

Because the blood gas sample is usually not measured at a pH of 7.4, it is necessary to calculate an adjustment to this pH, which must be done by manipulation of P_{CO_2} so that the metabolic component of interest is not altered. As P_{CO_2} is hypothetically moved up or down to adjust the pH, the hypothetic $[HCO_3^-]$ changes from its measured value as determined by the noncarbonic buffer slope:

$$\Delta[HCO_3^-] \cong -10 \times \Delta pH, \text{ or } -1 \text{ mmol/L per 0.1 pH unit rise.}$$

Example 1

Consider the situation in Table 7-2 where 12 mmol/L of excess acid was added to a patient's extracellular fluid and ventilation was maintained normal. The resultant blood gas measurements include pH, 7.2; P_{CO_2}, 40 mmHg; $[HCO_3^-]$, 14 mmol/L.

The pH must be adjusted up 0.2 units to 7.4, which requires a decrease in P_{CO_2}.

At pH $\cong$ 7.4, the hypothetic $[HCO_3^-]$ is adjusted by

$$\Delta[HCO_3^-] \approx -10 \times 0.2 = -2$$

The hypothetic $[HCO_3^-]$ equals the measured value of $14 - 2 = 12$

$$BE \cong [HCO_3^-] \text{ at } 7.4 - 24 \cong 12 - 24 \cong -12 \text{ mmol/L}$$

The negative base excess of 12 mmol/L is equal to the excess acid load added.

Example 2

Consider a patient with the measured values: pH, 7.1; P_{CO_2}, 95 mmHg; and $[HCO_3^-]$, 29 mmol/L.
The pH is adjusted up 0.3 units to 7.4.

$\Delta[HCO_3^-]$	$\cong -10 \times 0.3$	$\cong -3$
Hypothetic $[HCO_3^-]$	$\cong 29 - 3$	$\cong 26$
BE	$\cong 26 - 24$	$\cong 2$ mmol/L

While at first this patient may appear to have a significant metabolic alkalosis, which suggests partial compensation for the respiratory acidosis and therefore some chronicity, BE is small and within the normal limit of ± 2, so this suggests acute hypoventilation.

Note that as the pH is hypothetically corrected to 7.4, P_{CO_2} or $[HCO_3^-]$ may move in an abnormal direction. It is convenient to remember that, consistent with the hydration reaction for CO_2, the $[HCO_3^-]$ adjustment is always in the same direction as the P_{CO_2} change.

In the examples above, the measured HCO_3^- is hypothetically adjusted to a pH of 7.4 and compared with the normal value of 24 mmol/L. Alternatively, the same relationship can be used to adjust the normal HCO_3^- to the "normal" value expected at the measured pH and subtract the measured HCO_3^-. In Example 2, a "normal" HCO_3^- is calculated at pH 7.1 to be 27 mmol/L and the BE to be $29 - 27 \cong 2$ mmol/L. This is what happens visually on the Davenport diagram when the vertical distance of a point above or below the 10 sl line is assessed.

P_{CO_2} ratio closer to normal, even though the absolute values of both $[HCO_3^-]$ and P_{CO_2} are now abnormal. This response, and the opposite one in the case of a metabolic alkalosis, demonstrates ventilatory compensation for a primary metabolic acid–base disorder.

If the primary derangement is ventilatory in origin (e.g., respiratory acidosis with a high P_{CO_2}), the body responds by increasing $[HCO_3^-]$ and restoring the $[HCO_3^-]/P_{CO_2}$ ratio and pH toward normal. The compensatory response to respiratory alkalosis requires a decrease in serum HCO_3^-. These metabolic compensations for primary respiratory disorders involve both renal retention and excretion of HCO_3^- and physicochemical binding, which occurs in bone and intracellular proteins. The renal responses are mediated by upregulation or downregulation of HCO_3^- reabsorption in the proximal tubule. This occurs fairly rapidly, but the time course to completion of metabolic compensation is approximately 1–3 days, as opposed to the ventilatory compensations, which are immediate. Thus, respiratory acid–base disturbances can be divided into those that are uncompensated and therefore likely to be of short duration (i.e., acute) and those that are compensated (chronic) processes. This is not possible for metabolic acid–base disturbances, because their normal ventilatory compensation develops concurrently.

Davenport Diagram

In general, compensations for primary acid–base alterations do not completely restore pH to 7.4. The primary acid–base disorders and their mechanisms and limits of compensation can be displayed in one of several graphic formats. The Davenport diagram is a commonly used visual display of acid–base relationships (Figure 7-1) and is a graphic representation of the Henderson–Hasselbalch equation in which any point shows a potentially coexisting combination of the three variables.

Respiratory disorders are shown by moving from the normal central point to higher or lower values of P_{CO_2}. The sloping line that passes through the center shows the 10 sl buffer value of the noncarbonic buffers and thus indicates the expected values for pH and $[HCO_3^-]$ as P_{CO_2} rises or falls in a pure respiratory acidosis or alkalosis. Vertical displacements above or below this line indicate that a metabolic disorder (either primary or compensatory) has caused an excess or

deficit of base in the ECF. If no compensation occurred for a primary metabolic disorder, the values would follow the line that represents $P_{CO_2} = 40$. The Davenport diagram is a convenient way to visualize the paths of primary disorders and their compensation. Figure 7-2 shows, for example, the development of an acute respiratory acidosis with subsequent metabolic compensation. Figure 7-3 shows the range of values seen in common acid–base disorders and illustrates the usual limits of compensation. Several numerical formulas have been developed to calculate these expected compensatory changes (Box 7-2), but it should be noted that these could only estimate a point within the range of observed values.

Clinical Acid–Base Disorders

Respiratory Acidosis

Hypoventilation is defined as alveolar ventilation inadequate for metabolic demand and is indicated by an elevation of arterial P_{CO_2} above the normal 40 ± 3 mmHg (at sea level; it is lower at altitude). It results from an inadequate drive to breathe, from mechanical impairments of the chest wall or lung parenchyma, or most commonly from severe airflow limitation (e.g., asthma or chronic obstructive pulmonary disease [COPD]).

An elevated Pa_{CO_2} defines the presence of respiratory acidosis regardless of the arterial pH.

Acute Respiratory Acidosis

Acute respiratory acidosis is identified by high Pa_{CO_2}, a fall in pH, and an increase in $[HCO_3^-]$ that approximates 1 mmol/L for each 0.1 decrement in pH (i.e., BE ≈ 0). On the Davenport diagram, the values follow the 10 sl line to the left

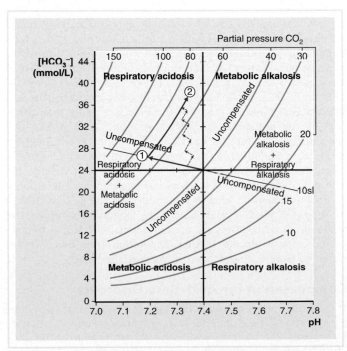

FIGURE 7-2 Compensation for a respiratory acidosis. Rapid development of hypoventilation, in which carbon dioxide partial pressure rises from 40 to 70 mmHg, would follow the 10 sl line of acute respiratory acidosis to point 1. If this level of hypoventilation were maintained for days, metabolic compensation would increase HCO_3^- and improve the pH toward point 2. More likely, a progressive decline in ventilation over days might follow the stuttering, dotted path to the same end point.

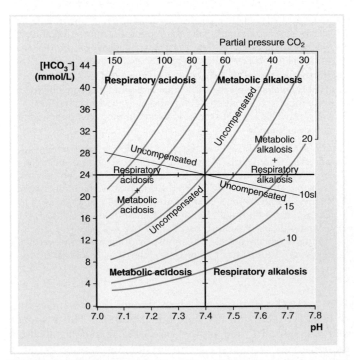

FIGURE 7-1 Davenport diagram. This graphic display plots plasma HCO_3^- against plasma pH, with lines of equal carbon dioxide partial pressure (P_{CO_2}) curving across the graph (intermediate values of P_{CO_2} can be interpolated along vertical lines).

that exceeds 1 mmol/L for each 0.1 decrement in pH (i.e., BE > 2). On the Davenport diagram, the values are in the left upper quadrant above the 10 sl line (see Figure 7-3). Metabolic compensation probably begins within hours by the redistribution of HCO_3^- from bone and intracellular stores. Over the course of a few days, renal retention of HCO_3^- can produce nearly complete compensation for moderate elevations of Pa_{CO_2} and bring the pH very near to 7.4 (see Figures 7-2 and 7-3). At higher levels of Pa_{CO_2}, renal tubular reabsorption of HCO_3^- is not sufficient to restore the normal $[HCO_3^-]/P_{CO_2}$ ratio, and the pH remains increasingly acid. As shown in Figure 7-3, the range of observed chronic values is quite wide and thus not well estimated by numerical rules. Patients with fully compensated respiratory acidosis may be quite stable despite considerable elevations of Pa_{CO_2}. Accordingly, the decrement in pH is a better indication of clinical risk.

Respiratory Alkalosis

Hyperventilation is defined as alveolar ventilation in excess of metabolic demand and is indicated by a fall in arterial P_{CO_2} below the normal 40 ± 3 mmHg. It results from an excessive drive to breathe, which may result from pain or anxiety, but is also stimulated by hypoxemia and the derangements of many pulmonary diseases, including mild to moderate asthma, pulmonary emboli, pulmonary hypertension, and interstitial pulmonary fibrosis; by systemic illnesses, including head injury, shock, and bacteremia; and by ingestion of aspirin. Respiratory alkalosis is easily induced by excessive mechanical ventilation.

A low Pa_{CO_2} defines the presence of respiratory alkalosis regardless of the arterial pH.

Acute Respiratory Alkalosis

Acute respiratory alkalosis is identified by a low Pa_{CO_2}, a rise in pH, and a decrease in $[HCO_3^-]$ that approximates 1 mmol/L per 0.1 increment in pH (i.e., BE ≈ 0). On the Davenport diagram, the values follow the 10 sl line to the right (see Figure 7-3). The empirical data plotted in Figure 7-3 show that patients who have more severe degrees of acute hyperventilation may have somewhat lower $[HCO_3^-]$ values than expected for the immediate effects of noncarbonic buffers. The change in $[HCO_3^-]$ may also be estimated as a fall of 2 mmol for each 10 torr decrease in Pa_{CO_2} (see Box 7-2).

Chronic Respiratory Alkalosis

Chronic respiratory alkalosis is identified by a low Pa_{CO_2}, a variable but small increase in pH, and a decrease in $[HCO_3^-]$ that exceeds 1 mmol/L per 0.1 increment in pH (i.e., BE < −2). On the Davenport diagram, the values are in the right lower quadrant below the 10 sl line (see Figure 7-3). The mechanisms of metabolic compensation described earlier, but in the reverse direction, can produce almost complete compensation to a pH near 7.4 (see Figure 7-3) when hyperventilation is sustained, as, for example, in those living at high altitudes or in patients with restrictive lung disease.

Metabolic Disorders

Metabolic Acidosis

Metabolic acidosis is defined by a decrement in $[HCO_3^-]$ greater than that expected for the pH effect alone and is quantified by calculation of a base deficit or negative BE. A negative BE defines the presence of a component of metabolic acidosis regardless of the arterial pH.

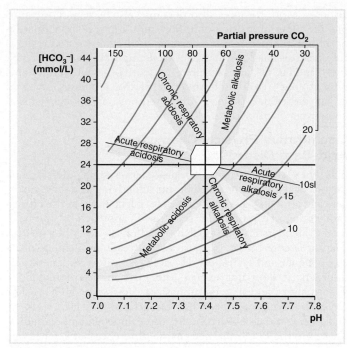

FIGURE 7-3 Typical limits of compensation are conveniently displayed on the Davenport diagram. (Modified with permission from Hornbein TF: Acid–base balance. In Culver BH, ed: The respiratory system. Seattle: University of Washington Publication Services; 2006. Data from Goldberg M, Greene SB, Moss ML, *et al*: Computer based instruction and diagnosis of acid-base disorders. JAMA 1973; 223:269–275.)

BOX 7-2 Numerical Estimates for Acute and Chronic Acid–Base Disorders

Respiratory Acidosis
Acute: The increase in HCO_3^-
        = 0.1 × the increase in Pa_{CO_2} above 40 or
        = 1 mEq for each 0.1 pH unit below 7.4
Chronic: The increase in HCO_3^-
        = 0.3 × the increase in Pa_{CO_2} above 40

Respiratory Alkalosis
Acute: The decrease in HCO_3^-
        = 0.2 × the decrease in Pa_{CO_2} from 40 or
        = 1 mEq for each 0.1 pH unit above 7.4
Chronic: The increase in HCO_3^-
        = 0.4 × the decrease in Pa_{CO_2} from 40

Metabolic Acidosis
Expected respiratory compensation:
    1 mmHg decrease in Pa_{CO_2} for each mEq decrease in HCO_3^- below 24

Metabolic Alkalosis
Expected respiratory compensation:
    0.7 mmHg increase in Pa_{CO_2} for each mEq increase in HCO_3^- above 24

(see Figure 7-3). The small change in $[HCO_3^-]$ may also be approximated as a rise of 1 mmol for each 10 torr increment in Pa_{CO_2} (see Box 7-2).

Chronic Respiratory Acidosis

Chronic respiratory acidosis is identified by a high Pa_{CO_2}, a variable decrement in pH, and an increase in $[HCO_3^-]$

Two general types of metabolic acidosis occur—those that result from excess acid accumulation with the subsequent loss of HCO_3^- through ventilation, as described earlier, and those that result from a primary loss of HCO_3^- from the body. Examples of excess acid include the following:

- Production of lactic acid when tissue oxygen demand outstrips supply, as in exercising muscle, low cardiac output states, or conditions of low arterial oxygen content
- Ketoacidosis associated with insulin deficiency
- Inadequate excretion of acid in acute or chronic renal failure

Bicarbonate loss may occur from defects in renal tubular function and from intestinal secretions in diarrhea. Although the base deficit quantifies the net acidosis from any of these causes, it does not differentiate between the two types, which is done by calculating the unmeasured anions, or "anion gap." Ionic balance must be maintained in the ECF, so the sum of the positive ions (mainly Na^+ and K^+) must equal the sum of the negative ions (Cl^-, HCO_3^-, and unmeasured anions). The difference, $(Na^+ + K^+) - (Cl^- + HCO_3^-)$, gives the anion gap (although K^+ is often ignored in the clinical calculation) and is normally less than 8–12. The anion gap remains normal with primary HCO_3^- losses, because these are typically balanced by retention of Cl^-, but is increased by the accumulation of the unmeasured anions left behind when excess acid (other than HCl) is buffered by the bicarbonate system.

Metabolic Alkalosis

Metabolic alkalosis is defined by an increase in $[HCO_3^-]$ greater than expected for the pH effect alone and is quantified by calculation of a positive BE. A positive BE defines the presence of a metabolic alkalosis, regardless of the arterial pH.

Metabolic alkalosis is most commonly caused by loss of acid through gastric secretions (vomiting or gastric suction) or by retention of HCO_3^- with diuretic therapy. Both are associated with chloride depletion, with a decrease in serum chloride concentration roughly equivalent to the increase in plasma $[HCO_3^-]$.

Respiratory Compensation

Respiratory compensation for primary metabolic disorders is rapid but does not result in complete compensation (see Figure 7-3). Respiratory drive is stimulated by low pH, so hyperventilation in response to an acid stimulus can result in more than a doubling of alveolar ventilation (driving $PaCO_2$ to < 20 mmHg). Metabolic alkalosis generally results in moderate degrees of hypoventilation, with $PaCO_2$ rarely exceeding 60 mmHg unless pulmonary abnormalities are present as well. The hypoxemia associated with hypoventilation when breathing air provides a ventilatory drive to limit a further rise in PCO_2. Figure 7-3 shows that the maximum extent of ventilatory compensation observed with a chronic metabolic acidosis or alkalosis results in a pH that is approximately halfway between that which would have existed in the absence of any ventilatory compensation (at $PaCO_2 = 40$ mmHg) and complete compensation (pH = 7.4). Metabolic acid–base derangements of shorter duration show less complete compensation, presumably related to the rate of readjustment of brain ECF acid–base balance.

Combined Disorders

Not all acid–base disorders fit neatly into the primary and compensatory patterns described. Combined primary disorders may occur, such as an acute cessation of ventilation (asphyxia) that causes both respiratory and metabolic (lactic)

acidoses. More complex disorders may also be seen. For example, the superimposition of a short-term increase in ventilation or of diuretic therapy on a chronic, well-compensated respiratory acidosis may result in an alkalemic pH. The blood pH, PCO_2, and HCO_3^- are sufficient to identify the net components present, but a full understanding of the processes involved in an individual patient often requires additional clinical knowledge or prior data.

Quantitative Physical Chemistry of Acid–Base Disorders

In recent years there has been renewed interest in understanding the physical chemistry mechanisms underlying acid–base disorders and applying this at the bedside, particularly in the critical care setting. Although the "traditional" approach on the basis of the Henderson–Hasselbalch equation as described in this chapter is convenient, because of the ready availability of its components, and accurately describes respiratory and metabolic disorders, it does not explain the mechanisms of metabolic abnormalities and it overemphasizes the role of HCO_3^-. The physical chemistry approach considers pH and HCO_3^- to be dependent variables, driven by three independent variables. These are the PCO_2, the net charge difference between strong cations and anions (those fully dissociated at physiologic pH, such as Na^+, K^+, Ca^{++}, Mg^{++}, Cl^-, and lactate), and the total concentration of weak acids (predominantly albumin and phosphate). The quantitative application of this approach requires measurement of these additional variables and computerized solution of six simultaneous equations, so it has not been conducive to routine clinical work; further discussion is beyond the scope of this chapter. Its potential value lies in providing more information about the cause of metabolic acidosis than possible with the simple anion gap, in better accounting for the role of hypoalbuminemia, and in explaining the acid–base effects of large infused volumes of saline or other fluids.

CONTROL OF VENTILATION

Neural Control

The control of ventilation involves a process of central rhythm generation, with the rate and depth of breathing adjusted by a combination of mechanical and chemical stimuli, along with higher central nervous system inputs. The rhythmicity of breathing is thought to result from complex interactions among cells in regions of the medulla and pons. The medulla contains two dense, bilateral aggregations of neurons that have respiratory-related activity. The dorsal respiratory group lies in the dorsomedial medulla and is associated with the ventrolateral nucleus of the solitary tract. The ventral respiratory group lies in the ventrolateral medulla and is associated with the retrofacial nucleus, nucleus ambiguus, and nucleus retroambigualis. Outputs from these neurons descend through the ventral and lateral columns of the spinal cord to phrenic and intercostal motoneurons to control the diaphragm and intercostal muscles. Another important respiratory area is located in the dorsolateral pons, associated with the nucleus parabrachialis medialis, and is commonly called the pneumotaxic center. This region seems to play a role in switching between the inspiratory and expiratory phases.

Although the average ventilation level is normally set predominantly by chemical stimuli, mechaniconeural receptors may also modify the ventilatory pattern. Although these receptors can be demonstrated in animals, their roles in humans are less clear. They include the following:

- Slowly adapting pulmonary stretch receptors located in the airways with vagal afferents that are stimulated by increases in lung volume. For example, when functional residual capacity is raised or when lung volume is held at its end-inspiratory level, a reduction in respiratory frequency results primarily from prolongation of the expiratory period (inflation reflex of Hering–Breuer). A reduction in activity of these receptors with lung deflation stimulates inspiratory onset (deflation reflex) and may contribute to the tachypnea that accompanies atelectasis.
- Rapidly adapting pulmonary stretch receptors concentrated near the carina and central bronchi, also with vagal afferents, are stimulated both mechanically and chemically to generate the cough reflex.
- C-fiber endings attached to unmyelinated afferent fibers are found close to the pulmonary capillaries, where they have been called type J (juxtapulmonary capillary) receptors and are also present in the bronchi in proximity to the bronchial circulation. Both types of C-fiber endings are stimulated by endogenously produced substances, including histamine, some prostaglandins, bradykinin, and serotonin, and may have a role in conditions such as asthma, pulmonary venous congestion, and pulmonary embolism. C-fiber endings also are mechanically sensitive and can be activated by lung hyperinflation.
- Musculoskeletal afferents stimulated by the stretching of skeletal muscle increase ventilation and may contribute to the initial hyperpnea of exercise.

Chemical Stimuli

The influence of ventilation on the levels of carbon dioxide and oxygen in the blood is described in Chapter 5. In turn, these levels are sensed and modulate neural inputs to the respiratory centers to complete a feedback loop by adjusting respiratory rate and tidal volume. Receptors responsive to changes in levels of oxygen, carbon dioxide, and pH are located peripherally in the aortic and carotid bodies and in the central nervous system on the brain side of the blood–brain barrier.

Peripheral Chemoreceptors

The carotid bodies lie close to the carotid bifurcation on either side of the neck, and the aortic bodies lie near the aortic arch. Each of these receives an extremely high blood flow relative to their size, which results in tissue blood–gas partial pressures very close to the arterial level. Arterial oxygen partial pressure, rather than oxygen content, is the principal chemical stimulus to these peripheral receptors. Experiments in which blood oxygen content is lowered by anemia or carbon monoxide administration show little or no change in peripheral chemosensor output when PaO_2 is not reduced simultaneously. Receptor neural output is minimal above a PaO_2 of 200 mmHg, increases gradually with lower levels, and increases much more rapidly below a PaO_2 of 60 mmHg.

The peripheral chemoreceptors are also sensitive to arterial pH. A decrease in pH (acidemia) increases the firing rate and stimulates ventilation, whereas an increase in pH has the opposite effect. $PaCO_2$ stimulates the peripheral receptors, in addition to its pH effect. These two chemical stimuli, hypoxia and acidity, interact and are more than additive in their combined influence on chemoreceptor discharge and ventilation.

Central Chemoreceptors

Chemosensitive areas have been demonstrated near the ventrolateral surface of the medulla in the cat and rat. The stimulus to this receptor seems to be primarily the pH or hydrogen ion content of brain ECF, and, again, acidosis increases the ventilatory signal. The stimulus is similar with pH reduction of either respiratory or metabolic origin, but because the blood–brain barrier is much more permeable to carbon dioxide than to HCO_3^-, the effect of respiratory acid–base disturbances is much more immediate.

Interaction of Chemical Stimuli

The acute ventilatory increase in response to hypoxia seems to be mediated entirely by the peripheral receptors, whereas hypoxia, if anything, depresses central chemosensor output. The response is initially attenuated by the effect of hypocapnic alkalosis on both peripheral and central chemoreceptors, but if hypoxia persists, such as at altitude, and metabolic compensation occurs, the ventilation can increase further.

The ventilatory response to an acute rise in $PaCO_2$ results primarily (approximately 80%) from the central chemoreceptors, with the remainder attributable to peripheral chemoreceptors. For the same arterial pH change, the ventilatory response to respiratory acidosis is greater than that seen with metabolic acidosis. This results from a difference in central chemoreceptor activity because of the effect of the blood–brain barrier. Carbon dioxide, like other gases, readily crosses the blood–brain barrier, so that brain ECF PCO_2 is similar to that in blood, but most ions, including H^+ and HCO_3^-, cross the blood–brain barrier much more slowly. Respiratory acidosis stimulates both peripheral and central chemoreceptors as the carbon dioxide crosses the blood–brain barrier to acidify brain ECF. The resultant ventilatory response reflects the sum of the signals from both receptors. With metabolic acidosis, the peripheral chemoreceptor response is similar to that with carbon dioxide, but because the hydrogen ion does not readily reach the central chemosensor, central stimulation does not occur. Instead, the hypocapnia that results from peripheral chemoreceptor stimulation creates a central nervous system alkalosis, and the resultant ventilatory response reflects the net effect of an increased peripheral drive partially offset by a decreased central drive.

Although the blood–brain barrier is poorly permeable to H^+ and HCO_3^-, redistribution of these ions does occur over several hours. The blood–brain barrier and choroid plexus may regulate ECF composition of the brain, much as the kidney does for the rest of the body. However, equilibrium across the blood–brain barrier may develop over hours, whereas renal adjustments may require days.

Measurement of Ventilatory Drive

The classic methods of measuring ventilatory drive alter the stimulus (PCO_2 or PO_2) and measure the response in ventilation per minute. A major drawback to these methods is that they depend on normal lungs and chest wall. Because ventilation is the index of response, any mechanical impairment of the breathing apparatus (restrictive or obstructive disease) tends to reduce the measurement. An attempt to make more meaningful measurements in patients who have lung disease led to the development of the mouth occlusion pressure technique, in which the inspiratory pressure developed against a shutter transiently closed during the first 100 msec of a tidal breath ($P_{0.1}$) is taken as an index of respiratory center output.

This technique tends to parallel phrenic nerve traffic, but its accuracy may be reduced in severe COPD, where the time constant for transmission of an inspiratory pressure change to the mouth may be prolonged and where hyperinflation may disadvantage the diaphragm.

Ventilatory Pattern

The total ventilation per minute is the product of the tidal volume and the respiratory frequency ($\dot{V}E = VT \times f$). The ventilatory pattern can be further described by measurement of the time during inspiration in relationship to the total tidal cycle (T_I/T_{TOT}), and the average inspiratory flow rate is given by VT/T_I. Ventilation is typically measured by use of a mouthpiece and nose clips, but these tend to alter the pattern. To avoid this, research studies may use calibrated magnetometers or inductance belts.

Resting Partial Pressure of Arterial Carbon Dioxide

Human alveolar ventilation is normally regulated to maintain Pa_{CO_2} between 37 and 43 mmHg at sea level. In the absence of serious mechanical impediments to ventilation, a Pa_{CO_2} above this range may be interpreted as reflecting low respiratory drive, whereas a low Pa_{CO_2} in a spontaneously breathing individual reflects increased drive.

Carbon Dioxide Response Curves

Carbon dioxide is introduced into the inspired gas to raise Pa_{CO_2} or, alternately, endogenous carbon dioxide is built up by rebreathing from a closed system while the increase in ventilation is monitored. Both are done with a high inspired oxygen level to eliminate the influence of fluctuations in Pa_{O_2}. In the physiologic range of Pa_{CO_2}, a straight line is obtained in a plot of minute ventilation versus Pa_{CO_2} (Figure 7-4). The slope of this line, a measurement of the sensitivity of the respiratory system to Pa_{CO_2}, is normally 2–5 L/min per mmHg Pa_{CO_2}. A decrease in this slope in the absence of ventilatory impairment is an indication of a decreased respiratory drive.

Hypoxia Response Curves

Changes in ventilation in response to decreasing arterial oxygen partial pressures tend to follow a hyperbolic curve (Figure 7-5). The response is quite modest at Pa_{O_2} levels in the high-normal range, but $\dot{V}E$ increases sharply as Pa_{O_2} falls below 60 mmHg. If Pa_{CO_2} is allowed to decrease as ventilation increases, the response is attenuated by the offsetting pH effect, so carbon dioxide may be progressively added to maintain isocapnic conditions. The alinearity makes it difficult to express drive numerically, but a left shift or flattening of the curve is interpreted as decreased hypoxic drive. When the results of such a test are plotted as ventilation versus arterial oxygen saturation, the inverse relationship is typically linear. This is a coincidental outcome of the two curvilinear relationships, because the signal for ventilation is Pa_{O_2}, not Sa_{O_2}. The range of hypoxic sensitivity among normal individuals is wide.

Because the hypoxic drive is rather modest for Pa_{O_2} greater than 60 mmHg, it is generally held that the carbon dioxide response is mainly responsible for maintaining the level of ventilation in normal humans at sea level. The range of measured drives among normal individuals is wide, largely determined genetically, and hypoxic and hypercapnic drives do not correlate well with each other. The ventilatory sensitivities to carbon dioxide and to hypoxia tend to decrease with age and are depressed by anesthetics, sedatives, and narcotics. The impact of a low ventilatory drive is most likely to become manifest when the system is stressed by high ventilatory demand or by the increased work of airflow obstruction.

Ventilatory Loading

Respiratory drive may be further examined by studying the response of subjects to an imposed external load, such as an added inspiratory resistance or a threshold of negative pressure. With an added load, normal subjects typically show a decreased ventilatory response to hypercapnia or hypoxia but an increase in neural drive, as reflected by phrenic activity or mouth occlusion pressure. Similarly, with advanced COPD,

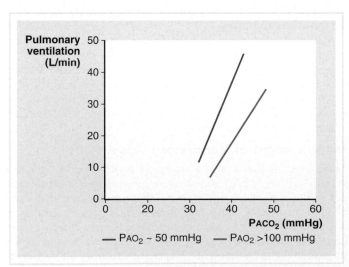

FIGURE 7-4 Ventilatory response to inhaled carbon dioxide at two different levels of alveolar partial pressure of oxygen (Pa_{O_2}). Minute ventilation increases as Pa_{CO_2} (and with it, Pa_{CO_2}) is elevated. The slope showing ventilatory sensitivity to Pa_{CO_2} increases with the added stimulus of low Pa_{O_2}.

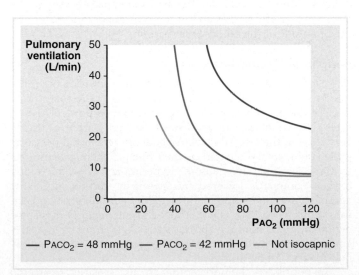

FIGURE 7-5 Ventilatory response to hypoxia. Minute ventilation increases in a nonlinear fashion as Pa_{O_2} is decreased (with constant Pa_{CO_2}). The response is greater with the added stimulus of higher P_{CO_2}. The lowest line shows a diminished response when P_{CO_2} is permitted to fall (not isocapnic) as hyperventilation is stimulated by hypoxia. (Modified from Hlastala MP, Berger AJ: Physiology of respiration. 2nd ed. New York: Oxford University Press; 2001:156.)

ventilatory responses to chemical stimuli are reduced, but $P_{0.1}$ values tend to be high. A potential contributor to hypercapnia in COPD and asthma is a failure to perceive or respond to the added load.

SUGGESTED READINGS

Berger AJ, Hornbein TF: Control of breathing. In Patton HD, *et al.*, eds: Textbook of Physiology, vol 2, 21st ed. Philadelphia: WB Saunders; 1989:ch 54.

Calverley PMA: Control of breathing. In Hughes JMB, Pride N, eds. Lung Function Tests: Physiologic Principles and Clinical Application, London: WB Saunders; 1999:107–120.

Davenport HW: The ABC of Acid-Base Chemistry, 6th ed. Chicago: The University of Chicago Press; 1974.

Hlastala MP, Berger AJ: Physiology of Respiration, 2nd ed. New York: Oxford University Press; 2001:134–179.

Morgan TJ: Clinical review: The meaning of acid-base abnormalities in the intensive care unit—effects of fluid administration. Crit Care 2005; 9:204–211.

Story DA: Bench-to-bedside review: A brief history of clinical acid-base. Crit Care 2004; 8:253–258.

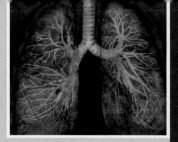

8 Physiology and Testing of Respiratory Muscles

THEODOROS VASSILAKOPOULOS • CHARIS ROUSSOS

INTRODUCTION

The respiratory muscles are the only muscles, along with the heart, that have to work continuously, though intermittently, to sustain life. They have to repetitively move a rather complex elastic structure, the thorax, to achieve the entry of air into the lungs and thence effect gas exchange. Their great number mandates that they should interact properly to perform their task despite their different anatomic location, geometric orientation, and motor innervation. They should also be able to adapt to a variety of working conditions and respond to many different chemical and neural stimuli. This chapter describes some aspects of the respiratory muscles' function that are relevant to the understanding of the way the respiratory muscles accomplish the action of breathing and how their function can be tested in the laboratory.

FUNCTIONAL ANATOMY

The Intercostal Muscles

The intercostal muscles are two thin layers of muscle fibers occupying each of the intercostal spaces. They are termed external and internal because of their surface relations, the external being superficial to the internal. The muscle fibers of the two layers run approximately at right angles to each other: The *external intercostals* extend from the tubercles of the ribs dorsally to the costochondral junctions ventrally, and their fibers are oriented obliquely, downward, and forward, from the rib above to the rib below. The *internal intercostals* begin posteriorly, as the posterior intercostal membrane on the inner aspect of the external intercostal muscles. From approximately the angle of the rib, the internal intercostal muscles run obliquely, upward, and forward from the superior border of the rib and costal cartilage below to the floor of the subcostal groove of the rib and the edge of the costal cartilage above, ending at the sternocostal junctions. All the intercostal muscles are innervated by the intercostal nerves.

The external intercostal muscles have an inspiratory action on the rib cage, whereas the internal intercostal muscles are expiratory. An illustrative clinical example of the "isolated" inspiratory action of the intercostal muscles is offered by patients who have *bilateral diaphragmatic paralysis*. In these patients, inspiration is accomplished solely by the rib cage muscles. As a result, the rib cage expands during inspiration, and the pleural pressure falls. Because the diaphragm is flaccid and no transdiaphragmatic pressure can be developed, the fall in pleural pressure is transmitted to the abdomen, causing an equal fall in the abdominal pressure. Hence the abdomen moves paradoxically inward during inspiration, opposing the inflation of the lung (Figure 8-1). This paradoxic motion is the cardinal sign of diaphragmatic paralysis on clinical examination and is invariably present in the supine posture, during which the abdominal muscles usually remain relaxed during the entire respiratory cycle. However, this sign may be absent in the erect posture.

The Diaphragm

The floor of the thoracic cavity is closed by a thin musculotendinous sheet, the diaphragm, the most important inspiratory muscle, accounting for approximately 70% of minute ventilation in normal subjects. The diaphragm is anatomically unique among the skeletal muscles in that its fibers radiate from a central tendinous structure (the central tendon) to insert peripherally into skeletal structures. The muscle of the diaphragm falls into two main components on the basis of its point of origin: the crural (vertebral) part and the costal (sternocostal) part. The crural part arises from the crura (strong, tapering tendons attached vertically to the anterolateral aspects of the bodies and intervertebral disks of the first three lumbar vertebrae on the right and two on the left) and the three aponeurotic arcuate ligaments. The costal part of the diaphragm arises from the xiphoid process and the lower end of the sternum and the costal cartilages of the lower six ribs. These costal fibers run cranially so that they are directly apposed to the inner aspect of lower rib cage, creating a *zone of apposition*.

The shape of the relaxed diaphragm at the end of a normal expiration (functional residual capacity, FRC) is that of two domes joined by a saddle that runs from the sternum to the anterior surface of the spinal column (Figure 8-2). The motor innervation of the diaphragm is from the phrenic nerves, which also provide a proprioceptive supply to the muscle. When tension develops within the diaphragmatic muscle fibers, a caudally oriented force is applied on the central tendon and the dome of the diaphragm descends; this descent has two effects. First, it expands the thoracic cavity along its craniocaudal axis and consequently the pleural pressure falls. Second, it produces a caudal displacement of the abdominal visceral contents and an increase in the abdominal pressure that in turn results in an outward motion of the ventral abdominal wall. Thus, when the diaphragm contracts, a cranially oriented force is being applied by the costal diaphragmatic fibers to the upper margins of the lower six ribs that has the effect of lifting and rotating them outward (insertional force; see Figure 8-2). The actions mediated by the changes in pleural and abdominal pressures are more complex: if one assumes that the diaphragm is the only muscle acting on the rib cage, it seems that it has two opposing effects when it contracts.

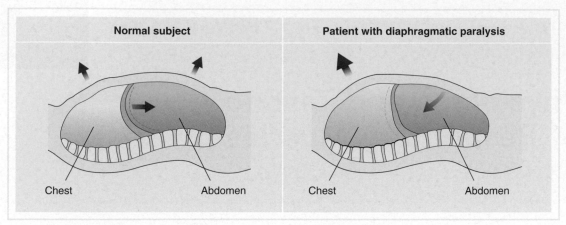

FIGURE 8-1 Schematic demonstration of normal abdominal and rib cage movement *(left panel)* and the paradoxical abdominal motion of isolated diaphragmatic paralysis *(right panel)*. The diaphragm at resting end-expiration is shown as a solid line and after inspiration as a dashed line. In the normal subject *(left)*, the diaphragm moves caudally, and in the patient with diaphragmatic paralysis *(right)*, the diaphragm moves in a cephalad direction. The anterior abdominal wall moves inward instead of outward.

On the upper rib cage, it causes a decrease in the anteroposterior diameter, and this expiratory action is primarily because of the fall in pleural pressure (see Figure 8-2). On the lower rib cage, it causes an expansion. In fact this is the pattern of chest wall motion observed in *tetraplegic patients* with transection injury at the fifth cervical segment of the spinal cord or below, who have complete paralysis of the inspiratory muscles except for the diaphragm. This inspiratory action on the lower rib cage is caused by the concomitant action of two different forces, the "insertional" force already described and the "appositional" force.

THE NECK MUSCLES

The Sternocleidomastoids

The sternocleidomastoids arise from the mastoid process and descend to the ventral surface of the manubrium sterni and the medial third of the clavicle. Their neural supply is from the accessory nerve. The action of the sternocleidomastoids is to displace the sternum cranially during inspiration, to expand the upper rib cage more in its anteroposterior diameter than in its transverse one, and to decrease the transverse diameter of the lower rib cage. In normal subjects breathing at rest, however, the sternocleidomastoids are inactive, being recruited only when the inspiratory muscle pump is abnormally loaded or when ventilation increases substantially. Therefore, they should be considered as accessory muscles of inspiration.

The Scalenes

The scalenes are composed of three muscle bundles that run from the transverse processes of the lower five cervical vertebrae to the upper surface of the first two ribs. They receive their neural supply mainly from the lower five cervical segments. Their action is to increase (slightly) the anteroposterior diameter of the upper rib cage. Although initially considered as accessory muscles of inspiration, they are invariably active during inspiration. In fact, seated normal subjects cannot breathe without contracting the scalenes even when they reduce the required inspiratory effort by reducing tidal volume. Therefore, scalenes in humans are primary muscles of inspiration, and their contraction is an important determinant of the expansion of the upper rib cage during breathing.

The Abdominal Muscles

The abdominal muscles with respiratory activity are those constituting the ventrolateral wall of the abdomen (i.e., the rectus abdominis ventrally and the external oblique, internal oblique, and transverses abdominis laterally). They are innervated by the lower six thoracic nerves and the first lumbar nerve. As they contract, they pull the abdominal wall inward, thus increasing the intraabdominal pressure. This causes the diaphragm to move cranially into the thoracic cavity, increasing the pleural pressure and decreasing lung volume. Thus, their action is expiratory. Expiration is usually a passive process but can become active when minute ventilation has to be increased (e.g., during exercise) or during respiratory distress. Expiratory muscle action is also essential during cough.

TESTING RESPIRATORY MUSCLE FUNCTION

Muscles have two functions: to develop force and to shorten. In the respiratory system, force is usually estimated as pressure and shortening as lung volume change. Thus, quantitative characterization of the respiratory muscles usually relies on measurements of volumes and pressures.

Vital Capacity

Vital capacity (VC) is an easily obtained measurement with spirometry, which, when decreased, points to respiratory muscle weakness. The VC averages approximately 50 mL/kg in normal adults. However, VC is not specific and may be decreased because of both inspiratory and expiratory muscle weakness and restrictive lung and chest wall diseases. A marked fall (>30%) in VC in the supine compared with the erect posture (which in the normal individual is 5–10%) is associated with severe bilateral diaphragmatic weakness.

Maximal Static Mouth Pressures

Measurement of the maximum static inspiratory ($P_{I,max}$) or expiratory ($P_{E,max}$) pressure that a subject can generate at the mouth is a simple way to estimate inspiratory and expiratory muscle strength. These are measured at the side port of a

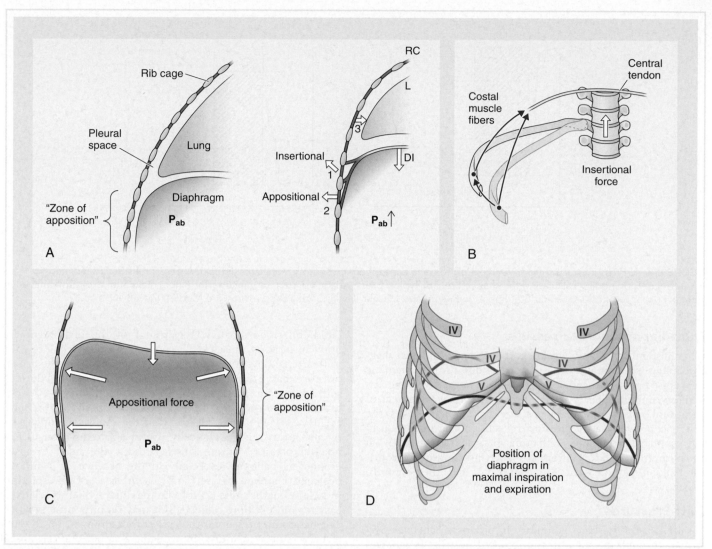

FIGURE 8-2 Actions of the diaphragm. **A,** Zone of apposition and summary of diaphragm's actions. When the diaphragm contracts, a caudally oriented force is being applied on the central tendon and the dome of the diaphragm descends (DI). Furthermore, the costal diaphragmatic fibers apply a cranially oriented force to the upper margins of the lower six ribs that has the effect of lifting and rotating them outward (*insertional force, arrow 1*). The zone of apposition makes the lower rib cage part of the abdomen, and the changes in pressure in the pleural recess between the apposed diaphragm and the rib cage are almost equal to the changes in abdominal pressure. Pressure in this pleural recess rises rather than falls during inspiration because of diaphragmatic descent, and the rise in abdominal pressure is transmitted through the apposed diaphragm to expand the lower rib cage (*arrow 2*). All these effects result in expansion of the lower rib cage. On the upper rib cage, isolated contraction of the diaphragm causes a decrease in the anteroposterior diameter, and this expiratory action is primarily caused by the fall in pleural pressure (*arrow 3*). **B,** Insertional force; **C,** appositional force; **D,** shape of the diaphragm and the bony thorax at maximum inspiration and expiration.

mouthpiece that is occluded at the distal end. A small leak is incorporated to prevent glottic closure and buccal muscle use during inspiratory or expiratory maneuvers. The inspiratory and expiratory pressure must be maintained, ideally for at least 1.5 sec, so that the maximum pressure sustained for 1 sec can be recorded (Figure 8-3). The pressure measured during these maneuvers (Pmo) reflects the pressure developed by the respiratory muscles (Pmus), plus the passive elastic recoil pressure of the respiratory system including the lung and chest wall (Prs) (Figure 8-4). At FRC, Prs is 0 so that Pmo represents Pmus. However, at residual volume (RV), where $P_{I,max}$ is usually measured, Prs may be as much as 30 cm H_2O, and thus makes a significant contribution $P_{I,max}$ of up to 30% (or more if Pmus is decreased). Similarly, $P_{E,max}$ is measured at total lung capacity (TLC), where Prs can be up to 40 cm H_2O. Clinical

measures and normal values of $P_{I,max}$ and $P_{E,max}$ do not conventionally subtract the elastic recoil of the respiratory system. Normal values are available for adults, children, and the elderly. The tests are easy to perform and are well tolerated. However, the measurements exhibit significant between-subject and within-subject variability, as well as learning effect (values obtained improve as subjects become accustomed to the maneuvers). The normal ranges are wide, so that values in the lower quarter of the normal range are compatible both with normal strength and with mild or moderate weakness. However, a $P_{I,max}$ of −80 cm H_2O usually excludes clinically important inspiratory muscle weakness. Values less negative than this are difficult to interpret, and more detailed studies are required. A normal $P_{E,max}$ with a low $P_{I,max}$ suggests isolated diaphragmatic weakness.

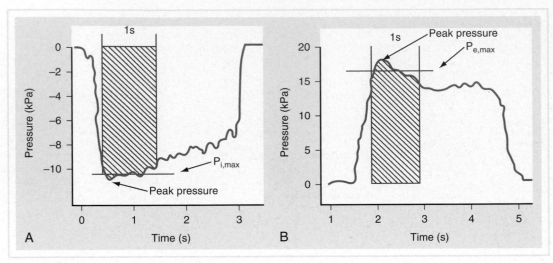

FIGURE 8-3 A, Pressure tracing from a subject performing a maximum inspiratory maneuver (*PImax*). A peak pressure is seen, and the 1-sec average is determined by calculating the *shaded area.* **B,** Typical pressure tracing from a subject performing a maximum expiratory maneuver (*PEmax*). (Adapted from ATS/ERS: Statement on Respiratory Muscle Testing. Am J Respir Crit Care Med 2002; 166:518–624.)

Transdiaphragmatic Pressure

When inspiratory muscle weakness is confirmed, the next diagnostic step is to unravel whether this is due to diaphragmatic weakness, because the diaphragm is the most important inspiratory muscle. This is accomplished by the measurement of maximum transdiaphragmatic pressure (Pdi,max). Pdi,max is the difference between gastric pressure (reflecting abdominal pressure) and esophageal pressure (reflecting intrapleural pressure) on a maximum inspiratory effort after the insertion of appropriate balloon catheters in the esophagus and the stomach, respectively.

Sniff Pressures

A sniff is a short, sharp voluntary inspiratory maneuver performed through one or both unoccluded nostrils. It achieves

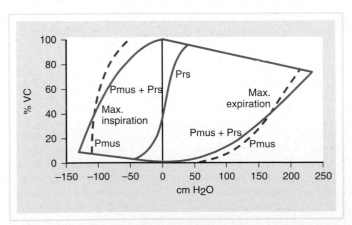

FIGURE 8-4 Relationship of muscle and respiratory pressures at different lung volumes. Vertical axis, lung volume as a percentage of vital capacity (%VC). Horizontal axis, alveolar pressure in cm H_2O. The *broken lines* indicate the pressure contributed by the muscles. Pmus, pressure developed by the respiratory muscles; Prs, pressure of the respiratory system. (Adapted from Agostoni E, Mead J: Statics of the respiratory system. In Fenn WO, Rahn H, eds: Handbook of physiology: respiration, Vol. 1, Section 3. Washington, DC: American Physiology Society; 1964:387–409.)

rapid, fully coordinated recruitment of the diaphragm and other inspiratory muscles. The nose acts as a Starling resistor, so that nasal flow is low and largely independent of the driving pressure that is the esophageal pressure. Pdi measured during a sniff (Pdi,sn,max) reflects diaphragm strength, and Pes reflects the integrated pressure of the inspiratory muscles on the lungs (Figure 8-5). Pressures measured in the mouth, nasopharynx, or one nostril give a clinically useful approximation to esophageal pressure during sniffs without the need to insert esophageal balloons, especially in the absence of significant obstructive airway disease. To be useful as a test of respiratory muscle strength, sniffs need to be maximal, which is relatively easy for most willing subjects, but may require some practice. The nasal sniff pressure is the easiest measurement for the subject. Pressure is measured by wedging a catheter in one nostril by use of foam, rubber bungs, or dental impression molding (Figure 8-6). The subject sniffs through the contralateral unobstructed nostril. There is a wide range of normal values, reflecting the wide range of normal muscle strength in different individuals. In clinical practice, Pdi,sn,max values greater than 100 cm H_2O in males and 80 cm H_2O in females are unlikely to be associated with clinically significant diaphragm weakness. Values of maximal sniff esophageal or nasal pressure numerically greater than 70 cm H_2O (males) or 60 cm H_2O (females) are also unlikely to be associated with significant inspiratory muscle weakness. However, these reflect the integrated pressure of all the inspiratory muscles, and it is possible that there could be a degree of weakness of one or more of these muscle groups that would not be detected at this level. In chronic obstructive pulmonary disease, nasal sniff pressure tends to underestimate sniff esophageal pressure because of dampened pressure transmission from the alveoli to the upper airway but can complement $P_{I,max}$ in excluding weakness clinically.

Electrophysiologic Testing

The next diagnostic step consists of determining whether weakness is due to muscle, nerve, or neuromuscular transmission impairment. This requires the measurement of Pdi in response to bilateral supramaximal phrenic nerve electrical or magnetic stimulation, with concurrent recording of the elicited

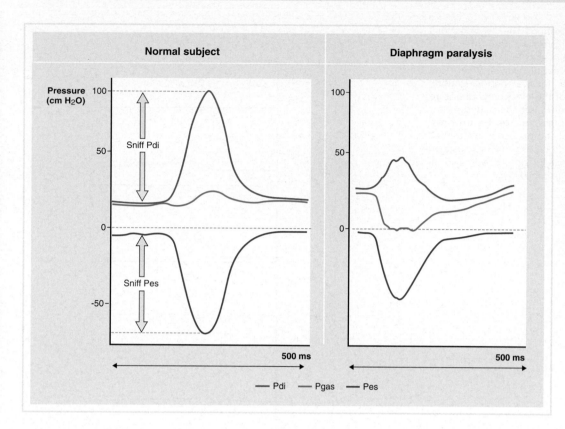

FIGURE 8-5 Examples of the sniff maneuver. Left panel shows a recording from a healthy subject. Note that the esophageal (pleural) pressure change is subatmospheric, whereas the intraabdominal pressure becomes more positive. Measurement conventions for the sniff esophageal (Sn Pes) and sniff transdiaphragmatic pressures (Sn Pdi) are illustrated. The right panel shows an example from a patient with bilateral diaphragmatic paralysis. Note that there is now a negative pressure change in the abdominal compartment, because the diaphragm fails to prevent pressure transmission from the thorax.

electromyogram (EMG) of the diaphragm (called the compound muscle action potential, CMAP) with either surface or esophageal electrodes (Figure 8-7). If the phrenic nerve is stimulated, the diaphragm contracts. This contraction is called a twitch. If the stimulus is intense enough, all phrenic fibers are activated synchronously giving reproducible results. The intensity of the twitch increases with the frequency of stimulation. If multiple impulses stimulate the phrenic nerve, the contractions summate to cause a tetanic contraction. Thus, if both phrenic nerves are stimulated with various frequencies (1, 10, 20, 50, and 100 Hz) at the same lung volume with closed airway (to prevent entry of air and thus changes in lung volume and initial length of the diaphragm), the isometric *force-frequency curve* of the diaphragm is obtained (Figure 8-8). (It should be noted that the usual rate of motor nerve discharge during voluntary muscle contraction in humans is between 5 and 15 Hz, and, because of the steep shape of the force-frequency curve in this range, small alterations in the

discharge rate cause significant changes in the force produced. Maximum voluntary contractions, such as the $P_{I,max}$ are achieved with discharge rates higher than 50 Hz, but cannot be sustained for long. Stimulation of the phrenic nerve with high frequencies is technically difficult to achieve (because of displacement of the stimulating electrode by local contraction of the scalene muscles and movement of the arm and shoulder because of activation of the brachial plexus). Therefore, the transdiaphragmatic pressure developed in response to single supramaximal phrenic nerve stimulations at 1 Hz, called the *twitch Pdi*, is commonly measured.

Although technically demanding, this approach has the great advantage of being independent of patient effort/motivation. This also allows for the measurement of *phrenic nerve conduction time* or *phrenic latency* (i.e., the time between the onset of the stimulus and the onset of CMAP [Mwave] on the diaphragmatic EMG) (Figure 8-7, *B*). A prolonged conduction time suggests nerve involvement.

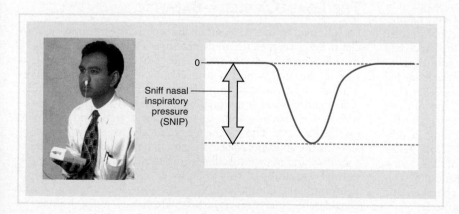

FIGURE 8-6 The sniff maneuver, which makes use of a nasal bung and an adapted pressure meter. **A,** Measurement setup. The meter returns a numerical value that is the amplitude of the pressure swing between atmospheric (0) pressure and the nadir. **B,** The trace produced. The meter returns a numerical value that is the amplitude of the pressure swing between atmospheric (0) pressure and the nadir.

FIGURE 8-7 Electrophysiologic testing: The "twitch Pdi." **A,** The twitch transdiaphragmatic pressure (Pdi) after magnetic/electrical stimulation. **B,** A detailed (enlarged) view of a compound muscle action potential (M wave), where the latency (time from stimulus to muscle depolarization), the duration, and the amplitude of the electromyogram are evident. *a.u.,* Arbitrary units; *L-CMAP,* left compound motor action potential; *Pes,* esophageal pressure; *Pga,* gastric pressure; *R-CMAP,* right compound motor action potential. (Adapted from Vassilakopoulos T, Roussos C: Neuromuscular respiratory failure. In Slutsky A, Takala R, Torres R, eds. Clinical Critical Care Medicine. St. Louis: Mosby, 2006.)

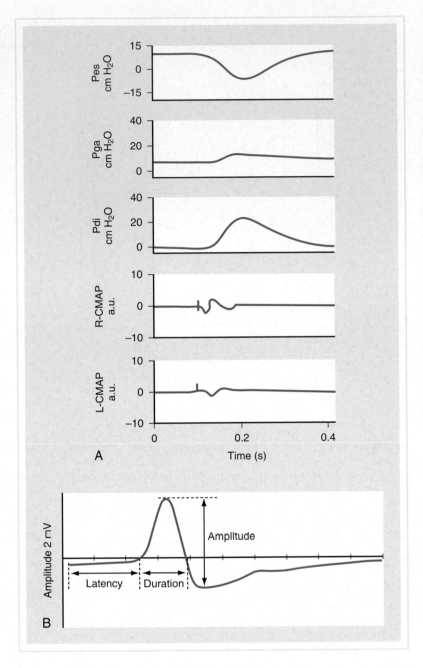

However, electrophysiologic testing also has shortcomings. Although the conduction time or latency is prolonged in neuropathies that are predominantly demyelinating, it may be preserved in neuropathies that are predominantly axonal despite substantial diaphragm weakness. Moreover, when the preceding technique is used, it is important that costimulation of the brachial plexus be avoided, otherwise the action potential recorded from surface electrodes may originate from muscles other than the diaphragm. This problem is compounded if the phrenic nerve is stimulated by use of a magnetic technique. Classically, an axonal neuropathy is characterized by the finding of preserved latencies with diminished CMAP. Lack of CMAP after nerve stimulation is an indication of paralysis with the lesion located proximal to or at the neuromuscular junction. Decreased twitch Pdi in the face of normal CMAP is characteristic of contractile dysfunction that resides within the muscle.

PHYSIOLOGY: THE ABILITY TO BREATH: THE LOAD/CAPACITY BALANCE

For a human to take a spontaneous breath, the inspiratory muscles must generate sufficient force to overcome the elastance of the lungs and chest wall (lung and chest wall elastic loads), as well as the airway and tissue resistance (resistive load). This requires an adequate output of the centers controlling the muscles, anatomic and functional nerve integrity, unimpaired neuromuscular transmission, an intact chest wall, and adequate muscle strength. This can be schematically represented by considering the ability to take a breath as a balance between inspiratory load and neuromuscular competence (Figure 8-9). Under normal conditions, this system is polarized in favor of neuromuscular competence (i.e., there are reserves that permit considerable increases in load). However, for a human to

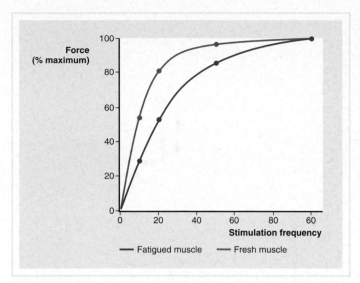

FIGURE 8-8 Force-frequency relationship of *in vivo* human respiratory muscles. The force-frequency curve of the fresh muscle is shown in red, and the relationship after a fatiguing task is shown in blue; a disproportionate force loss at low stimulation frequencies is observed. (Adapted from Moxham J, Wiles CM, Newham D, Edwards RHT: Ciba Found Symp 1981; 82:197–212.)

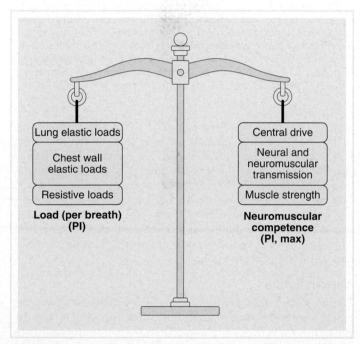

FIGURE 8-9 Balance between inspiratory load and neuromuscular competence. The ability to take a spontaneous breath is determined by the balance between the load imposed on the respiratory system (pressure developed by the inspiratory muscles; PI) and the neuromuscular competence of the ventilatory pump (maximum inspiratory pressure; PI, max). Normally, this balance weighs in favor of competence, permitting significant increases in load. However, if the competence is, for whatever reason, reduced below a critical point (e.g., drug overdose, myasthenia gravis), the balance may then weigh in favor of load, rendering the ventilatory pump insufficient to inflate the lungs and chest wall. (Adapted from Vassilakopoulos T, Roussos C: Neuromuscular respiratory failure. In Slutsky A, Takala R, Torres, eds. Clinical Critical Care Medicine. St. Louis: Mosby, 2006.)

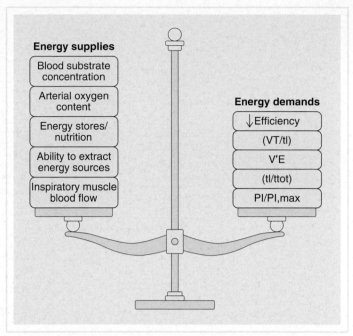

FIGURE 8-10 Balance between energy supplies and energy demands. Respiratory muscle endurance is determined by the balance between energy supplies and demands. Normally, the supplies meet the demands, and a large reserve exists. Whenever this balance weighs in favor of demands, the respiratory muscles ultimately become fatigued, leading to inability to sustain spontaneous breathing. *VT/tl,* Mean inspiratory flow (tidal volume/inspiratory time); *tl/ttot,* duty cycle (fraction of inspiration to total breathing cycle duration); *PI/PI, max,* inspiratory pressure/maximum inspiratory pressure ratio; *V'E,* minute ventilation. (Adapted from Vassilakopoulos T, Roussos C: Neuromuscular respiratory failure. In Slutsky A, Takala R, Torres, eds. Clinical Critical Care Medicine. St. Louis: Mosby, 2006.)

breathe spontaneously, the inspiratory muscles should be able to sustain the aforementioned load over time as well as adjust the minute ventilation in such a way that there is adequate gas exchange. The ability of the respiratory muscles to sustain this load without the appearance of fatigue is called endurance and is determined by the balance between energy supplies and energy demands (Figure 8-10).

Energy supplies depend on the inspiratory muscle blood flow, the blood substrate (fuel) concentration and arterial oxygen content, the muscle's ability to extract and use energy sources, and the muscle's energy stores. Under normal circumstances, energy supplies are adequate to meet the demands, and a large recruitable reserve exists (see Figure 8-10). Energy demands increase proportionally with the mean pressure developed by the inspiratory muscles per breath (PI) expressed as a fraction of maximum pressure that the respiratory muscles can voluntarily develop ($P_I/P_{I,max}$), the minute ventilation (V_E), the inspiratory duty cycle (T_I/T_{TOT}), and the mean inspiratory flow rate (V_T/T_I) and are inversely related to the efficiency of the muscles. Fatigue develops when the mean rate of energy demands exceeds the mean rate of energy supply (i.e., when the balance is polarized in favor of demands).

The product of T_I/T_{TOT} and the mean transdiaphragmatic pressure expressed as a fraction of maximal ($P_{di}/P_{di,max}$) defines a useful "tension-time index" (TTI_{di}) that is related to the endurance time (i.e., the time that the diaphragm can

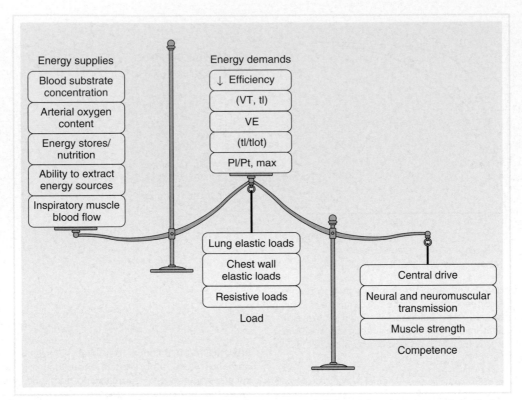

FIGURE 8-11 System of two balances: load and competence, energy supplies and demands. The system of two balances, incorporating the various determinants of load, competence, energy supplies, and demands is represented schematically. The PI/PI, max, one of the determinants of energy demands (see Figure 8-10) is replaced by its equivalent: the balance between load and neuromuscular competence (see Figure 8-9). In fact, this is the reason the two balances are linked. When the central hinge of the system moves upward or is at least at the horizontal level, a balance exists between ventilatory needs and neurorespiratory capacity, and spontaneous ventilation can be sustained. In healthy persons, the hinge moves far upward, creating a large reserve. For abbreviations, see legends to Figures 8-9 and 8-10. (Adapted from Vassilakopoulos T, Roussos C: Neuromuscular respiratory failure. In Slutsky A, Takala R, Torres R, eds. Clinical Critical Care Medicine. St. Louis: Mosby, 2006.)

sustain the load imposed on it). Whenever TTI_{di} is smaller than the critical value of 0.15, the load can be sustained indefinitely; but when TTI_{di} exceeds the critical zone of 0.15–0.18, the load can be sustained only for a limited time period, in other words, the endurance time. This was found to be inversely related to TTI_{di}. The TTI concept is assumed to be applicable not only to the diaphragm but also to the respiratory muscles as a whole:

$$TTI = P_I/P_{I,max} \times T_I/T_{TOT}$$

Because endurance is determined by the balance between energy supply and demand, TTI of the inspiratory muscles has to be in accordance with the energy balance view. In fact, as Figure 8-4 demonstrates, $P_I/P_{I,max}$ and T_I/T_{TOT}, which constitute the TTI, are among the determinants of energy demands; an increase in either that will increase the TTI value will also increase the demands. But what determines the ratio $P_I/P_{I,max}$? The nominator, the mean inspiratory pressure developed per breath, is determined by the elastic and resistive loads imposed on the inspiratory muscles. The denominator, the maximum inspiratory pressure, is determined by the neuromuscular competence (i.e., the maximum inspiratory muscle activation that can be voluntarily achieved). It follows, then, that the value of $P_I/P_{I,max}$ is determined by the balance between load and competence (see Figure 8-9). But $P_I/P_{I,max}$ is also one of the determinants of energy demands (see Figure 8-10); therefore, the two balances (i.e., between load and competence and energy supply and demand) are in essence linked, creating a

system (Figure 8-11). Schematically, when the central hinge of the system moves upward, or is at least at the horizontal level, spontaneous ventilation can be sustained indefinitely (see Figure 8-11). The ability of a subject to breathe spontaneously depends on the fine interplay of many different factors. Normally, this interplay moves the central hinge far upward and creates a great ventilatory reserve for the healthy individual. When the central hinge of the system, for whatever reason, moves downward, spontaneous ventilation cannot be sustained, and ventilatory failure ensues.

Hyperinflation

Hyperinflation (frequently observed in obstructive airway diseases) compromises the force-generating capacity of the diaphragm for a variety of reasons: First, the respiratory muscles, like other skeletal muscles, obey the length-tension relationship. At any given level of activation, changes in muscle fiber length alter tension development. This is because the force-tension developed by a muscle depends on the interaction between actin and myosin fibrils (i.e., the number of myosin heads attaching and thus pulling the actin fibrils closer within each sarcomere). The optimal fiber length (Lo) where tension is maximal is the length at which all myosin heads attach and pull the actin fibrils. Below this length (as with hyperinflation, which shortens the diaphragm), actin-myosin interaction becomes suboptimal, and tension development declines. Second, as lung volume increases, the zone of apposition of the diaphragm decreases in size, and a larger fraction of

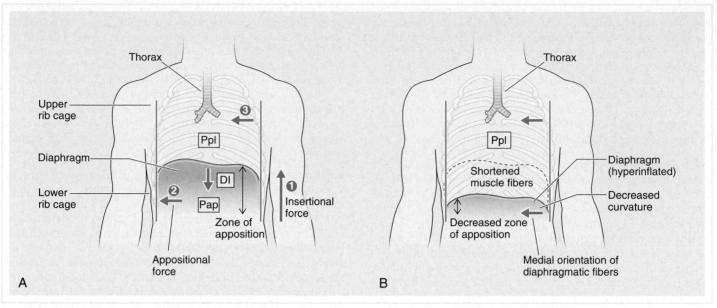

FIGURE 8-12 Consequences of hyperinflation on the diaphragm. **A,** Normal actions of the diaphragm as in Figure 8-2. **B,** Deleterious effects of hyperinflation on the diaphragm.

the rib cage becomes exposed to pleural pressure. Hence, the diaphragm's inspiratory action on the rib cage diminishes. When lung volume approaches total lung capacity, the zone of apposition all but disappears (Figure 8-12), and the diaphragmatic muscle fibers become oriented horizontally internally (Figure 8-12, *B*). The insertional force of the diaphragm is then expiratory, rather than inspiratory, in direction. This explains the inspiratory decrease in the transverse diameter of the lower rib cage in subjects with emphysema and severe hyperinflation (Hoover's sign). Third, the resultant flattening of the diaphragm increases its radius of curvature (Rdi) (see Figure 8-12, *B*) and, according to Laplace's law, Pdi = 2Tdi/Rdi, diminishes its pressure-generating capacity (Pdi) for the same tension development (Tdi).

RESPIRATORY MUSCLE RESPONSES TO CHANGES IN LOAD

Acute Responses

Increased Load

Respiratory Muscle Fatigue. Fatigue is defined as the loss of capacity to develop force and/or velocity in response to a load that is reversible by rest. Thus, fatigue may be present before the point at which a muscle is unable to continue to perform a particular task (task failure). In applying this concept to the inspiratory muscles, one could conclude that they may be fatigued before there is hypercapnia because of their inability to continue to generate sufficient pressure to maintain alveolar ventilation.

Fatigue should be distinguished from weakness in which reduced force generation is fixed and not reversed by rest, although the presence of weakness may itself predispose a muscle to fatigue. The site and mechanisms of fatigue remain controversial. Theoretically, the site of fatigue may be located at any link in the long chain of events involved in voluntary muscle contraction leading from the brain to the contractile machinery. A widely used convention is to classify fatigue as central fatigue, peripheral high-frequency fatigue, or peripheral low-frequency fatigue.

Central Fatigue. Central fatigue is present when a maximal voluntary contraction generates less force than does maximal electrical stimulation. If maximal electrical stimulation superimposed on a maximal voluntary contraction can potentiate the force generated by a muscle, a component of central fatigue exists. This procedure applied to the diaphragm consists of the *twitch occlusion test* that may separate central from peripheral fatigue. This test examines the transdiaphragmatic pressure (Pdi) response to bilateral phrenic nerve stimulation superimposed on graded voluntary contractions of the diaphragm. Normally, the amplitude of the Pdi twitches in response to phrenic nerve stimulation decreases as the voluntary Pdi increases. During Pdi,max, no superimposed twitches can be detected. When diaphragmatic fatigue is present, superimposed twitches can be demonstrated. A number of experiments have suggested that a form of central diaphragmatic "fatigue" may develop during respiratory loading so that, at the limits of diaphragmatic endurance, a significant portion of the reduction in force production is due to failure of the central nervous system to completely activate the diaphragm. Central fatigue may be caused by a reduction in the number of motor units that can be recruited by the motor drive or by a decrease in motor unit discharge rates or both. The observed decreased central firing rate during fatigue may, in fact, be a beneficial adaptive response preventing the muscle's self-destruction by excessive activation.

Peripheral Fatigue. Peripheral fatigue refers to failure at the neuromuscular junction or distal to this structure and is present when muscle force output falls in response to direct electrical stimulation. This type of fatigue may occur because of failure of impulse propagation across the neuromuscular junction, the muscle surface membrane or the t tubules (transmission fatigue), impaired excitation—contraction coupling, or failure of the contractile apparatus of the muscle fibers (because of alterations in metabolism or changes in contractile proteins).

Peripheral fatigue can be further classified into *high-frequency* and *low-frequency fatigue* on the basis of the shape of the muscle force-frequency curve (Figure 8-8). High-frequency fatigue results in depression of the forces generated by a muscle in response to high-frequency electrical stimulation (50–100 Hz), whereas low-frequency fatigue results in depression of force generation in response to low-frequency stimuli (1–20 Hz). Low-frequency fatigue can occur in isolation, but high-frequency fatigue is invariably associated with some alterations in muscle force generation at lower frequencies.

High-Frequency Fatigue. During artificial stimulation of a motor neuron, especially at high frequencies, muscle force declines rapidly in association with the decline in CMAP amplitude. This response, known as "high-frequency fatigue" (see Figure 8-8), is attributed to transmission fatigue. The site of this type of fatigue may be located postsynaptically (from a decrease in sarcolemmal membrane endplate excitability or a reduction in action potential propagation into the t tubular system) or presynaptically (probably in fine terminal filaments of the motor nerve or less frequently from depletion of synaptic transmitter substance). Teleologically, transmission block could be beneficial in some instances by protecting the muscle against excessive depletion of its ATP stores, which would lead to rigor mortis. Normal subjects breathing against high-intensity inspiratory resistive loads develop high-frequency fatigue, which resolves very quickly after cessation of the strenuous diaphragmatic contractions.

Low-Frequency Fatigue. All processes that link the electrical activation of the muscle fiber and the various metabolic and enzymatic processes providing energy to the contractile machinery are called excitation-contraction coupling processes. Impaired excitation contraction coupling is thought to be responsible when the loss of force is not accompanied by a parallel decline in the electrical activity. This type of fatigue is characterized by a selective loss of force at low frequencies of stimulation (low-frequency fatigue) (see Figure 8-8) despite maintenance of the force generated at high frequencies of stimulation, indicating that the contractile proteins continue to generate force provided that sufficient calcium is released by the sarcoplasmic reticulum. The mechanism of this type of fatigue is not understood. It may occur because of a reduced level of calcium availability caused by alterations in sarcoplasmic reticulum function or a reduction in the calcium sensitivity of the myofilaments (troponin binding site) at submaximal calcium concentrations (because of high hydrogen and phosphate ion concentration). These defects would reduce the force developed at low-frequency stimulation. In contrast, at higher stimulation frequencies, a relatively normal force can be generated when the interior of the fiber is saturated with calcium.

This type of fatigue is characteristically long lasting, taking several hours to recover. Low-frequency fatigue occurs during high-force contractions and is less likely to develop when the forces generated are smaller, even if these are maintained for longer time periods, thereby achieving the same total work. As previously stated, fatigue develops when the mean rate of energy demands exceeds the mean rate of energy supply to the muscle (see Figure 8-10), resulting in depletion of muscle energy stores, pH changes from lactate accumulation, and excessive production of oxygen-derived free radicals. However, the exact interplay of all these factors is not yet identified in either the diaphragm or the

other skeletal muscles. Accordingly, low-frequency fatigue occurs in the diaphragm of experimental animals during cardiogenic or septic shock. Low-frequency fatigue has also been found in the diaphragm and sternocleidomastoid of normal subjects after they breathed against very high inspiratory resistance or after sustaining maximum voluntary ventilation (for 2 min) (Figure 8-13).

The clinical relevance of respiratory muscle fatigue is difficult to figure out, because the measurements that are required for fatigue detection are hard to apply in situations where fatigue is likely present (such as during acute hypercapnic respiratory failure).

Inflammation and Injury. Strenuous diaphragmatic contractions (induced by resistive breathing, which accompanies many disease states such as COPD and asthma) initiate an inflammatory response consisting of elevation of plasma cytokines and recruitment and activation of white blood cell subpopulations. These cytokines are produced within the diaphragm secondary to the increased muscle activation. Strenuous resistive breathing results in diaphragmatic ultrastructural injury (such as sarcomere disruption, necrotic fibers, flocculent degeneration, and influx of inflammatory cells) in both animals and humans. The mechanisms involved are not definitely established but may involve intradiaphragmatic cytokine induction, adhesion molecule upregulation, calpain activation, and reactive oxygen species formation. Cytokines are also essential in orchestrating muscle recovery after injury by enhancing proteolytic removal of damaged proteins and cells (through recruitment and activation of phagocytes) and by activating satellite cells. Satellite cells are quiescent cells of embryonic origin that reside in the muscle and are

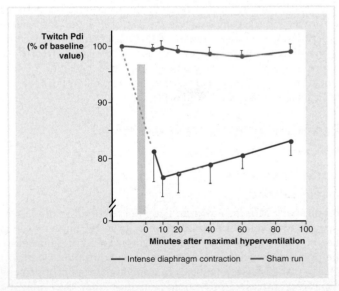

FIGURE 8-13 Demonstration of low-frequency fatigue of the diaphragm in normal subjects. The mean twitch tension (twitch transdiaphragmatic pressure; Tw Pdi) is shown before and at intervals up to 90 min after intense diaphragmatic contraction (in this case, a 2-min period of maximal normocapnic hyperventilation) in nine healthy adults (*blue symbols*). Data in the same subjects after a sham ("normal breathing") run are shown in red. A significant decline in Tw Pdi is observed that has only partially recovered at 90 min, which confirms the presence of low-frequency diaphragmatic fatigue. (Data from Hamnegård C-H, Wragg SD, Kyroussis D, *et al*: Diaphragm fatigue following maximal ventilation in man. Eur Respir J 1996; 9:241–247.)

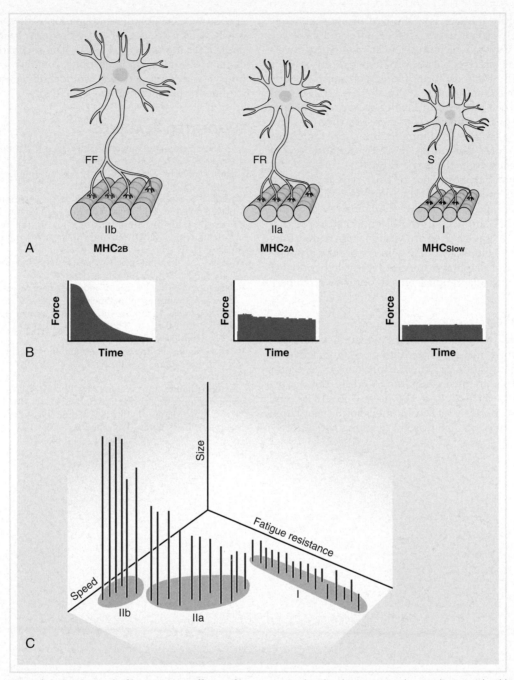

FIGURE 8-14 Properties of skeletal muscle fiber types. Different fiber types in the diaphragm muscle are distinguished by size, myosin heavy chain content, contractile characteristics (force and speed of contraction), and fatigue resistance (type S, slow; type FR, fast-twitch, fatigue resistant; and type FF motor units, fast-twitch, fatigable), as well as myosin heavy chain (MHC) isoform expression (MHCSlow, MHC2A, and MHC2B). **A,** Size; **B,** force; **C,** size, speed of contraction, fatigue resistance. (Adapted from Mantilla CB, Sieck GS: Mechanisms underlying motor unit plasticity in the respiratory system. J Appl Physiol 2003; 94:1230–1241; and Jones DA: Skeletal muscle physiology. In Roussos C, ed: The Thorax, 2nd ed. New York: Marcel Dekker; 3–32).

transformed into myocytes, when the muscle becomes injured, to replace damaged myocytes.

Chronic Responses

Increased Load

Plasticity and Adaptation. The respiratory muscles are plastic organs that respond to chronic changes of the load they are facing and thus of their activity with structural and functional changes/adaptations.

COPD is the paradigm of a disease with chronically increased respiratory muscle load. A major adaptation of the respiratory muscles is fiber type transformation. The myosin heavy chain component of the myosin molecule constitutes the basis for the classification of muscle fibers as either (type I) or (type II) (Figure 8-14, *A*). Myosin heavy chain exists in various isoforms, which in increasing order of maximum shortening velocity are myosin heavy chain (MHC) I, IIa, and IIb, the latter being the faster (Figure 8-14, *C*). The diaphragm in healthy humans is composed of approximately 50% type I fatigue-resistant fibers, 25% type IIa, and 25% type IIb. There are two ways in which muscles can modify their overall MHC phenotype: preferential atrophy/hypertrophy of fibers containing a specific MHC isoform and actual transformation from one fiber type to another. In COPD, there is a transformation of type II to type I fibers, resulting in a great predominance of type I fatigue-resistant fibers. This increases the resistance of the diaphragm to fatigue development, but at the same time compromises the force-generating capacity, because type I fibers can generate less force than type II fibers.

Adaptation is not only restricted to fiber type transformation. In an animal model of COPD (emphysematous hamsters), the number and the length of sarcomeres decrease, resulting in a leftward shift of the length-tension curve, so that the muscle adapts to the shorter operating length induced by hyperinflation. These alterations may help restore the mechanical advantage of the diaphragm in chronically hyperinflated states. In humans, this adaptation seems to occur by sarcomere length shortening.

Inactivity-Unloading

Respiratory muscles do not only adapt when they function against increased load but also when they become inactive, as happens during denervation or when a mechanical ventilator undertakes their role as force generator to create the driving pressure permitting airflow into the lungs. Inactivity and unloading of the diaphragm caused by mechanical ventilation is harmful, resulting in decreased diaphragmatic force-generating capacity, diaphragmatic atrophy, and diaphragmatic injury, which are described by the term *ventilator-induced diaphragmatic dysfunction (VIDD)*. The mechanisms are not fully explained, but muscle atrophy, oxidative stress, structural injury, and muscle fiber remodeling contribute to various extents in the development of VIDD.

SUGGESTED READINGS

ATS/ERS: Statement on Respiratory Muscle Testing. Am J Respir Crit Care Med 2002; 166:518–624.

Laghi F, Tobin M: Disorders of the respiratory muscles. Am J Respir Crit Care Med 2003; 168:10–48.

Mantilla CB, Sieck GS: Invited review: Mechanisms underlying motor unit plasticity in the respiratory system. J Appl Physiol 2003; 94:1230–1241.

Orozco-Levi M: Structure and function of the respiratory muscles in patients with COPD: impairment or adaptation? Eur Respir J 2003; 22:Suppl.46, 41s–51s.

Roussos C, Zakynthinos S: Fatigue of the respiratory muscles. Intensive Care Med 1996; 22:134–55.

Vassilakopoulos T: Ventilator-induced diaphragmatic dysfunction: The clinical relevance of animal models. Intensive Care Med 2007 (in press).

Vassilakopoulos T, Roussos C: Neuromuscular respiratory failure. In Slutsky A, Takala R, Torres R, eds. Clinical Critical Care Medicine. St. Louis: Mosby, 2006:275–282.

Vassilakopoulos T, Roussos C, Zakynthinos S: The immune response to resistive breathing. Eur Respir J 2004; 24:1033–1043.

Vassilakopoulos T, Zakynthinos S, Roussos C: Respiratory muscles and weaning failure. Eur Respir 1996; J9:2383–2400.

Vassilakopoulos T, Zakynthinos S, Roussos C: Muscle function: Basic concepts. In Marini JJ, Slutsky A, eds. Physiologic Basis of Ventilator Support. New York: Marcel Dekker; 1998:103–152.

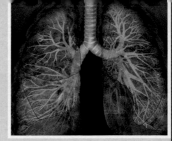

9 Pulmonary Function Testing

SCOTT E. EVANS • PAUL D. SCANLON • BRUCE H. CULVER

INTRODUCTION

Pulmonary function testing (PFT) includes a number of direct and indirect measurements that assist in the characterization of respiratory physiology. These studies play an essential role in the diagnosis and management of patients with or at risk for respiratory disease. They provide the clinician objective assessments, which may be correlated with highly subjective symptoms, such as dyspnea. Their quantitative results also allow for longitudinal monitoring of patients' respiratory health, particularly when respiratory symptoms correlate poorly with disease severity and progression. By themselves, they do not provide specific diagnoses, but in many situations they can meaningfully inform the clinician of the patterns and extent of the underlying process.

INDICATIONS FOR PULMONARY FUNCTION TESTING

As endorsed by the American Thoracic Society, lung function tests should facilitate the description of respiratory dysfunction, assessment of disease severity, and estimation of prognosis in lung disease. They are established as essential diagnostic criteria for specific disorders, including asthma. When used for monitoring patient progress, they allow assessment of both beneficial and untoward effects of therapy, as well as monitoring the natural course of the disease. Lung function testing can provide longitudinal surveillance after patient exposures to environmental insults, radiation therapy, and pulmonary toxic medications. Furthermore, they are sensitive to various extrapulmonary disorders, including neuromuscular, cardiovascular, and inflammatory processes.

The benefit of screening asymptomatic patients without specific risk factors remains controversial. However, physician-initiated screening of select asymptomatic populations seems to allow the identification of preclinical lung diseases, which, in turn, may allow early intervention while these diseases remain most treatable. The third National Health and Nutrition Examination Survey (NHANES III) and the Lung Health Study confirmed the ability of lung function tests to identify presymptomatic lung disease in smokers. These data, along with observations that abnormal PFT results influence smokers to seek medical treatment and to attempt smoking cessation, prompted recommendations for the performance of office-based screening spirometry for current smokers 45 years of age or any smoker with respiratory complaints. In addition to the use of screening and symptom-indicated spirometry, these documents also endorse spirometry as a tool for global health assessment.

SPIROMETRY

Spirometry is the most fundamental element of lung function testing. It directly measures the volume of air exhaled or inhaled by a subject as a function of time. Thus, the reported values from spirometric tests may be measures of volume (liters) or flow (liters/second).

Most spirometric values are obtained during a forced expiratory vital capacity (FEVC) maneuver, requiring the subject to forcefully expel air from a point of maximal inspiration (total lung capacity, TLC) to a point of maximal expiration (residual volume, RV). Table 9-1 lists the functional measurements possible from the forced expiratory maneuver; the most important ones are the forced vital capacity (FVC), the forced expired volume in the first second (FEV_1), and the FEV_1/FVC ratio.

During expiration, flow is determined by the driving airflow pressure—the difference between the intraalveolar pressure (i.e., the pleural pressure (ppl) and elastic recoil pressure [pel]) and the ambient atmospheric pressure at the mouth and the resistance to flow imposed by the airways. Because the increasing intrapleural pressures produced during forceful expiration may exceed the intraluminal pressure of the airways, the FEVC maneuver may result in increased airway resistance compared with the airway pressures generated during a relaxed expiratory maneuver (the so-called slow-VC maneuver; see Figure 4-3). The increased airways resistance associated with the FEVC maneuver results in decreased flows in some patients and has recently prompted the American Thoracic Society (ATS) and the European Respiratory Society (ERS) to jointly recommend the use of the slow VC relative to the FEV_1 to establish the presence of obstructive lung disease.

Laboratories vary in their use of the FEV_1/VC ratio to identify and evaluate airflow obstruction. Some use the FEV_1/FVC, and others the FEV_1/VC. This is because the VC (slow/relaxed) is often greater than FVC, and almost never less, so substituting FEV_1/VC for FEV_1/FVC will result in an overestimation of the severity of obstruction.

The forced inspiratory vital capacity (FIVC) maneuver requires forced maximal inhalation from RV to TLC. Like the slow VC, in some subjects with obstructive lung disease, the FIVC may be somewhat less prone to induce airways closure and airtrapping than the FEVC.

In addition to the absolute values, the FEVC and the FIVC maneuvers can be plotted graphically to enhance their diagnostic yield and as a quality assurance tool. As shown in Figure 9-1, plotting the FEVC maneuver with volume versus time can provide information about the performance quality of the test. Conversely, if plotted with flow versus volume exhaled, FEVC

TABLE 9-1 **Definitions of Common Spirometric Values**

Reported Value	Description	Interpretation
VC	Vital capacity Volume of air displaced by maximal exhalation or maximal inhalation maneuver	Typically preserved in obstruction, but reduced in restriction.
FVC	Forced vital capacity Volume forcefully exhaled from maximal inhalation (TLC) to maximal exhalation (RV), the FEVC maneuver	Pattern similar to VC, although more likely to be reduced in obstruction than VC. Used to grade severity of restriction.
FEV_1	Forced expiratory volume in one second Volume exhaled in 1st second of FEVC maneuver	Reduction typical of medium to large airways obstruction. Used to grade severity of obstruction.
FEV_1/FVC	Ratio of FEV_1 to FVC	Reductions indicative of airway obstruction.
FEF_{25-75}	Forced expiratory flow (25–75%) Mean expiratory flow rate in the middle half of FEVC maneuver	Sensitive but nonspecific indicator of small airways obstruction. Poorly reproducible, varies with effort and time of expiration.
FIVC	Forced inspiratory vital capacity Maximum volume forcefully inhaled from maximal exhalation, the FIVC maneuver	Inspiratory flows reduced in extrathoracic airways obstruction, correlate with MVV.
MVV	Maximum voluntary ventilation Estimate of one minute's maximal air displacement extrapolated from repeated inspiratory and expiratory efforts	Disproportionate reductions relative to FEV_1 may indicate upper airways obstruction, muscle weakness, or poor performance.
PEF	Peak expiratory flow Maximal sustained airflow achieved during the FEVC maneuver	Worsening may correlate with asthma exacerbations. Sometimes helpful in assessing subject effort.

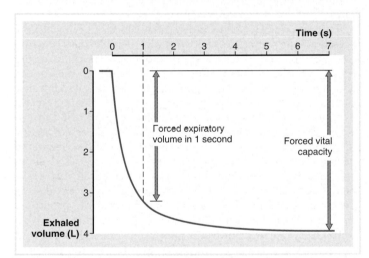

FIGURE 9-1 Normal forced expiratory spirogram plotted as exhaled volume versus time. The forced expiratory volume at 1 sec (FEV_1) and forced vital capacity (FVC) are indicated by arrows. In this example, FEV_1 is 3.35 L, FVC is 4 L, and the FEV_1/FVC ratio is 84%. (Modified with permission from Culver BH: Pulmonary function testing. In Kelly WN, ed: Textbook of Internal Medicine. Philadelphia: JB Lippincott; 1988.)

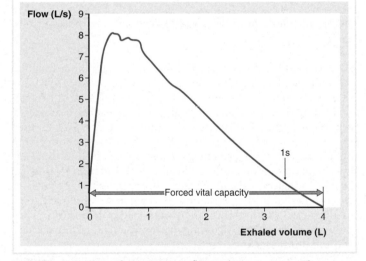

FIGURE 9-2 Normal expiratory flow-volume curve. The same forced expiratory volume maneuver shown in Figure 9-1 is plotted here as a flow-volume curve. The airflow rate reaches a peak early in the exhalation, then decreases progressively until airflow ceases at residual volume.

may provide a more comprehensive view of a subject's respiratory mechanics and facilitate the identification of maneuver errors, as well as subtle physiologic abnormalities (Figure 9-2).

An additional flow measurement commonly reported from the spirogram is the average forced expiratory flow rate between 25 and 75% of the exhaled VC (FEF_{25-75}), formerly referred to as the maximum midexpiratory flow rate. This measurement shows wider variability than does FEV_1 or the FEV_1/FVC ratio, both within and between individuals. When this variability is appropriately accounted for, the FEF_{25-75} is

no more sensitive than the FEV_1/FVC ratio for the detection of airflow limitation.

The peak expiratory flow rate achieved during the FVC maneuver cannot be accurately calculated from a spirogram display but is readily seen on the flow-volume display and can be calculated by microprocessors. It can show considerable effort-to-effort variability, even when FEV_1 and FVC measurements are nearly identical. A peak flow measurement can also be obtained by simple hand-held devices, which are useful for interval follow-up and for home management of patients who have reactive airway disease, but they are less accurate and less sensitive than spirometry for screening. Whereas spirographic flow measurements are obtained over a time interval or volume interval, measurements from the flow-volume display or current microprocessors can be reported at specific lung volumes. Maximum flow rates at 50% and 75% of exhaled volume are commonly reported, but nomenclature varies, and the latter is often designated as the flow rate at 25% of remaining VC.

Bronchodilator Response

Spirometry is often performed before and after the administration of a bronchodilator. Usually, this involves the inhalation of a β_2-agonist, such as albuterol, although ipratropium bromide can be substituted for albuterol. The ATS defines a significant response as an increase in either FEV_1 or FVC, which are both >12% of the baseline value *and* >200 mL. Of these, changes in the FEV_1 correlate more closely with reversibility of airflow obstruction, because the FVC may increase merely because of longer expiratory effort. However, an isolated FVC increase that does not solely result from an increased expiratory time may indicate a reduction in "airtrapping" and can be interpreted as a bona fide bronchodilator response. As many as 30% of patients that do not respond to one bronchodilator will respond to another agent. Bronchodilator responsiveness can vary over time, with > 50% of individuals changing from positive to negative response or vice versa.

The response to bronchodilator is clinically relevant for several reasons. A significant response in the setting of asthma can justify the confident use of appropriate medications, and the demonstration of benefit may be psychologically important to promoting patient compliance with medications. However, the lack of a bronchodilator response does not always suggest sustained bronchodilator therapy will confer no benefit. In chronic obstructive pulmonary disease (COPD), responsiveness to bronchodilator and bronchoconstrictor correlate with worse decline in lung function over time, and, thus, this information may be helpful in directing intensive therapy. Finally, improvement in flows after bronchodilators may facilitate the identification of occult airflow obstruction, when the baseline spirometry may have been otherwise interpreted as low-normal or may reveal a restrictive abnormality.

Bronchoprovocation

Spirometry performed before and after bronchoprovocation challenge is also useful in identifying airways hyperreactivity. Most protocols require at least a 15–20% decrease in FEV_1 after inhalation of methacholine or histamine aerosol to consider a bronchoprovocation challenge positive. Asthma is not absolutely excluded by a negative methacholine challenge, because other stimuli may precipitate bronchospasm in some asthmatic individuals. In these cases, well-equipped laboratories offer protocols to perform spirometry before and after other challenges, such as exercise or cold air exposure. Bronchoprovocation challenge is typically requested to identify occult asthma, as seen with episodic cough, wheeze, or chest tightness without airflow obstruction noted on baseline spirometry. It is important to recall that bronchoprovocation challenges can be positive in nonasthmatic conditions, as well. Common examples include gastroesophageal reflux, allergic rhinitis, COPD, and after viral lower respiratory tract infections.

Reference Standards

A variety of reference equations are available to determine expected normal spirometric values. In all accepted standards, height, gender, age, and ethnicity are included. The predictions in all cases are derived from cross-sectional population studies, thus they are subject to cohort effects. It is imperative that each laboratory select for itself a reference standard that is congruent with the demographics of its patient population. The most recent statement from the ATS and ERS recommends the use of the NHANES III reference equations for patients aged 8–80 in the United States. No recommendation is made for European laboratories, although the European Community for Coal and Steel (1993) values are widely used.

Lung Volumes

Spirometry is a vital element of lung function testing, measuring volumes of inhaled and exhaled air. It cannot determine the total amount of air in the chest at full inspiration (TLC), the amount of air remaining in the lungs at the end of quiet (tidal) expiration (functional residual capacity, FRC), or the amount of air remaining after maximal expiration (RV; see Figure 4-2). To determine these "static lung volumes," one of three methods must be used. Although each has technical limitations, all are physiologically sound methods capable of providing accurate results.

Inert Gas Dilution

The inert gases include helium, argon, and neon. They have very low solubility in blood, so are not taken up by pulmonary capillary blood and remain within the lungs. Taking advantage of these properties, the inert gas dilution technique allows for calculation of lung volumes by determining the dilution of a known concentration of inert gas in the chest. The subject breathes from a water-sealed spirometer containing a known volume and concentration of gas (usually 10–15% helium; Figure 9-3). Oxygen is supplemented to account for metabolic use, carbon dioxide is absorbed from the system to maintain a steady state, and a nose clip prevents escape of the test gases. The patient is "turned in" the system as close to FRC as possible and breathes tidally with occasional VC maneuvers to allow optimal distribution of the gas mixture within the lungs. Once a new steady-state gas concentration is achieved, lung volumes are calculated by use of the equation $C_1V_1 = C_2V_2$. Most often, FRC is determined by direct measurement of the concentration, and TLC and RV are calculated as FRC plus inspiratory capacity or FRC minus expiratory reserve volume.

Inert gas dilution is well suited to patients who cannot undergo plethysmography because of physical constraints or claustrophobia. The primary drawback of this method is that it assumes even gas distribution in the lungs, which may not be the case in obstructive lung diseases, noncommunicating cavities, or pneumothoraces. In these circumstances, the FRC and the consequent measurement of TLC may be underestimated. This is especially the case in emphysema where the wash in of the He/O_2 mixture into large alveolar spaces is too slow.

Nitrogen Washout

Although helium can be "washed in" to measure lung volumes, nitrogen can be "washed out." The lung is normally filled with air containing approximately 80% nitrogen (16% O_2, some H_2O, and ~5% CO_2). This test calculates lung volumes by having the subject breathe 100% oxygen and collecting the exhaled air by means of a one-way valve (Figure 9-4). The subject continues to breathe nitrogen-free oxygen until the resident nitrogen has been "washed out," as indicated by

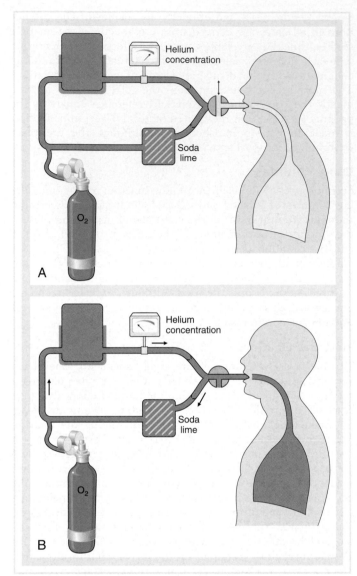

FIGURE 9-3 Lung volume measurement by helium dilution. **A,** The spirometer and circuit are prepared with a known gas volume and concentration of helium. **B,** The subject breathes through the circuit, as carbon dioxide is absorbed and oxygen consumption is replaced, until a new lower helium concentration is established. The unknown lung volume added to the circuit when the valve was turned is calculated from the dilution of the initial helium concentration: $[He]_{initial} \times Vol_1 = [He]_{final} \times (Vol_1 + FRC)$.

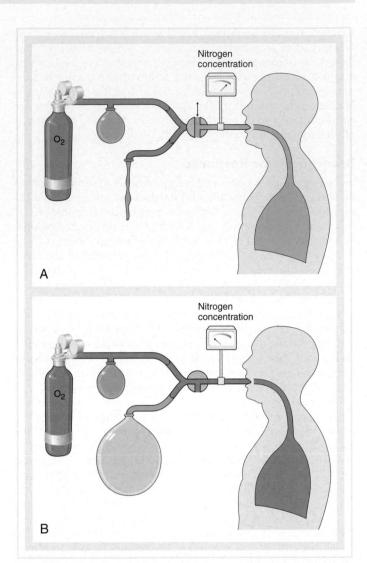

FIGURE 9-4 Lung volume measurement by nitrogen washout. **A,** Before the test, as the subject breathes air, the lungs are filled with 80% nitrogen and the collection system is flushed free of nitrogen. **B,** The subject inhales 100% oxygen and exhales into the collection bag until the exhaled N_2 concentration approaches zero. The total volume of the bag and its final N_2 concentration are measured, and the unknown initial lung volume (including valve and mouthpiece dead space) is calculated: $[N_2]_{bag} \times Vol_{bag} = 0.80 \times FRC$.

concentrations of nitrogen reaching a target value. The total collected nitrogen is then analyzed, and knowledge of the original concentration can be used to calculate the original lung volume. Like the inert gas dilution technique, this method underestimates the lung volumes of patients with uneven gas distribution, as in COPD. This effect can be partly overcome by extending the test time to 15–20 min (normal tests last 3–4 min), but this is often impractical for laboratories and may be unpleasant for patients.

Body Plethysmography

Boyle's law states that, given constant temperatures, the product of the pressure and the volume of a gas will remain constant ($P_1V_1 = P_2V_2$; Figure 9-5). Plethysmography harnesses

this principle to calculate static lung volumes by measuring mouth pressure changes during compression and rarefaction of the intrathoracic air of a subject enclosed in a sealed box. The pulmonary blood flow ensures isothermic thoracic gas. This approach not only allows for direct measurement of multiple volumes, but it allows for rapidly repeated measurements, unlike inert gas techniques that require that the patient reequilibrate. This test is also sensitive to all thoracic air, so noncommunicating areas of the lung, such as emphysematous bullae, are accounted for in the measurements.

INTERPRETATION OF LUNG VOLUME ABNORMALITIES

Inspiration is limited at TLC when the maximum inspiratory force that can be applied by the chest muscles and diaphragm

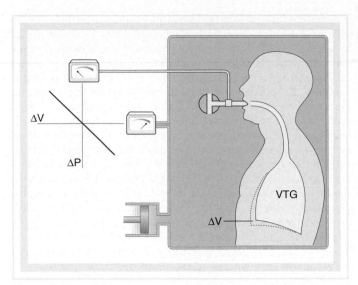

FIGURE 9-5 Lung volume measurement by body plethysmography. As the subject makes panting efforts against a closed airway shutter valve, the product of pressure and thoracic gas volume (VTG) stays constant (Boyle's law). Thus, $P_B \times V_{TG} = (P_B - \Delta P) \times (V_{TG} + \Delta V)$. Solving for VTG yields: $V_{TG} = P_B (\Delta V/\Delta P) - \Delta V$. Because ΔV is very small relative to VTG, it is ignored, so $V_{TG} = P_B (\Delta V/\Delta P)$. ΔP is obtained directly from the airway pressure transducer, and ΔV is obtained from the pressure change in the plethysmograph after calibration by cycling a known volume with a piston pump. VTG is obtained from the slope of this relationship plotted during the panting maneuver.

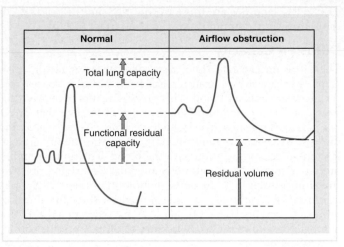

FIGURE 9-6 Severe airflow obstruction is associated with an increase in residual volume. Prolonged expiratory airflow may continue until the subsequent inhalation, and alveolar gas is trapped behind narrowed and closed airways. The functional residual capacity at which tidal breathing occurs is also increased, and total lung capacity may be high as well. (Modified with permission from Culver BH: Pulmonary function testing. In Kelly WN, ed: Textbook of Internal Medicine. Philadelphia: JB Lippincott; 1988.)

is opposed equally by the increasing recoil force of the lungs as they are distended to higher volumes. Usually, TLC is limited primarily by the elastic properties of the lungs, because variations in muscle strength have only a small effect on total chest expansion until weakness becomes quite marked. Parenchymal restrictive diseases reduce lung compliance, so greater distending pressure is required to achieve any volume change and, eventually, lower TLC. The displacement of intrathoracic gas volume by effusions, edema, intravascular volume, and inflammatory cells also contributes to a reduction in measured lung gas volumes. Except for pleural effusions, these quantities are relatively small and are outweighed by the frequently associated changes in lung elastic properties.

The minimum lung volume, or RV, is determined by a combination of two factors. The first is the amount of squeeze the chest wall and abdominal muscles can provide, and this is the dominant factor determining the RV in youth. The second factor is airway closure. With progressive age and the normal loss of tissue elastic recoil forces, the lung volume at which small airways close and trap remaining gas behind them increases, and this becomes the dominant factor in determining RV.

Restrictive Disease

Restrictive lung diseases are defined as those that cause a significant decrease in TLC. In most parenchymal infiltrative processes, this is accompanied by parallel decrements in FRC, RV, and VC, although a reduction in only RV may be seen in early stages of disease as increased tissue recoil delays airway closure. Obesity shows a different pattern, in that the primary effect is on the relaxed end-expiratory volume or FRC. The large abdomen and heavy chest wall reduce the outward recoil

of the thoracic cage, which opposes the inward recoil of the lung parenchyma and maintains normal FRC. However, RV is determined by airway closure and is little affected, and the TLC achievable by use of maximum inspiratory force is only minimally reduced until obesity becomes extreme. Thus, the typical spirogram in obesity shows an FRC that approaches RV (i.e., the expiratory reserve volume is markedly reduced), but with a relatively large inspiratory capacity and a near-normal TLC and VC.

Obstructive Disease

Obstructive diseases cause airway closure that stops exhalation at a higher lung volume because of the combined effects of airway inflammation and loss of tissue recoil on luminal caliber. This results in a progressive increase in RV (Figure 9-6), because increasing amounts of gas are trapped behind closed airways. These patients breathe at an increased FRC because of the combined effects of a decrease in lung recoil force from emphysema and the need to increase luminal caliber to minimize the resistive work of airflow. The TLC is normal to high, which again reflects the loss of lung recoil forces. Because RV increases to a greater extent than does TLC, the VC decreases with severe airway obstruction.

Reference Standards

As with spirometry, standing height is the strongest predictor of lung volumes. Ethnicity should be considered in predicting normal lung volumes. African American subjects have values for TLC, VC, and RV that are, on average, approximately 12% smaller than Caucasian subjects of equal height. Asian subjects are considered to have smaller differences from white subjects, particularly if raised on Western diets. The reasons for these differences are not entirely clear, but it is notable that most prediction models were derived from relatively small samples, many of which underrepresent African American and Asian populations. The recommended reference for

TLC, FRC, and RV are those of the ATS and ERS (2005) or the European Community for Coal and Steel (1993).

Diffusion Capacity

The diffusion capacity (D_L), also called transfer factor, measures the capacity to transfer gas from alveolar spaces into the alveolar capillary blood. This process occurs by passive diffusion and is a function of the pressure difference that drives gas, the surface area over which exchange takes place, and the resistance to gas movement through the membrane and into chemical combination with the blood. The units are milliliters per minute per millimeter mercury of driving pressure (mL/min/mmHg). (In SI units, 1 mole/min/kPa = 2.896 mL/min/mmHg.) Carbon monoxide is used for the clinical test of diffusing capacity (D_LCO) because its extreme avidity for hemoglobin allows the back pressure to diffusion to be considered negligible.

In the widely used single-breath method, the subject exhales to RV, then takes a VC inhalation of the test gas, which contains a low level of carbon monoxide (0.3%) and an inert gas (e.g., 10% helium). After holding at full inspiration for 8–10 sec, the subject exhales quickly. The initial portion of the expirate, which includes anatomic dead space, is discarded, and a sample of the subsequent alveolar gas is collected or measured. The reduction in helium concentration in the alveolar sample allows calculation of the alveolar volume at TLC into which carbon monoxide was distributed and of the initial carbon monoxide concentration after its dilution by the resident RV. The final concentration of carbon monoxide measured in the exhaled alveolar sample allows calculation of the volume of carbon monoxide transferred out of alveoli and a calculation, for which an exponential decline is assumed, of the mean carbon monoxide driving pressure during the breath-holding period. An effective residence time is calculated from the breath-holding period plus a portion of the time of inspiration and sample collection.

A significant problem with the diffusing capacity measurement is that numerous variations in the handling of small correction factors (for gas conditions, apparatus dead space, timing measurement, and so on) can cumulatively cause the calculated value to vary substantially. Although reproducibility within a laboratory can be acceptable, the accuracy of comparisons between laboratories or to published normal standards is much less consistent, as reflected by published predicted values that vary by 20% or more. It is essential that each laboratory choose prediction equations that are appropriate to the nuances of its equipment and technique.

Although diffusion is often thought of as a function of alveolar membrane thickness, the dominant factor is usually the capillary blood volume, which influences both the surface area available for exchange and the volume of blood and hemoglobin available to accept carbon monoxide. The influence of hemoglobin concentration (Hb) can be accounted for by theoretical or empirical correction factors. The rate of blood flow is not important, because carbon monoxide is taken up even by stagnant blood (or extravasated blood, in the case of pulmonary hemorrhage), but the recruitment of capillaries during high-flow conditions such as exercise or with congenital left-to-right shunt increases the measured diffusing capacity. The lower limit of normal (LLN) needs to be determined according to the same principles described earlier for spirometry.

Many laboratories also report the diffusing capacity as a ratio to the alveolar volume (D_L/V_A). This is also called the transfer coefficient (K_{CO}). The implication is that loss of lung volume caused by mechanical abnormalities is accompanied by a parallel loss of diffusion capacity. This, however, is not the case with a voluntary limitation of inspiration, in which capillaries remain perfused and D_L/V_A rises, or with pneumonectomy, in which capillaries are recruited in the remaining lung and D_L/V_A is again high. Diffusing capacity is commonly reduced in parenchymal inflammatory diseases, primarily because of the loss of available capillaries. The most common pattern in diseases such as sarcoidosis and interstitial fibrosis is for D_L to be reduced and D_L/V_A to be slightly low or "normal," as volume is also lost. Both D_L and D_L/V_A are low with the loss of capillary surface area and blood volume in emphysema and in diseases that are primarily vascular, such as vasculitis, recurrent emboli, and pulmonary hypertension. Clinical interpretation of diffusion abnormality should be based primarily on the D_L, with small, published correction factors available for (Hb) and lung volume, rather than the D_L/V_A ratio.

Tests of Gas Distribution

Abnormalities of spirometry and airflow rate reflect overall narrowing of airways, but most lung diseases affect airways irregularly, which leads to abnormalities of gas distribution that may be more sensitive indicators of early airway disease.

CLOSING VOLUME

As lung volume decreases, the smaller, intraparenchymal airways decrease in caliber until they close at low lung volume, and ventilation to or from alveoli beyond these points of closure ceases. Because there is a vertical gradient in the pleural pressure that surrounds the lungs (when subjects are supine, standing, sitting, or in either lateral decubitus position), the lung is less distended in dependent regions than it is higher in the thorax. In late exhalation, dependent airways close (and these areas reach their regional RV), whereas air continues to flow from the upper portions of the lung until they too close, and overall RV is reached. The beginning of this wave of ascending airway closure can be detected by physiologic tests and is termed *closing volume*. Closing volume is usually expressed as a percentage of VC. That is, a closing volume of 20% means that airway closure can be detected during a slow exhalation when 20% of the VC remains before reaching RV (Figure 9-7). Alternately, when RV is measured, this can be added to closing volume, and the sum, termed the *closing capacity*, is expressed as a percentage of TLC.

Both these measures have been used as tests of early airway dysfunction in the natural history of COPD. Abnormalities can be detected in a high percentage of smokers, but the diagnostic usefulness is limited, because this includes many who do not go on to develop progressive airflow limitation. On an individual patient basis, the closing volume is most helpful in its relationship to the lung volume at which tidal breathing occurs. When airway closure occurs at a volume below FRC, the airways are open throughout the lungs during tidal breathing, but when airway closure occurs above FRC, the affected alveoli are underventilated. Because the dependent regions are well perfused, this creates a region with a low ventilation/perfusion ratio, which contributes to hypoxemia. This occurs when the closing volume is increased by normal aging, COPD, and the effect of peribronchial edema in left ventricular failure. Similar consequences follow when FRC is reduced by recumbent posture or by obesity.

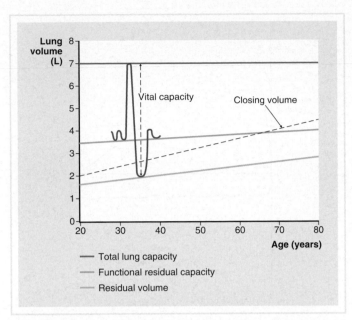

FIGURE 9-7 Effects of age on the normal spirogram. Residual volume progressively increases, with an associated small reduction in vital capacity. The functional residual capacity (FRC) increases slightly, but the closing volume, at which dependent airways cease to ventilate, increases more steeply and exceeds the normal FRC in older ages. (Modified with permission from Culver BH, Butler J: Alterations in pulmonary function. In Andres R, Bierman E, Hazzard W, eds: Principles of geriatric medicine. New York: McGraw-Hill; 1985.)

Arterial Blood Gas Measurement

Measurement of pH, P_{CO_2}, and P_{O_2} in arterial blood is commonly included in the complete pulmonary function assessment of patients suspected of having lung disease. Both pH and P_{CO_2} are directly measured, and the accompanying bicarbonate concentration is calculated from the Henderson–Hasselbalch equation. (The value of this "calculated" data must not be discounted; it is every bit as accurate as the pH and P_{CO_2} measurements from which it is derived.)

An increase in arterial P_{CO_2} means that alveolar ventilation is low relative to carbon dioxide production, because total ventilation is low, the effective alveolar ventilation is reduced by excessive wasted ventilation, or the carbon dioxide production level has increased without a concomitant increase in ventilation. The matching of ventilation to the needed carbon dioxide elimination is a function of both mechanical capabilities and ventilatory drive. Most patients who have hypercapnia have severe mechanical impairments, but those who also have relatively low drive are more likely to retain carbon dioxide. Patients who have an FEV_1 greater than 1 L rarely retain carbon dioxide unless lack of drive is a major factor. Despite the airflow obstruction present during an acute asthma attack, multiple stimuli tend to increase drive and ventilation. However, when obstruction becomes extreme, again with an FEV_1 approximately 1 L or less for an adult, the development of acute hypercapnia is likely. Most parenchymal restrictive diseases tend to be associated with mild hyperventilation, presumably from mechanical stimuli to the respiratory centers, until the functional abnormalities become very severe.

The normal P_{CO_2} remains in a narrow range (approximately 40 mmHg at sea level) throughout life, but the normal P_{O_2} diminishes progressively with age, and the decline is more marked when measured in the supine position. In both cases, this reflects the progressive increase in closing volume with age (see Figure 9-7). Abnormal reductions in P_{O_2} are caused by hypoventilation, as reflected by an increase in P_{CO_2}, or by the combined effects of pulmonary blood flow to poorly ventilated areas (low $\dot{V}/\dot{Q}$ ratio) and right-to-left shunting. Diffusion abnormalities, unless extremely severe, rarely contribute to a low P_{O_2} among patients at rest. The low P_{O_2} commonly seen in patients who have diffusion abnormalities reflects the concomitant presence of $\dot{V}/\dot{Q}$ abnormalities associated with their disease. Diffusion limitation may make a small contribution to the reduction in P_{O_2} observed during exercise, but again, the major component is a worsened effect of the $\dot{V}/\dot{Q}$ abnormalities.

SPECIAL TESTING

Upper Airway Obstruction

Obstruction in the central airways (e.g., tracheal tumor or stenosis) affects the expiratory flow-volume relationship in a different way than does the more common peripheral airway obstruction of COPD. The latter has its predominant effect late in expiration, with slowing of terminal flow rates, so that peak flow tends to be relatively maintained, whereas the remaining flow-volume curve becomes progressively convex toward the horizontal axis (Figure 9-8). Central obstructions have their primary effect early, which results in a truncated, flat-topped flow-volume curve (Figure 9-9), reflecting a steady effort against a constant resistance. In the latter portion of expiration, the decreasing lung volume and airway caliber shift the site of major resistance to the more peripheral airways, so that the latter portion of the flow-volume curve is normal.

When a central obstruction is in the extrathoracic airway and has some variability (e.g., vocal cord paralysis), its effect is much greater during inspiratory flow than expiratory flow.

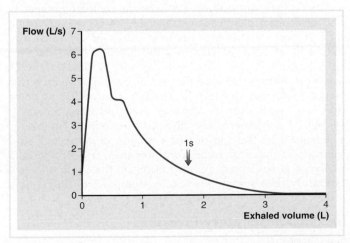

FIGURE 9-8 Expiratory flow-volume curve of chronic airflow obstruction. Airflow rates are markedly reduced at mid to lower lung volumes, with a curve that is convex to the horizontal axis. In this example, just under 50% of the vital capacity has been exhaled in 1 sec. (Modified with permission from Culver BH: Pulmonary function testing. In Kelly WN, ed: Textbook of internal medicine. Philadelphia: JB Lippincott; 1988.)

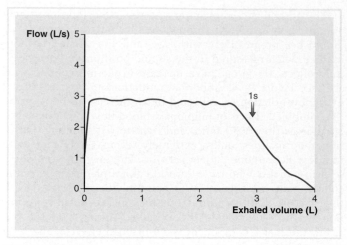

FIGURE 9-9 Expiratory flow-volume curve shows the pattern typical of central airway obstruction. Peak flow is markedly truncated, but the flow rates at low lung volume are unaffected. Despite the dramatic effect on the flow-volume curve, the FEV_1/FVC ratio is only modestly affected (71% in this example). (Modified with permission from Culver BH: Pulmonary function testing. In Kelly WN, ed: Textbook of internal medicine. Philadelphia: JB Lippincott; 1988.)

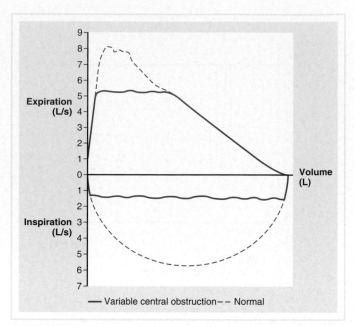

— Variable central obstruction – – Normal

FIGURE 9-10 Flow-volume loop showing both forced expiratory and inspiratory airflows. The expiratory peak flow is somewhat truncated, consistent with a mild central obstruction during exhalation, whereas inspiratory flow is markedly reduced compared with the normal curve. This pattern is typical of a flexible, extrathoracic obstruction such as that caused by paralyzed vocal cords. (Modified with permission from Culver BH: Pulmonary function testing. In Kelly WN, ed: Textbook of internal medicine. Philadelphia: JB Lippincott; 1988.)

The negative intraluminal pressure generated during inspiration narrows the airway, which exacerbates the obstruction, whereas during expiration, the positive airway pressure below the site of obstruction tends to distend the airway, which reduces the abnormality. These lesions are assessed by recording on the flow-volume display the maximum-effort inspiratory flow pattern, as well as that during expiration, to complete a flow-volume "loop." The normal inspiratory flow pattern has a hemicircular shape with peak inspiratory flow at midvolume that consistently exceeds midvolume expiratory flow (Figure 9-10).

Maximum Voluntary Ventilation

The maximum voluntary ventilation (MVV) maneuver requires maximal inspiratory and expiratory effort over 12–15 sec to estimate the subject's maximum ventilatory capacity. This episode of panting is extrapolated to 60 sec and is generally reported in liters. An individual's MVV (in 1 min) should be at least 30–40 times the baseline FEV_1 but may be reduced by upper airway obstruction, respiratory muscle weakness, obstructive lung disease, or poor maneuver performance. Although the test is relatively nonspecific, it correlates well with exercise capacity and subjective reports of dyspnea. Furthermore, the diagnostic usefulness of the test is enhanced by the appropriate selection of adjunctive studies, such as maximal respiratory pressures, if neuromuscular weakness is suspected, or inspection of the inspiratory and expiratory flow-volume curves, if attempting to differentiate the location of airflow obstruction.

Maximal Respiratory Pressures

See Chapter 8.

OXIMETRY

By use of noninvasive pulse oximetry, arterial oxyhemoglobin saturation can be estimated at rest and after standardized exercise such as stepping, a 6-min walk, or shuttle test. Desaturation measured at either time point is a sensitive indicator of gas exchange abnormalities. Oximetry has also been used to screen for opportunistic pneumonias in patients with AIDS and is helpful in titration of supplemental oxygen therapy.

EXHALED NITRIC OXIDE IN LABORATORY ASSESSMENT OF ASTHMA

Asthma is recognized as a disease characterized by airway obstruction along with the presence of airways hyperresponsiveness to contractile stimuli and airway inflammation.

The challenge in the laboratory assessment of asthma is in identifying evidence of inflammation or airway hyperresponsiveness in patients without baseline airways obstruction and in distinguishing asthma as a cause of airways obstruction from other causes.

Measurement of exhaled nitric oxide has been shown to correlate well with the presence of eosinophilic mucosal inflammation in patent with asthma.

NO has been shown to be increased in patients with asthma and to be reduced by therapy with inhaled corticosteroids. It is also increased in viral respiratory tract infections, lupus erythematosus, hepatic cirrhosis, and lung transplant rejection. It is reduced or variable in COPD, cystic fibrosis, and HIV infection with pulmonary hypertension. It is decreased both acutely and chronically by cigarette smoking. Of all these conditions, measurement of exhaled NO (eNO) has been most widely applied for the diagnosis and management of asthma. The normal value for eNO from the mouth is 3–7 parts/billion (ppb). The upper limit of normal, used to distinguish normals from patients with asthma, has been variously reported between 15 and 30 ppb. Methods have also been developed for measuring nasal eNO as an indicator of allergic rhinitis.

The role of measurement of eNO is evolving as the device becomes more available, the scientific basis for its use in clinical practice becomes better defined, and clinicians increasingly recognize the test.

SUGGESTED READINGS

ATS/ERS recommendations for standardized procedures for the online and offline measurement of exhaled lower respiratory nitric oxide and nasal nitric oxide, 2005. Am J Respir Crit Care Med 2005; 171(8):912–930.

Calverley PM, *et al*: Bronchodilator reversibility testing in chronic obstructive pulmonary disease. Thorax 2003; 58(8):659–664.

Ferguson GT, *et al*: Office spirometry for lung health assessment in adults: A consensus statement from the National Lung Health Education Program. Chest 2000; 117(4):1146–1161.

MacIntyre N, *et al*: Standardisation of the single-breath determination of carbon monoxide uptake in the lung. Eur Respir J 2005; 26(4):720–735.

Mannino DM, *et al*: Obstructive lung disease and low lung function in adults in the United States: data from the National Health and Nutrition Examination Survey, 1988–1994. Arch Intern Med 2000; 160(11): 1683–1689.

Miller MR, *et al*: Standardisation of spirometry. Eur Respir J 2005; 26(2): 319–338.

Miller MR, *et al*: General considerations for lung function testing. Eur Respir J 2005; 26(1):153–161.

Payne DN, *et al*: Relationship between exhaled nitric oxide and mucosal eosinophilic inflammation in children with difficult asthma, after treatment with oral prednisolone. Am J Respir Crit Care Med 2001; 164(8 Pt 1): 1376–1381.

Pellegrino R, *et al*: Interpretative strategies for lung function tests. Eur Respir J 2005; 26(5):948–968.

Smith AD, *et al*: Use of exhaled nitric oxide measurements to guide treatment in chronic asthma. N Engl J Med 2005; 352(21):2163–2173.

Wanger J, *et al*: Standardisation of the measurement of lung volumes. Eur Respir J 2005; 26(3):511–522.

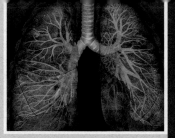
10 Exercise Testing

DARRYL Y. SUE • KATHY E. SIETSEMA

Exercise stresses the cardiac, pulmonary, and other systems by providing an additional metabolic load. Physiological testing during exercise observes how well these systems cope with this added load, measuring, in effect, how much reserve the subject or patient has. Simple tests that use exercise include examining the patient while walking down a hallway or going up a flight of stairs. A standardized test that requires little equipment measures the distance a patient can walk in 6 min. Electrocardiograms obtained during exercise are useful for detection of coronary artery disease and for subsequent risk assessment, especially when combined with myocardial imaging.

Cardiopulmonary exercise testing refers to an exercise test during which oxygen uptake and carbon dioxide output are measured from respired air. Additional monitoring or imaging procedures may be added. Success in maintaining homeostasis depends on close and timely coupling of the heart, systemic and pulmonary circulations, and ventilatory function. From the pattern, time course, and magnitude of gas exchange variables, a great deal can be inferred about the function and capacity of these organ systems (Table 10-1).

PHYSIOLOGY OF EXERCISE GAS EXCHANGE

During exercise, the movement of the body comes from muscular contraction, and the metabolic cost of the exercise is related to the external work done over time (work rate) expressed as watts. Increments in work rate can be accurately measured for some kinds of exercise, notably arm or leg exercise with a stationary cycle. Estimates of work rate can be made for other forms of exercise, but the complex ergonomic relationships of walking, for example, make these less precise. Although meaningful, the amount of external work is an imperfect reflection of the metabolic and cardiopulmonary capacity of the individual. However, the consumption of oxygen ($\dot{V}O_2$) and the production of carbon dioxide ($\dot{V}CO_2$) can be readily and noninvasively measured (Figure 10-1).

Muscular contraction accomplishing external work uses energy in the form of adenosine triphosphate (ATP), either preaccumulated or concurrently generated from a variety of metabolic pathways. These pathways generally oxidize carbohydrate or fat located in, or delivered to, the exercising muscles and, therefore, require a continuous supply of oxygen. Pathways requiring oxygen to generate ATP are aerobic, but ATP can also be produced anaerobically (without oxygen) through glycolysis (Figure 10-2), albeit at greater cost of substrate and production of lactic acid.

Higher levels of work require increased rates of ATP production that, in turn, require greater substrate use. Although it is inconvenient or impossible to measure substrate use, $\dot{V}O_2$ and $\dot{V}CO_2$ can be determined. The body stores some O_2 in the form of oxymyoglobin or as additional O_2 that can be extracted from hemoglobin, but the amount of stored O_2 available is small. Therefore, with exercising muscles consuming oxygen, there must be rapid uptake of oxygen from the atmosphere, and this can be measured from respired gas. Similarly, the increased CO_2 produced from metabolism of substrate accumulates in tissues and blood, but, when carried to the lungs, is quickly exhaled and measurable. This important concept is illustrated in Figure 10-1.

$\dot{V}O_2$ measured from exhaled breath is a reflection of the ability of the heart and circulation to carry oxygen to the muscles and deoxygenated blood away from the muscles, the capacity of the lung to exchange O_2 between the alveoli and the pulmonary capillaries, and the ability of blood to carry and off-load oxygen (indicating adequate hemoglobin concentration, and normal oxyhemoglobin dissociation).

Most energy required for sustained muscular exercise is derived from oxidative (i.e., aerobic) metabolism. But in each individual, there is a work rate or metabolic rate for each group of exercising muscles (leg exercise, for example) above which aerobic metabolism alone is unable to provide sufficient ATP to meet demands. This level depends on oxygen delivery. Continued exercise at or above this rate will depend on generating additional ATP from anaerobic glycolysis. Glycolysis produces far less ATP than aerobic metabolism for the same amount of glucose (the mandatory substrate for glycolysis), and lactic acid is also formed as a by-product. Lactic acid is highly dissociated at body pH, and the hydrogen ion reacts with bicarbonate, producing CO_2. As a result, the onset of lactic acidosis can be detected from gas exchange measurements as an increase in $\dot{V}CO_2$ above that produced by concurrent aerobic metabolism (Figure 10-3).

METHOD OF CARDIOPULMONARY EXERCISE TESTING

During most cardiopulmonary exercise tests, the patient usually performs an increasing work rate task (incremental or continuous) on a cycle or treadmill ergometer until they are no longer able to continue. Accordingly, these are symptom-limited tests, and measurements throughout the test and at maximum effort are reported. For diagnostic purposes, the goal is for a patient with symptoms during exertion or exercise limitation to reproduce the symptoms or reach the limit of exercise to determine the cause and magnitude of the problem. Other goals might be to quantify exercise limitation or grade severity of disease. Exercise of the legs is preferred because the larger muscle mass compared with the arms results in a higher $\dot{V}O_2$, thereby providing a greater stress to the heart, lungs, blood, and pulmonary and systemic circulations.

TABLE 10-1 Questions Asked During Cardiopulmonary Exercise Testing

Question	Variable(s)	Abnormal, if
Does the patient have an abnormal limitation to exercise? How severe is this limitation?	Peak $\dot{V}O_2$	Peak $\dot{V}O_2$ is low compared with that predicted for age, gender, and size.
Is the patient's exercise capacity limited by ventilatory capacity?	Highest minute ventilation during exercise ($\dot{V}E$) compared with maximum voluntary ventilation (MVV) at rest	A small difference between $\dot{V}E$ and MVV suggests ventilatory limitation to exercise.
Is the patient potentially limited by heart disease?	Highest heart rate compared with predicted for age; O_2 pulse ($\dot{V}O_2$/HR)	A maximum exercise heart rate much lower than predicted (non-beta-blockade) suggests either a "noncardiac" reason for exercise limitation or chronotropic incompetence. Low peak $\dot{V}O_2$/HR suggests cardiac or cardiovascular disease.
Is a problem with delivery of O_2 contributing to exercise limitation?	Lactic acidosis threshold; $\dot{V}O_2$ vs work rate slope	A low lactic acidosis threshold compared with that predicted or a low $\dot{V}O_2$ vs work rate slope suggest impaired O_2 delivery from anemia or cardiovascular disease.
Does the patient have areas of high ventilation/perfusion ratio?	V_D/V_T; $P(a\text{-}ET)CO_2$ difference at peak exercise. $\dot{V}E/\dot{V}CO_2$ at nadir	High $\dot{V}E/\dot{V}CO_2$ at nadir, high V_D/V_T and/or $P(a\text{-}ET)CO_2$ difference >0 at end exercise suggest increased contribution from high $\dot{V}A/\dot{Q}$ regions.
Does the patient have areas of low ventilation/perfusion ratio?	PaO_2 or O_2 saturation by pulse oximetry; alveolar-arterial PO_2 difference	Low or decreasing PaO_2 or O_2 saturation, or high $P(A\text{-}a)O_2$ result from contribution of low $\dot{V}A/\dot{Q}$ regions during exercise.

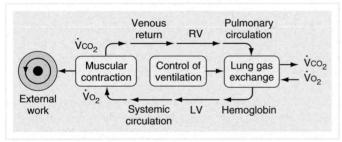

FIGURE 10-1 Link between consumption of O_2 and production of CO_2 by the exercising muscles while performing "external work" on a cycle ergometer. The delivery of O_2 from the atmosphere to the muscle (mitochondria) requires exchange across the lung, binding to adequate hemoglobin, convective transport by the heart and systemic circulation, and diffusion into the muscles from the systemic capillaries. Similarly, CO_2 evolved by the muscles returns in the venous blood and is eliminated by the lungs. Normal function maintains remarkable homeostasis under exercise stress. Limitation of any part(s) of the overall system limits peak O_2 uptake measured from respired gas.

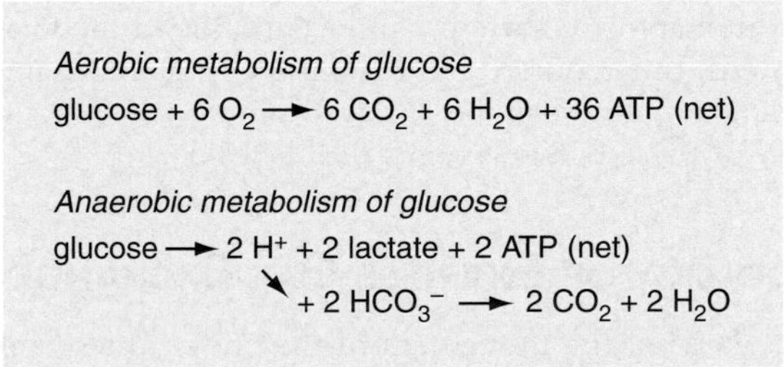

A large amount of data can be collected from cardiopulmonary exercise testing systems. The most robust and best-characterized variables are the peak $\dot{V}O_2$, which is the conventional expression of exercise capacity, and the peak minute ventilation ($\dot{V}E$) and heart rate. Important derived variables include the O_2 pulse ($\dot{V}O_2$/HR), the lactic acidosis threshold, and the $\dot{V}E/\dot{V}CO_2$ and $\dot{V}O_2$/work rate.

EXERCISE GAS EXCHANGE

1. *Peak $\dot{V}O_2$.* If a subject or patient is able to exercise to a point where symptoms limit further exercise, the peak $\dot{V}O_2$ has important functional and physiologic meaning. $\dot{V}O_2$ is calculated from respired gas as:

Aerobic metabolism of glucose

glucose + 6 O_2 ⟶ 6 CO_2 + 6 H_2O + 36 ATP (net)

Anaerobic metabolism of glucose

glucose ⟶ 2 H^+ + 2 lactate + 2 ATP (net)

⟶ + 2 HCO_3^- ⟶ 2 CO_2 + 2 H_2O

FIGURE 10-2 Aerobic metabolism of glucose results in energy production (ATP) along with CO_2 and H_2O. In the mitochondria, oxygen serves as an acceptor for electrons, which give up their energy to high-energy phosphate bonds of ATP. Aerobic metabolism requires a continuous supply of O_2, which is transported from the atmosphere. Anaerobic metabolism does not require O_2, but is less efficient (fewer ATP per molecule of glucose) and produces lactic acid, with additional CO_2 made from buffering of hydrogen ion by bicarbonate.

$$\dot{V}O_2 = \dot{V}E \times (FIO_2 - FEO_2^*)$$

where $\dot{V}E$ is minute ventilation, FIO_2 is inspired O_2 fraction, and FEO_2^* is expired O_2 fraction adjusted to account for the difference between inspiratory and expiratory minute ventilation.

However, $\dot{V}O_2$ is also a "cardiovascular" variable that can be represented as:

$$\dot{V}O_2 = \dot{Q} \times (CaO_2 - C\bar{v}O_2)$$

where $\dot{Q}$ is cardiac output, CaO_2 is arterial O_2 content, and $C\bar{v}O_2$ is mixed venous oxygen content. Both arterial and mixed venous O_2 contents are determined by O_2 saturation (related to PO_2) and hemoglobin concentration.

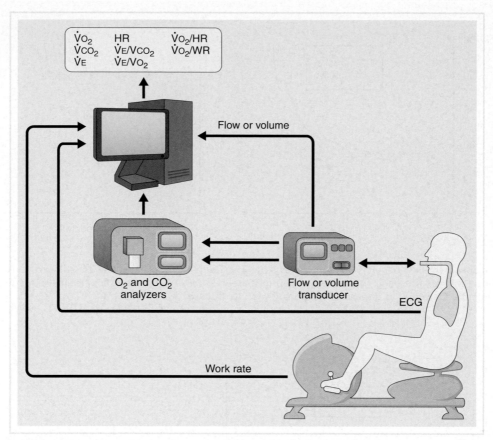

FIGURE 10-3 A typical cardiopulmonary exercise testing system. The subject cycles an ergometer that has an adjustable calibrated brake, thereby allowing the subject to perform a measured work rate (watts). The subject exhales through a flow or volume transducer connected to a computer. Expired O_2 and CO_2 are measured with rapidly responding analyzers. The computer integrates these data and calculates the gas exchange variables of interest. Customized software produces graphs and tables of data needed for interpretation.

Thus, if peak $\dot{V}O_2$ is reduced compared with normal (i.e., that predicted for an individual of that height, gender, and age), the reduced peak $\dot{V}O_2$ could be due to reduced capacity to ventilate (i.e., a low $\dot{V}E$), circulate blood (i.e., a low $\dot{Q}$), transfer O_2 from the lungs (i.e., a low PaO_2), carry O_2 in the blood (i.e., anemia), or deliver O_2 to the exercising muscles (i.e., abnormal circulation or abnormal circulatory control).

Peak $\dot{V}O_2$ is useful for characterizing cardiovascular fitness, determining whether there is any abnormal limitation to exercise, predicting outcome in chronic diseases such as heart failure, and predicting postoperative complications from thoracic and abdominal surgery.

2. $\dot{V}E/\dot{V}CO_2$ is termed the ventilatory equivalent for CO_2, the amount of ventilation required per liter of CO_2 output. It is a marker of efficiency of CO_2 elimination by the lungs. $\dot{V}E/\dot{V}CO_2$ is determined by these variables:

$$\dot{V}E(BTPS)/\dot{V}CO_2(STPD) = 863/(PaCO_2 \times [1 - VD/VT])$$

where $\dot{V}E$ (BTPS) is expressed at body temperature, saturated; $\dot{V}CO_2$ (STPD) at standard temperature and pressure, dry; $PaCO_2$ is in mmHg; and VD/VT is the ratio of dead space/tidal volume.

An increase in $\dot{V}E/\dot{V}CO_2$ is expected with hyperventilation (reflected by a low $PaCO_2$) or if there is an increase in VD/VT. Distinguishing one from the other requires arterial blood

gas measurement. $\dot{V}E/\dot{V}CO_2$ is increased in patients with chronic congestive heart failure, pulmonary vascular disease, and pulmonary airway or interstitial diseases.

Because $\dot{V}E/\dot{V}CO_2$ generally decreases to a nadir during incremental exercise and then subsequently rises, measuring $\dot{V}E/\dot{V}CO_2$ at its nadir is useful. Normal values increase slightly with age but are approximately 24–29. A related variable is the slope of $\dot{V}E$ versus $\dot{V}CO_2$ during incremental exercise; a high slope has similar meaning (Figure 10-4).

3. *Lactic acidosis threshold (Figure 10-5).* Numerous studies have linked the lactic acidosis threshold to insufficient O_2 delivery to the exercising muscle, including earlier and more severe lactic acidosis when O_2 flow is disrupted by decreased blood flow, anemia, carbon monoxide, or other factors. The onset of anaerobic metabolism occurring at a lower-than-expected work rate or lower-than-expected $\dot{V}O_2$ indicates impaired O_2 delivery or consumption.

Measuring lactate in the blood is invasive, but the lactic acidosis threshold can be determined from identifying the point of exercise at which an increased rate of CO_2 output is observed relative to the output occurring before the onset of anaerobic metabolism (see Figure 10-5). A low lactic acidosis threshold, expressed as %-predicted peak $\dot{V}O_2$, suggests a disorder of O_2 delivery during exercise, and it may occur in patients with heart disease, vascular

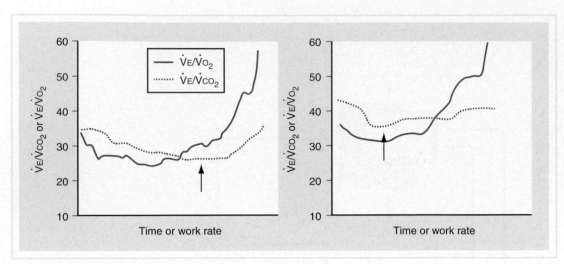

FIGURE 10-4 In a normal subject (*left panel*), V̇E/V̇CO₂ reaches a nadir value that is approximately 26–28 (*arrow*). The right panel shows a patient with chronic heart failure. The nadir for V̇E/V̇CO₂ is approximately 35 (*arrow*), reflecting inefficient ventilation. Similar increases in V̇E/V̇CO₂ may be seen in patients with lung disease or pulmonary vascular disease.

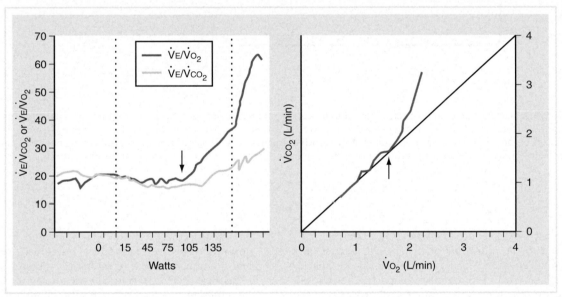

FIGURE 10-5 Evidence of onset of lactic acidosis (lactic acidosis threshold, expressed as V̇O₂) can be seen by the increase in V̇E relative to V̇O₂ (*left panel, solid line, arrow*). This reflects V̇E "tracking" increased CO₂ produced by buffering of hydrogen ion by bicarbonate added-to CO₂ from aerobic metabolism. Thus, V̇E/V̇CO₂ is relatively unchanged at this point. The increase in V̇CO₂ can also be clearly seen when plotted against V̇O₂ in the right panel (*arrow*). The diagonal line is the line of identity.

disease, or anemia. Normal values average approximately 55% of predicted peak V̇O₂, and values less than 40% of predicted peak V̇O₂ are usually abnormal. The normal lactic acidosis threshold is a higher percentage of predicted peak V̇O₂ in women and those of advanced age.

4. *V̇O₂ versus work rate (Figure 10-6).* The quantitative relationships between ATP use and muscular work, and between V̇O₂ and ATP production, are relatively fixed. When a patient exercises on the cycle ergometer without added resistance, the work rate and V̇O₂ are functions of the weight of the legs and cycling rate. When resistance on the ergometer is increased and the patient cycles at the same rate, the increase in V̇O₂ is directly proportional to the increase in work rate, with a highly predictable value of approximately 10.1 mL/min/watt (the variable ergonomics of treadmill walking make this determination

much less predictable). If the V̇O₂ versus WR slope is appreciably less than 10.1, disorders of O₂ delivery are likely; less O₂ is taken up for the same work rate, and, therefore, anaerobic metabolism is likely contributing to ATP generation. Cardiovascular disorders limiting O₂ delivery usually cause a decreased slope of V̇O₂ versus work rate.

5. *Electrocardiogram.* Twelve-lead electrocardiograms can identify rhythm disturbances or significant ST-segment changes consistent with exercise-induced myocardial ischemia. At times, ST-depression may be associated with a decrease in the slope of V̇O₂ versus work rate, possibly reflecting decreased O₂ delivery because of myocardial ischemia.

6. *Arterial blood gases (ABGs).* Pulse oximetry is commonly used to estimate arterial O₂ saturation during exercise, but measuring ABGs has an increased sensitivity for detecting a

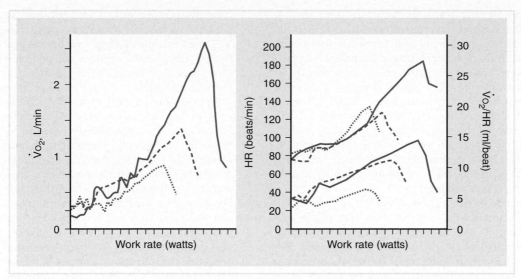

FIGURE 10-6 Examples of $\dot{V}O_2$ versus work rate for a normal subject (*solid line*), a patient with COPD (*dashed line*), and a patient with dilated cardiomyopathy (*dotted line*) during progressive cycle exercise. These *typical* patterns show a lower peak $\dot{V}O_2$ for the patients compared with normal; in this example, the patient with cardiomyopathy has a lower peak $\dot{V}O_2$ at a lower work rate than the others. The same three subjects are shown in the right panel for heart rate (*top three curves*) and O_2 pulse ($\dot{V}O_2/HR$, *bottom curves*). The lower and flatter O_2 pulse is characteristic of cardiomyopathy; in the COPD patient, further increase in HR and O_2 pulse may be constrained by ventilatory limitation at the end of symptom-limited exercise.

fall in arterial PaO_2 during exercise, identifying hyperventilation as a cause of increased $\dot{V}E/\dot{V}CO_2$, confirming lactic acidosis, and calculating alveolar-arterial PO_2 difference ($P[A\text{-}a]O_2$), dead-space/tidal volume ratio (VD/VT), and arterial-end tidal PCO_2 difference ($P[a\text{-}ET]CO_2$). High values of the latter two variables often reflect increased areas of high ventilation/perfusion ratio; increased $P(A\text{-}a)O_2$ reflects the existence of low ventilation-perfusion units.

In normal subjects breathing air during exercise, PaO_2 does not appreciably change, but $PaCO_2$ decreases in response to lactic acidosis. The $P(A\text{-}a)O_2$ increases, sometimes to as much as 30 mmHg at sea level. VD/VT and the $P(a\text{-}ET)CO_2$ fall during exercise, reflecting increasing homogeneity of lung ventilation and perfusion in normal subjects.

PATTERNS OF GAS EXCHANGE DURING EXERCISE

Although individual variables have demonstrated utility for addressing specific questions, the pattern of gas exchange variables may often be more characteristic of particular disorders. For patients with unexplained dyspnea or exercise intolerance, or in those with multiple possible disorders contributing to exercise limitation, features of these patterns may be very helpful with respect to establishing the cause of the problem.

The following describes patterns seen in some patients undergoing symptom-limited incremental exercise on a cycle ergometer.

1. *Normal.* Normal subjects will note dyspnea or fatigue at the end of exercise, but will reach peak $\dot{V}O_2$ predicted and predicted maximum HR. The maximum $\dot{V}E$ will be much less than the maximum voluntary ventilation (MVV) measured at rest. The lactic acidosis threshold will occur at more than 40% of the predicted peak $\dot{V}O_2$ and generally will be 55–60% of this value. The $\dot{V}O_2$ will increase with work rate

at approximately 10 mL/min/watt. Patients who have early and subtle heart or lung diseases may have normal gas exchange; the most sensitive indicators may be small abnormalities of arterial blood gases. As is true for pulmonary function testing, serial assessment of exercise function may identify decrements in measurements while still within the normal range.

2. *Lung disease.* Patients with obstructive or restrictive lung disease have mechanical constraints to increasing their ventilation. They often have ventilation-perfusion mismatching that decreases ventilatory efficiency resulting in a higher $\dot{V}E$ for any given $\dot{V}CO_2$ and decreases in oxygenation efficiency that result in an increased $P(A\text{-}a)O_2$. Thus, maximum exercise and peak $\dot{V}O_2$ are low, ventilatory reserve is small (i.e., small difference between MVV and peak $\dot{V}E$), and $\dot{V}E/\dot{V}CO_2$ is high throughout exercise, especially at its nadir value. In most patients with airway disease, delivery of oxygen is not markedly impaired, so lactic acidosis threshold may be normal. During exercise, patients with restrictive lung disease characteristically breathe at a higher frequency with lower tidal volume. Arterial blood gases may verify gas exchange abnormalities, chiefly a fall in PaO_2, increases in $P(A\text{-}a)O_2$, and a high VD/VT. Oxygen delivery may also be impaired because of secondary pulmonary vascular disease, with features similar to patients with intrinsic heart disease.

3. *Heart disease.* Patients with a cardiomyopathy (systolic and/or diastolic dysfunction) who are unable to increase stroke volume normally during exercise have a low maximum exercise capacity and a peak $\dot{V}O_2$ lower than normal. Because oxygen delivery is compromised by low stroke volume, the lactic acidosis threshold is abnormally low and the slope of $\dot{V}O_2$ versus HR may be reduced. Peak HR may be normal or may be reduced because of chronotropic incompetence or beta-adrenergic blockers. Even so, the increase in $\dot{V}O_2$ is usually limited disproportionally to any limitation

in HR increase, so that the peak $\dot{V}O_2/HR$ (i.e., the O_2 pulse) is less than normal. The rate of rise of $\dot{V}O_2/HR$ is flat throughout exercise. In patients with ischemia that develops during exercise, the pattern of gas exchange variables may be relatively normal until the onset of ischemia. At that point, there may be ST-segment changes, a decrease in the rate of rise of $\dot{V}O_2$ versus work rate, and a flattening of the O_2 pulse slope. A characteristic feature of heart failure is an increase in the nadir value of $\dot{V}E/\dot{V}CO_2$ and an increase in the slope of $\dot{V}E$ versus $\dot{V}CO_2$. This probably reflects heterogeneous perfusion of the lungs, resulting in increased regions of high ventilation-perfusion that contribute to exertional dyspnea.

4. *Pulmonary vascular disease.* These disorders may have features of impaired cardiovascular function (i.e., right ventricular dysfunction and increased pulmonary vascular resistance) and lung disease (manifested by abnormal pulmonary gas exchange). If mild, only subtle abnormalities of VD/VT, $P(A\text{-}a)O_2$, and $P(a\text{-}ET)CO_2$ may be found. More severely affected patients have reduced peak $\dot{V}O_2$, low lactic acidosis threshold (reflecting O_2 delivery problems), high $\dot{V}E/\dot{V}CO_2$, high HR, and low O_2 pulse because of low stroke volume, and a low and sometimes flattening $\dot{V}O_2$ versus work rate slope. Abnormal arterial blood gases during exercise are common. On occasion, sudden and severe arterial oxygen desaturation occurs during exercise, indicating the opening of a patent foramen ovale with abrupt onset of right-to-left shunting of venous blood.

5. *Other patterns.* Obese patients often have exercise limitation, but distinction must be made between decreased capacity of the heart and lungs and decreased ability to perform external work. Normal values for peak $\dot{V}O_2$ and lactic acidosis threshold are based on height or ideal weight to reflect the capacity of the heart and lungs. A normal obese subject may have normal values for exercise gas exchange, but an increased proportion of O_2 uptake, for example, is used to move the larger legs and torso. Therefore, a smaller proportion can be devoted to external work.

Anemia obviously will impair O_2 delivery and can result in low peak $\dot{V}O_2$ and lactic acidosis threshold; it contributes to decreased exercise tolerance from any cause. Peripheral vascular disease may manifest itself as claudication; in addition, impaired O_2 delivery to exercising muscle may result in a shallow $\dot{V}O_2$ versus work rate slope. Low peak $\dot{V}O_2$ will be seen in someone making little or submaximal effort; support for this conclusion may include normal ECG, normal lactic acidosis threshold, and normal arterial blood gases.

CLINICAL APPLICATION OF CARDIOPULMONARY EXERCISE TESTING

Cardiopulmonary exercise testing has wide application, ranging from determining the etiology of unexplained dyspnea or exercise intolerance to making accurate measurements of aerobic capacity in elite athletes, but several clinical areas have been particularly influenced.

1. *Chronic heart failure (cardiomyopathy).* The functional status of patients with heart failure correlates closely with peak $\dot{V}O_2$ and lactic acidosis threshold. Patients with peak $\dot{V}O_2 < 10\text{--}15$ mL/min/kg are severely limited; those < 10 mL/min/kg, very severely limited. Patients with NYHA

class III averaged only 17 ± 3 mL/min/kg in one study. Of patients referred for potential cardiac transplantation, a peak $\dot{V}O_2 > 14$ mL/min/kg had excellent 2-year survival, whereas those < 14 mL/min/kg did much poorer. This finding has led to inclusion of peak $\dot{V}O_2$ as an important determinant of transplant eligibility. A high slope of $\dot{V}E$ versus $\dot{V}CO_2$ is associated with higher early mortality, a lactic acidosis threshold <11 mL/min/kg is associated with worse outcome, and combinations of these variables with peak $\dot{V}O_2$ have been used to predict survival and response to therapy.

2. *Preoperative risk assessment.* The parallels between the stress of major surgery and exercise are striking; both require increases in blood flow, ventilation, and oxygen delivery. For patients with limited cardiopulmonary function, exercise testing is an objective way of determining capacity to withstand surgery. In patients undergoing pulmonary resection, higher peak $\dot{V}O_2$ has been associated with fewer postoperative complications and death. Those with peak $\dot{V}O_2 > 15\text{--}20$ mL/min/kg have few complications, whereas patients with a peak $\dot{V}O_2 < 10$ mL/min/kg might be considered as having very high risk. Similar results for elective abdominal surgery have been reported. Some investigators have found that the combination of peak $\dot{V}O_2$ and $\dot{V}O_2$ at the lactic acidosis threshold have better predictive value than either alone.

Cardiopulmonary exercise testing seems most valuable in identifying patients who can tolerate surgery when, by other tests, they would be judged inoperable. Accordingly, patients with marginal pulmonary function who are considering lung resection should have an exercise test. Better-than-expected peak $\dot{V}O_2$ would be reassuring; a low peak $\dot{V}O_2$ would portend very high risk and might help justify a nonoperative course.

3. *Pulmonary rehabilitation.* In patients with chronic obstructive pulmonary disease, exercise capacity is often a component of prognostic scoring systems; peak $\dot{V}O_2$ is an independent predictor of outcome even when FEV_1 and age are considered. Exercise capacity may be related to both lung and cardiovascular reserve, as well as to the nutritional and functional status of the skeletal muscles in these patients. Reduced exercise capacity identified a subgroup of patients with emphysema who benefited from surgical lung-volume reduction surgery.

Cardiopulmonary exercise testing can be used to help measure improvement during rehabilitation, to adjust the "exercise prescription," to help ensure safety of new participants, and to identify coexisting cardiovascular disorders that might interfere with rehabilitation.

4. *Impairment evaluation.* Exercise capacity is a fundamental component of impairment assessment. The amount of $\dot{V}E$ needed to perform a given degree of exercise is often poorly predictable from resting measurements alone. Thus, even if spirometry and lung volume measurements are abnormal, the amount of impairment is difficult to estimate. Similarly, if pulmonary function is normal, exercise testing may identify more subtle findings supporting a claim of impairment with subsequent disability. Exercise testing may be particularly helpful in attribution of impairment in the presence of more than one disorder. Some guidelines recommend assessment of peak $\dot{V}O_2$ in determination of impairment when resting studies are inconclusive or inconsistent with symptoms.

PRINCIPLES OF INTERPRETATION

When performing a cardiopulmonary exercise test on a patient, specific questions should be addressed (Box 10-1). This will help determine the type of test, the likelihood that exertional complaints will be reproduced, the need for arterial blood gas or cardiac imaging during the exercise test, and the duration and intensity of the work rate stress. Most often, a symptom-limited test to the patient's maximum work rate will be chosen. Normal values have been published for all of the relevant exercise gas exchange variables, including peak $\dot{V}_{O_2}$, heart rate, minute ventilation, and lactic acidosis threshold. The pattern and magnitude of changes in arterial blood gases can be compared with normal responses. As with interpretation of pulmonary function tests, there must be assessment of the technical quality of the data and the adequacy of the patient's effort.

The reason why the patient stopped exercising (during a symptom-limited test) is essential for interpretation, because symptoms of chest pain, claudication, dyspnea, joint or muscle pain, or other discomfort can be correlated with gas exchange variables.

Interpretation of a cardiopulmonary exercise test should focus on identifying the cause, if any, of exercise limitation, weighing the relative contributions if more than one cause is identified, and relating the patient's performance to his or her complaints.

BOX 10-1 Typical Clinical Questions Addressed by Cardiopulmonary Exercise Testing

A patient has symptoms during exercise that are difficult to explain from results of resting pulmonary function tests, echocardiogram, and chest roentgenogram. What is causing exertional dyspnea or exercise intolerance?

A patient will be undergoing thoracic or abdominal surgery. What is the patient's postoperative risk?

A patient complains of inability to perform exercise. How much is he or she limited?

A patient has a known diagnosis of cardiomyopathy. How severe is the heart failure and is he or she a likely candidate for cardiac transplantation?

A patient has elements of heart failure and lung disease. How much is each contributing to exercise intolerance?

A patient will be starting a pulmonary or cardiac rehabilitation program. What would be an appropriate amount of exercise to prescribe as a starting point for rehabilitation?

A patient has emphysema. Will he or she possibly benefit from lung volume reduction surgery?

SUGGESTED READINGS

American Medical Association: Guides to the evaluation of permanent impairment, 5th ed. Cocchiarella L, Andersson GBJ, eds. Chicago: American Medical Association; 2001.

American Thoracic Society; American College of Chest Physicians: ATS/ACCP Statement on cardiopulmonary exercise testing. Am J Respir Crit Care Med 2003; 167:211–277.

Arena R, Myers J, Abella J, Peberdy MA: Influence of heart failure etiology on the prognostic value of peak oxygen consumption and minute ventilation/carbon dioxide production slope. Chest 2005; 128:2812–2817.

Beckles MA, Spiro SG, Colice GL, Rudd RM; American College of Chest Physicians: The physiologic evaluation of patients with lung cancer being considered for resectional surgery. Chest 2003; 123(1 Suppl):105S–114S.

Berry MJ, Adair NE, Rejeski WJ: Use of peak oxygen consumption in predicting physical function and quality of life in COPD patients. Chest 2006; 129:1516–1522.

Celli BR, Cote CG, Marin JM, et al: The body-mass index, airflow obstruction, dyspnea, and exercise capacity index in chronic obstructive pulmonary disease. N Engl J Med 2004; 350:1005–1012.

Wasserman K, Hansen JE, Sue DY, et al: Principles of Exercise Testing and Interpretation, 4th ed., Philadelphia: Lippincott Williams and Wilkins; 2005.

Yasunobu Y, Oudiz RJ, Sun XG, et al: End-tidal P_{CO_2} abnormality and exercise limitation in patients with primary pulmonary hypertension. Chest 2005; 127:1637–1646.

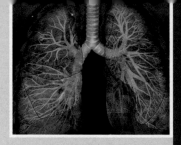

11 Host Defenses

CHUNG-WAI CHOW • THEO J. MORAES • GREGORY P. DOWNEY

INTRODUCTION

The epithelial surface of the lung is the largest in the body and is continuously exposed to a variety of potentially pathogenic microorganisms, allergens, particulate pollutants, and other noxious agents. An intricate defense system has evolved over time to protect the lungs from these pathogens while preserving lung function (Figure 11-1). These defense mechanisms can be divided into an innate (nonspecific) response and an adaptive or acquired (specific) response.

The innate immune response is evolutionarily conserved to provide immediate (seconds to minutes) host defense in a nonspecific manner. Only vertebrates have an additional adaptive immune system that is directed at specific pathogens or molecules. Although the two systems work in concert to protect the host, they have several distinct features. With rare exception, the innate immune system depends on proteins and signaling pathways that exist in a fully functional form, does not require priming, and is not strengthened with subsequent exposures. By contrast, the adaptive immune response requires time (days to weeks; see Figures 11-2 and 11-3) to ramp up to full capacity, is specific to the pathogen (and even to specific molecular determinants of the pathogen), and has memory to provide for stronger responses with subsequent attacks ("anamnestic response").

Together these systems provide a formidable force to combat invading pathogenic microbes as indicated by the rarity with which healthy humans succumb to lung infections. Specific components of the innate and adaptive host defense mechanisms are reviewed in this chapter.

STRUCTURAL DEFENSES

With a lung surface area in adults of $70\,m^2$ that comes into contact with roughly 10,000 L of air a day, the lung is confronted with constant threats from microbes. In addition to inhaled pathogens, there are high bacterial concentrations in oropharyngeal secretions (10^8/mL), and aspiration of these may also pose a serious risk for invasive infection (aspiration pneumonia). Therefore, the lung has developed a series of structural barriers that are designed both to minimize the number of microbes entering the lungs and to hasten their clearance before an infection can be established (see Table 11-1).

Particle size is an important factor determining the degree of penetration in the lung (see Table 11-2). Very large particles are filtered by vibrissae (nasal hairs). Particles approximately 30 μm in size are removed in the nasal airway where turbulent airflow results in prolonged air–mucosa contact with subsequent particle impaction. Most particles between 10 and 30 μm will also impact on the turbinates and nasal septum,

carina, or within the larger bronchi. The branching nature of the airways provides two additional mechanisms of protection: (1) the secondary, tertiary, and quaternary carinae force particles to impact on the mucosa, thus preventing further penetration into the lung; and (2) reduced airflow with increased airway branching allows gravity to sediment most particles larger than 2 μm. Particles less that 0.2–0.5 μm tend to stay suspended as aerosols and are exhaled. Much smaller particles (<0.1 μm) may be deposited as a result of Brownian motion (bombardment with gas molecules).

Thus, only particles roughly between 2 and 0.2 μm will reach the alveoli. Unfortunately, most bacteria are from 0.5–2 μm in size and, when inhaled, may reach the terminal bronchioles where they have the potential to establish an infection. Some exceptionally pathogenic bacteria require exceedingly small numbers (e.g., only 2–50 organisms) to establish infection.

In addition to particle size, other factors such as shape, charge, and state of hydration may influence the depth of penetration. For example, timothy grass, or *Alternaria*, can penetrate deeper into the lung than expected given their physical size.

Nares

The efficiency of the nose in filtering inspired air and trapping aerosolized particles has been highlighted by inhaled drug delivery studies that demonstrate enhanced pulmonary drug deposition with mouth inhalers compared with mask inhalers. Nasal congestion and increased mucus production also serve to trap unwanted particles or microbes and prevent them from going further into the airways.

In addition to filtration, the nose functions to warm and humidify inspired air, thus protecting cells from physical stress and ensuring optimal performance of the mucociliary system. Olfaction is also protective, because sniffing allows potentially harmful gases to be detected before they contact the lower airways.

However, as noted previously, the upper respiratory tract may be a source of infection when aspiration of small amounts of upper airway secretions compromises the host. Microbial colonization is normal, and although potential pathogens can be isolated from the nasopharynx of healthy hosts, normally resident flora competitively inhibit the growth of pathogens.

Cough/Sneeze

Mechanical or chemical stimulation of receptors in the nose, larynx, trachea, or elsewhere in the respiratory tree may produce bronchoconstriction to prevent deeper penetration of irritants and may also trigger the cough or sneeze reflex to expel particles deposited in the airways (see Table 11-3). The cough reflex aids the mucociliary transport to remove trapped particles.

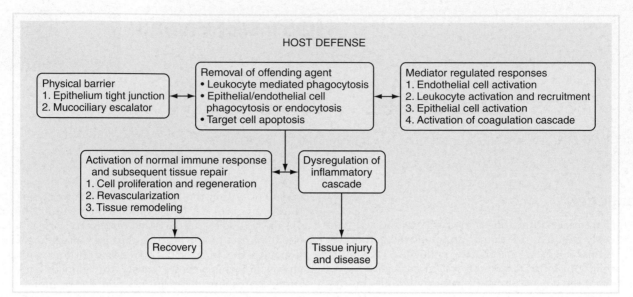

FIGURE 11-1 Host defense. The pulmonary host defense system is composed of multiple components, including physical barriers such as the nose and mucous layer that lines the airways. Mechanisms also exist to remove offending microbial pathogens or noxious particles, either directly by phagocytosis or endocytosis or indirectly by mediator-regulated responses. Activation of the immune and inflammatory responses will usually facilitate resolution of the injury and recovery of the host. However, if these immune and inflammatory responses are excessive or unregulated, tissue injury and disease ensue.

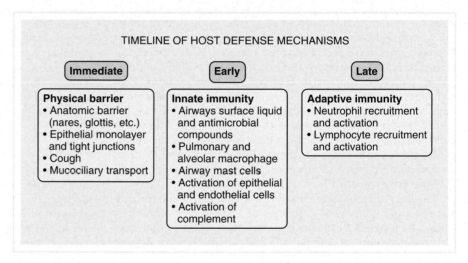

FIGURE 11-2 Timeline of host defense mechanisms. The immediate, early (seconds to hours), and late (hours to days) mechanisms that serve to protect the lung are illustrated.

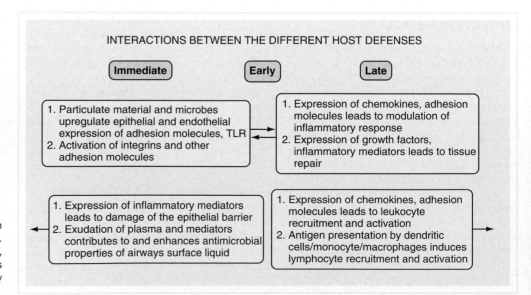

FIGURE 11-3 Interactions between the different host defense mechanisms. Interactions between the immediate, early, and late host defense mechanisms augment the immune and inflammatory response. *TLR*, Toll-like receptor.

TABLE 11-1 Structural Defenses of the Airway

Structure	Functions
Nose	Filters air Warms and humidifies air Sediments particles Olfaction Sneeze reflex
Glottis	Protects from GI and nasopharyngeal contamination Cough reflex
Mucociliary escalator	Traps foreign particles Facilitates physical removal of particles
Epithelium	Barrier to microbes Mucociliary escalator Production of antimicrobial factors Cytokine production Adhesion molecule expression

TABLE 11-2 Effect of Particle Size on Penetration into Airways

Particle size	Fate
>>> 30 μm	Filtered by vibrissae
> 30 μm	Nasopharyngeal (NP) impaction
10–30 μm	NP, tracheal, and large bronchial impaction
2–10 μm	Sedimentation in airways
0.2–2 μm	Reach alveoli
0.2–0.5 μm	Exhaled
<0.2 μm	Exhaled or deposited (Brownian motion)

TABLE 11-3 Phases to Cough/Sneeze

Inspiratory phase	Deep inspiration, usually 1–2 times tidal volume.
Compression phase	Begins with closure of the glottis and contraction of respiratory muscles resulting in the generation of high intrathoracic pressure (up to 100–200 cm H_2O in adults).
Expressive phase	Glottis opens and airflow as high as 25,000 cm/sec occurs (partly helped by compression of airway cross section).
Relaxation phase	Respiratory muscles relax, and temporary bronchodilation occurs.

Mucus is usually brought to the carina by the cilia and then expelled by coughing from this location. Disruption of the cough reflex and impaired mucociliary clearance (e.g., in smokers or patients with bronchiectasis) result in a predisposition to pneumonias.

Glottis

The digestive tract and the respiratory tract share both an embryologic origin and an opening with the external world (the mouth). The glottis protects the lungs from the possibility of contamination of the airways with digestive tract materials.

However, small amounts of aspiration do occur from the nasopharynx and oro-pharynx or esophagus in healthy individuals, usually without pathological consequences. However, frequent aspiration or episodes of aspiration of large amounts of material, as is seen in individuals with glottic dysfunction, can lead to bacterial pneumonia and chemical pneumonitis.

Respiratory Epithelium

The pulmonary epithelium is a highly effective barrier to microbes. Conducting airways are lined with pseudostratified columnar epithelial cells that become cuboidal as the branches extend to the alveoli. Formation of apical junctional complexes composed of intercellular tight junctions and adherens junctions separates the epithelial monolayer into apical (luminal) and basolateral sides that form an important barrier to the passive passage molecules and microbes from the airway lumen/alveolar space.

In addition to this important physical barrier function, the epithelial cells and the other structural cells of the airway epithelium, goblet cells, serous cells, basal cells, and Clara cells are integral to the normal function of the mucociliary escalator, the production of a variety of antimicrobial molecules, and the initiation of an inflammatory response (see Figure 11-4).

Mucociliary Escalator (see Table 11-4)

The airway epithelium is lined from the trachea to the respiratory bronchioles by the airway surface liquid (ASL), a 5–25-μm-thick surface film the primary function of which is to trap and facilitate the physical removal of foreign particles, as well as to provide an environment conducive for the activity of antimicrobial molecules.

ASL is the result of secretions by glands, serous cells, and of plasma transudation (see Table 11-5). The inner low viscosity periciliary sol facilitates the coordinated beating action of the cilia that propels the outer viscous mucous blanket toward the mouth, thus facilitating the removal of trapped pathogens or particles by expectoration or ingestion. The viscous mucus is composed of mucopolysaccharides, produced predominantly by submucous glands in the larger airways, with increasing contributions from goblet cells and Clara cells as airway generation increases.

Dysfunction of the ASL is seen in conditions such as asthma and chronic bronchitis in which excessive mucus is produced, resulting in airway obstruction. In cystic fibrosis, defects in ion transport are thought to reduce ASL volume, thus increasing viscosity. This impairs mucociliary clearance and predisposes to bacterial colonization, highlighting the importance of the antimicrobial function of normal ASL.

The cilia are integral to respiratory system defense and are present from the upper airways down to the terminal bronchioles. There are approximately 200 cilia per ciliated cell. Each is approximately 6-μm long and 0.2 μm in diameter and is arranged longitudinally to coordinate a beating activity of 500–1500 bpm, which serves to efficiently propel the mucous layer. Dysregulation of the ciliary function predisposes to pneumonia and is most evident in bronchiectasis, whether from genetic causes such as primary ciliary dyskinesia and cystic fibrosis or from acquired defects such as sequelae of pulmonary infections, including pulmonary tuberculosis.

Although these structural components of the respiratory system are not formally considered to be part of the "immune" system, they are, nonetheless, an important and early component of the microbial defense systems of the lung.

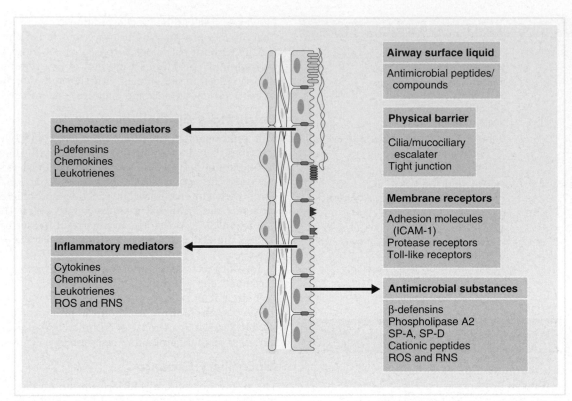

FIGURE 11-4 Epithelial cell defense mechanisms. The pulmonary epithelial monolayer functions as a highly effective defense system. The different mechanisms are illustrated, including the airway surface liquid that contains potent antimicrobial compounds, the mucous layer, junctions between the epithelial cells, and surface receptors expressed by the epithelial cells. *ROS,* Reactive oxygen species; *RNS,* reactive nitrogen species; *ICAM,* intracellular adhesion molecule; *SP-A,* surfactant associated protein A; *SP-D,* surfactant associated protein D.

TABLE 11-4 Mucociliary Escalator		
Properties	**Function**	**Dysfunction in Diseases**
Present from trachea down to level of respiratory bronchioles 200 cilia/ciliated cells Each cilia 6 μm long and 0.2 μm in diameter Thickness of layer: 5–25 μm Inner layer: low viscosity, periciliary solutes Outer layer: viscous mucous blanket	Traps foreign particles and transports them up and out of respiratory; tract rate (small airways): 0.5–1.0 mm/min; rate (large airways and nose): 5–20 mm/min Antimicrobial compounds	Smokers—decreased no. of ciliated cells and depressed cilia functions Bronchiectasis 1-degree ciliary dyskinesis Stents

TABLE 11-5 Airway Surface Liquid		
Composition	**Function**	**Dysfunction in Diseases**
Secretions from glands and goblet cells Plasma transduction	Antimicrobial properties because of low pH and secreted antimicrobial compounds	Cystic fibrosis Asthma COPD

TABLE 11-6 Cells Mediating Host Defense and the Inflammatory Response		
	Immune Cells	**Non-Immune Cells**
Early phase	Monocyte/macrophages Eosinophils Mast cells Neutrophils Natural killer cells	Endothelial cells Epithelial cells
Late phase	Lymphocytes Dendritic cells	Endothelial cells Epithelial cells Fibroblasts Mesenchymal cells

SPECIFIC CELL RESPONSES

Diverse cell populations contribute to the host defense system of the lung. In addition to the pulmonary epithelium, these include other structural cells of the lung, the pulmonary vascular endothelium and fibroblasts, resident leukocytes, and, at later stages of immune responses, recruited immune cells (see Table 11-6). These are reviewed in the following.

Epithelial Cells (see Table 11-7)

The contribution of the pulmonary epithelium is not limited to its roles as a structural barrier and in facilitation of mucociliary clearance. Respiratory epithelial cells actively participate in the modulation of inflammation and are capable of mounting an

TABLE 11-7 Immunomodulatory Molecules Secreted by Airway Epithelial Cells

Inflammatory mediators	Cytokines Chemokines Leukotrienes Calprotectin
Chemotactic mediators	LL-37/CAP-18 β-Defensins Chemokines Leukotrienes
Antimicrobial substances	β-defensins LL-37/CAP-18 Lysozyme Lactoferrin SLPI (secretory leukocyte proteinase inhibitor) Elafin Calprotectin Phospholipase A2 SP-A, SP-D Anionic peptides

immune response by internalization of organisms and secretion of cytotoxic and antimicrobial peptides. Epithelial cells are induced by bacterial components, such as LPS, and by cytokines such as tumor necrosis factor (TNF)-α and IL-1β to express various gene products (by the NFκB and IκB signaling pathways) that modulate the inflammatory response (Figure 11-4). These include:

1. Cytokines such as TNF-α, IL-1β
2. Chemokines that include macrophage inflammatory protein (MIP)-2, CXC chemokines, monocyte chemoattractant protein (MCP)-1, IL-7, IL-8, IL-15
3. Nitric oxide (NO$^•$) and reactive nitrogen species (ONOO$^{•-}$)
4. Adhesion molecules such as β-integrins and ICAM-1
5. Toll-like receptors such as TLR-2 and TLR-4
6. TNF-α receptors, TNFR1 and TNFR2
7. Growth factor receptors such as EGFR (epidermal growth factor receptor) and PDGFR (platelet derived growth factor receptor)
8. Plasminogen activator receptors

In addition to these molecules, pulmonary epithelial cells also express a number of antimicrobial mediators that are unique to the lung. These include the surfactant proteins SP-A and SP-D (members of the collectin family) and the β-defensins, potent antimicrobial peptides.

Endothelial Cells

Endothelial cells play a pivotal role in the regulation of host defense and propagation of the inflammatory response. Like epithelial cells, endothelial cells also form tight junctions that separate the endothelial monolayer into apical and basal surfaces and prevent passive movement of particles and molecules. In addition to this physical barrier, activated endothelial cells modulate the expression of numerous proteins involved in different pathways that contribute to host defense. These include the following:

1. Reactive nitrogen and oxygen species, including nitric oxide, peroxynitrite, superoxide (O$_2^{•-}$), and hydrogen peroxide (H$_2$O$_2$), which are cytotoxic to microorganisms and cells

2. Inflammatory cytokines such as TNF-α, IL-1β, and IL-6, as well as chemokines such as IL-8, RANTES, and MIP-1, which activate and recruit leukocytes
3. Cytokine and chemokine receptors such TFNR1 and IL-1R
4. Adhesion molecules, including ICAM-1, ICAM-2, PECAM, VCAM-1, E-selectin, and P-selectin, which have differential binding specificities for different leukocyte populations
5. Toll-like receptors (TLR)
6. Procoagulants and protease activated receptors
7. Proteases
8. Leukotrienes and prostaglandins
9. Growth factors such as vascular endothelial growth factor (VEGF) and transforming growth factor (TGF)-β
10. Alterations in the cytoskeleton and in intercellular (junctional) proteins to allow for leukocyte transmigration and changes in vascular permeability

Fibroblasts

Although fibroblasts are classically viewed as structural cells and passive responders to exogenous influences, they are actually integral to the regulation of host defense. Fibroblasts synthesize extracellular matrix proteins such as collagen that is required to maintain the structural integrity of the lung during normal tissue turnover and tissue repair after infection and injury. They also express matrix-degrading proteases such as matrix metalloproteinases and cytokines such as IL-1 and TNF that play important roles in leukocyte recruitment and activation.

Immune Cells (Table 11-8)

Several leukocyte populations play distinct and vital roles in host defense in the lung and can be broadly classified as those that are normal residents of the lung (mast cells, monocyte/macrophages, dendritic cells) and those recruited in response of infection in injury (neutrophils and lymphocytes).

MONOCYTES/MACROPHAGES

Macrophages are present within the interstitial tissues, alveolar spaces, and on mucosal surfaces throughout the body. They function to provide:

1. Constant immune surveillance
2. Orchestration of the immune response
3. A bridge between the innate and adaptive arms of the immune system.

Macrophages are derived from myeloid precursors in bone marrow, spleen, and fetal liver. Precursor cells, termed monocytes, leave the vascular space in response to chemokines or other tissue-specific homing factors. The environment of the destination heavily influences the function of macrophages such that macrophages resident in different tissues display different patterns of function.

In response to infection or injury, the resident tissue macrophages can contribute to the innate immune response by phagocytosis, as well as expression of a variety of inflammatory and antimicrobial compounds, the pattern of which is differentially regulated by the microenvironment of the different tissues. Moreover, subsets of macrophages (dendritic cells, discussed later) function in antigen recognition, processing, and display to cells of the adaptive immune system (lymphocytes).

TABLE 11-8 Leukocyte Defense Mechanisms

Immune Cell	Primary Role(s)	Primary or Unique Inflammatory Mediators
Neutrophils	Kill and eliminate invading organisms	Reactive oxygen and nitrogen species Proteolytic enzymes and cationic proteins TNF-α, IL-1β, IL-6
Macrophages	Immune surveillance Kill and contain invading microorganisms Removal of particulate matter Antigen presentation	TNF-α, IL-1β, IL-6 TGF-β ICAM-1 Reactive oxygen and nitrogen species
Mast cells	"Antennae" of immune response	Granule release (mediated by Fcε receptors) TLRs PAF, leukotrienes, and prostaglandins IL-1, IL-3, IL-4, IL-5, IL-6, IL-8, IL-10, IL-13, IL-16, TNF-α, VEGF, TGF-β, MIP-1α, and MCP-1
Dendritic cells	Antigen presentation	TNF-α, IL-1β
Eosinophils	Allergic response Removal of parasites	Eosinophils specific granules Cationic proteins Major basic protein Eosinophil peroxidase Eosinophil-derived neurotoxin Lipid mediators—leukotriene C4 and PAF

Mast Cells

Mast cells are key elements in the innate immune system and have been termed the "antenna" of the immune response. Mast cells are located throughout the body in close proximity to epithelial surfaces, near blood vessels, nerves, and glands, placing them at strategic locations for detecting invading pathogens. In addition, mast cells express a number of receptors that allow them to recognize diverse stimuli.

In sensitized individuals, IgE is bound to Fcε receptors (FcεRI) on the mast cell surface, and binding of antigen to surface-bound IgE results in mast cell activation. Thus, multiple stimuli (foreign antigens) may trigger the same class of receptor. However, there is specificity in this system as a result of multiple signal transduction pathways that are differentially activated on the basis of antigen size, receptor location, number, and subtype.

In addition, human mast cells also express toll-like receptors (TLRs), TLR-1, TLR-2, TLR-6, and TLR-4. TLRs are pattern recognition receptors that recognize specific molecular patterns of microorganisms. Expression of TLRs, in combination with other receptors, allows the mast cell to recognize many potential pathogens and mount a specific response. Importantly, mast cells are capable of releasing many immune modulating molecules that stimulate inflammation, and the adaptive immune response can polarize T-cell subpopulations toward TH1 or TH2 subtypes. Mast cell products include the following:

1. Preformed mediators that are granule-associated (such as histamine)
2. Mediators synthesized *de novo* (such as leukotriene C4, platelet activating factor, and prostaglandin D2)
3. A vast array of cytokines and chemokines, including IL-1, IL-3, IL-4, IL-5, IL-6, IL-8, IL-10, IL-13, IL-16, TNF-α, VEGF, TGF-β, MIP-1a, and MCP-1.

In summary, the strategic location of mast cells in the body, their diversity of receptors, and cytokines indicate an important role for mast cells in regulating innate and adaptive immunity.

Dendritic Cells

Dendritic cells function as "conductors" of the immune response. These cells, resident within tissues, develop *in vivo* from hematopoietic precursor cells. Dendritic cells bind, internalize, and process antigens and then display them on their surface in conjunction with human leukocyte antigen (HLA) molecules. These antigens are then "presented" to cells of the adaptive immune system (lymphocytes) along with other requisite activation signals resulting in activation of lymphocytes, a pivotal process in the adaptive immune response.

Eosinophils (see Figure 11-5)

Eosinophils are considered to be effector cells of allergic responses and of parasite elimination. These bone marrow–derived cells contain four distinct granule cationic proteins:

1. Major basic protein
2. Eosinophil peroxidase
3. Eosinophil cationic protein
4. Eosinophil-derived neurotoxin

During allergic inflammation, eosinophils release granule contents, as well as inflammatory mediators including lipid mediators such as leukotriene C4 and platelet-activating factor, that may cause dysfunction and destruction of other cells.

Polymorphonuclear Neutrophils (PMNs)

The primary function of PMNs in the innate immune response is to contain and kill invading microbial pathogens. PMNs merit particular mention in pulmonary host defense as the pulmonary microvascular endothelium preferentially recruits this leukocyte population in response to infection and inflammation (see Figure 11-6) by the expression of adhesion molecules and chemokines that target PMNs. PMNs achieve their antimicrobial function through a series of rapid and coordinated

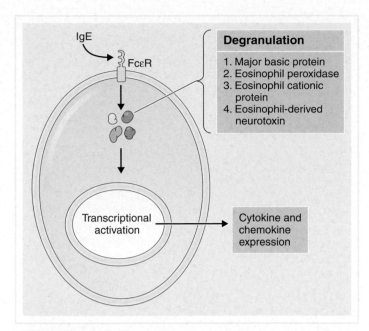

FIGURE 11-5 Defense mechanisms mediated by eosinophils and basophils. IgE-mediated degranulation induces release of four distinct granule cationic proteins from eosinophils that can modulate the inflammatory response and display antihelminthic properties. Eosinophils and basophils are also capable of releasing cytokines and chemokines in a stimulus-specific manner.

responses that culminate in phagocytosis and destruction of the pathogens (Figure 11-7). PMNs have a potent antimicrobial arsenal that includes the following:

1. Oxidants
2. Powerful proteolytic enzymes (proteinases)
3. Cationic peptides

Oxidants such as O_2^- and H_2O_2 are produced by a multi-component enzyme termed the phagocyte NADPH oxidase. Granules within the cytoplasm of PMNs contain potent proteinases and cationic proteins that can digest a variety of microbial substrates. These compounds are released directly into the phagosome, compartmentalizing both the pathogen and the cytotoxic products (Figure 11-8).

ANTIMICROBIAL MOLECULES (Table 11-9)

Antimicrobial molecules are expressed by multiple cell types and play important roles in destruction and removal of pathogens. The important factors that have been shown to impede microbial growth and infection in the context of host defense of the lung are discussed in the following.

Antimicrobial Components in the ASL

The acidic pH (6.4–7.3) of the ASL is inhibitory to microbial proliferation, as well as providing an optimal environment for the activity of the antimicrobial molecules found in the ASL. Important among these are lactoferrin and lysozymes.

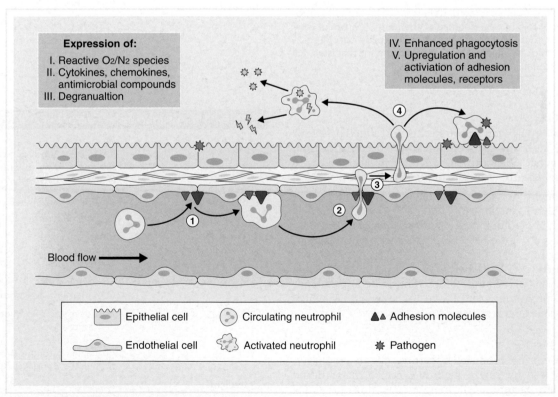

FIGURE 11-6 Leukocyte recruitment in airways and alveolar spaces. Contact with noxious agents or pathogens induces activation and enhanced expression of adhesion molecules on the apical surface of vascular endothelial cells (1) that facilitate leukocyte adhesion, recruitment, and activation; (2) leukocytes then transmigrates across the endothelium, through the interstitial tissues, and across the epithalamium and into the airspace; (3) leukocytes and the epithelial cells may become activated during these processes, leading to enhanced inflammatory cytokine and chemokine production (4).

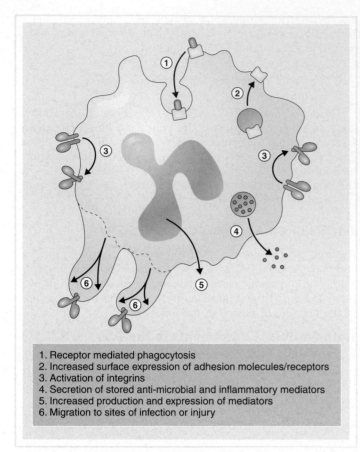

1. Receptor mediated phagocytosis
2. Increased surface expression of adhesion molecules/receptors
3. Activation of integrins
4. Secretion of stored anti-microbial and inflammatory mediators
5. Increased production and expression of mediators
6. Migration to sites of infection or injury

FIGURE 11-7 Neutrophil-mediated defense mechanisms. Neutrophils play a central role in host defense of the lung by virtue of their different defense mechanisms, including their ability to phagocytose pathogens and, by oxidative and proteolytic mechanisms, kill the invading bacteria.

Primary granules

β-Glucuronidase
Cathepsins
Defensins
Elastase
Lysozyme
Myeloperoxidase
N-acetyl-β-glucosaminidase
Proteinase-3

Secondary granules

CD11b   hCAP-18
CD66   Histaminase
Cytochrome b588 Heparanase
FMLP-R   Lactoferrin
Collagenase   Lysozyme
Gelatinase   Vitamine B$_{12}$
               binding protein

NADPH Oxidase

O2$^-$ H2O2

FIGURE 11-8 Neutrophil-derived products. O_2^- and H_2O_2 are produced by a multicomponent enzyme termed the phagocyte NADPH oxidase that is expressed by neutrophils (PMNs) and macrophages. Leukocytes also contain unique secretory granules called the primary and secondary granules that release potent proteolytic enzymes and cationic proteins that can digest a variety of microbial substrates.

Lactoferrin

Lactoferrin is an iron-binding protein that is secreted by serous epithelial cells and PMN that competes with bacteria for iron, thus inhibiting bacterial growth. Lactoferrin also possesses other antimicrobial properties, including the following:

1. Enhancement of PMN function—motility, adherence, superoxide production
2. Inhibition of biofilm formation of *Pseudomonas aeruginosa*
3. The ability to injure bacterial membranes with resultant release of LPS
4. Modulation of LPS activity by competitively binding LPS and thus preventing LPS binding protein from binding and promoting an LPS-CD14 interaction, which would result in cell activation.

Lysozyme

Lysozyme is an enzyme produced by serous cells, macrophages, and PMN that can hydrolyze peptidoglycan, a major ligand in gram-positive bacterial cell membranes, thus providing defense against gram-positive bacterial infections. Lysozyme also aids in the defense against gram-negative bacteria and acts synergistically with lactoferrin, secretory leukoprotease inhibitor (SLPI), and LL-37 (an antimicrobial peptide) to provide multiple mechanisms for bacterial destruction and removal.

TABLE 11-9 Antimicrobial Factors in ASL

Lactoferrin	Binds iron Inhibits bacterial growth Enhances PMN function Modulates LPS activity
Lysozyme	Hydrolyses peptidoglycan
Fibronectin	Binds to bacteria
Complement	Opsoninization Chemotactic Bacterial lysis
Immunoglobulin A and G	Opsoninization Complement activation
Defensins	Pore formation in microbial membranes Chemotactic Promotes cytokine production Stimulates dendritic cells
Cathelicidins	Modulates LPS Chemotactic Stimulates dendritic cells
Collectins	Binds carbohydrate domains of organisms, with reduced virulence and increased phagocytosis

COMPLEMENT

Complement proteins are sequentially activated in a cascade encompassing three distinct pathways: (1) the classic antibody–antigen complex–dependent pathway, (2) the alternate pathway that is initiated by foreign/microbial products, and (3) a recently identified pathway that is initiated by mannose-binding lectin (MBL), a member of the collectin family, and a related family of proteins called ficolins, which are present in the lung. Complement proteins exude from plasma into airways in response to inflammation and are also produced by macrophages, type II pneumocytes, and fibroblasts. Specific complement components have important roles in host defense. These include the following:

1. C5a—recruits PMN into the lung and enhances PMN-mediated microbial killing
2. C3a—a potent anaphylatoxin, also stimulates mucus production from goblet cells and enhanced LPS-induced synthesis of TNF and IL-1 by adherent phagocytes while decreasing synthesis in nonadherent cells
3. C5a–C9 complex—also known as the membrane attack complex (MAC), which creates pores in cell membranes, effectively killing bacteria.

Multiple complement components can function as opsonins aiding phagocytosis of foreign particles (Figure 11-9). Importantly, hereditary deficiency of specific components of the complement pathway results in recurrent respiratory tract infections.

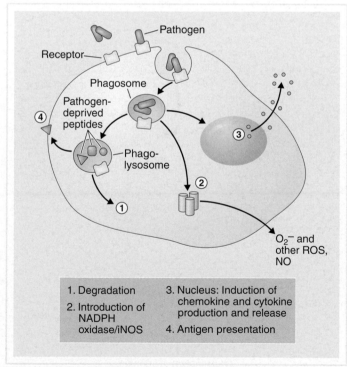

FIGURE 11-9 Immune defense mechanisms mediated by receptor-mediated phagocytosis and signaling. Internalization of pathogens or particulate matter induces multiple host defense mechanisms, including (1) degradation of the offending agent, (2) induction of the NAPDH oxidase (neutrophils and macrophages) or iNOS, (3) induction of chemokine and cytokine expression, and (4) antigen presentation (particularly in dendritic cells and macrophages).

ANTIMICROBIAL PEPTIDES

There are a number of antimicrobial peptides in the airways, and these can be classified conveniently into three groups on the basis of structural motifs: defensins, cathelicidins, and histatins.

Defensins

Defensins are single-chain strongly cationic peptides that have a broad spectrum of antimicrobial activity against gram-positive bacteria, gram-negative bacteria, fungi, and viruses. They work synergistically with other host defense molecules such as lysozyme and lactoferrin. The antimicrobial activities of defensins include the ability to form pores in target membranes, to interfere with protein synthesis, and to directly damage DNA. Defensin activity is influenced by the salt concentration of the ASL, with higher concentrations decreasing its antimicrobial activity.

Defensins are defined by the presence of six cysteines and three intramolecular disulfide bridges and are classified into three different subgroups: α, β, and θ defensins. Only α and β defensins are relevant to humans. The first four human α defensins (HD 1–4) are produced by neutrophils and are found in the airways, and the other two (HD 5, 6) are found in the small intestine and female urogenital tract. Of the 28 human β defensins identified, 6 (HBD 1–6 are mainly expressed by epithelial cells. HBD 2–4 are inducible in response to a variety of stimuli, including bacterial and viral infection, IL-1, TNF, and LPS. The levels of HD 1–4 are increased in inflammatory processes as a result of release by activated neutrophils.

In addition to their direct antimicrobial properties, defensins also contribute to host defense in other ways. These include the following:

1. Enhanced airway epithelial cells bacterial binding, cytotoxicity, and cytokine production
2. Chemotactic for monocytes and immature dendritic cells
3. Direct binding to CCR6 receptors on dendritic cells, thus linking the innate immune system to adaptive immunity (β-defensins)
4. Down-regulation of the inflammatory response by increasing SLPI release from airway epithelial cells and inhibiting the complement cascade.

Cathelicidins

The only human cathelicidin is LL-37, a peptide with a broad spectrum of antimicrobial activity that acts synergistically with lysozyme and lactoferrin. LL-37 is stored as a precursor, hCAP-18, in specific granules and is also secreted by mast cells and the respiratory epithelium. Other host defense activities of LL-37 include the following:

1. Neutralization of LPS
2. Chemotactic for neutrophils, eosinophils, mast cells, and T lymphocytes
3. Direct interaction with dendritic cells to form TH1 cells
4. Mast cell degranulation
5. Induction of cytokine and chemokine expression by epithelial cells and monocytes
6. Induction and angiogenesis
7. Induction of epithelial wound healing

Histatins

Histatins are a family of cationic histidine-rich peptides that are strongly antifungal and may have LPS neutralizing properties. Histatins are present in saliva and play an important role in preventing oral infections. They have not been isolated from airway secretions.

Collectins

The collectins, or collagenous C-type lectins, are a family of polypeptides that bind collagenous carbohydrates. Collectin proteins that play a role of pulmonary host defense include MBL and the surfactant proteins, A (SP-A) and D (SP-D). The collectins have antimicrobial activity against viruses, as well as bacteria, by binding to conserved carbohydrate domains of organisms and particles. As discussed previously, MBL can also activate the complement cascade and has also been shown to induce inflammatory mediator production from monocytes.

Together these groups of antimicrobial molecules in the ASL function to destroy or inhibit microbes before they have a chance to proliferate and compromise the host. If pathogens evade the structural defenses outlined previously and then survive the previously described antimicrobial properties of the ASL, they can come into contact with host cell membranes, which allows for interaction with toll-like receptors.

TOLL-LIKE RECEPTORS

Toll-like receptors (TLRs) function primarily as pattern recognition receptors that recognize conserved molecular patterns in microbial pathogens, called pathogen-associated molecular patterns (PAMPs), which are not normally found in the host (see Table 11-10). The 10 human TLRs share a protein structure characterized by an extracellular domain with a number of leucine-rich repeats (LRRs) and a cytoplasmic domain containing a toll/interleukin 1 receptor homology domain (TIR). They are highly expressed by leukocytes and in tissues in contact with the external environment, such as the lung. Cellular expression of TLRs is modulated by microbial stimuli.

TLR activation after binding of its cognate ligand triggers signal transduction pathways that ultimately lead to altered gene expression. The signaling pathway after recruitment of MyD88 is conserved for all TLRs (see Figure 11-10). Binding of MyD88 to the activated TLR leads to recruitment of IL-1 receptor–associated kinase (IRAK) and IRAK autophosphorylation. TNF-receptor–associated factor-6 (TRAF-6) links with this complex and activates IκB kinase (IKK). IKK phosphorylates IκB, leading to its dissociation from NF-κB. NF-κB then translocates to the nucleus to activate gene transcription. Specificity of TLR signaling is maintained in part by suppressors of cytokine signaling (SOCS; discussed later).

TABLE 11-10	Toll-Like Receptors and Their Ligands
Receptor	**Reported Ligands**
TLR-1	Heterodimerization with TLR-2
TLR-2	Peptidoglycan and lipoteichoic acid (components of gram-positive bacteria) LPS Bacterial lipoproteins (components of *Borrelia burgdorferi*) Components of mycobacterial cell walls Mannuronic acid polymers (components of *Pseudomonas aeruginosa*) Glycosylphosphotidylinositol lipid (components of *Trypanosoma cruzi*) Phenol soluble modulin (from *Staphylococcus epidermidis*) Soluble tuberculosis factor (19-kDa lipoprotein secreted by *Mycobacterium tuberculosis*) Whole bacteria (heat-killed *Listeria monocytogenes*)
TLR-3	Ds-RNA
TLR-4	LPS Mannuronic acid polymers (components of *Pseudomonas aeruginosa*) RSV fusion protein Endogenous inflammation related products (HSP 60, HSP 90, fibronectin)
TLR-5	Flagellin
TLR-6	Heterodimerization with TLR-2
TLR-7	Antiviral compounds
TLR-8	Antiviral compounds
TLR-9	CpG dinucleotides
TLR-10	?

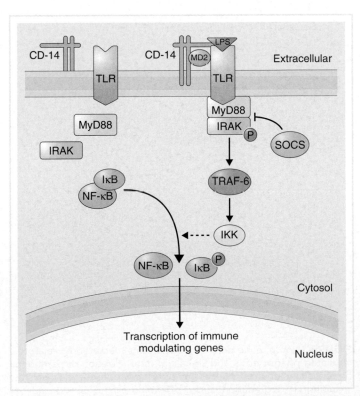

FIGURE 11-10 Toll-like receptor (TLR) signaling. The classical signaling pathway triggered by TLRs involves MyD88/IRAK and TRAF-6, leading to transcriptional regulation of immune and inflammatory genes.

TLR-4

TLR-4 is the prototypical and most extensively studied of the TLRs. It recognizes lipopolysaccharide (LPS, endotoxin), mannuronic acid polymers (components of *Pseudomonas aeruginosa*), and the F protein of the respiratory syncytial virus (RSV). Unlike the other TLRs, TLR4 also recognizes several endogenously derived molecules, including heat shock protein (HSP) 60, HSP 70, and fibronectin.

TLR-2

TLR-2 has a large number of reported ligands. These include components of gram-positive and gram-negative bacteria, mycobacteria, the protozoan parasite *Trypanosoma cruzi*, and zymosan, a yeast wall component. Additional ligands include secreted factors from *Staphylococcus epidermidis* and *Mycobacterium tuberculosis*, as well as whole bacteria (heat-killed *Listeria monocytogenes*). TLR-2 does not recognize these PAMPs in isolation but rather forms heterodimers with TLR-6 and TLR-1, thus contributing to the diversity and specificity of TLR-2–mediated immune response.

TLR-3

TLR-3 is activated by double-stranded (ds)–RNA, a marker of viral infection, and, through the activation of NF-κB, triggers the production of type I interferons. Because TLR-3 is found only on the plasma membrane, it is believed that ds-RNA comes into contact with TLR-3 after the lysis of infected cells and release of ds-RNA into the extracellular milieu.

TLR-5

TLR-5 recognizes a highly conserved cluster of 13 amino acid residues in flagellin, the structural component of flagellae found in many pathogenic bacteria. This interaction triggers an innate response, resulting in cytokine production from leukocytes and dendritic cell activation and maturation.

TLR-9

TLR-9 binds to unmethylated CpG DNA and triggers a predominantly TH1-weighted immune response. Bacteria do not methylate their DNA, whereas vertebrates do. Specifically, unmethylated CpG dinucleotides are present at high frequencies in most bacterial genomes, whereas in the human genome, these dinucleotides are suppressed, methylated, and flanked by bases that are immune neutralizing. TLR-9 is believed to be localized on an organelle membrane within the cytosol, thus facilitating its interaction with bacterial DNA.

Other TLRs

TLR-1 and TLR-6, as mentioned previously, interact with TLR-2 and function as a complex that recognizes a broad range of antigens. TLR-10 is related to TLR-1 and TLR-6, but its role remains to be clarified. TLR-7 and TLR-8 recognize antiviral compounds. This may seem paradoxical; however, it is likely that these compounds show clinical efficacy by mimicking uncharacterized viral antigens and thus stimulating an immune response.

TABLE 11-11   Cytokines, Chemokines, and Their Functions

Cytokine	Function	Other Clinical Roles
TNF-α	Proinflammatory Neutrophil activation in ARDS	Proximate cytokine released in response to inflammatory stimulus
IL-1β	Proinflammatory Neutrophil activation in ARDS Upregulation of adhesion molecules on leukocytes, endothelium, and a/w epithelium	One of first cytokines to be released in response to inflammatory stimulus
IL-6	Proinflammatory Leukocyte activation Promotes proliferation of myeloid progenitor cells Induces pyrexia Acute phase reactant	Circulating levels are a marker of severity of acute respiratory distress syndrome of different etiologies
IL-10	Antiinflammatory Inhibits release of TNF-α, IL-1β, and IL-6 from monocyte/macrophages Stimulates the production of IL-1ra and soluble p75 TNF receptor	
GM-CSF	Alveolar macrophage function Lung host defense Surfactant homeostasis	Low circulating levels associated with poor prognosis in sepsis
PAF	Acts by means of receptors on platelets, leukocytes, and endothelial cells Increases vascular permeability Leukocyte recruitment Primes and triggers leukocyte secretion	
ICAM-1	Leukocyte recruitment and retention	Increased in inflammation
C5a	Product of classical and alternate complement cascade Potent anaphylatoxin and chemoattractant Acts by means of C5aR Can be both proinflammatory and antiinflammatory	
Substance P	Neuropeptide that acts by means of its receptor NK1R Proinflammatory and associated with development of lung injury	

SOCS

Specificity of TLR signaling may be explained by differential inhibition of TLRs by the suppressors of cytokine signaling (SOCS) family of proteins. SOCS are intracellular proteins that negatively regulate cytokine-induced signal transduction pathways by direct inhibition of the receptor and associated kinases. SOCS also down-regulate signaling by targeting receptor-associated molecules for lysosomal degradation. Several SOCS, including SOCS1 and SOCS3, are induced by TLR-2 signaling and by other PAMPs associated with TLR-4 and TLR-9. In animal studies, SOCS1 deficiency results in exaggerated responses to LPS and displays reduced LPS tolerance compared with wild-type litter mates. Furthermore, SOCS-3 has been shown to directly inhibit production of nitric oxide, TNF-α, IL-6, and GM-CSF in response to LPS in mouse macrophages. Together, these studies indicate an important role for SOCS in modulating cellular responses to LPS (see Figure 11-10).

INFLAMMATORY MEDIATORS

Cytokines (see Table 11-10)

Cytokines are soluble, low-molecular-weight proteins that play important roles in host defense by regulating the inflammatory response and are expressed not only by leukocytes but also by endothelial cells, epithelial cells, and fibroblasts. Expression and secretion of cytokines are transcriptionally regulated and can be quickly enhanced after cell stimulation.

Signaling through cognate receptors, cytokines exert distinct responses in specific cell populations, stimulating some populations to activate, proliferate, and differentiate while having an inhibitory effect on other cells types. In this way, cytokines play a major role in regulating the intensity and duration of the inflammatory response. The cytokines that play important roles in inflammation, particularly in the early proinflammatory phase, include TNF-α, IL-1β, IL-6, and IL-10. Significant elevations of these cytokines are observed in generalized inflammatory states and particularly in gram-negative sepsis.

Chemokines (Table 11-12)

Chemokines are 8–10-kD glycoproteins that, although structurally related to cytokines, are distinct from them as a result of their ability to bind and signal G-protein–coupled receptors. Chemokines are both chemotactic and cellular activating factors for leukocytes and can be classified into four groups on the basis of their amino acid structure. The two primary groups that play an important role in host defense are the CC chemokines (e.g., MCP-1, MIP-1α, and RANTES [regulated on *activation, normal T cell expressed and secreted*]), which are chemotactic for monocytes, lymphocytes, basophils, and eosinophils and the CXC chemokines (e.g., IL-8, GRO-α [growth related oncogene α], and ENA-78 [epithelial-derived neutrophil-activating peptide]), which act primarily on neutrophils.

The chemokine receptors are structurally related seven-transmembrane spanning proteins that transmit their signals

TABLE 11-12 Chemokine Families

Family	Members	Function
CXC	IL-8 MIP-2 GRO ENA-78 NAP-2	Chemotactic and stimulatory to neutrophils
CC	MCP-1 MCP-2 MCP-3 RANTES MIP-1α MIP-1β	Chemotactic and activation of: Monocytes Lymphocytes Eosinophils Basophils Mast cells
C	Lymphotactin	
CXXXC	Fractalkine	

through heterotrimeric G proteins. Like cytokines, the effect of chemokine activation results in diverse physiologic responses that are cell- and stimulus-specific. The binding specificity of individual chemokine receptors is determined by a region in the amino terminus of the protein. Some receptors are highly specific, whereas others bind multiple chemokines of both CC and CXC families. Differential regulation and expression of the chemokines receptor in different cell types plays an important role in determining the biologic result of chemokine activation.

SUMMARY

It is apparent that the lung has multiple lines of defense against microbial pathogens and noxious environmental agents. These include physical barriers such as mucus and soluble factors such as antimicrobial peptides and proteins produced by epithelial cells, as well as leukocytes of the innate and adaptive immune systems. It is this diversity and redundancy that enables the lung to thwart infection under most circumstances.

SUGGESTED READINGS

Bals R, Hiemstra PS: Innate immunity in the lung: How epithelial cells fight against respiratory pathogens. Eur Respir J 2004; 23(2): 327–333.

Gurish MF, Boyce JA: Mast cells: ontogeny, homing, and recruitment of a unique innate effector cell. J Allergy Clin Immunol 2006; 117(6): 1285–1291.

Kyd JM, Foxwell AR, Cripps AW: Mucosal immunity in the lung and upper airway. Vaccine 2001; 19(17–19):2527–2533.

Lambrecht BN, Prins JB, Hoogsteden HC: Lung dendritic cells and host immunity to infection. Eur Respir J 2001; 18(4):692–704.

McCormack FX, Whitsett JA: The pulmonary collectins, SP-A and SP-D, orchestrate innate immunity in the lung. J Clin Invest 2002; 109(6): 707–712.

Moraes TJ, Zurawska JH, Downey GP: Neutrophil granule contents in the pathogenesis of lung injury. Curr Opin Hematol 2006; 13(1):21–27.

Proud D: The role of defensins in virus-induced asthma. Curr Allergy Asthma Rep 2006; 6(1):81–85.

Zaas AK, Schwartz DA: Innate immunity and the lung: defense at the interface between host and environment. Trends Cardiovasc Med 2005; 15(6):195–202.

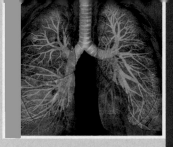

12 Bronchoscopy

ANIL VACHANI • DANIEL H. STERMAN

INTRODUCTION

The first bronchoscopy was performed by Gustav Killian in 1897. Technologic advances during the next century facilitated development of bronchoscopy as a pivotal diagnostic and therapeutic tool in pulmonary medicine. Although a number of bronchoesophagologists contributed to refinement of the technique based on the use of a rigid instrument, the advent of flexible fiberoptic bronchoscopy, pioneered by Ikeda in 1967, opened new horizons to clinicians. At the end of the 1980s, the development of videobronchoscopy significantly improved imaging quality and data storage. Thereafter, several other bronchoscopic applications have been developed for both diagnostic and therapeutic purposes.

This chapter is an overview of bronchoscopy and related techniques. After a general discussion of bronchoscopy and associated instrumentation, applications of the technique and patient preparation are considered. Specific indications for diagnostic and therapeutic bronchoscopy are discussed. Finally, safety factors related to bronchoscopy, contraindications, and complications of the technique are reviewed.

TYPES OF BRONCHOSCOPY AND GENERAL INSTRUMENTATION

Rigid Bronchoscopy

The initial bronchoscope, developed by Killian and further perfected by Chevalier Jackson, was a rigid metal tube that permitted either spontaneous or mechanical ventilation. Over the decades, rigid bronchoscopes of various lengths and sizes, which are adaptable for diverse applications in children and adults, have become available. Today, the flexible bronchoscope has, to a large extent, replaced the rigid bronchoscope for most diagnostic and some therapeutic indications.

Both rigid and flexible modern systems are equipped with optic capabilities for airway observation alone. With the rigid bronchoscope, various types of telescopic rods, equipped with circumferential illumination, permit direct and magnified visualization (Figure 12-1). Specially designed telescopes allow viewing not only directly forward but also at oblique and lateral angles. Various diagnostic and therapeutic accessories can be inserted through the rigid bronchoscope while the patient remains ventilated. Rigid bronchoscopy allows a number of therapies such as laser photoresection, endobronchial stents, balloon dilation, electrocautery, argon beam coagulation, and cryotherapy to be performed safely and effectively. The rigid scope can also be used for the passage of a flexible bronchoscope, which may be necessary for dealing with tortuous airways or distal lesions.

Flexible Bronchoscopy

The flexible bronchoscope is used in most bronchoscopic procedures. Although initial flexible bronchoscopes used fiberoptic systems, most scopes now use a charged coupled camera at the tip that allows transmission of digital images to a monitor. The main advantages of flexible bronchoscopes include their ease of manipulation and greater flexibility, allowing a more complete evaluation of the tracheobronchial tree than rigid bronchoscopy (Figure 12-2).

The flexible bronchoscope varies from ultrathin devices, allowing for endoscopy in infants and neonates, to larger, adult-sized therapeutic scopes. The working channel of the bronchoscope can be used for aspiration of secretions and for various diagnostic or therapeutic accessories. The most commonly used ancillary diagnostic instruments include biopsy forceps, biopsy needles, bronchial brushes, and various catheters and balloons (Figure 12-3). The use of endobronchial ultrasound probes is discussed in Chapter 14.

Biopsy forceps are available in various sizes, have smooth or serrated edges, and can have a small needle between the cups for stabilization. The use of smooth edges may reduce tissue trauma and the concomitant risk of bleeding. Lesions not accessible to direct forceps biopsy can be approached with a bronchial brush. This device consists of a rigid central wire surrounded by brushes of various sizes and shapes. To-and-fro movement of the brush against the adjacent tissue produces minor trauma but enables collection of ample specimens for cytologic or microbiologic analysis. Uncontaminated specimens from the lower respiratory tract can be collected with a brush protected by an additional sheath and tip. Needles of various sizes can be used to obtain both cytologic and histologic material from transbronchial lesions (e.g., lymph nodes, mediastinal masses) or from endobronchial and submucosal lesions.

PATIENT PREPARATION AND MONITORING DURING BRONCHOSCOPY

All patients undergoing bronchoscopy should undergo a complete prebronchoscopy evaluation, including a medical history, physical examination, and chest imaging (Box 12-1). Although routine laboratory tests are not required, each evaluation should be individualized on the basis of patients' underlying conditions and the diagnostic and therapeutic procedures planned.

Most fiberoptic bronchoscopies are performed after patient premedication with sedative agents. Most frequently a combination of a short-acting benzodiazepine (e.g., midazolam) and a narcotic agent (e.g., fentanyl) is used. The sedatives

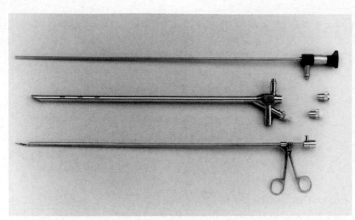

FIGURE 12-1 A typical rigid bronchoscope (*middle*) with Hopkins rod rigid telescope (*top*) and optical biopsy forceps. (Courtesy of Beamis.)

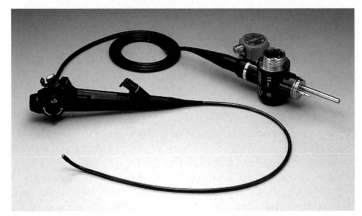

FIGURE 12-2 Flexible bronchoscope. The flexible distal tip permits easy maneuverability in all lobar and segmental bronchi. (Courtesy of Olympus Corporation.)

> **BOX 12-1 Prebronchoscopy Checklist**
>
> 1. Is there an appropriate indication for bronchoscopy?
> 2. Has there been a previous bronchoscopy?
> 3. If the answer to the preceding question is yes, were there any problems or complications?
> 4. Does the patient (and close relative[s] if patient is unable to communicate) fully understand the goals, risks, and complications of bronchoscopy?
> 5. Does the patient's medical history (allergy to medications or topical anesthesia) and present clinical condition pose special problems or predispose to complications?
> 6. Are all the appropriate tests completed and the results available?
> 7. Are the premedications appropriate and the dosages correct?
> 8. Does the patient require special consideration before bronchoscopy (e.g., corticosteroids for asthma, insulin for diabetes mellitus, or prophylaxis against endocarditis) or during bronchoscopy (e.g., supplemental oxygen, extra sedation)?
> 9. Is the plan for postbronchoscopy care appropriate?
> 10. Are all the appropriate instruments and personnel available to assist during the procedure and to handle the potential complications?

Adapted from Prakash UBS, Cortese DA, Stubbs, SE: Technical solutions to common problems in bronchoscopy. In Prakash UBS, ed: Bronchoscopy. New York: Raven; 1994. Copyright Mayo Foundation.

---

with minimal anesthesia and later under general anesthesia, the recent trend has been to perform the procedure with patients either breathing spontaneously or ventilated with a jet ventilator, often under total intravenous anesthesia (TIVA) with drugs such as propofol and remifentanil. With appropriate monitoring, good oxygenation and adequate ventilation can be ensured.

Success of bronchoscopy, whether diagnostic or therapeutic, depends, in large part, on proper preparation of the patient, including relief of anxiety, muscle relaxation, cough suppression, and adequate anesthesia. Time spent in achieving these goals will be well worth it in reducing the risks of complications and in increasing the ease of performance of the procedure.

are generally administered along with an anticholinergic medication (e.g., atropine or glycopyrrolate) to reduce the risk of vasovagal reactions and to minimize airway secretions. Local anesthesia of the upper airway, larynx, and tracheobronchial tree is achieved with inhaled or bronchoscopically instilled lidocaine. Although rigid bronchoscopy was performed initially

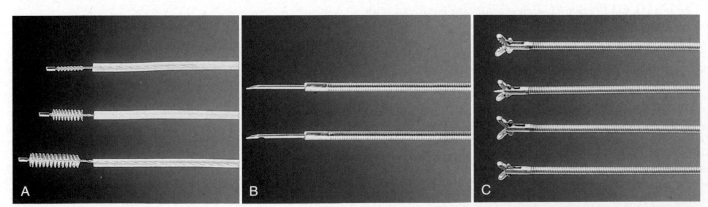

FIGURE 12-3 Bronchoscopy brushes **(A)**, needles **(B)**, and biopsy forceps **(C)** are available in various sizes and types. (Courtesy of Olympus Corporation.)

TECHNIQUE

The flexible bronchoscope is usually inserted nasally, orally, or through an endotracheal tube or a tracheostomy stoma. When necessary, it can also be inserted through a rigid bronchoscope. The nasal route is often preferred, because the nasal passage serves as a stent for the bronchoscope and allows for somewhat better control during airway inspection. When the oral route is used, a "bite block" should be inserted to prevent the patient from biting and damaging the scope. Supplemental oxygen should be administered to prevent hypoxemia, which is fairly common during bronchoscopy, particularly in patients with underlying lung disease.

The bronchoscopic evaluation should begin with a thorough examination of the upper airway, as well as the integrity and function of the larynx. The vocal cords should be examined for any abnormalities, such as polyps or tumors, and evaluated for paralysis during phonation.

Once the upper airway inspection is completed, a systematic evaluation of the lower respiratory tract should be performed, beginning with an evaluation of the trachea and then all segmental bronchi. The integrity of the airways should be assessed, with special attention paid to dynamic changes in airway caliber during either relaxed breathing or forced expiration and coughing. Flexible bronchoscopy is superior to rigid bronchoscopy for this assessment. Relaxation and prolapse of the membranous portion of the trachea and main bronchi secondary to destruction of elastic connective tissue may account for exacerbations of expiratory airflow obstruction. On the other hand, finding localized, posttraumatic chondromalacia has very different therapeutic implications. On the basis of these bronchoscopic determinations, open surgical versus bronchoscopic therapeutic correction may be chosen.

It is important to distinguish among normal anatomy, anatomic variations without clinical significance, and frankly pathologic conditions. These considerations have important implications regarding potential diagnostic and therapeutic approaches. For example, finding an abnormal branching of a bronchus may be of no clinical significance. On the other hand, such an abnormality could explain symptoms of frequent infections caused by impaired ventilation and drainage of the affected area. Bronchoscopy is particularly useful in documenting posttraumatic or postsurgical changes in bronchial integrity, such as bronchial rupture, tracheoesophageal or bronchopleural fistulas, or anastomotic complications after reconstructive or lung transplantation surgery. Similarly, bronchoscopy can be used to document tracheal injuries occurring in critically ill patients after prolonged intubation or tracheostomy. Although tracheal injuries have decreased in incidence over past decade, they are still an important cause of complications in these patients. These complications include tracheal stenosis, tracheomalacia, and tracheoinnominate fistula formation. Complications specific to the use of percutaneous tracheotomy include flaps of cartilage protruding into the tracheal lumen and extraluminal placement of the tracheostomy tube.

A thorough evaluation of the mucosal surface is an important part of the bronchoscopic examination. The most common abnormality is the change in mucosal coloration, with prominent hypervascular areas seen in patients with chronic bronchitis. The presence of granulation tissue can be due to reaction to a foreign body. Inflammatory mucosal reactions, although not very characteristic, should raise the possibility of mycobacterial infection, nonspecific viral and nonviral infections, and other

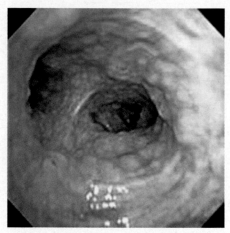

FIGURE 12-4 Endobronchial sarcoidosis. Bronchoscopy demonstrates edematous airways with a "cobblestone" appearance often seen in endobronchial sarcoidosis. (Courtesy of Meeta Prasad, MD.)

granulomatous diseases, such as sarcoidosis (Figure 12-4). Ulcerations of the mucosa are more characteristic of Wegener's granulomatosis or malignancy. Loss of the usual mucosal luster and presence of a roughened surface may be an early sign of an infiltrative or neoplastic process.

The trachea and bronchi are surrounded by mediastinal and parenchymal structures. Developmental or pathologic changes in these organs may be noted during bronchoscopic evaluation. An enlarged goiter or thymus can compress upper airways, resulting in airflow obstruction. Lymphadenopathy may produce structural changes, including widening of the carina caused by subcarinal involvement and compression of other bronchi—as, for example, in the right-middle-lobe syndrome. Calcification of peribronchial lymph nodes may result in erosion of the bronchial wall and formation of a broncholith. These lesions are potential sources of obstruction, infection, or dangerous hemoptysis.

After the bronchoscopic inspection of the airways and surrounding structures has been performed, appropriate samplings should be obtained from the abnormalities identified. Aspirated secretions can be sent for microscopy and for cultures to determine the offending organism in cases of infection or suspected infection. Endobronchial lesions can be sampled with cytology brushes, biopsy forceps, or needles. Bronchoscopic lung biopsy can be performed for either focal abnormalities or diffuse lung diseases (Figure 12-5). For small or focal lesions, fluoroscopy helps guide the placement of the forceps in the periphery of the lung and improves the diagnostic yield of biopsies. The use of fluoroscopy also obviates the need for routine chest radiography after lung biopsy. In the case of diffuse lung disease, such as sarcoidosis, use of fluoroscopy has not been demonstrated to improve the diagnostic yield of transbronchial biopsies. Fluoroscopy is useful, however, in providing information regarding the proximity of the forceps to the pleura and in more rapidly establishing the diagnosis of complications (e.g., pneumothorax). Transbronchoscopic needle aspiration (TBNA) and biopsy (TBNB) permit sampling of peribronchial lymph nodes. These transbronchial approaches provide cost-effective diagnostic modalities with less risk and a lower complication rate than mediastinoscopy (see Chapter 17).

A useful bronchoscopic sampling technique is bronchoalveolar lavage (BAL) (Figure 12-6). BAL is safe, even in critically ill patients, when biopsy or brushings are not recommended

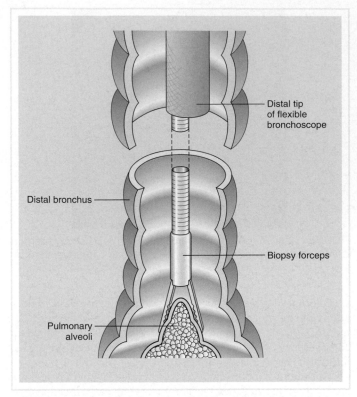

FIGURE 12-5 The mechanism by which bronchoscopic lung biopsy is obtained. The biopsy forceps pinches off the lung tissue located between two branches of terminal bronchi.

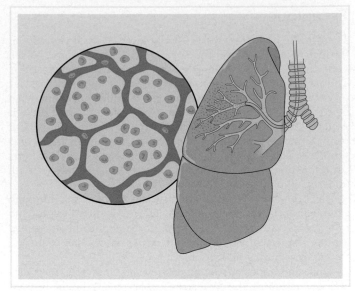

FIGURE 12-6 Bronchoalveolar lavage (BAL) is performed by wedging the tip of the flexible bronchoscope in the segmental bronchus leading to the parenchymal abnormalities detected by imaging techniques. Normal saline, 100–150 mL, in aliquots of 10–50 mL, is instilled through the bronchoscope channel and suctioned back into a container for analysis.

because of the risk of bleeding. Normal saline solution, devoid of any bacteriostatic material, is instilled into distal airspaces through the "wedged" bronchoscope and then aspirated through the instrument's suction channel. The fluid collected in this manner is analyzed for gross appearance to detect possible alveolar hemorrhage. The fluid may also be subjected to a variety of tests, depending on the clinical circumstances: microbiologic testing, specific cytologic analysis and cell count, immunologic parameters, presence of various biochemical mediators related to pathologic processes, tissue markers, polymerase chain reaction, electron microscopy, flow cytometry, and DNA probes. The diagnostic yield of BAL very much depends on specific patient characteristics, the underlying pathologic process, and many technical factors.

INDICATIONS FOR DIAGNOSTIC BRONCHOSCOPY

There are many potential indications for both diagnostic and therapeutic bronchoscopy, many of which are listed in Boxes 12-2 and 12-3. The most common reason for bronchoscopy remains the evaluation of a lung mass or nodule. Other major indications include the evaluation of pulmonary infiltrates, evaluation of opportunistic infections in immunocompromised hosts, hemoptysis, suspected foreign body, and treatment of airway complications related to neoplasms in the tracheobronchial tree. Some of these indications are discussed in the following sections.

BOX 12-2 Indications for Diagnostic Bronchoscopy

Cough
Hemoptysis
Wheeze and stridor
Abnormal chest radiograph
Pulmonary infections
Diffuse interstitial lung disease
Intrathoracic lymphadenopathy or mass
Bronchogenic carcinoma
Metastatic carcinoma
Esophageal and mediastinal tumors
Foreign body in the tracheobronchial tree
Tracheobronchial strictures and stenoses
Airway burns
Thoracic trauma
Vocal cord paralysis
Bronchopleural fistula
Tracheoesophageal fistula
Assessment of endotracheal tube placement or complications
Assessment of airway anastomosis

Chronic Cough

Chronic cough remains one of the most common reasons for patients to seek medical attention. Although flexible bronchoscopy is frequently used in the evaluation of chronic cough, its role has not been clearly defined, particularly in patients without other indications for the procedure. The routine use of bronchoscopy in chronic cough has a diagnostic yield of <5%. Chronic cough that is associated with localizing symptoms,

BOX 12-3 Indications for Therapeutic Bronchoscopy

Hemoptysis
Atelectasis
Foreign body removal
Neoplasms of the tracheobronchial tree
   Bronchoscopic removal
   Laser therapy
   Argon plasma coagulation
   Brachytherapy
   Stent placement
Strictures and stenoses
   Bronchoscopic dilation
   Laser therapy
   Balloon dilation
   Stent replacement
Lung lavage (pulmonary alveolar proteinosis)
Bronchoscopic drainage
   Lung abscess
   Mediastinal or bronchogenic cysts
Thoracic trauma
Endotracheal tube placement

such as hemoptysis, a focal wheeze, or an abnormal imaging study, is much more likely to lead to a specific diagnosis by bronchoscopy. In nonsmokers with normal chest imaging, the most likely causes of cough are asthma, gastroesophageal reflux disease, and rhinitis. Bronchoscopy can be considered if these etiologies have been effectively ruled out by a combination of empiric treatment and diagnostic testing, including the use of spirometry, bronchoprovocation tests, sinus imaging, and esophageal pH probes.

Evaluation of Hemoptysis

Hemoptysis is a common clinical symptom and one of the most frequent indications for bronchoscopic evaluation. The most common causes of scant hemoptysis include chronic bronchitis, tuberculosis, and bronchiectasis, whereas massive hemoptysis, usually defined as bleeding of >200 mL in a 24-h period, is most often due to tuberculous cavities, lung cancer, mycetomas, or lung abscess (see Chapter 24). Bronchoscopy can be of help in localizing the site and cause of bleeding. Although the timing of the procedure should be dictated by clinical circumstances, studies have shown that early bronchoscopy (within 48 h) is more likely to demonstrate active bleeding and allow for the determination of the bleeding site. Chest imaging, with either chest X-ray (CXR) or CT scan, can assist in the localization of the bleeding site and, in stable patients without massive hemoptysis, should precede a bronchoscopy. In patients with a normal CXR, the prevalence of malignancy is approximately 5%, which in most cases is visible by CT scan. The yield of bronchoscopy in patients with a normal CT scan is extremely low, and a conservative approach consisting of observation and serial imaging should be considered.

In cases in which the site of bleeding is not readily apparent, examination with an ultrathin bronchoscope may be beneficial in identifying the source of bleeding in a peripheral airway. Beyond its role as a diagnostic tool, bronchoscopy can often

be used to perform various therapeutic procedures in patients with hemoptysis (see following).

Pulmonary Infections

Bronchoscopy is a useful technique in the diagnosis of pulmonary infections, allowing for the collection of respiratory samples for evaluation with special stains and culture. Respiratory samples can be collected by one or more techniques, including bronchial wash, BAL, protected specimen brush (PSB), and bronchoscopic lung biopsy (Table 12-1).

Bronchoscopy is not indicated for the diagnosis of community-acquired pneumonia, which is currently treated empirically with appropriate antibiotic therapy. Bronchoscopy is likely to be useful in cases of nonresolving pneumonia, ventilator-associated pneumonia (VAP), or immunocompromised patients with new infiltrates. Nonresolving pneumonia is defined as lack of improvement or worsening of symptoms despite a minimum of 10 days of antibiotic therapy or failure of radiographic abnormalities to resolve after 2–3 months. The causes of nonresolving pneumonia are myriad and include inadequate antibiotic therapy, resistant or highly virulent organisms, impaired host defenses, obstructing endobronchial lesions, or a noninfectious etiology. Although controversial, bronchoscopy should be considered in these patients.

Ventilator-Associated Pneumonia

Ventilator-associated pneumonia is defined as a pneumonia occurring more than 48 h after intubation and initiation of mechanical ventilation. Intubated patients are at increased risk for pneumonia because of the impairment in mucociliary clearance caused by the endotracheal tube. These patients are also often on broad-spectrum antibiotics, placing them at greater risk for infection with resistant organisms. Recent guidelines support the use of either a quantitative or semi-quantitative strategy (e.g., tracheal aspirates) in the diagnosis of VAP. Two quantitative bronchoscopic methods that are particularly useful are BAL and PSB. The threshold for diagnosis of VAP with PSB is 10^3 colony-forming units (CFU) per milliliter. PSB seems to have higher specificity than sensitivity for the presence of VAP—a positive result greatly increases the likelihood of pneumonia being present. For quantitative BAL, a threshold of 10^4 or 10^5 CFU per milliliter is used for the diagnosis of pneumonia. The detection of pneumonia by quantitative BAL culture has a sensitivity of 40–90% and a specificity of 45–100%. Because a larger proportion of lung parenchyma is sampled with BAL, this may be a better method than PSB for the diagnosis of VAP. Techniques incorporating molecular testing in addition to microbiologic cultures are currently being evaluated.

Mycobacterial Infections

In cases in which pulmonary tuberculosis is suspected, the initial diagnostic evaluation should consist of serial examination of sputum for the presence of acid-fast bacilli (AFB) in stained smears. Ideally, induced sputum samples should be obtained. If sputum studies are negative and tuberculosis is still suspected, bronchoscopy with BAL and biopsy should be performed. Both induced sputum collection and bronchoscopy should be performed with appropriate infection control precautions to minimize the risk of nosocomial transmission. A bronchoscopy may cause the patient to produce sputum

TABLE 12-1 Bronchoscopic Techniques and Applications in Respiratory Infections	
Bronchoscopic Techniques	**Clinical Applications**
Bronchoscopy (visualization)	1. Assessment of mucosal, intraluminal, and extraluminal pathology 2. Evaluation of endobronchial tuberculosis, mycoses, viral vesicles (in AIDS) 3. Invasive tracheobronchial aspergillosis, candidiasis, and others 4. Follow-up of endobronchial disease (tuberculosis, etc.)
Bronchial washing	Culture of mycobacteria, fungi, and viruses, and Pneumocystis smears
Bronchoalveolar lavage	Culture of all organisms, especially for identification of mycobacteria, fungi, cytomegalovirus, and other viruses, and Pneumocystis smears
Protected specimen brushing	Culture and aerobic and anaerobic bacteria
Nonprotected bronchial brushing	Stains and culture for mycobacteria, fungi, Pneumocystis, and viruses
Endobronchial biopsy	1. Mucosal lesions caused by mycobacteria, fungi, protozoa, etc. 2. Removal of obstructing lesions responsible for infection (tumor, foreign body, etc.) 3. Drainage of lung abscess, piecemeal removal of mycetomas (aspergillomas and other fungus balls)
Bronchoscopic needle aspiration	1. Stains and culture of extrabronchial lymph nodes for identification of mycobacteria and fungi 2. Drainage of bronchogenic cyst and instillation of sclerosing agent
Bronchoscopic lung biopsy	Stains and culture of all organism, especially for identification of *Pneumocystis jiroveci*, mycobacteria, and fungi; also detection of parasitic lung infections
Rigid or flexible bronchoscope	Insertion of tracheobronchial prosthesis (stent) to overcome airway obstruction caused by intrinsic stenosis (post-tuberculous or fungal), extrinsic compression caused by mediastinal fibrosis due to histoplasmosis

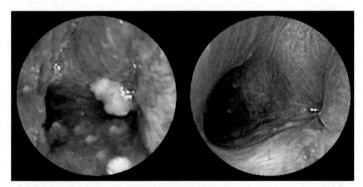

FIGURE 12-7 Endobronchial tuberculosis involving distal trachea and main bronchi. Figure on left was obtained before chemotherapy, and the posttherapy appearance is shown on the right. Endobronchial tuberculosis is commonly mistaken for bronchogenic carcinoma.

for several days afterwards; ideally, these specimens should also be collected and analyzed. The utility of bronchoscopy varies widely in the literature with reported diagnostic yields of 50–95%. The yield in patients with miliary TB, in whom sputum smears are frequently negative, is approximately 70%. Bronchoscopy is also useful in tuberculosis presenting as an endobronchial lesion or with mediastinal and hilar adenopathy, in which case diagnostic tissue can be obtained with TBNA (Figure 12-7). The yield of diagnostic procedures, including bronchoscopy, will likely improve as newer nucleic acid amplification techniques are incorporated into everyday practice (see Chapter 31).

Immunocompromised Patients

Pulmonary infections represent the most common complication and an important cause of mortality in immunocompromised patients. This is an increasingly common occurrence

given the expanding use of aggressive chemotherapeutic regimens and the ever-expanding number of solid organ and hematopoietic stem cell transplantations that are being performed. The differential diagnosis of pulmonary infiltrates is broad; however, most cases are caused by infectious agents, including bacterial, fungal, viral, and mycobacterial pathogens. Bronchoscopy is the most commonly used diagnostic procedure in these patients and should be performed as early as possible, because a delay in diagnosis of greater than 5 days has been shown to significantly increase mortality in these patients.

The sensitivity of bronchoscopy varies, depending on the population studied and the specific etiology. In non-HIV patients, the yield of BAL for *Pneumocystis jiroveci* is approximately 80% compared with the >95% yield observed in HIV-positive individuals. This difference is due to the much lower organism load present in non-HIV subjects. Although empiric therapy is often initiated in patients suspected of *P. jiroveci* infection, bronchoscopy should be performed in most cases to confirm the diagnosis. Bronchoscopy also has a high diagnostic yield for cytomegalovirus (CMV); however, because CMV cultures from BAL are not specific, the diagnosis of CMV pneumonia should be limited to patients with pathologic evidence of CMV infection demonstrated by the presence of CMV inclusion bodies on BAL or biopsy. Although bronchoscopy is also useful for the diagnosis of aspergillosis, the sensitivity is approximately 50%—disease is often peripheral and patchy and thus not easily diagnosed by BAL or bronchoscopic biopsy. Overall, in immunocompromised patients with infiltrates, bronchoscopy is successful in establishing the diagnosis in more than 80% of cases.

Human Immunodeficiency Syndrome

The introduction of HAART (highly active antiretroviral therapy) has led to a sharp decline in the incidence of opportunistic infections in patients with HIV disease. Nevertheless, infectious complications remain one of the most common indications for bronchoscopy in this population. *Pneumocystis* pneumonia remains the most frequent serious opportunistic infection in patients with HIV. Bronchoscopy with BAL remains the preferred diagnostic procedure for this disease, although in select centers, the use of sputum induction has had a relatively high diagnostic yield and may avoid the need for bronchoscopy. Bronchoscopic biopsy may increase the diagnostic yield of BAL. Empiric therapy is often initiated in patients with suspected *Pneumocystis* infection and can impair the diagnostic yield of BAL if not performed within 24 h. In patients receiving pentamidine prophylaxis, the diagnostic yield is decreased unless the upper lobes are sampled. Several PCR assays have been tested on BAL, induced sputum, and oral wash specimens; these have generally been more sensitive but less specific than traditional microscopic methods.

Bronchoscopy also plays an important diagnostic role in HIV-positive patients with infections caused by *Mycobacteria*, including tuberculosis, atypical bacterial pneumonias, and various fungal infections. Kaposi's sarcoma, caused by HHV8, can present with violaceous endobronchial plaques that typically occur at airway bifurcations; pulmonary parenchymal involvement is characterized by lymphangitic infiltration of tumor leading to the development of nodules and masses.

BRONCHOGENIC CARCINOMA

Diagnosis

Bronchoscopy is most commonly performed in the evaluation of patients with lung cancer. Bronchoscopy remains the most commonly used modality for the diagnosis of bronchogenic carcinoma and plays an important role in staging. Centrally located lesions can generally be approached with flexible bronchoscopy with minimal risk. Central tumors can present as exophytic mass lesions, with partial or total occlusion of the bronchial lumen, as peribronchial tumors with extrinsic compression of the airway, or with submucosal infiltration of tumor. The changes with peribronchial tumors or with submucosal infiltration are often subtle—the airways should be examined closely for characteristic changes such as erythema, loss of bronchial markings, and nodularity of the mucosal surface.

Central lesions are usually sampled with a combination of bronchial washes, bronchial brushings, and endobronchial biopsies. The yield of endobronchial biopsies is highest for exophytic lesions, with a diagnostic yield of approximately 80%. Three to four biopsies are likely adequate in this situation. Attempts should be made to obtain the biopsies from areas of the lesion that seem viable. Endobronchial needle aspiration (EBNA) to obtain a "core" biopsy from centrally located tumors should be considered, particularly if the lesion appears necrotic. For submucosal lesions, EBNA can be performed by inserting the needle into the submucosal plane at an oblique angle, and in patients with peribronchial disease causing extrinsic compression, the needle should be passed through the bronchial wall into the lesion. For all of these indications, EBNA has been shown to increase the diagnostic yield of conventional sampling methods.

Peripheral lesions are usually sampled with a combination of bronchial wash, brushes, transbronchial biopsy, and TBNA. The diagnostic yield of bronchoscopy for peripheral lesions depends on a number of factors, including lesion size, the distance of the lesion from the hilum, and on the relationship between the lesion and bronchus. The yield of bronchoscopy for lesions smaller than 3 cm varies from 14–50% compared with a diagnostic yield of 46–80% when the lesion is larger than 3 cm. The presence of a bronchus sign on chest CT predicts a much higher yield of bronchoscopy for peripheral lung lesions. In these cases, fluoroscopic guidance should be used to ensure proper positioning of the diagnostic accessory (Figure 12-8).

Several newer methods have been developed for the evaluation of peripheral lung lesions, including endobronchial ultrasound (EBUS) (see Chapter 14) and electromagnetic navigation bronchoscopy (ENB). ENB is based on virtual bronchoscopy and real-time 3D CT images and uses an electromagnetic board placed under the bronchoscopy table (Figure 12-9). This allows a steerable probe with a position sensor allowing its position to be displayed in real time. Preliminary studies suggest that this technique improves the diagnostic yield of bronchoscopy for peripheral lung lesions.

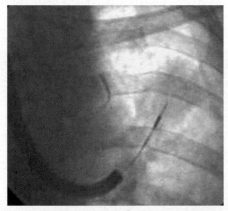

FIGURE 12-8 Bronchoscopic lung biopsy with fluoroscopic guidance. Fluoroscopy assists in the placement of the diagnostic accessory for small or focal lesions and improves the diagnostic yield.

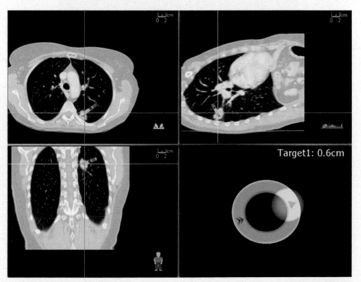

FIGURE 12-9 Electromagnetic navigation bronchoscopy. Representative images from a bronchoscopy by use of electromagnetic guidance. The parenchymal lesion is visible in sagittal, coronal, and axial views. (Courtesy of SuperDimension, Inc.)

Staging

Bronchoscopy is an important modality for establishing the stage of lung cancer. In patients with potentially resectable tumors, a thorough airway examination helps confirm the absence of a concomitant, radiographically occult lesion. For lesions that involve the central airways, it is important to document the extent of disease and the degree of involvement of mainstream bronchi and main carina.

TBNA has emerged as a valuable tool for the evaluation of enlarged or metabolically active mediastinal lymph nodes (Figure 12-10). The procedure is particularly useful for patients who are marginal or poor surgical candidates; in these patients, more invasive approaches, such as mediastinoscopy or mediastinotomy, may be obviated. TBNA has proven particularly useful with the use of rapid onsite evaluation, where a cytopathologist present in or near the bronchoscopy suite can evaluate obtained specimens in real time (see Chapter 14).

Several precautions should be observed during the performance of TBNA to minimize the risk of false-positive results. The bronchoscope should be introduced into the bronchial tree without suction, and TBNA should be performed before inspection of the distal airway and before any other sampling procedures. N3 nodes should be sampled first, followed by N2 and N1 nodes.

Because of a high false-negative rate (~25%), a negative result with TBNA should prompt consideration of more invasive staging methods (i.e., mediastinoscopy). A positive TBNA is more likely in the presence of significant adenopathy on CT scanning, endoscopically visible tumors, subcarinal lymph nodes greater than 2 cm in diameter, or an abnormal-appearing carina. The use of image guidance with TBNA, such as CT fluoroscopy, ENB, or EBUS, is promising and may provide higher diagnostic yields with TBNA.

Autofluorescence

The development of autofluorescence bronchoscopy (AFB) has improved the detection of dysplasia, carcinoma *in situ*, and invasive carcinoma of the central airways (Figure 12-11). AFB systems rely on the principle that infiltrating tumors disturb the fluorescence characteristics of normal tissue. Fluorophores, substances responsible for fluorescence, are variously concentrated within organs and may change according to prevailing conditions. When the bronchial tree is illuminated with blue light (442 nm in wavelength), subepithelial fluorophores within normal tissues emit light with a higher fluorescence intensity compared with preneoplastic or neoplastic lesions especially in the green region of the emission spectrum. Reasons for the weaker green fluorescence in dysplasia, carcinoma *in situ*, and microinvasive carcinoma include epithelial thickening, tumor hyperemia, and reduced fluorophore concentrations. Thus, the intensity of the emitted light is weaker, and the composition is altered in favor of the red spectrum.

Several recent studies have evaluated the utility of AFB as a screening tool for dysplasia or carcinoma of the central airways in comparison with white light bronchoscopy (WLB). These studies have included patients at high risk (e.g., asbestos exposure, smokers), with known or suspected lung cancer, and after surgical resection for lung tumors. Although the sensitivity for detecting high-grade dysplasia or carcinoma *in situ* was increased twofold to sixfold on average, the question of whether screening bronchoscopy improves cancer survival remains unanswered. Furthermore, there is no accepted algorithm for the management of the lesions identified by AFB. Finally, significant interobserver variability among AFB endoscopists and histopathologists also exists.

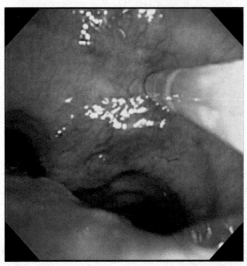

FIGURE 12-10 Transbronchial needle aspiration (TBNA) of a precarinal lymph node.

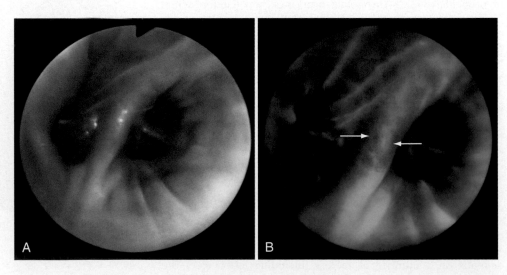

FIGURE 12-11 White light and autofluorescence images of severe dysplasia. Standard white light bronchoscopy demonstrates normal appearing mucosa. Fluorescence endoscopy demonstrates abnormal appearing tissue (*reddish brown area*), which was confirmed as severe dysplasia by histologic evaluation. (Courtesy of Xillix Technologies Corporation.)

DIFFUSE LUNG DISEASES

A wide range of acute and chronic pulmonary disorders is capable of causing diffuse interstitial lung diseases, with more than 150 distinct clinical entities. These processes include infection, neoplasm, pulmonary edema, alveolar hemorrhage, alveolar proteinosis, occupational lung diseases, drug-induced disease, and various types of interstitial lung diseases. In general, patients with diffuse lung disease have undergone a high-resolution CT, which helps to narrow the differential diagnosis and in some cases is virtually diagnostic of certain disorders. In many cases, it is still necessary to obtain samples for cytologic and histologic evaluation to confirm a specific diagnosis and to help exclude other possible disorders.

The most common bronchoscopic procedures used to help establish the diagnosis in diffuse lung disease are BAL and bronchoscopic lung biopsy. The findings of HRCT can be used to determine the best location for BAL or lung biopsy. In truly diffuse disease, the right middle lobe or lingula are the best locations for BAL; these sites are easily accessed and have good fluid retrieval. BAL should be performed with a total of 100–200 mL of saline instilled in multiple aliquots, with a return of 5–10% of the fluid. It is important to obtain a reasonable sampling of the alveolar spaces for the necessary cellular analysis.

Certain findings on BAL can be suggestive or virtually diagnostic of a number of interstitial lung diseases (Table 12-2). It is important that the BAL findings are correlated with the clinical and HRCT findings. For example, specific characteristics of the freshly retrieved lavage fluid can support the diagnosis of alveolar hemorrhage, pulmonary alveolar proteinosis, microlithiasis, or lipid aspiration. In patients with suspected eosinophilic pneumonia, a high eosinophil count is diagnostic, and in cases of pulmonary Langerhans' cell histiocytosis, BAL flow cytometry should be performed to evaluate for CD1a cells.

In a number of disorders, BAL findings may be suggestive, but additional diagnostic procedures will likely be required. These include diseases such as sarcoidosis, hypersensitivity pneumonitis, and organizing pneumonia. Bronchoscopic lung biopsy should be considered in situations in which the

diagnosis has not been established by HRCT and BAL. In many situations, bronchoscopic lung biopsy can establish the diagnosis and avoid the need for surgical lung biopsy (Box 12-4). For example, in pulmonary sarcoidosis, the diagnosis is usually established by a combination of BAL and biopsy findings. The BAL can be used to exclude the presence of tuberculosis and fungal infections and can demonstrate the characteristic high CD4/CD8 ratio seen in sarcoidosis, whereas bronchoscopic biopsy specimens should demonstrate the classic finding of noncaseating granulomas. In general, bronchoscopic biopsy should be performed from several affected areas, and at least five to six specimens should be taken. The sensitivity for sarcoidosis is only approximately 60–70%, and many patients require further invasive testing, such as surgical lung biopsy. Recently, the use of TBNA has been extended to the diagnosis of sarcoidosis, especially in patients with mediastinal adenopathy. The addition of TBNA to transbronchial biopsy can provide the diagnosis in more than 85% of sarcoidosis cases.

Bronchoscopy has a limited role in the diagnosis of idiopathic interstitial fibrosis (IPF). There is a nonspecific increase in BAL levels of neutrophils, eosinophils, and, less commonly, lymphocytes. Bronchoscopic biopsy is limited by the small size of the specimen obtained and the lack of histologic preservation because of mechanical crushing of the tissue. In the cases in which the diagnosis of IPF is probable or definite on the basis of clinical and HRCT criteria, bronchoscopy (and surgical lung biopsy) is not required. In situations in which the HRCT findings are "nondiagnostic," a bronchoscopy should be considered to evaluate for the presence of other potential etiologies. If the specific diagnosis cannot be established on the basis of BAL and bronchoscopic biopsy findings, a surgical lung biopsy should be considered.

SPECIAL BRONCHOSCOPIC TECHNIQUES

Ultrathin Bronchoscopy

Bronchoscopes with small external diameters (<3 mm), otherwise known as ultrathin bronchoscopes, were developed to deal with specific clinical situations, such as performing bronchoscopy in pediatric patients, investigating peripheral lung lesions, and evaluating tracheobronchial stenoses. The external diameter of traditional bronchoscopes is generally 5–6 mm and, therefore, cannot easily examine beyond fourth to fifth

---

BOX 12-4 Pulmonary Disease in which Bronchoscopic Lung Biopsy Provides High Diagnostic Yield

Sarcoidosis
Hypersensitivity pneumonitis
Pulmonary Langerhans' cell histiocytosis
Pulmonary alveolar proteinosis
Lymphangitic metastasis
Diffuse pulmonary lymphoma
Diffuse alveolar cell carcinoma
Pneumocystis jiroveci infection
Mycobacterial infection
Mycoses
Cytomegalovirus infection
Pneumoconioses
Lung transplant rejection

TABLE 12-2 Bronchoalveolar Lavage in Diffuse Interstitial Disease

Disorder	BAL Observation
Pulmonary hemorrhage	Progressive increase in RBCs with sequential aliquots; hemosiderin-laden macrophages
Pulmonary alveolar proteinosis (PAP)	Grossly cloudy, milky appearance; positive PAS stain
Eosinophilic pneumonia	Eosinophilia >25%
Sarcoidosis	CD4/CD8 ratio > 3.5
Pulmonary Langerhans' cell histiocytosis	CD1a positive cells > 5%
Hypersensitivity pneumonitis	Lymphocytosis; decreased CD4/CD8 ratio
Lipid pneumonia	Oily material that layers above aqueous phase
RBILD/DIP	Brown macrophages

order bronchi in adults. The use of ultrathin bronchoscopes with small working channels allowing for BAL and the use of a cytology brush have demonstrated promise in the diagnosis of peripheral lung lesions. The newest generation of ultrathin scopes has larger channels that can accommodate forceps and larger cytology brushes.

Virtual Bronchoscopy

Virtual bronchoscopy (VBS) is a novel radiographic reconstruction technique that exploits the versatility of helical CT by transforming axial CT data into simulated three-dimensional intraluminal views of the airways. This form of perspective rendering has benefited enormously from continued advances in computing technology and is currently capable of providing images which in many ways mimic those obtained during conventional bronchoscopy (Figure 12-12). Although VBS has yet to find its place in routine clinical practice, it has nonetheless proven useful in the evaluation and management of a wide range of pulmonary diseases involving the tracheobronchial tree, including bronchogenic carcinoma, benign airway stenoses, tracheomalacia, lung transplantation, and bronchiectasis. By providing the bronchoscopist with a "virtual camera" inside the patient's tracheobronchial tree, images and perspectives unattainable by conventional bronchoscopy are readily available with VBS. These include examination of airways distal to a completely occluded bronchus, retroflexion of the bronchoscope, and *en face* views. Current limitations of VBS include its inability to adequately characterize mucosal abnormalities, identify subtle submucosal disease, or visualize small endobronchial lesions. Needless to say, VBS can never replace conventional bronchoscopy insofar as it is incapable of allowing biopsy or therapeutic intervention.

THERAPEUTIC BRONCHOSCOPY TECHNIQUES

Since the introduction of bronchoscopy, the technique has been used not only for observation but also for treatment of local airway disorders. As with any clinical intervention, the guiding rule for treatment always remains, "If I can do no good, I will at least do no harm."

RIGID BRONCHOSCOPIC DEBULKING OR BALLOON DILATATION

The ideal tool for rapid reestablishment of airway patency in endoluminal obstruction is the rigid bronchoscope. Rigid bronchoscopes have beveled tips, which are ideal for coring through large tumors in the airways and for dilating strictures, and they have large internal diameters, which facilitate débridement of tumors, evacuation of clots, and ventilation. Despite advances in other adjunctive endoscopic techniques, rigid bronchoscopic recanalization remains the treatment of choice for life-threatening tracheobronchial obstruction.

Balloon dilation has become an attractive alternative to dissection with a blunt rigid bronchoscope in less urgent cases of obstruction caused by malignant tumors. High-pressure angioplasty catheters with various balloon lengths and diameters were commonly used in the past. There are now balloons designed specifically for tracheobronchial use (i.e., controlled radial expansion [CRE] balloon, Boston Scientific Corp., Cambridge, MA) that are expandable to specific diameters by application of defined atmospheric pressure. These are inserted through the working channel of the bronchoscope under fluoroscopic and/or direct visual guidance. The balloon, filled with saline or radiopaque contrast media, is inflated at the site of the stenosis until a smooth, uniform lumen of predictable diameter is attained. This technique is often used in combination with bronchoscopic laser therapy and placement of a tracheobronchial stent for the treatment of airway stenosis (Figure 12-13).

Balloon bronchoplasty has also been used successfully to treat other disorders, including endobronchial tuberculosis, fibrosing mediastinitis, and strictures associated with lung transplantation or prolonged intubation. It is less successful when used alone to treat stenosis accompanied by extrinsic airway compression and is not beneficial and, indeed, contraindicated in patients with tracheobronchomalacia.

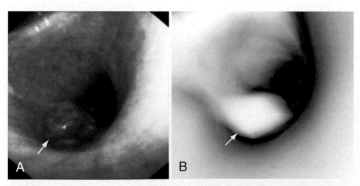

FIGURE 12-12 Endoluminal lesion obstructing the superior segment of the left lower lobe in a patient with metastatic melanoma. The visualization of this lesion (*white arrow*) by FB (*top left*, **A**) and virtual bronchoscopy (*top middle*, **B**). (From Finkelstein SE, Schrump DS, Nguyen DM: Comparative evaluation of super high-resolution CT scan and virtual bronchoscopy for the detection of tracheobronchial malignancies. Chest 2003; 124;1834–1840.)

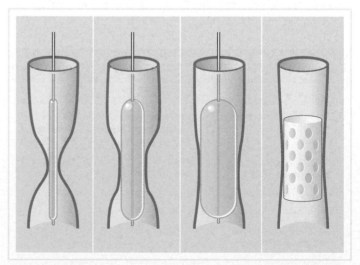

FIGURE 12-13 Bronchoscopic balloon dilatation of tracheal stenosis, diagrammatic depiction. This can be accomplished with a flexible or rigid bronchoscope by use of graduated dilating balloons. After optimal dilation, a silicone stent (placed with a rigid bronchoscope) relieves airway obstruction.

Although in most cases, balloon dilation is performed while the patient is under general anesthesia, treatment of many airway lesions (e.g., short fibrotic strictures) can be accomplished with the use of a flexible bronchoscope while the patient is under conscious sedation. Complications of balloon dilation of airway lesions include bronchospasm, chest pain, mucosal laceration, airway perforation, bleeding, postprocedure airway edema, pneumothorax, and pneumomediastinum.

ENDOBRONCHIAL LASER THERAPY

Perhaps the most widely known technique in interventional pulmonology is laser bronchoscopy. Lasers produce a beam of monochromatic, coherent light that can induce tissue vaporization, coagulation, hemostasis, and necrosis. Although primarily useful in the ablation of endoluminal malignant tumors, bronchoscopic laser therapy is also beneficial for the treatment of other tracheobronchial disorders, including inflammatory strictures, obstructive granulation tissue, amyloidosis, and benign tumors such as hamartomas and lipomas.

Since the initial report of endobronchial laser ablation of an obstructive neoplasm by Laforet in 1976, several types of lasers have become available for the management of tracheobronchial obstruction. The carbon dioxide (CO_2) laser, used mainly by otolaryngologists, allows shallow penetration of tissue (to a depth of 0.1–0.5 mm) and highly precise cutting, but it has minimal hemostatic properties and traditionally was used through a rigid bronchoscope. Recently developed technology has facilitated the delivery of CO_2 laser energy by means of unique reflective fiberoptic probes (OmniGuide, Inc., Cambridge, MA), allowing applications with flexible laryngoscopy and bronchoscopy. The CO_2 laser, with its fine control of tissue ablation, is ideal for the management of laryngeal lesions (webs, vocal cord nodules, etc.). Interventional pulmonologists primarily use the neodymium:yttrium-aluminum-garnet (Nd:YAG) laser, which provides deeper penetration of tissue (to a depth of 3–5 mm), superior photocoagulation, and improved hemostasis, but with less precision in cutting. Photocoagulation with an Nd:YAG laser can be performed through a rigid or flexible bronchoscope, but rigid bronchoscopy remains the preferred method for the treatment of patients who have respiratory distress caused by severe tracheobronchial obstruction or active intraluminal bleeding.

The use of a laser in the tracheobronchial tree requires careful consideration of the anatomic location and configuration of the lesion. If the lesion is in close proximity to the esophagus or the pulmonary artery, endobronchial laser therapy poses a risk of fistula formation. Use of laser therapy in a patient with tracheobronchial narrowing caused by extrinsic compression may result in perforation of the airway. In addition, prolonged obstruction of the airway (for more than 6 weeks) may lead to refractory atelectasis, cavitary pneumonia, or bronchiectasis, minimizing the benefits of endobronchial recanalization. The potential for airway recanalization in the setting of long-standing endoluminal obstruction can be assessed by bronchography or by perfusion scanning.

Although endobronchial laser therapy is generally safe and well tolerated, it may be complicated by cardiac arrhythmias, perforation of the airway, pneumothorax, hemorrhage, hypoxemia, or endobronchial fire (ignition of the bronchoscope or endotracheal tube). In rare cases, pulmonary edema or fatal pulmonary venous gas embolism has been reported. Patients with standard silicone endotracheal tubes or silicone tracheobronchial stents and those who require high concentrations of supplemental oxygen are at increased risk for endobronchial fire. Fortunately, the overall risk is less than 0.1%. The overall rate of mortality attributable to endoscopic laser therapy is quite low, not exceeding 0.3–0.5% in several large series.

Success rates and complications directly related to laser therapy are not different when the procedure is performed with the patient under general anesthesia through the rigid bronchoscope or under topical anesthesia and conscious sedation through a flexible bronchoscope. Nd:YAG laser photoablation therapy has demonstrated a single-modality recanalization rate of >90% for endobronchial obstruction of large central airways but is less successful with peripheral lesions or with associated extrinsic airway compression. Laser therapy may improve the chances of successful weaning from mechanical ventilation in patients with advanced endoluminal lung cancer presenting in respiratory failure. In addition, photocoagulation with an Nd:YAG laser is an invaluable treatment for patients with airway obstruction caused by benign endoluminal tumors.

ENDOBRONCHIAL CRYOTHERAPY AND ELECTROCAUTERY

Cryotherapy and electrocautery are excellent, cost-effective alternatives to laser therapy for the management of tracheobronchial obstruction. The depth of penetration and resulting injury are, however, much more difficult to control. As with the Nd:YAG laser, both electrocautery and cryotherapy can be administered through a rigid or flexible bronchoscope. The effects of electrocautery on tissue are similar to those of the Nd:YAG laser, with tissue destruction induced by intense coagulation and vaporization. Argon plasma coagulation (APC) is similar to electrocautery except that it uses argon gas to conduct the electrical current rather than a contact probe. APC has a depth of penetration of only a few millimeters and is, therefore, more suitable for the treatment of superficial and spreading lesions. Cryotherapy probes induce tissue necrosis through hypothermic cellular crystallization and microthrombosis. Specially designed probes are inserted through the bronchoscope until they contact the target tissue. Through the channel in the probe, liquid nitrous oxide or liquid nitrogen is introduced, resulting in the rapid creation of an "ice ball" (approximate temperature of $-20°C$) at the end of the tip. This freezing effect is maintained for approximately 20 sec; the area is then rewarmed, resulting in thawing. Treatment of an endobronchial lesion with a cryoprobe requires several freeze–thaw cycles.

Cryotherapy and electrocautery have been used successfully to relieve airway obstruction caused by benign tracheobronchial tumors, polyps, and granulation tissue. These techniques—cryotherapy in particular—may be superior to lasers for distal lesions because of the lower risk of airway perforation. Similarly, carcinoma *in situ* and mucosal dysplasia may be adequately treated with cryotherapy or electrocautery alone, although multiple treatments may be required for optimal results. Cryotherapy is a safe treatment for infiltrative lesions of the airway, and according to anecdotal reports, it has proved beneficial in patients with posttransplantation anastomotic stenosis and in those with foreign-body aspiration. Interestingly, cryotherapy may be the premier bronchoscopic modality for the removal of endobronchial blood clots and mucus plugs.

Endobronchial cryotherapy is generally not effective for paucicellular lesions that are relatively impervious to freezing, such as fibrotic stenoses, cartilaginous or bony lesions, and lipomas. Furthermore, endobronchial cryotherapy, unlike either laser therapy or electrocautery, is inefficient in achieving rapid relief of symptomatic airway obstruction. The most common serious complication of both electrocautery and cryotherapy is hemorrhage because of disruption of endobronchial tumor without full coagulation of distal tissue and tumor vessels. The estimated incidence of clinically significant bleeding in patients treated with electrocautery is 2.5%.

ENDOBRONCHIAL BRACHYTHERAPY

Brachytherapy is the local treatment of tumors with radiation delivered internally through implanted radioactive seeds or in an adjacent fashion with inserted wires. This technique ensures the delivery of a maximal therapeutic dose of radiation to the tumor with a minimal effect on normal surrounding tissues. Endobronchial brachytherapy involves the bronchoscopic insertion of a thin, hollow "afterloading" catheter through or parallel to a malignant obstruction under fluoroscopic guidance (Figure 12-14). A radioactive implant is then inserted into the catheter and left in position for a predetermined period (2–40 h, depending on the dose rate).

In 1922, Yankauer reported the use of rigid bronchoscopic brachytherapy for the palliation of airway obstruction caused by malignant tumors. Modern techniques, including the use of flexible bronchoscopes, polyethylene afterloading catheters, and iridium-192 implants, were first described in 1983. Since the development of techniques involving high dose-rate delivery in the 1980s, endobronchial brachytherapy has become a particularly attractive option for outpatient treatment of peribronchial tumors.

Relief of airway obstruction is the primary goal of endobronchial brachytherapy, although curative treatment may be attempted in conjunction with external-beam radiation in selected patients. Brachytherapy is safest and most effective for central airway lesions, although in one study, small peripheral tumors proved to be more responsive than bulkier central tumors. Among patients with obstruction caused by malignant tumors, rates of recanalization range from 60–90%, with decreased dyspnea, cessation of hemoptysis, and relief of cough

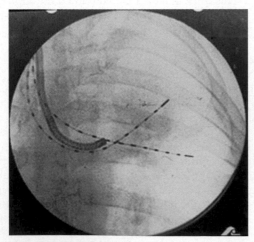

FIGURE 12-14 Placement of two brachytherapy catheters under fluoroscopic guidance.

in most cases. Brachytherapy has also been used for the prevention and treatment of airway stenosis related to recurrent growth of granulation tissue in patients with lung transplants.

Endobronchial brachytherapy may require multiple treatments to be effective. It is generally used as an adjunct to either Nd:YAG photocoagulation or conventional external-beam irradiation in an effort to achieve both rapid and sustained recanalization in patients with obstruction because of malignant tumors. Brachytherapy may also be administered in conjunction with the placement of an endobronchial stent in patients with extrinsic compression of the airways because of malignant tumors. Brachytherapy works best with submucosal and peribronchial malignant disease.

Serious complications of brachytherapy include massive hemoptysis and fistula formation, secondary to necrosis of the airway wall and adjacent vascular structures. Because of the risk of fatal hemorrhage, every effort should be made to rule out the involvement of central vessels before treatment is administered. The incidence of serious complications varies widely, with rates as low as 0–10% in some of the largest studies and as high as 30–40% in smaller studies.

PHOTODYNAMIC THERAPY

Photodynamic therapy (PDT) is currently approved by the U.S. Food and Drug Administration for the palliation of airway obstruction caused by malignant tumors and as an alternative to surgery in selected patients with minimally invasive central lung cancer. PDT works on the principle that certain compounds, such as hematoporphyrin derivatives (Photofrin®) or amino-levulinic acid (ALA), function as photosensitizing agents, rendering malignant cells susceptible to damage from monochromatic light. Tumor necrosis occurs as a result of cellular destruction through the generation of oxygen-free radicals or by ischemic necrosis mediated by vascular occlusion resulting from thromboxane A_2 release. The selective effect of PDT on malignant cells is thought to be due to the greater uptake and retention of photosensitizing agents in neoplastic cells compared with normal cells—with the exception of cells of the reticuloendothelial system, particularly those in the skin. This relative tumor selectivity effect seems to be most pronounced approximately 24–48 h after infusion of the photosensitizing agent. For this reason, bronchoscopic treatment of target lesions is often performed 1–2 days after the agent has been injected. Given the delayed onset of action of PDT, it is not useful in patients with acute respiratory distress from tracheobronchial obstruction. Follow-up "toilet" bronchoscopies are often required to débride necrotic tissue.

Ideal candidates for PDT include patients with airway obstruction caused by malignant polypoid endobronchial masses, with minimal extrinsic airway compression, and patients with minimally invasive tumors of the central airways. Although surgical resection remains the treatment of choice for early lung cancer, some patients refuse surgery or are deemed inoperable because of high surgical risk. PDT may represent an appropriate alternative. Response rates are highest in patients with small tumors and minimal depth of penetration. In patients with bulky tumors, endobronchial PDT may substantially reduce the obstruction, with objective increases in spirometric measurements and subjective improvements in dyspnea and the quality of life. Metastatic tumors have also been treated successfully with PDT. Complications include increased skin photosensitivity and hemoptysis resulting from extensive tumor necrosis. Cutaneous photosensitivity, similar to that seen with sunburn, occurs in 0–20% of patients according to published series and can be obviated by adequate sunlight precautions. Sensitivity to sunlight after Photofrin administration can persist for 6 weeks or longer.

TRACHEOBRONCHIAL STENTING

The medical term "stent" refers to any device designed to maintain the integrity of hollow tubular structures, such as the coronary arteries and the esophagus. Anecdotal reports of attempts to implant stents in the tracheobronchial tree date back to 1915. The Montgomery T tube, designed in the 1960s, was the first reliable, dedicated airway stent. However, stent implantation in the lower trachea and bronchi did not become standard medical practice until Dumon's 1990 report on the safety and ease of placement of a dedicated airway stent made of silicone.

There are two main types of endobronchial stents in use today: tube stents made of silicone or plastic, and self-expandable metallic stents (SEMS). Silicone stents are placed by means of rigid bronchoscopy with the patient under general inhalational, or more commonly total intravenous, anesthesia. Silicone stents are relatively inexpensive (~$200–$300 USD) compared with SEMS (~$1800 USD) and are easier to remove from the airway; they provide protection from tumor ingrowth and cause minimal irritation to adjacent normal tissues. In one large single center series, the complications of silicone stents included a 5% migration rate, a 10% incidence of granulation tissue formation, and a 27% incidence of partial stent occlusion by inspissated secretions. Bifurcated silicone and composite stents are also available for the palliation of distal tracheal and main carinal lesions. These stents have been effectively used in the management of carinal compression associated with malignant tumors, tracheoesophageal fistulas, and tracheobronchomalacia. Custom silicone stents can be designed by the treating bronchoscopist to deal with unique anatomic problems such as stump-related bronchopleural fistula after pneumonectomy. Unlike silicone stents, SEMS can be placed with the use of a flexible bronchoscope, and they are less likely to migrate and are more likely to preserve normal mucociliary clearance. However, if metal stents are misplaced in the airway, rigid bronchoscopy is often required for their removal. In addition, mucosal inflammation and the formation of granulation tissue are common at the proximal and distal ends of metal stents, and endoscopic intervention may be required to restore airway patency. For all these reasons, SEMS are not recommended for most patients with nonmalignant airway stenosis, particularly in the tracheal location, unless all other treatment options, including silicone stenting, have been obviated. One exception may be the development of postoperative dehiscence of the bronchial anastomosis in lung transplantation, in which temporary insertion of uncovered SEMS across the region of dehiscence has been used to induce focal granulation tissue formation, which can then facilitate wound healing.

Endobronchial stents have a critical role in multimodality endoscopic approaches to both benign and malignant stenoses of the airways. Stenoses caused by locally advanced bronchogenic carcinoma, for example, can be treated with a combination of endoscopic laser therapy and stent implantation to preserve the improvement in airway lumen diameter achieved by the ablative technique by preventing tumor ingrowth

(Figure 12-15). Stent placement can also be used to maintain airway patency after endobronchial brachytherapy or can be combined with laser therapy and balloon dilation in the endoscopic management of fibrotic strictures. Most large studies of the results of endobronchial stent placement have demonstrated impressive efficacy. Dumon and colleagues reported excellent clinical outcomes and few complications with the use of silicone stents in patients with extrinsic airway compression caused by malignant tumors, but a lower success rate among patients with tracheal stenosis caused by other disorders. Success rates, broadly defined as symptomatic relief, have ranged in limited studies between 78% and 98%, although none of the early trials used objective measures such as the LCSS to determine efficacy. In two small studies of patients who were intubated because of respiratory failure because of unresectable tracheobronchial and mediastinal disease, stent placement facilitated extubation in most patients.

The benefits of stent placement seem to persist in patients who survive for a period of several months or years after device implantation. Long-term follow-up data, however, are based on patients with benign disease, because the mean follow-up period in patients with airway compression because of malignant tumors does not usually exceed 3–4 months because of limited survival from the underlying disease. Some authors have reported poor long-term results with the use of metal stents in patients with fibroinflammatory stenosis caused by nonmalignant disorders. In addition, there have been case reports of massive hemorrhage associated with the use of stents in patients with extrinsic compression attributable to aneurysmal dilatation or congenital malformations of the aorta.

INDICATIONS FOR THERAPEUTIC BRONCHOSCOPY

Therapeutic bronchoscopy is most commonly performed for aspiration of retained secretions and mucous plugs and for the treatment of airway obstruction. The indications for therapeutic bronchoscopy are listed in Box 12-3, and many of these are discussed in the following.

Endoluminal Airway Obstruction

Endoluminal obstruction of the tracheobronchial tree may result from various benign and malignant processes. The most common cause of endobronchial obstruction is advanced bronchogenic carcinoma. In patients with inoperable tumors of the central airways, restoration of airway patency may provide palliation and may even prolong life, particularly in the case of impending respiratory failure.

Signs and symptoms of central airway obstruction vary but often include wheezing, cough, stridor, hoarseness, hemoptysis, and chest pain. A careful pretreatment evaluation should be performed to distinguish symptoms attributable to focal tracheobronchial lesions from those related to underlying diffuse airflow obstruction, parenchymal lung disease, or both. Mild-to-moderate tracheal stenosis, for example, may contribute only marginally to the degree of dyspnea experienced by a patient with severe chronic obstructive lung disease. Although pulmonary function testing and thoracic imaging techniques such as chest CT and magnetic resonance imaging may be useful in the evaluation of a patient with suspected obstruction of the central airway, bronchoscopy, either rigid or flexible, remains the diagnostic "gold standard." Increasingly, however,

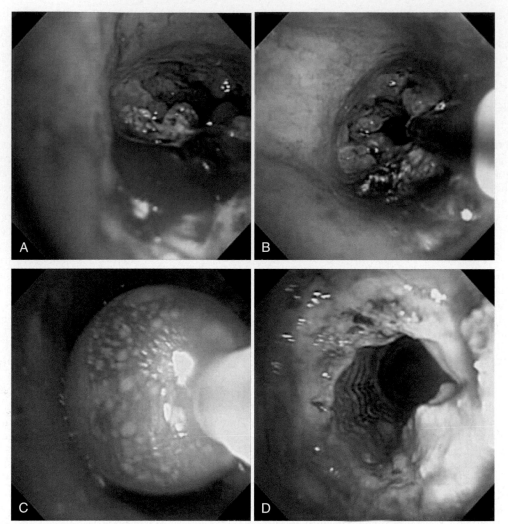

FIGURE 12-15 **(A)** Endoluminal tumor with extrinsic compression treated with a combination of **(B)** bronchoscopic laser therapy, **(C)** balloon bronchoplasty, and **(D)** stent placement.

3-dimensional reconstruction CT imaging—so-called virtual bronchoscopy—is being applied as a reliable noninvasive method of assessing the nature and extent of airway obstruction.

The bronchoscopic approach to the management of endoluminal obstruction depends on the location of the lesion, the presence or absence of associated extrinsic compression, and the degree of clinical urgency (Table 12-3). Rigid-bronchoscopic debulking, with adjunctive laser therapy or electrocautery, is recommended when airway recanalization must be performed on an emergency basis. If endobronchial obstruction is accompanied by marked extrinsic compression, the placement of a stent may be beneficial (Figure 12-16).

The complexity of a lesion is equally important in determining the best approach to resection. Tracheal webs, for example, are often managed by laser resection alone; whereas complex fibrotic strictures may warrant the combination of rigid-bronchoscopic or balloon dilation, laser resection, and stent placement. For focal tracheal stenoses in low-risk patients, surgical resection and primary reanastomosis should remain the treatment of choice.

Extrinsic Airway Compression

Extrinsic airway compression usually results from malignant involvement of structures adjacent to the central airways, such as mediastinal lymph nodes or the esophagus, but it may be associated with a benign process, such as fibrosing mediastinitis, tuberculosis, aneurysmal dilatation of the aorta, or sarcoidosis. The clinical signs and symptoms of extrinsic airway compression often mimic those of endobronchial obstruction. The diagnosis is established on the basis of bronchoscopic detection of marked airway narrowing in the absence of an endoluminal mass. Contrast-enhanced CT, and increasingly EBUS (balloon-sheathed radial probe), has an important adjunctive role in identifying anatomic structures external to the narrowed lumen.

Therapeutic options in the management of extrinsic airway compression are limited. Ablative endoscopic approaches such as laser therapy, cryotherapy, PDT, and electrocautery are contraindicated because of the lack of demonstrable benefit and risk of airway perforation. Although some patients with

TABLE 12-3 Bronchoscopic Therapies

Therapy	Type of Lesion	Type of Bronchoscope	Rapidity of Positive Result	Repeatability of Therapy
Mechanical débridement	Endoluminal or submucosal	Rigid or flexible (rigid preferable)	+ + + +	+
Laser	Endoluminal	Rigid or flexible (rigid preferable)	+ + + +	+ + + +
Argon plasma	Endoluminal	Rigid or flexible	+ + + +	+ + + +
Brachytherapy	Endoluminal or submucosal	Flexible	+	+
Cryotherapy	Endoluminal	Rigid or flexible	+ +	+ + +
Balloon dilation	Endoluminal or submucosal with extraluminal compression	Rigid or flexible (rigid preferable)	+ + + +	+ + + +
Photodynamic therapy	Endoluminal	Flexible	+ +	+ + +
Electrocautery	Endoluminal	Rigid or flexible	+ + +	+ + + +
Stent	Endoluminal with extraluminal compression	Rigid or flexible (Dumon stent requires rigid bronchoscope; Wall stents and Gianturco stents require fluoroscopy)	+ + + +	+ + +

+ + + +, Most rapid or repeatable.

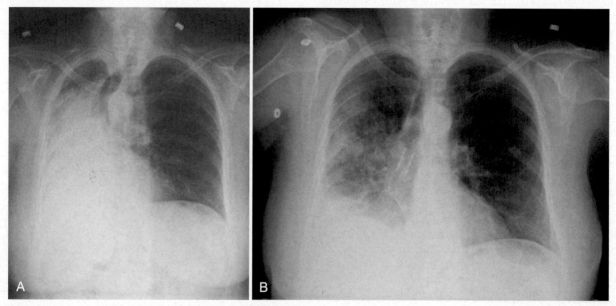

FIGURE 12-16 A, Chest radiograph of an obstructing small-cell carcinoma in right main stem causing right lung atelectasis and mediastinal shift. **B,** Imaging after rigid bronchoscopic debulking of the lesion and placement of a Dumon silicone stent. (Courtesy of Colin Gillespie, MD.)

malignant disease may benefit from endobronchial brachytherapy, tracheobronchial stent placement is the palliative treatment of choice for patients with symptomatic extrinsic airway compression.

Tracheobronchomalacia

Diffuse or focal tracheobronchomalacia is perhaps the most challenging disorder encountered by the interventional pulmonologist. Cartilaginous tracheobronchomalacia, as seen in patients with postintubation injury or relapsing polychondritis, reflects a loss of the structural integrity of the trachea or mainstem bronchi because of destruction of the airway's cartilaginous rings. Membranous, or crescentic, tracheobronchomalacia (also known as EDAC—excessive

dynamic airway collapse) is manifested by airway collapse during exhalation as a result of laxity of the membranous portion of the trachea and main bronchi and is usually seen in patients with long-standing chronic obstructive pulmonary disease. Focal tracheobronchomalacia may be a complication of long-standing intubation or an anastomotic complication after lung transplantation. Tracheobronchomalacia is best diagnosed on the basis of flexible bronchoscopy, with the patient breathing spontaneously (Figure 12-17), although dynamic CT scanning, with images obtained on inspiration and expiration, is often helpful.

The endoscopic treatment of choice for patients with diffuse tracheobronchomalacia is the insertion of a standard or bifurcated silicone tracheobronchial stent. This intervention is more likely to be successful in patients with the cartilaginous

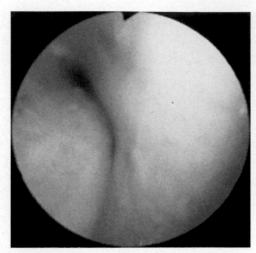

FIGURE 12-17 Tracheal buckling. Bronchoscopic examination revealed localized upper tracheal buckling on hyperflexion of the neck. Symptoms cleared after three tracheal rings were resected. Pathologic analysis showed localized tracheomalacia.

type of tracheobronchomalacia than in those with the membranous type. Patients with membranous tracheobronchomalacia may benefit from a trial of stenting with a silicone endoprosthesis. For those who benefit in terms of decreased respiratory symptoms and improved pulmonary function, surgical plication and/or buttressing of the posterior membrane can be performed often with good results and with facilitation of stent removal. For many patients with focal tracheomalacia, particularly from postintubation injury, surgical resection and primary reanastomosis is the best therapeutic option. An alternative treatment for selected patients with diffuse tracheobronchomalacia is the "pneumatic stent" provided by noninvasive ventilatory techniques such as continuous positive airway pressure.

There are also unpublished reports of the use of Nd:YAP (yttrium-aluminim-perovskite) laser, which has more thermal than ablative properties, for photocoagulation of the posterior membrane of the distal trachea and the membranous portion of the proximal mainstem bronchi to induce scarring and retraction of the submucosal tissues with resultant decrease in EDAC. This intervention carries the potential risk of airway perforation and fistulization.

CONTROL OF HEMOPTYSIS

In cases of hemoptysis, bronchoscopy may be of value not only for diagnosis, but frequently for emergency management of endobronchial bleeding as well (Box 12-5). Because of difficulties with visualization, instruments with large and maximally effective suction channels should be used. Rigid bronchoscopy is generally preferred with massive bleeding, when the need to remove large clots is anticipated.

When continuous suctioning of blood fails to clear the airways, other means can be used. An iced saline solution can be instilled along with vasoactive drugs, such as epinephrine, to induce spasm of the bleeding vessels. The bronchoscope itself can also be used to stem the bleeding by tamponade of the bleeding site or to occlude the lumen of the bronchus from which the bleeding originates. The same effect, perhaps with better local control, can be achieved with bronchoscopic balloon catheters (Figure 12-18). Specially designed catheters

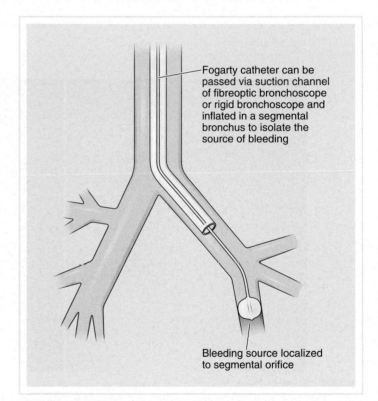

Fogarty catheter can be passed via suction channel of fibreoptic bronchoscope or rigid bronchoscope and inflated in a segmental bronchus to isolate the source of bleeding

Bleeding source localized to segmental orifice

FIGURE 12-18 Placement of a Fogarty balloon catheter under bronchoscopic guidance to control massive hemorrhage from a segmental or lobar bronchus. (From Lordan JL, Gascoigne A, Corris PA: The pulmonary physician in critical care: illustrative case 7: assessment and management of massive hemoptysis. Thorax 2003; 58:814–819.)

have been developed for introduction through the working channel of the flexible bronchoscope, several permitting subsequent removal of the scope while the tamponading balloon remains in place, as well as the potential for suctioning beyond the balloon for clearance of blood from distal airways. Another effective method for control of visible sources of bleeding, particularly from endobronchial neoplasms, is Nd:YAG laser photocoagulation.

Recent reports have demonstrated the benefit of endobronchial packing, by both flexible and rigid bronchoscopy, with oxidized regenerated cellulose (Surgicel), which performs multiple roles, including local tamponade and isolation at the segmental/subsegmental bleeding site, absorption of blood, and promotion of endobronchial clot formation by induction of fibrin polymerization. This procedure may obviate the need for bronchial artery embolization or other more invasive procedures.

REMOVAL OF FOREIGN BODIES

Foreign body (FB) aspiration is more likely to occur in children than in adults, with most occurring in children younger than 3 years. In children the obstruction most often involves a mainstem bronchus, whereas in adults most foreign bodies are wedged distally, most commonly in the right lower lobe. Before the development of bronchoscopy, most FB aspirations resulted in high morbidity and mortality, commonly from postobstructive pneumonia. Until the introduction of the flexible bronchoscope, all FB removals were accomplished with the rigid bronchoscope. Even at present, the rigid bronchoscope remains the tool of choice for the removal of foreign bodies, especially in children. The advantage of the rigid instrument resides in its larger access channel, permitting use of larger and more adaptable retrieval tools and its ability to simultaneously provide and maintain ventilation. In adults, flexible bronchoscopy is the most common initial diagnostic tool for FB aspiration and allows for successful removal of the FB in most cases.

Various types of instruments have been developed for use with bronchoscopy for the removal of FB, including grasping forceps, balloon catheters, retrieval baskets, snares, and magnetic extractors. The choice of instrument depends on the specifics of the type of FB and its location in the tracheobronchial tree. Grasping forceps may be helpful in the retrieval of hard objects with an irregular surface. Smooth objects or organic material (e.g., nuts, food particles) may require the use of expandable baskets or a combination of balloon catheters, suction devices, and grasping forceps. Fogarty balloon catheters are used frequently to dislodge the FB and bring it proximally into the trachea before removal with other instruments.

Special attention should be paid to the period after removal of the foreign body, because serious complications can occur. Patients should be observed closely for any signs of hemoptysis, subcutaneous emphysema, or subglottic edema. Trauma inflicted during the extraction or forceful manipulation of instruments greatly accentuates the risk of postoperative complications, particularly if oversized instruments are used or if the bronchoscopy is prolonged.

ASPIRATION OF SECRETIONS

According to a survey of bronchoscopists in the United States, removal of retained secretions is cited as a leading indication for therapeutic bronchoscopy. Bronchoscopic aspiration of secretions may be indicated in patients presenting with weakness of respiratory muscles (e.g., because of underlying neuromuscular disease or the postoperative state) or disorders leading to recurrent aspiration of food or excessive upper-airway secretions. In critically ill or mechanically ventilated patients, removal of secretions and mucous plugs usually can be rapidly achieved with the flexible bronchoscope. A flexible scope with a large-diameter suction channel should be chosen for this procedure. The nature of the retained material—its consistency

and viscosity—may dictate frequent bronchoscopies to relieve segmental or lobar atelectasis because of inspissated mucous plugs. Underlying pulmonary diseases, such as bronchiectasis, may aggravate the retention of airway secretions. Bronchoscopic aspiration of secretions should not be considered "routine" in the postoperative period or in other conditions in which good chest physiotherapy and maintenance of adequate pulmonary toilet could be more effective.

Two specific disorders are worth highlighting in the context of therapeutic bronchoscopy: pulmonary alveolar proteinosis (PAP) and allergic bronchopulmonary aspergillosis (ABPA). In PAP, BAL has been used for therapeutic clearance of alveolar material, although the standard approach is whole-lung lavage that uses double-lumen endotracheal tube intubation. In ABPA, lavage with saline solution may be insufficient to remove tenacious impactions (described as "plastic bronchitis"). In these circumstances, use of bronchoscopic forceps or snare may prove helpful.

CLOSURE OF BRONCHIAL FISTULAE

Flexible and/or rigid bronchoscopy can be a useful intervention in confirming the diagnosis of suspected bronchopleural fistula (BPF) and specifying its precise location. Depending on the location and the size of the fistula, bronchoscopic procedures can be attempted with the goal of occlusion and sealing of the BPF. Simple tamponade by use of the body of the flexible bronchoscope or a balloon catheter provides only temporary relief. Many different techniques for more permanent closure have been used, including introduction of bronchial mucosal irritants (e.g., silver nitrate, with the object of stimulating reactive granulation tissue formation). Several potentially useful agents have been described, including Gelfoam, autologous blood patch, cryoprecipitate, and thrombin injection to create fibrin clot. In addition, laser photocoagulation surrounding small, proximal BPF has been reported to be beneficial as has the placement of one-way endobronchial valves for more peripheral BPF. Small bronchial openings in an otherwise normal bronchus after thoracic surgery respond much better, with a higher rate of success of bronchoscopic sealing. It is much more difficult to achieve good obliteration of a fistula if it is infected or is due to an underlying malignancy.

BRONCHOSCOPIC TREATMENTS FOR COMMON "BENIGN" LUNG DISEASES

One of the major advances in therapeutic bronchoscopic use over the past decade has been the development of experimental bronchoscopic interventions for highly prevalent lung diseases such as asthma and emphysema.

Bronchoscopic Treatments for Emphysema

Bronchoscopic treatments for emphysema have been in development by industry and academia for the past 10 years. The risks of lung volume reduction surgery (LVRS) ("reduction pneumoplasty") in which diseased portions of emphysematous lung are resected through median sternotomy or videothoracoscopy, including a perioperative mortality of 5% or greater, as well as substantial perioperative morbidity, have spurred the development of minimally invasive approaches for palliation of dyspnea in patients with emphysema. These novel bronchoscopic approaches currently in clinical study include airway occlusion with silicone plugs (i.e., Endobronchial Watanabe Spigot [EWS]); insertion of one-way bronchial valves (Emphasys, Spiration); creation of artificial noncompressible communications ("bypass tracts") between cartilaginous airways and emphysematous parenchyma (Airway Bypass, Broncus, Inc.); and biologic restructuring of emphysematous lung parenchyma to induce tissue fibrosis, atelectasis, contraction, and thereby lung volume reduction. The latter approach was inspired by numerous case reports of "medical" lung volume reduction, in which patients with heterogeneous emphysema achieved significant clinical and physiologic improvements in lung function after receiving external beam radiation therapy for an upper lobe non-small cell carcinoma or after developing infection/inflammation in an upper-lobe bulla resulting in fibrosis and contraction of the bullous lung tissue after resolution of the infectous/inflammatory process.

The major advantage of the bronchial valve approach for palliation of emphysema is the potential for reversibility—the valves are generally removable with minimal risk to the patient within several months of the insertion. Even the Airway Bypass™ procedure is potentially reversible with removal of the transbronchial stents or with allowance/induction of occlusion by granulation tissue. One of the major downsides of the biologic approach to lung volume reduction is the permanent destruction of lung tissue, with no option for reversibility in the event of worsening lung function. The bane of bronchial valves in the treatment of emphysema is collateral ventilation, which inhibits induction of atelectasis and thereby prevents successful lung volume reduction. Nonetheless, the results of a randomized, double-blinded sham-controlled multicenter international trial of the Emphasys EBV for treatment of patients with severe upper-lobe predominant emphysema demonstrated that the study met both its primary efficacy endpoints showing statistically significant improvements in lung function and exercise tolerance, both at 6 months. The study also met its primary safety endpoint, a composite of major complications at 6 months.

Novel Bronchoscopic Treatment for Moderate-to-Severe Asthma

Chronic asthma is a major cause of morbidity and mortality in, and also a major contributor to, rapidly rising health care costs. Bronchial thermoplasty is a new bronchoscopic procedure that delivers controlled thermal energy to the bronchial wall of conducting airways, with the intent to inhibit airway smooth muscle contractile function. This offers the potential to attenuate bronchoconstriction occurring during asthma exacerbations. Bronchial thermoplasty is performed by use of the Alair® System (Asthmatx, Inc.) consisting of a single-use radiofrequency device that delivers thermal energy to the bronchial wall during an outpatient bronchoscopic procedure. All accessible upper and lower lobe airways, ranging from 3–10 mm in diameter, are treated during the procedure. Pilot studies in patients with mild-to-moderate asthma demonstrated that bronchial thermoplasty was generally well tolerated with some decrease in airway hyperresponsiveness after treatment and no evidence of long-term airways obstruction at 1–2 year follow-up. Side effects were common but were transient and self-limited; the most frequent were cough and wheeze (transient asthma exacerbation). The results of the randomized, multicenter AIR (Airway Intervention with Radiofrequency) trial were recently published, demonstrating

decreased moderate and severe asthma exacerbations in the group undergoing bronchial thermoplasty compared with those patients treated with standard medical treatment alone. The results of a randomized, sham-controlled multicenter U.S. trial are pending, as accrual has completed.

SAFETY FACTORS IN BRONCHOSCOPY

Bronchoscopy is a specialized procedure that requires extensive training. Familiarity with both the physiology and anatomy of the airways and other intrathoracic structures is essential. As with any other procedure, analysis of the risk/benefit ratio helps reduce the complication rate. Mild sedation, muscular relaxation, and anterograde amnesia increase patient cooperation and permit quicker and less traumatic procedures. During and shortly after the procedure, appropriate monitoring of hemodynamic parameters (heart rate, rhythm, and blood pressure), oxygenation, and ventilation contributes to the safety of bronchoscopy. Last, but not least, proper knowledge and application of safety standards and maintenance procedures decrease the cost of bronchoscopy.

In general, bronchoscopy is a safe and well-tolerated procedure. There are few absolute contraindications to bronchoscopy. Bronchoscopy should not be performed in patients with severe refractory hypoxemia, unstable cardiac disease, or life-threatening arrhythmias. Bronchoscopic lung biopsy should be performed with caution in patients with moderate-to-severe pulmonary hypertension.

COMPLICATIONS OF BRONCHOSCOPY

Complications are generally due to inappropriate preparation of patients before bronchoscopy, effects of local or general anesthesia, and manipulation of various instruments. Appropriate training and experience of the bronchoscopist and supporting team are crucial in reducing the rate of complications.

Anesthesia and Related Blood Gas Abnormalities

Approximately half of the life-threatening complications of diagnostic bronchoscopy are associated with premedication and use of topical anesthesia. The major complications include respiratory depression, hypoventilation, hypotension, and syncope. Risk is significantly increased in the elderly and in those with serious concomitant illnesses, including cardiovascular disease, chronic pulmonary disease, renal and hepatic dysfunction, seizures, and altered mental status. If there is underlying organ dysfunction, doses of sedative agents and topical anesthetics should be adjusted. Conscious sedation techniques by use of short-acting benzodiazepines (e.g., midazolam), which offer significant anterograde amnesia but less muscle relaxation, have reduced the incidence of potentially dangerous hypotension and respiratory depression.

Inadequate topical anesthesia potentiates coughing, gagging, and patient discomfort and increases the risk of injury during bronchoscopy. However, topical anesthetics such as lidocaine, the most frequently used agent, are absorbed systemically through the respiratory mucosa, increasing the risk of cardiac or CNS toxicity. These complications are more likely to occur in patients with underlying low cardiac output, hepatic dysfunction, and oropharyngeal candidiasis. Another, less frequent complication of excessive lidocaine use is methemoglobinemia and tissue hypoxia.

Introduction of the bronchoscope frequently results in a decrease in oxygenation and in hypoventilation, with demonstrable increases in $PaCO_2$. In patients with underlying chronic lung disease, severe hypoxemia may occur, triggering life-threatening cardiac arrhythmias. All patients should, therefore, be monitored continuously (ECG, blood pressure, O_2 saturation, and, if indicated, expiratory CO_2 concentration). Use of supplemental oxygen during the procedure should be routine.

Significant oxygen desaturation may occur during BAL. The degree of desaturation is directly related to the duration of the procedure and the volume of lavage fluid used. Return to the prebronchoscopy level of O_2 saturation may be prolonged after removal of the bronchoscope, and supplemental O_2 should be continued throughout the procedure and during the postbronchoscopy observation period.

Fever and Infection

A variety of pulmonary procedures, including bronchoscopy, have been reported to cause transient bacteremia. However, there are no data demonstrating a link between bronchoscopy and increased risk of infective endocarditis. For high-risk patients (e.g., prosthetic valve, previous endocarditis, congenital heart disease), the American Heart Association does not recommend the use of prophylactic antibiotics before bronchoscopy unless the procedure involves incision of the respiratory tract mucosa. Antibiotic prophylaxis should be considered, however, in high-risk patients who are undergoing a procedure to treat an active infection, such as drainage of an abscess.

Transient fever after bronchoscopy is fairly common and generally does not require any therapy. However, persistent fever in the setting of progressive radiographic infiltrates necessitates antibiotic therapy. The incidence of fever is increased in the elderly, in those with underlying chronic pulmonary disease or documented endobronchial obstruction, and in those with bronchoscopic interventions for malignancy. The incidence of fever and extension of pulmonary infiltrates increase with the volume of BAL fluid and the total number of pulmonary segments lavaged. The incidence of post-bronchoscopic infection is higher in immunocompromised hosts and those with chronic suppurative lung disease, such as cystic fibrosis.

Airway Obstruction and Perforation

The advent of interventional bronchoscopy has resulted in complications not ordinarily seen with diagnostic bronchoscopy. Inappropriate use of lasers has resulted in endobronchial burns and bronchial perforations associated with catastrophic bleeding, pneumomediastinum, or pneumothorax. Endobronchial edema may also occur as a result of laser thermal effects.

As noted previously, airway stent insertion is associated with several complications. Stents may not be properly adapted to the diameter of the airway, resulting in either incomplete stent deployment or stent migration, possibly engendering life-threatening airway obstruction. The presence of this palliative endoprosthesis in the airway may predispose to difficulties with secretion clearance and accumulation of inspissated mucus. Placement of SEMS may result in severe local airway reactions, particularly at the edges of the device, producing granulation tissue, hemorrhage, or bronchial perforation.

Pneumothorax

Pneumothorax after transbronchial biopsy occurs in approximately 4% of cases, even when the procedure is done under fluoroscopic guidance. The impact of fluoroscopy on the incidence of pneumothorax remains controversial. Uncontrolled studies have not found a difference in the incidence of pneumothorax after transbronchial biopsy when performed with and without fluoroscopy.

The incidence of pneumothorax is increased, however, in immunocompromised hosts. This is likely due to the increased risk of pneumothorax associated with *Pneumocystis* infection. The risk is also elevated in mechanically ventilated patients, with peripheral lung biopsies, and in the presence of bullous lung disease. The risk of pneumothorax does not seem to be related to the size of the bronchoscopic biopsy forceps. In case of a significant pneumothorax, a chest tube should be inserted immediately to avoid oxygen desaturation and/or tension physiology.

Hemorrhage

One of the most frequently reported complications related to bronchoscopy is hemorrhage. Patients with uremia or with underlying bleeding disorders, especially those caused by platelet dysfunction or thrombocytopenia, have an increased risk of bleeding during bronchoscopy. Bronchoscopic lung biopsy should not be performed if the platelet count is $<50,000/mm^3$, and aggressive interventional procedures (laser therapy, bronchoplasty, or stent placement) are probably safe only with platelet counts $>75,000/mm^3$. Manipulation of the bronchoscope, mechanical trauma, vigorous suctioning, endobronchial brushing, and biopsy may result in bleeding during bronchoscopy. In one large series, the overall rate of bleeding after transbronchial biopsy was 4.7%, although the risk of severe bleeding (defined as the need for a bronchus-blocker, application of fibrin, critical care admission, or blood transfusion) was less than 1%. Hemorrhage can also occur with inadvertent perforation of pulmonary vessels during transbronchial needle aspiration or biopsy.

SUMMARY

Technologic advances in bronchoscopy continue to improve our ability to perform minimally invasive, accurate evaluations of the tracheobronchial tree and to perform an ever-increasing array of diagnostic, therapeutic, and palliative interventions. The role of both diagnostic and therapeutic bronchoscopy will continue to evolve as further improvements are made in bronchoscopes, accessory equipment, and imaging technologies. Therapeutic bronchoscopy may soon be used to provide treatment for conditions that have been traditionally treated with surgery. The major challenge in the adoption of the many new bronchoscopic techniques into routine clinical practice is the need for well-designed studies to delineate the appropriate use of these interventions and to better define their limitations.

SUGGESTED READINGS

Beamis JF Jr, Mathur PN, Mehta AC, eds: Interventional pulmonary medicine. New York: M. Dekker; 2004.
Bolliger CT, Mathur PN, Beamis JF, *et al*: ERS/ATS statement on interventional pulmonology. Eur Respir J 2002; 19:356–373.

Cox G, Thomson NC, Rubin AS, *et al*: AIR Trial Study Group: Asthma control during the year after bronchial thermoplasty. N Engl J Med 2007; 356:1327–1337.

Ernst A, Silvestri GA, Johnstone D: ACCP Interventional/Diagnostic Procedures Network Steering Committee: Interventional pulmonary procedures. Guidelines from the American College of Chest Physicians. Chest 2003; 123:1693–1717.

Mehta AC, Prakash UBS, Garland R, *et al*: American College of Chest Physicians and American Association for Bronchology Consensus Statement: Prevention of flexible bronchoscopy-associated infection. Chest 2005; 128:1742–1755.

Seijo LM, Sterman DH: Medical progress: Interventional pulmonology. N Engl J Med 2001; 344:740–749.

Simoff MJ, Sterman DH, Ernst A, eds: Thoracic endoscopy: Advances in interventional pulmonology. Malden, Mass: Blackwell, Futura; 2006.

Wang K-P, Mehta AC, Turner JF Jr, eds: Flexible bronchoscopy. Malden Mass: Blackwell Scientific; 2004.

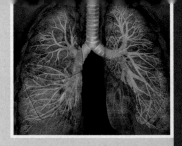

13 Thoracentesis and Closed Pleural Biopsy

STEPHEN G. SPIRO

INTRODUCTION

Pleural effusions are most commonly caused by malignancy and infection—in particular parapneumonic and tuberculous—and may need to be investigated by means of closed pleural biopsy if an initial aspirated sample is negative for malignant cytology or an obvious infection. Most malignant causes are diagnosed on the cytologic examination of a 20-mL aliquot of the effusion, which can be aspirated by inserting a needle through the chest wall with the patient under local anesthesia. In cases of tuberculosis, the fluid rarely yields acid-fast bacilli when direct smears are examined, but it is predominantly lymphocytic and usually has a reduced glucose content. Pyogenic infection or parapneumonic effusions may be milky and have a purulent appearance, may show a lesser shade of turbidity, or even may be clear but contain neutrophils. Empyemas tend to appear creamy and sometimes have a fecal smell. The rare chylous effusion is paler and more milky in appearance.

INDICATIONS AND CONTRAINDICATIONS

If the initial pleural aspiration is not diagnostic, it should be repeated, and a closed pleural biopsy should be performed at the same time. The biopsy is especially useful in cases of suspected tuberculosis, because the pleural histologic examination may yield granulomata in up to 50% of cases. Pleural biopsy adds 2–10% to the yield of cytology for malignancy and is particularly important in the diagnosis of mesothelioma. Current practice in the evaluation of pleural disease would advocate a thorax CT as the next test after negative pleural aspiration. If the pleura appears abnormal with localized thickening or masslike areas, a CT-guided pleural biopsy would be the investigation of choice. If the pleura showed no specific features, closed biopsy is appropriate.

TECHNIQUE

A variety of needles are available. The Cope needle was introduced in 1958, but the Abrams needle remains the most popular. The Raja needle is a modification of the Abrams needle and was introduced in 1993. Tru-Cut biopsy needles are used under ultrasound control by radiologists to produce a core of tissue from obviously thickened pleural tissues for histologic examination. Finally, biopsy specimens can be taken from the parietal pleura with forceps during the course of a thoracoscopy, usually as a video-assisted thoracoscopic procedure.

Positioning the Patient

The patient should sit upright, leaning forward with arms folded across the chest, and leaning onto a pillow that rests on the bed table. Position the patient's head also leaning forward onto the pillow for several minutes to allow comfortable breathing. The folding of the patient's arms lifts the scapula upward and outward and prevents them from impeding the procedure.

Anesthesia

After cleaning the skin, introduce 1% plain lidocaine (lignocaine) into the posterior axillary line with as small a needle as possible. Once the skin is anesthetized, a longer No. 1 needle is advanced. Push out lidocaine continuously and aim to advance beneath the rib until the pleura are penetrated and fluid can be drawn back into the attached syringe (Figure 13-1). At this stage, use a second syringe that contains 1% lidocaine to widen the area of anesthesia, keeping the skin entry site as the apex of an imagined pyramid of anesthesia. Always withdraw the needle back to just under the skin before advancing it at a new angle. The best practice is to use a new syringe of lidocaine once the pleural cavity has been entered, because malignant pleural effusions can seed along the needle track from the pleura. A total of 10 mL of 1% lidocaine should be sufficient to anesthetize the chest wall of most patients.

Incision

Next, make a stab incision with a No. 11 scalpel blade along the intended biopsy track. This easily can be widened and extended down to the pleural surface by blunt dissection with a pair of straight Spencer–Wells forceps (Figure 13-2).

Use of the Abrams Needle

The Abrams needle contains an inner stylus, which is removed and not used. The inner of the two remaining cylinders has a cutting edge that, when pulled back, opens a triangular aperture on the outer sheath of the needle and allows fluid to enter the inner cannula (Figure 13-3). To open or close the window in the outer sheath, the ferrule is rotated clockwise or counterclockwise, respectively (Figure 13-4). The ferrule lies in line with the closed aperture when turned clockwise as far as it can go. The hub of the needle is attached to a three-way tap with a hose to drain fluid for collection and to a large syringe with a Luer lock fitting.

The knob on the ferrule of the inner sheath must be in line with the needle aperture. With the aperture closed, use

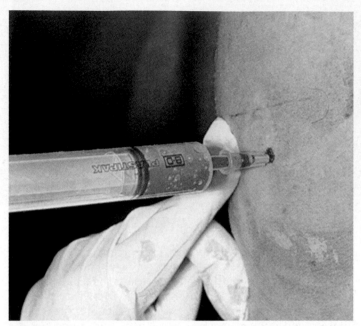

FIGURE 13-1 Infiltration of chest wall with local anesthetic. The needle penetrates the pleura, and fluid is aspirated back into the syringe.

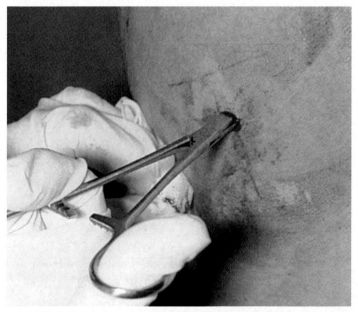

FIGURE 13-2 A blunt dissection down to and into the pleural cavity. The forceps are opened gently and pushed forward to tease apart the muscle fibers.

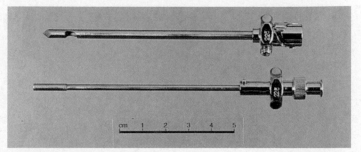

FIGURE 13-3 The inner and outer sheaths of an Abrams needle showing the aperture in the outer sheath. The tip of the inner sheath cuts the biopsy specimen.

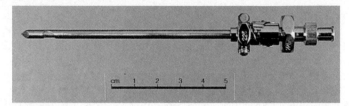

FIGURE 13-4 Needle assembled showing the ferrule that is rotated to cut the specimen.

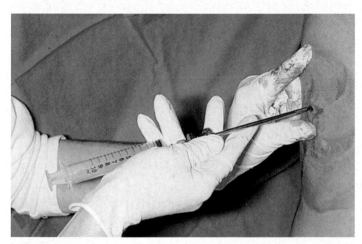

FIGURE 13-5 Gentle insertion of the closed needle into the pleural cavity. The needle, with aperture closed, should enter the pleural space with only gentle, rotating pressure by the hand of the operator.

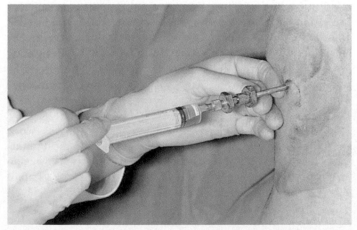

FIGURE 13-6 Fluid is withdrawn into the syringe with the needle aperture open. A three-way tap system can be added if fluid is to be collected for laboratory testing.

a rotating action to push the needle gently through the chest wall into the pleural cavity (Figure 13-5). Blunt dissection (see "Incision," earlier in this chapter) enables the needle to pass easily and prevents it from bursting into the pleural cavity, thus avoiding the risk of trauma. The needle point is blunt, which also limits potential damage, for example, a pneumothorax.

Once the pleural cavity has been entered, open the needle and withdraw fluid (Figure 13-6). Collect samples of 20 mL and eject them into specimen containers by use of a three-way tap. After collecting the pleural fluid samples, attach the needle directly to a 20-mL syringe and then tilt it so that the

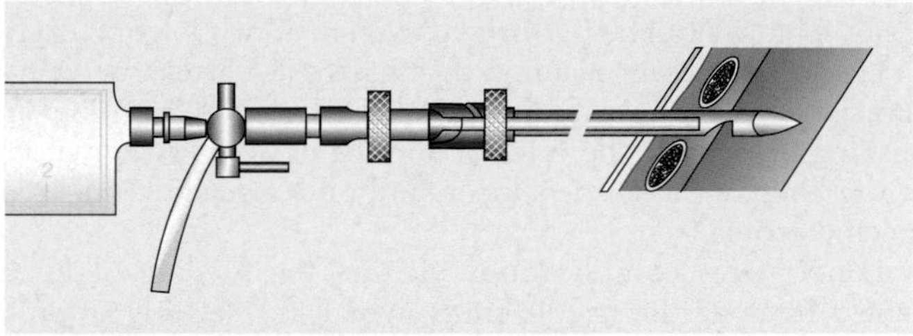

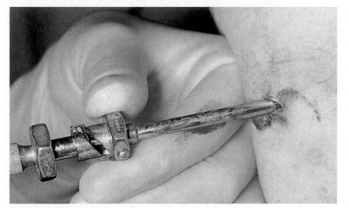

FIGURE 13-7 Biopsy position of the needle.

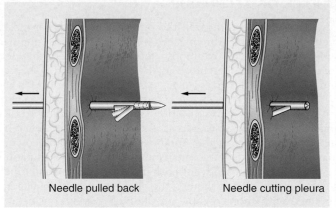

Needle pulled back   Needle cutting pleura

FIGURE 13-9 Method of biopsy with a Raja needle. The flap impinges on the pleura as the needle is pulled back and cuts off a piece of pleura on closure.

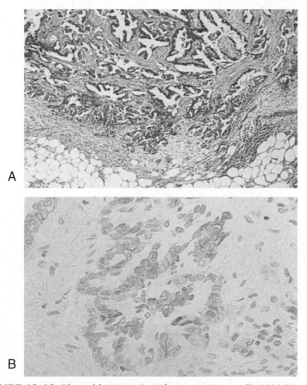

FIGURE 13-8 Taking a pleural biopsy by rotating the ferrule to close the aperture. Pull the entire apparatus sharply out of the chest.

A

B

FIGURE 13-10 Pleural biopsy. **A,** Adenocarcinoma; **B,** AUA1 immunostaining positive for adenocarcinoma.

aperture is felt snagging the pleural surface. When lateral pressure is exerted as the needle is slowly pulled back, the pleura is pushed into the aperture (Figure 13-7). While tension is maintained, twist the ferrule closed (Figure 13-8) and pull the needle out of the chest cavity sharply. Then, open the needle over either saline or formal saline (saline plus formaldehyde) and squirt the biopsy sample into a container or tease it off with a needle. Perform several biopsies at various clock positions, apart from the positions between 10 PM and 2 AM (to avoid damaging an intercostal nerve or vessel lying in the bed of the rib above). One biopsy sample should be placed into saline for culture for *Mycobacterium tuberculosis* and the others into formal saline.

The Abrams system is relatively easy to use and is recommended as the most effective method of obtaining pleural fluid drawn by the needle and three-way tap, as well as for biopsy specimens.

The Raja Needle

The Raja needle is a modification of the Abrams system; it has a biopsy flap that opens once the pleural cavity is entered, and the inner sheath is pulled back. The flap fixes onto the parietal pleural surface and, when closed, cuts off a piece of pleura (Figure 13-9). Comparisons with the more readily available Abrams needle have suggested a higher diagnostic yield.

SPECIMEN HANDLING

Always take important biopsy specimens directly to the laboratory. To prevent contamination of the fluid by additional bleeding, remove it for investigation before taking a biopsy. Send the fluid for routine bacterial culture, direct smear and culture for tuberculosis, cytology, and protein and glucose

estimation (together with a serum glucose sample). Measurement of pleural fluid amylase and rheumatoid factor should be requested if necessary.

Between four and six biopsies are usually taken and sent in formal saline for histologic examination and in normal saline for culture.

Pleural biopsy is very successful in the identification of tuberculosis, but less so for malignancy (Figure 13-10). Needle biopsies increase the yield for finding tuberculosis, especially if the biopsy sample is also sent for culture. In malignancy, needle biopsy has a 50% sensitivity compared with pleural fluid cytology but adds a little to the overall yield. Needle biopsy is, however, very useful for mesothelioma, which cannot easily be distinguished from adenocarcinoma in pleural fluid cytology.

CHOICE OF TECHNIQUE

Few studies have compared the different methods for closed pleural biopsy. The Abrams needle remains the most popular, and if an average of five biopsy specimens is taken, the yield (usually tumor or tuberculosis) is 60%. A comparison of the Raja and Abrams needles gives a diagnosis in approximately 80% and 50% of biopsies, respectively. Comparing the Abrams needle with the Tru-Cut biopsy needle demonstrates similar results, and use of fiberoptic thoracoscopes for biopsies in general is superior to the use of the Abrams needle. Rigid thoracoscopy may be even better. A comparison of cytology, closed pleural biopsy, and thoracoscopy for both malignant disease and tuberculosis shows that although the highest diagnostic yield is obtained with thoracoscopy, needle biopsy adds considerably to the number of cases diagnosed on examination of the pleural effusion, making thoracoscopy unnecessary in 74% of malignant and 61% of cases of tuberculosis (Figure 13-11).

COMPLICATIONS

Very few complications of closed-needle biopsy have been reported. Pneumothorax is uncommon, because the needle point is blunt and only a small amount of fluid need be present for a biopsy to be taken. Provided the two pleural surfaces part easily, a biopsy can be performed even in a "dry" pleural cavity.

Hemorrhage can occur if the intercostal artery or vein is damaged by taking a biopsy at the 12-o'clock position and pushing up against the inferior surface of a rib. A hematoma of the chest wall can develop rapidly but usually requires no specific action.

Longer-term complications include the seeding of malignant cells along the needle track, which is relatively common in malignant effusions. Should this occur, a single fraction of radiotherapy controls the developing nodule in most cases.

PITFALLS AND CONTROVERSIES

In the case of a large pleural effusion, enough fluid should be aspirated both for testing and to make the patient more comfortable. It is becoming common to insert intercostal tubes into large effusions and then drain them completely. In these cases, pleural fluid samples may have been sent to the laboratory without any biopsy having been taken. Although additional fluid can easily be obtained from the chest tube if the fluid examinations are negative, a new incision will have to be made for a closed pleural biopsy. Furthermore, once an intercostal drain is inserted, the patient may need to remain in the hospital in discomfort for some days while awaiting results, and then further interventions across the chest wall may be required.

A preferred course is to aspirate approximately 1 L of fluid from a large effusion and send samples to the laboratory. The patient may then be able to go home and await results. If all results are negative, the procedure should be repeated and, ideally a CT scan performed, followed by the appropriate type of pleural biopsy. If results are still negative and there is no systemic or other obvious cause for the effusion, a thoracoscopy should be performed with biopsies taken from the parietal pleura under direct vision. Even this may not provide a diagnosis, but, in experienced hands, thoracoscopy adds approximately 10–30% to the overall yield of closed biopsy and cytology diagnoses.

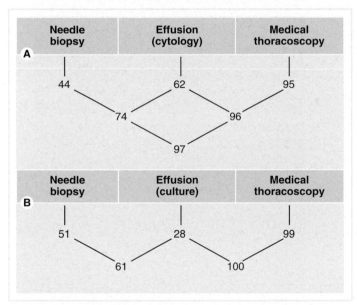

FIGURE 13-11 Sensitivity (%) for cytology and histology. **A,** Sensitivity for cytology and histology combined for the different biopsy techniques in 208 malignant pleural effusions. **B,** Sensitivity for cytology and histology in the diagnosis of 100 tuberculous pleural effusions by use of the different diagnostic techniques. (From Loddenkemper R: Thoracoscopy—state of the art. Eur Respir J 1998; 11:213–221.)

SUGGESTED READINGS

Loddenkemper R, Boutin C: Thoracoscopy: Diagnostic and therapeutic indications. Eur Respir J 1993; 6:1544–1555.

McLeod DT, Ternouth I, Nkanza N: Comparison of the Tru-Cut biopsy needle with the Abrams punch for pleural biopsy. Thorax 1989; 44: 794–796.

Mungall IPF, Cowen PN, Cooke NT, et al: Multiple pleural biopsy with the Abrams needle. Thorax 1980; 35:600–602.

Ogirala RG, Agarwal V, Vizioli LD, et al: Comparison of the Raja and the Abrams pleural biopsy needles in patients with pleural effusions. Am Rev Respir Dis 1993; 47:1291–1294.

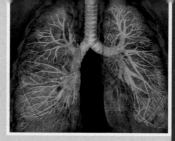

14 Transbronchial and Esophageal Ultrasound-Guided Biopsy of the Mediastinum

FELIX J.F. HERTH

INTRODUCTION

The analysis of mediastinal masses, for example, enlarged mediastinal lymph nodes in patients with lung cancer, is of major clinical importance. Radiologic imaging has been proven to be unreliable in the diagnosis of these structures. Histologic proof of the diagnosis often requires invasive procedures such as mediastinoscopy or mediastinotomy, thoracoscopy, or even thoracotomy. These procedures are not only burdensome for patients but they also have limitations in their reach, require hospitalization, and are, therefore, accompanied by high costs. The development of endoscopic ultrasound has opened up new diagnostic possibilities.

Endoscopic ultrasound-guided fine-needle aspiration biopsy (EUS-FNA) was originally developed for gastrointestinal diseases. However, it very soon became apparent that a considerable part of the mediastinum can be reached and tissue sampled by this method. Endoesophageal EUS-guided biopsy of lesions in the mediastinum is a minimally invasive diagnostic method that can spare patients from much more aggressive and risky methods. At present, both cytology and histology can be obtained by EUS guidance, which has broadened the range of applications for EUS even further. The main indications of EUS-guided biopsy in the mediastinum is, at present, staging of non-small-cell lung cancer (NSCLC), diagnosis of lymph nodes of unknown nature, staging of a wide range of cancers if CT has demonstrated enlarged mediastinal lymph nodes, and accurate differentiation between specific cancers or lymphomas (EUS-guided histology).

The endobronchial ultrasound system has been commercially available since 1999 and is being gradually introduced into bronchoscopic practice. This has broadened the range for the bronchoscopist and augmented the diagnostic possibilities for bronchial and mediastinal pathosis.

Today, two different systems are available. The endobronchial mini-probes, which are usable through the working channel of the normal scope, and in 2005 the endobronchial ultrasound-guided transbronchial needle aspiration (EBUS-TBNA) scope became available.

ENDOBRONCHIAL ULTRASOUND MINI-PROBES

The imaging in ultrasound is different from the processes in X-ray imaging. It is the difference in resistance of different tissues to the ultrasound waves that is more complex and only partly dependent on its water content. The different impedance of soft tissues has made ultrasound an indispensable diagnostic tool in medicine.

Instruments that are used for gastrointestinal applications could not be applied inside the airways because of their diameter. For application inside the central airways, therefore, a flexible catheter for the probes with a balloon at the tip was developed (Figure 14-1), which allows circular contact for the ultrasound, providing a complete 360-degree image of the parabronchial and paratracheal structures (Figure 14-2). As the balloon is providing enhancement of the ultrasound, penetration of the waves produced by 20-MHz probes is increased. Thus, under favorable conditions, structures at a distance of up to 4 cm can be visualized. The probes can be used with flexible bronchoscopes that have a biopsy channel of at least 2.6 mm.

EARLY LUNG CANCER

In small radiologically invisible tumors, decision for local endoscopic therapeutic intervention depends on their intraluminal and intramural extent within the different layers of the wall (Figure 14-3). In contrast to radiologic imaging, very small tumors of a few millimeters diameter can be analyzed reliably by endobronchial ultrasound and differentiated from benign lesions. Combination of EBUS with autofluorescence bronchoscopy has proven to be very accurate in prospective studies and has become the basis for curative endobronchial treatment of malignancies in some institutions, by use of photodynamic therapy, coagulation, or brachytherapy.

ADVANCED CANCER

In preoperative staging, EBUS allows detailed analysis of intraluminal, submucosal, and intramural tumor spread that can be essential for a decision on resection margins. EBUS proved especially useful in the diagnosis of mediastinal tumor involvement of, for example, the great vessels such as the aorta, vena cava, main pulmonary arteries, and of the esophageal wall, which is frequently impossible by conventional radiology. In one trial it was shown that differentiation of external tumor invasion from compression only of the tracheobronchial wall by EBUS was highly reliable (94%) compared with CT imaging (51%). The sensitivity of EBUS versus CT was 89% vs

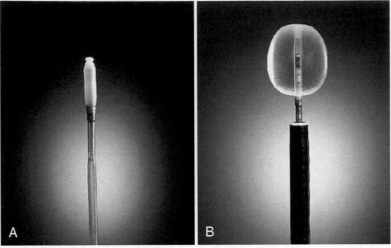

FIGURE 14-1 The EBUS miniprobe **(A)** inserted in a normal bronchoscope with inflated balloon tip **(B)**.

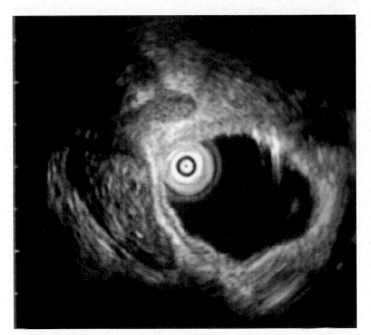

FIGURE 14-2 A 360-degree scanning view in the lower left main stem bronchus. The bronchial wall is visible and a lymph node in position 10 left.

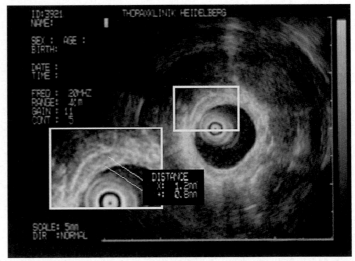

FIGURE 14-3 The normal-sized bronchial wall in a normal and a zoomed range.

25% and the specificity was 100% vs 89% in the superiority of the ultrasound technique in the differentiation between airway infiltration and compression by tumor (Figure 14-4). Thus, many patients considered to have nonresectable tumors with conventional imaging because of apparent T4 tumor invasion could be curatively resected after EBUS examination.

PERIPHERAL LESIONS

For the histologic diagnosis of peripheral intrapulmonary lesions, bronchoscopic transbronchial biopsy (TBNA) under fluoroscopic or CT guidance is the standard procedure.

This demands expensive X-ray equipment in the bronchoscopy suite or coordination with the radiology department and risks exposure to radiation for patient and staff.

In a prospective study, we were able to show that those lesions could be approached by EBUS guidance with the same success rate of approximately 75%. Recently, these data have been confirmed by another group of Japanese bronchoscopists who also achieved a diagnostic yield of 75% by use of the miniprobe as a guidance tool for the forceps.

Another trial is aiming to asses the yield of EBUS-guided TBB in fluoroscopic invisible solitary pulmonary nodules. Fifty-four patients with a solitary pulmonary nodule (SPN)

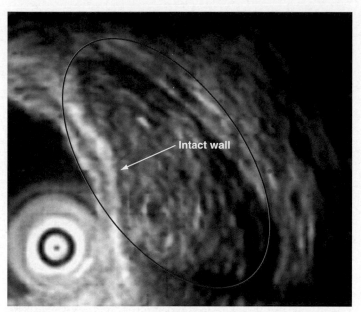

FIGURE 14-4 On a CT, a tumor in the right upper lobe was seen. With the help of EBUS, it can clearly shown that the tumor (marked in red) respected the tracheal wall.

that could not be visualized with fluoroscopy were examined. In 48 (89%) cases, the lesion could be reached with EBUS, and in 38 (70%) cases, the biopsy established the diagnosis. The mean nodule size was 2.2 cm. Clearly, these techniques need to be compared with transthoracic CT-guided biopsies of SPNs.

INDICATIONS AND RESULTS FOR EBUS-TBNA

Accurate lymph node staging is the main indication for the EBUS-TBNA-scope, because it can provide a diagnosis and cancer staging at a single procedure. The EBUS-TBNA samples nodes in the paratracheal regions and also the aortopulmonary window. However, EUS (see later) samples nodes alongside the esophagus and within the abdomen (Figure 14-5). These two techniques, therefore, are complementary and between them gain access to a far greater area within the mediastinum than a surgical approach by mediastinoscopy.

The ultrasonic bronchoscope is introduced through an endotracheal tube under visual control or under local anesthesia to the area of interest, mostly on an outpatient basis. The bronchoscope is inserted orally with additional sedation, usually 2 mg midazolam. Patients must be monitored for ECG,

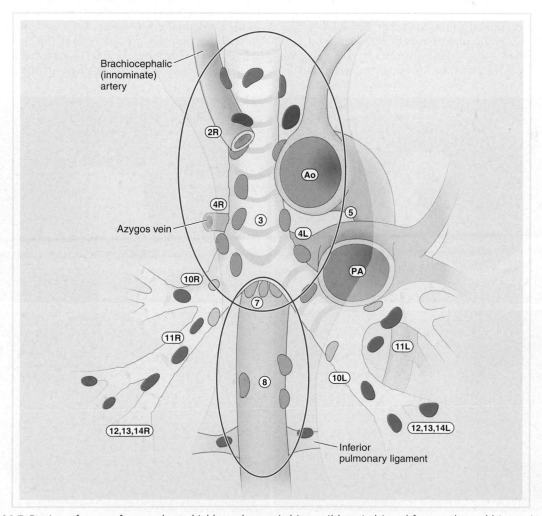

FIGURE 14-5 Region of access for transbronchial bronchoscopic biopsy (*blue circle*) and for esophageal biopsy (*red circle*).

pulse oximetry, and blood pressure. Images can be obtained from direct contact of the probe against the airway wall or by attaching a balloon to the probe tip and inflating it with saline.

Because the balloon is designed not to over inflate, it will not occlude the central airway, and no technical difficulties have been reported when the balloon was used.

When a lesion is outlined, a 21-gauge full-length steel needle is introduced through the biopsy channel of the endoscope. Power Doppler examination is used immediately before the biopsy to avoid unintentional puncture of vessels between the wall of the bronchi and the lesion (Figure 14-6). Under real-time ultrasonic guidance, the needle will be placed in the lesion. Suction is applied with a syringe, and the needle is moved back and forth inside the lesion.

Several studies have been published on this procedure. Yasufuku and colleagues examined 70 patients with mediastinal ($n = 58$) and hilar lymph nodes ($n = 12$).

The sensitivity, specificity, and accuracy of EBUS-TBNA in distinguishing benign from malignant lymph nodes were 95.7%, 100%, and 97.1%, respectively. There were no complications.

The largest trial to date reported results in 502 patients; 572 lymph nodes were punctured, and 535 (94%) yielded a diagnosis. Biopsies were taken from all reachable lymph node stations. Mean (SD) diameter of the nodes was 1.6 cm (0.36 cm), and the range was 0.8–3.2 cm.

Sensitivity was 92%, specificity was 100%, and the positive predictive value was 93%. As in all other trials, no complications occurred.

Another study examined the accuracy of EBUS-TBNA in sampling nodes <1 cm in diameter. Of 100 patients, 119 lymph nodes between 4 and 10 mm were detected and sampled. Malignancy was detected in 19 patients but missed in 2 others; all diagnoses were confirmed by surgical biopsy or exploration. The mean (SD) diameter of the sampled lymph nodes was 8.1 mm. The sensitivity of EBUS-TBNA for detecting malignancy was 92.3%; the specificity was 100%; and the negative predictive value was 96.3%. Again, no complications occurred. Thus, EBUS-TBNA can sample even small mediastinal nodes, avoiding unnecessary surgical exploration in one of five patients who have no CT evidence of mediastinal disease. Potentially operable patients with clinically nonmetastatic NSCLC may benefit from presurgical EBUS-TBNA biopsies as a final staging procedure before thoracotomy.

ENDOESOPHAGEAL ULTRASOUND

Esophageal endoscopic ultrasound is performed with devices that are used in gastroenterologic practice (Figure 14-7). Currently, there are both radial and linear ultrasound probes available. EUS enables an anatomic visualization of the esophagus and its surrounding structures. It is possible to obtain tissue samples of lesions that lie adjacent to the esophagus by puncturing the target lesion under ultrasound guidance. The material obtained in this way is suitable for cytologic and molecular-biologic diagnosis, for example, polymerase chain reaction (PCR) analysis for *Mycobacterium tuberculosis*.

For esophageal ultrasound-guided fine-needle aspiration biopsy (EUS-FNA), only a linear ultrasound probe is used. The procedure is performed in an outpatient setting and does not require any specific preparations. The patient is positioned in the left lateral position and, after spraying a local anesthetic to the pharynx, the procedure is performed under conscious sedation. The ultrasound probe is advanced into the distal part of the esophagus until the left lobe of the liver is visualized.

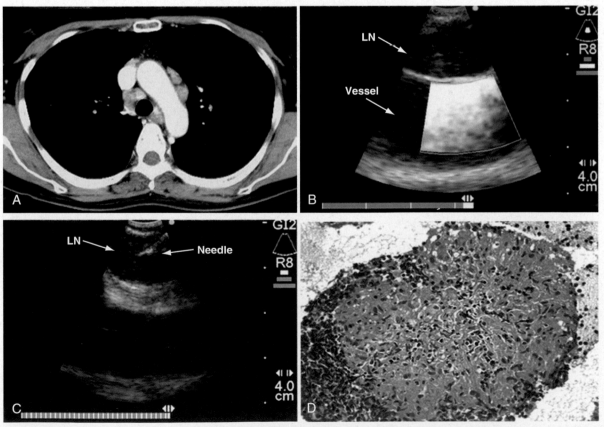

FIGURE 14-6 Enlarged lymph node in the upper mediastinum (**A**), with the power Doppler the vessels are clear to see (*LN*, lymph node) (**B**) and the real-time puncture process was started (**C**). **D,** The histologic result shows a sarcoidosis.

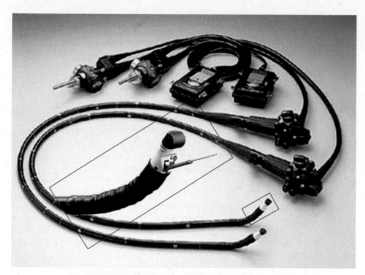

FIGURE 14-7 The EUS-FNA scopes.

There are no absolute contraindications for an endoscopic investigation of the upper gastrointestinal tract, although esophageal strictures and diverticulae increase the risk of perforation. The complication rates of EUS-FNA are between 0.5 and 2%.

The theoretical advantages of this new diagnostic procedure—compared with radiologic and surgical alternatives—are several. EUS-FNA is more sensitive in the identification of mediastinal lymph nodes than chest imaging and allows a real-time controlled sample. In comparison with the surgical alternatives, EUS-FNA is less invasive, is performed on an outpatient basis, and is more cost-effective.

In assessing the mediastinum, EBUS-TBNA and EUS-FNA are complementary. EBUS-TBNA provides good access to the pretracheal and paratracheal lymph node stations, whereas EUS-FNA is more suitable in assessing paraesophageal lymph nodes, as well as lymph nodes in the aorta pulmonary window and the ligamentum pulmonale.

From this landmark, the scope is withdrawn stepwise while making circular movements enabling the investigator to visualize most parts of the mediastinum. Location, size, and echo features of lesions are determined. It is recommended that these findings be recorded and stored.

The registered lymph nodes are anatomically classified according to the Naruke classification. Suspicious lesions can be punctured smoothly through the wall of the esophagus under real-time ultrasound guidance (Figure 14-8). An on-site evaluation of the punctured material by a cytologist is recommended. In the hands of an experienced investigator, EUS-FNA of the mediastinum takes approximately 30 min to perform.

RESULTS OF EUS-FNA

More than 50 studies on EUS-FNA have reported sensitivities of 0.61 ± 1.00 (median, 0.90) and specificities of 0.71 ± 1.00 (median, 1.00). As an example, a study of 84 patients selected for EUS-FNA by CT evaluated the clinical impact of EUS-FNA. In 18 of 37 patients (49%), a thoracotomy or mediastinoscopy was avoided as a result of EUS-FNA.

In another study, 242 consecutive patients with suspected ($n = 142$) or proven ($n = 100$) lung cancer and enlarged (>1 cm) mediastinal lymph nodes on chest CT underwent EUS-FNA. This prevented 70% of scheduled surgical procedures, because it demonstrated lymph node metastases. These included non-small-cell lung cancer metastases (52%), direct tumor invasion of the mediastinum (T4) (4%), tumor invasion and lymph

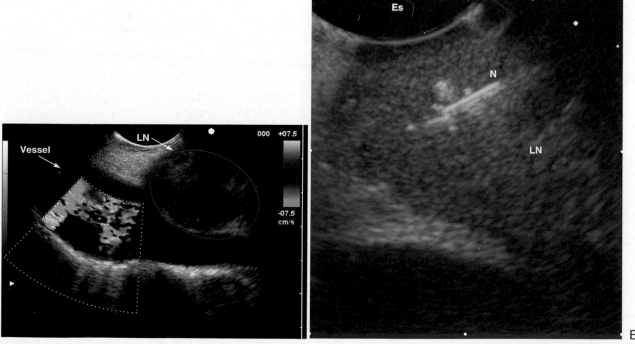

FIGURE 14-8 A, Enlarged lymph node in the upper mediastinum (marked in red). With the help of the Doppler mode, the vessels are visible. **B,** Enlarged image of a real-time EUS-FNA. *LN,* Lymph node; *Es,* esophageal; *N,* needle.

node metastases (5%), small-cell lung cancer (8%), or benign diseases (1%).

SUMMARY

The novel diagnostic methods of endobronchial ultrasound-guided transbronchial needle aspiration and transesophageal ultrasound-guided fine-needle aspiration enable ultrasound-controlled mediastinal tissue sampling. Implementation of these techniques will drastically alter lung cancer staging algorithms in the near future. Thanks to its minimally invasive approach, excellent safety record, accuracy, and diagnostic reach, complete endoscopic staging of the mediastinum, left lobe of the liver, celiac axis, and left adrenal gland is now possible, providing evidence of disease stage with one investigation.

SUGGESTED READINGS

Annema JT, Rabe KF: State of the art lecture: EUS and EBUS in pulmonary medicine. Endoscopy 2006; 38(S1):118–122.

Annema JT, Versteegh MI, Veselic M, Voigt P, Rabe KF: Endoscopic ultrasound-guided fine-needle aspiration in the diagnosis and staging of lung cancer and its impact on surgical staging. J Clin Oncol 2005; 23:8357–8361.

Falcone F, Fois F, Grosso D: Endobronchial ultrasound. Respiration 2003; 70:179–194.

Hawes RH, Fockens P: How to perform EUS in the esophagus and mediastinum. In Hawes RH, Fockens P, eds. Endosonography. Philadelphia: WB Saunders; 2006:57–72.

Herth F, Becker HD: Endobronchial ultrasound of the airways and the mediastinum. Monaldi Arch Chest Dis 2000; 55:36–45.

Herth FJ, Eberhardt R, Vilmann P, Krasnik M, Ernst A: Real-time, endobronchial ultrasound-guided, transbronchial needle aspiration: a new method for sampling mediastinal lymph nodes. Thorax 2006; 61:795–798.

Herth FJ, Ernst A, Eberhardt R, Vilmann P, Dienemann H, Krasnik M: Endobronchial ultrasound-guided transbronchial needle aspiration of lymph nodes in the radiologically normal mediastinum. Eur Respir J 2006; 28:910–914.

Herth FJ, Rabe KF, Gasparini S, Annema JT: Transbronchial and transesophageal (ultrasound-guided) needle aspirations for the analysis of mediastinal lesions. Eur Respir J 2006; 28(6):1264–1275.

Larsen SS, Krasnik M, Vilmann P, et al: Endoscopic ultrasound guided biopsy of mediastinal lesions has a major impact on patient management. Thorax 2002; 57:98–103.

Vilmann P: Endoscopic ultrasonography-guided fine-needle aspiration biopsy of lymph nodes. Gastrointest Endosc 1996; 43:S24–S29.

Yasufuku K, Chiyo M, Koh E, et al: Endobronchial ultrasound guided transbronchial needle aspiration for staging of lung cancer. Lung Cancer 2005; 50:347–354.

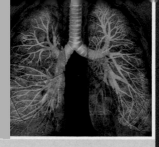

15 Percutaneous Biopsy Procedures

PENNY SHAW • FABIAN SEBASTIAN

INTRODUCTION

This section describes the equipment and techniques available to obtain diagnostic tissue from predominantly solid lesions within the chest by use of the percutaneous transthoracic route. The common lesions and sites biopsied are summarized in Figure 15-1, and the most frequent method of biopsy by site is summarized in Figure 15-2. The technique and its indications are different from those required to diagnose more diffuse intrapulmonary disease. The latter, which includes conditions such as idiopathic pulmonary fibrosis, requires a transbronchial lung biopsy or an open lung biopsy through a minithoracotomy or video-assisted thoracoscopy.

Imaging plays an important role in confirming and identifying the site of the lesion, its size, and the quality of the surrounding lung tissue. It is also used to assess the extent of the pathology and the presence of other diseases. The radiologist determines whether the lesion is suitable for transthoracic biopsy and identifies the optimum site for biopsy and under which imaging modality it should be performed. The choice of needle depends on risk factors, whether histology or cytology is required, and personal preference.

PERCUTANEOUS BIOPSY OF INTRAPULMONARY LESIONS

Indications and Contraindications

Transthoracic needle biopsy is an established and accepted technique for the diagnosis of malignant masses or nodules, with a sensitivity of 90–97%. The technique was previously limited by the low specificity for benign disease, but this has improved with needle placement under computed tomographic (CT) guidance and the use of coaxial transthoracic needle biopsy with an automated cutting needle. The main indication is in patients with cancer to establish cell type in inoperable advanced disease with negative sputum cytology and bronchoscopy. It is also widely used when there are solitary or multiple masses with a known extrathoracic malignancy to confirm metastatic disease. During staging of a thoracic malignancy, a contralateral pulmonary nodule or mediastinal, hepatic, or adrenal mass may be discovered. For assessment of operability, it is then of paramount importance to biopsy such lesions. It is also an established technique for confirming a Pancoast tumor. However, biopsy of a solitary mass or nodule is more controversial. If there is a high clinical and radiologic index of suspicion that the lesion is malignant, and the patient is otherwise operable, the patient may go straight to surgery. However, if a solitary mass is thought clinically and radiologically to be benign, a biopsy (preferably a core biopsy) is performed. Fine-needle aspiration (FNA) or biopsy for microorganisms

is increasingly being used in the diagnosis of consolidation or masses, especially in immunocompromised patients. Hilar and mediastinal lesions may also be biopsied percutaneously, which may be of particular value as an alternative to transbronchial biopsy, mediastinoscopy, or transesophageal biopsy.

The contraindications are largely relative and are summarized in Table 15-1. Biopsy of a lesion in patients with very poor lung function is possible, provided the lesion lies peripherally and a "safe" route that does not traverse the lung parenchyma is identified (usually with CT). When performing the biopsy, care should be taken to avoid a pneumothorax, which could be life threatening. A coagulation screen is performed if risk factors are present, for example, if the patient has hepatic metastases, has a history of alcohol ingestion, or is taking warfarin or aspirin. A prothrombin time <15–16 sec and an international normalized ratio <1.4 are acceptable. Some hydatid lesions have been biopsied, but there is still an increased and probably unacceptable risk of an anaphylactic reaction in this group of patients.

Techniques

Needles

Many different needles are available but are generally either fine needles for aspiration for cytology or cutting needles that produce a core of tissue for histology. Fine needles include the Westcott, Chiba, and Franseen needles and those that have a corkscrew appearance, such as the Rotex needle (Figure 15-3). They are usually 20 to 23 gauge and provide a specimen for cytology or culture. More flexible, 22-gauge needles can be difficult to position. The Westcott needle has an added advantage in that small fragments of tissue are frequently obtained in addition to the aspirate, in the small "notch" or slotted opening just proximal to the needle tip. This provides cores for histologic examination in approximately 50% of biopsies.

Aspirates should be obtained only if there is local cytologic expertise available. Ideally, the cytologist attends the biopsy to ensure that an adequate specimen is obtained. Larger cutting needles (18- or 20-gauge) provide a core for histologic examination and have greater rigidity, allowing greater control in placement. Commonly used cutting needles have a spring-loaded mechanism that fires the inner notched stylet and outer cutting cannula when a button is pushed; examples include the Bard Biopty biopsy system (Figure 15-4) and the Bauer Temno biopsy device (Figure 15-5). The "gun" or handle of the Bard system is reusable, and the needle is disposable.

Various sizes are available (14-, 18-, or 20-gauge needles), and a core of tissue is consistently produced. The "throw" of the gun is usually 10 or 20 mm, so lesions ideally need to be at least this size. The 20-mm throw produces better cores.

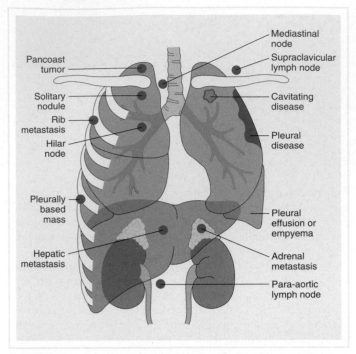

FIGURE 15-1 Common sites for needle or core biopsy techniques.

TABLE 15-1 Contraindications to Needle Biopsy	
Type of Contraindication	Comment
Relative	Uncooperative patient: Uncontrollable cough Inability to lie prone or supine Poor lung function/chronic obstructive pulmonary disease (forced expiratory volume in 1 second <40% of predicted normal or multiple bullae) Pneumonectomy Bleeding disorder Pulmonary hypertension Small nodules, <5-mm diameter Hydatid disease (because of the risk of anaphylactic reaction)
Absolute	Arteriovenous malformation with high pulmonary artery pressure

Historically, it has been suggested that cutting needles are associated with a higher complication rate than fine needles. A recent review of UK lung biopsy practice analyzed data from 5444 biopsies and found no difference between the two methods, a conclusion supported by other studies. The pneumothorax rate is related to the number of pleural passes made, which can be reduced by use of a coaxial system that has an 18- or 19-gauge, thin-walled introducer needle through which a fine needle can be passed, or by performing a fine-needle core biopsy. Fluid introduced into the pleural space can also be used to provide a safer route in some patients. The choice of needle takes into account the risk to the patient, the approach, and personal choice of the radiologist.

Image Guidance

Fluoroscopy has been superseded by CT as the imaging modality for percutaneous biopsy, allowing precise positioning of the needle within the lesion (Figure 15-6) and avoidance of vascular structures. Ultrasound guidance, used when the lesion is

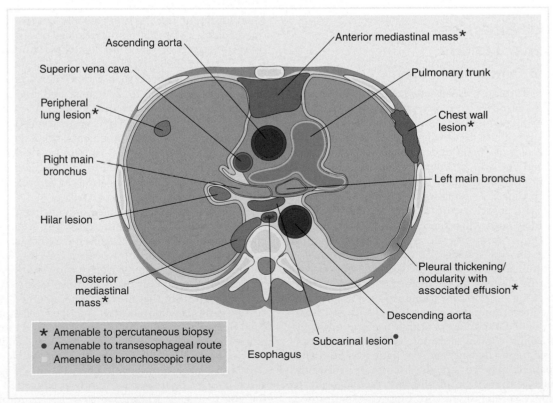

FIGURE 15-2 Common methods for biopsy according to site.

Needle name	Design	
Westcott	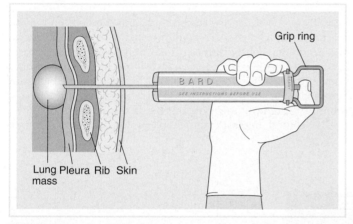	Slotted tip for small core
Chiba		25-degree bevel
Rotex		Tapered screw with cutting edges and outer cutting cannula
Franseen		Trephine

FIGURE 15-3 Needle tip design.

FIGURE 15-4 The Bard Biopty system. The needle is introduced into the patient so that the tip reaches the area in which biopsy will be performed.

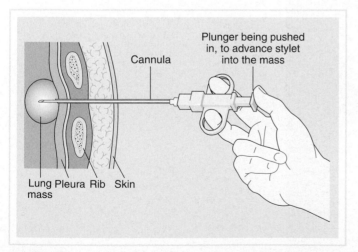

FIGURE 15-5 Use of the Bauer Temno biopsy instrument. The stylet is positioned within the lesion to be biopsied by pushing the plunger. The advantages are that the instrument requires one hand only, is lightweight, is easy to use under computed tomographic (CT) guidance, and produces a 2-cm core.

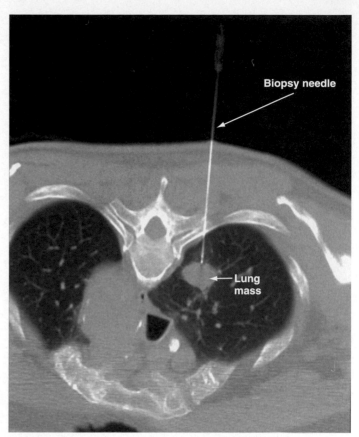

FIGURE 15-6 Lung biopsy. Biopsy of a small intrapulmonary lesion with a Wescott needle.

large and pleurally based, has the added advantage of not involving radiation.

A patient being considered for a percutaneous lung biopsy should undergo an initial staging CT examination of the thorax, providing the precise anatomic localization required to plan the procedure. The approach should ideally cover the shortest distance from the skin surface to the region of interest, avoiding fissures, while still allowing the patient to be placed in a position that will be comfortable for approximately 20 min. The latter consideration is particularly important, because often the patients referred for this procedure are elderly or frail and breathless at rest.

Role of PET-CT in Guiding Biopsy

Positron emission tomography (PET) is rapidly becoming an established technique in the evaluation and staging of oncology patients. In lung cancer, it provides information regarding the pulmonary nodule or mass, mediastinal disease, and extrathoracic metastases. The positron-emitting agent most frequently used is 18 F-fluoro-2-deoxyglucose (FDG). The imaging technique is based on the higher rate of glucose metabolism within neoplastic cells compared with surrounding normal tissue. FDG accumulates at these regions of increased glycolysis, which are imaged by the PET camera. In recent years, the development of PET cameras combined with CT (PET-CT) has allowed more precise anatomic localization of these FDG-avid foci.

The use of PET in oncology patients both upstages and downstages disease in conjunction with other imaging techniques.

It also provides valuable information regarding disease activity for the planning of biopsy procedures.

Potential pitfalls in its sensitivity relate to the fact that a sufficient amount of metabolically active tissue is required for a PET diagnosis, making the imaging of lesions smaller than 1 cm unreliable. False-negative results may occur with tumors with relatively low metabolic activity, such as carcinoid tumors and alveolar cell cancers. False-positive results are produced by inflammatory conditions such as bacterial pneumonia, abscess, tuberculosis, and active sarcoidosis. These false-positive results are caused by increased granulocyte activity.

This technique is being increasingly used to aid needle placement, particularly in identifying active foci within thickened pleura and pulmonary lesions obscured by atelectasis on CT (Figure 15-7).

Procedure

The patient should be fasted and informed consent taken by the person performing the biopsy. The more frequently occurring complications namely pneumothorax (possibly requiring a chest drain) or hemoptysis is explained to the patient. Overnight admission in the hospital may rarely be required. The patient is informed that more than one biopsy sample is usually needed. Sedation may be necessary in fragile or high-risk patients, and intravenous access should be obtained. An electrocardiograph and pulse oximeter are necessary if sedation is used. With the patient comfortably positioned on the CT table, radiopaque markers approximately 0.5–1 cm apart are placed over the region of interest, and a short scan covering the area is performed in inspiration.

Once the location of the target lesion is confirmed from the images obtained, the optimal skin entry site for the needle and the route to the lesion is planned by selecting an appropriate level. A mark is made on the patient's skin at this point. The procedure is undertaken under full sterile conditions. Lidocaine (lignocaine) 1% (10 mL) or 2% (5 mL) should be administered, taking care that the lung parenchyma and visceral pleura are not punctured but that the pleura is anesthetized. The patient should be warned that it is not always possible to anesthetize the pleura fully because of the risk of pneumothorax from the anesthetic needle.

A slight "give" is felt when the biopsy needle enters the pleural space. The needle is advanced either in suspended respiration or in small rapid movements during the same phase of gentle respiration to reduce trauma to the lung parenchyma. The progression of the needle toward the lesion and the final position of its tip are intermittently checked by repeating the initial scan as required. Accurate placement of the needle tip is essential and may take time with small nodules. Once the needle is in position, the central stylet is removed, and a finger is placed over the hub to prevent air embolism. A syringe is attached, suction applied, and gentle to-and-fro movements are made to obtain an aspirate, aiming the needle in slightly different directions. Pressure is released before the needle is withdrawn, or the specimen will be pulled back into the syringe. Saline (2–5 mL) can be injected into and then aspirated from a localized infiltrate before withdrawal to attempt to identify microorganisms. If the lesion is cavitating or has central necrosis, the biopsy must be taken from its periphery.

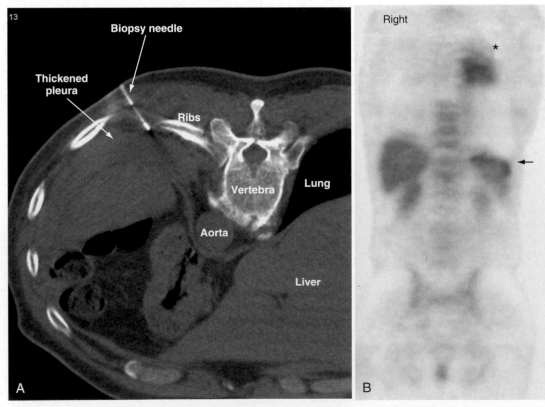

FIGURE 15-7 Pleural biopsy under computed tomographic (CT) guidance. **A,** Oblique route of pleural biopsy under CT guidance by use of the PET scan for localization. Metastatic disease was confirmed. **B,** PET scan demonstrating activity in left pleural base (*arrow*) and uptake in the primary tumor in the left upper lobe (*).

The specimen is dealt with immediately. The number of passes will vary, but on average one to three will be required (fewer if the patient is at high risk). The aim is to obtain a diagnosis, but the safety of the patient is paramount.

Specimen Handling

The aspirated material is smeared onto slides, with some fixed in alcohol and the rest air-dried. A saline wash of the needle is also taken. Larger cores of tissue are placed in formalin unless fresh tissue is required (if lymphoma or infections are suspected). Advanced cytologic procedures such as flow cytometry for lymphoma, estrogen receptor status for metastatic breast carcinoma, and immunocytochemistry for malignancies are useful. It is essential that the specimen reach the laboratory promptly.

Patient Aftercare

After lung biopsy, patients are monitored in the hospital for 4–5 h after the procedure. A "biopsy-side-down" position should be maintained whenever possible and talking, laughing, or coughing should be discouraged. Heart rate, respiratory rate, and blood pressure should be monitored for 2–3 h. In general, patients should undergo chest radiography at 1 and 4 h after the procedure. If the mass is large and pleurally based and if the patient remains asymptomatic, no chest radiograph is required.

Complications

The risk to the patient should always be weighed against the benefits of the procedure (Table 15-2). Deaths after aspiration are rare (1 in 5000–10,000 biopsies) and result from cardiac arrest, air embolism, tension pneumothorax, or hemorrhage.

If the patient has dyspnea at the end of the procedure, an immediate scan will detect even a small pneumothorax. Approximately 88% of pneumothoraces requiring intervention will be detected immediately and the remainder after 1 h. Patients may experience sharp chest pain as it occurs. Most pneumothoraces are small (<2 cm on chest X-ray); however, some require treatment with a chest drain. The frequency of this complication lies in the range of 0–17%. The pneumothorax rate with fine-needle aspiration and cutting needle biopsy is surprisingly similar, being in the range of 3–42%. Lying the patient with the puncture site dependent can reduce the pneumothorax rate. Drainage through a one-way valve (Heimlich valve) is useful in emergency situations and in patients who are recovering, because it allows the patient to remain ambulatory. Aspiration with an 18-gauge catheter attached to a three-way tap also reduces the need for chest tube placement in many patients. If the chest X-ray film is satisfactory or if the patient remains well with a small but static pneumothorax at 4 h, then they can go home with instructions to return if they become symptomatic, because a delayed or expanding pneumothorax is a rare complication. The patient may then require hospitalization and treatment. If a conservative line of management is followed, then, high flow oxygen (10 L/min) should be administered whenever possible, because this has been shown to increase the rate of pneumothorax reabsorption by up to four times.

Tension pneumothorax occurs within minutes and is a medical emergency. They are rare but occur in patients with emphysema.

Hemoptysis occurs in approximately 4–5% of biopsies. It is more common in patients with pulmonary hypertension and is often preceded by a cough. Hemoptysis usually resolves rapidly and rarely requires treatment, but, if massive, may be life threatening.

Air embolism is rare but should be considered if the patient breathes deeply and collapses. Coughing at the time of needle insertion suggests this possibility. Needles should always be removed during uncontrollable coughing to reduce this risk and also hemorrhage. Treatment includes administration of 100% oxygen, placement of the patient head down in a left lateral decubitus position, and transfer to a hyperbaric unit if available.

Pitfalls and Controversies

The yield in malignant disease is high (sensitivity of 90–95%) whether a fine-needle aspirate or cutting needle is used and even if the nodules are small. If no specific diagnosis is made, the biopsy should be repeated. This will enable an additional 5–10% of patients with undiagnosed but potentially curable malignancy to be identified.

The technique of fine-needle aspiration has been limited by a low rate of diagnosis of benign disease (sensitivity 20–50%), which has been improved (>70%) by obtaining core biopsies for histologic examination by use of coaxial systems and cutting needles, for example, in cryptogenic organizing pneumonia, Wegener's granulomatosis, and some infections.

Diagnostic difficulties still occur in lesions with a high level of fibrosis, for example, metastatic breast carcinoma and Hodgkin's disease. Excessive mucus production as in bronchoalveolar carcinoma can also interfere with the diagnosis.

Biopsy of a solitary mass with suspected malignancy in a patient who is potentially operable remains controversial. The argument against performance of a biopsy is that the patient still requires surgery, and, therefore, the management is not altered by the procedure. The advantages are that the patient is better informed and the operation is better planned and faster as frozen sections are avoided.

MEDIASTINAL BIOPSIES

Mediastinal biopsies can be performed by mediastinoscopy; thoracoscopy; anterior mediastinotomy; percutaneously, if

TABLE 15-2 Complications of Needle Biopsy	
Type	**Complication**
Early complications	Pneumothorax, 5–50% Hemoptysis, 5–10% Hemorrhage, 10–40% Air embolism, rare
Late complications	Tumor seeding, extremely rare Empyema Bronchopleural fistula
Increased risk of pneumothorax	If the patient has: • chronic obstructive pulmonary disease/bullae • uncontrollable coughing during the procedure • a small central lesion Or if: • multiple pleural passes are made • fissure is crossed • procedure is prolonged

the mediastinal mass abuts the chest wall anteriorly or posteriorly; or with a transesophageal approach for central subcarinal or aortopulmonary nodes.

Percutaneous Route

Techniques

Percutaneous mediastinal biopsies can be performed with CT or ultrasonographic (US) guidance. A contrast-enhanced CT examination is required to delineate the position of large vessels. For ultrasound-guided procedures, a 3.5–7.5 MHz curvilinear or linear probe is used to locate the lesion and identify a safe route; color Doppler is used to locate vessels.

Large mediastinal masses abutting the chest wall provide a biopsy route avoiding the lung parenchyma (Figure 15-8). A safe route may be provided with smaller masses by use of a transpleural approach through an existing effusion or

pneumothorax, or the patient can be positioned in the lateral decubitus position, which causes a slight shift of the mediastinum, providing an extrapulmonary route. An approach through an effusion can be created by injecting saline into the pleural space, or into the mediastinum, allowing access for large-bore extrapleural biopsy. These alternative approaches reduce the incidence of complications.

Either the single-needle or coaxial-needle technique is used. Core biopsies are necessary for primary mediastinal tumors, lymphomas, and thymomas.

Limitations and Complications

The extrapleural access to the target lesion often varies with breathing and may rarely result in inadvertent introduction of the biopsy needle into the lung/pleura. Breathing may cause small lesions to move out of the biopsy plane. Biopsy is

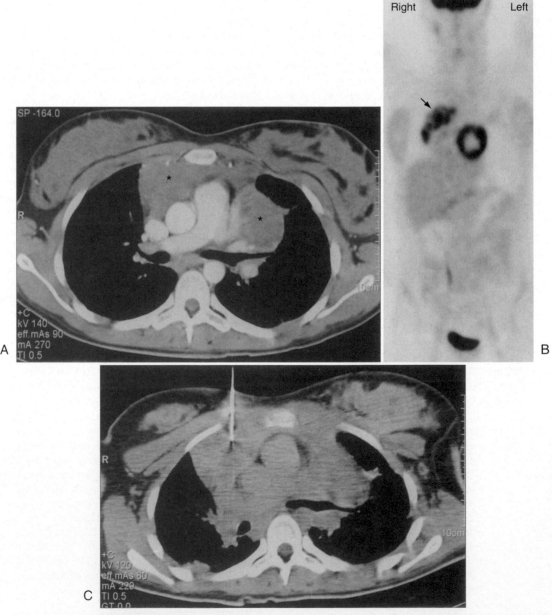

FIGURE 15-8 Mediastinal biopsy. **A,** Young patient with extensive mediastinal adenopathy after treatment for Hodgkin's disease. Note the right- and left-sided adenopathy *(asterisks)*. **B,** The PET scan guided the mediastinal biopsy, because activity was present in the right side of the mediastinal mass *(arrow)*. **C,** Actual biopsy under CT guidance. Recurrent Hodgkin's lymphoma was confirmed.

preferably carried out under CT guidance enabling a parasternal approach to avoid the internal mammary vessels, which could result in serious hemorrhage. A paravertebral approach may rarely injure paravertebral vessels, azygous vein, intercostal nerves and vessels, and spinal nerves.

Mediastinal Abscesses and Collections

Mediastinal abscess is a life-threatening condition with high mortality. Percutaneous aspiration or catheter drainage of mediastinal abscesses secondary to esophageal perforation may be a useful alternative to surgery. A Seldinger technique is used; a 17- or 18-gauge needle is introduced into the mediastinal abscess under CT guidance. After confirming its position, a guidewire is introduced through the needle, which is then removed and the tract dilated over the guidewire. The drain is then introduced over the guidewire. Usually 10–12 F drains are used. This technique is valuable in patients with advanced collections and if unfit for surgery.

PLEURAL AND CHEST WALL BIOPSIES

Pleural biopsies are performed under ultrasound guidance if there is an accompanying pleural effusion. Once the site of biopsy has been identified, the depth of the parietal pleura is judged by aspirating pleural fluid during administration of local anesthesia. The biopsy needle is placed half a centimeter proximal to the pleural fluid and then "fired," so that the core of tissue obtained will contain the full thickness of the pleura and the needle tip passes into the pleural fluid. Core biopsies are essential for pleural masses to differentiate mesothelioma from metastatic adenocarcinoma. Usually at least three to seven cores are obtained. If the pleura is not very thickened, multiple passes may be necessary. If there is no pleural fluid, the pleural biopsy is performed under CT guidance. The optimum route is one that runs along the main axis of the pathology (i.e., an oblique biopsy tract), allowing more of the lesion to be sampled but with less risk of a pneumothorax (Figure 15-9). Radiologists favor the 18-gauge Bard Biopty biopsy system or Temno cutting needles. Specimens are sent for microbiologic and histologic examination.

Image-guided cutting needle pleural biopsy has a sensitivity of 88%, specificity of 100%, and an overall accuracy of 91% for malignant disease.

EXTRATHORACIC BIOPSY

Lesions may be identified in the liver, adrenal glands, lymph nodes, or bones during staging of patients with bronchogenic carcinoma. If appearances suggest metastases (often with the aid of CT-PET scans), it is essential to perform a biopsy to confirm inoperability (Figure 15-10).

Biopsies of hepatic lesions are preferably performed under ultrasound guidance, where they are easily imaged and biopsy is rapid. Core biopsies are obtained.

Biopsies of adrenal lesions are usually performed under CT guidance (Figure 15-11). It may be necessary even then to traverse the hepatic or pulmonary parenchyma to enter the adrenal mass. If the mass is on the side opposite the primary carcinoma, the pulmonary parenchymal route should be avoided, because a pneumothorax could delay surgery.

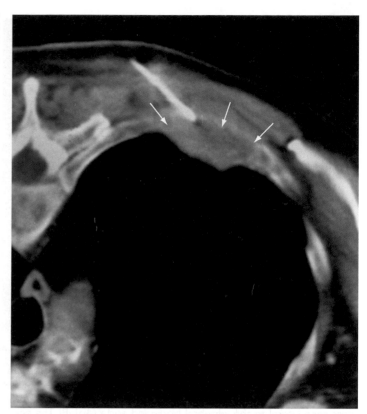

FIGURE 15-9 Biopsy of a rib metastasis. Non-small-cell carcinoma was confirmed on this "safe" biopsy, performed under CT guidance.

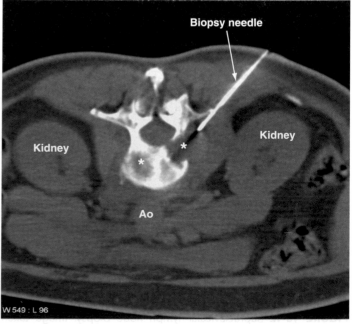

FIGURE 15-10 Biopsy of lytic vertebral body lesion (*) (Ao, Aorta).

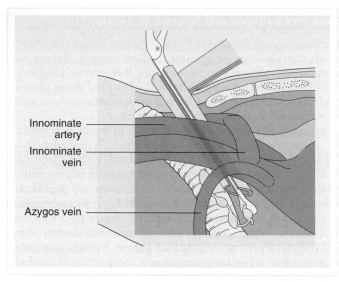

FIGURE 17-3 Path of the cervical mediastinoscope.

Anterior Mediastinotomy

Anterior mediastinotomy, also known as the Chamberlain procedure, is a technique that provides access to the anterior mediastinum. It is typically used to sample lymph nodes in the aortopulmonary window and paraaortic lymph nodes (stations 5 and 6, respectively, in the AJCC nomenclature). These nodal stations can also be accessed by extended cervical mediastinoscopy or left thoracoscopy. Although anterior mediastinotomy is to some extent more invasive than cervical mediastinoscopy, patients are usually able to leave the hospital on the same day of surgery.

Technique

A 3–4-cm transverse incision is usually made in the second interspace, just lateral to the lateral sternal border. The pectoral muscle can commonly be split in the line of its fibers without cutting through muscle. The intercostal muscle is then incised along the upper edge of the second costal cartilage. The internal mammary vessels, located medially, can usually be avoided and preserved. The mediastinal pleura is bluntly pushed laterally to avoid entry into the pleural space. The mediastinoscope is introduced to permit optimal lighting and visualization and obtain appropriate biopsies.

Occasionally, the mediastinal pleura is breached. A chest tube is generally not required if the visceral pleura has not been damaged. At the end of the procedure, a small catheter can be inserted into the pleural space through the mediastinotomy. The tube is pulled out once the overlying muscular tissues have been almost closed, with the anesthesiologist providing sustained positive-pressure ventilation to evacuate any residual intrapleural air.

Thoracoscopy

Minimally invasive access to the lung, pleural space, and mediastinum can be obtained by thoracoscopy. Also referred to as video-assisted thoracic surgery (VATS), this can be useful in the diagnosis of pleural pathology such as diffuse or focal thickening because of mesothelioma, pleural metastases, asbestos-related plaques, or benign inflammatory pleuritis. Thoracoscopy can also assist in the diagnosis and treatment of pleural fluid collections. In the staging of lung and esophageal cancer,

thoracoscopy can provide access, in a minimally invasive way, to the paratracheal, prevascular, aortopulmonary window, paraaortic, subcarinal, paraesophageal, and inferior pulmonary ligament lymph node groups (stations 2 to 9, respectively, in the AJCC nomenclature). Tumor invasion of local structures and overall resectability can also be assessed. Thoracoscopy is also used to obtain biopsies of lung tissue to assess discreet nodules or diffuse lung disease.

Thoracoscopy is most effectively done with single lung ventilation of the contralateral side by use of a double-lumen endotracheal tube or a bronchial blocker. This allows collapse of the lung on the operated side permitting adequate visualization and maneuverability within the pleural space. Dense pleural adhesions are, therefore, a contraindication for effective thoracoscopy as is the inability to tolerate single lung ventilation.

It should be noted that although thoracoscopy is a form of minimally invasive surgery, it remains a high-risk procedure when performed in high-risk patients. Of particular note are patients with interstitial lung disease requiring lung biopsy to tailor treatment options. These patients usually have severe respiratory compromise before thoracoscopy. They are sometimes already on mechanical ventilation, and a significant proportion of these patients have elevated pulmonary arterial pressures. In the experience published from the Mayo Clinic, patients with interstitial lung disease undergoing thoracoscopic lung biopsy had an operative mortality of just less than 6%.

Technique

Thoracoscopy is performed by use of single lung ventilation of the contralateral side. The patient is positioned in the lateral position similar to the positioning used for a posterolateral thoracotomy. When thoracoscopy is done for drainage and evaluation of a pleural effusion, a single 1-cm port is usually sufficient. It is placed in the sixth or seventh interspace in the anterior axillary line. Through this port, the camera and a thin suction tip or biopsy forceps can be introduced and maneuvered. For most other applications, one or two additional 1-cm ports are required and are commonly positioned separately along the fourth or fifth interspace, in the line of a potential posterolateral thoracotomy (Figure 17-4). In this

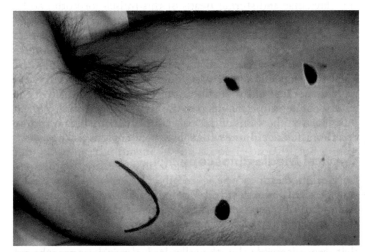

FIGURE 17-4 Location of thoracoscopic port sites. One port is placed at the seventh interspace in the anterior axillary line. Further ports may be required and are usually placed along the line of a potential posterolateral thoracotomy incision at the level of the fifth interspace.

way, conversion to thoracotomy simply requires extending the incision between these two upper port sites. The anterior port can be converted to a 5–7-cm "access" port for removal of a lobectomy specimen if the procedure requires conversion to a VATS lobectomy in the case of a biopsied lung nodule found to be an invasive primary lung cancer.

Whereas biopsy for diagnosis of interstitial lung disease requires only defining several areas of representative pathology, wedge resection of an indeterminate pulmonary nodule first necessitates precise localization of the lesion. This is usually done with the surgeon's finger introduced through one of the thoracoscopy incisions (Figure 17-5). It is clearly easier to locate larger and peripherally located lesions. Smaller or deeper lesions may not be accessible and may require conversion to open thoracotomy. Recent experience has been initially promising with radiotracer guidance (technetium 99m) to locate small pulmonary lesions not otherwise discernible thoracoscopically.

Once the area to be biopsied has been located, an endoscopic stapling device can be inserted through a thoracoport and used to perform a wedge resection (Figure 17-6). Once the specimen has been resected, it should be removed from the pleural cavity within an endoscopic specimen retrieval bag to avoid port site contamination. A more economical alternative is to use a surgical glove introduced through one of the port sites and held open with two Kelly clamps.

The biopsy specimen should be processed initially on a sterile back table in the operating room. In the case of diffuse lung infiltrates, the staple line can be excised and used for microbiology culture testing, whereas the remainder of the specimen is sent to pathology for histologic evaluation. When an indeterminate lung nodule is excised, a small portion should be kept for microbiology cultures should the evaluation of the rest of the nodule suggest a nonmalignant diagnosis.

After all biopsies have been taken, the pleural cavity should be reassessed for any bleeding or other injury. Special attention should be paid to the staple lines and port sites. Once hemostasis is ascertained, a single 28 Fr chest tube is introduced through the initial thoracoport in the seventh interspace anteriorly. It is guided posteriorly, and care is taken to avoid

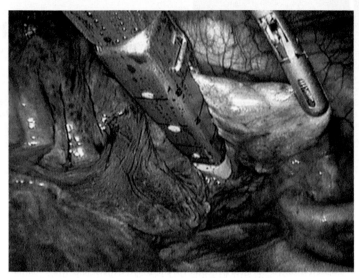

FIGURE 17-6 Use of endoscopic stapler during thoracoscopic surgery.

placement within the fissure. Barring a significant air leak, this tube can usually be removed within 12–24 h and the patient discharged from the hospital on the day after surgery.

Open Thoracotomy

Although open thoracotomy is a commonly performed procedure for thoracic surgeons, it is at the far end of the spectrum of morbidity for thoracic surgical procedures performed only for diagnostic purposes. It is, therefore, usually the least preferred option. There are, however, several situations in which this procedure is indicated and serves as the best diagnostic modality available. These include patients who, because of a fused pleural space or the inability to withstand single lung ventilation, cannot safely undergo thoracoscopy.

Frequently, patients referred for open lung biopsy are critically ill and have significant pulmonary compromise, often requiring mechanical ventilatory assistance. Although open lung biopsy is generally a very accurate diagnostic tool, most studies do not show a survival benefit in critically ill patients with diffuse lung disease even when a biopsy directs a change in therapy. Special care should be taken to assess the risk of such a procedure and its likely diagnostic yield in the specific patient's situation.

Technique

Usually, the patient undergoing thoracotomy for diagnostic purposes is placed in the lateral position, with both arms flexed forward at the shoulder. The incision is made transversely approximately one to two fingerbreadths beneath the scapular tip. This provides access to the fourth, fifth, or sixth interspace. Alternately, the patient is positioned supine, and an anterolateral thoracotomy is performed just beneath the mammary fold in the fourth or fifth interspace. As with the thoracoscopic approach, pulmonary resection is most commonly performed with the assistance of surgical stapling devices. At the end of the procedure, before closing the wound, a single 28 Fr chest tube is inserted through a separate incision in an interspace beneath the main thoracotomy incision. It is guided into the pleural space and positioned posteriorly. It will remain until drainage of air or fluid ceases.

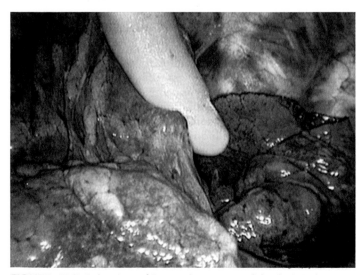

FIGURE 17-5 Palpation of intrapulmonary nodule during thoracoscopic surgery.

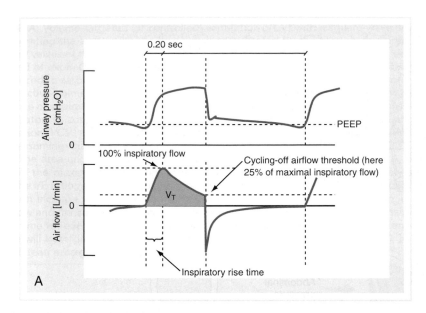

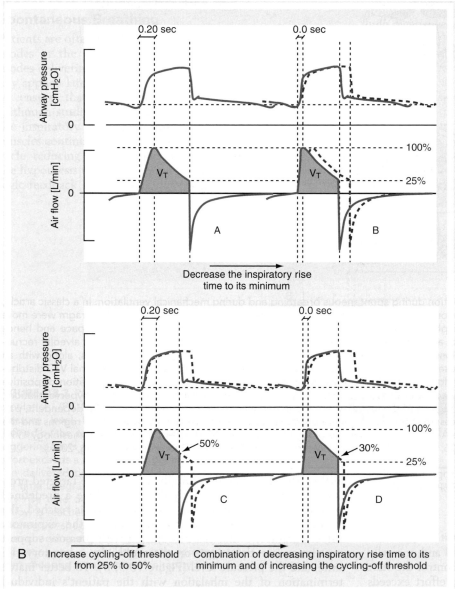

FIGURE 18-5 A, Pressure support ventilation (PSV). The delivered tidal volume (V_T) is calculated by integrating the area under the flow curve, as indicated by the blue shaded area. The inspiratory rise time defines how fast the maximal airflow (100%) is achieved. Thereafter, the inspiratory airflow continuously decreases because, once the pressure target is reached, maintaining this level requires progressively less air to flow into the lungs. As soon as the cycling-off airflow threshold (i.e., a preset percentage of maximal air flow) is reached, the ventilator ceases to deliver inspiratory flow, and the expiratory valve is opened to allow passive exhalation. **B,** Changes in the parameters of pressure support ventilation result in characteristic changes of the pressure and volume curves. Panels *A–D* demonstrate isolated changes of parameters assuming that all other ventilatory parameters and the mechanical characteristics of the respiratory system remain unchanged. *A,* PSV breath with an inspiratory rise time of 0.20 sec. *B,* After reducing the inspiratory rise time to its minimum, the peak inspiratory flow and consequently also the cycling-off airflow threshold are both reached earlier. Decreasing the inspiratory rise time results in a shorter inspiratory time while the V_T remains unchanged. Note that although the inspiratory rise time is decreased to 0 sec, the peak inspiratory flow is reached with a small delay. *C,* Increasing the cycling-off airflow threshold from 30% to 50% similarly shortens the inspiratory time; however, V_T decreases in this case. *D,* A combination of a maximal decrease in the inspiratory time and a moderate increase in the cycling-off airflow threshold shortens the inspiratory time, while the loss in V_T is only minimal. Such an approach can be used to achieve a prolongation of the expiratory time in patients at risk for dynamic hyperinflation because of expiratory flow limitation (e.g., patients with COPD; see also Figure 18-19).

Analogous to all pressure-targeted ventilation modes, pressure support ventilation does not guarantee a specific V_T or minute ventilation. Changes in V_T and minute ventilation can be achieved by adjusting the level of pressure support and/or the cycling-off criteria.

Difficulties with Conventional Modes of Assistance to Spontaneous Breathing

Although the use of assistance to spontaneous breathing early in the course of the disease process has a number of theoretical advantages, implementing such a strategy in clinical practice is not always easy. It is sometimes assumed that assisting spontaneous breathing will decrease respiratory effort; however, unless the ventilator settings are selected to satisfy the patient's demand, such a mode can actually result in the opposite. Ideally, assistance should be delivered in synchrony and in proportion to the patient's actual respiratory demand (i.e., both the timing and magnitude of the assist delivered by the ventilator are synchronized to the patient's inspiratory effort).

Whereas important improvements in the trigger-on characteristics and the cycling-off characteristics of ventilators have been made, ideal synchrony between the ventilator and the patient has not been achieved with most modes of ventilation and patient–ventilator asynchrony is common (Figure 18-6). Patient–ventilator asynchrony may result in increased inspiratory and expiratory muscle activity and may introduce an unnecessary burden in patients whose respiratory muscles are already under stress. Technologies that allow delivery of assistance in proportion to the patient's demand on a breath-by-breath basis have only recently been developed (see proportional assist ventilation [PAV] and neural adjusted ventilatory assist [NAVA] later).

Variables that can be adjusted to improve synchrony between the patient and the ventilator include the trigger-on threshold, the inspiratory rise time or flow rate, and the cycling-off airflow threshold. The mechanisms used to initiate

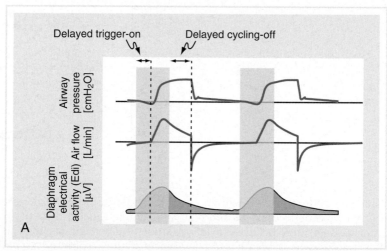

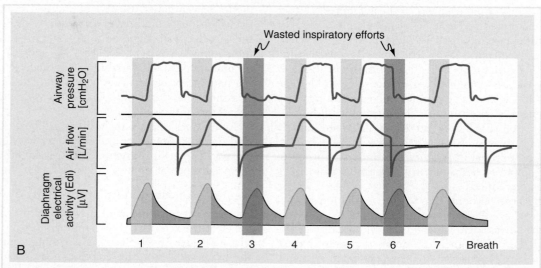

FIGURE 18-6 Examples of patient-ventilator asynchrony. **A,** Both the initiation and the termination of the assist delivered by the ventilator are delayed compared with the patient's respiratory demand, as reflected by the electrical activity of the diaphragm (*Edi*). Note that the neural expiration normally starts at approximately 70–80% of the maximum Edi. **B,** The ventilator delivers assist in response to the breathing efforts 1 and 2, whereas effort 3 fails to trigger the ventilator. Wasted inspiratory efforts frequently occur when settings for the trigger threshold are inadequate, when excessive inspiratory efforts are required because of auto-PEEP, when delay in cycling-off is excessive, or when the respiratory muscles are too weak to translate a neural inspiratory effort into an effective breath.

(Continued)

FIGURE 18-6 cont'd, C, Auto triggering may occur when the generation of airflow or negative pressure in the expiratory limb of the ventilatory circuit is not related to an inspiratory effort (e.g., transmission of pressure oscillations because of cardiac activity, leaks in the ventilator circuit). Auto triggering often occurs when the trigger-on threshold is set at a level that is too sensitive. **D,** Short cycles. Delivery of assist by the ventilator is prematurely terminated and immediately resumed as the patient makes an inspiratory effort. For example, short cycles may occur when the airflow is impeded by a high resistance within the ventilator circuit (e.g., secretion in the endotracheal tube or in the trachea) or when the patient actively blocks inspiratory airflow that might be delivered in excess of the patient's demand.

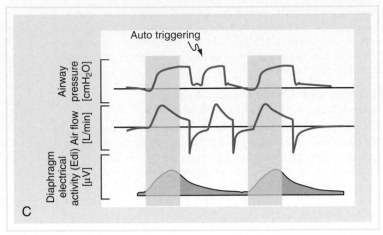

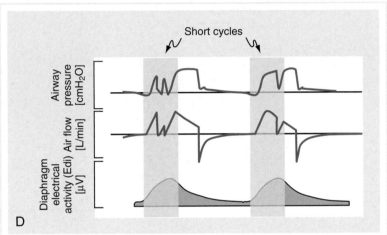

a breath (trigger-on) detect changes in airflow or in pressure in the ventilatory circuit. Hence, negative deflections of short duration (pneumatic trigger mechanisms) may be detectable in the airway pressure and/or flow tracings when a breath is triggered by the patient's effort. Delivery of the assistance is either terminated after a predefined time has elapsed (time-cycled) or after a prespecified cycling-off airflow threshold (flow-cycled) has been reached (see Figure 18-5). Rise time refers to the time required by the ventilator to increase the inspiratory airflow from zero to peak. As demonstrated in Figure 18-7, the rise time changes the slope of the pressure increase during early inspiration. Generally, rise time (or the inspiratory flow pattern) should be set to ensure that air is delivered rapidly (fast increase in airway pressure) after initiation of a breath. By establishing an optimal inspiratory rise time, synchrony to the patient's respiratory demand can be optimized and work of breathing can be reduced.

The fact that conventional modes of ventilation always deliver a uniform, predefined level of assist but do not take into account the physiologic variability of the breathing pattern stimulated the development of modes that deliver pressure assistance in proportion to the patient's demand: proportional assist ventilation (PAV) and neurally adjusted ventilatory assistance (NAVA).

Proportional Assist Ventilation (PAV)

PAV, the first patient-triggered mode that adapted the level of assist to the patient's inspiratory effort, was introduced in 1987. With PAV, the ventilator delivers positive pressure

throughout inspiration in proportion to the inspiratory airflow and volume generated by the patient (Figure 18-8). The magnitude of unloading is based on measuring elastance and resistance of the respiratory system. Whereas with conventional modes of ventilation the V_T or the delivered P_{VENT} are relatively constant from breath to breath, with PAV only the relationship between delivered P_{VENT} and the inspiratory effort of the patient is constant, whereas V_T and the delivered P_{VENT} become dependent variables. Although PAV requires that the patient always assumes a portion of the respiratory work, this mode has been demonstrated to effectively unload the respiratory muscles.

Limitations of PAV include the necessity to determine elastance and resistance of the respiratory system (a task that is not easy to perform in spontaneously breathing patients) and the occurrence of runaway phenomena at high levels of assist.

Neurally Adjusted Ventilatory Assist (NAVA)

A new strategy of mechanical ventilation termed *NAVA* uses the electrical activity of the diaphragm (Edi) to control the ventilator (Figure 18-9). Because breathing signals originate from the brain and reach the diaphragm by means of the phrenic nerves, Edi represents the neural respiratory effort both with respect to timing and to amplitude. Because during NAVA, positive pressure is applied to the airway opening in direct proportion to the Edi amplitude, defining a target pressure or volume is not required. The patient's respiratory control mechanisms, including feedback from mechanoreceptors and chemoreceptors, adjust the Edi and hence regulate the pressure and delivered

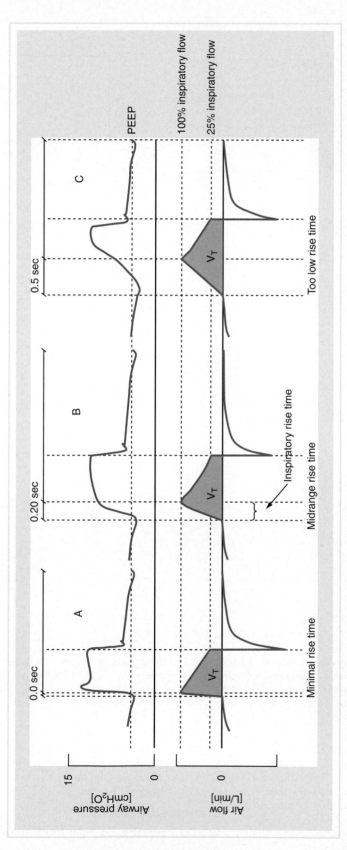

FIGURE 18-7 The rise time of the inspiratory flow is adjustable with most current ventilators. *A,* A pressure spike in early inspiration may indicate inspiratory flow in excess of the patient's demand or an obstruction in the central airways including the tracheal tube. *B,* No deformation of the inspiratory pressure waveform is visible with a midrange rise time. *C,* A concave deformation of the inspiratory pressure waveform indicates that the patient is making an inspiratory effort, because demand is higher than the flow provided by the ventilator. (Adapted from Branson RD, Campell RS: Respir Care 1998; 43:1045.)

FIGURE 18-8 Proportional assist ventilation (PAV) as volume assist. **A,** With PAV, the assist is delivered in proportion to inspiratory effort. The pressure delivered to the airways increases until the end of inspiration. **B,** An increase in volume assist results in a higher pressure delivered for the same tidal volume. Note that with PAV delivered as flow assist, the waveforms appear different, although the basic principles are very similar to PAV delivered as volume assist. (Adapted from Oczenski W [ed]. Atmen-Atemhilfen. Georg Thieme Verlag, 2006.)

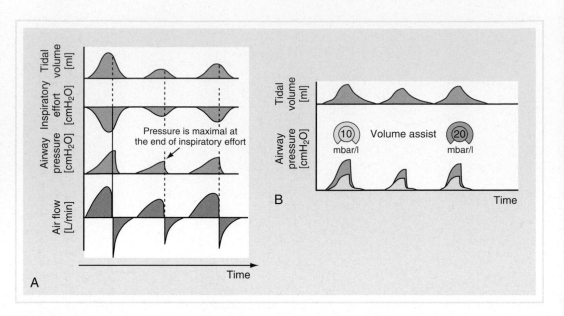

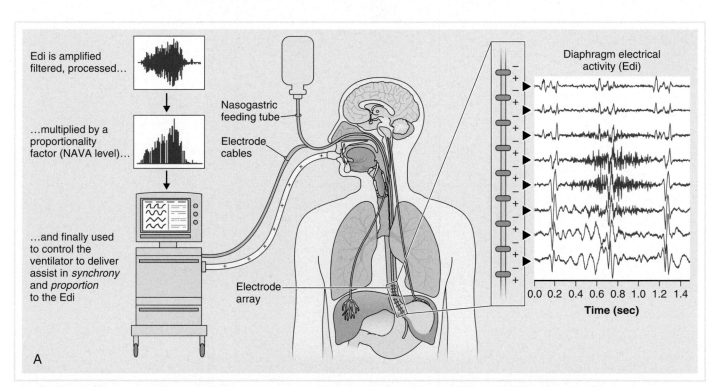

FIGURE 18-9 A, With neurally adjusted ventilatory assist (NAVA), the electrical activity of the diaphragm (Edi) is derived by use of an array of electrodes mounted on a nasogastric tube. The signals from each electrode pair on the array are differentially amplified, filtered, and multiplied by a proportionality factor (NAVA level) before the signal is used to control the pressure generated by the ventilator. Hence, with NAVA, the pressure delivered to the patient is synchronous and (virtually) instantaneously proportional to the patient's Edi. (Adapted from Sinderby C, et al. Nat Med 1999; 5[12]:1433–1436.)

volume. Animal data and one clinical study suggest that NAVA is applicable in the ICU environment, efficiently delivers assistance synchronous to the subject's demand, unloads the respiratory muscles, maintains gas exchange, and preserves cardiac performance during invasive ventilation and also during noninvasive ventilation even when an excessively leaky interface is used. NAVA does not require measurement of respiratory system mechanics, and run-away phenomena are unlikely.

PAV and NAVA both depend on the patient having an intact respiratory drive. Although the concept of delivering

assistance in proportion to the patient's demand is appealing, and although data from experimental and clinical studies are promising, these modes need to be tested in clinical trials to better define their indications and limitations.

Combined Modes

Airway Pressure Release Ventilation (APRV)

Airway pressure release ventilation (APRV) is a mode of mechanical ventilation that was introduced to improve oxygenation in spontaneously breathing patients (Figure 18-10).

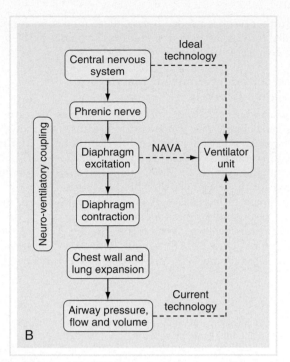

B

FIGURE 18-9 cont'd, B, Neuromechanical coupling and control of the ventilator. Chain of steps necessary to transform central respiratory drive into an inspiration (neuromechanical coupling) that ultimately results in delivery of assist by the ventilator (neuroventilator coupling). The current technology requires transmission of the electrical excitation into a contraction of the respiratory muscles (e.g., the diaphragm) and in generation of a pneumatic signal (pressure or flow at the airway opening) that is sufficient in magnitude to exceed the trigger-on threshold of a sensor within the ventilator. With neurally adjusted ventilatory assist (*NAVA*), the Edi is used to control the ventilator. Hence, with NAVA, control of the ventilator is independent of the force generated by the respiratory muscles and is also independent of leaks in the ventilator circuit. (Adapted from Sinderby C, *et al*: Nat Med 1999; 5:1433–1436.)

With APRV, the pressure in the ventilator circuit alternates between a high and a lower level (normally the high pressure level is of longer duration than the lower pressure level) and spontaneous breathing is allowed in any phase of the cycle. The high- and low-pressure levels, the rate of change between the two levels, the respiratory system compliance, and the airway resistance to flow are the main determinants of the "mechanical ventilation" portion with APRV, whereas the complementary "spontaneous breathing" portion mainly depends on the patient's respiratory drive. In contrast to continuous positive airway pressure (CPAP), APRV interrupts P_{VENT} briefly to augment spontaneous minute ventilation and thereby increases alveolar ventilation and CO_2 removal without increasing the work of breathing. Spontaneous efforts during APRV are not actively assisted except for those breaths that happen to occur during the change from the lower to the upper pressure level. Total minute ventilation with APRV is the sum of the mechanical, pressure-controlled ventilation and the complementary spontaneous breathing. APRV *without* spontaneous breathing is essentially the same as PCV.

APRV has a number of interesting features. First, APRV overcomes shortcomings inherent in many modes of assisted spontaneous breathing related to triggering-on and cycling-off the ventilator by simply avoiding inspiratory and expiratory valves in the ventilator circuit. However, the time-cycled release and reestablishment of the high P_{VENT} is not synchronized to the patient's breathing efforts and, therefore, may result in patient–ventilator asynchrony. Second, the application of CPAP recruits some atelectatic areas, increases lung volume, and allows spontaneous breathing to occur on a portion of the pressure/volume curve where impedance to airflow is low and only a small transpulmonary pressure change is required to produce the V_T. Third, APRV maintains P_{VENT} at high levels for a prolonged time. As alveoli are continually recruited along the inspiratory limb of the pressure/volume curve, recruitment may be more efficient with APRV than

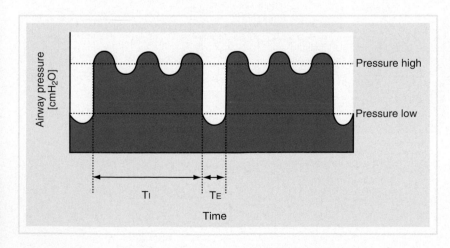

FIGURE 18-10 With airway pressure release ventilation (APRV), two levels of continuous positive airway pressure are delivered by the ventilator. The high pressure level is maintained until the inspiratory time (T_I) has elapsed; the pressure is then changed to the lower pressure level, usually for a short period of time (T_E, typically 0.5–1.5 sec), before the high-pressure level is resumed. The duration of T_I and T_E is defined by the caregiver. Spontaneous breathing is allowed in any phase of the cycle. Because the pressure release periods are of short duration, a residual expiratory positive airway pressure (intrinsic PEEP) will be maintained in the lung compartments with a high time constant (slow passive exhalation), preventing end-expiratory collapse of these lung regions. While preventing end-expiratory collapse of the lungs, this helps improve oxygenation as a result of a better match between ventilation and perfusion, periodic release of the airway pressure assists in removal of carbon dioxide.

with shorter application of positive pressure (e.g., with pressure support ventilation).

Bilevel Positive Airway Pressure (BiPAP) Ventilation

With BiPAP ventilation, two levels of continuous positive pressure are used similar to APRV, and unrestricted spontaneous breathing is allowed on both pressure levels (Figure 18-11, *A*). Optionally, assistance to spontaneous breathing efforts can be provided at the lower pressure level (Figure 18-11, *B*), at the higher pressure level, or at both levels. The transition from the low-pressure to the high-pressure level is coordinated with the patient's breathing effort. The abbreviations Bi-Vent, DuoPAP, and Bi-level used by ventilator manufacturers are synonymous to BiPAP.

Despite the theoretical advantages of APRV and BiPAP, trials showing clinically relevant benefits are currently lacking and further work is needed before these modes can be recommended for specific patient conditions or phases in the process of mechanical ventilation.

Synchronized Intermittent Mandatory Ventilation (SIMV)

SIMV combines volume- or pressure-targeted breaths at a caregiver-defined rate (mandatory breaths) with unassisted spontaneous breathing (Figure 18-12). Because ideally the mandatory breaths should be synchronized to the patient's own breathing effort, SIMV requires that the ventilator settings for the trigger-on threshold are adequate.

The main differences between SIMV and BiPAP are that SIMV does not allow spontaneous breathing during the mandatory breaths, whereas spontaneous breathing is possible during all phases with BiPAP; as well, with SIMV, all mandatory breaths are volume- or pressure-targeted, whereas BiPAP

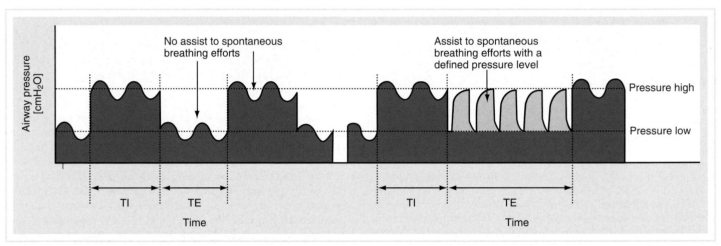

FIGURE 18-11 A, With bi-level positive airway pressure (BiPAP) ventilation, two levels of continuous positive airway pressure are delivered by the ventilator. The pressure levels and the relationship between T_I and T_E are both defined by the caregiver. **B,** Delivery of assist to individual spontaneous breathing efforts is optional and can be combined with BiPAP to compensate for the additional inspiratory work imposed by the flow resistance of the endotracheal tube. Of note, changes between the lower and the higher pressure levels are synchronized to the patient's efforts. The major difference between BiPAP and APRV is the longer duration at the low-pressure level with BiPAP, and hence a higher probability of derecruitment of lung regions. (Adapted from Oczenski W [ed]. Atmen-Atemhilfen. Georg Thieme Verlag, 2006.)

FIGURE 18-12 Synchronized intermittent mandatory ventilation (SIMV) with unassisted spontaneous breathing between two volume-targeted breaths. Within a short period before starting the next mandatory breath, a trigger window allows synchronization of the controlled breath to the patient's breathing effort. When the patient's breathing effort does not exceed the trigger-on threshold during this trigger window, the ventilator will deliver a mandatory breath (either volume or pressure targeted as defined by the caregiver) after the maximal time interval for intermittent mandatory ventilation (*IMV*) has elapsed. This time interval is defined by the preset rate for IMV. (Adapted from Oczenski W [ed]. Atmen-Atemhilfen. Georg Thieme Verlag, 2006.)

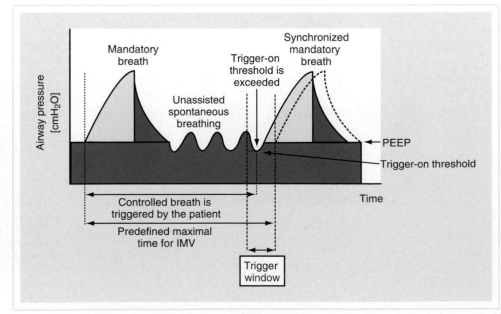

provides only pressure-targeted breaths. Despite its name, similar concerns regarding the delivery of ventilator assistance in synchrony and in proportion to the patients demand as with all pneumatically triggered modes of mechanical ventilation apply for SIMV.

Pressure-Regulated Volume Control (PRVC) and Volume Support (VS)

These modes use either a pressure-targeted ventilation (for PRVC) or a pressure support ventilation (for VS) to achieve a predefined V_T. Basically, both modes first deliver a test breath at a low-pressure level, measure the achieved V_T, and calculate the necessary adjustments in the inspiratory pressure to achieve the targeted V_T in the subsequent breath. The same procedure is repeated for every breath. It has been suggested that these modes might be useful in weaning the patient from the ventilator on the basis of the rationale that the stronger the respiratory muscles (e.g., the higher the share of the V_T produced by the inspiratory effort of the patient) the lower the level of assistance needed by the ventilator. The major concern with both PRVC and VS is that if the patient's breathing efforts increase because of an increased respiratory demand (e.g., hypoxemia, fever, increased metabolism), the level of assistance will paradoxically decrease. Also, spontaneous breathing patterns in critically ill patients are often highly variable, and the required V_T may vary on a breath-by-breath basis. Again, PRVC and VS are designed such that the level of assist paradoxically decreases during periods of high demand, and vice versa.

Modes That Facilitate Spontaneous Breathing

Continuous Positive Airway Pressure (CPAP)

With CPAP, a caregiver-defined level of positive pressure is maintained by the ventilator while the patient is breathing spontaneously (Figure 18-13). Of note, because the patient's breathing efforts are not assisted with CPAP, the patient must have adequate respiratory drive and adequate respiratory muscle function. CPAP helps to increase and maintain the functional residual capacity (FRC) and, hence, to increase the lung units available for gas exchange (reduction of intrapulmonary right-to-left shunt), prevent end-expiratory airway collapse, and counter the effects of auto-PEEP or intrinsic PEEP.

Positive End-Expiratory Pressure (PEEP)

PEEP refers to the airway pressure (relative to atmospheric pressure) at the end of a breath. PEEP can be applied with most ventilation modes. Patients with respiratory failure from asthma or chronic obstructive pulmonary disease who require mechanical ventilation have increases in functional residual capacity (FRC), and alveolar pressure at the end of exhalation that exceeds atmospheric pressure (i.e., auto-PEEP or intrinsic PEEP), thereby increasing the inspiratory work of breathing (in a spontaneously breathing patient). Applying PEEP counters the effect of auto-PEEP on work of breathing. Patients with the acute respiratory distress syndrome (ARDS), acute lung injury (ALI), or hypoxemic respiratory failure from obesity have a reduced FRC that leads to alveolar and/or airway collapse. In these patients, PEEP is used to restore FRC, to recruit regions with collapsed alveoli or airways, to prevent derecruitment of open alveoli, to redistribute fluid within the lung, and to make dependent lung regions available for ventilation. All these effects can improve the match between ventilation and perfusion, improve oxygen saturation, and decrease the need for high fractions of inspired oxygen.

Prevention of cyclic, partial lung collapse at the end of exhalation with PEEP also allows breathing to occur within a more favorable range of the pressure-volume curve, and thereby to reduce the work of breathing.

PEEP has also been used in patients with flail chest to stabilize the chest wall.

All of the aforementioned beneficial effects of PEEP are lost and adverse or even harmful effects may occur when excessive levels of PEEP are used. For example, excessive PEEP may increase dead space by overdistending alveoli and concomitantly decreasing alveolar capillary blood flow or may add to the hyperinflation of the lungs in patients with COPD or asthma. High levels of PEEP may reduce pulmonary blood flow by impeding venous return, thereby increasing pulmonary vascular resistance (i.e., decreasing cardiac output in the face of constant pulmonary arterial and venous pressure translates to an increased pulmonary vascular resistance). If pulmonary vascular pressures are kept constant relative to the level of PEEP, however (as will be the case unless cardiac output decreases), the effect of increasing lung volume on pulmonary vascular resistance is small. Of note, the effects of PEEP on cardiac performance are more pronounced during hypovolemia and can partially be reversed by ensuring adequate intravascular fluid volume.

In the past, PEEP was used mainly to increase oxygenation, thereby improving oxygen transport; however, there has been a change in the rationale underlying the use of PEEP, with a greater focus on its use to minimize cyclic airspace opening and closing (i.e., atelectrauma) and hence to decrease ventilator-induced lung injury, rather than simply to improve oxygenation.

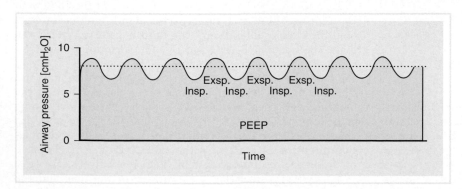

FIGURE 18-13 With continuous positive airway pressure (CPAP), a caregiver-defined level of pressure within the ventilatory circuit is maintained. Changes in the airway pressure because of inspiration and expiration are constantly compensated for by pressure generated by the ventilator.

TABLE 18-1 Combinations of Inspiratory Oxygen Fraction (FiO_2) and Positive End-Expiratory Pressure (PEEP) in Patients with Acute Lung Injury or Acute Respiratory Distress Syndrome to Achieve the Oxygenation Goals*

FiO_2	PEEP (cmH_2O)
0.3	5
0.4	5
0.4	8
0.5	8
0.5	10
0.6	10
0.7	10
0.7	12
0.7	14
0.8	14
0.9	14
0.9	16
0.9	18
1.0	18
1.0	20
1.0	22
1.0	24

* Partial pressure of arterial oxygen (PaO_2) of 55–80 mmHg or oxyhemoglobin saturation measured by pulse oximetry (SpO_2) of 88%–95%. (Adapted from ARDSnet, *N Engl J Med* 2000; 342:1301–1308.)

Given the current lack of tools to monitor both alveolar overdistention and collapse, and given the heterogeneity of the distribution of most disease processes within the lung, identification of the "best PEEP" level is not straightforward in clinical practice, and, in fact, the gravitational gradient in pleural pressure and end-expiratory lung volume that exists in both normal subjects and patients requiring mechanical ventilation implies that there cannot be a single level of PEEP that is "best" for all regions of the lung. Pending further clarification, a pragmatic approach for daily clinical practice in patients with ALI is to adhere to the algorithm used in the large ARDSnet trial (Table 18-1) and to carefully observe the effect of changes in PEEP on parameters such as blood oxygenation, cardiac performance, and expiratory flow limitation. Of note, in patients with stiff chest walls (e.g., massive ascites), higher levels of PEEP are warranted.

PRINCIPLES OF RESPIRATORY SYSTEM MECHANICS RELEVANT TO MECHANICAL VENTILATION

Adjusting ventilator parameters to the patient's individual condition and interpreting pressure and airflow tracings requires an understanding of the fundamental principles of respiratory system mechanics in ventilated patients. Although these general principles apply to the entire respiratory system, regional inhomogeneities (e.g., lower end-expiratory lung volumes, airway closure, and/or atelectasis in dependent regions) and regional differences in disease processes result in ventilation is never distributed uniformly within the lungs in mechanically ventilated patients. The compliance of a specific alveolar region and the resistance of the associated airways ultimately determine the portion of the V_T received by a particular lung region.

Airway Resistance and Lung Elastance

To a simplified approximation, the patient–ventilator can be considered as an in-series mechanical system that consists of a resistive element (semiflexible ventilator tubing + rigid endotracheal tubing + flexible central airways) and an elastic element (lung-thorax compartment). During inflation, the pressure applied to the tube inlet (P_{VENT}) is equal to the sum of the pressure required to overcome the resistive elements (P_{RESIST}) and the pressure required to distend the lung and chest wall (P_{ELAST}). The flow through the resistive element is a function of the difference in pressure between the tube inlet and the tube outlet (P_{RESIST}) and the resistance of the tubing system (i.e., flow [L/min] = P_{RESIST} [cmH_2O]/resistance [$cmH_2O \times min/L$]). For example, forcing air at a low flow rate through a large-bore tube requires less pressure than if a high flow is applied to a small bore tube. Because P_{RESIST} is used to overcome the resistive element, only P_{ELAST} is applied across the respiratory system (i.e., the lungs and the chest wall). Figure 18-14 demonstrates the relationship between P_{VENT} and the pressure within the central airways (P_{AW}) throughout a respiratory cycle.

P_{ELAST} is made up of two components: the pressure required to distend the lung and the pressure required to distend the chest wall (which includes both the ribcage and the diaphragm and, as such, includes the abdomen). The elastance (1/Compliance = Applied pressure [P_{ELAST}] divided by the applied V_T) of the chest wall (E_{CW}) and of the lung (E_L) are mechanically in series, and their sum equals the elastance of the entire respiratory system (E_{RS}). In clinical practice, P_{VENT} measured either at the airway opening or in the ventilator circuit is considered to be the "driving pressure," and P_{VENT} is usually used to assess the propensity for induction of VILI. Such an approach has important shortcomings, however, and might be misleading. P_{VENT} is referenced to ambient pressure and, therefore, reflects the pressure gradient across the entire respiratory system (i.e., across both the lung and the chest wall). The key variable defining the degree of lung distention and the propensity for induction of VILI, however, is only the pressure across the lung (i.e., the transpulmonary pressure [P_L]).

The relative stiffness (or elastance) of the lung and the chest wall define what proportion of P_{AW} is used to distend the chest wall and what proportion is used to distend the lung (Figure 18-15). For example, if the elastance of the chest wall is twice that of the lung, then two thirds of P_{AW} is used to distend the chest wall and only one third is used to distend the lung. The fractions E_L/E_{RS} and E_{CW}/E_{RS} determine how P_{AW} is apportioned between the lung ($P_L = P_{AW} \times E_L/E_{RS}$) and the chest wall ($P_{CW} = P_{AW} \times E_{CW}/E_{RS}$). Predicting P_L on the basis of P_{AW} without information on the elastance of the lung and the chest wall is not possible. Furthermore, lung and chest wall elastance vary among individuals and may also change over time during critical illness (e.g., with accumulation of edema or ascites). Although calculating the elastance of the entire respiratory system (E_{RS}) is relatively easy ($E_{RS} = P_{VENT}/V_T$), calculating the elastance of the lung and the

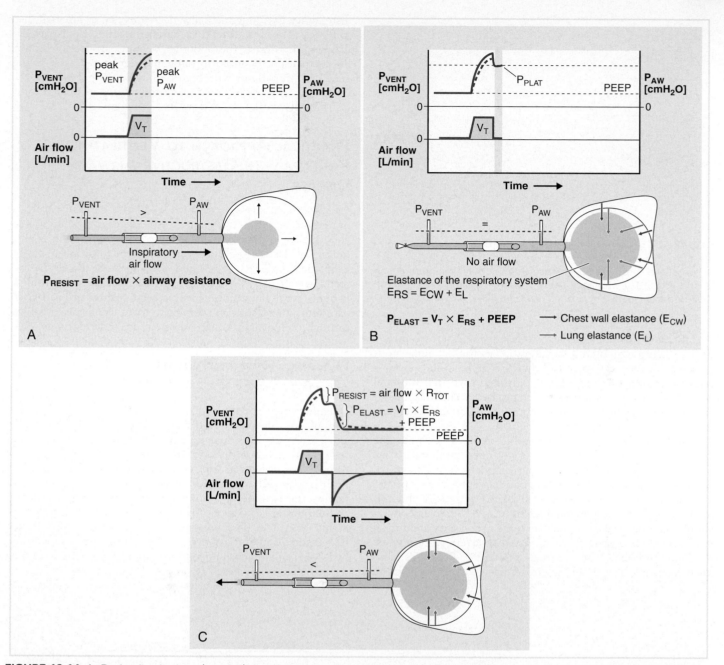

FIGURE 18-14 A, During inspiration, the ventilator generates pressure (P_{VENT}) to force a predefined volume of air (V_T) in a predefined time into the lungs of the patient. The pressure loss over the total resistance of the endotracheal tube and of the central airways (P_{RESIST}) defines what proportion of the P_{VENT} reaches the central airways (P_{AW}). **B,** Because the pressure within the respiratory system and the central airways equilibrates when the inspiratory and expiratory valves are closed, assessment of the respiratory system elastance (E_{RS}) is possible during an end-inspiratory hold. For a given V_T, the E_{RS} defines the plateau pressure (P_{PLAT}) at the end of inspiration. Note that because of the inhomogeneity of the time constants among different lung regions, the duration of the end-inspiratory plateau (normally approximately 10% of the breath cycle) is often too short for sufficient equilibration of the pressure across all lung regions. Hence, an end-inspiratory hold of longer duration (e.g., >5 sec) is necessary to adequately assess respiratory system mechanics. **C,** The expiration is passive (not actively supported by the ventilator) and driven only by the elastic recoil of the lungs and the chest wall.

chest wall separately is unfortunately not straightforward and requires knowledge of P_L. Figure 18-16 illustrates the intrabreath changes in P_L during unassisted spontaneous breathing and during volume-targeted ventilation.

P_L equals the difference between the alveolar pressure (P_{ALV}) and the pleural pressure (P_{PL}). Because P_{VENT} closely approximates P_{ALV} during an end-inspiratory and end-expiratory airway occlusion, P_L can be calculated as $P_L = P_{VENT} - P_{PL}$ after performing an occlusion of the airways. Because direct

measurement of P_{PL} is invasive, and because the pressure in the lower one third of the esophagus closely approximates the pressure of the adjacent pleura, measurement of P_{es} (by means of inflatable latex balloons) can be used to estimate P_{PL}. Hence, P_L can be estimated as $P_L = P_{VENT} - P_{es}$ (with a number of caveats such as the effect of mediastinal weight on P_{es} in a supine patient, gravitational gradients, and spatial heterogeneity of P_{PL}). Accordingly, the use of Pes to approximate P_{PL} is not widely used currently in routine clinical practice.

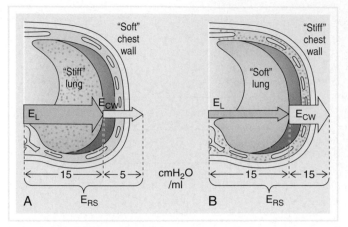

FIGURE 18-15 The total respiratory system elastance (E_{RS}) equals the sum of its components: E_{RS} = elastance of the lungs (E_L) + elastance of the chest wall (E_{CW}). The same E_{RS} may arise from a high E_L and a low E_{CW} elastance **(A)** or from identical E_L and E_{CW} **(B)**. (Adapted from Gattinoni L, et al: Crit Care 2004, 8:350–355.)

Patients with ALI or ARDS may have an increase in E_{RS} that is mainly attributed to an alteration in the E_L. Some studies suggest, however, that the increase in E_L results from a large portion of the lung being fluid-filled such that the tidal volume delivered now fills the ventilated lung to a higher end-inspiratory lung volume (requiring a higher distending pressure, which is reflected in a greater E_L). An increase in E_{RS} could also be due to an increase in the E_{CW}. Of note, the chest wall in this context comprises not only the thoracic cage but also its caudal boundary, the diaphragmatic-abdominal compartment. E_{CW} is increased in patients with severe obesity, chest wall injury, surgical dressings, ascites, and major abdominal surgery. For example, in a patient with ALI associated with abdominal surgery, E_{CW} may increase when intraabdominal hypertension (e.g., bowel edema, ascites) develops, even when the lung mechanics are normal. Assuming P_{VENT} remains unchanged in the patient described previously, the pressure

distending the lung actually decreases as a greater share of P_{VENT} is used to distend the chest wall (i.e., to displace the diaphragm towards the abdomen). Thus, arbitrarily limiting P_{VENT} to a specific uniform value may not be necessary to prevent VILI in patients with high E_{CW} but may potentially even cause harm by leading to marked reductions in tidal volume, insufficient ventilation, and severe hypoxemia.

PRACTICAL APPROACH TO VENTILATING PATIENTS WITH OBSTRUCTIVE AIRWAY DISEASE

An increase in airway resistance leading to expiratory airflow limitation and gas trapping is the major pathophysiologic abnormality in patients with asthma or COPD. With healthy lungs, the elastic recoil forces are sufficient to promote passive exhalation until FRC is reached. Partial loss of the elastic lung recoil in patients with COPD further aggravates this problem. Patients with limitation of expiratory airflow often activate expiratory muscles in an attempt to force the inspired volume through the partially collapsed or constricted central airways.

DYNAMIC HYPERINFLATION AND AUTO-PEEP

Dynamic hyperinflation occurs when expiratory flow has not emptied alveoli to their resting FRC valves by the end of exhalation. The residual positive pressure within the lungs referenced to atmospheric pressure or to PEEP applied through a ventilator is referred to as auto-PEEP (or as intrinsic PEEP). Although auto-PEEP usually implies dynamic hyperinflation, the two are not synonymous, because lung volume at end-expiration can be normal when expiratory muscles are highly activated. The presence of auto-PEEP results in the underestimation of mean pressure within the lung as measured by P_{VENT}, and hence in misinterpretation, if assessment of lung mechanics is solely based on P_{VENT}.

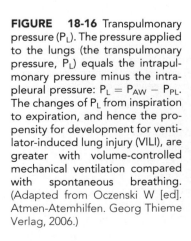

FIGURE 18-16 Transpulmonary pressure (P_L). The pressure applied to the lungs (the transpulmonary pressure, P_L) equals the intrapulmonary pressure minus the intrapleural pressure: $P_L = P_{AW} - P_{PL}$. The changes of P_L from inspiration to expiration, and hence the propensity for development for ventilator-induced lung injury (VILI), are greater with volume-controlled mechanical ventilation compared with spontaneous breathing. (Adapted from Oczenski W [ed]. Atmen-Atemhilfen. Georg Thieme Verlag, 2006.)

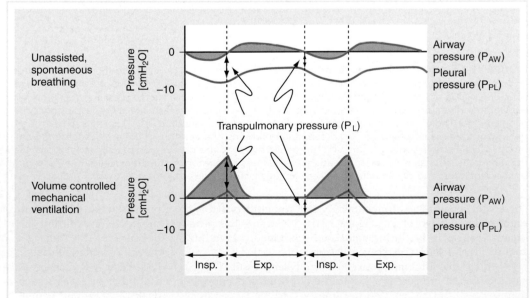

Classically, dynamic hyperinflation is present in patients with COPD, where the unstable airways collapse during exhalation (Figure 18-17), and in patients with asthma, where increased bronchomotor tone impedes exhalation. Exacerbation of the disease process such as bronchospasm in asthma or bronchitis with thickening of the mucosa in COPD worsens the condition. Of note, auto-PEEP may also develop in patients with more restrictive disease processes such as ARDS where intrapulmonary time constants are widely inhomogeneous or when low V_T at high ventilatory rates are used. A narrow diameter or kinked endotracheal tube, inspissated secretions, an obstructed filter in the expiratory limb of the ventilatory circuit, a highly variable respiratory rate, or tachypnea further predispose to the development of auto-PEEP.

Persistent airflow at the end of exhalation, especially in combination with consistent failure to trigger the ventilator with inspiratory efforts, should heighten the suspicion of the presence of dynamic hyperinflation. Measurement of auto-PEEP requires equilibration of the pressure across the entire lung during occlusion of the expiratory valve at end-expiration (Figure 18-18), ideally performed during muscle paralysis (but paralysis should not usually be undertaken solely to make this measurement). Measurement of auto-PEEP during spontaneous breathing is difficult and often unreliable, because the inspiratory and expiratory efforts interfere with the procedure, and studies have shown that expiratory muscle contraction can occur. These contractions may be difficult to detect clinically.

Dynamic hyperinflation can markedly increase the oxygen cost of breathing in a spontaneously breathing patient (Figure 18-19). Because the compliance of the respiratory system is lower at high lung volumes, more energy is required to expand the lungs. Furthermore, with dynamic hyperinflation the patient needs to produce large pleural pressure swings to overcome the auto-PEEP before pressure in the ventilator circuit decreases below the applied PEEP level and before pneumatic trigger systems located in the ventilator can be excited. Because generation of force by the inspiratory muscles is impaired during hyperinflation (decreased resting length of the diaphragm requires a higher than normal respiratory drive to lower pleural pressure), triggering the ventilator becomes challenging for patients with COPD and especially for those who have weakness or fatigue of the respiratory muscles (both of which are difficult to distinguish from the effects of trying to inhale at near-TLC).

Dynamic hyperinflation increases resistance of the inferior vena cava and increases pleural and juxtacardiac pressures, thereby impeding venous return to the right atrium leading to a decrease in cardiac output. For example, in patients with obstructive airway disease, the combination of sedative and paralytic agents with auto-PEEP may add to the markedly reduced arterial blood pressure frequently seen after tracheal intubation and institution of positive-pressure ventilation. In the presence of auto-PEEP, absolute (as opposed to relative) cardiac filling pressures may be elevated, leading to the false interpretation that the ventricular filling is adequate or even high, whereas, in fact, transmural cardiac pressures (and hence end-diastolic volumes) are low because intrathoracic pressure is also elevated. Recognition that auto-PEEP and not cardiac dysfunction is the main cause of impaired cardiac performance under such circumstances is important, because treatment strategies are markedly different.

Inappropriate settings during mechanical ventilation can worsen dynamic hyperinflation, especially when high ventilatory rates and/or high V_T resulting in excessive minute ventilation are used, when the assist is delivered asynchronous to the patient's demand (Figure 18-20), or when PEEP levels higher than those needed to counterbalance auto-PEEP are used.

The main goals in ventilating a patient with obstructive airway disease are to maintain adequate gas exchange and to decrease the oxygen cost of breathing, while simultaneously minimizing iatrogenic complications such as barotrauma (e.g., pneumothorax), worsening dynamic hyperinflation, and inducing respiratory muscle weakness because of excessive rest or drug-related myopathy (e.g., corticosteroids and neuromuscular blocking agents). The first approach to minimizing dynamic hyperinflation is to decrease the resistance in the expiratory airways by removing any mechanical obstruction in the airways (including the ventilator circuit) and by treating bronchospasm and airway inflammation. The most effective and abrupt way to decrease auto-PEEP is to reduce minute ventilation, although this may lead to an increase in an already elevated arterial PCO_2 ($PaCO_2$). Alternatively, adding extrinsic PEEP (Figure 18-21) will abruptly and markedly decrease the work of breathing, thereby reducing CO_2 production and lowering the $PaCO_2$ even if alveolar ventilation is unchanged. Because patients with COPD with chronically elevated $PaCO_2$ levels retain sufficient bicarbonate to normalize arterial pH, minute ventilation should not be adjusted to maintain a normal $PaCO_2$. In addition, the inspiratory phase should be shortened (thereby allowing maximum time for exhalation) as demonstrated in Figures 18-19 and 18-20. Of note, the variability in the duration of the expiratory phase and, hence, in the expired volume per breath increases when switching from a controlled mode of ventilation to a mode that delivers assistance to spontaneous breathing. This may result in modification of the degree of dynamic hyperinflation on a breath-by-breath basis and can induce patient–ventilator asynchrony because of wasted inspiratory efforts, especially when high levels of assist are used (see Figure 18-6).

The principles of a ventilatory strategy in acute asthma are very similar to those described previously. Adjusting the ventilatory rate to low frequencies while accepting hypercapnic acidosis (a pH of as low as 7.20) is normally well tolerated in these patients, and such an approach helps minimize hyperinflation.

PRACTICAL APPROACH TO VENTILATING PATIENTS WITH RESTRICTIVE PULMONARY DISEASE

A decrease in lung compliance and in FRC is the major pathophysiologic abnormality in patients with restrictive pulmonary disease processes such as pulmonary fibrosis, interstitial pneumonias, sarcoidosis, bronchiolitis obliterans organizing pneumonia, and those with ALI and ARDS.

The challenge in ventilating patients with restrictive diseases is to provide adequate oxygenation, while at the same time not causing further lung injury. Although mechanical ventilation clearly leads to improved survival in patients with ALI/ARDS, the ability to improve survival in patients with other restrictive processes (particularly idiopathic pulmonary fibrosis) is limited at best. The approach is one of maintaining adequate oxygenation while trying not to overinflate the lung at end-inhalation (see later).

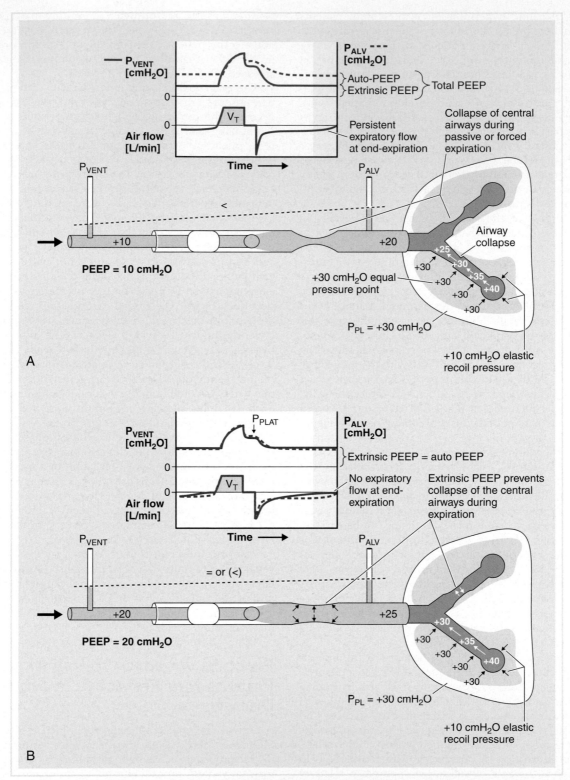

FIGURE 18-17 A, Ideally there is no airflow at the end of the expiration, and hence alveolar pressure (P_{ALV}) is in equilibrium with the pressure in the ventilator (P_{VENT}), and the respiratory system has returned to its functional residual capacity (FRC). Unstable airways collapse during passive or during forced expiration when the pressure surrounding the airways exceeds the intraluminal pressure, resulting in expiratory flow limitation. Consequently, air may be trapped within the lung, and a pressure gradient between the alveoli (P_{ALV}) and the ventilator circuit (P_{VENT}) may be established (auto-PEEP) if the expiratory phase is too short to allow complete exhalation. **B,** Application of extrinsic PEEP partially counters the collapse of the airways, reduces the resistance to expiratory airflow, and may help with triggering of the ventilator by the patient. Note that peak and plateau pressure did not change, because extrinsic PEEP partially replaced auto-PEEP without adding to it. Note that expiratory flow may be impeded when an extrinsic PEEP level in excess of the auto-PEEP level is used.

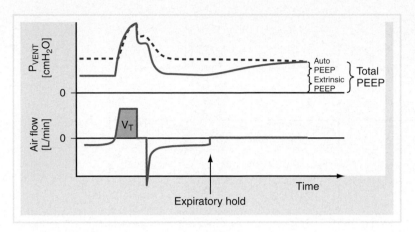

FIGURE 18-18 Expiratory hold technique to estimate the level of auto-PEEP. The exhalation valve is closed during an expiratory hold. When the expiratory flow equals zero, airway pressure rises to the auto-PEEP level. After reopening the expiratory valve, flow continues, and the additional exhaled volume equals the volume of trapped gas. Of note, inspiratory and expiratory muscle activity interferes with the measurement of intrinsic PEEP. (Adapted from MacIntyre NR: Prob Respir Care 1991; 4:45.)

COMPLICATIONS

Complications and side effects of intubation and/or of invasive mechanical ventilation include upper airway trauma (e.g., vocal cord injury), aspiration of gastric contents, barotrauma (e.g., pneumothorax or pneumomediastinum), disruption of normal host defense mechanisms, reduction in the ability to heat and humidify inspired gases, local tracheal ischemia induced by the cuff of the endotracheal tube, impairment of communication and of swallowing, and the perceived need by health care providers for sedatives and occasionally neuromuscular blocking drugs. Although a cuffed endotracheal tube helps prevent gross aspiration, pharyngeal secretions that pool at the top of the cuff may still seep into the lungs and increase the probability of nosocomial pneumonia developing.

An endotracheal tube greatly impairs the patient's inherent cough mechanisms by preventing closure of the glottis.

Mechanical ventilation itself can induce or aggravate lung injury that is clinically, functionally, and histologically indistinguishable from ALI/ARDS. Also, applying positive pressure to the lungs may impact cardiac performance and result in hemodynamic compromise.

VENTILATOR-INDUCED LUNG INJURY (VILI)

Diseased lungs are more susceptible to the development of VILI compared with healthy lungs. VILI can also initiate and propagate cascades (e.g., upregulation of a systemic inflammatory

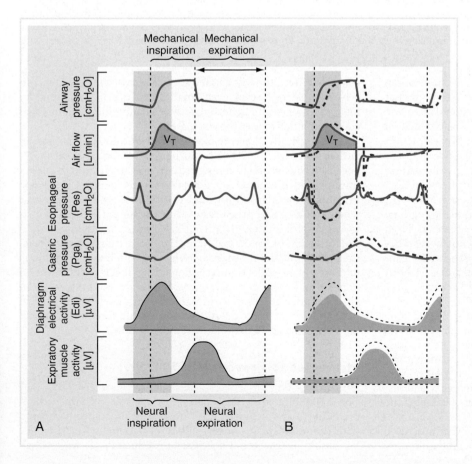

FIGURE 18-19 A, Demonstration of delivery of assist with pressure support ventilation (PSV) in a patient with expiratory flow limitation resulting in dynamic hyperinflation. There is substantial asynchrony (delayed triggering-on and cycling-off) between the assist delivered by the ventilator and the patient's (neural) respiratory demand as reflected by the electrical activity of the diaphragm (Edi). The high amplitudes for the Edi and for esophageal pressure (Pes) deflections indicate that the inspiratory muscles are highly active during delivery of pressure by the ventilator, whereas the high amplitudes for the expiratory muscle activity and for the gastric pressure (Pga) deflections indicate that the patient uses his expiratory muscles to counter delivery of pressure by the ventilator during neural expiration. **B,** After optimizing the trigger-on threshold, delivery of assist starts earlier (requiring less inspiratory effort) and also ceases earlier (requiring less activation of the expiratory muscles).

(Continued)

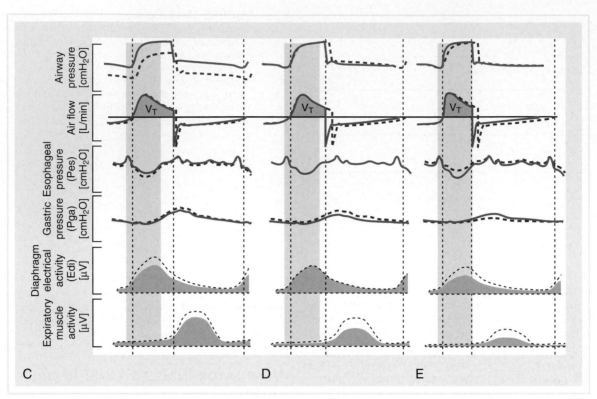

FIGURE 18-19 cont'd, C, Adjusting the level of extrinsic PEEP to compensate for auto-PEEP allows earlier detection of the inspiratory effort by the ventilator (see Figure 18-21) and helps to further reduce the inspiratory workload. **D,** Increasing the cycling-off airflow threshold results in earlier termination of the assist. Hence, expiratory muscle activity can be reduced. Note that the ventilator inspiratory time, as well as the delivered tidal volume (V_T), decreases when the cycling-off airflow threshold is increased, whereas the expiratory time increases (provided the respiratory rate remains unchanged). **E,** When the inspiratory rise time is reduced, the peak inspiratory flow and, therefore, the cycling-off airflow threshold are both reached earlier, and the inspiratory time is further shortened. After completion of all steps as demonstrated in **B–E,** ventilator assist is delivered in synchrony with the patient's neural respiratory demand, and unloading of the inspiratory muscles is achieved as reflected by minimization of the amplitudes for Edi and for Pes deflections. Expiration is driven only by the elastic recoil of the lung and the chest wall, as reflected by minimization of the amplitudes for expiratory muscle activity and for Pga deflections.

response) that ultimately culminate in multiple system organ failure (MSOF) (Figure 18-22). A ventilatory strategy that uses low V_T and limited P_{VENT} is not only protective to the lung but also has the potential to reduce the incidence of MSOF. Exposure to excessive mechanical stresses can result in damage to lung tissue and cell integrity from two primary factors, namely, overdistention of the lung (i.e., volutrauma) or repetitive airspace recruitment and derecruitment (atelectrauma). The critical feature defining induction of VILI because of volutrauma seems to be the degree of regional lung distention, rather than the absolute P_{VENT} reached. High pressures per se in the respiratory system do not necessarily result in VILI. For example, trumpet players repeatedly generate very high airway pressures (>150 cmH$_2$O) without lung damage developing because there is no excessive lung distention.

Alveolar overdistention and shear forces can stimulate lung and immune cells to produce and release inflammatory cytokines and chemokines (i.e., biotrauma). Biotrauma encompasses the release of numerous biologic (including inflammatory) mediators into the pulmonary interstitial and alveolar spaces. Concomitant disruption of lung tissue and cell integrity and disruption of lung epithelial and endothelial barriers facilitates the spillover of lung-derived inflammatory mediators, endotoxin, and even bacteria into the bloodstream, resulting in initiation, exacerbation, or propagation of a systemic inflammatory

response. Given the vast aerated surface area of the lung, it is conceivable that release of even small quantities of inflammatory mediators per cell could lead to a large quantity of mediators that could potentially enter the circulation.

The typically heterogeneous distribution of disease in patients with ALI/ARDS puts them at a high risk of VILI, because the consolidated lung regions are susceptible to atelectrauma, and the better or normally aerated regions are prone to volutrauma. Barotrauma and volutrauma are likely to occur when volumes and pressures meant for the entire lung (e.g., a V_T of approximately 10 mL × kg^{-1}) are forced into only a small portion of functional lung (the "baby lung"). In addition, shear forces at the interface between the open and closed lung units result in atelectrauma when PEEP levels insufficient to prevent end-expiratory alveolar collapse are used. Hence, ideally, a ventilatory strategy in patients with ALI/ARDS should prevent both alveolar overdistention during lung inflation and alveolar collapse at the end of lung deflation.

Strategies to Prevent VILI in Daily Clinical Practice

The ARDSNet study demonstrated that a V_T of 6 mL × kg^{-1} predicted body weight (PBW) decreased mortality compared with the use of 12 mL × kg^{-1} PBW in patients with ALI. This V_T should be lowered if necessary to reduce P_{PLAT} to less than

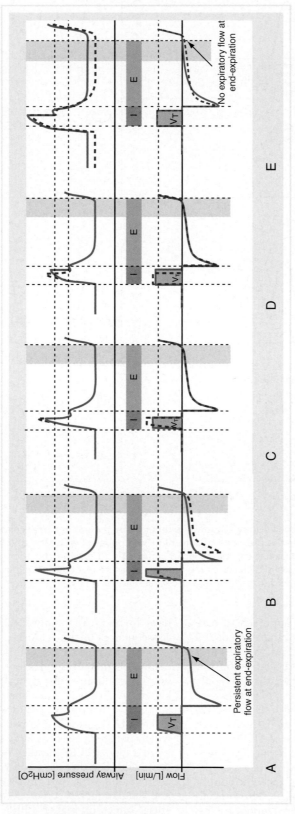

FIGURE 18-20 Adjustment of ventilatory parameters with volume-targeted ventilation in a patient with expiratory flow limitation and dynamic hyperinflation. **A,** Baseline condition with persistent flow at end-expiration. **B,** Shortening the inspiratory phase by reduction of the I/E relationship allows longer expiration provided the ventilatory rate remains unchanged. A higher maximal inspiratory airflow, and hence a higher peak pressure, during inspiration is required to force the same tidal volume (V_T) into the lungs in a shorter period of time. Of note, a high inspiratory flow may result in a moderate increase in the respiratory rate that requires careful monitoring of the net effect on the duration of the expiration. **C** and **D,** Decreasing the inspiratory rise time (here from 5% to 0% of the respiratory cycle) and shortening the time of the inspiratory pause at end-inspiration (here from 10% to 5% of the respiratory cycle) allows more time to deliver the tidal volume and hence results in lower maximal flow and lower peak pressure. **E,** Increasing the extrinsic PEEP partially counteracts the dynamic collapse of airways during expiration and diminishes the impedance to expiratory flow.

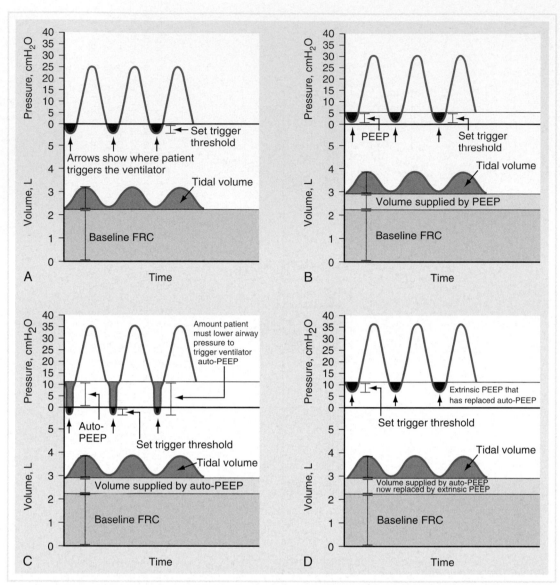

FIGURE 18-21 **A** and **B,** Without auto-PEEP, a small inspiratory effort is required by the patient to exceed the predefined trigger-on threshold (here 1–2 cmH_2O below extrinsic PEEP). **C,** In the presence of auto-PEEP, the patient first needs to lower alveolar pressure to overcome auto-PEEP before the pressure in the ventilator circuit can be reduced sufficiently to exceed the trigger threshold below extrinsic PEEP. **D,** Applying extrinsic PEEP brings the trigger threshold closer to the alveolar pressure level at end-expiration. Now only a small inspiratory effort is required to exceed the trigger-on threshold. (Adapted from Howman SF: Hosp Phys 1999: 26–36.)

$30\ cmH_2O$. It is important in applying this approach to base V_T on the PBW. The PBW of a male patient can be calculated as $50 + 0.91 \times$ (cm of height $- 152.4$) and the PBW of a female patient can be calculated as equal to $45.5 + 0.91 \times$ (cm of height $- 152.4$). Although mechanical ventilation is only one of multiple factors contributing to the pathogenesis of MODS, clinical trials have clearly shown that lung-protective mechanical ventilation decreases mortality in patients with ARDS and is associated with a lower incidence of MODS.

In a number of studies, the authors used *permissive hypercapnia* (i.e., allowing the $PaCO_2$ to increase if necessary to maintain a sufficiently low V_T,) if there was no specific contraindication (e.g., increased intracranial pressure). The concept is that the detrimental effects of the acute hypercapnia are less than the use of higher V_T. How one treats the accompanying respiratory acidosis is still a matter of debate, but decreases in pH to ~7.25 are usually well tolerated and likely do not

have to be treated unless there are detrimental physiologic consequences of the acidosis.

Some suggest that a ventilatory strategy that keeps P_{PLAT} below $30\ cmH_2O$ is sufficient to ensure lung protection. The safe upper limit of P_{PLAT} in patients with ALI/ARDS is not known. A recent *post hoc* analysis demonstrated that lowering P_{PLAT} to $< 30\ cmH_2O$ may lower mortality.

How to adjust PEEP in patients with ARDS continues to be widely debated. A recent large study found no effect on mortality of a higher PEEP strategy (approximately $13\ cmH_2O$) compared with one that used a PEEP of approximately $8\ cmH_2O$ in combination with lung-protective, volume-, and pressure-limited ventilation, but some have suggested that a potentially beneficial effect of higher PEEP in some (recruitable) patients might have been negated by a detrimental effect occurring in others (i.e., nonrecruitable). Pending further clarification of how to define optimal PEEP levels in individual patients, a

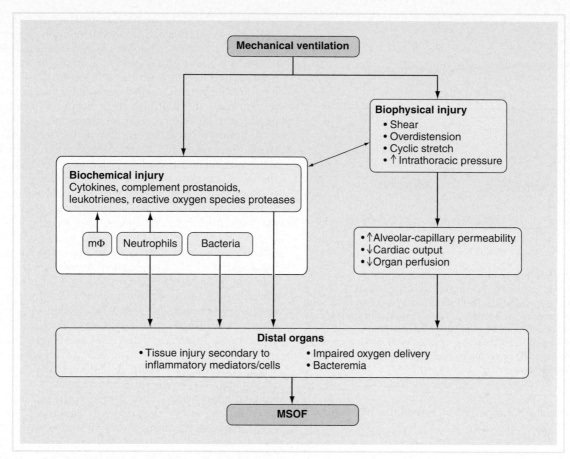

FIGURE 18-22 Postulated mechanisms whereby mechanical ventilation may contribute to multiple system organ failure (*MSOF*). (Adapted from Slutsky AS, Tremblay LN: Am J Respir Crit Care Med 1998; 157:1721–1725.)

pragmatic approach for daily clinical practice is to adhere to the algorithm used in the large ARDSnet trial (see Table 18-1).

Determining optimal ventilator setting in patients with ALI/ARDS must take into account changes in the disease process over time. Defining and maintaining optimal ventilatory settings in an individual patient is always a continuous, iterative process of evaluation, intervention, and reevaluation.

Lung Recruitment

Recruitment maneuvers can decrease the heterogeneities present in the lung, improve gas exchange, and potentially mitigate VILI by reducing cyclical airspace opening and closing. Recruitment refers to the process of reopening collapsed alveoli by transiently increasing P_{VENT}. This can be accomplished by maintaining a static P_{VENT} of 40 cmH$_2$O for 40 sec or by increasing PEEP transiently. Although animal studies seem to indicate that recruitment maneuvers are effective in decreasing VILI, human data indicating improved clinical outcomes are not available. This may be because recruitment maneuvers are likely to be effective in patients who have "recruitable" lungs, and none of the studies to date have stratified patients on the basis of their lung recruitability. If recruitment maneuvers are used, it is important to monitor for adverse effects such as hypotension, barotraumas, and arrhythmias.

Alternative Approaches to Lung Recruitment

Prone positioning and high-frequency ventilation (HFV) represent alternative ways of attaining lung recruitment. Placing patients with ARDS prone improves PaO$_2$ in approximately 70% of patients. Prone positioning may also decrease VILI by improving the homogeneity of end-expiratory lung volume. Randomized controlled trials have not demonstrated reductions in mortality with prone ventilation, but all are flawed by either suboptimal design (e.g., the use of prone positioning only 6 h/day, instituting it late) or small sample sizes.

HFV refers to a number of ventilatory modes, including high-frequency positive pressure ventilation (HFPPV), high-frequency jet ventilation (HFJV), high-frequency flow interruption (HFFI), and high-frequency oscillatory ventilation (HFOV), all of which use substantially higher ventilatory frequencies (i.e., in the range of 1–25 Hz) and much lower V_T than conventional modes (Figure 18-23). During HFV, the V_T is typically less than the dead space and gas transport is accomplished by various aspects of convection and diffusion. With HFV, a high mean P_{VENT} is used to recruit alveoli and maintain lung volume above FRC. Thus, in contrast to controlled modes of ventilation, HFV maintains lung volume at a relatively constant level and uses very small V_T to accomplish ventilation. Intermittent sighs or sustained inflations are optionally used to recruit collapsed lung regions and to avoid atelectasis.

HFV is a potentially interesting ventilatory approach in patients with ARDS, because the small V_T and the small pressure excursions allow the use of a relatively high mean P_{VENT} without overdistending the lungs or allowing cyclic collapse to occur. Recent clinical studies in infants and adults with ARDS suggest that HFV may be as effective as conventional

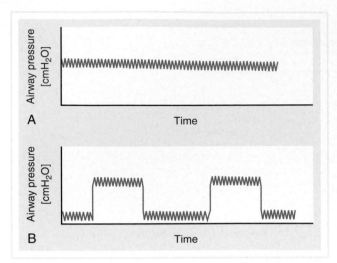

FIGURE 18-23 With high-frequency ventilation (HFV), extremely small tidal volumes (typically 1–3 mL/kg) are applied at very high ventilatory rates (typically 60–1500/min, equivalent to 1–25 Hz). HFV allows maintenance of a relatively high mean airway pressure, whereas tidal excursions, and hence alveolar recruitment and derecruitment, are minimized. HFV can be applied with either a constant mean airway pressure **(A)** or with alternating between a lower and a higher mean airway pressure **(B)**.

mechanical ventilatory support, but no studies have demonstrated that it reduces mortality.

HEART–LUNG INTERACTIONS DURING MECHANICAL VENTILATION

The heart is the nonpulmonary organ most directly affected by mechanical ventilation. Positive-pressure ventilation and PEEP help improve arterial oxygenation, but also decrease return of blood to the right ventricle. Tidal inflation is accompanied by a transient reduction in left ventricular afterload, leading to an increase in arterial blood pressure and in left ventricular stroke volume. The effect is generally trivial except in patients with profound reductions in ejection fraction. Although some suggest that increasing lung volume increases pulmonary vascular resistance (thereby increasing right ventricular afterload), others find that the effect is trivial except at the highest lung volumes in patients with high pulmonary arterial pressures.

During spontaneous breathing, periodic reduction of intrathoracic pressure combined with simultaneous compression of the intraabdominal vascular beds facilitates return of venous blood to the heart.

WEANING FROM MECHANICAL VENTILATION

"Weaning" is often used interchangeably with "liberation" from mechanical ventilation and refers to the transition from full ventilatory support to resumption of unassisted spontaneous breathing by the patient.

All mechanically ventilated patients should be allowed to progress to spontaneous breathing at the earliest possible time, because unnecessary prolongation of ventilation renders the patient at risk of adverse events such as ventilation-associated

pneumonia, VILI, or perhaps respiratory muscle atrophy. On the other hand, premature discontinuation of ventilatory support when a patient is not yet ready to assume the entire work of breathing also entails potential harm, including complications related to reintubation. Conventional weaning predictors measure the patient's ability to breathe without assistance but do not assess the ability to clear respiratory tract secretions or protect the lower airways from aspiration.

Initiation of weaning requires that the patient can and will trigger the ventilator, a prerequisite that often can only be achieved when the level of sedation is reduced and/or when the $PaCO_2$ is allowed to increase by reducing the minute ventilation. It is not surprising that protocolized interruption of sedation on a daily basis reduces the total time spent on mechanical ventilation. Before commencing weaning, clinicians must believe that the patient has a reasonable likelihood of being able to breathe on his or her own. Although measuring a variety of physiologic variables may help guide this decision, the process often entails a "trial and error" component. Careful monitoring of the patient's comfort, gas exchange, respiratory mechanics, and hemodynamics during a trial of spontaneous breathing is mandatory. The protocolized use of spontaneous breathing trials (SBT) is recommended to identify patients who are likely to be able to breathe spontaneously without assistance (Figure 18-24). An SBT is a process that allows patients to breathe spontaneously with minimal or no ventilatory support for a predefined period of time (e.g., 30 min) to assess the patient's readiness for extubation. A range of criteria to initiate an SBT as recently recommended by a consensus conference are summarized in Box 18-1 (for details, see MacIntyre NR et al: Chest 2001; 120 [Suppl]: 375–395), but each patient must be evaluated for specific factors that might modify the recommendation or mandate an alternate approach.

A formal SBT is often not required after short-term ventilation (e.g., in patients ventilated for less than 24 h as, for example, in the postoperative period), whereas a SBT should be performed on a daily basis during a daily interruption of sedation in those patients who fulfill certain criteria (see Box 18-1). Conventionally, an SBT is performed by use of a minimal level of assist (i.e., 0–7 cmH$_2$O, preferably 0 cmH$_2$O), a FiO$_2$ of 0.5, and a PEEP level of 5–7.5 cmH$_2$O. An initial brief period of spontaneous breathing can be used to assess the capability of continuing onto a formal SBT. The criteria used to assess patients' readiness to continue tolerance during SBTs are the respiratory pattern, the adequacy of gas exchange, hemodynamic stability, and subjective comfort. Tolerating a SBT for 30–120 min should prompt discontinuation of the ventilator. Removal of the artificial airway is a separate consideration and is based on assessing airway patency and the ability of the patient to protect the airway.

When an SBT fails, the cause should be determined. Once reversible causes for failure are corrected, and if the patient still meets the criteria listed in Box 18-1, subsequent SBTs should be performed at least every 24 h. Patients who fail an SBT trial should receive a stable, nonfatiguing, comfortable form of ventilatory support. Anesthesia/sedation strategies and ventilator management aimed at early extubation should be used in postsurgical patients. Weaning protocols designed for nonphysician health care professionals should be developed and implemented by ICUs. Protocols aimed at optimizing sedation should also be developed and implemented.

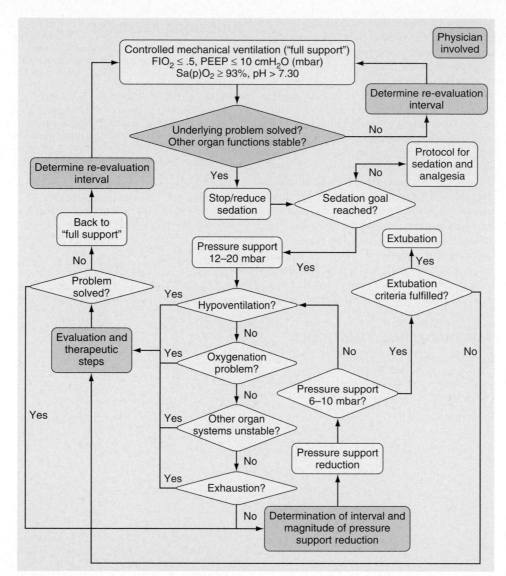

FIGURE 18-24 Example of a protocol to inform the process of gradual reduction in the assist level during weaning. (Adapted from Jakob SM *et al*: J Crit Care 2007; 22[3]:219–228.)

Tracheotomy should be considered after an initial period of stabilization on the ventilator when it becomes apparent that the patient will require prolonged ventilator assistance. Unless there is evidence for clearly irreversible disease (e.g., high spinal cord injury or advanced amyotrophic lateral sclerosis), a patient requiring prolonged mechanical ventilatory support for respiratory failure should not be considered permanently ventilator-dependent until 3 months of weaning attempts have failed. Weaning strategies in the patients requiring prolonged mechanical ventilation should be slow paced and should include gradual lengthening of self-breathing trials.

PITFALLS AND CONTROVERSIES

Better understanding of the potential harm of mechanical ventilation, of the interaction between the patient and the ventilator, and of the importance of optimizing treatment processes associated with mechanical ventilation (e.g., sedation and weaning protocols) have fostered the development of many technical and conceptual improvements in recent years. Nevertheless, further advances are required in numerous areas such as developing ventilatory strategies that individualize ventilation to the specific patient at a specific point in time and that minimize VILI and its systemic consequences, improving alternate approaches to protecting the lung during mechanical ventilation, in improving patient-ventilator interactions, and in preventing respiratory muscle deconditioning during mechanical ventilation. Current controversies include the precise role of recruitment maneuvers and ways to individualize PEEP levels, as well as the indications for invasive versus noninvasive ventilation.

Although further research is likely to provide us with new insights, an important challenge for researchers and clinicians alike is to identify elements of the current knowledge that can be incorporated into daily clinical management to improve the outcome of patients who require ventilatory assistance. In general, a protocolized approach is more likely to result in a lasting improvement of care for ventilated patients. Implementing such protocols requires adequate resources, and institutions must make a commitment not only to develop protocols but also to the iterative process of implementation, reassessment, and refinement.

WEB RESOURCES FOR GUIDELINES/PROTOCOLS

http://ardsnet.org provides information on completed and on future research projects related to various aspects of ARDS.

http://www.ccmtutorials.com/rs/mv/index.htm provides an illustrative tutorial on mechanical ventilation.

SUGGESTED READINGS

Acute Respiratory Distress Syndrome Network: Ventilation with lower tidal volumes as compared with traditional tidal volumes for acute lung injury and the acute respiratory distress syndrome. N Engl J Med 2000; 342:1301–1308.

dos Santos CC, Slutsky AS: The contribution of biophysical lung injury to the development of biotrauma. Annu Rev Physiol 2006; 68:585–618.

Fan E, Needham DM, Stewart TE: Ventilatory management of acute lung injury and acute respiratory distress syndrome. JAMA 2005; 294:2889–2896.

MacIntyre NR, Cook DJ, Ely EW Jr, et al: Evidence-based guidelines for weaning and discontinuing ventilatory support: a collective task force facilitated by the American College of Chest Physicians; the American Association for Respiratory Care; and the American College of Critical Care Medicine. Chest 2001; 120(Suppl):375–395.

Slutsky AS, Brochard L, eds: Mechanical ventilation. Update in intensive care and emergency medicine. Heidelberg: Springer Verlag Berlin; 2004.

Tobin MJ: Advances in mechanical ventilation. N Engl J Med 2001; 344(26):1986–1996.

Tobin MJ, ed: Principles and Practice of Mechanical Ventilation. 2nd ed. New York: McGraw-Hill Professional; 2006.

Tremblay LN, Slutsky AS: Ventilator induced lung injury: From the bench to the bedside. Intensive Care Med 2006; 32(1):24–33.

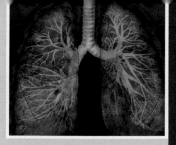

19 Noninvasive Mechanical Ventilation

INDERJIT K. HANSRA • NICHOLAS S. HILL

Noninvasive ventilation is mechanical ventilation administered without an invasive artificial airway. Since the first description of a prototype negative-pressure "tank" ventilator 150 years ago, many types of noninvasive ventilators have been developed. Tank ventilators, like the iron lung, were the mainstay of mechanical ventilatory assistance during the polio epidemics that occurred from the 1920s to the 1950s. By the 1960s, invasive positive-pressure ventilation became the preferred treatment of acute respiratory failure. Noninvasive ventilators, mainly of the negative-pressure type, continued to be used sporadically for chronic respiratory failure until the early 1980s. After the introduction of nasal ventilation during the late 1980s, however, noninvasive positive-pressure ventilation became the preferred mode for assisting patients with respiratory failure.

RATIONALE FOR THE USE OF NONINVASIVE VENTILATION

Invasive mechanical ventilation has proved to be effective and reliable, but use of an endotracheal airway involves potential complications. These complications may be categorized as:

1. Traumatic complications (e.g., hemorrhage, tracheal laceration, vocal cord paralysis)
2. Complications related to bypassing the airway defense system (interfering with cough, mucociliary action)
3. Discomfort (e.g., pain, interference with communication and swallowing)

These complications apply to acute translaryngeal intubations and chronic tracheostomies. Furthermore, airway invasion serves as a continual irritant, increasing mucus production and necessitating intermittent suctioning. By avoiding these complications, noninvasive ventilation has the potential of improving patient outcomes, enhancing patient satisfaction, and reducing the cost of care. It must be emphasized, however, that patients who receive noninvasive ventilation must be selected carefully (see later).

TECHNIQUES AND EQUIPMENT

Noninvasive Positive Pressure Ventilation

Noninvasive positive-pressure ventilation (NPPV) consists of a positive-pressure ventilator connected by tubing to a mask or an "interface" that applies positive air pressure to the nose, mouth, or both.

Interfaces

Nasal Masks. Nasal masks are the most commonly used interfaces for treating chronic respiratory failure because they are convenient and permit normal speech and swallowing. Manufacturers offer numerous modifications of the three basic types of nasal mask:

- Standard nasal continuous positive airway pressure (CPAP) masks
- Nasal "pillows" or "seals"
- Custom-fitted masks

Standard nasal CPAP masks consist of clear plastic triangular domes that fit over the nose (Figure 19-1). A soft cuff makes contact with the skin around the perimeter of the nose to form an air seal. These masks must be properly fitted to minimize pressure over the bridge of the nose, which may cause redness, skin irritation, and occasionally ulceration. Thin silicone flaps are used to create an effective air seal with minimal strap tension, and forehead "spacers" are used to minimize pressure on the bridge of the nose. Strap systems that hold the masks in place are also important for patient comfort. "Minimasks" that fit over the tip of the nose and nostrils are designed to minimize claustrophobia, and gel-containing seals have been introduced in recent years to enhance patient comfort.

Nasal pillows or seals consist of small rubber cones that are inserted directly into the nostrils (Figure 19-2). These are useful for patients with nasal bridge irritation or ulceration, because they make no contact with the bridge of the nose. Some patients alternate between different types of masks as a way of minimizing discomfort.

Although kits for custom molding are available commercially, they require time and skill for successful application and are rarely used because a suitable commercially available mask can almost always be found.

Oronasal Masks. Oronasal (full face) masks cover both the nose and the mouth (Figure 19-3) and can reduce the amount of air leaking through the mouth, which may limit the efficacy of nasal masks. For this reason, they are the preferred interface for treating acute respiratory failure, but they interfere with speech and eating more than nasal masks do, have more dead space, and are less comfortable than nasal masks for chronic use. The Total Face Mask™, seals around the perimeter of the face and may enhance comfort compared with standard oronasal masks. Concerns have been raised about the risk of aspiration if the patient vomits or asphyxiation if the ventilator fails, so recommended masks come with quick-release straps and antiasphyxia (nonrebreathing) valves.

Helmet. The helmet is not yet approved by the Food and Drug Administration for noninvasive ventilation in the United States but has been used in Europe. A clear plastic cylinder that fits

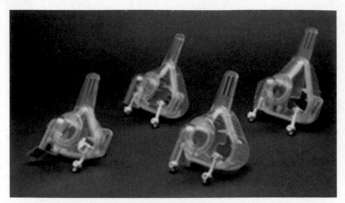

FIGURE 19-1 Standard nasal masks. Various sizes of standard nasal mask are available, ranging from small (*left*) to large (*right*).

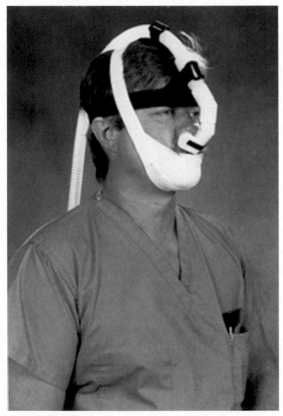

FIGURE 19-2 Nasal pillows. These avoid placing pressure on the bridge of the nose. The chinstrap helps keep the mouth closed, reducing air leakage.

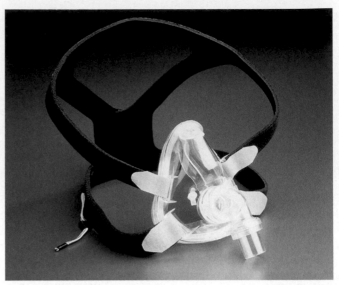

FIGURE 19-3 Oronasal facemask. The headgear (consisting of straps) is shown as though it were wrapped around the head. This mask has a very soft silicone seal and a rapid-release mechanism, and the exhalation valve is in the upper portion of the mask to minimize rebreathing.

over the head, it seals around the neck and shoulders with straps under the axillae. It is more comfortable and reduces facial ulcerations compared with a full-face mask but costlier and less efficient at CO_2 removal. It is best suited for applying CPAP but needs high flow rates to minimize rebreathing, creating much more noise than with a full-face mask (100 vs 70 dB, respectively).

Oral Interfaces. Commercially available oral interfaces use a mouthpiece inserted into a lip seal that is strapped tautly around the head to minimize air leakage; there is also a strapless type that has flanges that fit inside and outside the lips. For daytime use, the mouthpiece can be mounted on a

gooseneck device on a wheelchair, permitting patients to remain mobile while receiving ventilatory assistance. Strapless mouthpieces that are custom fitted by an orthodontist can be easily expectorated if necessary, even by patients with severe neuromuscular disease. These devices have been used for 24-h ventilatory support in patients with neuromuscular disease, some of whom have little or no measurable vital capacity.

Ventilators

NPPV may be administered by use of volume-limited or pressure-limited modes on critical care ventilators (i.e., those designed mainly for invasive ventilation in the acute setting), ventilators designed specifically for acute applications of noninvasive ventilation, or portable positive-pressure ventilators designed mainly for noninvasive ventilation in the home. The choice of ventilator depends largely on practitioner preferences and patient needs. For example, simple, portable, pressure-limited ventilators are frequently preferred, because they lack sophisticated alarm systems that may needlessly interrupt sleep in patients requiring only nocturnal ventilatory assistance at home. In other situations, the enhanced alarm and monitoring capabilities of critical care ventilators may be preferred for acute applications. For chronic use in the home, simplicity and portability are important features.

Critical Care Ventilators. Many of the microprocessor-controlled ventilators currently used in critical care units can be adapted for noninvasive ventilation. Either volume-limited or pressure-limited modes may be selected, although most practitioners prefer pressure support ventilation, which has been rated by clinicians as better tolerated. The responses of these ventilators to the air leaks that inevitably occur with NPPV may be problematic, sometimes necessitating modifications in the masks or disabling of the alarms. Some newer critical care ventilators have noninvasive ventilation modes that automatically improve leak tolerance, disable alarms, and permit adjustments to limit inspiratory time. As long as the patient is critically ill, however, alarms should be disabled only in a closely monitored setting such as a critical care or stepdown unit.

Portable Volume-Limited and Hybrid Ventilators. Portable volume-limited ventilators (Figure 19-4) are commonly used to administer NPPV to patients with chronic respiratory failure. The ventilators are usually set in the assist/control mode to allow for spontaneous patient triggering, and the backup rate is usually set slightly below the spontaneous patient breathing rate. Currently available volume-limited ventilators have more alarm and pressure-generating capabilities than do most portable pressure-limited ventilators, and they may be better suited to patients who need continuous ventilation or those with severe chest wall deformities or obesity who need high inflation pressures. So-called hybrid ventilators have recently been introduced that offer both pressure- and volume-limited modes, some no larger than a laptop computer.

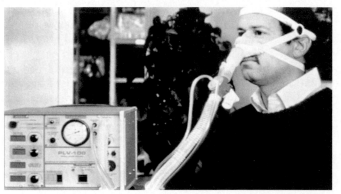

FIGURE 19-4 Typical volume-limited portable ventilator configured to deliver nasal ventilation.

Pressure-Limited Ventilators. The use of portable ventilators that deliver pressure assist or pressure support ventilation (often referred to as bilevel devices) has increased in recent years. These deliver a preset inspiratory positive airway pressure (IPAP) that can be combined with positive end-expiratory pressure (PEEP) (Figure 19-5). The difference between the IPAP and PEEP is the level of inspiratory assistance, or pressure support. Pressure support modes provide sensitive inspiratory triggering and expiratory cycling mechanisms, potentially allowing excellent patient–ventilator synchrony, reducing diaphragmatic work, and improving patient comfort. Because these devices are lighter (2–10 kg), are more compact (<0.02–5 m^3), and have fewer alarms than critical care or portable volume-limited ventilators, they are preferred for patients requiring only nocturnal support in the home. Most have limited IPAP and oxygenation capabilities (up to 20–35 cm H_2O, depending on the ventilator) and lack alarms or battery backup systems. Unless appropriately modified, they have limited use in the acute setting, although newer versions designed specifically for acute applications have sophisticated alarms and oxygen blenders.

Unlike volume-limited ventilators, bilevel devices are able to adjust inspiratory airflow to compensate for air leaks, potentially providing better support of gas exchange during leakage. Because they use a single tube with a passive exhalation valve, however, rebreathing can interfere with the ability to augment alveolar ventilation. This rebreathing problem can be minimized by use of masks with in-mask exhalation valves, nonrebreathing valves, or PEEP pressures of 4 cm H_2O or greater; the last option ensures higher bias flows during exhalation.

Negative-Pressure Ventilation. Negative-pressure ventilators are used much less frequently today than in the past, but some centers in Italy and Spain still use them, mainly for

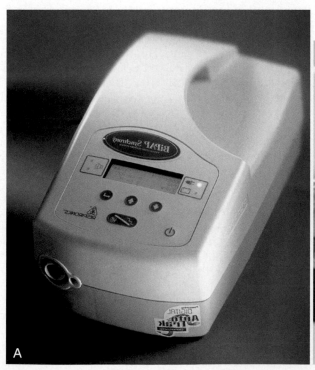

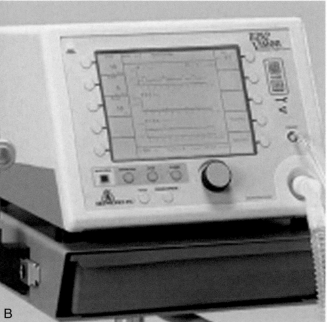

FIGURE 19-5 Typical bilevel-type portable pressure-limited ventilators. **A,** This device is designed for portability and convenience in the home. **B,** This device has an oxygen blender and graphics screen to facilitate in-hospital acute applications.

patients with acute exacerbations of chronic obstructive pulmonary disease (COPD). Negative pressure ventilators include tank ventilators (like the iron lung; Figure 19-6) and the smaller, more portable wrap or jacket ventilators (Figure 19-7) and cuirass or shell ventilators (Figure 19-8). The wrap ventilator consists of an impermeable nylon jacket suspended by a rigid chest piece that fits over the chest and abdomen. The cuirass ventilator is a rigid plastic or metal dome fitted over the chest and abdomen. Negative pressure ventilators expand the lungs by intermittently applying a subatmospheric pressure to the chest wall and abdomen, and expiration occurs passively by elastic recoil of the lung and chest wall. The tank is the most efficient and the cuirass the least efficient of these ventilators. Although these ventilators were commonly used to support

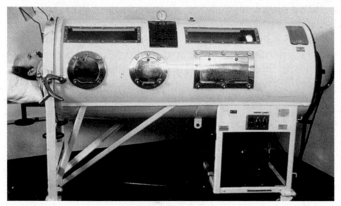

FIGURE 19-6 Iron lung. Tank-type negative-pressure ventilator that was widely used during the polio epidemics.

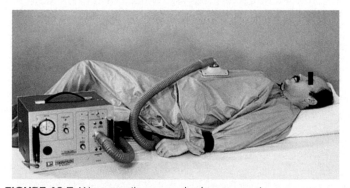

FIGURE 19-7 Wrap ventilator attached to a negative-pressure generator. Note the contour of the rigid plastic chest piece, which suspends the wrap above the chest and abdomen.

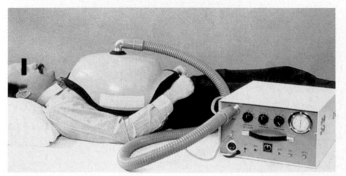

FIGURE 19-8 Chest cuirass attached to a negative pressure generator.

patients with chronic respiratory failure in the past, this is no longer the case because of their tendency to exacerbate or even induce obstructive sleep apnea in patients with neuromuscular disease.

Other Types of Ventilatory Assistance. Although technically not forms of "mechanical" ventilation, diaphragm pacing and glossopharyngeal breathing are ventilatory methods used in selected patients to enhance independence from mechanical ventilation. Diaphragm pacers consist of a radiofrequency transmitter and antenna that signal a surgically implanted receiver and electrode to stimulate the phrenic nerve. An intact phrenic nerve and diaphragm are usually required for successful application, but intercostal nerve implantation can be used when the phrenic nerves are damaged. Patients with high spinal cord quadriplegia, especially children, are the main users of pacers, allowing them freedom from invasive positive-pressure ventilation.

Glossopharyngeal, or "frog," breathing uses intermittent gulping motions of the tongue and pharyngeal muscles to force air into the trachea. The technique can be used to provide freedom from mechanical ventilation for up to several hours, even in severely compromised patients. Use is limited to patients who have intact upper airway musculature, normal (or near normal) lungs and chest walls, and the ability to learn the technique. Good candidates include those with high spinal cord injuries, those with postpolio syndrome, and selected patients with other neuromuscular diseases.

ACUTE APPLICATIONS OF NONINVASIVE VENTILATION

Established Indications

Chronic Obstructive Pulmonary Disease

Earlier observations that NPPV reduces the work of breathing in patients with respiratory disease led investigators to hypothesize that it would be useful for ventilatory support of patients with acute respiratory deterioration in whom respiratory muscle fatigue was developing. This hypothesis has now been confirmed in patients with COPD. Two recent meta-analyses of multiple randomized, controlled trials confirmed that NPPV reduces respiratory rate, improves dyspnea and gas exchange, and lowers mortality compared with standard therapy. In these analyses, the intubation rate in those receiving NPPV was approximately 20%, down from the 50% rate seen in controls. European studies have demonstrated that NPPV also reduces hospital length of stay, but this has not been confirmed in North America, where length of stay tends to be much shorter than in Europe. Other studies have demonstrated that COPD complicated by pneumonia responds well to NPPV, that NPPV can be used to permit early extubation in selected patients with COPD who require initial intubation, and that patients with mild exacerbations are not helped by NPPV, probably because they are not sufficiently ill to benefit from ventilatory assistance. The evidence is so strong for the initial use of NPPV for appropriately selected patients with COPD exacerbations that many now consider it a standard of care.

Acute Pulmonary Edema

The beneficial effects of positive pressure have long been known in patients with acute pulmonary edema. It improves compliance and oxygenation by increasing functional residual capacity and opening collapsed air spaces. At least four randomized, controlled trials have demonstrated that noninvasive CPAP alone improves dyspnea and oxygenation and lowers intubation rates in patients with acute pulmonary edema. One trial showed abbreviated intensive care unit stays compared with oxygen-treated controls, but no study has shown a reduction in mortality. More recently, several studies evaluated the efficacy of noninvasive ventilation (i.e., inspiratory assistance with pressure support superimposed on PEEP) compared with either oxygen therapy or CPAP alone. Although noninvasive ventilation has benefits similar to those previously demonstrated for CPAP, its superiority over CPAP alone has not been convincingly established, and one study raised the possibility that the myocardial infarction rate may be higher in those receiving noninvasive ventilation. More recently, a number of meta-analyses on these studies have confirmed the benefits of CPAP and even showed a significant reduction in mortality. Noninvasive ventilation performed as well as CPAP, but not better, and no increase in the myocardial infarction rate was apparent. Accordingly, CPAP alone is generally regarded as the initial noninvasive modality of choice, but noninvasive ventilation should be substituted if patients treated with CPAP remain dyspneic or hypercapnic.

Acute Respiratory Failure in Immunocompromised Patients

Immunocompromised patients (those with *Pneumocystis jiroveci* pneumonia and those who have received solid-organ or bone marrow transplants) often have poor outcomes when they need invasive mechanical ventilation. Nosocomial infections and fatal bouts of septicemia are common complications in this setting, and those with hematologic malignancies may have fatal airway hemorrhages develop caused by thrombocytopenia and platelet dysfunction. Accordingly, avoiding intubation by use of noninvasive ventilation is an attractive alternative. Randomized trials on patients with acute respiratory failure related to solid organ transplantation and hematologic malignancy have demonstrated reduced intubation and mortality rates compared with controls. Thus, noninvasive ventilation should be considered early during the development of respiratory failure in immunocompromised patients as a way to avoid intubation and its attendant mortality.

Other Possible Indications

Table 19-1 lists non-COPD causes of acute respiratory failure that may be treated with noninvasive ventilation in appropriately selected patients. As might be expected, other diseases with airflow limitation as an important manifestation (e.g., cystic fibrosis) seem to respond favorably, although randomized trials are lacking. A recent randomized trial treating acute asthma exacerbations in the emergency department indicated that noninvasive ventilation improves FEV_1 more rapidly and lowers the hospitalization rate compared with sham ventilation.

Hypoxemic respiratory failure encompasses a diverse category of conditions, including acute respiratory distress syndrome, acute pneumonia, trauma, and acute pulmonary edema. With the exception of the last diagnosis and pneumonia in COPD or immunocompromised patients, however, evidence supporting the use of noninvasive ventilation is limited, and it should be applied selectively and with caution in these patients.

Other broad categories of respiratory failure that are increasingly being treated with noninvasive ventilation include

TABLE 19-1 Non-COPD Causes of Acute Respiratory Failure and General Categories of Patients Treated with Noninvasive Positive-Pressure Ventilation

Obstructive Diseases	Hypoxemic Respiratory Failure
Asthma (B)	ARDS (C)
Cystic fibrosis (C)	Pneumonia (B*)
Upper airway obstruction (C)	Acute pulmonary edema (A†)
	Trauma (C)
Restrictive Diseases	**Others**
Kyphoscoliosis (C)	Immunocompromised patients (A)
Neuromuscular disease (C)	Postoperative respiratory failure (B)
Obesity hypoventilation syndrome (C)	Facilitation of extubation (A*)
	Extubation failure (B‡)
	Do-not-intubate patients (C)

Letters in parentheses indicate level of evidence: A, multiple controlled trials; B, single supportive controlled trial; C, uncontrolled trials, case reports.
*For COPD patients only.
†Strongest evidence for continuous positive airway pressure of 10 to 12 cmH2O.
‡Conflicting data.
ARDS, Acute respiratory distress syndrome; *COPD*, chronic obstructive pulmonary disease.

postoperative patients, patients with extubation failure, and those in whom a decision has been made not to intubate. Noninvasive ventilation or CPAP alone can improve oxygenation and reduce complications compared with oxygen therapy in patients undergoing major abdominal or bariatric surgery, and noninvasive ventilation reduces the need for reintubation and mortality in patients in whom respiratory failure develops after lung resection surgery. Noninvasive ventilation also reduces the need for intubation in patients at high risk for extubation failure, especially in hypercapnic patients with COPD or congestive heart failure (CHF), but not if it delays a needed intubation. Noninvasive ventilation can be used with considerable success for "do-not-intubate" patients who have COPD exacerbations or acute pulmonary edema. It is less successful, however, in those with an underlying malignancy or acute pneumonia. Although noninvasive ventilation is generally reserved for patients with reversible diagnoses, it may occasionally be appropriate for terminally ill patients to alleviate respiratory distress or to provide additional time to settle affairs. In these situations, patients and their families and caregivers should clarify the goals (life support vs palliation) and be prepared to stop if the goals are not being met.

Time Demands on Medical Personnel

The advantages of NPPV over conventional therapy for acute respiratory failure may be offset by excessive time demands on medical personnel. Earlier reports raised this as a potential problem, but it may have been related to a lack of experience with the technique. Nurses rate NPPV as no more demanding than conventional therapy, and they spend no more time with patients receiving NPPV than with controls. Respiratory therapists tend to spend more time with NPPV patients than with conventionally treated patients during the first 8 h of use, but not subsequently.

TABLE 19-2 Characteristics of Patients Successfully Treated with Noninvasive Positive-Pressure Ventilation

Cooperative
Intact neurologic function
Able to coordinate breathing with ventilator
Moderately high (but not very high) APACHE II scores
Intact dentition
Less air leakage (often through the mouth) than in patients who fail
Able to control secretions
Hypercapnic, but not severely so
Acidemic, but not severely so (pH > 7.10)
Reduced respiratory rate and gas exchange within first 2 hours

TABLE 19-3 Selection Guidelines for Use of Noninvasive Positive Pressure Ventilation in Patients with Acute Respiratory Failure

Identify Patients at Risk of Needing Ventilatory Assistance

Clinical criteria
  Moderate to severe respiratory distress
    Increased dyspnea
    Tachypnea (respiratory rate > 24/min)
    Use of accessory muscles
    Paradoxical breathing pattern
  Blood gas criteria
  $Pa_{CO_2} > 45$ mmHg (> 6.0 kPa) and pH < 7.35, or
    $Pa_{O_2}/F_{IO_2} < 200$

Exclude Patients Who Would Be More Safely Managed Invasively

Respiratory arrest
Medically unstable
  Shock states
  Unstable cardiac status
    Acute severe ischemia or infarction
    Uncontrolled life-threatening arrhythmias
  Active severe upper gastrointestinal bleeding
Uncooperative or agitated
Unable to protect airway
  Excessive secretions
  Severe cough or swallowing impairment
Severe facial trauma

Appropriate, Reversible Cause for Respiratory Failure (As in Table 19-1)

These findings indicate that NPPV initially requires more time to administer, but as patients and medical practitioners become familiar with the technique, time demands rapidly diminish.

Determinants of Success

Factors predicting the success of NPPV are shown in Table 19-2. In summary, these predictors indicate that patients most likely to benefit have advanced, but not catastrophic, respiratory failure. The predictors also suggest that there is a window of opportunity for the implementation of NPPV during which success is most likely. NPPV should be started when patients have evidence of acute respiratory distress and high Acute Physiology and Chronic Health Evaluation II (APACHE II) scores, but not too late, when they are approaching respiratory arrest, have advanced carbon dioxide retention and acidemia, have higher APACHE II scores, and are unable to cooperate. In a recent prospective multicenter study, SAPS II scores of <34 and a Pa_{O_2}/F_{IO_2} ratio >175 after the first hour of noninvasive ventilation were predictors of NPPV success. Although there is no evidence that establishes the efficacy of NPPV to treat acute respiratory distress syndrome (ARDS), an attempt might be considered if these parameters are met.

Selection Guidelines

Selection guidelines for the use of NPPV in acute respiratory failure on the basis of selection criteria used in randomized, controlled trials are shown in Table 19-3. In the two-step process, patients are identified as those at risk of needing ventilatory assistance (and possibly intubation) on the basis of clinical and blood gas indicators. Patients with mild respiratory distress are apt to do well without ventilatory assistance.

The second step is to exclude those who would be at higher risk of complications if they were managed noninvasively. Exclusions are listed in Table 19-3 and include patients who are too medically unstable or uncooperative, those with frank or imminent cardiopulmonary arrest, and those who cannot protect their airway. Obtundation is not necessarily an exclusion. Patients with hypercapnic coma (Glasgow Coma Scale < 8) secondary to acute respiratory failure have success and mortality rates with NPPV that are equivalent to those of similar noncomatose patients. Adherence to the guidelines helps ensure the safe administration of noninvasive ventilation, but patients are still at risk for deterioration and should be monitored closely until stabilized. Delay of needed intubation by excessively prolonging failed attempts at noninvasive ventilation can add to morbidity and should be avoided.

The underlying cause and potential reversibility of the acute respiratory deterioration are also important considerations in patient selection. In this regard, NPPV may be viewed as a way to assist the patient during a critical interval of hours or days, allowing time for other therapies such as bronchodilators, corticosteroids, or diuretics to act. Severe, less reversible forms of respiratory failure that will likely require prolonged periods of ventilatory support, such as acute respiratory distress syndrome, should be managed with invasive ventilatory support.

LONG-TERM APPLICATIONS OF NONINVASIVE VENTILATION

Restrictive Thoracic Disease

A few weeks of nocturnal nasal NPPV consistently improves gas exchange and symptoms in patients with chronic respiratory failure caused by restrictive thoracic disease (e.g., severe neuromuscular disease, kyphoscoliosis) and in patients with the obesity-hypoventilation syndrome. Although no studies have compared nasal and mouthpiece NPPV, mouthpiece NPPV may be used for long-term ventilatory support in patients with severe neuromuscular disease who have virtually no measurable vital capacity.

Temporary withdrawal of nocturnal nasal ventilation from patients with chronic respiratory failure caused by restrictive thoracic disease results in worsening nocturnal gas exchange, daytime symptoms, and poorer sleep quality. These findings provide strong evidence that NPPV is effective in reversing nocturnal hypoventilation and improving symptoms in these patients. In addition, long-term follow-up studies on several hundred patients by use of NPPV for 3–5 years observed high rates of NPPV continuation (and hence survival) among patients with postpolio syndrome, most myopathies, and kyphoscoliosis. Survival is less favorable for patients with more rapidly progressive neuromuscular diseases such as amyotrophic lateral sclerosis (ALS), but NPPV seems to extend survival in these patients as well. In a randomized trial of NPPV for patients with ALS, those with intact bulbar function had improvements in quality of life, sleep-related symptoms, and a 205-day survival advantage compared with controls, whereas those with impaired bulbar function experienced no survival advantage but did improve symptomatically. Thus, NPPV should be offered to patients with ALS who have respiratory insufficiency develop, especially those with orthopnea or daytime hypercapnia, which were predictors of a favorable response. These findings establish NPPV as the ventilatory modality of first choice in treating chronic respiratory insufficiency in restrictive thoracic diseases.

Although the long-term efficacy of NPPV for patients with restrictive thoracic disease seems to be well established, the optimal time for initiation is unclear. Most authorities recommend starting at the onset of symptoms associated with nocturnal hypoventilation, but before the occurrence of daytime hypoventilation. This is partly for pragmatic reasons, because patients comply better if motivated by the desire for symptom relief and awaiting the onset of daytime hypercapnia can increase the risk of respiratory arrest.

Chronic Obstructive Pulmonary Disease

The most controversial long-term application of noninvasive ventilation has been in patients with severe, but stable, COPD. During the early 1980s, investigators theorized that the respiratory muscles in patients with severe COPD may be chronically fatigued and might benefit from intermittent rest. Early trials found that intermittent daytime sessions that used negative pressure wrap ventilators improved daytime gas exchange and inspiratory and expiratory muscle strength in patients with severe COPD. Longer-term controlled studies failed to demonstrate the same favorable effects of intermittent negative-pressure ventilation, however. In addition, patients with COPD tolerated the wrap ventilators poorly, using them for less time daily than recommended, and they had trouble sleeping during ventilator use.

The disappointing results with negative-pressure ventilators stimulated interest in the use of NPPV for severe COPD, but these studies have yielded conflicting results as well. In a 3-month crossover trial, only 7 of 19 patients with severe COPD improved, and this improvement was limited to tests of neuropsychological function; it was not apparent relative to nocturnal or daytime gas exchange, sleep quality, pulmonary function, exercise tolerance, or symptoms. In contrast, a similar study of 18 patients found that NPPV improved nocturnal and daytime gas exchange, total sleep time, and quality-of-life scores. The substantial difference in the baseline characteristics of patients entering these trials may explain the conflicting results. Patients entering the favorable study had greater hypercarbia ($PaCO_2$ 56 vs 46 mmHg) and more nocturnal oxygen desaturation, despite having less severe airway obstruction (FEV_1 0.81 vs 0.54 L) than did patients entering the unfavorable trial. These findings support the hypothesis that the subgroup of patients most likely to benefit from NPPV is that with substantial daytime carbon dioxide

retention (>50–55 mmHg) and nocturnal oxygen desaturation. A recent controlled trial of patients with COPD with chronic retention ($PaCO_2$ >50 mmHg) demonstrated less increase in $PaCO_2$, less deterioration of quality of life, and a trend toward fewer hospital days after 2 years of nocturnal NPPV compared with oxygen-treated controls.

These studies suggest that, compared with oxygen therapy alone, NPPV maintains gas exchange and quality of life and probably reduces the need for hospitalization in patients with severe stable COPD who have substantial carbon dioxide retention. Adherence to the therapy remains a major challenge, however.

Obesity Hypoventilation

Obesity hypoventilation syndrome (OHS) is the combination of hypercapnia and obesity (BMI >30) in the absence of other causes for hypoventilation such as hypothyroidism or neuromuscular disease. Obesity has reached epidemic proportions in many Western countries, and OHS has become a very common reason for initiating NPPV. Predisposing factors for OHS include upper airway resistance caused by anatomic narrowing, impairment of respiratory system mechanics related to the obesity, blunted central ventilatory drive, and deficiency of or resistance to the respiratory stimulant, leptin. Approximately 90% of patients with OHS have underlying obstructive sleep apnea (OSA) and may respond to CPAP treatment alone. Some of these patients have persisting hypoventilation despite CPAP therapy and are candidates for NPPV, which enhances nocturnal alveolar ventilation, resets the respiratory center sensitivity for CO_2, and lowers daytime $PaCO_2$.

NPPV also relieves clinical symptoms such as morning headache, daytime hypersomnolence, and edema; improves quality of life; and reduces the need for hospitalization in patients with OHS. The high inspiratory impedance encountered in some very obese individuals may necessitate high inflation pressures to adequately treat OHS. The mean inspiratory and expiratory pressures in one study on patients with an average BMI of 42 were 18 and 7 cm H_2O, respectively. Evidence and guidelines to assist with the decision between CPAP and NPPV are lacking, but most clinicians start with CPAP alone if OSA is present (and NPPV if not), and switch to NPPV if hypoventilation fails to improve within the first few months.

Selection Guidelines

A number of characteristics permit the selection of appropriate patients with chronic respiratory failure to receive NPPV (Table 19-4). The combination of mild to moderate daytime carbon dioxide retention (usually an indication of more severe nocturnal retention) and symptoms attributable to hypoventilation and associated poor sleep quality is a clear indication, as is symptomatic nocturnal hypoventilation even in the absence of daytime carbon dioxide retention. Secondary considerations include a history of repeated hospitalizations for bouts of respiratory failure.

Patients should be excluded from consideration if they are unable to protect their airway adequately because of swallowing impairment or excessive secretions, particularly if combined with a weakened cough mechanism. If such patients desire aggressive support, they are usually more safely managed with invasive ventilation.

The patient's diagnosis is also an important consideration. Those with stable or slowly progressive neuromuscular diseases or chest wall deformities are the best candidates. Others,

TABLE 19-4 Guidelines for Initiating Noninvasive Ventilation in Patients with Chronic Respiratory Failure*

Restrictive Thoracic Disorders

1. Symptomatic despite optimal medical therapy† (e.g., morning headaches, daytime hypersomnolence, chronic fatigue) and

2. Gas exchange disturbance:
   - Chronic CO_2 retention ($Paco_2 > 45$ mmHg) or
   - Nocturnal hypoventilation (as evidenced by O_2 saturation < 88% for > 5 consecutive minutes while breathing room air), intact neurologically, or

3. Severe pulmonary dysfunction:
   - FVC < 50% predicted or
   - Maximal inspiratory pressure < 60 cmH$_2$O or

4. Other considerations:
   - Repeated hospital admissions for hypercapnic respiratory failure

Chronic Obstructive Pulmonary Disease

1. Symptomatic despite optimal medical therapy (including oxygen supplementation, if indicated) and

2. Gas exchange disturbance:
   - Chronic CO_2 retention ($Paco_2 \geq 52$ mmHg) and
   - Nocturnal hypoventilation (as evidenced by O_2 saturation < 89% for $\geq$ 5 consecutive minutes while breathing usual FIO_2) and

3. Obstructive sleep apnea (OSA) excluded (on clinical grounds; sleep study needed only if clinically indicated); if OSA present, CPAP indicated initially

4. Other considerations:
   - Repeated hospital admissions for hypercapnic respiratory failure

*Based on Medicare guidelines for reimbursement of noninvasive ventilation. These guidelines do not recognize repeated hospital admissions as a reason for reimbursement, and appeal may be necessary if that is justification.

†Oxygen therapy alone may exacerbate CO_2 retention and should be avoided in hypercapnic patients with restrictive thoracic disorders.

such as those with central hypoventilation or obstructive sleep apnea who have had a trial of nasal CPAP fail, are also acceptable candidates. Patients with rapidly progressive neuromuscular processes, particularly if there is upper airway involvement, are poor candidates. Selection criteria used by Medicare to guide reimbursement for patients with chronic airway obstruction are listed in Table 19-4. Because of the numerous studies showing no benefit among patients with COPD with daytime carbon dioxide levels of 40–45 mmHg, the threshold for carbon dioxide retention is higher in these patients than in those with restrictive thoracic disease ($Paco_2 \geq 52$ mmHg).

APPLICATION OF NONINVASIVE POSITIVE PRESSURE VENTILATION

Initiation

Techniques for initiating NPPV are similar in the acute and long-term settings, except that the level of urgency differs. Initiation must be tailored for each individual patient under both circumstances. In the acute setting, the interface and the ventilator must be selected rapidly. Accordingly, it is advisable to attach a "mask bag" containing a variety of types and sizes

of nasal and oronasal masks and straps to a noninvasive ventilation cart or to initially use masks that will fit most individuals and can be rapidly applied. In the chronic setting, it is also useful to have a variety of interfaces readily available, but mask interchanges can be made over periods of days to weeks rather than minutes. In both settings, implementation by experienced practitioners who can impart a sense of confidence and reassurance is helpful.

Evidence and experience indicate that, in the acute setting, the oronasal mask is usually preferred because it has the advantage of controling mouth leaks better than nose masks. The nasal mask is rated by patients as more comfortable for long-term application, so transitioning from an oronasal to a nasal mask should be contemplated after the first few days if NPPV is going to continue. Proper mask fit is also important. Selection of a mask that is too large should be avoided, because this necessitates excessive tightening of the straps to minimize air leakage. With regard to ventilator selection, both pressure-limited and volume-limited ventilators have been used with similar success rates. In the acute setting, pressure-limited ventilators specifically designed for noninvasive ventilation that offer oxygen blenders and display waveforms are gaining popularity; likewise, in the long-term setting, pressure-limited ventilators (bilevel type) have seen increasing use. Portable volume-limited ventilators are used mainly for patients with a continuous need for mechanical ventilation because of their enhanced alarm capabilities.

To begin NPPV, the mask should be placed on the patient's face and ventilation started. Cooperative patients may feel more comfortable if they hold the mask themselves. Initial ventilator settings should be relatively low to enhance patient comfort and acceptance, but inspiratory pressure or tidal volume should be adjusted upward as tolerated to provide adequate ventilatory assistance. Typical initial settings on pressure-limited ventilators are 8–12 cmH$_2$O for inspiratory and 4–5 cmH$_2$O for expiratory pressures (pressure support of 5–10 cmH$_2$O and PEEP of 4–5 cmH$_2$O), with subsequent adjustments as needed to alleviate respiratory distress (increased inspiratory pressure) or to counterbalance auto-PEEP, treat hypoxemia, or eliminate obstructive apnea (increased expiratory pressure). The difference between the two (pressure support) should be adequate to reduce ventilatory effort. In some patients, higher levels of IPAP or PEEP may be so effective in reducing the inspiratory work of breathing that the additional benefit of IPAP cannot be discerned. For volume ventilation, initial tidal volumes range from 10–15 mL/kg to compensate for air leaks. The ventilator is usually set to allow patient triggering (assist/control mode). The ventilator backup rate is set at the spontaneous breathing rate if the aim is to assume the patient's breathing and minimize the work of respiratory muscles; it is set slightly below this level to encourage spontaneous breathing. Once the patient seems to be synchronizing with the ventilator, the head straps can be tightened. These should be adjusted to minimize air leakage, particularly into the eyes, but the practitioner should still be able to slip one or two fingers under the strap. Most manufacturers have developed ways to minimize facial trauma, such as forehead cushions and soft silicon seals, and these should be used as recommended. Humidification is not needed in the acute setting for short-term use (<6–12 h) but probably enhances comfort for longer-term applications. Oxygen supplementation is adjusted to maintain the desired oxygen saturation. It is administered by means of the blender on critical care ventilators and some bilevel ventilators, or directly through a cannula connected to the mask or T-connector in the ventilator tubing when other bilevel ventilators are used.

Adaptation and Monitoring

In the acute setting, the first 1–2 h are critical in achieving successful adaptation. Coaching and encouragement are usually required to assist the patient in keeping the mouth shut during nasal ventilation and in adopting a breathing pattern that achieves synchronization with the ventilator and reduction of breathing effort. Instructions such as "Try to take slow, deep breaths and let the machine breathe for you" may be helpful. Also, judicious administration of low doses of sedatives such as midazolam may be helpful in enhancing patient acceptance.

Ventilators designed to administer noninvasive ventilation often lack sophisticated monitoring capabilities, but even when critical care ventilators are used for noninvasive ventilation in the acute setting, monitoring by means of the ventilator may be inaccurate or even misleading because of air leaks. Accordingly, close bedside monitoring is essential until the patient's respiratory status stabilizes. Although NPPV can easily be administered on general medical wards, the acuteness of the patient's illness and the need for close monitoring should dictate the site of administration. Acutely ill patients should be treated in an intensive care or stepdown unit until their condition stabilizes, regardless of whether they are treated with invasive or noninvasive ventilation.

Achieving patient comfort (or at least minimizing discomfort), tolerance, and reduced respiratory effort is the most important initial goal, so frequent bedside assessments are obligatory. Oxygen saturation is monitored continuously, with oxygen supplementation titrated to achieve a target such as 92% or greater. Patient synchrony with the ventilator, respiratory and heart rates, and sternocleidomastoid muscle activity are monitored closely. Blood gases are also monitored as clinically indicated. Inspiratory pressures or tidal volumes (target 6–7 mL/kg) are usually adjusted upward as tolerated to bring about desired improvements in $Paco_2$. Some suggest that this is best achieved by increasing expiratory rather than inspiratory pressures, reducing the $Paco_2$ by reducing the inspiratory work of breathing associated with auto-PEEP.

In the chronic setting, adaptation usually takes much longer than in the acute setting, mainly because the patient must learn to sleep with the ventilator being used. The patient is instructed to initiate noninvasive ventilation at home for 1- or 2-h trial periods during the daytime and then try to fall asleep with the device at bedtime. The patient is encouraged to leave the equipment on as long as tolerated but is allowed to remove it if desired. During this period, frequent contact with an experienced home respiratory therapist helps ensure proper use and adjustment. Some patients successfully sleep through the night within days of initiation, but others require several months to become accustomed to the machine. Occasional patients are unable to adapt successfully to NPPV, usually because of mask intolerance. In these cases, trials with alternative noninvasive ventilators, such as negative pressure or abdominal ventilators, may be successful, as long as the patient has no more than mild obstructive sleep apnea.

Patients should be seen every few weeks by a physician during the initial adaptation period. At the time of office follow-up, symptoms and physical signs should be assessed for evidence of nocturnal hypoventilation or cor pulmonale. Spirometry is indicated, particularly in patients with progressive neuromuscular syndromes. Daytime arterial blood gases or pulse oximetry

and end-tidal Pco_2 ($Petco_2$) levels should be obtained at the time of visit or when symptoms worsen. Although there is no consensus on the ideal level, daytime $Petco_2$ values ranging from approximately 40–55 mmHg are usually associated with good control of symptoms. Nocturnal monitoring by use of oximetry, multichannel recorders, or full polysomnography is also useful after adaptation to noninvasive ventilation to ensure the adequacy of oxygenation and ventilation.

Commonly Encountered Problems and Possible Remedies

NPPV is safe and well tolerated in most properly selected patients. The most commonly encountered problems are related to the interface or to air pressure or flow (Table 19-5). Patients often complain of mask discomfort, which can be alleviated by minimizing strap tension or trying different mask sizes or types. The most common error is to select a mask that is too large, necessitating excessive strap tension to minimize leaks. For acute applications, patients may be anxious and have difficulty synchronizing their breathing efforts with the ventilator. Adjustments in ventilator mode (to pressure support, which usually enhances synchrony) and in inspiratory and expiratory pressures, plus judicious use of sedation, may help. In patients with severe COPD who have intrinsic PEEP, increases in expiratory pressure may facilitate triggering.

Excessive air pressure leading to sinus or ear pain is another common complaint, alleviated by lowering the pressure temporarily and then gradually raising it again as tolerance improves. Patients may also complain of dryness or congestion of the nose or mouth. For dryness, nasal saline or gels or efforts to reduce air leaks may help. Heated, flow-by humidifiers may also be helpful, particularly in dry climates or during winter. For nasal congestion, inhaled corticosteroids or decongestants or oral antihistamine–decongestant combinations may be used.

Other commonly encountered problems include erythema, pain, and ulceration on the bridge of the nose related to pressure from the mask seal. Minimizing strap tension, by use of artificial skin, or switching to alternate masks such as nasal pillows can alleviate this problem. Gastric insufflation is

TABLE 19-5	Adverse Side Effects and Complications of Noninvasive Positive-Pressure Ventilation
Mask-related	Discomfort Nasal bridge redness, ulceration Anxiety, claustrophobia Acne-like skin rash
Related to airflow or pressure	Nasal or oral dryness or congestion Eye irritation Sinus or ear pain Gastric insufflation Air leakage Sleep arousals
Related to ventilator type	Asynchrony; inability to sense inspiration or expiration Inability to compensate for leaks Rebreathing
Major complications	Failure to tolerate or ventilate, need for intubation (25–33%) Aspiration pneumonia Pneumothorax

common, but it is usually not severe, probably because inflation pressures are low compared with those used with invasive ventilation.

Air leaking through the mouth (with nasal masks), through the nose (with mouthpieces), or around the mask (with all interfaces) is inevitable during NPPV. Nasal and oronasal masks, particularly if too large, may leak air into the eyes, causing conjunctival irritation. Refitting or reseating the mask usually addresses this problem. Pressure-limited devices compensate for air leaks by maintaining inspiratory airflow during leaking; tidal volumes on volume-limited ventilators must be adjusted by the practitioner to compensate. To reduce air leaking through the mouth, patients are coached to keep the mouth shut or use chinstraps or oronasal masks. Air leakage occurs during most sleep in many patients, but fortunately, gas exchange is usually well maintained. Leaks may still contribute to arousals and poor sleep quality, however, and ventilatory assistance may occasionally be compromised. In this case, options include trials of alternative interfaces or ventilators or, if these fail, tracheostomy. Major complications of noninvasive ventilation, such as aspiration and pneumothorax, are unusual if patient selection guidelines are observed.

CONCLUSION

Noninvasive ventilation, mainly in the form of NPPV, has established itself as an important ventilator modality. In the acute setting, NPPV is preferred to invasive positive-pressure ventilation for selected patients with COPD exacerbations because of reduced morbidity and mortality, the possibility of reduced costs, and enhanced patient comfort. NPPV is also suitable for initial mechanical ventilatory assistance in patients with a variety of other forms of acute respiratory failure, including those with acute pulmonary edema or an immunocompromised status, as long as selection guidelines are observed. These guidelines are designed to identify patients at risk of needing mechanical ventilatory assistance while excluding those who are too ill to be safely managed noninvasively. Also, the cause of the patient's respiratory failure should be one that is anticipated to be reversed within a few days.

NPPV is also considered the ventilatory modality of first choice for a variety of causes of chronic respiratory failure, including neuromuscular diseases, chest wall restrictive processes, and central and obesity hypoventilation. Here, NPPV offers comfort, convenience, and cost advantages over invasive positive-pressure ventilation. Ideal candidates should require

only intermittent ventilatory assistance and have intact upper airway function, but NPPV has been successfully applied even in patients requiring continuous assistance and those with bulbar dysfunction.

The efficacy of NPPV has not been firmly established in patients with chronic respiratory failure because of COPD, but patients with substantial hypercarbia and nocturnal oxygen desaturation seem to be the ones most likely to benefit.

If NPPV fails in patients with chronic respiratory failure, alternative forms of noninvasive ventilation, such as negative pressure ventilators, pneumobelts, or rocking beds, may still occasionally be effective.

SUGGESTED READINGS

Antonelli M, Conti G, Esquinas A, et al: A multiple-center survey on the use in clinical practice of noninvasive ventilation as a first-line intervention for acute respiratory distress syndrome. Crit Care Med 2007; 35(1): 18–25.

Bach JR, Alba AS, Saporito LR: Intermittent positive pressure ventilation via the mouth as an alternative to tracheostomy for 257 ventilator users. Chest 1993; 103:174–182.

Bourke SC, Bullock RE, Williams TL, et al: Noninvasive ventilation in ALS: Indications and effect on quality of life. Neurology 2003; 61: 171–177.

Bourke SC, Tomlinson M, Williams TL, et al: Effects of non-invasive ventilation on survival and quality of life in patients with amyotrophic lateral sclerosis: a randomized controlled trial. Lancet Neurol 2006; 5:140–147.

Esteban A, Frutos-Vivar F, Ferguson ND, et al: Noninvasive positive-pressure ventilation for respiratory failure after extubation. N Engl J Med 2004; 350:2452–2460.

Ferrer M, Valencia M, Nicolas JM, et al: Early noninvasive ventilation averts extubation failure in patients at high risk: a randomized trial. Am J Respir Crit Care Med 2006; 173:164–170.

Gonzalez Diaz G, Alcaraz AC, Talavera JCP, et al: Noninvasive positive-pressure ventilation to treat hypercapnic coma secondary to respiratory failure. Chest 2005; 127:952–960.

Hill NS: Noninvasive ventilation in chronic obstructive pulmonary disease. Resp Care 2004; 49(1):72–89.

Lightowler JV, Wedjicha JA, Elliott MW, Ram FS: Non-invasive positive pressure ventilation to treat respiratory failure resulting from exacerbations of chronic obstructive pulmonary disease: Cochrane systematic review and meta-analysis. BMJ 2003; 326:177–178.

Majid A, Hill NS: Noninvasive ventilation for acute respiratory failure. Curr Opin Crit Care 2005; 11:77–81.

Masip J, Roque M, Sanchez B, et al: Noninvasive ventilation in acute cardiogenic pulmonary edema. JAMA 2005; 294:3124–3130.

Mehta S, Hill NS: Noninvasive ventilation—State of the art. Am J Respir Crit Care Med 2001; 540–577.

Nava S, Gregoretti C, Fanfulla F, et al: Noninvasive ventilation to prevent respiratory failure after extubation in high-risk patients. Crit Care Med 2005; 33:2465–2470.

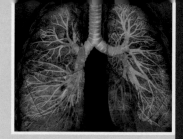

20 Airway Management

JEANINE P. WIENER-KRONISH • DAVID W. SHIMABUKURO

INTRODUCTION

The decision to instrument the airway is made in response to one or more of three circumstances: (1) failure of oxygenation, (2) failure of ventilation, or (3) for protection of the airway. The medical provider responsible for securing the airway must know the advantages and problems of the various available techniques for airway management and rapidly integrate these concepts for the patient who needs immediate assistance. Adverse outcomes occur with failure to restore ventilation, failure to recognize an esophageal intubation, or massive aspiration by the patient in association with intubation. Death or hypoxic brain damage occurs when airway management is poorly performed. Closed claim analyses have determined that, in many instances, there is an associated failure to recognize the scope of the clinical problem and/or a failure to act in a timely manner.

INDICATIONS AND CONTRAINDICATIONS

The most common indication for definitive airway management with endotracheal intubation is respiratory failure (i.e., failure of oxygenation and/or ventilation) and the need to deliver positive-pressure ventilation. This can be manifested by hypoxia, hypercapnia, or excessive work of breathing. Other indications include protection for the lungs from aspiration of gastric contents or blood in patients with neurologic compromise leading to an inability to protect the airways, insurance of airway patency in facial or airway trauma and/or swelling of upper airway structures, and the need to administer deep sedation/general anesthesia. The only contraindication to airway management is if doing so violates a competent patient's wishes.

TECHNIQUES

General Considerations

The initial approach to management of the airway is to obtain a history of any prior airway problems and to recognize situations that are associated with difficulty securing an airway. Patients who have a restricted oral opening, a small pharyngeal space, a noncompliant submandibular tissue, limited atlantooccipital flexion/extension, or partial airway obstruction from masses or redundant tissue can be difficult to manage. Mask ventilation may be particularly difficult in obese patients, edentulous patients, those with full beards, or those who have partial airway obstruction.

Special Considerations

There are a number of special considerations when managing an airway. Patients who are at an increased risk of aspiration (nausea/vomiting, postprandial, obese, pregnant, hiatal hernia, significant gastroesophageal reflux, intraabdominal pathology) require Sellick's maneuver during direct laryngoscopy (Figure 20-1). Alternately, they can be intubated while awake or lightly sedated.

Repeated attempts at emergency tracheal intubations (i.e., more than two attempts) is associated with increased morbidity and with cardiac arrests (Mort TC: Anesth Analg 2004; 99:607–13). Therefore, after two attempts at tracheal intubation with conventional laryngoscopy, other techniques should be considered, such as the use of a laryngeal mask airway (LMA). Patients who are hypotensive from acute myocardial ischemia or infarction (cardiogenic shock), hypovolemia (hypovolemic shock), or sepsis (septic shock) requiring vasopressor therapy to maintain an adequate perfusion pressure have a higher incidence of preintubation death. These patients do not tolerate increases or decreases in heart rate or blood pressure. Accordingly, medications and techniques that maintain normal hemodynamics need to be used.

Patients who have aneurysms do not tolerate rapid alterations in their blood pressure, which increases the risk of rupture. Therefore, as in those with shock, medications and techniques that maintain normal hemodynamics must be used. Irrespective of underlying diseases, before managing a patient's airway, certain sedatives, paralytics, vasopressors, and vasodilators should be readily available.

Airway Management Paradigms

Six broad types of airway management include noninvasive ventilation, awake intubation, intubation with spontaneous ventilation, intubation with neuromuscular paralysis, emergent nonsurgical airway management, and surgical airway management.

Noninvasive Ventilation

Patients may maintain adequate oxygenation and ventilation if assisted with continuous positive airway pressure or bilevel positive airway pressure. Both can be delivered either nasally, with a full-face mask or head chamber. Contraindications to these techniques include ventilatory or hemodynamic instability, a requirement for sedation, inability to handle upper airway secretions, severe hypoxia, risk of aspiration, or inability to wear a tight mask.

Awake Intubation

Ideally, patients should be intubated awake. However, most would find the experience to be very unpleasant and quite traumatic. Regardless, this is the preferred method in those with difficult airways, because the patients can continue to spontaneously ventilate and oxygenate. Approaches for awake intubation range from blind nasal, which does not require

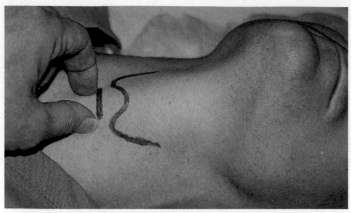

FIGURE 20-1 Sellick maneuver. The cricoid cartilage is identified by palpation below the thyroid cartilage. Firm pressure is placed on this structure to occlude the esophagus. Pressure is maintained until after intubation, and airway control is documented by auscultation of the lung fields and end tidal CO_2.

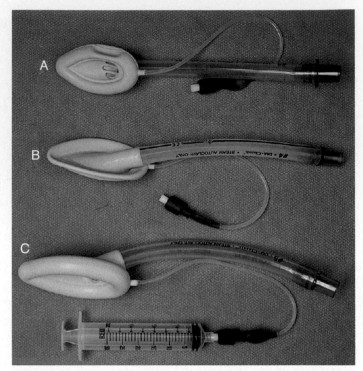

FIGURE 20-2 Laryngeal mask airway (LMA). Available in sizes 1–5. Note the slits to allow ventilation and placement of an endotracheal tube by means of a fiberoptic bronchoscope. There are several techniques for proper insertion. Commonly, the LMA is placed slightly inflated, with the tongue and mandible gently pulled anteriorly, with continuous pressure straight posteriorly until it "slides" in place. Position is confirmed after full inflation by the ability to ventilate the patient, as noted by chest rise and auscultation. Most adults will accept a size 4 or 5. **A,** Number 3, partially inflated. **B,** Number 4, completely deflated. **C,** Number 5, completely inflated.

laryngeal visualization, to direct laryngoscopy, which uses topical anesthesia, fiberoptic laryngoscopes, or fiberoptic bronchoscopes.

Intubation with Spontaneous Ventilation

Sedative agents administered as a bolus can maintain spontaneous ventilation, yet permit direct laryngoscopy or the placement of an LMA (Figure 20-2). The LMA rests in the posterior hypopharynx, displacing the tongue anteriorly while keeping the glottis open. Once inflated, the LMA provides a seal to allow limited positive-pressure ventilation if needed. Because it sits above the larynx, it does not protect against aspiration of gastric contents. A fiberoptic bronchoscope can be passed through an LMA for placement of an endotracheal tube (Figure 20-3).

Intubation with Neuromuscular Paralysis

Intubation with neuromuscular paralysis is the most common method used for direct laryngoscopy, because relaxation of the masseter muscle facilitates visualization of the glottis (see Figure 20-3). Loss of spontaneous respiration means the practitioner must obtain immediate airway control or ensure adequate ventilation by mask. When this option is selected, the provider must have an alternate plan, because the larynx is not always visualized.

A rapid sequence approach is undertaken in patients thought to have an airway that can be easily controlled by direct laryngoscopy and are at significant risk for aspiration of gastric contents. The patient is preoxygenated with 100% oxygen by full-face mask to increase the alveolar PO_2. A sedative agent (hypnotic) and a short-acting muscle relaxant are administered sequentially (Table 20-1). At the same time, an assistant applies pressure to the cricoid cartilage (the only complete ring in the tracheobronchial tree) by means of Sellick's maneuver, which occludes the esophagus and decreases the risk of aspiration of gastric contents (see Figure 20-1). This external pressure is maintained until the airway is secured by tracheal intubation. The goal is rapid definitive control of the airway. New antagonists will be available in the near future that will be able to reverse nondepolarizing neuromuscular blockade. This will allow the rapid reversal of neuromuscular blockade in

patients and, therefore, may allow more frequent use of these drugs without the fear of prolonged paralysis.

Emergent Nonsurgical Airway Management

Transtracheal catheter oxygenation or transtracheal jet ventilation is used in emergent situations in which one or several approaches have failed and improvement in oxygenation is imperative (Figure 20-4). This technique is usually only able to achieve minimally acceptable levels of oxygenation but does provide time for more definitive measures to obtain an airway. Emergency cricothyroidotomy is not technically difficult (based on Seldinger technique) and can be accomplished quickly with readily available equipment. Single-use, sterile kits are commercially available.

Percutaneous tracheotomy is also based on the Seldinger technique. It should ideally be done with the aid of direct visualization through a fiberoptic bronchoscope in the trachea. It is technically more difficult and requires more time than a cricothyroidotomy. Regardless, oxygenation and ventilation are easily achieved once the tracheotomy tube is properly placed (Figure 20-5).

Surgical Airway Management

Surgical access, emergent or nonemergent, is necessary when laryngeal visualization cannot be achieved and a definitive airway cannot be established. A surgical cricothyroidotomy

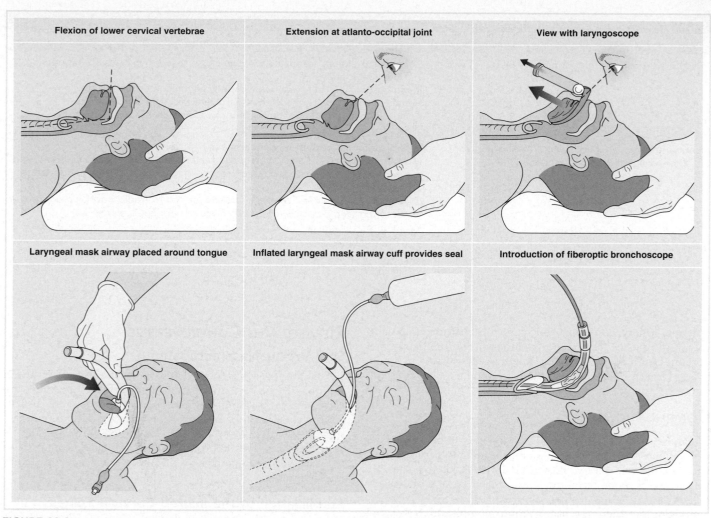

FIGURE 20-3 Airway management techniques. Correct positioning is important to optimize the view during direct laryngoscopy. Flexion of the lower cervical spine brings the trachea in line with the pharynx, and extension at the atlantooccipital joint aligns the trachea with the oral cavity. The laryngoscope is usually introduced from the right side of the mouth. The tongue is displaced leftward into the mandible by traction in an anterocaudal direction (arrow) to reveal the glottis. The laryngeal mask airway (LMA) is placed manually around the tongue in an unconscious patient. The LMA cuff seats around the glottis and, when inflated, provides a seal to allow spontaneous or limited positive pressure ventilation. The LMA cuff also lies over the esophagus, which allows the possibility of gastric inflation, regurgitation, and pulmonary aspiration. A fiberoptic bronchoscope may be introduced through the mouth or nose and used to traverse the larynx. (A bronchoscope can also go through the LMA.) An endotracheal tube is then guided over the bronchoscope into the trachea.

requires more skill than a percutaneous approach but allows for direct visualization of anatomy to ensure proper placement (see Figure 20-4). An open surgical tracheotomy is not an option in an emergency, because it is very time consuming. It should be performed only by physicians trained in this procedure. Surgical airways can be performed with the patient awake with local anesthesia.

Considerations in the Choice of Airway Control

A number of considerations affect the choice of airway control. Whether all structures are seen by laryngoscopy or by bronchoscopy, any visualization is preferable to blind techniques when placement of the endotracheal tube must be precise (i.e., when oxygenation is low, the patient is unstable, or the patient is soiling the airway).

Techniques that maintain the patient's spontaneous ventilation give the clinician time, and the opportunity, to try different approaches. Practitioners must be able to achieve ventilation by mask if paralytic agents are being administered, but the relaxation of glottic structures that occurs with paralysis may make mask ventilation more difficult. Fiberoptic approaches usually take longer than 3 min and, accordingly, should not be the first choice in extremely emergent situations. When these approaches are selected, alternative methods, which include laryngeal mask airways, should be available to deal rapidly with acute deteriorations. New or unfamiliar techniques should not be tried in emergency situations that require immediate action or in situations that involve critically ill patients who have limited respiratory or ventilatory reserve.

If the approach selected is unsuccessful, proper judgment dictates abandonment of the procedure, aiding the patient with mask ventilation as necessary, and either obtaining help or trying another approach. The patient must be oxygenated. Remember, only 3 min is available to achieve oxygenation when the patient stops breathing. Transtracheal ventilation or cricothyroidotomy should be attempted instead of repeated

TABLE 20-1   Common Agents Used for Airway Control

Drug			Dosage (mg/kg)	Comments
Sedative drugs		Thiopental	3–5	Cardiac depression, vasodilatation, can cause severe hypotension during hypovolemic states
		Propofol	1.5–2.5	Rapid onset and offset, vasodilates, easily contaminated, affirm sterility
		Etomidate	0.2–0.3	Hemodynamic stability, myoclonus, associated adrenal suppression
		Ketamine	0.5–2 mg IV 4–6 mg IM	Analgesic, sympathetic stimulant, bronchodilator, causes dysphoria
Neuromuscular blocking agents		Midazolam	0.5–0.25 mg	Vasodilatation, hypotension, dangerous in hypovolemic states
		Succinylcholine	1–2	Most rapid onset, lasts <5 minutes; contraindicated in hyperkalemia, burns, and chronic neural injuries; associated with malignant hyperthermia and masseter spasm in children
		Vecuronium	0.07–0.1	Clinical duration 30 minutes; higher dose required for rapid onset; associated with prolonged paralysis in corticosteroid-dependent patients
		Rocuronium	1–1.5	Rapid onset, but clinical duration 20 minutes; associated with prolonged paralysis in corticosteroid-dependent patients
		Cisatracurium	0.2–0.35	Slightly delayed onset, clinical duration 30 minutes; metabolism via plasma cholinesterase

attempts at laryngoscopy. Clinicians who instrument the airway must practice transtracheal ventilation and/or cricothyroidotomies until they can obtain an emergency airway in 3 min or less (Figure 20-6).

COMPLICATIONS

The most serious complication is the inability to perform mask ventilation or to oxygenate a patient, leading to cardiac arrest and anoxic brain injury. Prolonged intervals of hypoxia can be caused by poor technique, resulting in a lack of oxygen delivery.

In addition, there are other serious complications as well. Oral and tracheal mucosal damage arise from intubation attempt(s). Blades, stylets, and other objects in the airway can damage the airway mucosa and cause life-threatening hemorrhage. These risks are increased in the patient who has coagulopathies or friable mucosa (e.g., mucositis). Dental damage can also occur. Stylets should never protrude beyond the distal end of the endotracheal tube, because tracheal disruption can occur.

Transtracheal needles or catheters can lead to massive and life-threatening subcutaneous emphysema and/or pneumothorax. Tracheotomy tubes may be misplaced into nontracheal structures, resulting in subcutaneous emphysema and life-threatening hypoxemia. Also, the distal end of the endotracheal tube may inadvertently be placed in the right mainstem bronchus with consequent single lung ventilation. The position of all endotracheal and tracheotomy tubes should be confirmed by radiograph or by direct visualization and withdrawn sufficiently to sit above the carina.

Tracheotomies can lead to bilateral pneumothoraces secondary to the surgical site's proximity to the apices of the lungs. Damage to the veins in the neck can also occur with the possibility of severe hemorrhage. Newly placed tracheotomy tubes should not be replaced by inexperienced clinicians because of the difficulty in finding the proper position in the trachea and the danger of creating a false passage. A reasonable option for the management of a dislodged fresh tracheotomy includes orotracheal intubation for airway control, followed by the elective replacement of the tracheotomy tube as a surgical procedure.

PITFALLS AND CONTROVERSIES

Oral Versus Nasal Intubation

The nasal approach is somewhat easier than the oral because of the broader curve that the oral endotracheal tube must traverse before reaching the glottis. Nasal intubations usually require smaller tubes and topical application of local anesthesia mixed with a vasoconstrictor for the nasal mucosa to prevent bleeding. This approach should be avoided in patients who have coagulopathies or in those who have sustained midface trauma.

Stabilization of the Injured Cervical Spines

The risk of catastrophic neurologic injury makes it imperative that any lateral displacement of the cervical spine be avoided in patients who are suspected of having sustained traumatic cervical spine injuries. Although gentle manual stabilization may be all that is available, it must be appreciated that this stabilization does not fully immobilize the head during the atlantooccipital extension that occurs with direct laryngoscopy. The placement of a halo jacket on such a patient fully protects their cervical spine. Fiberoptic or blind nasal techniques should be used for situations in which full neck extension cannot be tolerated.

Ventilation After a Failed Rapid Sequence Induction

When the trachea cannot be intubated during a rapid sequence maneuver, the external pressure on the cricoid cartilage should be maintained. Ventilation with small rapid breaths maintains airway pressure at a low level so the pressure that compresses the esophagus is not exceeded.

Management of Regurgitation during Mask Ventilation

Positive pressure in the airway forces regurgitated gastric contents from the hypopharynx into the trachea and can cause acute lung injury. Appropriate management includes maintenance of cricoid pressure and rapidly placing the patient in the Trendelenburg position. The bulk of the gastric contents are removed by manual clearance or by suctioning. If conditions

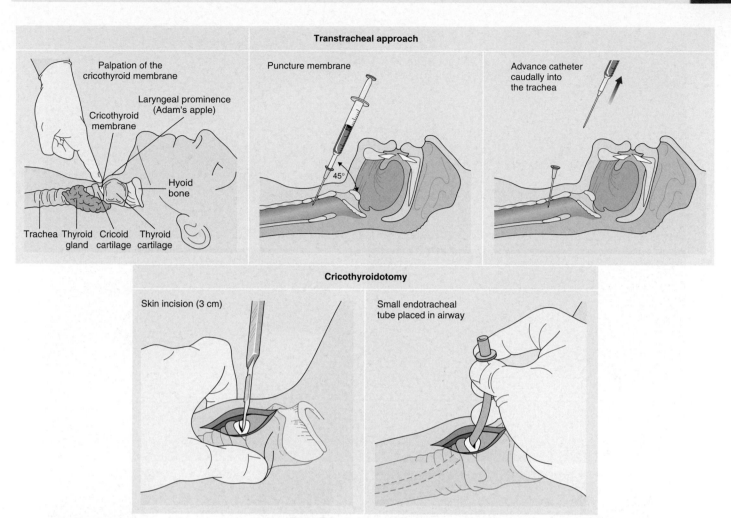

FIGURE 20-4 Transtracheal ventilation and cricothyroidotomy. The initial maneuver with either technique is palpation of the cricothyroid membrane below the laryngeal prominence of the thyroid cartilage. In the transtracheal approach, the membrane is punctured with a catheter while aspirating for air. The catheter is advanced caudally into the trachea after removing the needle. The catheter is then attached to noncompliant tubing connected to an oxygen delivery system. Exhalation is passive, either through the oropharynx or by detachment from the oxygen supply. To perform a cricothyroidotomy, a 3-cm vertical skin incision is made below the thyroid notch; the cricothyroid membrane is then cut and distended with a finger, and a small endotracheal tube is placed in the airway.

allow, immediate direct laryngoscopy should be performed to inspect the vocal cords, with intubation of the trachea and suctioning of the airway before resumption of positive-pressure ventilation. If continued mask ventilation is necessary, small, gentle breaths are administered to limit gastric insufflation and the migration of gastric material into the distal airways.

Aspiration Prophylaxis

Aspiration prophylaxis is a prudent measure in the high-risk patient (e.g., full stomach, morbid obesity, gastroesophageal reflux, parturients). Antacids should be administered immediately before endotracheal intubation, because they rapidly increase the gastric pH above 2.5. Animal studies demonstrate aspiration of particulate antacids is associated with the development of severe pneumonitis; thus, nonparticulate antacids, such as 30 mL of sodium citrate, are recommended. Although the administration of sodium citrate increases the gastric fluid volume, additional animal studies suggest that pulmonary injury is worse after the aspiration of small quantities of low pH fluid compared with the aspiration of larger quantities of high pH fluid. H_2-Receptor antagonists and proton-pump

inhibitors take longer to act and do not affect the preexisting gastric contents. They are of little value in the acute situation.

Size of Endotracheal Tube

For the average adult man, an 8.0-mm internal diameter (ID) endotracheal tube is appropriate, whereas a 7.5-mm ID tube is used for women. For pediatric patients, tube size selection is based on age by use of the formula ID = (age + 16)/4. Depending on coexisting diseases and indications for endotracheal intubation, noncuffed endotracheal tubes may be preferable in those children younger than 12 years old. Tubes at least one size larger and smaller should always be available to accommodate individual anatomic variations.

Type of Blade

Laryngoscope blades come in a variety of styles and sizes. The most commonly used blades include the curved Macintosh and the straight Miller blades. The curved blades are inserted into the vallecula, immediately anterior to the epiglottis, which is then flipped out of the visual axis to expose the larynx. The Miller blade is inserted past the epiglottis, which is simply

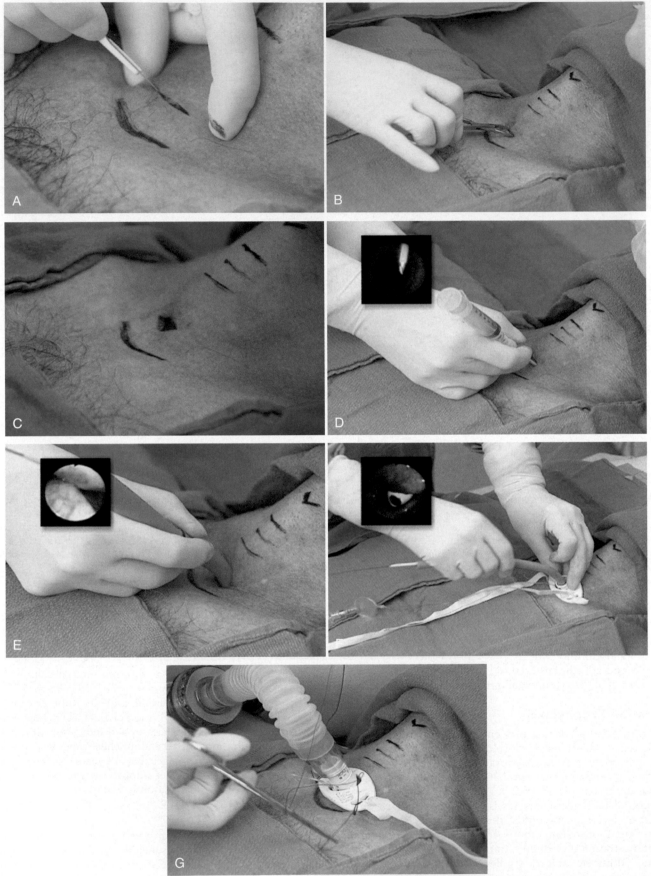

FIGURE 20-5 For legend, see page 273.

FIGURE 20-5 Bedside percutaneous dilatational tracheotomy. To perform a bedside percutaneous tracheotomy, a 1- to 2-cm horizontal skin incision is made at the level between the first and second or second and third tracheal rings (**A**). By use of a blunt clamp, the tissue is dissected to the level of the trachea (**B, C**). An introducer needle with an attached syringe filled with fluid is placed into the trachea. Placement is confirmed by aspiration of air or bubbling of fluid in the syringe or by direct visualization with fiberoptic bronchoscopy (**D**). The syringe is removed, and a J-tipped guidewire is advanced through the needle; the needle is then removed. Serial dilators are placed over the guidewire into the trachea to widen the opening (**E**). The final dilator contains the tracheotomy tube. Once the tracheotomy tube is placed, the final dilator with guidewire is removed, and the tube is sutured and tied into place (**F, G**). (Courtesy of Cook Critical Care, Bloomington, Indiana.)

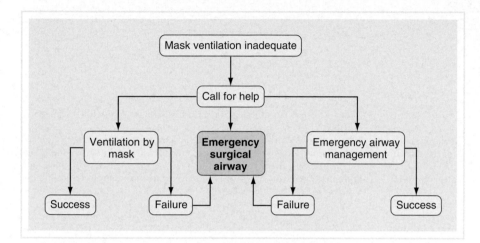

FIGURE 20-6 Emergency airway algorithm. If mask ventilation is insufficient, assistance from other personnel should be obtained to perform a jaw thrust and to place an oral airway. If these attempts fail, the provider must obtain an emergent airway (laryngeal mask airway, retrograde intubation techniques, transtracheal ventilation) or a surgical airway. (Adapted from the American Society of Anesthesiologists.)

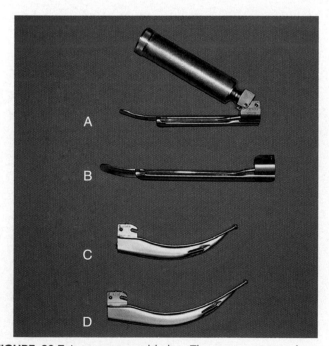

FIGURE 20-7 Laryngoscope blades. The most common laryngoscope blades are the Miller and Macintosh blades. **A,** Miller 2. **B,** Miller 3. **C,** Macintosh 3. **D,** Macintosh 4. In the average adult male, a Miller 2 or Macintosh 3 blade is best.

lifted out of the way of the glottis. Many clinicians believe the Macintosh blade is technically easier because the wider blade prevents intrusion of the tongue into the visual field. However, in difficult situations (i.e., anteriorly situated larynx, large epiglottis), the straight blade frequently affords improved visualization (Figure 20-7).

Positioning the Obese Patient

The proper "sniff" position (neck flexion, head extension) should be achieved before attempts at direct laryngoscopy. In the obese patient, this requires elevating and supporting the shoulders by the placement of towels or blankets. In addition to elevating the head to optimize the visual axis, this maneuver also creates more room for head extension (Figure 20-8).

Acute Asthma, Cardiac Ischemia, or Hypertension in the Patient with a Full Stomach

To avoid increasing bronchospasm, ischemia, or hypertension, a deep level of sedation or anesthesia should be achieved before laryngoscopy. Intubation attempts during "light" planes of anesthesia or sedation may cause dangerous sympathetic responses or intense bronchospasm. However, the risk of aspiration is increased with an increased depth of sedation.

An alternative approach is to test the ease of mask ventilation while administering cricoid pressure when the patient is awake. Small doses of sedation are then administered while gentle mask ventilation with cricoid pressure is continued. Tidal volumes are kept small to maintain low pharyngeal pressures. The depth of sedation can be titrated to maintain stable heart rate and blood pressure. Muscle relaxation should be used. Laryngoscopy may be achieved in two stages. On the first view of the glottis, the cords and trachea may be sprayed with lidocaine (lignocaine). Subsequent ventilation for 1 min allows time for the local anesthetic to take effect. The patient's hemodynamic response is observed during the initial laryngoscopy to determine the adequacy of sedation. Marked sympathetic responses indicate the need for further sedation or for other autonomic agents before repeat laryngoscopy and placement of the endotracheal tube.

FIGURE 20-8 Positioning the obese patient. With the obese patient in the supine position, neck movement and access with a laryngoscope are hindered by fat. When the same patient is positioned with the shoulders elevated and the occiput further elevated so that the head assumes a "sniffing" position, access to the airway is facilitated.

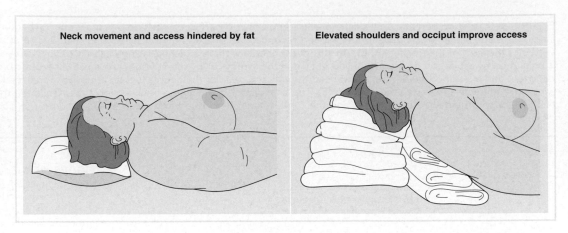

Neck movement and access hindered by fat

Elevated shoulders and occiput improve access

SUGGESTED READINGS

American Society of Anesthesiologists Task Force on Management of the Difficult Airway: Practice guidelines for management of the difficult airway. Anesthesiology 1993; 78:597–602.

Benumof JL: Laryngeal mask airway: indications and contraindications. Anesthesiology 1992; 77:843–846.

Jaber S, Amraoui J, Lefrant J-Y, Arich C, Cohendy R, Landreau L, Calvet Y, Cappdevila X, Mahamat A, Eledjam J-J: Clinical practice and risk factors for immediate complications of endotracheal intubation in the intensive care unit: A prospective multiple-center study. Crit Care Med 2006; 4:2355–2361.

Miller RD, ed: Anesthesia, 5th ed. Philadelphia: Churchill Livingstone; 2000.

Schwartz DE, Matthay MA, Cohen NH: Death and other complications of emergency airway management in critically ill patients. Anesthesiology 1995; 82:367–376.

Walz JM, Zayaruzny M, Heard SO: Airway management in critical illness. Chest 2007; 131:608–620.

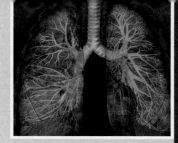

21 Preoperative Pulmonary Evaluation

COENRAAD F.N. KOEGELENBERG • ANDREAS H. DIACON • CHRIS T. BOLLIGER

Major surgery carries a definite risk that is accentuated in patients with underlying comorbidities. Postoperative pulmonary complications are more frequent than cardiac complications, prolong hospital stay by an average of 1–2 weeks, and undoubtedly contribute to perioperative morbidity and mortality. The reported frequency of postoperative pulmonary complications varies from very rare occurrences to almost 70%. This wide range is due to patient selection, procedure-related risk factors, and differing definitions for postoperative complications. Ensuring that measures are in place to anticipate and prevent these events remains paramount. This chapter reviews the changes in pulmonary physiology that occur with anesthesia and surgery; briefly describes the typical pulmonary complications arising from surgery; reviews the preoperative functional assessment; and concludes with a rational and practical approach to preoperative evaluation of patients undergoing various major surgical interventions.

PERIOPERATIVE PULMONARY PATHOPHYSIOLOGY

Postoperative pulmonary complications follow as extensions of perioperative pulmonary physiology. These physiologic alterations are summarized in Table 21-1 and discussed below.

Pulmonary gas exchange can deteriorate during the perioperative periods by several mechanisms. Placing a normal subject in a supine position leads to changes in all lung volumes except tidal volume. The vital capacity (VC) decreases by 2–5%, total lung capacity (TLC) by 7–10%, closing volume (CV) by 10%, residual volume (RV) by 40%, and functional residual capacity (FRC) by up to 20%. These changes occur without evidence of airflow obstruction. The addition of a general anesthetic worsens the restrictive ventilatory defects: the FRC may drop by 25% after an uncomplicated procedure. This fall is accentuated with a thoracotomy or sternotomy (drop in lung volumes by 30%). Upper abdominal surgery (drop in FRC by up to 50% for up to a week) particularly predisposes patients to postoperative complications. The fact that these changes persist well after the reversal of anesthesia indicates that changes in lung and chest wall mechanics occur as a result of the surgery itself, with diaphragmatic dysfunction likely to be the major contributor. The cause of this phenomenon remains to be fully explained. Direct injury to the diaphragmatic muscle during surgical manipulation has been implicated as a mechanism, but measurements of transdiaphragmatic pressure during maximal phrenic nerve stimulation also suggest that decreased efferent neural activity is involved. Inhibitory reflexes involving pain and other stimuli to sympathetic, vagal, or splanchnic receptors have all been implicated as possible mechanisms.

The reduction in FRC reduces the effective lung volume available for gas exchange. As FRC falls, it converges on the closing capacity (CC), and eventually leads to the point where dependent regions of lung may become atelectatic (creating a shunt) or may open for only a portion of the tidal breath, so that they become relatively hypoventilated in proportion to their perfusion (resulting in ventilation/perfusion [$\dot{V}/\dot{Q}$] mismatching), ultimately leading to hypoxemia. Factors that significantly contribute to atelectasis during the perioperative phase include decreased mucociliary clearance as a result of inhaled anesthetic agents, a depressed cough reflex (caused by pain and opiates), and neuromuscular blockade. Volatile anesthetics attenuate hypoxic pulmonary vasoconstriction that may worsen $\dot{V}/\dot{Q}$ mismatching.

Intraoperative and postoperative arterial hypoxemia and hypercapnia are frequently encountered. Immediately after surgery, the residual effects of anesthesia are responsible and result in depression of normal $\dot{V}/\dot{Q}$ matching. Beyond the first day, the restrictive changes noted earlier, particularly the low FRC, become important. Hypoventilation, increased dead space ventilation with rapid and/or shallow breathing, and decreased mixed venous oxygen saturation because of low cardiac output, anemia, and arterial desaturation and increased peripheral oxygen consumption all contribute to the impairment of gas exchange.

Central respiratory depression is not uncommon during the postoperative period. Opiates and related drugs may cause suppression of respiratory drive and attenuation of the normal responses to hypoxia and hypercapnia.

POSTOPERATIVE PULMONARY COMPLICATIONS

A detailed discussion of pulmonary complications is beyond the scope of this chapter (see Box 21-1). Atelectasis complicated by hypoxemia and nosocomial sepsis is common, whereas clinically significant pulmonary embolism, gastric aspiration, and acute lung injury (and acute respiratory distress syndrome) all carry a significant morbidity and mortality.

RISK FACTORS

Patient-Related Preoperative Risk Factors

Several well-defined risk factors have been identified and are summarized in Box 21-2. *Cigarette smokers* have an increased risk for postoperative pulmonary complications even in the

TABLE 21-1 Pulmonary Pathophysiology During Surgery and General Anesthesia

Functional residual capacity (FRC)	↓ 25% with lower abdominal surgery ↓ 30% with thoracic surgery ↓ 50% with upper abdominal surgery
Diaphragmatic impairment	Multifactorial
Inhibition of cough and mucus clearance	Inhaled anesthetics, opiates Pain
Atelectasis	↓ Lung volumes (FRC) Diaphragmatic impairment Inhibition of cough (pain, opiates) ↓ Mucociliary clearance
Impairment of gas exchange	Shunt caused by atelectasis Ventilation/perfusion mismatch secondary to hypoventilation and pulmonary vasoconstriction
Depression of ventilatory control	Opiates

BOX 21-1 Postoperative Pulmonary Complications

General Complications

Atelectasis
Nosocomial infections
  Bronchitis
  Pneumonia
Respiratory failure/hypoxemia
Pulmonary embolism
Gastric aspiration
Acute lung injury/acute respiratory distress syndrome
Bronchospasm
Exacerbation of underlying lung disease
Obstructive sleep apnea

Specific to Thoracic Surgery

Nerve injuries
  Phrenic nerve
  Recurrent laryngeal nerve
Pleural effusion
Bronchopleural fistula with prolonged air leaks
Empyema
Postpneumonectomy pulmonary edema
Sternal wound infection and dehiscence
Postpneumonectomy syndrome
Pulmonary torsion

BOX 21-2 Patient-Related Risk Factors for Postoperative Pulmonary Complications

Smoking ++
Chronic pulmonary disease ++
  (particularly chronic obstructive pulmonary disease)
Diminished general health status ++
  (American Society of Anesthesiologists Class > 2; see
  Table 21-2)
Poor nutritional and metabolic status +
  (including albumin < 30 g/L and urea > 30 mg/dL)
Advanced age +/−
Obesity +/−

++, Strong predictors; +, moderate predictors; +/− little evidence of increased risk.

absence of overt lung disease. The relative risk of pulmonary complications among smokers varies from 1.4–4.3, being highest in those who smoke during the 2 months before surgery. Although many smokers and ex-smokers have apparent normal lung function, most have hypersecretion of mucus and impairment in mucociliary clearance. With superadded pain, opiates, impaired cough, and atelectasis, the burden of pooled secretions is a major risk factor for respiratory infections and hypoxemia. Several studies suggest that smoking cessation must occur as long as 4–8 weeks before surgery for the complication rate to fall to that of nonsmokers. A prospective study of 200 smokers awaiting coronary bypass grafting found a lower risk of pulmonary complications among those who had stopped smoking at least 8 weeks before surgery than among those who had continued smoking up to their surgery (14.5% vs 57.1%).

Chronic obstructive lung disease is an important patient-related risk factor for postoperative pulmonary complications. Unadjusted relative risks of postoperative pulmonary complications range from 2.7–6.0. Because there is a definite correlation between preoperative lung functions and the rate and severity of pulmonary complications in patients with chronic obstructive pulmonary disease (COPD), attempts to improve lung function should be undertaken. Measures may include intensive preoperative bronchodilator therapy, smoking cessation, and a short course of systemic corticosteroids (particularly in patients who are not at their real or anticipated optimal baseline). The indiscriminate use of preoperative antibiotics is generally discouraged. Elective surgery should be deferred if an acute exacerbation is present. Despite the increased risk with obstructive lung disease, there seems to be no prohibitive level of pulmonary function below which surgery is absolutely contraindicated (apart from pulmonary resection, as discussed later).

Although an increased rate of postoperative pulmonary complications would be expected in patients with *asthma*, no evidence exists to confirm this. In fact, well-controlled asthma (free of wheezing, peak flows >80% of predicted, or personal best) has been shown not to carry any added risk. A short course of perioperative corticosteroids, if required, does not increase the incidence of infection or other postoperative complications in patients with asthma.

TABLE 21-2 American Society of Anesthesiologists Classification of Preoperative Risk

ASA Class	Systemic Disturbance	PPC (%)	Mortality (%)
1	Healthy patient with no disease outside of the surgical process	1.2	<0.03
2	Mild to moderate systemic disease caused by the surgical condition or by other pathologic processes, medically well-controlled	5.4	0.2
3	Severe disease process that limits activity but is not incapacitating	11.4	1.2
4	Severe incapacitating disease process that is a constant threat to life	10.9	8
5	Moribund patient not expected to survive 24 h with or without an operation	NA	34%
E	Suffix to indicate emergency surgery for any class	Increased	Increased

PPC, Postoperative pulmonary complications; NA, not applicable.

General health status, as per the American Society of Anesthesiologists (ASA) classification (see Table 21-2), is strongly predictive of postoperative pulmonary complications. Given the fact that the criteria for assigning ASA class include the presence of a systemic disease that affects activity or is a threat to life, patients with significant preexisting lung disease would be expected to have a higher ASA class. In fact, an ASA class >2 confers an almost 5-fold increase in risk. The Goldman cardiac risk index (see later) also performs well for pulmonary complications, because heart and lung diseases often overlap.

Metabolic disturbances adversely affect the respiratory system and contribute to a high rate of complications. Malnutrition (albumin <30 g/L, odds ratio = 2.5) reduces ventilatory drives to hypoxia and hypercapnia, contributes to respiratory muscle dysfunction, impairs immunity, and alters lung elasticity. However, no evidence exists to suggest that nutritional intervention attenuates the risk. A blood urea (BUN) greater than 30 mg/dL carries an odds ratio of 2.3 for postoperative complications.

Advanced age often appears in univariate analyses as a moderate risk factor but fades to insignificance once confounding issues such as coexisting comorbidities are considered. When data are stratified according to the ASA class, the overall perioperative mortality for classes II–V is the same in all age groups. Age alone should not be given predictive weight in decision making, nor should it be grounds to withhold surgery.

Obesity was once assumed to be a risk factor for postoperative pulmonary complications, but a number of recent studies found no difference in the pulmonary complication rates between obese and nonobese patients. Obstructive sleep apnea, often associated with obesity, may worsen during the postoperative phase.

Intraoperative Risk Factors

Box 21-3 lists intraoperative risk factors. The *surgical site* is of key importance. Risk increases as the incision approaches the diaphragm: upper abdominal and thoracic procedures carry the highest risk (ranging from 5–40%), probably because of related diaphragmatic impairment. In abdominal surgery, vertical incisions carry slightly greater morbidity than horizontal incisions. Video-assisted thoracoscopic and laparoscopic procedures have approximately one tenth the pulmonary complication rates of open procedures. Procedures outside the thorax or abdomen carry a very low risk.

There is a threefold to fourfold increase in postoperative pulmonary complications in patients who undergo *lengthy procedures* (longer than 3 h) compared with those having shorter

---

BOX 21-3 Intraoperative Risk Factors for Postoperative Pulmonary Complications

Site: Thoracic and upper abdominal procedures
Emergency procedures
Prolonged anesthesia (>3 h)
General anesthesia (vs spinal or local anesthesia)
Long-acting neuromuscular blockers (e.g., pancuronium)
Large intraoperative blood transfusion requirements

---

operations. An increased rate of pulmonary complications is also associated with prolonged neuromuscular blockade secondary to long-acting nondepolarizing agents (e.g., pancuronium). Accordingly, shorter-acting vecuronium or atracurium are the preferred intraoperative neuromuscular blockers. The use of epidural and spinal anesthesia may reduce complication rates, because anesthesia up to a T4 level does not alter lung mechanics to the same extent as general anesthesia. Regional anesthetic techniques have an even lower risk.

PREOPERATIVE FUNCTIONAL ASSESSMENT

Cardiac Impairment

Perioperative myocardial infarctions (MI) occur in 1.4% of patients older than the age of 40. Among patients preselected to undergo preoperative myocardial perfusion scanning, the risk is much higher: MI occurs in almost 7%. Patients with underlying peripheral or cerebrovascular disease also have an increased risk.

The history, physical examination, and electrocardiogram must be integrated to develop an *initial estimate of perioperative cardiac risk*. The American College of Cardiology/American Heart Association (ACC/AHA) guidelines on perioperative cardiovascular evaluation for noncardiac surgery states that three components must be assessed to estimate cardiac risk: patient-specific clinical parameters, exercise capacity, and surgery-specific risk (Figure 21-1).

A detailed *history* of the patient's symptoms and exercise capacity and a complete physical *examination* are essential for risk assessment. Further special investigations should be guided by the clinical evaluation and only performed if the results would have an impact on patient care.

A *preoperative resting electrocardiogram (ECG)* is recommended in patients with a recent episode of possible ischemic

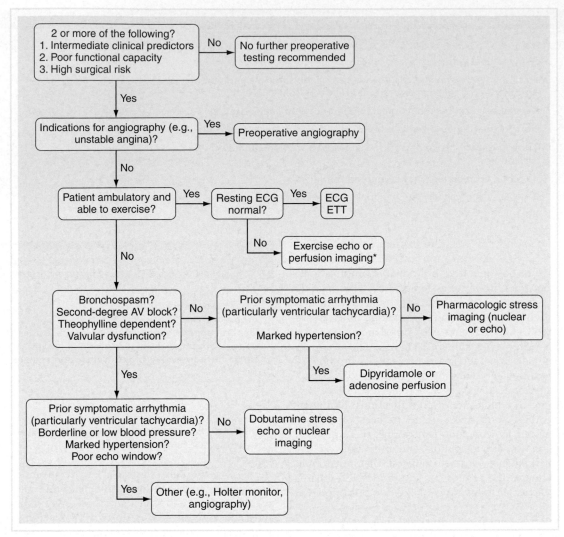

FIGURE 21-1 ACC/AHA guidelines: stepwise approach to preoperative cardiac assessment. Testing is only indicated if the results will impact care. Subsequent care may include cancellation or delay of surgery, coronary revascularization followed by noncardiac surgery, and intensified care. *In the presence of a left bundle branch block (LBBB), vasodilator perfusion imaging is preferred. *ECG*, Electrocardiogram; *ETT*, exercise tolerance test. (Reproduced with permission from Eagle KA, Berger PB, Calkins H, *et al*: ACC/AHA guideline update on perioperative cardiovascular evaluation for noncardiac surgery. J Am Coll Cardiol 2002; 39:542).

chest pain, patients with known ischemic or other cardiac disease, those with diabetes mellitus or who are older than 70 years, and in patients undergoing an intermediate or high-risk surgical procedure. A resting preoperative ECG is also recommended in asymptomatic men older than age 45 and women older than age 55 years in the presence of risk factors for atherosclerosis.

The *type and timing of surgery* significantly affect the risk of perioperative cardiac complications. Emergency surgery is associated with particularly high risk, as is major vascular surgery.

To simplify the prediction of risk, Goldman *et al* identified and validated six independent predictors of major cardiac complications—the *revised Goldman cardiac risk index* (Box 21-4). The risk of major cardiac complications varies according to the number of risk factors, ranging from 0.4% with no risk factors to 5.4% with three or more risk factors. This index should

identify patients who may benefit most from *further evaluation and definitive preoperative management.*

Exercise ECG testing is usually the preferred stress test because the actual exercise tolerance is considered an even more important predictor of outcome than ischemic ECG changes. Exercise ECG testing can also incorporate perfusion imaging or echocardiography. The main indications for stress testing are patients deemed to be at high risk for ischemic heart disease, patients at intermediate risk plus poor or indeterminate functional status, a history consistent with coronary disease, or high-risk surgery. Stress testing has a very high negative predictive value for postoperative cardiovascular events, but a low positive predictive value. It is, therefore, more useful for reducing estimated risk (if negative) than for identifying patients at very high risk. Among patients who cannot exercise sufficiently to reach the target heart rate, the two most widely used alternatives are *thallium myocardial perfusion imaging (MPI)*

BOX 21-4 Revised Goldman Cardiac Risk Index (RCRI): Six Independent Predictors of Major Cardiac Complications**

1. High-risk type of surgery
2. History of ischemic heart disease
   a. History of myocardial infarction MI (within 6 mo)
   b. Positive exercise test
   c. Current complaint of ischemic chest pain
   d. Use of nitrate therapy
   e. Pathologic Q waves on ECG
   (Not included: prior coronary revascularization procedure unless one of the other criteria for ischemic heart disease is present)
3. History of cardiac failure
4. History of cerebrovascular disease
5. Diabetes mellitus requiring treatment with insulin
6. Preoperative serum creatinine >2.0 mg/dL (177 μmol/L)

and *dobutamine echocardiography*. *Resting transthoracic echocardiography (TTE)* or *ambulatory ECG monitoring* may add predictive information in certain patients undergoing noncardiac surgery.

Pulmonary Reserve

A detailed *history and physical examination* are critical components of the preoperative risk assessment. A history suggesting undiagnosed chronic lung disease should be determined, including decreased exercise tolerance, unexplained dyspnea, and cough with or without sputum production. Symptoms of sleep apnea must be explained. Preexisting lung disease, recent respiratory tract infection or exacerbation, and the smoking status should be noted. The physical examination should be directed toward evidence of chronic obstructive lung disease, particularly decreased breath sounds, a prolonged expiratory phase, or wheezes. Clinical evidence suggesting deep venous thrombosis should be sought.

There is considerable controversy and unfortunately little evidence regarding the role of routine preoperative *pulmonary function testing* (PFT) for risk stratification, apart from lung resection (see later) and before coronary artery bypass. The prohibitive spirometric threshold below which the risks of surgery are unacceptable is unknown, and some studies suggest that PFTs is in fact inferior to the history and physical examination in predicting postoperative pulmonary complications. Furthermore, the 2006 American College of Physicians guideline recommends that preoperative spirometry should not be used routinely for risk stratification. Therefore, spirometry should be reserved for patients who are thought to have undiagnosed COPD, those with COPD or asthma who may not be at their best baseline (according to clinical evaluation), and patients with clinically unexplained dyspnea or exercise intolerance. Pulmonary function testing should never primarily be used to deny surgery.

The routine use of *arterial blood gas analysis* is also discouraged. No evidence suggests hypercapnia to be independently associated with an elevated risk. Hypoxemia has also not been identified as a significant independent predictor of

complications in clinical studies. Nevertheless, the American College of Physicians has recommended preoperative arterial blood gas analysis in patients undergoing coronary bypass surgery or upper abdominal surgery with a history of smoking or dyspnea and in all patients undergoing pulmonary resection.

Chest X-rays add very little to the preoperative risk assessment of healthy individuals. Studies of routine preoperative chest radiographs demonstrated that only 1–3% of these films yielded abnormalities that actually impacted on the preoperative evaluation or management. The prevalence of abnormal chest radiographs increases with age. With the scarcity of evidence, it is no wonder that opinions and practices vary considerably from institution to institution. Most authorities would perform routine chest radiographs in patients with known cardiopulmonary disease and in those older than 50 years of age undergoing high-risk surgical procedures.

Formal exercise testing has been studied most extensively in preparation for lung resection surgery (see later). There are no convincing data to support the routine use of this modality in the evaluation of patients before general surgery.

Arozullah evaluated and validated a *multifactorial risk index* for postoperative respiratory complications by use of a prospective cohort model that included both derivation and validation cohorts from a large Veterans Administration database. Point values were awarded to various preoperative predictors (Table 21-3), which, in turn, gave a weighted postoperative pneumonia and respiratory failure risk index (Table 21-4).

Combined/Multifactorial Assessment

A combined *Cardiopulmonary Risk Index (CPRI)* was proposed by Epstein for pulmonary resection candidates. He suggested a 10-point CPRI, with 4 points awarded to various cardiac parameters (comparable to the Goldman Risk Index) and 6 points to pulmonary parameters (obesity; smoking; wheezing, productive cough; $FEV_1/FVC < 0.7$; and $P_aCO_2 > 45$ mmHg 6 kPa). In the original series, it was found that patients with a combined score greater than 4 were 17 times more likely to have postoperative pulmonary complications develop than those with a score less than 4; no complications occurred in patients with a score of 2 or less. This CPRI unfortunately failed at predicting complications in multiple subsequent studies and reviews (which included patients undergoing general thoracic and upper abdominal surgery) and has thus not gained general acceptance. A further limitation of this index is the requirement for PFTs and arterial blood gas analysis in all cases.

A simple, objective, and reproducible test of the combined function of lung, heart, and proximal muscle endurance is *the 6-minute walk distance (6-MWD)*. The unit of measurement is total distance covered during 6 min (in meters). Level of dyspnea during the test may be assessed by use of the Borg scale. The 6-MWD (performed according to the American Thoracic Society Guidelines) is validated for the assessment and follow-up of both chronic obstructive lung disease and diffuse parenchymal lung disease. A walk distance of less than 200 meters is associated with significant impairment, but there is little prospective evidence to correlate this modality with postoperative complications.

TABLE 21-3 Postoperative Pneumonia and Respiratory Failure Risk Index Scoring

Preoperative Risk Factor	Point Value Postoperative Pneumonia	Respiratory Failure
Type of surgery		
Abdominal aortic aneurysm repair	15	27
Thoracic	14	21
Upper abdominal	10	14
Neck	8	11
Neurosurgery	8	14
Vascular	3	14
Age		
>80 yr	17	6
70–79 yr	13	6
60–69 yr	9	6
50–59 yr	4	4
Functional status		
Totally dependent	10	7
Partially dependent	8	7
Weight loss >10% in past 6 mo	7	—
History of chronic obstructive pulmonary disease	5	6
General anesthesia	4	—
Impaired sensorium	4	—
History of cerebrovascular accident	4	—
Blood urea nitrogen level		
<2.98 mmol/L (<8 mg/dL)	4	—
2.97–7.85 mmol/L (8–21 mg/dL)	0	—
7.95–10.7 mmol/L (22–30 mg/dL)	2	—
>10.7 mmol/L (>30 mg/dL)	3	8
Transfusion >4 units	3	—
Emergency surgery	3	11
Steroid use for chronic condition	3	—
Current smoker within 1 yr	3	—
Alcohol intake >2 drinks per day in past 2 wk	2	—
Albumin <3.0 g/dL (<30 g/L)	—	9

Adapted from Arozullah AM, Daley J, Henderson WG, Khuri SF: Multifactorial risk index for predicting postoperative respiratory failure in men after major non-cardiac surgery. Ann Surg 232:242–250, 2000. Arozullah AM, Khuri SF, Henderson WG, Daley J: Development and validation of a multifactorial risk index for predicting postoperative pneumonia after major noncardiac surgery. Ann Intern Med 135:847–857, 2001.

PRACTICAL APPROACH TO PREOPERATIVE EVALUATION

Surgery in General

A detailed history and physical examination remain paramount for preoperative risk assessment in evaluating patients for potential postoperative pulmonary complications. Specific attention should be paid to symptoms that suggest the possibility of underlying (occult) lung disease, including exercise intolerance, cough, and unexplained dyspnea. Risk factors for postoperative complications should be actively sought.

A stepwise approach, suggested by Smetana and based on evidence presented in this chapter, is given in Figure 21-2.

A high-risk patient will benefit from strategies to reduce pulmonary complications, which may include preoperative medical interventions, the reconsideration of the indications for surgery, and the use of alternative anesthetic techniques (e.g., spinal or epidural anesthesia).

Lung Resection Surgery

Pulmonary resection remains a high-risk procedure. The morbidity and mortality depend not only on the patient risk profile (see Box 21-2) but also on the extent of resection. A lobectomy, for example, carries a mortality of 2–3% and a pneumonectomy 4–6%. Validated evidence-based guidelines (see Figure 21-3) fortunately exist that should standardize the preoperative approach to these patients, who often have significant cardiac and pulmonary (tobacco-related) comorbidity. In distinct contrast to the marginal use of pulmonary function testing and imaging in the preoperative evaluation for surgery not involving lung resection, these modalities provide a solid quantitative foundation for risk stratification before pulmonary resection.

The *clinical evaluation* of the patient should focus on respiratory and cardiovascular pathology. Airflow limitation should be optimized before further evaluation and cardiac disease identified and managed either medically or surgically. The initial *pulmonary function evaluation* should include at least an FEV_1, FVC, and DL_{CO} (diffusing capacity for carbon monoxide). Values greater than 80% of predicted for FEV_1 and DL_{CO} are associated with an uncomplicated surgical course for resection up to a pneumonectomy. All other candidates, unless grossly impaired, should undergo a formal *exercise test*. Measurement of maximal oxygen consumption ($\dot{V}O_2max$) in a progressive, incremental cycle ergometry or treadmill test has proved helpful in risk assessment, because the measurement integrates a number of relevant physiologic and functional aspects (see Chapter 10). Several studies have shown that patients with a $\dot{V}O_2max$ greater than 20 mL/kg/min (or greater than 75% of predicted) tolerate pulmonary resection up to a pneumonectomy, and that patients with a $\dot{V}O_2max$ of greater than 15 mL/kg/min are candidates for lobectomies. Values of less than 10 mL/kg/min (or less than 40% of predicted) are predictive of major postoperative complications and disability, and hence constitute a high risk for lung resection.

Further evaluation according to a validated *algorithm* (see Figure 21-3) necessitates the estimation of the relative contribution of the tissue earmarked for resection (that can range from a wedge resection to segmentectomy, or a lobectomy up to a pneumonectomy) by means of the predicted postoperative (PPO) values for FEV_1, DL_{CO}, and $\dot{V}O_2max$ (see Figure 21-3, "Split Function"). The PPO values of these parameters are equal to their preoperative values × (1−fractional contribution of tissue earmarked for resection). There are three acceptable ways of estimating the relative functional contribution or split lung function (and thus to calculate the PPO values): anatomic calculation, quantitative CT scanning, or split perfusion scanning.

Anatomic calculations of the PPO values are by far the simplest: the number of patent (or functional) segments that are due for resection is subtracted from the total number of segments (19), and this value is divided by 19 to give a fraction. The FEV_1–PPO is estimated to be equal to the preoperative FEV_1 × ([19-patent segments removed]/19). For a right upper lobectomy, FEV_1–PPO would be equal to the preoperative

TABLE 21-4 Risk Class Assignment by Postoperative Pneumonia and Respiratory Failure Risk Index Score

Risk Class	Postoperative Pneumonia Risk Index (Point Total)	Predicted Probability Pneumonia (%)	Respiratory Failure Risk Index (Point Total)	Predicted Probability Respiratory Failure (%)
1	0–15	0.2	0–10	0.5
2	16–25	1.2	11–19	2.2
3	26–40	4.0	20–27	5.0
4	41–55	9.4	28–40	11.6
5	>55	15.3	>40	30.5

Adapted from Arozullah AM, Daley J, Henderson WG, Khuri SF: Multifactorial risk index for predicting postoperative respiratory failure in men after major non-cardiac surgery. Ann Surg 232:242–250, 2000; Arozullah AM, Khuri SF, Henderson WG, Daley J: Development and validation of a multifactorial risk index for predicting postoperative pneumonia after major noncardiac surgery. Ann Intern Med 135:847–857, 2001.

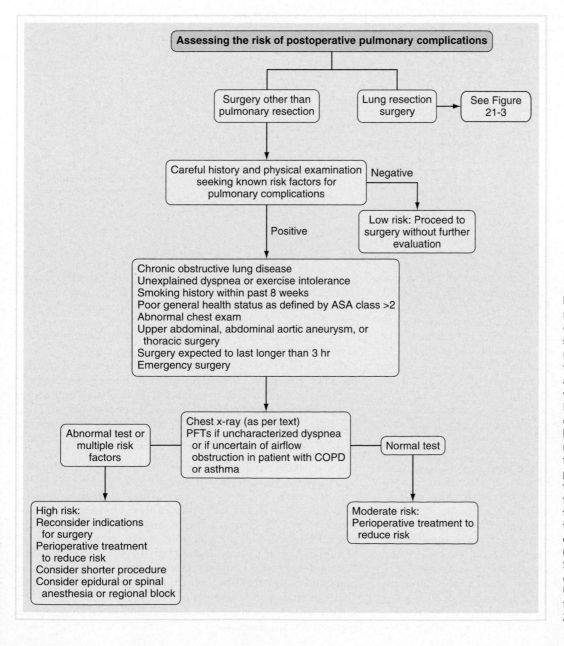

FIGURE 21-2 Assessing the risk of postoperative pulmonary complications after general surgery. Note that patients undergoing pulmonary resection are excluded from this algorithm, because separate validated algorithms exist (see Figure 21-3 and text for details). A high-risk patient will benefit from strategies to reduce pulmonary complications, which may include preoperative medical interventions, the reconsideration of the indications for surgery, and the use of alternative anesthetic techniques (e.g., spinal, epidural, or local anesthesia). (Adapted with permission from Smetana G: Evaluation of preoperative pulmonary risk. In UpToDate, Rose BD, ed: Waltham, MA 2006. Copyright 2006 UpToDate, Inc.)

FIGURE 21-3 Algorithm for the assessment of cardiorespiratory reserve and operability of candidates for lung resection. Patients undergo successive steps from top to bottom until they either qualify for varying extents of resection or are deemed high risk. A safety loop for patients with possible cardiac disease detected on exercise testing (signs or symptoms of myocardial ischemia) is shown by the dashed line in the upper left-hand corner. Split lung function testing allows a more accurate estimate of predicted postoperative (PPO) function (see text for details). This is usually calculated by means of anatomic calculations, CT scan, or the use of split perfusion scanning. Note that all percentages refer to percentages of predicted. Care must be taken to understand that PPO calculations by implication take the calculated extent of resection into account, and that this may vary from a wedge resection to a lobectomy up to a pneumonectomy. ($\dot{V}O_2$max, maximal oxygen consumption; FEV_1, forced expiratory volume in 1 sec; ppo, predicted postoperative value; DL_{CO}, carbon monoxide diffusing capacity). (Reproduced from Schuurmans MM, Diacon AH, Bolliger CT: Functional evaluation before lung resection. Clin Chest Med 2002; 23:159–172.)

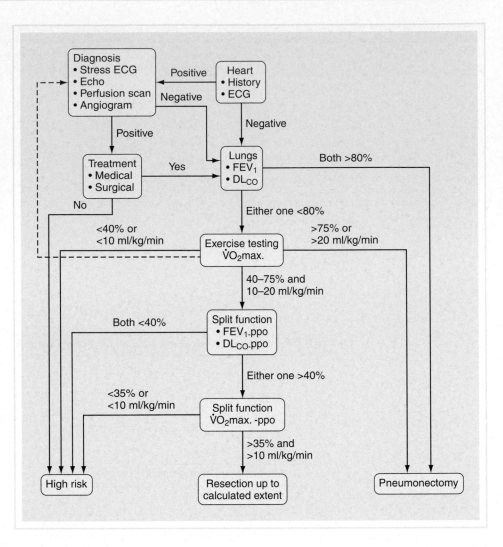

$FEV_1 \times (16/19)$, provided that the segments are all patent. For example, if a patient with an actual preoperative FEV_1 of 2.20l (59.9% of a predicted 3.70l) undergoes this procedure, then the FEV_1–PPO will be $2.20 \times 16/19 = 1.85l$ (50% of a predicted 3.70l). The DL_{CO}–PPO and the $\dot{V}O_2$–PPO are calculated in a similar fashion. Anatomic calculations have been shown in prospective studies to overestimate functional loss (i.e., there may be minimal or no functional loss after removal of destroyed lung parenchyma). It is thus worthwhile to perform these calculations in each pulmonary resection candidate, because patients who are deemed operable by means of anatomic calculations of their PPOs will generally not require radiologic calculations.

Calculated values for PPO on the basis of perfusion scans (with technetium 99m-labeled macroaggregates) have been prospectively shown to correlate the best with actual postoperative values ($R = 0.92$ for FEV_1). This technique, however, is relatively complex and requires a higher degree of expertise. Relative function is estimated by means of three-dimensional calculations that are derived from anterior, posterior, and oblique views. Densitometric calculations on the basis of CT scans are marginally less accurate than perfusion scans ($R = 0.91$) but are the preferred method in many centers (after anatomic calculations) given their availability and the fact that most lung resection candidates invariably have a preoperative

(e.g., staging) chest CT scan. Once again, calculations are based on the relative volume of lung resected. Modern software that allows three-dimensional reconstruction can simplify the calculations.

Once a candidate is deemed operable, it remains imperative to appreciate that "resection up to the calculated extent" (see Figure 21-3) refers to the extent that was used in estimating the PPO values (i.e., wedge resection to pneumonectomy). It is also important to keep in mind that an algorithm only serves as a guide, and that common sense still needs to prevail (e.g., subjecting a patient with an FEV_1 and a DL_{CO} <30% of predicted to a formal exercise test is unlikely to alter his or her "high-risk" status).

Lung volume reduction surgery for end-stage emphysema has, to an extent, redefined the limits of lung resection. Many patients with preoperative FEV_1 and diffusing capacity between 20% and 40% of predicted have benefited from targeted removal of the most emphysematous lung regions. The general tolerability of the procedure confirms the conservative nature of the previously mentioned thresholds and the fact that removal of the most diseased regions may permit better function of other regions. It remains to be determined whether tumor resection in conjunction with lung volume reduction surgery will be as successful as resection after conventional segmental approaches.

PITFALLS AND CONTROVERSIES

Arguably the greatest pitfall in the preoperative evaluation of lung resection candidates is an overreliance on certain absolute FEV_1 values as exclusive cutoffs (e.g., excluding patients with an $FEV_1 < 1.0$ l/sec from surgery). Current evidence and validated algorithms clearly favor the use of predicted postoperative values (given as percentages of predicted) for FEV_1, DL_{CO}, and $\dot{V}O_2$max.

An interesting, yet controversial, development has been the revival of simple stair climbing as a low-cost alternative to assess exercise capacity and operative risk. A large prospective study by Brunelli showed a significant correlation between the ability to climb to a 20.6-meter elevation and an uncomplicated surgical course. The major advantage of stair climbing lies in its availability, simplicity, brevity, and in the familiarity of the patients with this form of exercise. Although stair climbing may one day obviate the need for formal exercise testing in most surgical candidates, it remains unclear which parameter (maximum altitude vs speed of ascent) or which cutoffs values will be validated.

WEB-BASED READING

The ACC/AHA Practice Guidelines on Perioperative Cardiovascular Evaluation for Noncardiac Surgery is available on the Web sites of the American College of Cardiology (www.acc.org) and the American Heart Association (www.americanheart.org).

The American College of Physicians' Guidelines on the Risk Assessment for and Strategies to Reduce Perioperative Pulmonary Complications for Patients Undergoing Noncardiothoracic Surgery are available at www.acponline.org/clinical/guidelines/index.html

SUGGESTED READINGS

Arozullah AM, Khuri SF, Henderson WG, Daley J: Development and validation of a multifactorial risk index for predicting postoperative pneumonia after major noncardiac surgery. Ann Intern Med 2001; 135:847–857.

Bolliger CT, Guckel C, Engel H, et al: Prediction of functional reserves after lung resection: comparison between quantitative computed tomography, scintigraphy, and anatomy. Respiration 2002; 69(6):482–489.

Bolliger CT, Kendal R, Koegelenberg CF: Preoperative assessment for lung cancer surgery. Curr Opin Pulm Med 2005; 11(4):301–306.

Brunelli A, Al Refai M, Monteverde M, et al: Stair climbing test predicts cardiopulmonary complications after lung resection. Chest 2002; 121 (4):1106–1110.

Colice GL, Shafazand S, Griffin JP, et al: Physiologic evaluation of the patient with lung cancer being considered for resectional surgery. Chest 2007; 132:161S–177S.

Eagle KA, Berger PB, Calkins H, et al: ACC/AHA guideline update for perioperative cardiovascular evaluation for noncardiac surgery-executive summary: A report of the American College of Cardiology/American Heart Association Task Force on Practice Guidelines (Committee to update the 1996 Guidelines on Perioperative Cardiovascular Evaluation for Noncardiac Surgery). J Am Coll Cardiol 2002; 39:542.

Lawrence VA, Cornell JE, Smetana GW: Strategies to reduce postoperative pulmonary complications after noncardiothoracic surgery: Systematic review for the American College of Physicians. Ann Intern Med 2006; 144(8):596–608.

Qaseem A, Snow V, Fitterman N, et al: Risk assessment for and strategies to reduce perioperative pulmonary complications for patients undergoing noncardiothoracic surgery: A guideline from the American College of Physicians. Ann Intern Med 2006; 144(8):575–580.

Smetana GW: Preoperative pulmonary evaluation. N Engl J Med 1999; 340:937.

Smetana GW, Lawrence VA, Cornell JE: Preoperative pulmonary risk stratification for noncardiothoracic surgery: Systematic review for the American College of Physicians. Ann Intern Med 2006; 144 (8):581–595.

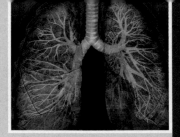

22 Cough

SURINDER S. BIRRING • IAN D. PAVORD

INTRODUCTION

Cough is a reflex that occurs when afferent nerve receptors are stimulated by inhaled, aspirated, or endogenous substances. The most sensitive sites for initiating cough are the larynx, the carina, and the points of bronchial branching. Cough receptors are also present in extrapulmonary structures, including the esophagus, diaphragm, and stomach. A broad group of "rapidly adapting 'irritant' receptors" (RARs) found in the larynx and tracheobronchial tree can be stimulated by a wide range of stimuli, including cigarette smoke, ammonia, ether vapor, acid and alkaline solutions, hypotonic and hypertonic saline, and mechanical stimulation by direct contact, mucus, or dust; all these stimuli can provoke cough. Another closely related fiber is the slowly adapting stretch receptor (SAR) that terminates inspiration and initiates expiration when the lungs are at an adequate level of inflation. SARs may also influence cough. C-fiber receptors, which have thin nonmyelinated vagal afferent fibers, are found in the laryngeal, bronchial, and alveolar walls. They are relatively insensitive to mechanical stimulation and lung inflation but are exquisitely sensitive to chemicals such as bradykinin, capsaicin, and acid pH. Stimuli that are known to cause cough in human subjects such as capsaicin, bradykinin, and citric acid activate C-fiber afferents, particularly those located in the bronchi. Afferent nerve fibers pass to a central cough receptor in the medulla triggering a forced expiratory maneuver against a closed glottis followed by glottal opening and high-velocity expiration.

Cough is an important defense mechanism that clears the airways of secretions and prevents entry of foreign bodies and irritants to the lower respiratory tract. It is a universal experience in health but also a nonspecific presenting feature of most respiratory conditions and a number of nonrespiratory conditions. Acute cough is one of the most common presenting symptoms to a general practitioner. Most cases result from viral and bacterial upper respiratory tract infections, are self-limiting, and do not require further evaluation, but a small proportion of patients have persistent cough that requires specialist opinion. Chronic cough is arbitrarily defined as a cough greater than 8 weeks in duration. It is present in 3–10% of the general population and is responsible for between 10 and 20% of respiratory outpatient referrals. Chronic cough with significant sputum production is likely to be due to intrapulmonary disease such as chronic bronchitis or bronchiectasis. A chronic dry or minimally productive cough may be due to extrapulmonary factors; the cough is likely to be due to abnormal sensitization of the cough reflex secondary to the effects of local inflammation on sensory nerve endings. Chronic cough is often perceived as a trivial problem but can be a disabling symptom associated with impairment of quality of life and distressing symptoms such as musculoskeletal chest pains, syncope, incontinence, disturbed sleep, and social embarrassment.

The key to successful management is establishing a clear diagnosis and applying effective treatment for long enough to reset the activity of cough receptors at a more physiologic level. Important pitfalls include atypical presentations, the presence of multiple etiologies, and inadequate therapy of the underlying disorder. The fact that evidence for the efficacy of specific therapies in chronic cough is largely based on expert opinion or uncontrolled trials and there is a scarcity of randomized controlled trials with well-validated outcome measures to guide the clinician presents further difficulty. Nevertheless, a systematic approach on the basis of the so-called anatomic diagnostic protocol does seem to be successful, and various series have reported a high rate of treatment success even in tertiary referral populations. There is a general consensus that the cause of most cases of chronic cough in patients with no other respiratory symptoms or signs and normal spirometry and chest radiography is asthma, eosinophilic bronchitis, gastroesophageal reflux, rhinitis, or a combination of these. Many of these conditions can be recognized clinically, and successful diagnosis and management are often possible without recourse to expensive or invasive investigations. This review will primarily focus on isolated chronic cough, because this is a common and difficult diagnostic problem for both primary and secondary care physicians.

DIFFERENTIAL DIAGNOSIS

The causes of cough can be conveniently divided into acute and chronic (Table 22-1 and Box 22-1). An acute cough is arbitrarily defined as a cough of less than 3 weeks duration. Infectious and allergic conditions are by far the most common etiologies. Most acute coughs related to viral upper respiratory tract infection resolve by 3 weeks, but a small proportion becomes persistent and requires further evaluation.

Most conditions implicated in causing chronic cough such as chronic obstructive pulmonary disease, lung cancer, foreign bodies, pulmonary tuberculosis, sarcoidosis, idiopathic pulmonary fibrosis, and heart failure will be obvious after clinical assessment, spirometry, and a chest radiograph. Thus, most patients referred for investigation of chronic cough are nonsmokers and have normal findings on physical examination and chest radiography. Most present with a nonproductive or minimally productive cough, and 60–75% will be female. There is a tendency for cough to first present around the time of menopause. The most common conditions implicated in causing chronic cough in these patients are listed in Table 22-1.

TABLE 22-1 Common Conditions Implicated in Causing Chronic Cough

Diagnosis	Approximate Incidence (%)
Rhinitis	25–30
Asthma/eosinophilic bronchitis	20–25
Gastroesophageal reflux	15–20
Postviral cough	5–10
Chronic bronchitis	5–10
Bronchiectasis	5–10
ACE inhibitor–induced cough	5–10
Unexplained	5–20

ACE, Angiotensin-converting enzyme.

BOX 22-1 Common Causes of Acute Cough

Upper respiratory tract infections
Acute sinusitis
Allergic rhinitis
Asthma

TABLE 22-2 An Initial Evaluation of a Patient with Chronic Cough

History	Cough: onset, duration, character, triggers Sputum (volume, character) Smoking, occupation Upper respiratory tract infection Drug history (ACE inhibitors) Asthma: breathlessness, wheeze, nocturnal symptoms, atopy Gastroesophageal reflux: reflux associated symptoms Rhinitis: postnasal drip, sinusitis, throat clearing, nasal congestion Adverse quality of life: musculoskeletal chest pains, incontinence, syncope, social embarrassment, anxiety, disturbed sleep
Examination	Clubbing External nasal: polyps Oropharyngeal: signs of postnasal drip, tonsillar enlargement Chest: signs of airflow obstruction, crackles
Investigations	Chest radiograph Spirometry ± bronchodilator reversibility Serial peak expiratory flow Full blood count and eosinophil differential cell count
Optional investigations	Methacholine challenge test, induced sputum, allergen skin tests Sinus X-ray/CT sinus 24-hour esophageal pH and manometry CT chest/bronchoscopy in selected patients Polysomnography Quality of Life Questionnaires Cough monitoring
Treatments	Directed at cause(s)

ACE, Angiotensin-converting enzyme; CT, computerized tomography.

PATIENT EVALUATION

An initial assessment of a patient with chronic cough is directed at finding a specific cause, assessing severity, and initiating trials of treatment. A careful history and physical examination are paramount to the evaluation of a patient with chronic cough (Table 22-2). Details of the factors surrounding the onset of cough and associated symptoms and a careful assessment of the upper airways and the respiratory system is particularly important. Basic initial investigations should include up-to-date chest radiograph, spirometry, and bronchodilator reversibility if appropriate. An abrupt onset of coughing while eating or chewing should raise the possibility of an inhaled foreign body, and the onset of cough shortly after introduction of angiotensin-converting enzyme (ACE) inhibitor therapy suggests ACE-inhibitor associated cough. The presence of significant quantities of sputum, hemoptysis, systemic symptoms, prominent breathlessness, wheeze, or abnormal physical signs increases the probability of intrinsic lung disease and should trigger appropriate investigations, which may include a high-resolution CT scan of the chest and a bronchoscopy even if there are no suggestive findings with more simple investigations. The onset of cough with symptoms suggesting an upper or lower respiratory tract infection raises the possibility of a postinfectious cough; prominent whoops, a very troublesome nocturnal cough, and cough associated with vomiting are all associated with pertussis, a condition that it increasingly recognized in school-age children and adults. Otherwise, there is little evidence that information on the timing, nature, complications, and potential aggravating factors is predictive of the underlying cause of the cough.

The history and physical examination are often unremarkable, in which case the evaluation of a patient focuses on the recognition of corticosteroid responsive conditions (i.e., asthma and eosinophilic bronchitis) and extrapulmonary factors that

may be aggravating the cough such as rhinitis and gastroesophageal reflux. One approach to the assessment of patients with chronic cough is outlined in Figure 22-1. There is emphasis on early recognition of corticosteroid responsive cough, which can be detected easily in most cases with appropriate investigations and/or treatment trials. In contrast, the management of patients with nonasthmatic cough can be complex, time-consuming, and expensive; it is often associated with disappointing response to specific therapy. It must be emphasized that it is far from clear whether extrapulmonary factors implicated in causing cough are aggravating a preexisting tendency to cough or are the underlying cause of the cough. Several factors suggest the former, including the tendency for nonasthmatic chronic cough to affect middle-aged women and the frequent clinical observation that interventions against potential causes of chronic cough often help, but rarely cure, the cough. Our view is that it is best to have no preconceptions about the underlying causal factors in nonasthmatic cough and to view extrapulmonary factors such as rhinitis and gastroesophageal reflux as potential aggravating factors rather than causes of the problem. This model has the advantage of providing a basis for the incomplete response to the treatment of these conditions seen in many patients; it should also stimulate research into the cause and treatment of the underlying heightened cough reflex sensitivity.

A further difficulty in evaluating patients with nonasthmatic chronic cough is that there is a poor correlation between

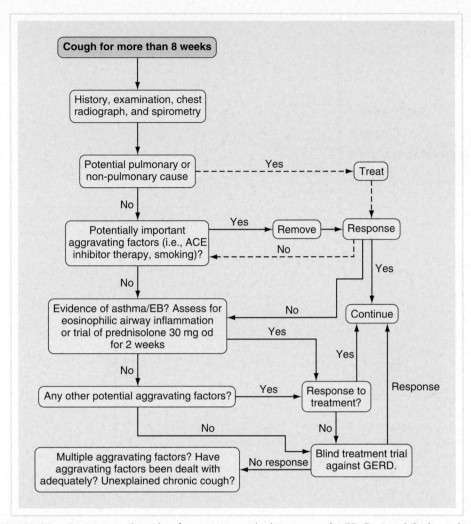

FIGURE 22-1 Diagnostic algorithm for patients with chronic cough. *EB, Eosinophilic bronchitis.*

the presence of symptoms or abnormalities on investigation of the potential aggravating factor and the success of treatment directed against that factor. Thus, the diagnosis is largely secured by demonstrating improvement in the cough after a suitable trial of treatment. Multiple potential aggravating factors are commonly present, which presents further difficulties. Treatment trials are more easily interpreted when combined with attempts to assess cough severity objectively before and after treatment. Suitable methods to do this include simple cough visual analog scores (0–100 mm; Figure 22-2), cough-specific health-related quality-of-life scores, 24-hour ambulatory cough monitoring, and evaluation of cough reflex sensitivity. Our approach is to regard a 15-mm change in visual analog score, 1.3 point change in Leicester Cough Questionnaire quality-of-life score, and a 2 doubling dose change C2 (concentration of capsaicin that causes 2 coughs) as evidence of a significant response to treatment. The remainder of this section focuses on the evaluation of the more common conditions implicated in causing chronic cough.

Cough Variant Asthma/Eosinophilic Bronchitis

Asthma is a condition characterized by airway hyperresponsiveness and inflammation that presents with variable symptoms of cough, dyspnea, and wheeze. A subgroup can present with an isolated chronic cough, known as cough variant asthma. Heightened cough reflex sensitivity is commonly seen in cough variant asthma but not in noncough predominant asthma. The airway inflammation in cough variant asthma is essentially similar to that seen in classical asthma. Typically, the cough is dry or minimally productive, it may occur nocturnally, after exercise or allergen and occupational exposure, although there are often no clinical clues. The key to diagnosing asthma is demonstrating variable airflow obstruction. Serial peak flow recordings and spirometry with bronchodilator response are routine first-line investigations but are often normal in cough variant asthma. Demonstration of airway hyperresponsiveness by bronchoprovocation testing is a more sensitive and specific index of variable airflow obstruction and can be the only abnormality seen. A blood eosinophilia and positive allergen skin prick testing or allergen-specific IgE provides supportive evidence for the presence of asthma. The diagnosis of cough variant asthma is usually confirmed with an improvement of cough with therapy.

Eosinophilic bronchitis is an increasingly recognized entity that presents with a corticosteroid responsive cough and is characterized by a sputum eosinophilia (Figure 22-3), heightened cough reflex sensitivity, but no evidence of variable airflow obstruction or airway hyperresponsiveness. Studies suggest that it is responsible for 10–15% of cases of chronic cough. The airway inflammation is similar to that seen in

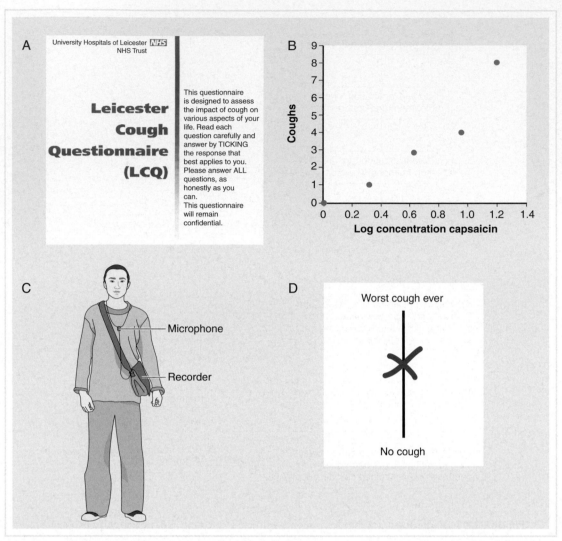

FIGURE 22-2 Cough severity assessment tools. **A,** Cough-specific health-related quality-of-life questionnaires; **B,** cough reflex sensitivity measurement; **C,** 24-h ambulatory automated cough frequency monitoring; and **D,** 100-mm cough visual analog scale.

asthma, although there is evidence that differences in airway physiology are due to the site of mast cell localization in the airway with infiltration of the epithelium occurring in eosinophilic bronchitis and infiltration of the airway wall smooth muscle occurring in asthma. It is important to recognize eosinophilic bronchitis, because it responds well to inhaled corticosteroids. This is best done by assessing airway inflammation by use of induced sputum or exhaled nitric oxide; if these techniques are not available, a trial of corticosteroid therapy is indicated irrespective of the presence of airway hyperresponsiveness.

Angiotensin-Converting Enzyme Inhibitor–Associated Cough

Approximately 8% of patients taking angiotensin-converting enzyme inhibitors develop a persistent cough. The risk is higher in females and is similar with all types of angiotensin-converting enzyme inhibitors. Excess cough is not seen with angiotensin-converting receptor antagonists. Increased airway concentrations of airway tussive mediators such as bradykinins and prostaglandins are thought to be responsible for heightened cough reflex sensitivity and cough in patients with angiotensin-converting enzyme inhibitor cough. The cough usually

resolves promptly after treatment withdrawal. Persistence may suggest asthma, the onset of which has been linked to the use of angiotensin-converting enzyme inhibitors.

Rhinitis/Upper Airway Cough Syndrome

Rhinitis, often associated with sinusitis and postnasal drip, is one of the most common conditions implicated as an aggravating factor in chronic cough. Allergy and infection are common causes of rhinitis and are thought to result in cough by mechanical stimulation from a postnasal drip and extension of local inflammation to the pharyngeal and laryngeal area where the cough receptors are most concentrated. Patients usually report nasal congestion, nasal discharge, facial pain, and may be aware of a postnasal drip and the need to frequently clear their throat. Careful examination of upper airways may reveal nasal quality to the voice, nasal polyps, sinus tenderness, and inflammation of the posterior pharyngeal wall with evidence of draining secretions. Investigations for rhinitis include nasal endoscopy and X-ray or CT scan of the sinuses, which may reveal mucosal thickening and fluid levels. An opinion from an ear, nose, and throat specialist opinion is helpful when there is diagnostic uncertainty or in the presence of severe disease.

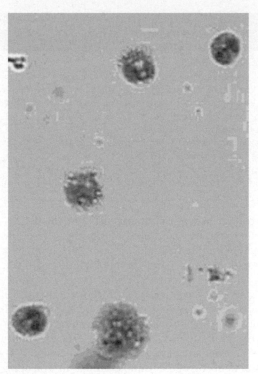

FIGURE 22-3 Sputum eosinophilia in eosinophilic bronchitis. Eosinophils are the cells with cytoplasmic granules stained bright red.

Gastroesophageal Reflux

Symptoms suggesting gastroesophageal reflux and abnormalities of esophageal function are common in patients with chronic cough of all age groups, and the frequent clinical observation that effective treatment of gastroesophageal reflux is associated with improvement of cough supports a causal association. The pathophysiology of gastroesophageal reflux–associated cough is poorly understood, but microaspiration of esophageal contents to the tracheobronchial tree and stimulation of a neural esophageal-tracheobronchial reflex are thought to be important. Gastroesophageal reflux–related cough is associated with the relaxation of the lower esophageal sphincter and often occurs during eating, talking, and on waking. Although most patients recognize heartburn, dysphagia, sore throat, globus, and dysphonia, up to a third of patients with gastroesophageal reflux–associated cough have no such symptoms. The investigations for gastroesophageal reflux such as 24-h esophageal pH studies have limited value in the investigation of cough, because they are poor predictors of response to therapy and are usually limited to patients with persistent cough despite adequate therapy or when considering more invasive therapy. Recent studies have suggested that esophageal dysmotility and nonacid gastroesophageal reflux may be aggravating factors for cough, but there are little data to support the routine evaluation of these conditions in the investigation of cough.

Other Causes of Cough

Community surveys suggest that most coughs related to upper respiratory tract infections resolve within 3 weeks. However, the cough can take several months to resolve in a small proportion of subjects. The infection in most cases remains unidentified but respiratory viruses *Mycoplasma pneumoniae*, *Chlamydia pneumoniae*, and *Bordetella pertussis* have been implicated in adults. Chronic bronchitis is a common cause of cough in smokers and may occur in nonsmokers with dusty occupations. Typically, patients have a productive morning cough. Other conditions recently reported to be associated with isolated chronic cough include asymptomatic enlarged tonsils, obstructive sleep apnea, and familial peripheral neuropathy.

Further Investigations

The use of fiberoptic bronchoscopy and high-resolution CT scanning should be reserved for patients with suggestive symptoms, signs or chest radiograph findings, or in those with no objective evidence of the more common causes of cough, because the investigations are invasive, expensive, and the diagnostic yield is low. Cough reflex sensitivity measurement has limited value in the validation of the presence of chronic cough in clinical practice because of the wide overlap of cough sensitivity between health and respiratory disease–causing cough. Ambulatory cough monitors have the advantage of providing objective evidence of the presence and intensity of cough, but routine use is hampered by automation difficulty of analysis of the recordings. Recent advances in recording devices and improved battery life have led to a renewed interest in cough monitor development, and they should be available for clinical use in the near future.

TREATMENT

Treatment directed at the specific cause of chronic cough is summarized in Table 22-3. By use of the anatomic diagnostic protocol, success rates of up to 95% in the management of chronic cough have been reported. The success rate goes down to approximately 80% in specialist cough clinics, possibly because of the complexity of cases referred. Reassessment of the patient after treatment and excluding additional aggravating factors or causes form an integral part of managing a patient with chronic cough. A common dilemma faced by physicians managing patients with chronic cough is that the diagnosis of cough often depends on successful trials of treatment, which, if unsuccessful, lead to the difficult question as to whether the underlying condition has not responded or is not responsible for the cough. In some situations, the use of objective tests to make a diagnosis and careful validation of the effect of therapy for the underlying condition should minimize this problem. Therapy for common causes of chronic cough are discussed in the following.

Rhinitis

Topical corticosteroids are the mainstay treatment for cough caused by rhinitis. Where nasal obstruction is prominent, initial additional treatment with topical decongestant sprays may be necessary, and antibiotics should be administered if infection is suspected. Topical ipratropium bromide is often helpful if rhinorrhea is prominent, and antihistamines are useful when sneeze and nasal itch is prominent and when there is coexisting atopy. Surgical treatment may be necessary when there are obvious anatomic abnormalities.

Cough Variant Asthma/Eosinophilic Bronchitis

Cough caused by asthma responds well to bronchodilators and inhaled corticosteroids. A response typically occurs within 1–2 weeks of starting therapy and reaches a maximum after

TABLE 22-3 Specific Therapy for Chronic Cough

Cause	Treatment
Rhinitis	Nasal corticosteroids Selected patients: topical ipratropium, topical decongestants, oral antihistamines, surgery
Asthma	Inhaled corticosteroids, as required inhaled bronchodilators, leukotriene antagonists
Eosinophilic bronchitis	Inhaled corticosteroids, oral corticosteroids in selected cases
GER-associated cough	Self-help measures: weight loss, smoking cessation, reduce alcohol intake, elevate head of bed, avoid eating within 2 h of bedtime Acid suppression: proton pump inhibitors Prokinetic agents: metoclopramide in selected patients Surgery: laparoscopic fundoplication in selected patients
Chronic bronchitis	Smoking cessation
ACE cough	Drug withdrawal; substitution of alternative if appropriate
Postviral cough	Observation
Bronchiectasis	Chest physiotherapy and postural drainage, antibiotics
Idiopathic chronic cough	Antitussives (dextromethorphan, codeine), nebulized lidocaine

GER, Gastroesophageal reflux; ACE, angiotensin-converting enzyme.

BOX 22-2 Common Pitfalls in the Management of Chronic Cough

- Incorrect diagnosis
- Not recognizing multiple causes of cough
- Lack of objective evidence for the diagnosis of asthma
- Prolonged and aggressive treatment may be required before cough improves
- Poor treatment compliance
- Post viral and gastroesophageal associated cough may take many months to resolve
- Inappropriate labeling of psychogenic cough
- Failure to assess the impact of cough on quality of life

sensitivity and airway inflammation. Organ-specific autoimmune diseases are common, suggesting that the airway abnormalities might have an autoimmune basis. They suffer considerable physical and psychological morbidity. Many patients with unexplained chronic cough are labeled with a diagnosis of psychogenic cough, although there is little evidence to support this view, and it is perhaps more likely that any abnormal illness behavior is secondary to the adverse impact of cough on psychosocial aspects of quality of life. When evaluating a patient with unexplained cough, it is important to recognize common pitfalls in managing chronic cough (Box 22-2). Therapy for idiopathic chronic cough is disappointing and is largely limited to nonspecific antitussive therapy such as dextromethorphan, codeine, and drugs with weak evidence of benefit such as baclofen and nebulized local anaesthetics (lidocaine, mepivacaine). There is, therefore, a large unmet need for better antitussive treatment in these patients. Referral to a respiratory physiotherapist or speech therapist for cough management advice may be of some help.

CONCLUSION

All pulmonary and many nonpulmonary conditions can be present with cough. Most will be evident after a simple clinical assessment that includes a history, physical examination, a chest radiograph, and a spirogram. Cough that remains unexplained after such an assessment is a common reason for referral to secondary care. Potential causes include asthma, eosinophilic bronchitis, rhinitis, and gastroesophageal reflux. Satisfactory outcomes can be achieved in most patients with a management strategy that includes targeted investigations and carefully controlled treatment trials. However, complete cure is not always possible, particularly in patients with cough thought to be due to extrapulmonary factors, and a significant minority of predominantly middle-aged women have unexplained chronic cough. Whether this reflects failure to identify important causes or inadequate treatment of established factors is unclear.

SUGGESTED READINGS

Birring SS, Berry M, Brightling CE, Pavord ID: Eosinophilic bronchitis: Clinical features, management and pathogenesis. Am J Respir Med 2003; 2(2):169–173.

Birring SS, Brightling CE, Symon FA, Barlow SG, Wardlaw AJ, Pavord ID: Idiopathic chronic cough: Association with organ specific autoimmune disease and bronchoalveolar lymphocytosis. Thorax 2003; 58:1066–1100.

Birring SS, Matos S, Patel RB, Prudon B, Evans DH, Pavord ID: Cough frequency, cough sensitivity and quality of life in patients with chronic cough. Resp Med 2006; 100:1105–1109.

8–10 weeks. Leukotriene antagonists are also helpful in cough variant asthma. The duration of asthma therapy remains unclear, but return of the cough on gradual withdrawal of therapy suggests long-term therapy may be necessary. Patients with cough variant asthma often have coexisting rhinitis or postnasal drip, and a complete response may not be seen until all potential aggravating factors are treated. Treatment of cough caused by eosinophilic bronchitis is with inhaled corticosteroids. Rarely oral corticosteroids are required to suppress eosinophilic airway inflammation and cough.

Gastroesophageal Reflux

Gastroesophageal reflux–associated cough is managed with self-help measures such as weight reduction, avoidance of tight clothing, elevation of headrest during sleep, reduced alcohol and tobacco intake, and drug therapy for acid suppression. Proton pump inhibitors are the most effective treatment for gastroesophageal reflux–associated cough. Anecdotal evidence suggests that high-dose therapy for at least 3 months is often required before the cough improves. Prokinetic agents such as metoclopramide may have a role in some cases. The role of antireflux surgery is unclear.

UNEXPLAINED CHRONIC COUGH

Cough remains unexplained after extensive investigations and treatment trials in up to 20% of patients. These patients are predominantly middle-aged females; they have objective evidence of airway abnormalities including increased cough reflex

Birring SS, Prudon B, Carr AJ, Singh SJ, Morgan MD, Pavord ID: Development of a symptom specific health status measure for patients with chronic cough: Leicester Cough Questionnaire (LCQ). Thorax 2003; 58(4):339–343.

Chung KF: Assessment and measurement of cough: The value of new tools. Pulm Pharmacol Ther 2002; 15(3):267–272.

Fuller RW, Jackson DM: Physiology and treatment of cough. Thorax 1990; 45(6):425–430.

Gibson PG, Dolovich J, Denburg J, Ramsdale EH, Hargreave FE: Chronic cough: eosinophilic bronchitis without asthma. Lancet 1989; 1(8651): 1346–1348.

Irwin RS, Corrao WM, Pratter MR: Chronic persistent cough in the adult: The spectrum and frequency of causes and successful outcome of specific therapy. Am Rev Respir Dis 1981; 123(4 Pt 1):413–417.

Irwin RS, Baumann MH, Bolser DC, Boulet LP, Braman SS, Brightling CE, et al: Diagnosis and management of cough, executive summary: ACCP evidence-based clinical practice guidelines. Chest 2006; 129 (1 Suppl):1S–23S.

Irwin RS, Madison JM: The diagnosis and treatment of cough. N Engl J Med 2000; 343(23):1715–1721.

Morice AH, Fontana GA, Sovijarvi AR, Pistolesi M, Chung KF, Widdicombe J, O'Connell F, Geppetti P, Gronke L, De Jongste J, Belvisi M, Dicpinigaitis P, Fischer A, McGarvey L, Fokkens WJ, Kastelik J: ERS Task Force: The diagnosis and management of chronic cough. Eur Respir J 2004; 24(3):481–492.

Morice AH, Kastelik JA, Thompson R: Cough challenge in the assessment of cough reflex. Br J Clin Pharmacol 2001; 52(4):365–375.

Morice AH, McGarvey L, Pavord I: British Thoracic Society Cough Guideline Group: Recommendations for the management of cough in adults. Thorax 2006; 61(Suppl 1):i1–24.

Widdicombe JG: Neurophysiology of the cough reflex. Eur Respir J 1995; 8(7):1193–1202.

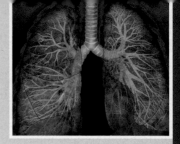

23 Dyspnea

JOANNA C. PORTER

INTRODUCTION/DEFINITION

Dyspnea is a clinical term derived from the Greek δυσ- (dys-) + πνοη (breath, breathing), literally "difficulty breathing," and describes a situation in which a subject is conscious of shortness of breath that is either inappropriate for the degree of exertion and/or distressing. Few patients will use the word dyspnea, and most will talk of being "short of breath," "out of breath," or "breathless," meaning that the demands put on their respiratory system are not being met by it. Dyspnea, one of the most common reasons for presentation to casualty departments, usually indicates serious disease of the heart and/or lungs and is an independent predicator of mortality. Breathlessness, like pain, is a powerful atavistic symptom, which delivers a harsh warning to modify behavior. It is such a strong deterrent that many people with severe disease give up their normal activities to avoid the sensation and become "respiratory invalids." In the worst cases, dyspnea becomes unavoidable, occurring even on minimal exertion and eventually at rest. The sensation of dyspnea is strongly influenced by many other nonphysiologic factors, so that for a given respiratory work load, the perception of dyspnea and the change in behavior this generates will vary between individuals. An inappropriate response to a given respiratory demand is thought to play a role in diseases as diverse as near fatal asthma and hyperventilation syndrome. Because of this, it is essential to appreciate the complexity of dyspnea, which begins with an understanding of the control of breathing.

CONTROL OF BREATHING

Breathing is regulated by both involuntary brainstem and voluntary cortical responses. It is an automatic and rhythmic act, initiated by respiratory control centers in the medulla (ventral and dorsal respiratory groups) and the pons (pontine respiratory group). These hindbrain areas project through bulbospinal projections to the spinal respiratory motor neurons, which also receive input from the motor cortex. The entire respiratory cycle takes place without conscious awareness, but this can be overridden by cortical input to allow talking, eating, coughing, and holding of breath. Respiratory motor output innervates the respiratory muscles to expand the chest wall and inflate the lungs and is constantly fine-tuned by sensory afferents feeding back information from various central and peripheral receptors that include central chemoreceptors in the medulla (which respond to H^+ and are considered to be CO_2 sensors) and peripheral chemoreceptors in the carotid and aortic bodies (which become increasingly sensitive to H^+ as O_2 falls). In addition, sensations are relayed by the vagus and cranial nerves from mechanoreceptors in the airways and lung: slowly adapting stretch receptors, rapidly adapting irritant receptors, and C fibers that respond to increases in interstitial pressure; chest wall: spindle muscle and joint receptors; and diaphragm: Golgi receptors. These signals are relayed to the medulla and to higher brain centers where the processing is influenced by situational, behavioral, and psychological cues. The result is that breathing is adjusted to maintain blood–gas and acid–base homeostasis, and adjustments can be made to brainstem respiratory motor output to allow for changes in respiratory muscle function. One important feature is that motor output is also "copied" to the sensory cortex, so called corollary discharge, resulting in conscious awareness of respiratory motor activity.

MECHANISM OF DYSPNEA

Many different contributing factors play a role in the sensation of dyspnea, and these include the work of breathing, mismatch between motor output and afferent input, and changes in the respiratory reserve, which are discussed later.

In general, an increase in the work of breathing will make people feel short of breath, especially if this occurs at rest or with a light physical work load. This may happen during hypoxia, acidosis, or when respiratory muscles are weakened. There is an additional theory, supported clinically, that dyspnea occurs when there is mismatch between the perceived effort of breathing (motor output) and the integrated incoming information from receptors throughout the respiratory system that give information on acid base, blood gases, airflow, airway pressures, and the movement of the chest and lungs (afferent input). If this afferent input does not reflect a level of respiration consistent with the motor output, there is mismatch interpreted as dyspnea. This mismatch has been termed "neuromechanical" or "efferent-reafferent" dissociation and is a refinement of the original "length-tension inappropriateness" idea proposed by Campbell and Howell. As this mismatch increases, so does the dyspnea. This explains the dyspnea experienced when the respiratory muscles are not working as efficiently and, therefore, have to work harder for the same level of gas exchange, or in mechanically underventilated patients in which the drive to breathe is not satisfied, or during breath holding, where the drive to breath is voluntarily resisted.

It has been recognized for many years that these feelings of dyspnea, produced by the work of breathing and neuromechanical dissociation, will be felt more acutely when the respiratory system is working at near maximal with little spare capacity or reserve. This respiratory reserve is assessed by higher centers that use respiratory afferent input to compare current or alveolar ventilation (V_A) with the maximal achievable or maximal voluntary ventilation (MVV), described as V_A/MMV. The higher this ratio, the lower is the respiratory reserve ($1 - V_A$/MVV). In patients with an already low MMV, a small change in V_A can cause a large change in V_A/MVV and, therefore, a large perceived fall in the respiratory reserve. It seems to be the ratio of V_A/MVV that determines the severity of dyspnea.

As well as the various physiologic factors that contribute to dyspnea, there are powerful additional influences of central processing that explain why patients with similar cardiovascular limitations may experience very different symptoms. Considering all of these contributing factors, it can be appreciated that diseases may cause dyspnea in several ways, by increasing the drive to breathe, by mechanical limitations on the respiratory system, or by affecting an individual's perception. Many diseases (e.g., asthma) affect more than one category; there will be increased work of breathing because of airway narrowing, to maintain V_A; the lungs will be working at a further disadvantage because of hyperinflation, secondary to gas trapping, and so reducing MVV; there may be input from bronchial irritant receptors and further cortical effects because of anxiety.

The Neural Mechanisms of Dyspnea

There is no single area of the brain responsible for the experience of dyspnea; instead, diffuse areas are involved. Functional brain imaging during dyspnea, by use of PET and MRI scans, shows consistent activation of the limbic and paralimbic structures, particularly the anterior cingular cortex and the anterior insula. These are phylogenetically ancient areas of the brain that are activated by other alarm stimuli such as pain and thirst. The input is complicated, for example, the vagus nerve is implicated in both relief and worsening of dyspnea, depending on the receptors activated (Figure 23-1).

Throughout the range of intensity of dyspnea, from very mild to severe, patients use various descriptors to describe what they are experiencing. These divide roughly into three categories: chest tightness, air hunger, and increased effort. There is interest in whether the descriptors chosen can predict the disease involved. In patients, chest tightness is more associated with bronchoconstriction and stimulation of irritant airway receptors. Air hunger is associated with increased input from chemoreceptors as in chronic lung disease and C fibers stimulated by a rise in interstitial pressure as in pulmonary edema. Patients with heart disease may complain that they feel they are suffocating. These feelings are reduced when sensory receptors of the upper airways and face are stimulated by cold

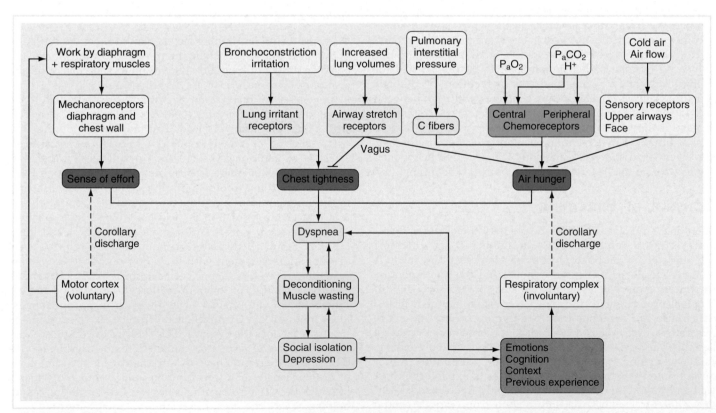

FIGURE 23-1 Mechanisms of dyspnea. Receptors in the respiratory muscles, lungs, upper airways, and face (*blue and green boxes*) relay information from various stimuli. These are experienced as sense of effort, chest tightness, and air hunger (*orange boxes*) and contribute to the sensation of dyspnea. The input from the vagus nerve is complex, because stimuli carried by the vagus can both increase and decrease dyspnea. Corollary discharge from the motor cortex and medullary respiratory complex (*dotted purple line*) also contribute to the sensation of dyspnea. Psychological factors (*pink box*) also influence symptoms and response to symptoms. Dyspnea causes a decrease in activity that leads to deconditioning and muscle wasting; this results in social isolation and depression, which further increases dyspnea and deconditioning, and a vicious circle is set in progress.

airflow. Increased work of breathing is more associated with dynamic hyperinflation and obesity, in which the work effort is increased because of poor mechanical efficiency of the lungs. The generation of these sensations that lead to dyspnea is shown diagrammatically in Figure 23-1.

DIFFERENTIAL DIAGNOSIS

The initial approach to diagnosis of dyspnea is usually determined by the quality and speed of onset of the symptoms.

Acute Dyspnea

Acute dyspnea developing over minutes to hours suggests potentially life-threatening involvement of the heart or lungs caused by a relatively small number of diseases and requires immediate attention (Figure 23-2). The diagnosis may be obvious as with an aspirated foreign body or laryngeal edema associated with anaphylaxis. Other conditions presenting with a sudden onset of shortness of breath are massive pulmonary embolus and pneumothorax. Dyspnea that has progressed over minutes to hours suggests asthma, acute exacerbation of chronic obstructive airways disease (COPD), or a cardiac event with left ventricular failure. An even longer onset of hours to days may be seen with subacute pulmonary emboli (PE), congestive cardiac failure (CCF), or infection. One sign that is not really dyspnea in the true sense is hyperventilation, which results in a low $PaCO_2$. This may be to compensate a metabolic acidosis caused, for example, by renal failure, diabetic acidosis, or lactic acidosis. Rarely, it can be the result of carbon monoxide or other form of poisoning. The hyperventilation syndrome (HVS), or psychogenic dyspnea, is a separate entity that is seen in the emergency room and can include dizziness, paresthesia, and fatigue that can be mimicked by reducing the arterial PCO_2 by voluntary hyperventilation. It is possible that patients are breathing at hyperinflated lung volumes and experience dyspnea (or chest discomfort) even when alveolar ventilation remains normal; this creates anxiety, further worsens the situation, and is most common among young women. HVS should be positively diagnosed and explained, which may aid resolution.

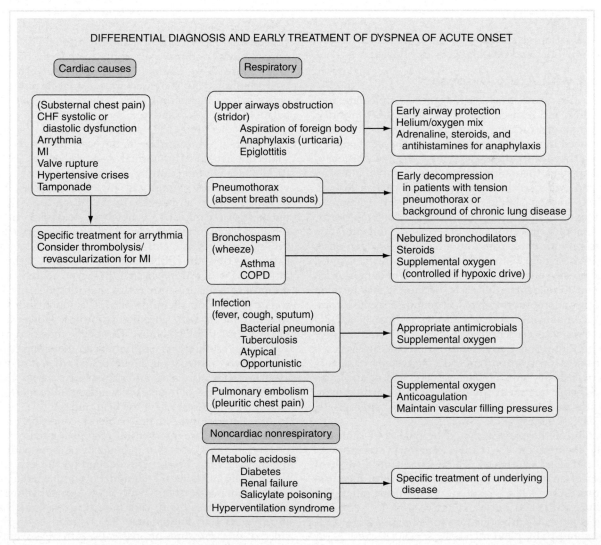

FIGURE 23-2 Differential diagnosis and early management of acute dyspnea. The diagnosis will be respiratory disease, cardiac disease, both, or neither. The main diagnoses are shown, with cardinal signs in parentheses. At all stages, resuscitation of the patient is the goal and may be necessary before a definitive diagnosis has been reached. *CHF,* Chronic heart failure.

Chronic Dyspnea

Chronic dyspnea is dyspnea lasting more than 1 month and is a very common symptom in those aged 55 and older. The underlying diagnosis is not determined by the duration or severity of dyspnea. Two thirds of cases are caused by cardiopulmonary disease and the differential diagnosis for chronic dyspnea is shown in Table 23-1. The most common causes are asthma, COPD, interstitial lung disease, and heart disease. There may be useful features in the history that help with the diagnosis (see Table 23-1). It is important to establish which organ system is involved, which usually means pulmonary or cardiac, both, or neither. In approximately one third of cases, there will be more than one cause. In reality, there are a small group of patients who remain breathless despite adherence to maximal therapy. It may be that another diagnosis has been overlooked or that there is a contribution from deconditioning or an emotional response to the illness. It is not uncommon for patients with longstanding disease to reduce their exercise level, resulting in increased breathlessness on minimal exertion and further reduction of exercise as a result of cardiovascular deconditioning.

Patient Evaluation

As for the evaluation of any patient, the sequence of history, physical examination, and investigations is followed.

The Patient with Acute Dyspnea

The patient with acute dyspnea may need immediate life-saving measures, and resuscitation of the patient is a priority. Upper airways obstruction, tension pneumothorax, and arrhythmias need immediate treatment often before the investigations have begun. In these cases, it is the recognition of symptoms and signs that is life saving. For example, a history of choking and evidence of stridor or poor tracheal airflow listening at the trachea should prompt immediate action to remove or bypass an upper airway obstruction. Pneumothorax, pulmonary embolus, infection, and other pleural inflammation may all present with chest pain; but a history of sudden onset of unilateral chest pain with shortness of breath, tachypnea, and reduced breath sounds should alert one to a pneumothorax. It is important to recognize this early, because it may develop into a tension pneumothorax that will require urgent decompression. Accompanying wheeze indicates asthma or COPD but can be seen with cardiac disease. Fever and sputum production suggest infection. Early identification of a cardiac cause for breathlessness is very important and is suggested by a history of heart disease, heavy substernal chest pain, and/or an abnormal ECG. Specific treatment should be given for arrhythmias, together with thrombolysis or intervention as appropriate, for ischemic heart disease.

Examination of the patient should be quick but thorough and usually focused on the cardiorespiratory system with obsessional detail to vital signs. There should be a frequent reassessment of an acutely ill dyspneic patient with measurements of consciousness level, respiratory rate, heart rate (HR), blood pressure (BP), and pulse oximetry.

The immediate early investigations for all patients are complete blood count (CBC) and metabolic screen. A chest X-ray may be arranged as a matter of urgency; careful attention should be paid to exclude a pneumothorax, more apparent when inspiratory and expiratory films are compared (Figure 23-3). This is particularly useful in cases with underlying lung disease, where a small pneumothorax may cause significant dyspnea and is easily missed on a conventional or portable inspiratory film. A normal chest X-ray does not exclude significant pathology and may be seen in PE and severe airways disease and also in the early stages of many lung diseases, in particular *Pneumocystis jirovecii*. The size of the cardiac silhouette on a posteroanterior film may show cardiomegaly associated with cardiac disease. A cardiac monitor and ECG provide essential information on both cardiac and lung disease (a tachycardia may be the only sign in a patient with pulmonary embolus). Note that current oximeters are inaccurate ($\pm2\%$), and may given false high readings with carboxy Hb or metHb. In some cases, desaturation on mild exertion (such as a short walk around the room) may be the only indicator of hypoxia and should be looked for. Any doubt or a low reading (<95% on air) should always prompt arterial blood gas tensions analysis (ABGs), which gives a more accurate reading of PaO_2, $PaCO_2$, and pH from which base excess (BE) is derived (Table 23-2). These may indicate type I (normocapnic) or type II (hypercapnic) respiratory failure and also allow calculation of the alveolar-arterial (A-a) difference or gradient. The A–a gradient is the difference between the alveolar PO_2 (calculated from the alveolar gas equation [see Chapter 5] and the arterial PO_2 (measured in arterial blood) and may contribute further diagnostic information (Figure 23-4). Normal A–a gradient values have not been well established but increase with age, may be different in pregnancy, and are higher on 100% O_2 than on room air. Several calculations, often unvalidated, are available to calculate the normal gradient (e.g., [age divided by 3] or [4 + age divided by 4] in mmHg). One estimate on the basis of a series of 80 normal subjects calculates the normal A–a gradient as 2.5 mmHg + (0.21 × age in years) mmHg. An important cause of tachypnea with normal pulse oximetry is a metabolic acidosis, the first sign of which may be an increase in the BE on the ABG measurements (to >−2 mEq/L). A metabolic acidosis in the setting of sepsis or hypotension is a marker of poor tissue perfusion, indicating severe disease, and requires immediate attention. Peak expiratory flow rate (PEFR) is an essential part of the evaluation of patients with asthma and COPD, even acutely. By contrast, for most patients presenting with acute dyspnea, immediate spirometry is seldom helpful, playing a much more important role in patients with chronic symptoms. However, the ratio of $FEV_1(mL)/PEFR(L/min)$ (Empey's index; normal value <10) is a very useful measurement in detecting patients with upper airway obstruction (Figure 23-5) when it may rise above 10. The index also gives an estimate of severity and is useful as a monitoring tool to give early indication of increasing upper airways obstruction (e.g., a tracheal tumor).

Any deterioration in the patient's condition or vital signs requires immediate intervention. Supplemental oxygen should be given in most cases, but judiciously in those with longstanding hypoxic lung disease who depend on the hypoxic drive to breathe. Bronchodilators should be administered to patients with asthma and patients with acute exacerbations of COPD but should be used with care in patients with cardiac disease. Intravenous rehydration may be required to increase right-sided filling pressures in patients with massive pulmonary embolus or septic shock who are poorly perfused, but early diuresis and/or vasodilatation may be the aim in patients with

TABLE 23-1 Differential Diagnosis of Dyspnea*

Disease(s)	History	Findings	Most Useful Initial Investigations	Further Studies
Asthma	Intermittent symptoms, triggers, atopy, allergic rhinitis, nasal polyps	Wheeze Prolonged expiration	Peak flow (PF) Reversible airways obstruction on spirometry	Serial PF readings Positive methacholine/allergen bronchoprovocation challenge Exhaled nitric oxide and sputum eosinophilia Serum IgG Improvement on asthma treatment of symptoms and tests
COAD	Cigarette smoking Sputum, cough	Wheeze Prolonged expiration	Nonreversible airway obstruction on spirometry	
Interstitial lung disease Pulmonary fibrosis Hypersensitivity pneumonitis	History of exposure to inorganic mineral, asbestos, nitrofurantoin, bleomycin, methotrexate, environmental or occupational allergens History of rheumatological disease	Finger clubbing Persistent crackles that do not clear with coughing	CXR Restriction on spirometry	High-resolution CT (HRCT) Pulmonary function testing (PFT)–decreased transfer factor (DLCO) IgG serum antibodies Diagnostic lung biopsy
Heart disease Cardiomyopathy (systolic and/or diastolic dysfunction) Ischemia Arrythmia Intracardiac shunt Pericarditis	History of hypertension, coronary artery disease, diabetes, orthopnea, paroxysmal nocturnal dyspnea	Tachycardia, raised JVP, s3 gallop rhythm, bibasal crepitations, pedal edema	BNP CXR ECG	Reduced ejection fraction (EF) or diastolic dysfunction on echocardiogram (ECHO) Reduced EF on radionuclide scan Positive cardiac stress test Positive cardiac catheterization study Holter monitor ECHO–valvular dysfunction, atrial tumors and pericardial disease
Postnasal drip syndrome	History of postnasal drip or throat clearing		–	PFT–Inspiratory slowing on flow volume loop
Bronchiectasis	Cough with sputum production Childhood infections Hypogammaglobulinemia Cystic fibrosis	Clubbing Crackles	Sputum and culture CXR	HRCT scan
Disease of the pleura and pleural space: effusion, pleural thickening, empyema mesothelioma, pneumothorax, fibrothorax	Pleuritic chest pain History of recent travel or operation	Reduced thoracic movements Decreased, absent breath sounds	CXR	Examination of pleural fluid and pleura (may be best done thoracoscopically) CT

Continued

Table 23-1 Differential Diagnosis of Dyspnea*—Cont'd

Disease(s)	History	Findings	Most Useful Initial Investigations	Further Studies
Pulmonary embolism	Hemoptysis, pleuritic chest pain, calf tenderness	Tachycardia May be signs of pulmonary hypertention (PHT—see below) Calf tenderness	D-dimers	Leg Dopplers Ventilation/perfusion ($\dot{V}/\dot{Q}$) scan CT with pulmonary angiogram (CTPA)
Opportunistic infections: protozoal (PCP), bacterial (TB, legionella), viral (CMV), fungal (aspergillus)	History of immunosuppression Fever Pleuritic chest pain Weight loss	Fever Coarse crepitations	CXR	CT scan Bronchoscopy (FOB) with bronchoalveolar lavage (BAL)
Pulmonary hypertension (primary and acquired)		Raised P2 (pulmonary component of second heart sounds), right ventricular heave (RVH), murmur	CXR	ECHO-raised pulmonary artery pressure (PAP) with tricuspid regurgitation (TR) Right heart catheter to confirm or diagnose less common causes
Obstruction of the large airways -Vocal cord paralysis -Laryngeal tumor -Tracheal stenosis -Endobronchial tumor -Inhaled foreign body		Airway obstruction: stridor or wheeze; lung collapse: unilateral reduced breath sounds	PF PFT-abnormal flow volume loop	Positive tomography or CT scan Laryngoscopy or bronchoscopy
Bronchiolitis obliterans	Bone marrow or lung transplant Connective tissue diseases Inhalation of toxic fumes Recent respiratory infection	Often unremarkable May be wheeze	CXR	CT-mosaic perfusion pattern PFTs Diagnostic lung biopsy
Deconditioning	Weight gain and decreased exercise			Exercise testing
Neuromuscular disease MND Myasthenia gravis	History of neuromuscular disease Generalized muscle weakness Bulbar weakness (choking on drinks)	Generalized muscle weakness, which may include the diaphragm	PF	PFTs-low maximum inspiratory and expiratory pressures Acetylcholine receptor antibodies Tension test Nerve/muscle biopsy Diaphragm dysfunction on ultrasound screening
Hematological and metabolic disease -Severe anemia -Liver cirrhosis -Hypothyroidism/ hyperthyroidism -Uremia and other acidaemias	History of metabolic or hematological disease		Complete blood count, liver function tests and biochemistry Thyroid function	Blood gases if acidosis suspected Further investigation of underlying disease
Psychogenic factors				Consistent exercise test; all other investigations normal

*This table shows the differential diagnosis of dyspnea in the approximate order in which they are encountered in the clinic, with the most common causes listed first. Initial consideration of history, physical examination, chest X-ray, ECG, and spirometry with routing blood tests and sputum culture often gives the result. If there is still some doubt, further appropriate studies are organized.

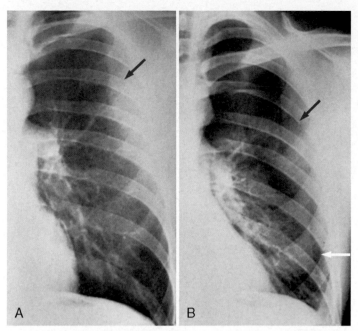

FIGURE 23-3 Inspiration **(A)** and expiration **(B)** films of a pneumothorax. **A,** With inspiration, the pneumothorax is difficult to visualize but is faintly seen in the upper thorax (*arrow*). **B,** With expiration, the pneumothorax is outlined against denser lung. It seems to be considerably larger than in the inspiration study (*arrows*). (From Masson RJ, Broaddus VC, Murray JF, Nadel JA: Murray and Nadel's Textbook of Respiratory Medicine, 4th ed. Philadelphia: Elsevier Saunders; 2005.)

cardiac disease and left ventricular failure. In severe cases, early involvement of anesthetic, intensive care, cardiology, and respiratory or thoracic surgical teams is recommended, depending on the underlying cause. Once the patient is stabilized, the pace of evaluation is similar to that for subacute or chronic dyspnea, and additional tests may be required to complete the diagnostic process, for example, lateral films of the neck to look for soft tissue shadowing and tracheal narrowing, and CT pulmonary angiography (CTPA) to exclude pulmonary emboli.

However, the division between acute and chronic dyspnea is not rigid; for example, asthma and infection can build up over weeks, pulmonary emboli may be subacute, and interstitial lung disease may present acutely.

THE PATIENT WITH CHRONIC DYSPNEA

In contrast to the acutely ill patient, there is usually more time to evaluate the patient with chronic dyspnea, and the initial step is to determine the organ system involved. In approximately two thirds of patients, the underlying cause is cardiopulmonary disease. The baseline assessment includes history, physical examination, and level 1 investigations (Table 23-3). The history should focus on the onset of symptoms, the quality and timing of the dyspnea (constant or episodic), associated symptoms (in particular wheeze), and the precipitating factors (allergens, position, exercise) and accompanying factors (such as cough and hemoptysis). Are there cardiac, rheumatologic, or gastrointestinal symptoms? Orthopnea or paroxysmal nocturnal dyspnea (PND) suggests cardiac disease, and wheeze in the early hours with cough suggests asthma. It is also important to assess the effect of shortness of breath on daily activities. Medical and surgical history and drug history are very important. Often, pulmonary disease such as TB may recur or malignancy may reappear in the lung. Occupational history may be important enough to be considered on its own, and the patient should provide a list of all their previous jobs and exposure to toxic materials and whether other workers were affected. In the case of asbestos-related lung disease, an occupational history of a cohabiter may be relevant if working clothes were brought home to be laundered. No history is complete without a smoking history and documenting, if the patient is no longer a smoker, when the patient gave up and after how long. Other features that may be important are a family history, household contacts with TB, travel history, risk factors for infection with HIV, exposure to pets, duvets/feathers and toxins, and known allergies. A history of recent long haul travel or an operation may be the only risk factor for PE. One important part of the history is to ask about previous chest X-rays, were they abnormal, where were they taken, and is it possible to obtain the films or copies of them?

TABLE 23-2 Arterial Blood Gas Readings: Normal Values and Alterations in Disease States

	Normal Values	Decreased In	Increased In
PaO_2	11–13 kPa or 80–100 mmHg	Hypoventilation Hypobaric O_2 Right to left shunt V/Q mismatch Alveolar-capillary diffusion problems	Hyperbaric oxygen
$PaCO_2$	4.7–5.9 mmHg or 35–45 mmHg	Metabolic acidosis Asthma Hyperventilation	Chronic COAD Hypoventilation
HCO_3	21–28 mMol/L	Metabolic acidosis	Metabolic alkalosis Chronic hypercapneic respiratory disease
BE	+/−2 mMol/L	Metabolic acidosis	Metabolic alkalosis Chronic hypercapneic respiratory disease
pH	7.36–7.44	Metabolic acidosis	Metabolic alkalosis Chronic hypercapneic respiratory disease
Saturation	>95%		

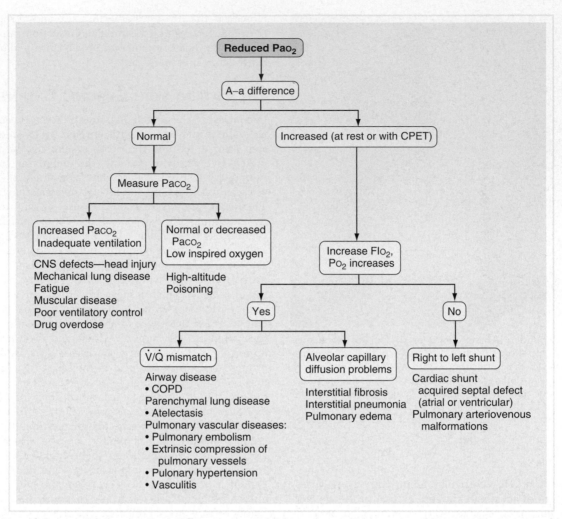

FIGURE 23-4 Use of the arterial-alveolar (A–a) difference in establishing the probable cause of hypoxia. The causes of hypoxia can be considered in five broad groups depending on the A–a gradient (normal or increased), the $Paco_2$ increased or decreased/normal, and, in those cases with an abnormal A–a gradient, whether the hypoxia is correctable by increasing inspired oxygen concentration (Flo_2). *CPET,* Cardiopulmonary exercise testing.

Examination of the respiratory system, including measurement of the quality and rate of breathing, may reveal various clues: clubbing of the digits—occurs in many different disorders such as chronic infiltrative and suppurative diseases of the lung, and bronchogenic carcinoma; wheeze—generalized or localized in airway narrowing:

- Prolonged expiration in the absence of a wheeze can be seen in some diseases of airway narrowing such as asthma.
- Crackles: fibrosis, interstitial edema, or infection, especially if they do not clear with coughing.
- A pleural friction rub: is heard in any disease in which the pleura is inflamed.
- Bronchial breathing: heard when breath sounds are transmitted from a large airway through consolidated lung.
- Stridor: wheeze heard over the trachea that suggests tracheal narrowing.

However, the absence of physical signs does not exclude the presence of significant lung disease. In addition, all the other systems should be fully examined with particular attention to the cardiovascular system for tachycardia, arrhythmia, added heart sounds and murmurs, peripheral edema, and bibasal pulmonary crepitations. Bruits may be heard over the abdomen in renal artery stenosis, a disease that can present with episodic PND.

After history taking and examination, the diagnosis may be apparent. Patients should have baseline investigation of CBC and biochemistry (with C-reactive protein) to exclude anemia, renal impairment, and undiagnosed infection. Pulse oximetry may show desaturation at rest or on exertion, in which case ABGs should be obtained. Sputum, if available, should be examined and sent for culture. Most patients will need a chest X-ray, and if there is a suggestion of cardiac disease or pulmonary hypertension with right ventricular strain, then an ECG.

The chest X-ray will offer a useful tool to decide on the next investigation (Table 23-3 and Figure 23-6). In reality, most patients presenting to respiratory physicians with significant symptoms and physiologic impairment will go on to have further imaging. High-resolution CT scanning (HRCT) is the investigation of choice for diffuse abnormalities (e.g., pulmonary

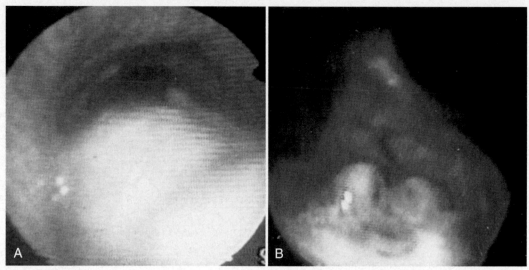

FIGURE 23-5 This young nonsmoker had slowly progressive dyspnea and wheeze over the previous 12 months and was initially treated for asthma. Stridor (heard by listening at the open mouth) was present. **A,** The tumor just about the carina at presentation. **B,** After bulk removal. The patient's peak expiratory flow (150 L/min) was disproportionately low compared with the forced expiratory volume in 1 sec (2.0 L), giving an Empey index of >13 and highly suggestive of upper airway obstruction. (Courtesy of Dr. P. V. Barber.)

TABLE 23-3 Investigation of Dyspnea*

Level 1 tests (appropriate for most patients)
Oximetry
Metabolic screen
Full blood count
CXR
ECG
Peak flow
Spirometry
Sputum culture
(Depending on clinical suspicion: brain natriuretic peptide [BNP],
  D-dimers)

Level 2 tests
Peak flow chart-serial measurements
PFTs
ABGs
Methacholine or allergen bronchoprovocation challenge (BPC)
High resolution CT
CT pulmonary angiogram
Ventilation/perfusion scan and/or leg Dopplers
ECHO
Bronchoscopy +/− bronchoalveolar lavage
Holter recording
Radionuclide cardiac scan

Level 3 (consulation with specialist)
Cardiac catheterization
Cardiopulmonary exercise test
Esophageal pH
Lung biopsy

*Level 1 tests are suitable for all patients, although D-dimer and BNP
  should be requested on clinical suspicion and according to local
  protocols. Level 2 tests are suitable in selected patients with a high
  index of suspicion. Level 3 tests should be arranged after discussion
  with a specialist.

fibrosis or bronchiectasis). Spiral CT scanning with contrast injection is the choice for exclusion or evaluation of suspected focal lesions. Lung function tests are very important in patients with chronic dyspnea. Simple spirometry, measuring forced expiratory flow (FEV_1) and force vital capacity (FVC), will distinguish between obstructive disease and restrictive disease. The classic obstructive diseases are asthma and COPD, and an increase of FEV_1 of >15% with bronchodilators indicates reversibility. Obstruction can also occur with any stenosing lesion in the tracheobronchial tree. A large number of diseases will cause restrictive lung function, and these include pleural and alveolar diseases, neuromuscular weakness, and thoracic cage abnormalities. Spirometry before and after exercise or after bronchoprovocation challenge with inhaled methacholine or allergen, under controlled conditions, may be useful in unmasking latent asthma; in these cases a fall of 20% in FEV_1 is considered diagnostic.

Most patients under investigation for chronic dyspnea will benefit from full pulmonary function tests (see Chapter 9). Total lung capacity (TLC) is reduced in restrictive disorders but is normal or even increased in obstructive disorders as a result of air trapping and lung destruction by emphysema. In restrictive disorders caused by lung parenchymal disease, all lung volumes are reduced equally, but in other restrictive diseases (such as neuromuscular disease or chest wall restriction), the residual volume (RV) and the RV/TLC ratio are increased. A decrease in the diffusion capacity of the lung for carbon monoxide (DL_{CO}) is a sensitive, but nonspecific, indicator of loss of surface area for alveolar gas exchange and occurs in a wide range of restrictive diseases involving the lung such as fibrosis, sarcoidosis, and drug toxicity. It can also be decreased in vascular diseases such as PE and increased in pulmonary

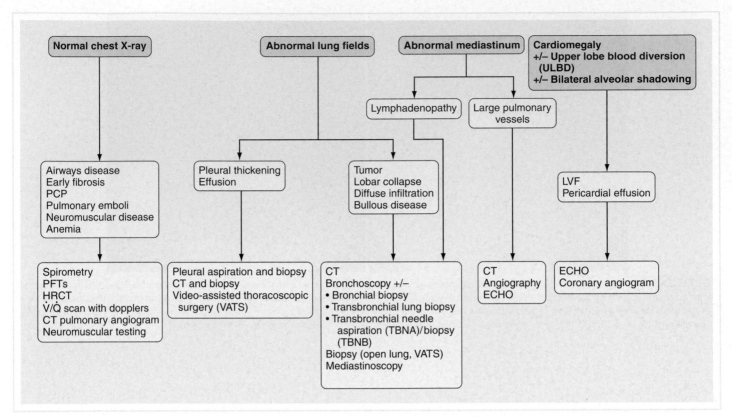

FIGURE 23-6 Chest radiograph in the differential diagnosis of dyspnea. The chest X-ray findings fall into four groups: Normal, abnormal lung fields, abnormal mediastinum, and cardiomegaly with upper lobe blood diversion. This is a simplified algorithm but illustrates the role of further investigations. The most appropriate investigation is guided by patient's presentation and probable diagnosis; in many patients this will involve further imaging of the chest, usually a CT scan.

hemorrhage (seen, for example, as part of a vasculitic disease). However, the normal range for DL$_{CO}$ is wide, so a normal value cannot exclude early disease. Maximum inspiratory and expiratory mouth pressures are a useful test of inspiratory muscle strength and should be measured in patients with suspected neuromuscular disease or in those with dyspnea, restricted lung volumes, normal chest X-ray, and normal HRCT scan. Flow volume loops may give a clue to the cause of breathlessness and are said to have a characteristic shape in upper airway stenosis (see Chapters 4 and 9).

If these preliminary tests are all normal, it is worth considering whether the disease is intermittent (e.g., asthma), are the tests too insensitive (early interstitial lung disease), is extrathoracic disease present (gastroesophageal reflux disease, GERD) or psychogenic dyspnea. Further investigations (see Table 23-3: stage 2 and stage 3) are carried out as indicated and with input from other relevant specialists. This will reveal most of the other causes. Even after this, there will be a small group of patients in whom a cause is not found. In one study of 72 patients with chronic dyspnea unexplained by stage 1 investigations who were referred to a respiratory unit, a cause was eventually found in 80%. Dyspnea was due to pulmonary disease in 36%, cardiac disease in 14%, and hyperventilation in 19% of patients. If patients remain breathless despite adherence to maximal therapy, it is important to consider other factors such as deconditioning or emotional factors.

Cardiopulmonary exercise testing (CPET) is useful in assessing patients with significant dyspnea when it is not clear whether the cause is cardiac or pulmonary. Patients are monitored during graded exercise and measurements made of respiratory rate, tidal volumes, blood gas tensions, expired gas concentrations, and HR and BP (Figure 23-7; see Chapters 9 and 10). Abnormalities may be picked up in patients who have normal physiology at rest. Exercise testing plays an important role not only in diagnosis but also to assess the impact of exercise on individuals to establish the need for supplementary oxygen and to evaluate the impact of therapy, including rehabilitation programs on patients with chronic lung disease.

SCALES TO MEASURE DYSPNEA

Because individuals vary in their response to a similar physiologic limitation as measured by PFTs, clinicians and researchers have sought other ways to measure dyspnea, and several semi-quantitative scales have been developed (Table 23-4). These scales were developed either as tools to help research or to evaluate individual patients and vary in the parameters that they measure. The simplest are subjective assessments, which rely on patient reporting. One-dimensional scales measure the intensity of one symptom at a given time. This can be by a stepwise scale (e.g., modified Borg, Figure 23-8) or a continuous visual analog scale (VAS, Figure 23-9) on which a patient marks the intensity of their symptom on a sliding scale between fixed descriptions. Both scales are able to mark changes caused by disease progression or treatment in a given

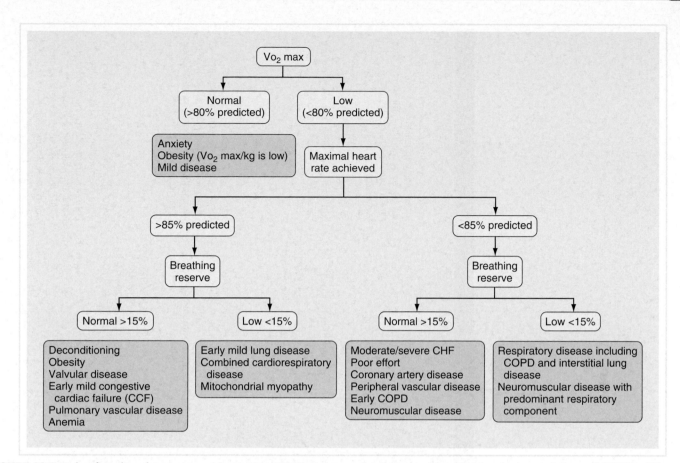

FIGURE 23-7 Role of cardiopulmonary exercise testing (CPET). An example of an algorithm to show the potential use of CPET in differential diagnosis of dyspnea. This algorithm is not fully comprehensive but demonstrates one way in which CPET, by evaluating $\dot{V}$ max, heart rate, and breathing reserve, can point to the relative contributions of cardiovascular, respiratory, and other factors in limiting exercise potential. In practice, different institutions will vary in the equipment and protocols they use and in the physiologic measurements taken. The situation is often complicated with varying contributions from multiple factors. Supervising and interpreting CPET requires expertise and experience (see ATS/ACCP statement on cardiopulmonary exercise testing). Breathing reserve (BR) is calculated as $(1 - V_E peak/MVV) \times 100$. Normal BR has a wide range but should be >15.

patient but are not useful for comparison between patients. The next type of scale identifies the activities that bring on dyspnea, examples are the Medical Research Council UK (MRC, Figure 23-10) dyspnea scale and the oxygen cost diagram (OCD; Figure 23-11). The MRC scale asks the patient to identify minimal conditions that cause symptoms. It is very easy to use, but because it is a stepwise scale, it does not pick up small differences and is only really useful as an initial staging tool. The OCD is more sensitive, because it lists several activities of increasing work requirement along a horizontal line. Other scales look at more variables: the baseline dyspnea index (BDI) is calculated by an observer and scores three parameters: the functional impairment caused by breathlessness, the magnitude of the task leading to breathlessness, and the magnitude of the effort leading to breathlessness at a baseline time point. The transition dyspnea index (TDI) can be used to evaluate changes in these parameters. The BDI and TDI are simple to use, they look at dyspnea as an isolated symptom, and give an idea of how patients are coping with their diseases. The BDI and TDI are not useful for comparing patients because individuals will have different expectations and may have adapted their behavior to suit their disease. Another set of tools looks at the effects of symptoms on

activities of daily living (ADL) and is valuable to highlight areas where patients can work to improve their quality of life. Again they are better for test-retest rather than comparison between patients. The best known is the St. George Respiratory Questionnaire (SGRQ), which looks at all the symptoms of airway disease. The chronic respiratory questionnaire (CRQ) assesses the impact of breathlessness on five activities that are selected by the patients as being most troublesome and has less value for measuring between patients. All of these scales rely on patient recall, and in some situations a more objective measurement is required. This has led to the development of exercise tests with graded work loads and immediate symptom reporting. The most widely used is the 6-min walk test (6 MWT), for which guidelines and reference values are available. Another test is the incremental shuttle walk test. The patient walks at an increasing pace until unable to keep up. These tests are easy to perform and do not require complicated apparatus. Other exercise tests require more equipment and can measure the maximum amount of work in watts that can be performed. Recording of HR, BP, and oximetry during exercise allows symptoms (by use of an MBS or VAS) to be equated with physiologic variables.

TABLE 23-4 Scales for Assessment of Dyspnea*

Evaluates	Type of Assessment	Examples	Pros	Cons	Uses
Symptom intensity	Scale with verbal descriptions Stepwise scale: Continuous scale:	Modified Borg Scale (MBS) (12-point scale using verbal descriptors) (Borg GV, 1982) Visual analogue scale (VAS)	Easy to use Adaptable Semi-quantitative	Not useful to compare patients	Response of individual patients to treatment/rehabilitation Can be adapted for symptoms other than dyspnea (e.g., cough or wheeze)
Magnitude of task causing dyspnea	Self-reporting Stepwise scale: Continuous scale:	Medical Research Council (MRC) scale (Fletcher CM, 1960) Oxygen cost diagram (OCD) (McGavin CR, 1978)	Simple to use Reasonably reproducible correlate well with each other	Not sensitive to small changes Lack of clear limits (MRC) Not all patients have tried activities of OCD	Useful in initial clinical evaluation but assumes patient is mobile
Magnitude of Task and effort causing dyspnea and the resulting functional impairment	Interviewed questionnaires	Baseline dyspnea index (BDI; dyspnea at a point in time). Transition dyspnea index (TDI) measures a change from baseline. (Mahler DA, 1984)	Multidimensional assessment Validity reported	Requires experienced observer interviewer Subjective and relies on patient recall Patients may avoid activities to prevent dyspnea Nonrespiratory disease and obesity may contribute to functional impairment	BDI useful for measuring baseline dyspnea TDI is a sensitive tool to evaluate change due to pharmacological or rehabilitative strategies or disease progression
Activities of daily living and dyspnea	Self-administered questionnaires	UCSDSOBQ (UCSD shortness of breath questionnaire) (Eakin EG, 1998) Pulmonary functional status and dyspnea questionnaire (PFDSQ) Pulmonary function status scale (PFSS)	Measure dyspnea during ADLs	Reliability and validity reported	Useful to assess dyspnea during common activities of daily living and to set goals for improvement Useful to evaluate changes in functional status after intervention or disease progression

Continued

Table 23-4 Scales for Assessment of Dyspnea*—Cont'd

Evaluates	Type of Assessment	Examples	Pros	Cons	Uses
Correlation of • Reported dyspnea and • Physiological measurements during a specific task and work load	Interviewed assessment during exercise or challenge such as • 6 min walk • Cycle ergometer • Methacholine BPC Using scales such as VAS or MBS together with physiological assessment		Quantifiable and immediate Objective and does not rely on self-reporting	Requires skilled operator, expensive and time consuming Qualitative but not between patients Focuses on physiological limitations rather than symptoms Exercise may be limited by nonrespiratory function	Very good for response of symptoms to treatment or rehabilitation in individual patients Allows symptoms to be correlated with measurable variables May not have much to do with functional status
Interaction between dyspnea and quality of life	Interviewed questionnaires	St. George's respiratory questionnaire (SGRQ)—self-administered assessment of • Symptoms • Activity • Impact (Jones PW, 1992) Chronic respiratory disease questionnaire (CRDQ) • Fatigue • Emotions • Control over disease (Guyatt GH, 1987)	Reasonably reproducible and correlate well with each other	SGRQ specific for airways diseases (COPD and asthma) but may be valid in others Demanding to use, require trained health personnel	Research and audit tools Unproven in routine clinical care but probably assess changes most clinically relevant to patients

*Various scales have been developed that measure different aspects of dyspnea. They vary in their uses and exam.

MODIFIED BORG SCALE

Grade	Description
0	Nothing at all
0.5	Extremely slight
1	Very slight
2	Slight
3	Moderate
4	Somewhat severe
5	Severe
6	
⑦	Very severe
8	
9	Very, very severe
10	Maximal

FIGURE 23-8 The modified scale for rating perceived exertion (Modified Borg Scale [MBS]). The MBS is used to assess the severity of symptoms during exertion, for example, during the 6-MWT or immediately after CPET. MBS is a modification of the Borg scale in which descriptors have a numerical equivalence; doubling of symptom severity is reflected by a doubling of graded score (e.g., "very severe—6" is roughly twice as bad as "moderate—3."

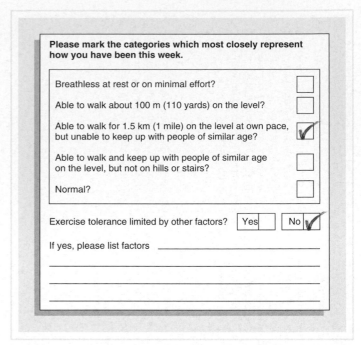

Please mark the categories which most closely represent how you have been this week.

Breathless at rest or on minimal effort? ☐

Able to walk about 100 m (110 yards) on the level? ☐

Able to walk for 1.5 km (1 mile) on the level at own pace, but unable to keep up with people of similar age? ☑

Able to walk and keep up with people of similar age on the level, but not on hills or stairs? ☐

Normal? ☐

Exercise tolerance limited by other factors? Yes ☐ No ☑

If yes, please list factors _____

FIGURE 23-10 UK Medical Research Council dyspnea grade. The dyspnea grade is useful for the initial assessment of patients' disability and is easily completed by a doctor, nurse, health visitor, or patient.

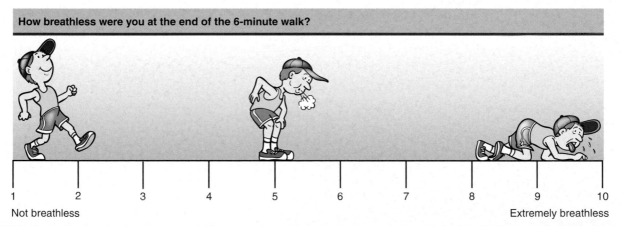

How breathless were you at the end of the 6-minute walk?

1   2   3   4   5   6   7   8   9   10
Not breathless   Extremely breathless

FIGURE 23-9 Example of a visual analog score. These can be adapted to any symptom and can be supplemented with anchoring verbal or visual descriptors as shown here.

Most clinical studies and patient assessments involve consideration of PFTs, with subjective and objective functional scores (e.g., transition dyspnea index [TDI] and 6-MWT, and SGRQ). One composite index that has been tested and validated is the BODE index from its components: *B*ody mass index, degree of airways *O*bstruction, modified MRC *D*yspnea score, and *E*xercise capacity on the basis of 6 MWT. This is scored from 0–10. The BODE index seems to be a better predictor of mortality in COPD than FEV_1 alone.

Treatment

The treatment of dyspnea begins with identification and treatment of the underlying cause. In the case of acute dyspnea, treatment is often instituted before full investigations have been completed. In most cases, the response to treatment is measured by an improvement in the patient's and physiologic markers. The treatment of chronic dyspnea may be a much harder process, requiring consideration not only of the underlying disease process but also of the physiologic, psychologic, and social limitations on quality of life.

In patients with chronic dyspnea, once medical treatment has been optimized, symptoms may still be improved by maneuvers that decrease respiratory drive, improve the efficiency of breathing, or reduce the central perception of dyspnea (Table 23-5). For example, supplemental oxygen can reduce respiratory drive, because oxygenation is achieved at lower V_A; respiratory and peripheral muscle function is improved; and the central perception of dyspnea may be reduced as the

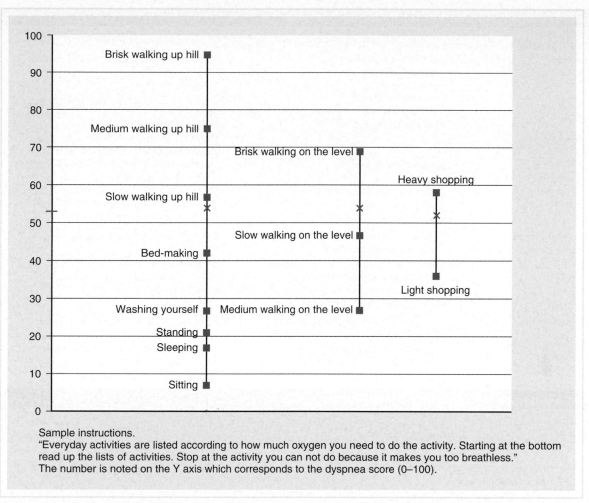

Sample instructions.
"Everyday activities are listed according to how much oxygen you need to do the activity. Starting at the bottom read up the lists of activities. Stop at the activity you can not do because it makes you too breathless."
The number is noted on the Y axis which corresponds to the dyspnea score (0–100).

FIGURE 23-11 The Oxygen Cost Diagram (OCD). The OCD assesses dyspnea severity by identifying the limits of physical exercise because of dyspnea. This diagram is based on the values for oxygen expenditure from McGavin CR *et al*: Dyspnea, disability, and distance walked: Comparison of estimates of exercise performance in respiratory disease. BMJ 1978 ; 2:241–243, from data presented in Durnin JGVA, Passmore R: Energy, work and leisure. London: Heinemann; 1967.

oxygen/air mixture passes over the face. Portable oxygen systems are becoming more freely available, are lighter and truly portable, making ambulatory oxygen much more available. Other methods to decrease symptoms are shown in Table 23-5.

One treatment modality increasingly recognized to be valuable is pulmonary rehabilitation (Table 23-6; see Chapter 42). Pulmonary rehabilitation is a formal structured approach to improve the quality of life in patients with chronic lung disease, and there is evidence that it can reduce dyspnea and increase exercise performance, which all contribute to reducing health-care costs. The major components of such a program are exercise training, nutrition, inspiratory muscle training, and improved ventilatory dynamics. To take one example, the exercise training probably works through a combination of effects: improving metabolic efficiency of muscles, so that less lactic acid is produced, as well as reducing patient sensitivity to dyspnea centrally.

As well as lifestyle changes, there is interest in pharmacologic agents that reduce dyspnea, but a side effect of all of these is to reduce respiratory drive. The most frequently used are opiates and benzodiazepines. Opiates have many side effects and do not have much of a role in chronic dyspnea but play a very important role in the breathlessness of some

terminal diseases. Benzodiazepines may be of use where excessive anxiety is a problem, but great care should be taken to minimize side effects. Locally delivered drugs such as nebulized local anesthetic lidocaine and/or opiates have not been shown to be of benefit except in terminal disease. Because of the side-effect profiles of the drugs that relieve dyspnea, their use in limited. Nonpharmacologic approaches to reduce the central perception of dyspnea include distraction (for example with music) or the use of relaxation techniques to reduce anxiety during attacks of dyspnea. Another approach is the use of cognitive behavioral therapy (CBT). CBT trains a patient to cope with their dyspnea by recognizing and reducing their feeling of anxiety or distress when they become short of breath. This allows a patient to do more with the same physiologic reserve.

The approach to the patient with severe chronic dyspnea involves distinct, but complementary, concepts. For example, a patient with severe COPD may need help to stop smoking, assessment of disease reversibility, and appropriate treatment with bronchodilators and inhaled steroids. Even when treatment has been maximized, hospital admissions may be further prevented by patient education; rapid recognition of, and intervention during, exacerbations; and by keeping influenza

TABLE 23-5 Treatment Approaches for Reducing Dyspnea

Aim	Therapy	Mechanism of Action
Reduce ventilatory demand (reduce V_E peak)	Treat airways disease: • Steroids • β2 agonist • Anticholinergics • Theophylline	Reduce airway resistance and ventilatory load
	Exercise training	Desensitization to dyspnea Prevents increase in lactic acid Resets peripheral mechanoreceptors
	Supplemental oxygen	Decreases hypoxic drive from peripheral chemoreceptors
	Drugs (anxiolytics, narcotics) Airflow over face Cognitive behaviour therapy	Depress hypoxic and hypercapneic drive (Role for inhaled lidocaine and/or opiates unproven except in terminal disease)
Reduce ventilatory impedence (improve efficiency of breathing)	Improve oxygen carrying potential of the cardiovascular system	Treat cardiovascular disease Correct anemia
	Breathing retraining: pursed lips and diaphragmatic breathing	Decrease the work of breathing
	Continuous positive airway pressure (CPAP) Lung volume reduction surgery	Reduce lung hyperinflation
Reduce muscle fatigue	Nutrition (enteral, parenteral, and supplements)	Increase muscle bulk and efficiency
	Inspiratory muscle training	Increase inspiratory muscle efficiency
	Partial ventilatory support	Rest muscles

TABLE 23-6 Strategies for Pulmonary Rehabilitation

Components of Program	Strategies and Aims	Notes

Patient education	• Smoking cessation
	• Breathing strategies
	• Management plan
	  -Recognize exacerbations
	  -Take appropritate action
	• Bronchial hygiene (selected patients)	

Exercise training	• Maximize medical therapy • 3 times per week • High intensity • Endurance and strength • Upper and lower extremities	• Avoid high intensity for patients with pulmonary hypertension • Continue LTOT during training • Supplemental oxygen for patients without hypoxemia may not affect clinical outcome • Respiratory muscle training and noninvasive positive pressure ventilation (NPPV) may help selected patients • Neuromuscular electrical stimulation (NMES) of peripheral muscle may help some bedbound patients • Teach energy conservation to patients with ILD and NMD
Optimize body composition	• Education, calorie meal planning and support • Help the obese to lose weight • Increase weight gain and fat-free mass (FFM) in others using nutritional supplementation and exercise	• Pharmacologic therapy (e.g., anabolic steroids, growth hormone, and megesterol acetate) still subject to clinical studies
Psychosocial support	• Supportive counseling • Training in stress management • Screen for anxiety and depression • Referral to mental health services for selected patients	
Physiologic assessment	Before rehabilitation may help with deciding on: • An exercise program • Need for supplemental oxygen • Contraindications to exercise During rehabilitation program will allow repeat evaluation of: • Symptom control • Ability to perform ADLs • Exercise performance (activity monitors, e.g., pedometer; 6 MWT, CPET) • Q of L (SGHQ, CRQ)	

and pneumococcal vaccines up to date. Supplemental oxygen and involvement in a pulmonary rehabilitation program may further improve quality of life. By keeping patients active, the spiral of decreased activity, leading to deconditioning, loss of self-esteem, social isolation, and anxiety/depression can be lessened or avoided. At this stage, the therapeutic process has evolved into attempts to make permanent changes to a person's style, physiology, and psychology and requires added commitment on the part of the individual, family, work place, and potential caregivers who will all need to accommodate changes in their responsibilities.

Web Resources for Guidelines/Protocols

http://www.lumetra.com/uploadedFiles/events/upcoming-events/dyspnea-best-practices.pdf

http://www.thoracic.org/sections/publications/statements/pages/pfet/sixminute.html

http://www.thoracic.org/sections/publications/statements/pages/pfet/methacholine1-21.html

http://www.mdcalc.com/aagrad (calculation of A-a gradient)

SUGGESTED READINGS

American Thoracic Society/American College of Chest Physicians: ATS/ACCP statement on cardiopulmonary exercise testing. Am J Respir Crit Care Med 2003; 167:1451–1452.

American Thoracic Society: Dyspnea. Mechanisms, assessment and management: A consensus statement. Am J Respir Crit Care Med 1998; 159:321–340.

American Thoracic Society/European Respiratory Society: American Thoracic Society/European Respiratory Society statement on pulmonary rehabilitation. Am J Respir Crit Care Med 2006; 173:1390–1413.

Celli BR, Cote CG, Marin JM, et al: The body-mass index, airflow obstruction, dyspnea, and exercise capacity index in chronic obstructive pulmonary disease. N Engl J Med 2004; 4:1005–1012.

Maisel AS, Krishnaswamy P, Nowak RM, et al: Rapid measurement of B-type natriuretic peptide in the emergency management of heart failure. N Engl J Med 2002; 347:161–167.

Manning HL, Schwartzstein RM: Pathophysiology of dyspnea. N Engl J Med 1995; 333:1547–1553.

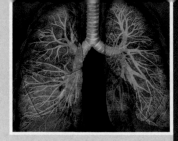

24 Hemoptysis

JOHN W. KREIT

Hemoptysis is defined as the expectoration of blood that results from hemorrhage into the lower respiratory tract. It can be caused by a wide variety of disorders and is a common reason for referral to a pulmonary specialist. The amount of blood expectorated can range from minimal streaking of the sputum to large volumes of pure blood and depends not only on the rate of bleeding but also on its location. For example, hemorrhage into the lung parenchyma or a distal airway may be accompanied by little or no hemoptysis, whereas even a relatively small amount of bleeding from a central airway may lead to a significant volume of expectorated blood.

Hemoptysis, by itself, does not usually lead to significant morbidity or mortality. Instead, it is typically important only as a sign of an underlying and often unrecognized disorder. Thus, hemoptysis is an extremely important symptom, and its cause must be determined by means of a thorough and orderly evaluation.

Massive hemoptysis is an uncommon, but potentially life-threatening, event because flooding of the airways and alveoli may quickly lead to respiratory failure. It requires rapid evaluation and emergent and specific therapy, so massive hemoptysis is usually considered as a distinct clinical entity and is discussed separately in a later section of this chapter.

DIFFERENTIAL DIAGNOSIS

A large number of disorders have been reported to cause hemoptysis, and the most important are listed in Table 24-1. Of these, bronchogenic carcinoma, bronchiectasis, bronchitis, and bacterial pneumonia are responsible for most cases. Table 24-2 lists the relative frequency of disorders causing hemoptysis in major series published since 1980. The significant variability, especially in the frequency of bronchiectasis, bronchitis, and tuberculosis, is probably due to differences in the time of publication, the patient population studied, and the diagnostic tests and criteria used. Figure 24-1 illustrates the percentage of patients with each diagnosis on the basis of pooled data from these studies.

Neoplasms

In most series, malignancy is the most common cause of hemoptysis, and bronchogenic carcinoma accounts for most of these cases. In patients with hemoptysis, the tumor typically involves a central airway (i.e., a main, lobar, or segmental bronchus) and is most commonly a squamous cell carcinoma. Much less commonly, hemoptysis is caused by a peripherally located carcinoma or by other primary pulmonary neoplasms, such as carcinoid tumor or hamartoma. Extrathoracic malignancies, especially melanoma and carcinoma of the breast,

colon, and kidney, may also cause hemoptysis because of their propensity to metastasize to the bronchi and trachea.

Bronchiectasis

In studies published before the early 1960s, bronchiectasis was often the most common cause of hemoptysis and frequently accounted for 25–35% of cases. In the subsequent decades, this number dropped dramatically to <5%. Although this decline was correctly attributed to the greater availability and effectiveness of antibacterial and antituberculous therapy, it was probably also caused by a marked decrease in the use of bronchography, the principal diagnostic modality of that era. Since the advent of high-resolution computed tomography, bronchiectasis has been diagnosed with increasing frequency, and recent studies indicate that it remains a very important cause of hemoptysis.

Acute Bronchitis

Hemoptysis is often attributed to an acute infectious bronchitis on the basis of compatible clinical or bronchoscopic findings, and this is a common final diagnosis in many series. Although acute bronchitis undoubtedly causes hemoptysis, the symptoms, signs, and bronchoscopic findings of this disorder are neither sensitive nor specific. In fact, several studies have demonstrated that the diagnosis of acute bronchitis is often made in patients with another source of bleeding. Thus, acute bronchitis must be considered a diagnosis of exclusion, and great care must be taken to search for other causes of hemoptysis.

Tuberculosis

Although tuberculosis remains relatively common in certain patient populations and geographic regions, successful methods of treatment and prevention have markedly reduced both its incidence and its importance as a cause of hemoptysis. Hemoptysis most commonly results from active disease, but it may also be caused by the sequelae of infection, particularly bronchiectasis, parenchymal cavitation, and mycetoma formation.

Bacterial Pneumonia

Hemoptysis may result from virtually any type of bacterial pneumonia but most often accompanies infection with *Streptococcus pneumoniae*. Other commonly implicated pathogens include *Klebsiella pneumoniae*, *Staphylococcus aureus*, *Pseudomonas aeruginosa*, and anaerobic organisms.

Miscellaneous Causes

Only a few of the conditions listed in Table 24-1 account for most of the remaining specific diagnoses made in patients with

TABLE 24-1 Causes of Hemoptysis

Common (≥5% each)	Nonbacterial pneumonia
Bronchogenic carcinoma	Broncholithiasis
Bronchiectasis	Foreign body aspiration
Bronchitis	Mitral stenosis
Bacterial pneumonia	Amyloidosis
Tuberculosis	Pulmonary arteriovenous
	malformation
Uncommon (1–4% each)	Pulmonary artery aneurysm
Pulmonary embolism	Endometriosis
Left ventricular failure	Pulmonary sequestration
Mycetoma	Alveolar hemorrhage
Nontuberculous mycobacterial	syndromes
infection	Goodpasture's syndrome
Traumatic or iatrogenic lung	Wegener's granulomatosis
injury	Microscopic polyarteritis
	Systemic lupus
Rare (<1% each)	erythematosus
Other primary lung neoplasms	
Metastatic neoplasms	

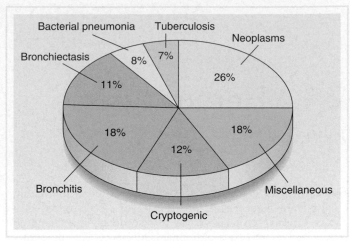

FIGURE 24-1 Final diagnosis in patients with hemoptysis. The approximate percentage of cases attributed to each diagnosis is shown.

hemoptysis. These disorders each account for 1–4% of cases and include pulmonary embolism, left ventricular (LV) failure, mycetoma, lung abscess, nontuberculous mycobacterial infection, and iatrogenic or traumatic lung injury.

Cryptogenic Hemoptysis

In almost all series, the cause of hemoptysis remains unknown in a significant percentage of patients. As shown in Table 24-2, the frequency of cryptogenic hemoptysis has varied widely, and this is presumably due to differences in diagnostic criteria and the extent of evaluation.

PATIENT EVALUATION

When a patient reports a history of expectorating blood, the first step must be to determine whether hemoptysis has actually occurred. That is, bleeding must be localized to the lower respiratory tract, and alternative sites, such as the nose, mouth,

pharynx, larynx, and gastrointestinal tract, must be excluded. Few patients have difficulty distinguishing between vomiting and expectorating blood, although specific questions may be required to elicit a report of nausea and retching. Distinguishing between an upper and a lower airway source of bleeding is occasionally more difficult, although this can usually be accomplished by a directed history and physical examination. Patients with hemoptysis almost always report that the expectoration of blood follows one or more episodes of coughing, whereas in those with an upper airway source, it is typically preceded by a feeling of blood pooling in the mouth or the need to "clear the throat." A history of epistaxis is also an important indicator of upper airway hemorrhage. Routine examination of the nose, mouth, and pharynx is important to rule out an obvious site of bleeding. A thorough examination that includes rhinoscopy and laryngoscopy is indicated when an upper airway source cannot be reliably excluded.

Once hemoptysis has been confirmed, a search must be made for its cause. This process begins with an initial evaluation

TABLE 24-2 Causes of Hemoptysis in Published Series

Series	Gong et al.	Santiago et al.	Johnston et al.	McGuiness et al.	Hirshberg et al.	Fidan et al.
Year(s)	1975-80	1974-81	1977-85	1991-92	1980-95	2000
Location	Los Angeles	Los Angeles	Kansas City	New York	Jerusalem	Istanbul
No. of cases	129	264	148	57	208	108
Neoplasms (%)	24	31	19	12	19	34
Bronchiectasis (%)	40*	1	1	25	20	25
Bronchitis (%)	40*	23	37	7	18	0
Pneumonia (%)	3	6	5	0	16	10
Tuberculosis (%)[†]	3	6	7	16	1	18
Cryptogenic (%)	11	22	3	19	8	0
Other (%)	19	11	26	21	18	13

*Bronchiectasis and bronchitis were combined in this series.
[†]Active and inactive disease.

that consists of a complete history and physical examination and a chest radiograph. This information is then used to determine what additional testing, if any, is required to establish a specific diagnosis.

Initial Evaluation

A thorough history and physical examination is the first step in identifying the cause of hemoptysis. Important symptoms, signs, and historic details that suggest one or more disorders are listed in Table 24-3. In some patients, such as those who have pulmonary embolism, LV failure, mitral stenosis, and traumatic or iatrogenic lung injury, the history and physical examination may provide the most important clues to the diagnosis.

As shown in Table 24-4, the chest radiograph may also yield important information about the underlying cause of hemoptysis. In fewer than 40% of patients, the chest radiograph is "localizing"—that is, it demonstrates a mass, cavity, infiltrate, lobar atelectasis, or other finding that is likely to be directly related to the cause of hemoptysis. In the remainder, the chest radiograph is either normal or demonstrates abnormal but nonspecific findings such as emphysema, interstitial fibrosis, minor atelectasis, or pleural thickening, a category

referred to as "nonlocalizing." This radiographic classification has important diagnostic and prognostic implications. Malignancy is found in almost 40% of patients with hemoptysis who have localizing findings on the chest radiograph. On the other hand, cancer is diagnosed in only approximately 6% of patients with normal or nonlocalizing chest radiographs, and almost all of these patients are current or former cigarette smokers older than 40 years of age.

Additional Testing

The history, physical examination, and chest radiograph are essential to reduce the number of possible causes of hemoptysis and often point toward specific disorders. This initial evaluation, however, yields a definite diagnosis in only a small percentage of patients. In most cases, additional testing is required, which most commonly consists of computed tomography (CT) and fiberoptic bronchoscopy (FOB).

Computed Tomography

Compared with conventional chest radiography, CT is clearly superior for imaging the peripheral and central airways, mediastinum, and lung parenchyma. Thus, it is not surprising that CT has been shown to be very useful in the evaluation of

TABLE 24-3 Important Clinical Features in Patients with Hemoptysis

Category	Feature	Disorder(s)
Historic	Cigarette smoking	Bronchogenic carcinoma
	Previously diagnosed malignancy	Metastatic malignancy
	Previously diagnosed pulmonary cardiac, pulmonary vascular, or systemic disease	
	Recent chest trauma or procedure	Traumatic/iatrogenic lung injury
	Risk factors for aspiration	Lung abscess, foreign body aspiration
Symptom	Purulent-appearing sputum	Bronchiectasis, bronchitis, pneumonia, lung abscess
	Pleuritic pain	Pneumonia, pulmonary embolism
	Paroxysmal nocturnal dyspnea, orthopnea	Left ventricular failure, mitral stenosis
	Fever	Pneumonia, lung abscess
	Weight loss	Bronchogenic carcinoma, other malignancy, tuberculosis, lung abscess
Sign	Bronchial breath sounds, egophony	Pneumonia
	Localized decrease in breath sounds, localized wheezing	Bronchogenic carcinoma, broncholithiasis, foreign body
	Coarse crackles, rhonchi	Bronchiectasis, bronchitis
	Pleural rub	Pneumonia, pulmonary embolism
	S3 gallop	Left ventricular failure
	Diastolic murmur	Mitral stenosis

TABLE 24-4 Important Radiographic Findings in Patients Who Have Hemoptysis

Radiographic Finding	Disorder(s)
Nodule(s) or mass(es)	Bronchogenic carcinoma or other neoplasm, lung abscess, Wegener's granulomatosis, fungal infection
Atelectasis	Bronchogenic carcinoma or other endobronchial neoplasm, broncholithiasis, foreign body
Hilar/mediastinal adenopathy	Bronchogenic carcinoma or other neoplasm, mycobacterial or fungal infection, sarcoidosis
Dilated peripheral airways	Bronchiectasis
Air-space consolidation	Pneumonia, alveolar hemorrhage, pulmonary contusion
Reticulonodular densities	Sarcoidosis, lymphangitic carcinoma
Cavity/cavities	Mycobacterial or fungal infection, mycetoma, lung abscess, bronchogenic carcinoma
Hilar/mediastinal calcification	Previous mycobacterial or fungal infection, broncholithiasis

patients with hemoptysis. In the presence of a normal or nonlocalizing chest radiograph, CT reveals an unsuspected cause of hemoptysis, most commonly bronchiectasis, in approximately one third of patients (Figure 24-2). CT may also demonstrate an endobronchial lesion (Figure 24-3) or an unsuspected parenchymal mass, nodule, or cavity (Figure 24-4). CT is also useful in more than half of all patients who have a localizing chest radiograph, either by revealing a new source of hemoptysis or by providing additional information about a previously recognized abnormality.

Fiberoptic Bronchoscopy

Since becoming widely available in the early 1970s, FOB has been used almost routinely in the evaluation of patients with hemoptysis. By combining endoscopic examination with brushings, washings, endobronchial and transbronchial biopsies, and

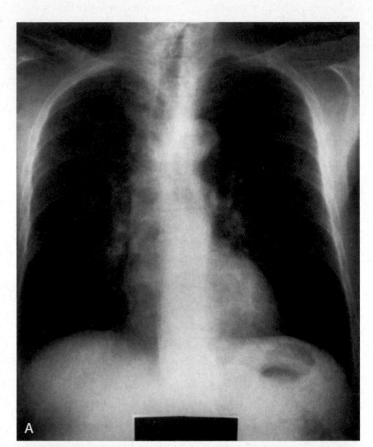

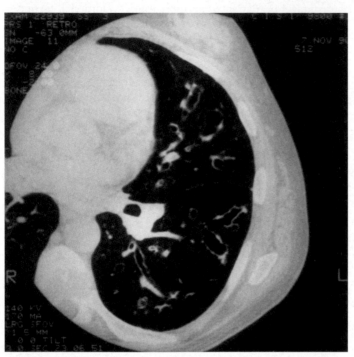

FIGURE 24-2 Computed tomography (CT) appearance of bronchiectasis. Dilated peripheral airways are clearly demonstrated by this high-resolution CT image.

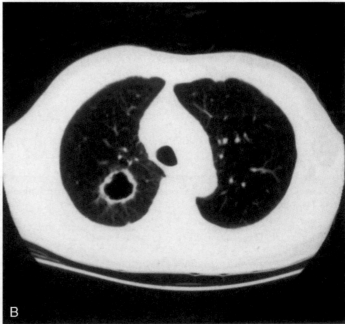

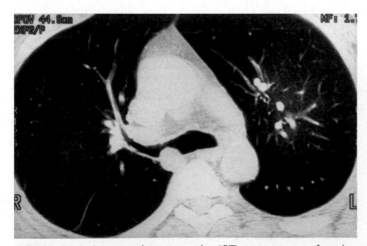

FIGURE 24-3 Computed tomography (CT) appearance of endobronchial mass. A bronchogenic carcinoma is clearly visible in the right main stem bronchus.

FIGURE 24-4 Chest radiograph and computed tomography (CT) in a patient who has a cavitary, squamous cell carcinoma. **A,** The cavitary lesion cannot be seen on the chest radiograph, but is clearly demonstrated by the CT scan **(B).**

transtracheal needle aspiration, FOB may be used to both identify the site of bleeding and determine a definitive diagnosis. FOB is most useful for diagnosing bronchogenic carcinoma and other endobronchial neoplasms (Figure 24-5), but it is far less effective at detecting other causes of hemoptysis. It follows that the yield of FOB is relatively high in patients with localizing chest radiographs and low in those whose chest radiographs are normal or nonlocalizing. The most common nonneoplastic diagnosis made by FOB is acute bronchitis, which is based on the presence of mucosal hyperemia and edema and purulent-appearing secretions. As previously discussed, however, these findings are nonspecific and are often unrelated to the actual cause of hemoptysis. When this diagnosis is excluded, a specific, nonneoplastic cause of hemoptysis is found by FOB in less than 10% of cases. The timing of FOB seems to be of little importance. Although the detection of active bleeding is more likely when FOB is performed during or shortly after an episode of hemoptysis, a delay in the procedure does not affect the diagnostic yield or patient management.

Computed Tomography versus Bronchoscopy

Five studies have compared the sensitivities of CT and FOB for detecting bronchogenic carcinomas and other neoplasms in patients with hemoptysis. All of these studies used conventional (nonhelical) single detector scanners, and most obtained high-resolution images through the central airways. Of a total of 83 patients with neoplasia, CT demonstrated all but one tumor found by FOB. On the other hand, 12 patients in these studies (14%) had neoplasms that were detected only by CT.

Over the past decade, CT technology has evolved from conventional, single detector scanning to multiple detector helical scanning, and this has been accompanied by a tremendous improvement in image quality and resolution. Reconstruction of multiple detector helical CT (HCT) data even allows the generation of three-dimensional images of the tracheobronchial tree, a technique referred to as "virtual bronchoscopy" (VB). Although these advancements would be expected to make CT an even more powerful tool, no studies have evaluated the efficacy of HCT or VB in patients with hemoptysis. Some information can be gleaned, however, from studies of VB in patients with a known endobronchial malignancy. With FOB as the "gold standard," a recent meta-analysis of published studies found VB to have a pooled sensitivity of 84% and a specificity of 75%. Not surprisingly, accuracy was found to decrease with the size of the endobronchial lesion and with airway caliber. On the other hand, several studies have demonstrated that VB can provide important information that cannot be obtained with FOB, such as identifying endobronchial lesions that are beyond the visual reach of FOB and characterizing the extent of an obstructing endobronchial mass.

DIAGNOSTIC ALGORITHM

On the basis of the preceding information, a suggested approach to the patient with hemoptysis is shown in Figure 24-6. If the initial evaluation yields a firm diagnosis, such as bacterial pneumonia or iatrogenic or traumatic lung injury, appropriate therapy is instituted. Alternatively, the initial evaluation may suggest a cause of hemoptysis that requires one or more specific tests. For example, an echocardiogram may confirm the presence of LV failure or mitral stenosis, pulmonary embolism may be diagnosed by means of a CT angiogram, and sputum cultures may be diagnostic in patients with tuberculosis. In all other patients, HCT is the most appropriate next step in the diagnostic evaluation. As discussed previously, CT often identifies an unsuspected cause of hemoptysis, even in patients whose chest radiograph is normal or nonlocalizing and may provide important information in patients who already have a

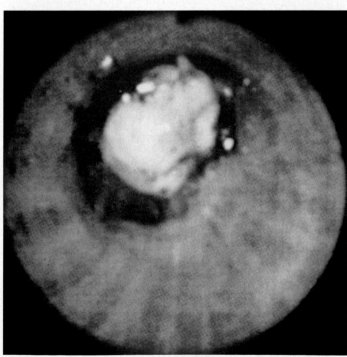

FIGURE 24-5 Bronchogenic carcinoma visualized through the fiberoptic bronchoscope. The tumor occludes the left upper lobe and is actively bleeding.

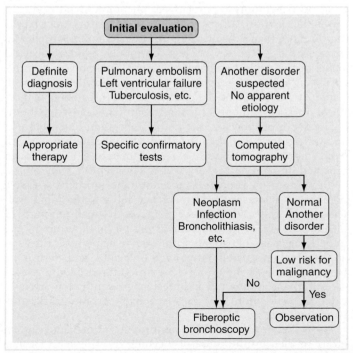

FIGURE 24-6 Diagnostic algorithm for patients who have hemoptysis.

presumptive diagnosis. For example, in patients with suspected bronchogenic carcinoma, CT provides vital information for staging and also provides a "road map" for bronchoscopy by defining the exact location of a parenchymal mass and enlarged mediastinal lymph nodes.

If CT suggests a disorder that is amenable to bronchoscopic diagnosis, such as neoplasm or infection, FOB is performed next in the diagnostic evaluation. Additional studies such as mediastinoscopy or surgical lung biopsy may be required if FOB is nondiagnostic. When CT is either normal or demonstrates another cause of hemoptysis, such as bronchiectasis, the role of FOB is less clearly defined. The absence of an endobronchial lesion on CT is associated with a low incidence of malignancy, and available data suggest that FOB may be safely omitted in nonsmokers younger than 40 years. Because CT occasionally fails to detect a small endobronchial lesion, FOB should be performed in all other patients.

MASSIVE HEMOPTYSIS

There is no generally accepted definition of massive hemoptysis, although the most commonly used criteria require the expectoration of between 200 and 600 mL of blood over 24 h. Any definition based on the amount of hemoptysis is, of course, arbitrary, especially because the volume of expectorated blood is often difficult to quantify.

From a clinical standpoint, it is more appropriate to define massive hemoptysis simply as bleeding that impairs ventilation and gas exchange and is, therefore, potentially life-threatening. Because hemoptysis-related morbidity and mortality depend not only on the volume of expectorated blood but also on the rate of bleeding, the ability of the patient to clear blood from the airways, and the extent and severity of any underlying lung disease, it is evident that the amount of hemoptysis needed to be considered "massive" will vary significantly from patient to patient.

Massive hemoptysis is relatively uncommon and occurs in fewer than 5% of patients with lower respiratory tract bleeding. In more than 90% of cases, massive hemoptysis originates from a bronchial artery or, less commonly, from a collateral vessel of the axillary, subclavian, internal mammary, or intercostal arteries. Although any of the disorders listed in Table 24-1 may potentially give rise to life-threatening hemorrhage, massive hemoptysis is most commonly caused by bronchiectasis, bronchogenic carcinoma, mycetoma, lung abscess, and tuberculosis (active or inactive). Overall, the risk of death from massive hemoptysis is approximately 20%, although reported mortality rates vary widely between 0% and 75%.

Because of its associated morbidity and mortality, massive hemoptysis is a respiratory emergency and requires rapid evaluation and therapy. Unlike patients with small amounts of bleeding in whom the emphasis is placed on determining the underlying cause, in patients with massive hemoptysis the goals are to maintain a patent airway and to localize and control the bleeding. Patients should be closely monitored in an intensive care unit, and intubation and mechanical ventilation are indicated if ventilation and gas exchange become sufficiently compromised.

Bronchoscopy should be performed immediately in an effort to identify the cause of bleeding or at least to localize the bleeding to a specific segment or lobe. Either rigid bronchoscopy or FOB may be used, depending largely on the clinical circumstances. Rigid bronchoscopy, with its large lumen, affords excellent airway control and suctioning capability and is ideally suited for patients with very rapid bleeding. Disadvantages include relatively poor visualization of the segmental and lobar bronchi and the need for general anesthesia. In most patients, FOB is the procedure of choice, because it can be performed rapidly, requires only light sedation, and allows excellent airway visualization. All patients with massive hemoptysis should be intubated before FOB. This optimizes airway control, allows effective suctioning should the rate of bleeding increase, and permits the bronchoscope to be easily removed and reinserted if the suction channel becomes occluded.

CT is also very effective in identifying both the cause and the site of bleeding in patients with massive hemoptysis and should be considered when bronchoscopy is nondiagnostic. CT may also provide additional information by predicting which patients have a nonbronchial systemic arterial source of bleeding and may even allow the visualization of bronchial and nonbronchial feeder vessels.

Localization of the bleeding site is important for two reasons. First, it provides a guide for therapy to control ongoing hemorrhage (see later). Second, in the setting of persistent, severe hemoptysis, it allows isolation of the bleeding site, which can be life saving, by preventing aspiration of blood throughout the tracheobronchial tree. Guided by the bronchoscope, a balloon catheter may be used to occlude a segmental or lobar airway. When bleeding can only be localized to one lung, a larger balloon may be inflated in a main stem bronchus, or the fiberoptic bronchoscope can be used to selectively intubate and ventilate the nonbleeding lung.

Once the bleeding site has been localized and a stable airway has been achieved, ongoing hemorrhage must be controlled. Guided by the results of bronchoscopy or CT, bronchial or other intrathoracic arteries may be visualized by use of selective arteriography and occluded with embolized, nonabsorbable material. Arterial embolization is successful in acutely controlling hemorrhage in 73–98% of patients. Emergent surgical resection is accompanied by a mortality rate that approaches 30% and is usually reserved for patients in whom arterial embolization is unsuccessful.

Once bleeding has resolved, either spontaneously or after embolization therapy, its cause, if not already identified, must be determined (see Figure 24-6). Specific treatment, such as antibacterial or antituberculous therapy, may successfully prevent further episodes of hemoptysis, but when effective medical therapy is not available, recurrent bleeding is common. As many as 40% of such patients will have recurrent and often life-threatening hemorrhage within 6 months, and therefore, these patients should be considered for elective surgical resection.

SUGGESTED READINGS

Goh P, Lin M, Teo N, et al: Embolization for hemoptysis: a six-year review. Cardiovasc Intervent Radiol 2002; 25:17–25.

Hirshberg B, Biran I, Glazer M, et al: Hemoptysis: etiology, evaluation, and outcome in a tertiary referral hospital. Chest 1997; 112:440–444.

Jones CM, Athanasiou T: Is virtual bronchoscopy an efficient diagnostic tool for the thoracic surgeon? Ann Thorac Surg 2005; 79:365–374.

Naidich DP, Funt S, Ettenger NA, et al: Hemoptysis: CT-bronchoscopic correlations in 58 cases. Radiology 1990; 177:357–362.

Swanson K, Johnson M, Prakash U, et al: Bronchial artery embolization: experience with 54 patients. Chest 2002; 121:789–795.

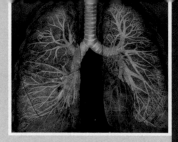

25 Chest Pain

RICHARD K. ALBERT

Chest pain is the most frequent new symptom reported by patients seen in outpatient clinics. Although it is an extremely nonspecific symptom (Table 25-1), it may be the presenting manifestation of a number of potentially life-threatening diseases. Accordingly, a complaint of chest pain always requires a thorough and careful investigation.

DIFFERENTIAL DIAGNOSIS

The pathophysiology of chest pain is understood for many, but not all, of the conditions with which it is associated.

Myocardial Ischemia

The chest pain associated with myocardial ischemia is attributed to an imbalance between myocardial oxygen (O_2) supply and demand. Most tissues can increase O_2 supply by increasing O_2 delivery, increasing O_2 extraction, or both. O_2 extraction by the myocardium is much greater than what occurs in other tissues, manifested by the O_2 content of coronary venous blood normally being much lower than that of blood coming from other muscles. Because the ability of the myocardium to increase O_2 extraction is limited (Table 25-2), the primary mechanism by which the heart increases O_2 delivery in response to increased demands is to increase coronary blood flow.

Coronary blood flow is determined by the driving pressure (i.e., the aortic pressure minus the left ventricular end-diastolic pressure) and the resistance in the coronary arteries. Chest pain can, therefore, be caused by conditions that increase myocardial O_2 demand (e.g., hypertension, hyperthyroidism, exercise) in the setting of a limited ability to increase O_2 supply, decrease mean aortic pressure (e.g., aortic stenosis), decrease O_2 delivery (e.g., anemia, hypoxemia), or increase the downstream pressure for coronary arterial flow (e.g., aortic and mitral valve disease, left or right ventricular hypertrophy, or dilatation). The importance of coronary arterial diameter is apparent in Poiseuille's law, which states that resistance is inversely related to the vessel radius taken to the fourth power, explaining why anything that might result in even a small change in coronary arterial diameter (e.g., coronary arterial spasm, thrombosis, atherosclerosis) can result in chest pain.

Pericardial Pain

The visceral pericardium has no pain fibers, and the pain fibers in the parietal pericardium are localized to the caudal (i.e., diaphragmatic) region. This sparse, localized distribution of pericardial pain fibers may explain why most noninflammatory causes of pericardial effusions (e.g., myocardial infarction, uremia) are not associated with chest pain and why inflammatory problems may cause pain only when the inflammation spreads to the visceral pleura.

Mitral Valve Prolapse

Mitral valve prolapse has frequently been included as one of the causes of chest pain, but this association is not supported by epidemiologic studies.

Pulmonary Pain

The lung parenchyma and the visceral pleura are insensitive to most painful stimuli. Pain can arise from the parietal pleura, the major airways, the chest wall, the diaphragm, and the mediastinal structures. Inflammatory conditions affecting the lung periphery or the peripheral portions of either hemidiaphragm cause chest wall pain when the process extends to the parietal pleura and stimulates the intercostal nerves. Inflammation of the parietal pleura that lines the more central portions of the diaphragm stimulates the phrenic nerves, with the result that the pain is referred to the ipsilateral neck or shoulder. The augmentation of pulmonary pain during inhalation is attributed to the stretching of the inflamed pleura.

Pulmonary Embolus

The pain associated with acute pulmonary embolus is thought to result from distention of the central pulmonary artery(ies). Pain occurring later in the illness is attributed to infarction of a peripheral segment of lung with resulting inflammation of the adjacent pleura.

Pulmonary Hypertension

The pain of chronic pulmonary hypertension is attributed to the disparity between right ventricular myocardial O_2 supply and demand.

Musculoskeletal Pain

Costochondral and chondrosternal articulations are common sites of anterior and anterolateral chest pain. The articulations of the second, third, and fourth ribs are most commonly involved. When accompanied by swelling, redness, and heat, the condition is referred to as Tietze's syndrome. Coughing or trauma can dislocate the costochondral junctions (most commonly those of the tenth through twelfth ribs). The pain resulting from intercostal neuritis most frequently results from cervical osteoarthritis. Intercostal neuritis is also seen with herpes zoster infection, in which the onset of pain may precede the typical rash by 1 or 2 days (Figure 25-1). Thoracic roots are most commonly involved. Subacromial bursitis, biceps or deltoid tendinitis, and arthritis of the shoulder can manifest as chest pain with extension to the shoulder and arm. The brachial plexus and subclavian artery can be compressed by a cervical rib (i.e., the thoracic outlet syndrome; Figure 25-2) or by spasm of the scalenus anticus muscle. The Pancoast

TABLE 25-1 Causes of Chest Pain

Cardiac system
Myocardial infarction
Myocardial ischemia
    Angina pectoris
    Variant angina
    Syndrome X (microvascular angina in setting of non-
        insulin-dependent diabetes mellitus, dyslipidemia, and
        central obesity)
    Myocarditis
Aortic dissection
Pericarditis (infections, Dressler's syndrome)
Aortic stenosis
Syphilitic aortitis
Takayasu's aortitis
Myocarditis
Hypertrophic cardiomyopathy

Pulmonary system
Pleurisy
Tracheobronchitis
Tumor
Pneumothorax
Pulmonary embolus (with or without infarction)
Pulmonary hypertension

Gastrointestinal system
Esophageal reflux
Esophageal dysmotility (i.e., spasm, achalasia, hyperactive
    lower sphincter)
Esophageal rupture
Peptic ulcer disease
Biliary colic
Pancreatitis
Splenic or hepatic flexure syndrome

Musculoskeletal conditions
Costochondritis
Subacromial bursitis
Biceps, supraspinitus, or deltoid tendinitis
Shoulder or spinal arthritis
Intercostal muscle cramps
Hyperabduction or strains of the anterior scalene or rectus
    abdominis muscles
Fibromyalgia
Slipping rib syndrome (pain at the costochondral juction,
    generally affecting the eighth, ninth, or tenth rib; may be
    post-traumatic)
Rib fractures
Sternal marrow pain (with acute leukemia)

Neurologic conditions
Neuritis-radiculitis (cervical compression, herpes zoster infection)
Brachial plexus involvement (cervical rib, spasm of the scalenus
    anterior, Pancoast's tumors)

Others
Breast inflammation
Chest wall tumors
Mondor's syndrome (thrombophlebitis of the superficial
    thoracic veins)
Diaphragm spasm
Mediastinal emphysema
Mediastinitis
Panic attacks
Hyperventilation syndrome

TABLE 25-2 Oxygen Extraction at Rest and Maximum Exercise

Rest	Body	Myocardium
Arterial oxygen content (mL/100 mL blood)	20	20
Venous oxygen content (mL/100 mL blood)	15	8
Oxygen extracted (mL/100 mL blood)	5	12
Extraction ratio	0.25	0.60
Maximum exercise		
Arterial oxygen content (mL/100 mL blood)	20	20
Venous oxygen content (mL/100 mL blood)	5	5
Oxygen extracted (mL/100 mL blood)	15	15
Extraction ratio	0.75	0.75
Increase in oxygen extraction (%)	300	125

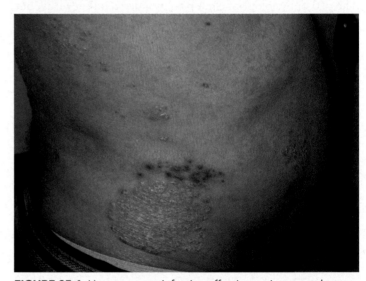

FIGURE 25-1 Herpes zoster infection affecting an intercostal nerve.

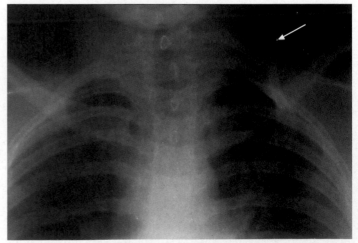

FIGURE 25-2 Chest radiograph showing compression of the left cervical nerve roots by a cervical rib (arrow).

syndrome (most commonly, but not exclusively, caused by bronchogenic carcinoma) may invade the C8, T1, and T2 nerve roots (Figure 25-3).

Esophageal Reflux or Dysmotility

The chest pain resulting from esophageal reflux or dysmotility (i.e., esophageal spasm, achalasia, hyperactive lower sphincter) results from acid irritation of the esophageal mucosa. Esophageal reflux or dysmotility accounts for the chest pain that

occurs in as many as 30% of patients with normal coronary arteriograms.

PATIENT EVALUATION

The approach to patients complaining of chest pain should initially focus on the potentially lethal causes of the symptom (Figure 25-4). Severe pain is more commonly associated with life-threatening causes, but any of these conditions may occur

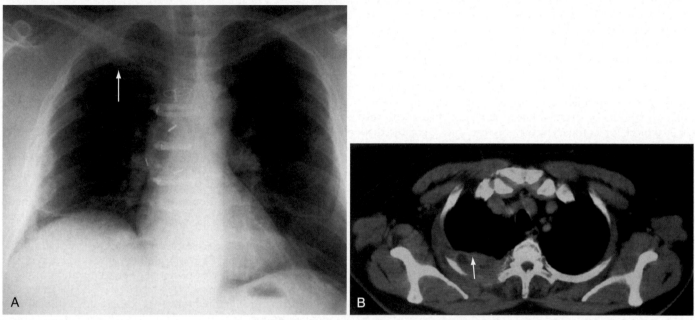

FIGURE 25-3 Pancoast tumor invading the C8, T1, and T2 nerve roots. **A,** Chest radiograph showing destruction of the posterior portion of the right second rib (*arrow*). **B,** Chest computed tomography (CT) scan showing necrotic tumor and rib destruction (*arrow*).

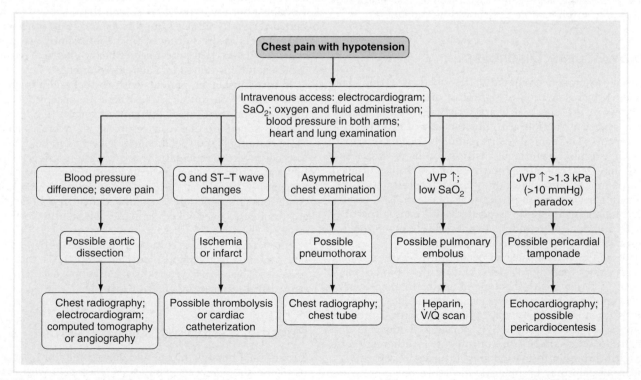

FIGURE 25-4 Evaluation algorithm for severely ill patient with chest pain. Therapeutic approach is determined by blood pressure and findings on brief examination of the neck, chest, and head. *JVP,* Jugular venous pressure; *SaO₂,* arterial oxygen pressure.

with minimal symptoms. Accordingly, patients are frequently treated as if the chest pain were life threatening until these more serious conditions can be excluded by studies that yield more specific information than what can be obtained at the time of the initial presentation.

Presentation

If the pain is acute and the patient is hypotensive, myocardial infarction, pulmonary embolism, pericardial tamponade, dissecting aneurysm, and tension pneumothorax should be considered first (see Figure 25-4). Less commonly, this clinical syndrome can result from a ruptured esophagus. In other patients, the approach is governed primarily by the history and physical examination, which are interpreted on the basis of actual or estimated prior probabilities for each of the conditions listed in Table 25-1. For example, a middle-aged man with one or more risk factors for coronary artery disease (e.g., hypercholesterolemia, diabetes, hypertension, obesity, smoking), who has exertional chest pain that abates with rest that is typical for coronary artery disease, has a greater than 90% probability of having myocardial ischemia as the cause of his symptoms. A similarly high risk is present for patients with exertional pain that occurs with ST depression, cardiac wall motion abnormalities, an increased or decreased blood pressure, an S4 gallop, or a systolic murmur indicative of ischemia-induced mitral regurgitation.

History

The onset, duration, location, radiation pattern, character, and intensity of the pain should be determined, as should the factors that precipitate or diminish it. Unfortunately, both the sensitivity and specificity of the history are low for many of the conditions that must be considered. For example, most episodes of electrocardiographically documented ischemia in patients with stable angina are asymptomatic. A history of cocaine and/or amphetamine use should be sought.

CARDIOVASCULAR DISORDERS

Myocardial ischemia is frequently described as a dull pain accompanied by a sensation of tightness, pressure, squeezing, or heaviness in the chest. It characteristically radiates down the ulnar aspect of the left arm, but radiation to the neck or jaw also occurs. The pain develops gradually; occurs in association with exertion, emotional distress, or large meals and abates within 2–10 min after the stressful activity is curtailed or within 5 min of administration of nitroglycerin.

The pain associated with myocardial infarction is of greater intensity; lasts longer; can be associated with nausea (particularly with inferior infarctions), diaphoresis, hypotension, or arrhythmias; and is not relieved by nitroglycerin.

Variant or Prinzmetal's angina occurs in the early morning and at rest rather than during stress and results from coronary artery spasm. Patients with this type of angina frequently have other vasomotor symptoms such as migraine headaches or Raynaud's phenomenon. Angina that occurs with a progressively lower degree of exertion is considered unstable and is thought to be secondary to rupture of an atherosclerotic plaque with thrombin formation and coronary vasospasm.

Pericardial pain may be pleuritic in nature but more commonly is steady, worsens when the patient is recumbent or lying on the left side, and improves when the patient sits up

and leans forward. The pain frequently radiates to the upper portion of the trapezius muscles. The pain can be pleuritic if the adjacent parietal pleura is involved in the inflammatory process. Pericardial pain can radiate to the shoulder, neck, flank, or epigastrium.

The pain of a dissecting aortic aneurysm begins abruptly, becomes extremely severe within seconds or minutes, and radiates to the back, abdomen, neck, flank, and legs. It is commonly described as "tearing" and may be seen in association with an acute cerebrovascular event; a cold, pulseless extremity; and aortic insufficiency. Unusually large amounts of analgesic agents are generally needed to provide relief.

PULMONARY INFLAMMATION AND CHEST WALL PROBLEMS

Many adjectives have been used to describe the pain resulting from conditions that cause pulmonary inflammation or chest wall problems, but the pain is almost always pleuritic in nature in that it increases with forced inhalation or exhalation (e.g., during coughing or sneezing), during spontaneous breathing, and when pressure is applied to the chest wall by bending or lying down. In response to the pleuritic or positional character of the pain, patients frequently limit their depth of inhalation and, accordingly, may complain of dyspnea rather than, or in addition to, pain.

An abrupt onset suggests a rib fracture, pneumothorax, or pneumomediastinum. A more gradual onset over a few minutes or hours is seen with bacterial pneumonia and pulmonary emboli; and a gradual onset (e.g., days or weeks) is more compatible with chronic infections (e.g., tuberculosis, fungal infections) or tumor.

Patients with chronic obstructive pulmonary disease who have an acute exacerbation of bronchitis develop frequently describe a burning type of chest pain that localizes in the substernal region. A similar symptom can occur in otherwise normal subjects in the setting of tracheobronchitis or during the hyperventilation that accompanies heavy exercise, particularly if the exercise is done in a cold environment.

In many instances, patients with costochondral pain or pain that results from muscle strains describe an episode of chest trauma or unusual upper extremity exercise (e.g., gardening, digging, scraping) that can result in an overuse syndrome. More commonly, no specific inciting event can be determined. The costosternal articulations are common "trigger sites" for the pain of fibromyalgia. Patients with this syndrome also have trigger sites in other locations (Figure 25-5). Musculoskeletal conditions are generally exacerbated by deep breathing and are frequently overlooked as causes of pleuritic or exercise-induced chest pain.

Intercostal neuritis is commonly described as being pleuritic. One potentially distinguishing characteristic is that patients may describe abrupt, shocklike sensations occurring in the same distribution as the pleuritic pain.

BURSITIS, TENDINITIS, AND ARTHRITIS

Subacromial bursitis, biceps and deltoid tendinitis, and arthritis of the shoulder can manifest as chest pain with extension to the shoulder and arm. In these conditions, the pain is worse with neck or shoulder movement but is not exercise related.

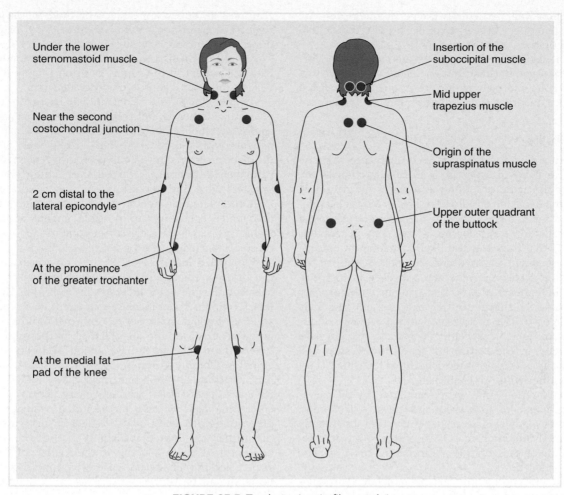

FIGURE 25-5 Tender points in fibromyalgia.

Labels on figure:

- Under the lower sternomastoid muscle
- Near the second costochondral junction
- 2 cm distal to the lateral epicondyle
- At the prominence of the greater trochanter
- At the medial fat pad of the knee
- Insertion of the suboccipital muscle
- Mid upper trapezius muscle
- Origin of the supraspinatus muscle
- Upper outer quadrant of the buttock

GASTROINTESTINAL DISORDERS

Like angina, the pain of esophageal reflux or dysmotility is located substernally; can radiate to the throat, neck, or left arm; and may be relieved by nitroglycerin. Unlike angina, however, the pain is rarely associated with exertion. Rather, it is exacerbated by bending, stooping, drinking alcohol, or lying supine and is frequently worse in the early morning in association with acidic gastric secretions. Chest pain from esophageal reflux or spasm typically lasts for 1 h or more and may be improved by sitting upright or by ingesting antacids or food. The history may also be positive for odynophagia, dysphagia, and/or regurgitation of undigested food.

The pain associated with peptic ulcer disease, biliary colic, or pancreatitis generally begins 1 or 2 h after eating. Pain associated with peptic ulcer disease may improve or worsen with eating. The pain associated with biliary colic and pancreatitis is frequently accompanied by nausea and vomiting.

Physical Examination

Although the physical examination may provide a number of clues to the cause of chest pain, the examination may be entirely normal even when the pain results from a life-threatening condition.

Shallow, more rapid respirations may suggest pleural inflammation or a musculoskeletal cause of pain. Cyanosis may suggest hypoxemia from a variety of pulmonary or cardiac problems. Xanthelasma and tuberous xanthomas suggest the presence of coronary disease.

In addition to the standard vital signs, blood pressure should be measured in *both* upper extremities, because a disparity would suggest aortic dissection. Heart rate and rhythm abnormalities suggest acute ischemia or pulmonary embolism. Fever points away from musculoskeletal pain and suggests pneumonia, pulmonary embolus, pancreatitis, or biliary obstruction. Patients with myocardial infarctions may be febrile, but the temperature rarely exceeds 38°C.

Elevated jugular venous pressure, abnormalities in the carotid upstroke, crackles, a pleural or pericardial rub, signs of parenchymal consolidation, gallop rhythms, paradoxical or fixed splitting or an increased intensity of the pulmonary component of the second heart sound, and cardiac murmurs have a high specificity for many of the cardiopulmonary disorders associated with chest pain, but the sensitivity of these physical findings is probably low because the physical examination may be entirely normal in patients with severe ischemia, pulmonary emboli, and many of the gastrointestinal causes of pain. The reduction in ventricular compliance that accompanies myocardial ischemia may be associated with an increase in left ventricular end-diastolic pressure sufficient to cause pulmonary edema.

Attempts should be made to reproduce or exacerbate the pain by moving the arms and shoulders and by thoroughly palpating the chest wall, particularly the peristernal region, the costochondral junctions, the subacromial bursae, the deltoid tendons, the shoulders, and the abdomen.

Intercostal neuritis is frequently associated with hyperalgesia or anesthesia over the distribution of affected intercostal nerves. Biliary colic and pancreatitis are frequently associated with right upper quadrant and midline abdominal tenderness, respectively.

Diagnostic Tests

Patients without a previous diagnosis of coronary artery disease are not likely to have an acute myocardial infarction as the explanation for the acute onset of chest pain if the pain does not radiate to the neck, left shoulder, or arm and if the electrocardiogram and serial serum troponins are normal. Although the finding of flat or downsloping ST-segment depressions greater than 0.1 mV increases the likelihood that an episode of chest pain is caused by myocardial ischemia, the tracing may be normal at rest, between attacks, or even in the presence of active ischemia. Up to 80% of patients with coronary disease have these ST changes during exercise, but they may also be found in up to 15% of patients with no evidence of disease at catheterization. Nonspecific ST-T wave changes have been documented in the setting of acute cholecystitis and esophageal spasm, as well as other conditions for which chest pain is a presenting symptom (Table 25-3).

Myocardial infarctions may be documented by ST elevations, the appearance of Q waves, and elevated troponins. Unfortunately, as many as 35% of patients who subsequently have a myocardial infarction may have normal electrocardiograms at the time of presentation. Accordingly, more specific testing may be needed.

Exercise thallium scintigraphy and radionuclide ventriculography demonstrate abnormalities in approximately 80% of patients with angina and in as many as 10% of patients who have normal coronary arteries. Other studies shown to be useful in the diagnosis of coronary artery disease include exercise two-dimensional echocardiography and dipyridamole thallium stress testing, but coronary arteriography continues to be the definitive study.

Chest radiographs should be obtained in all patients with chest pain unless a clear-cut musculoskeletal cause of the pain is evident on clinical evaluation. With myocardial ischemia or infarction, the chest radiograph may be entirely normal. Alternatively, it may reveal pulmonary edema, upper lobe vascular redistribution, valvular disease, or pericardial disease.

Radiographs may be normal in the setting of acute pulmonary emboli, although minor degrees of atelectasis, small effusions, a convex appearance of fluid in the costophrenic angle (i.e., Hampton's hump; Figure 25-6), or distention of the central pulmonary vessels may be seen.

A widened mediastinum or an apical effusion in films taken with the patient in the supine position (Figure 25-7) suggests the possibility of a ruptured aortic aneurysm.

Arterial blood gas tensions may be normal in the setting of myocardial ischemia, but respiratory alkalemia and respiratory and/or metabolic acidemia can occur in as many as 30% of patients with pulmonary edema, along with an increase in the alveolar-arterial oxygen tension difference (A-aDO2). Most patients with pulmonary emboli have acute respiratory alkalemia, and most (but not all) have an increased A-aDO2.

A complete blood count should be obtained, because anemia could contribute to possible angina and leukocytosis would support a diagnosis of pneumonia or other infectious cause of nonanginal chest pain.

Troponin T increases 4–12 h after myocardial infarction and is a better predictor of acute infarction than creatine kinase-MB, because the latter increases in both infarction and ischemia. Troponin T can increase as a result of rhabdomyolysis in absence of ischemia, however. A normal D-dimer excludes pulmonary embolism for all practical purposes in all patients except those believed to have a high likelihood of pulmonary embolus. Computed tomography of the heart to detect coronary artery calcification and magnetic resonance angiography to assess contractility and coronary artery narrowing are emerging diagnostic tests in the initial evaluation of patients presenting with chest pain. Radiation risks associated with the former and limited availability of the latter may prove to be important limiting factors to their wide applicability, however. Checking for the presence of cocaine metabolites in the urine should be routine in absence of a definitive alternate diagnosis.

TREATMENT

Pharmacotherapy for patients with myocardial infarctions or acute coronary syndromes (e.g., patients with unstable angina and those with myocardial infarctions but without non-ST-segment elevations) includes aspirin, nitrates, β-adrenergic blockers, and low-molecular-weight heparin. In patients with infarctions or with high risk of infarction (ST-segment depression, increased troponins, persistent chest pain, hemodynamic instability), a glycoprotein IIb/IIIa inhibitor is added. In some patients, angina may be improved by correction of anemia or treatment of hyperthyroidism. Relief of pain has been associated with reductions in oxygen consumption and circulating catecholamines. Invasive therapy includes percutaneous coronary stenting, balloon dilatation, thrombolytic therapy (in patients with infarctions only), and coronary arterial bypass grafting (CABG). Stenting is now used in most patients, and newer drug-eluting stents will likely increase their relative efficacy, because stent occlusion will be reduced. Recent data indicate that stenting offers no long-term mortality benefit over thrombolytic therapy, however.

The acute pericarditis occurring in the setting of large myocardial infarctions generally responds to aspirin. Nonsteroidal antiinflammatory agents or corticosteroids may be contraindicated, because these agents slow the rate at which myocardial scar formation occurs and, therefore, may be associated with an increased frequency of myocardial rupture. The pain associated with Dressler's syndrome (i.e., pericarditis developing

TABLE 25-3 Electrocardiographic Findings in Conditions Presenting with Chest Pain	
Condition	**Electrocardiographic Finding**
Acute cholecystitis	Inferior ST elevation
Pulmonary embolism	Inferior ST elevation
Dissecting aortic aneurysm	ST elevation ST depression
Pneumothorax	Poor R-wave progression Acute QRS axis shift
Pericarditis	ST elevation (generally diffuse)
Myocarditis	ST elevation

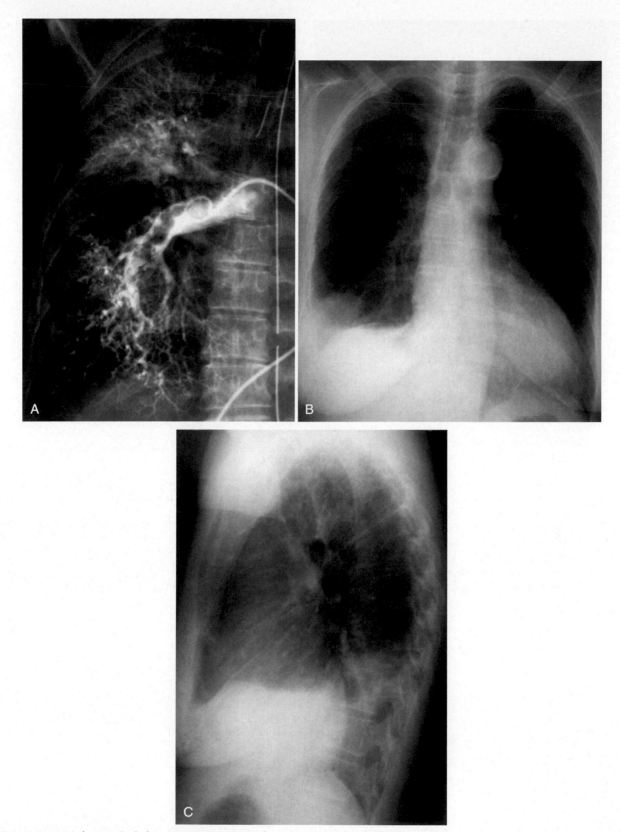

FIGURE 25-6 Hampton's hump. **A,** Pulmonary arteriogram of a patient with a pulmonary embolism showing a large thrombus in the right pulmonary artery. **B** and **C,** Chest radiographs of the same patient, showing a Hampton hump (i.e., lower lobe atelectasis taking a concave shape).

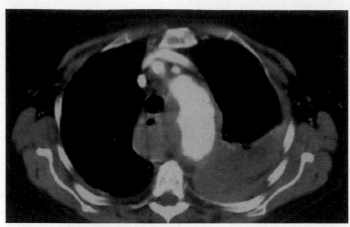

FIGURE 25-7 Aortic aneurysm. Chest computed tomography (CT) scan showing a dissecting aortic aneurysm.

1 or 2 months after an infarction in association with fever, leukocytosis, and elevations of antimyocardial antibodies) is treated with nonsteroidal antiinflammatory agents. Systemic corticosteroids may be needed in more severe cases.

The pain associated with pulmonary inflammation may respond to nonsteroidal antiinflammatory agents, although narcotics are occasionally needed. Right ventricular angina may be lessened by unloading the right ventricle with prostacyclin, prostacyclin analogs, endothelin-receptor antagonists, or calcium-channel blockers to dilate the pulmonary circulation. The pain associated with pneumothorax may be quickly replaced by that associated with the chest tube, and narcotics may be needed to circumvent limited chest wall excursions.

In addition to elevating the head of the bed (or by use of the reverse Trendelenburg position in markedly obese subject), the pain associated with esophageal reflux may also be reduced by avoiding food or liquid intake before reclining, eliminating substances known to reduce the lower esophageal sphincter pressure (e.g., coffee, chocolate, alcohol, mint), and the use of antacids, calcium-channel blockers, H_2-receptor antagonists,

metoclopramide, nitroglycerin, and/or proton-pump inhibitors. Gastroplasty may be indicated in selected patients. Whether this is best done endoscopically or by an open procedure is debated. Esophageal dysmotility has been treated with long-acting nitrates and calcium-channel blockers. Antacids, proton-pump inhibitors, H_2-antagonists, sucralfate, and treatment for *Helicobacter pylori* may be needed to eliminate the pain associated with peptic ulcer disease. The pain of pancreatitis generally requires narcotics. Meperidine is favored over other opiates, because it does not contract the sphincter of Oddi. Intractable pain is a common indication for surgical or invasive endoscopic approaches.

Patients with musculoskeletal pain can be treated with nonsteroidal antiinflammatory agents or the stretching exercises that are used in physical therapy. The chest pain associated with fibromyalgia may be improved by use of amitriptyline.

The pain associated with herpes zoster infections may be so severe as to require narcotics. Amitriptyline and fluphenazine have also been used, as have systemic corticosteroids.

SUGGESTED READINGS

Atar S, Barbagelata A, Birnbaum Y: Electrocardiographic diagnosis of ST-elevation myocardial infarction. Cardiol Clin 2006; 24:343–365.

Cayley WE Jr: Diagnosing the cause of chest pain. Am Fam Physician 2005; 72:2012–2021.

Eisnman A: Troponin assays for the diagnosis of myocardial infarction and acute coronary syndrome: where do we stand? Expert Rev Cardiovasc Ther 2006; 4:509–514.

Fletcher GF, Mills WX, Taylor WC: Update on exercise stress testing. Am Fam Physician 2006; 74:1749–1754.

Fox M, Forgacs I: Unexplained (non-cardiac) chest pain. Clin Med 2006; 6:445–449.

Haro LH, Decker WW, Boie ET, Wright RS: Initial approach to the patient who has chest pain. Cardiol Clin 2006; 24:1–17.

Jones JH, Weir WB: Cocaine-induced chest pain. Clin Lab Med 2006; 26:127–146.

Schoepf UJ, Savino G, Lake DR, Ravenel JG, Costello P: The age of CT pulmonary angiography. J Thoracic Imaging 2005; 20:273–279.

Tutuian R: Update in the diagnosis of gastroesophageal reflux disease. J Gastrointest Liver Dis 2006; 15:243–27.

Winters ME, Katzen SM: Identifying chest pain emergencies in the primary care setting. Prim Care 2006; 33:625–642.

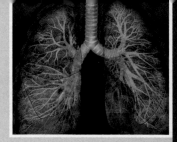

26 An Approach to the Diagnosis of Pulmonary Infection

MARK A. WOODHEAD

The clinical manifestations (both symptoms and signs) of respiratory tract disease are limited and not specific to the cause. The common symptoms of cough, dyspnea, and chest pain and the findings of lung crackles or wheezes can be caused by infection but also by many other diseases. It, therefore, requires some detective work to separate infection as a likely cause of illness from other possible causes and then to specifically identify and treat the likely causative pathogen or pathogens.

Chapters 27 through 29 describe in detail aspects of pneumonia caused by specific pathogens. The purpose of this chapter is to provide a framework from which to approach an individual patient who may have pulmonary infection. Such a patient may be assessed by posing a number of questions (Box 26-1). In this section each of these steps is examined in turn, although in clinical practice, a number of steps may be approached in parallel. Answers to the questions, "Is it infection" and "how severe is the illness" are perhaps the most important.

THE APPROACH

Is It Infection?

A careful history and physical examination are essential. However, there is no universally effective approach, and good clinical judgment is often essential (Table 26-1). Typically, a patient with pulmonary infection will be pyrexial and will have a cough characterized by purulent sputum. Rigors are even more specific to infection but only occur in more severe infections. An abrupt onset with pleuritic chest pain is a classical presentation in pneumonia but often is absent. Wheeze may be present in airway infections, and focal chest signs are common in pneumonia. The more specific pneumonia signs of bronchial breathing, egophony, and whispering pectoriloquy are rare. Unfortunately, in real life the presence of advancing age and immune suppression can mean that infection is present despite the absence of these signs, and underlying lung disease may mean that some of them are present in the absence of infection.

For these reasons a confident diagnosis of pneumonia is difficult outside the hospital, where the cardinal feature of consolidation on the chest radiograph may be difficult to obtain. Even this feature may have other causes, but in the context of symptoms and signs suggesting infection, this diagnosis is likely.

Very often the most important clinical questions are whether an antibiotic should be prescribed (i.e., is this a bacterial infection?) and should the patient be admitted to the hospital? Historically, sputum purulence and the raised peripheral blood white cell count were used to suggest bacterial infection. Inflammatory markers such as C-reactive protein may be more specific and sensitive than the white cell count, and the hormokine, procalcitonin, may be an even more accurate marker of the presence or absence of bacterial infection. However, it is too early to recommend its routine use today. The decision about hospital admission should mainly be guided by illness severity (see following text).

Identification of a microorganism should be the best way to confirm infection, but this, too, has a number of limitations.

What Type of Infection Is It?
Classification of Pulmonary Infections

The traditional anatomic classification of lung infection (e.g., upper respiratory, lower respiratory, pleural) forms a useful, but far from perfect, template on which to base this discussion. Although many infections are limited by anatomic boundaries (e.g., a lobar pneumonia), others do not fit easily into this classification schema (e.g., influenza virus infection).

The two main groups of acute adult pulmonary infections encountered in hospital practice are acute exacerbations of chronic obstructive pulmonary disease (see Chapter 39) and pneumonia (Chapters 27 and 28). A chest radiograph is the key to separating these two, as it is the most sensitive screening method for detecting pulmonary consolidation. The presence of focal crackles is the most common feature of underlying consolidation. A pleural rub, or features of pleural effusion, may coexist. Other less common features include diarrhea, hypotension, and, in the elderly, mental confusion, hypothermia, and urinary incontinence. When pneumonia is clinically suspected and the chest radiograph is normal, a chest CT scan may show changes in the lung parenchyma. However, other diseases may mimic pneumonia (Figures 26-1 to 26-4).

It is important to identify the likely type of pneumonia according to likely setting in which the infection was acquired (Table 26-2). The spectrum of pathogens differs in the three pneumonia types (i.e., community acquired, early, and late nosocomial).

Other roles for the chest radiograph include an enhanced ability to assess the extent of disease, to detect complications (e.g., cavitation, abscess, pneumothorax, pleural effusion), to detect additional or alternative diagnoses (e.g., bronchiectasis, pulmonary fibrosis, bronchial neoplasm), and sometimes to guide invasive investigation.

BOX 26-1 How to Approach the Patient Who May Have Pulmonary Infection

1. Is it infection?
2. What type of infection is it?
3. How severe is the illness?
4. What is the likely pathogen?
5. How do I identify the causative pathogen?
6. Is pathogen identification necessary?

TABLE 26-1 Features of Respiratory Infection and Alternative Causes

Feature	Pointer to Infection	Other Common Causes
Cough	Purulent sputum	Most other lung diseases
Temperature	Pyrexia Rigor	Bronchial carcinoma Pulmonary infarction
Sweats	Drenching and at night suggest TB	Septicemia Menopause
Chest signs	Features of consolidation	Bronchial carcinoma Any cause of alveolitis Pulmonary infarction
White cell count	Raised	Steroid therapy Bronchial carcinoma
C-reactive protein	Raised	Connective tissue disease
Chest radiograph	Focal shadowing	Bronchial carcinoma Any cause of alveolitis Pulmonary infarction

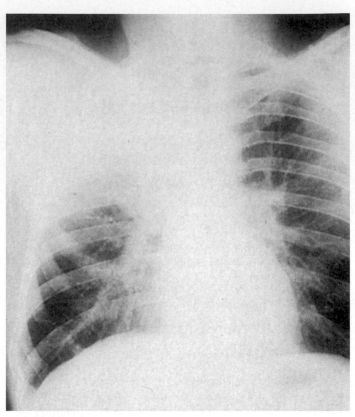

FIGURE 26-2 Pulmonary eosinophilia. Right upper lobe consolidation that mimics pneumonia.

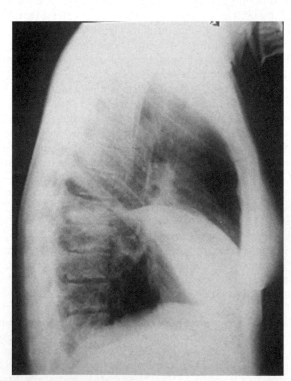

FIGURE 26-1 Mycoplasmal pneumonia. "Classic" homogeneous consolidation of the right middle lobe caused by a serologically confirmed infection of *Mycoplasma pneumoniae*.

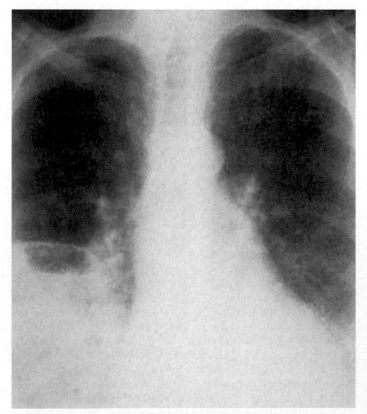

FIGURE 26-3 Pulmonary infarction. Cavitating right lower zone consolidation secondary to pulmonary infarction.

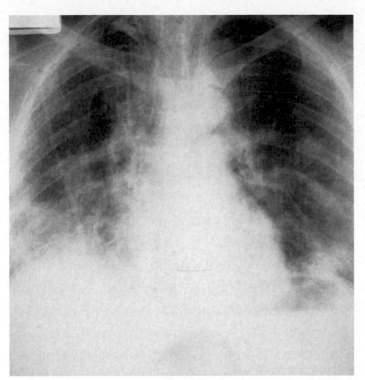

FIGURE 26-4 Drug-induced lung disease. Bilateral, patchy, predominantly basal consolidation secondary to bleomycin administration.

TABLE 26-2	Classification of the Pneumonias According to Likely Origin and Immune Status
Pneumonia Group	**Likely Pathogens**
Community-acquired	Gram-positive bacteria *Mycoplasma, Chlamydia, Coxiella* Common viruses (e.g., influenza)
Nosocomial, early	As for community-acquired
Nosocomial, late	Gram-negative enterobacteria *Staphylococcus aureus* Antibiotic-resistant bacteria
Immunocompromised	Opportunistic organisms

How Severe is the Illness?

The answer to this question guides the decisions about where to manage the patient (home or hospital; general ward, or intensive care unit) and may also guide specific investigations and treatment strategies.

In the patient with an exacerbation of COPD, measures of respiratory distress (e.g., respiratory rate) and gas exchange are the best markers of illness severity.

For patients with community-acquired pneumonia (CAP), those who die are usually severely ill at presentation, so the correct interpretation of presenting features is important. This information should be supplemented by the results of investigations as they emerge. Scoring systems have been developed as an aid to clinical judgment to assess CAP severity. The Pneumonia Severity Index (PSI) is a two-step severity score built from 20 clinical and laboratory features (Figure 26-5).

It has been validated in a number of studies mainly as a tool for keeping low-risk patients out of the hospital. The simpler CURB-65 index is also well validated and is based on just five clinical features (Figure 26-6). Comparisons of the two confirm the slightly greater accuracy of the PSI but simpler application of CURB-65. These scores are recommended in the most recent CAP management guidelines.

In nosocomial pneumonia (NP) and pneumonia in the immunocompromised patient, the importance of presenting features as opposed to features that develop during the course of the illness is less clearly defined than for those who have CAP. Prior or inappropriate antibiotic therapy, renal failure, prolonged mechanical ventilation, coma, shock, and infection with *Pseudomonas aeruginosa*, *Acinetobacter* species, and methicillin-resistant *Staphylococcus aureus* (MRSA) are additional markers of severe NP (Box 26-2).

High levels of lactate dehydrogenase that persist in peripheral blood, alveolar-arterial oxygen gradient greater than 4 kPa (>30 mmHg), and greater than 5% neutrophils in bronchoalveolar lavage (BAL) are markers of severe *Pneumocystis jirovecii* (formerly *Pneumocystis carinii*) infection in patients who have autoimmune deficiency syndrome.

What is the Likely Pathogen?

A wide range of microbial pathogens can cause pulmonary infection. In most patients, the cause of the infection is never identified. In those in whom a pathogen is found, a delay always occurs between the patient's presentation and the availability of culture results. Because therapy should be started immediately, it is helpful to identify markers that may help to determine the cause of infection and hence to direct therapy. Generally, information obtained at presentation may point to potential groups of pathogens rather than to individual pathogens, because few features are pathogen specific.

Airway infections are often of viral origin. When bacteria are present, *Haemophilus influenzae*, *Streptococcus pneumoniae*, and *Moraxella catarrhalis* are most frequently found, although such organisms may simply represent colonization rather than pathogens. These bacteria are important in bronchiectasis, in which for some patients *S. aureus* and *P. aeruginosa* may also be important. The latter two organisms are particularly important in patients who have cystic fibrosis. In patients who suffer from bronchiectasis, knowledge of previous sputum culture results may be helpful (see Chapters 33 and 46).

The range of potentially treatable pathogens that may cause pneumonia is much more diverse. Classification of the pneumonia according to the immune status of the patient and the likely origin of the infection (see Table 26-2) is helpful. Risk factors for unusual exposures (e.g., birds for psittacosis, grazing animals for Q fever) and immune compromise (e.g., unsuspected intravenous drug abuse or sexual contact for human immunodeficiency virus risk) must always be sought.

In CAP, the same pathogens are usually important regardless of age groups, with *S. pneumoniae* the most frequent cause (see Table 26-2). The exception is a lower incidence of *Mycoplasma* infection in the elderly. Gram-negative *Enterobacteriaceae* (e.g., *Escherichia coli*, *Proteus mirabilis*) may be more frequent in pneumonias in some elderly nursing home populations, and MRSA is now being recognized as a community pathogen in this setting. Only varicella-zoster virus pneumonia has specific clinical features (i.e., the vesicular rash).

All the pathogens encountered in the community setting can produce illnesses of varying severity, although legionella,

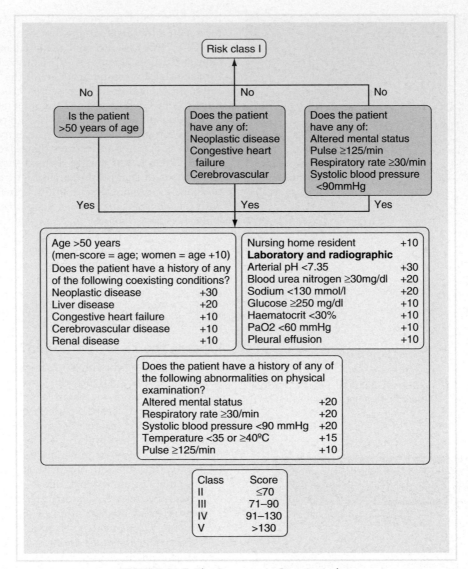

FIGURE 26-5 The Pneumonia Severity Index.

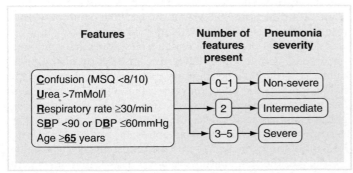

FIGURE 26-6 The CURB-65 score.

BOX 26-2 Severe Nosocomial Pneumonia

- Admission to the intensive care unit
- Respiratory failure (mechanical ventilation or the need for >35% oxygen to maintain an artificial oxygen saturation >90%)
- Rapid radiographic progression, multilobar pneumonia, or cavitating pneumonia
- Severe sepsis with hypotension and/or end-organ dysfunction:
  - Shock [systolic blood pressure <12.0 kPa (<90 mmHg) or diastolic blood pressure <7.9 kPa (<60 mmHg)
  - Requirement for vasopressors for >4 h
  - Urine output <20 mL/h or total urine output <80 mL/h in 4 h (without other explanation)
  - Acute renal failure that requires dialysis

staphylococcal, and gram-negative enterobacterial infections are more commonly found in severely ill patients (Table 26-3).

It may be helpful to retain the terms "atypical" and "typical" pneumonia to describe groups of pathogens (*atypical* referring to intracellular pathogens such as *Mycoplasma pneumoniae*, *Chlamydia pneumoniae*, and *Coxiella burnetii*, and *typical* referring to conventional bacteria such as *S. pneumoniae* and

H. influenzae), but recent studies have shown that a clinical distinction may not be helpful. *Legionella* pneumonia has been included in the "atypical" pneumonia group. In fact, the clinical features of this illness have much more in common with severe pneumococcal infection.

TABLE 26-3 Prediction of Microbial Etiology in Community-Acquired Pneumonia

Microorganism	Features that Occur More Frequently in Community-Acquired Pneumonia Caused by this Organism
Streptococcus pneumoniae	Abrupt illness onset
Haemophilus influenzae	Preexisting lung disease
Staphylococcus aureus	Concurrent influenza epidemic Radiographic cavitation Severe illness Intravenous drug abuse
Legionella species	Recent foreign travel Concurrent epidemic Countries that border the Mediterranean
Mycoplasma pneumoniae	Age <65 years
Chlamydia psittaci	Recent bird contact At-risk occupation
Coxiella burnetii	Animal contact (hoofed animals, cats, rabbits) At-risk occupation
Franciscella tularensis	Tick bites Rabbit contact
Brucella abortus	Cattle, sheep, goat, pig contact At-risk occupation (abattoirs, farming, veterinary work)
Gram-negative Enterobacteriaceae	Nursing home resident South Africa
Pseudomonas pseudomallei	Southeast Asia, northern Australia
Hantavirus pulmonary syndrome	Rodent contact
Tuberculosis	Nonindustrialized countries
Pneumocystis jirovecii	Risk factors for HIV Iatrogenic immune compromise

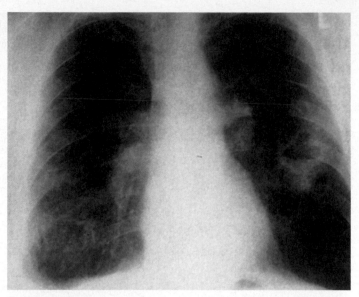

FIGURE 26-7 Cavitating pneumonia. Left midzone consolidation caused by anaerobic infection.

The range of pathogens that cause pneumonia in the immunocompromised patient, in addition to routine bacterial and viral infections, also includes infections by opportunistic organisms that are usually nonpathogenic in the immunocompetent host. Polymicrobial infections also occur more commonly in these patients. Prediction of likely pathogens is again imprecise, but attention should be paid to the nature and degree of the immunosuppression, time course of events, cytomegalovirus (CMV) status of donor and recipient, use of prophylactic therapies, and radiographic features (Table 26-4). Symptoms and signs, as in NP, are seldom helpful, although pancytopenia commonly accompanies CMV infections.

How Can the Causative Pathogen Be Identified?

Minimally Invasive Tests

Throat Swab. A throat swab may be used to identify some predominantly intracellular pathogens such as viruses, Mycoplasma, and Chlamydia, by direct immunofluorescence (Chlamydia, viruses) or cell culture. The yields are low and the methods often labor intensive, which means that in adults this is usually impractical, other than for research. In children, detection of respiratory syncytial virus by this method may be helpful.

Sputum. In many patients who have respiratory infection, this is easy to obtain. When not available, sputum production may be induced by administration of nebulized hypertonic saline—this is probably of value only for the detection of Mycobacterium tuberculosis or of P. jirovecii in immunocompromised patients. The value of examining sputum has been studied exhaustively, and its usefulness remains controversial. The main problem is that organisms identified in sputum may not be representative of what is happening in the lung. Second, bacteria may colonize the normally sterile airways when host defenses are compromised (e.g., by chronic bronchitis or intubation). The clinical illness may be attributed to these organisms when found in sputum even though another process (e.g., viral infection) is responsible.

Radiographic features also usually do not help to differentiate causative pathogens; however, cavitation occurs most commonly in staphylococcal, anaerobic (Figure 26-7), fungal, and tuberculous infections, and rarely with other pathogens.

It is helpful to distinguish NPs that develop within the first 5 days of hospitalization from those that develop thereafter. S. pneumoniae and H. influenzae are not uncommon within the first 5 days, but are rarely found after 5 days, when S. aureus (both methicillin-sensitive and methicillin-resistant strains), Acinetobacter species, and P. aeruginosa are the most commonly seen. No specific clinical or laboratory features allow an accurate prediction of the causative pathogen in NP; however, P. aeruginosa is less common in patients who have NP that developed outside the intensive care unit.

Bacterial antibiotic resistance is becoming increasingly important in both community-acquired and nosocomial pathogens. Patterns of resistance in community-acquired organisms are usually specific to that country, in nosocomial organisms often just to that institution. Knowledge of local resistance frequencies is, therefore, important in guideline empirical therapy.

TABLE 26-4 Predicting Microbial Etiology in Pneumonia in an Immunocompromised Host

Feature	Criteria	Organism
Nature of immunosuppression	B-cell dysfunction T-cell dysfunction Neutropenia	Bacterial Opportunist Bacteria Fungi
Severity on HIV infection	CD4 >200 CD4 <200	Bacteria Tuberculosis *Pneumocystis jirovecii* pneumonia (PCP) Other opportunists
Time course of events	0–1 month post-transplant 1–6 months post-transplant	Bacterial infection Opportunist
Cytomegalovirus (CMV) status	CMV⁺ donor to CMV⁻ recipient	CMV
Prophylactic therapy	PCP prophylaxis	PCP less likely + atypical presentations
Radiology	Focal consolidation Nodule Diffuse shadowing	Bacterial infection Lung abscess Fungi PCP CMV

Because some organisms are always pathogens (e.g., *Mycobacteria, Pneumocystis, Legionella*), their identification in sputum is always helpful. For other organisms, determination of the quality of the sputum sample is essential. Samples that contain 25 neutrophils and 10 or fewer squamous epithelial cells per high-power microscope field are considered to be representative of the lower respiratory tract. Other samples should be discarded unless the pathogens listed previously are being sought.

Various tests can be performed on sputum; Gram stain and routine culture are the best known (Figure 26-8). Visualization of an organism on Gram stain is more specific than culture but is less sensitive. Culture is important for the identification of antibiotic-resistant strains. In a patient who has CAP in which a predominant organism is identified within a purulent sputum sample, that organism is usually the cause of the pneumonia. Some organisms are identified in sputum only if appropriate stains are applied (e.g., *Pneumocystis*) or if culture is performed on specific media (e.g., *Legionella*, fungi).

Tracheal Aspirate. In NP, a tracheal aspirate can be obtained from the endotracheal tube. Even though the upper respiratory tract is bypassed, the frequency of colonization means that, as for sputum, microbiologic results from such a sample should be treated with caution. Culture results are often polymicrobial. Recent studies suggest that quantitative culture of tracheal aspirates may be as accurate as and less harmful than bronchoscopy in NP (see "Bronchoscopy," later in this chapter).

Blood Culture. Blood culture is readily available and highly specific if positive. Its drawback is its relative insensitivity, being positive in only 10–20% of hospitalized adult patients who have CAP. Its yield is even less in NP and very low in children.

Pleural Fluid. When present, pleural fluid should be sampled, because the results are highly specific. Lymphocytosis suggests the possibility of tuberculosis. Pleural pH, as well as cell content, may help in the diagnosis of empyema. Pleural biopsy for histologic and culture examination may assist the diagnosis of tuberculosis.

Urine. Enzyme-linked immunosorbent assay (ELISA) testing of urine for *Legionella* antigen is now the most frequent and rapid test for the diagnosis of *Legionella* infection. Minor drawbacks are that it is positive only in *Legionella pneumophila* serogroup I infection (>90% of cases of *Legionella* infection), that it may be negative if performed too early (antigen excretion begins approximately day 3 of clinical illness), and that antigen excretion may persist for up to 1 year after the clinical illness. Urine antigen tests for *S. pneumoniae* are probably more sensitive and specific than sputum examination, but their cost-effectiveness is uncertain.

Serology. In CAP, this is often the only method of diagnosis available for *Mycoplasma, Chlamydia, Coxiella, Legionella*, and viral infections. This approach does not usually help in immunocompromised hosts or in patients affected by nosocomial infections, unless *Legionella* is specifically suspected (e.g., during an ongoing epidemic). To establish such diagnoses, with certain exceptions, it is necessary to identify a fourfold rise in specific antibody titers to a titer of at least 1:128 between acute and convalescent samples. A single, high titer of 1:256 is presumptive evidence of infection. The need to wait for the second sample limits the clinical value of this method.

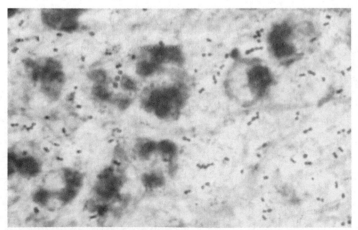

FIGURE 26-8 Sputum Gram stain. Gram-positive diplococci surrounded by degenerate neutrophils, which suggests pneumococcal infection.

Invasive Tests

Transtracheal Aspirate. The transtracheal aspirate obtained by passing a catheter through the cricothyroid membrane was used quite frequently in the past, but the risks of hemorrhage and subcutaneous emphysema have rendered it rarely used today.

Bronchoscopy. Bronchoscopy allows direct sampling from the lungs, but because the bronchoscope passes through the nasopharynx and upper airway, it is important to use an approach that minimizes contamination. It is most useful for patients who are not producing sputum. Other drawbacks are that the procedure and the associated local anesthetic and sedation may further compromise the patient's already altered ventilatory status; transbronchial biopsy may cause hemorrhage or pneumothorax; and the bronchoscope may also introduce infection. An advantage of BAL is that a wider area of the lung is sampled, but the risk of contamination is increased. Protected specimen brush (PSB) may be more specific, but it is less sensitive, because only a small area is sampled. Bronchoscopy has been the most commonly used technique for immunocompromised patients and those who have NP; it is most strongly validated in the former.

The use of bronchoscopic samples in the management of NP remains unclear; PSB sampling is probably better than BAL. Endotracheal aspirates may contain the same bacteria, and no outcome benefit has been conclusively shown. The technique cannot at present be recommended routinely.

In CAP, no evidence supports the routine addition of bronchoscopy to noninvasive sampling. It may be of value in the patient whose initial therapy fails.

Percutaneous Fine-Needle Aspiration. Percutaneous fine-needle aspiration is performed by inserting a 22-gauge needle percutaneously into consolidated lung tissue through an 18-gauge needle in the chest wall. It carries a risk of pneumothorax and lung hemorrhage, and it cannot be recommended other than for research purposes in the hands of those experienced in the technique.

Open Lung Biopsy. The value of open lung biopsy has not been systematically evaluated because of the potential risks. Anecdotally, it has helped in all three types of pneumonia when the patient has failed to respond to empirical therapy and when other tests have been unhelpful.

Other Techniques

Molecular biologic methods, especially polymerase chain reaction (PCR), are beginning to be used selectively for pathogen identification. The potential of this technique lies in its exquisite sensitivity; the test can detect the DNA of a single microorganism. This may also limit its potential, however, because the separation of commensal organisms from pathogens may not be possible. In the respiratory tract it is beginning to be used to detect noncommensal organisms such as viruses and fungi in respiratory samples and commensal organisms in normally sterile sites (e.g., blood, pleural fluid). Its other roles may be to detect multiple organisms at the same time in a single sample (so-called multiplex PCR) and to identify antibiotic resistance by detection of the specific gene defect that determines such resistance (e.g., rifampicin resistance in tuberculosis).

There is also interest in "near-patient" tests that rely on antigen or nucleic acid detection, usually with a colorimetric marker. These enable a microbiologic diagnosis at the bedside both in and outside the hospital. None are yet in routine use.

Is it Necessary to Identify the Causative Pathogen?

In some patients, it may be inappropriate to seek the causative pathogen because it is impractical, it is not cost-effective, and/or the potential risk to the patient outweighs any benefit. In the community, 95% or more of respiratory infections are managed empirically without investigation. The role for microbial investigations in this setting has yet to be determined, but these may be needed only when the patient fails to respond to initial therapy.

Microbial investigations on hospitalized patients are routine. However, in prospective studies of CAP in which intensive investigation is undertaken, pathogens are detected only in approximately 25–50% of patients, and the impact on treatment is small. Outcome benefit for bronchoscopic investigations in NP remains controversial. The reasons for the poor yield are multiple and relate to prior antibiotic therapy, inadequate sample collection, transport delays, and the use of insensitive laboratory methods that often depend on the presence of intact and viable organisms for a positive result. This may all change with the advent of newer microbiologic methods, but because empirical, broad-spectrum antibiotics are easy to give and patients who are not severely ill usually recover, it can be argued that airway infections or CAP microbial investigations should be limited (or not performed) in the mildly ill and used extensively only in the severely ill patient. In NP and the immunocompromised patient, microbial investigation may be more important, because it is often necessary to differentiate infective from noninfective pathology. Possible approaches in CAP, NP, and the immunocompromised patient are shown in Figures 26-9, 26-10, and 26-11, respectively.

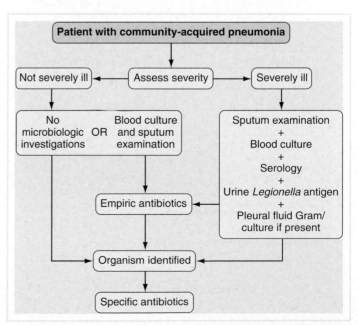

FIGURE 26-9 Diagnostic approach to the patient who has community-acquired pneumonia (CAP). A suggested algorithm to guide microbial investigation in CAP.

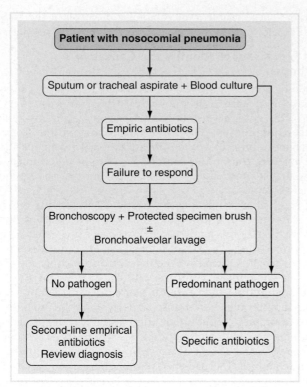

FIGURE 26-10 Diagnostic approach to the patient who has noso-comial pneumonia (NP). A suggested algorithm to guide microbial investigation in NP.

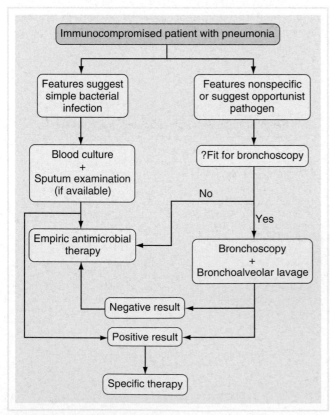

FIGURE 26-11 Diagnostic approach to pneumonia in an immuno-compromised patient (ICP). A suggested algorithm to guide micro-bial investigation in ICP.

Pitfalls and Controversies
Pitfalls
1. The symptoms and physical signs of respiratory infection are shared with other respiratory tract diseases.
2. The elderly, the very young, and the immunosuppressed may not manifest typical features of respiratory infection.
3. Bacteria present in respiratory secretions may be commen-sal rather than pathogenic.
4. Pneumococcal respiratory infections may usually still be treated by antibiotics to which a bacterium is resistant *in vitro* if used in an appropriate dose.

Controversies
1. Pneumonia cannot be diagnosed without a chest radiograph.
2. The distinction between typical and atypical pneumonias is clinically accurate and useful.
3. Routine sputum examination is useful in CAP.
4. Bronchoscopic sampling is useful in NP.

SUGGESTED READINGS
American Thoracic Society: Infectious Diseases Society of America guide-lines for the management of adults with hospital-acquired, ventilator-associated, and healthcare-associated pneumonia. Am J Respir Crit Care Med 2005; 171(4):388–416. www.thoracic.org.

Bartlett JG, Dowell SF, Mandell LA, *et al*: Practice guidelines for the man-agement of community-acquired pneumonia in adults. Infectious Diseases Society of America. Clin Infect Dis 2000; 31:347–382.

BTS Guidelines for the Management of Community Acquired Pneumonia in Adults. Thorax 2001; 56(suppl 4):IV1–IV64. www.brit-thoracic.org.

Mandell LA, Bartlett JG, Dowell SF, File TM Jr, Musher DM, Whitney C; Infectious Diseases Society of America: Update of practice guidelines for the management of community-acquired pneumonia in immuno-competent adults. Clin Infect Dis 2003; 37(11):1405–1433.

Niederman MS, Mandell LA, Anzueto A, *et al*: Guidelines for the manage-ment of adults with community-acquired pneumonia. Diagnosis, assess-ment of severity, antimicrobial therapy, and prevention. Am J Respir Crit Care Med 2001; 163:1730–1754.

Ramsdell J, Narsavage GL, Fink JB; American College of Chest Physicians' Home Care Network Working Group: Management of community-acquired pneumonia in the home: an American College of Chest Physi-cians clinical position statement. Chest 2005; 127(5):1752–1763. www.chestnet.org.

Woodhead M, Blasi F, Ewig S, Huchon G, Ieven M, Ortqvist A, Schaberg T, Torres A, van der Heijden G, Verheij TJ; European Respiratory Society; European Society of Clinical Microbiology and Infectious Diseases: Guidelines for the management of adult lower respiratory tract infections. Eur Respir J 2005; 26(6):1138–80. www.ersnet.org or www.escmid.org.

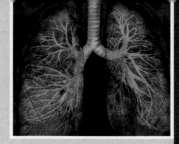

27 Bacterial Pneumonia

ANTOINE RABBAT • GÉRARD J. HUCHON

EPIDEMIOLOGY, RISK FACTORS, AND PATHOGENESIS

Community-acquired pneumonias (CAPs) are a major health care and economic problem because of their high morbidity and mortality and the direct and indirect costs of their management. Most patients with community-acquired bacterial pneumonia are managed in the community by general practitioners; the clinical diagnosis is usually uncertain for various reasons, including the difficulty of identifying CAP in patients with clinical findings indicative of a lower respiratory tract infection (LRTI) and the lack of sensitivity and specificity of laboratory and radiologic investigations. This uncertainty has an important clinical implication. CAP is often bacterial in origin and needs to be treated rapidly with an antibiotic, whereas other LRTIs are usually self-limited illnesses that do not require antibiotics. Because of the difficulty of excluding the diagnosis of CAP, however, most patients with LRTIs are given antibiotics. This results in excessive use of these drugs, which contributes to the resistance of bacteria to antibiotics.

Only a few studies have tried to document the frequency of CAP, and they suggest an incidence of 4.7–11.6 per 1000 and an association with increasing age. In adults older than 65 years, more than 915,000 episodes of CAP occur each year in the United States. Hospital admission rates for pneumonia vary from 22–51%. The mortality is higher in less-developed countries, in the young, and in the elderly, varying from 10–40 per 100,000 inhabitants in some Western European countries between 1985 and 1990. European prospective studies indicate an average mortality of 7% for patients admitted to the hospital, rising to 29% for those with severe pneumonia. CAP, together with influenza, remains the seventh leading cause of death in the United States.

Infection develops when defense mechanisms that enable the lower respiratory tract to remain sterile are overwhelmed, when there is an increase in the virulence of the infecting agent or the volume of the inoculum, or when systemic host defenses fail. Risk factors for the occurrence of pneumonia should not be confused with risk factors for the severity of pneumonia, even though many factors may be significant for both.

Age

Age is a risk factor for pneumonia independent of other risk factors; every year over 65 increases the risk of contracting pneumonia. The annual incidence of CAP in noninstitutionalized elderly people is estimated to be 25–44 per 1000, compared with 4.7–11.6 per 1000 in the general population. The risk of pneumonia caused by *Streptococcus pneumoniae* is higher in the elderly than in the general population. The frequency of hospital admissions as a result of severe infection also increases markedly with age, ranging from 1.6 per 1000 adults between 55 and 64 years to 11.6 per 1000 after 75. Age seems to be one of the main factors predictive of mortality caused by CAP: mortality caused by pneumonia or influenza has been evaluated at 9 per 100,000 in the elderly, rising to 217 per 100,000 in patients with one associated risk factor, and to 979 per 100,000 in those with more than one. This high mortality rate is associated with coexisting heart failure, cerebrovascular disease, cancer, diabetes mellitus, or chronic obstructive pulmonary disease (COPD).

Institutionalization

Both the frequency and the severity of pneumonia increase in institutionalized patients. Oropharyngeal colonization by gram-negative bacilli or *Staphylococcus aureus* may play a major role here, because the pathophysiology of pneumonia is attributed to contamination of the lower respiratory tract from microaspiration. Epidemics of viral infections are also frequent in this population. The main microorganisms isolated in institutionalized patients with pneumonia are, in decreasing frequency, *S. pneumoniae*, *S. aureus*, gram-negative bacilli, and *Haemophilus influenzae*. Because epidemiology and microbiology of pneumonia occurring in these patients are different from CAP, recent American Thoracic Society (ACS) guidelines have included such cases in health-care–associated pneumonia.

Alcoholism

Alcohol adversely affects many properties of the respiratory tract defense mechanism. It facilitates bacterial colonization of the oropharynx with gram-negative bacilli; impairs coughing reflexes; alters swallowing and mucociliary transport; and impairs the function of lymphocytes, neutrophils, monocytes, and alveolar macrophages. Each of these factors contributes to the reduced bacterial clearance from the airways found in these patients. The risks of alcoholism are compounded by the additional risks in the elderly, discussed earlier.

Infections caused by gram-negative bacilli and *Legionella pneumophila* occur more frequently in heavy drinkers. Bacteremia also seems to be more frequently associated with alcoholism. However, alcoholism is not a risk factor for pneumonia severity, except in the case of pneumococcal infection with leukopenia.

Nutrition

Susceptibility to infection is increased by a number of malnutrition-related phenomena, such as a decreased level of secretory immunoglobulin A, a failure in macrophage recruitment, and alterations in cellular immunity. As a result, the frequency of respiratory tract colonization by gram-negative bacilli is increased in patients with malnutrition, and the incidence and severity of respiratory infections are increased. Malnutrition acts in association with other comorbid conditions frequently found in patients with pneumonia, such as alcohol consumption, COPD, chronic respiratory failure, and neurologic disease.

Smoking

Smoking alters mucociliary transport, humoral and cellular defenses, and epithelial cell function and increases adhesion of S. pneumoniae and H. influenzae to the oropharyngeal epithelium. Accordingly, an increased proportion of patients admitted to the hospital with pneumonia are current smokers. Moreover, smoking predisposes to infection by influenza, L. pneumophila, and S. pneumoniae. However, smoking itself is not a risk factor for pneumonia severity.

Aspiration

The risk factors that predispose to aspiration are summarized in Table 27-1. Up to 50% of normal subjects aspirate oropharyngeal secretions during sleep. The prevalence increases to as much as 70% when consciousness is impaired by medications or neurologic disorders or when patients are intubated or have a tracheostomy. In normal subjects, the volume of material aspirated is small, the host is protected by the pulmonary defense mechanisms, and the episodes have no clinically detectable consequence. Even in urgent intubations, clinically apparent aspiration is as low as 3.5%.

Aspiration of gastric contents initially causes a chemical pneumonitis caused by the low pH of the fluid. Pneumonitis may be observed, however, even when the pH is relatively high (6 or higher). When this occurs, the lung injury is transient; when the pH is lower (<2.5), more persistent inflammatory and hemorrhagic bronchial damage may occur. Animal experiments suggest that the volume of material must exceed 1–4 mL/kg to cause inflammation. Atelectasis is frequent, occurs early, and likely arises from the deleterious effect of gastric acid on surfactant.

The diagnosis of aspiration pneumonia is generally restricted to patients who have a bacterial lung infection that occurs in association with a condition predisposing them to aspiration (see Table 27-1). Organisms encountered include a number of anaerobic bacteria (e.g., anaerobic streptococci and *Fusobacterium*, and *Bacteroides* species) and gram-negative enteric bacilli. Periodontal disease is found in many of these patients, and these pockets of gingivitis are thought to be the source of these pathogens.

Associated Diseases

Associated diseases are frequent in patients hospitalized with CAP, with rates ranging from 46–80%. Conditions encountered include COPD (13–53%), cardiovascular diseases (6–30%),

neurologic diseases (5–24%), and diabetes mellitus (5–16%). Pneumonia caused by S. pneumoniae, S. aureus, streptococcus B, and H. influenzae may occur after a viral infection (influenza), as well as in patients with COPD, neurologic diseases, and diabetes mellitus, which also favor the occurrence of pneumonia caused by gram-negative bacilli. Although associated diseases do not increase mortality in most studies, up to 70% of fatalities caused by pneumonia had a comorbid condition, versus 40% among survivors, and the risk of death is multiplied fivefold in association with cardiac disease.

Miscellaneous Factors

An increased frequency of S. pneumoniae pneumonia has been reported among soldiers (12 per 1000), painters (42 per 1000), South African gold miners, and after hospital admission within the preceding year. Previous hospital stay increases the risk of pneumonia caused by S. pneumoniae in particular. Being exposed to stagnant water or to domestic water supply systems may favor the development of Legionnaires' disease. A variety of medications may contribute to the development of pneumonia in elderly people, especially when associated with other risk factors: morphine and atropine interfere with mucociliary clearance, sedatives alter coughing and epiglottic function, and corticosteroids and the salicylates act on phagocytosis.

CLINICAL FEATURES

Diagnosis

The symptoms of pneumonia are not specific but generally include fever, possibly chills, and general uneasiness associated with a variety of respiratory and nonrespiratory symptoms such as cough, purulent sputum production, thoracic pain, dyspnea, coryza, pharyngitis, vomiting, myalgia, and headache. The classic signs of consolidation (dullness to percussion, crackles, increased tactile fremitus, and bronchial breathing) are found in only 33% of adults admitted to the hospital with radiographically confirmed CAP and in only 5–10% of adults with CAP in the community. Accordingly, radiographic consolidation is required for the diagnosis of pneumonia. Such a feature is present in approximately 40% of patients with LRTI and focal chest signs, in contrast to almost none when there are no focal signs. Because a chest radiograph is sometimes difficult to obtain rapidly, a clinical diagnosis is usual in the community, despite the lack of an agreed clinical definition of CAP. However, radiography has to be performed if there are risk factors for complications or if resolution does not begin after 2 or 3 days. There is usually an increase in the white cell count and erythrocyte sedimentation rate during the course of CAP. Table 27-2 suggests when to perform more extensive

TABLE 27-1 Conditions that Predispose to Aspiration Pneumonias		
Cause	Intrinsic	Extrinsic Including Iatrogenic
Neurologic disorders	Seizures, stroke, trauma, multiple sclerosis, Parkinson's disease, myasthenia gravis, pseudobulbar palsy, amyotrophic lateral sclerosis	Trauma, alcoholism, drug abuse, general anesthesia
Gastrointestinal disorders	Esophageal achalasia, stricture, tumor, diverticula, tracheoesophageal fistula, cardiac sphincter incompetency, protracted vomiting, bowel obstruction, gastric distention or delayed emptying	Upper gastrointestinal endoscopy, nasogastric tube
Respiratory disorders	Larynx incompetency (vocal cord paralysis), impairment of tracheobronchial mucociliary clearance	Endotracheal intubation, tracheostomy, pharyngeal anesthesia

TABLE 27-2 Clinical Indications for More Extensive Diagnostic Testing in Community-Acquired Pneumonia

Indication	Blood Culture	Sputum Culture	*Legionella* UAT	Pneumococcal UAT	Other
Intensive care unit admission	X	X	X	X	X*
Failure of outpatient antibiotic therapy	X	X	X	X	
Cavitary infiltrates	X	X			X†
Leukopenia	X	X	X	X	
Active alcohol abuse	X	X	X	X	
Chronic severe liver disease	X	X	X	X	
Severe obstructive/structural lung disease	X	X	X	X	
Asplenia (anatomic or functional)	X	X		X	
Recent travel (within past 2 weeks)	X	X†,‡	X	X	According to local epidemiology, X§
Positive *Legionella* UAT result		X‡	NA		
Positive pneumococcal UAT result	X	X		NA	
Pleural effusion	X	X	X	X	Thoracentesis and pleural fluid cultures

NA, Not applicable; *UAT*, urinary antigen test.
*Endotracheal aspirate if intubated, possibly bronchoscopy or nonbronchoscopic bronchoalveolar lavage.
†Fungal and tuberculosis cultures.
‡Special media for *Legionella*.
§See Table 27-3 for details.

diagnostic tests. Epidemiologic conditions related to specific pathogens in patients with community-acquired pneumonia are summarized in Table 27-3.

Typical versus Atypical Pneumonia

A traditional approach divides patients with pneumonia into those with typical and those with atypical manifestations, leading to the prescription of different antibiotics for each of these conditions. Typical pneumonia is characterized by an abrupt onset, high fever, chills, productive cough, thoracic pain, focal clinical signs, lobar or segmental radiographic findings, leukocytosis, and sputum Gram stain that is positive for bacteria, frequently of a single predominant type. Typical pneumonias are generally thought to be due to extracellular bacteria such as *S. pneumoniae*, *Streptococcus pyogenes*, and *H. influenzae*.

Atypical pneumonias are characterized by a progressive onset, fever without chills, dry cough, headache, myalgia, diffuse crackles, modest leukocytosis, interstitial infiltrates on chest radiograph, sputum Gram stain (and possibly culture) that is negative for bacteria, and possibly an upper respiratory tract infection. Atypical pneumonias are thought to be due to intracellular bacteria or to viruses. Unfortunately, pneumonia caused by viruses and intracellular bacteria may also present with symptoms and signs consistent with typical pneumonia and vice versa. Accordingly, many suggest that this classification scheme is of minor value.

Aspiration Pneumonia

Mendelson originally described the syndrome of aspiration of gastric contents in 1946 in 61 obstetric patients who had aspiration pneumonia develop after ether anesthesia. Manifestations begin very rapidly after the event and include cough (dry or with pink sputum because of bronchoalveolar hemorrhage), tachypnea, tachycardia, fever, diffuse crackles, cyanosis, and bronchospasm in some cases. Chest radiographs show extensive atelectasis and infiltrates, and arterial blood gas

tensions show hypoxemia and normocapnia or hypocapnia. In the most severe cases, the $Paco_2$ may be elevated, and a metabolic acidosis may be present.

A number of clinical features help distinguish aspiration pneumonia from other CAPs. Aspiration pneumonia tends to have a more insidious course, such that the patient may have an empyema, lung abscess, or necrotizing pneumonia at the time medical care is first sought. The sputum may be putrid because of anaerobic bacteria, and weight loss is common. Chest imaging commonly shows necrotizing infiltrates or multiple abscesses, typically located in dependent regions (Figure 27-1).

Lung Abscess

The incidence of pulmonary abscess has decreased over the last decade. Lung abscess is associated with several conditions, including poor dental status or periodontal disease, chronic alcoholism, intravenous drug use, and head and neck cancer. Lung abscess may complicate bronchiectasis (Figure 27-2) and the course of aspiration pneumonia in those with impaired consciousness, dysphagia and gastroesophageal reflux, or acute or chronic neurologic diseases, but it may also occur with bronchial obstruction by a foreign body or bronchial carcinoma.

Pulmonary abscesses are usually polymicrobial, with a predominant anaerobic flora such as *Streptococcus intermedius*, *Streptococcus salivarius*, *Streptococcus constellatus*, *Fusobacterium* species, *Prevotella* species, or *Bacteroides* species.

Clinical manifestations usually develop insidiously, particularly before necrosis develops. This period may last several weeks after an initial aspiration. When the lung abscess is diagnosed, patients may have lost weight and have a high fever, chills, putrid expectoration, and chest pain. Pleural involvement with an empyema is a frequent complication of lung abscess. Laboratory findings include a very high white cell count and considerable elevation of inflammatory and catabolic markers.

TABLE 27-3 Epidemiological Conditions Related to Specific Pathogens in Patients with Community-Acquired Pneumonia

Condition	Commonly Encountered Pathogen(s)
Elderly	*S. pneumoniae*, gram-negative bacilli, *H. influenzae*, *Staphylococcus aureus*, anaerobes, *Pseudomonas aeruginosa*, and *Legionella* species
Alcoholism	*Streptococcus pneumoniae* and anaerobes
COPD and/or smoking	*S. pneumoniae*, *Haemophilus influenzae*, *Moraxella catarrhalis*, *Legionella* species, *Pseudomonas aeruginosa*
Nursing home residency	*S. pneumoniae*, gram-negative bacilli, *H. influenzae*, *Staphylococcus aureus*, anaerobes, *Chlamydia pneumoniae*
Poor dental hygiene	Anaerobes
HIV infection—early stage	*S. pneumoniae*, *H. influenzae*, and *Mycobacterium tuberculosis*
HIV infection—late stage	*S. pneumoniae*, *H. influenzae*, *Pseudonomas aeruginosa*, *Mycobacterium tuberculosis*, *P. carinii*, *Cryptococcus*, *Histoplasma* species and *Aspergillus* species
Influenza active in community	Influenza, *S. pneumoniae*, *S. aureus*, *Streptococcus pyogenes*, and *H. influenzae*
Conditions that predispose to aspiration pneumonias (see Table 27-1)	Anaerobes
Structural disease of lung (bronchiectasis, cystic fibrosis, etc.)—early stage	*S. pneumoniae*, *S. aureus*, and *H. influenzae*
Structural disease of lung (bronchiectasis, cystic fibrosis, etc.)—late stage	*Pseudonomas aeruginosa*, *Burkholderia (Pseudomonas) cepacia*, *S. aureus*, and *Aspergillus* sp.
Injection drug use	*S. aureus*, anaerobes, *M. tuberculosis*, and *S. pneumoniae*
Airway obstruction	Anaerobes, *S. pneumoniae*, *H. influenzae*, and *S. aureus*
Travel to southwestern U.S.	*Coccidioides* species
Exposure to farm animals or parturient cats	*Coxiella burnetii* (Q fever)
Exposure to cooling towers, large air-conditioning systems, spas, hot tubs, humidifiers	*Legionella* species
Exposure to bats or soil enriched with bird droppings	*Histoplasma capsulatum*
Exposure to birds	*Chlamydia psittaci*
Exposure to poultry farm in area with previous H5N1 infection	*Influenzae H5N1*
Exposure to rabbits	*Francisella tularensis*

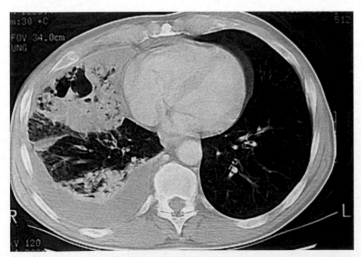

FIGURE 27-1 Necrotizing aspiration pneumonia. Chest computed tomography demonstrates involvement of the entire right middle lobe (which suggests pulmonary gangrene) and an effusion, which was found to be an empyema.

Radiologic features of lung abscess are typically a peripheral cavity more than 2 cm in diameter in the dependent lung regions. Computed tomography (CT) is useful to distinguish empyema with bronchopleural fistula from lung abscess.

Sputum Gram stain is often misleading. Bronchoscopic sampling such as bronchial aspirate, protected specimen brush, or bronchoalveolar lavage (BAL) should be performed onto anaerobic media. Percutaneous fluoroscopic or ultrasound or CT-guided fine-needle aspiration may be a useful diagnostic technique. Aspirates should be grown on anaerobic media, and samples should be sent rapidly to the laboratory for specific anaerobic cultures.

Specific Pathogens

Streptococcus Species

S. pneumoniae is the most common bacterium isolated from patients with CAP. It is a saprophyte of the respiratory tract, which can easily proliferate as soon as natural defenses decline (as with increasing age, alcoholism, diabetes, smoking, and immunosuppression). Classically, the onset is abrupt,

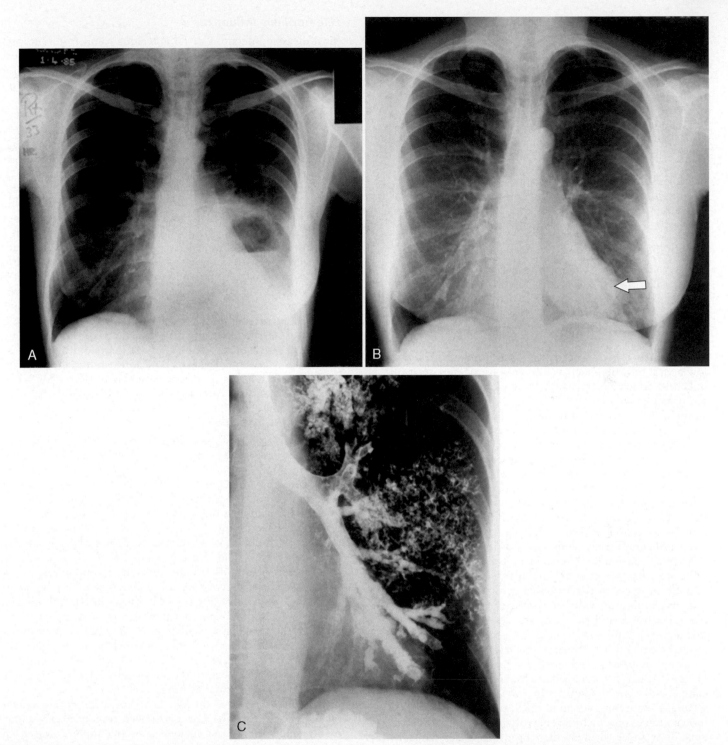

FIGURE 27-2 Left lower lobe pneumonia. **A,** Lung abscess associated with lower lobe pneumonia. **B,** Chest radiograph 3 months after resolution of the lung abscess, showing widened airways with thickened walls in the left lower lobe *(arrow)*. These bronchiectatic changes were consequent to the pneumonia. **C,** Fiberoptic bronchoscopic bronchogram of the left lower lobe, confirming gross dilatation of the airways typical of postinfective bronchiectasis.

characterized by intense and prolonged chills and considerable thoracic pain. Symptoms are rapidly progressive, with fever close to 40°C (104°F), tachycardia, and tachypnea; cough is common, as are oliguria and cyanosis. At this stage, a nasolabial herpes simplex lesion may develop, crackles are heard, and chest radiographs show homogeneous lobar or segmental consolidation. Without antibiotic treatment, cough persists and leads to rust-colored sputum. Leukocytosis is frequent, and blood cultures are positive in 10–20% of patients if these are obtained before antibiotic therapy. Arterial blood gas tensions show decreases in Pao_2 and $Paco_2$. A symptom recrudescence can occur after a few days; then the body temperature falls abruptly to 37° C (98.6° F) and an abundant diuresis occurs. Radiologic and physical signs characteristically improve rapidly and considerably. The rapid rate of multiplication of *S. pneumoniae*, together with the high risk of secondary complications (e.g., empyema, meningitis, septicemia), make any *S. pneumoniae* pneumonia a medical emergency.

Streptococcus species other than *S. pneumoniae* rarely cause pneumonia, but among these, *S. pyogenes* is most often involved, more in the young than in the elderly. Pneumonia caused by *S. pyogenes* occurs after viral infections such as measles, varicella, or rubella in infants and after influenza, measles, or varicella in adults. The clinical presentation is that of typical pneumonia. Pleural effusion and empyema frequently develop, and other complications include pneumothorax, pericarditis, mediastinitis, and bronchopleural fistula.

Staphylococcus Species

The severity of *Staphylococcus* infection is due to the prevalence of its resistance to multiple antibiotics and to lung tissue lysis as part of the infection, leading to bullae, rupture of bullae into the pleura (pneumothorax, pneumopyothorax), serious ventilatory defects, and septicemia. Staphylococcal infection occurs through the airways (inhalation, aspiration) or by hematogenous spread. Airborne contamination may follow a viral infection such as influenza or measles, or it may be linked to comorbidity (COPD, carcinoma, laryngectomy, seizure); hematogenous spread is the result of bacteremia (endocarditis, infective foci flowing into the bloodstream). Direct bloodstream infection caused by intravenous drug abuse is the most common cause in many inner-city hospital emergency departments. The clinical presentation may be unusual compared with typical pneumonia when the infection develops through vascular dissemination (e.g., dyspnea, cough, and purulent sputum might be masked by symptoms of endocarditis or the primary infective focus) or when the infection is causing a pleural effusion, empyema, or lung abscess. The chest radiograph may show two possible features: central or segmental consolidation secondary to aspiration or multiple infiltrates that are generally nodular early on and can subsequently progress to parenchymal consolidation with or without cavitation after vascular spread of the infection. Abscess, pleural effusion, and empyema are frequent, as well as septicemia. Overall outcome depends on associated diseases, spread of infection, and resistance of *Staphylococcus* to antibiotics.

Community-acquired methicillin-resistant *Staphylococcus aureus* (MRSA) has emerged as a frequent infectious agent associated with skin and soft-tissue infections in the community setting. Community-acquired MRSA can also cause severe pulmonary infections, including necrotizing pneumonia and empyema. It is more virulent than health-care–associated MRSA isolates. Community-acquired MRSA usually contains the gene encoding Panton-Valentine leukocidin and the SCC*mec* type IV element and belongs to the USA300 pulsed-field. Panton-Valentine leukocidin is a toxin that creates lytic pores in the cell membranes of neutrophils and induces the release of neutrophil chemotactic factors that promote inflammation and tissue destruction. Community-acquired MRSA is typically more susceptible to a wider class of antibiotics than health-care–associated MRSA. The optimal antibiotic treatment for Panton-Valentine leukocidin-positive community-acquired MRSA is unknown; however, antibiotics with activity against MRSA and the ability to inhibit toxin production may be optimal (linezolid or clindamycin for susceptible isolates).

Haemophilus Influenzae

Most invasive infections of *H. influenzae* result from encapsulated, typeable strains rather than from nonencapsulated, nontypeable strains. A history of upper respiratory tract infection is common. Small pleural effusions can occur, but empyema and cavitation are rare.

Mycoplasma Pneumoniae

Mycoplasma pneumoniae pneumonias usually occur in small epidemics, particularly in closed populations. The clinical presentation is commonly that of an atypical pneumonia, as described earlier. *M. pneumoniae* infections mimic, to some extent, the presentation of viral respiratory infections, but the incubation period is longer (10–20 days) than for viruses, and the fever is generally below 39°C (102.2°F). Within a few days, most symptoms improve, although the low-grade fever and cough frequently persist. A history of a preceding upper respiratory tract infection may be found in up to 50% of patients. A variety of extrapulmonary manifestations may be encountered, including arthralgia, cervical lymphadenopathy, bullous myringitis, diarrhea, immune hemolytic anemia, meningitis, meningoencephalitis, myalgia, myocarditis, hepatitis, nausea, pericarditis, skin eruptions, and vomiting. Diffuse crackles are occasionally heard. Infiltrates are usually localized in the lower lobes and regress very slowly over 4–6 weeks. Pleural effusions and mediastinal lymphadenopathy are rare.

Chlamydia Species

Psittacosis is a pneumonia caused by an intracellular bacterium, *Chlamydia psittaci*, which is responsible for ornithosis in the domestic fowl. *C. psittaci* can be transmitted to humans by inhalation from infected birds, including canaries, parakeets, parrots, pigeons, and turkeys. The clinical presentation is that of an atypical pneumonia. After 7–14 days' incubation, the onset might be abrupt. Fever of 38°–40°C (100.4°–104.0°F), possibly with chills, is associated with arthralgia, headache, myalgia, dyspnea, and thoracic pain. Cough may be severe, and sputum, if any, is usually mucoid. Splenomegaly and a macular rash are evocative of psittacosis. The radiologic appearance is variable but typically shows lower lobe infiltration. Hepatitis, phlebitis, encephalitis, myocarditis, renal failure, and intravascular coagulation are unusual complications. Despite the efficiency of antibiotics such as tetracycline and erythromycin, psittacosis is associated with a mortality of approximately 1%. Relapse is prevented by 2 weeks' treatment after return to a normal temperature.

Previously known as the TWAR agent, *Chlamydia pneumoniae* has been recognized as a pathogen responsible for pneumonia since 1985. The incidence of pneumonia caused by *C. pneumoniae* is uncertain. The clinical presentation is that of an atypical pneumonia in young adults; in the elderly, the course may be severe, particularly if comorbidities are present. Sore throat may precede the appearance of fever (37.7°–39°C [100°–102.2°F]) and a nonproductive cough. The chest radiograph shows subsegmental infiltrates, which usually clear over 2–4 weeks.

Legionella Pneumophila

Legionella species are aerobic gram-negative intracellular bacilli; approximately 30 species have been identified, the most common being *L. pneumophila*. Water and air-conditioning systems are their natural reservoirs; spreading of the bacilli occurs by air, but no transmission between human beings has been reported. *L. pneumophila* infection may cause an asymptomatic seroconversion, a single episode of pyrexia, and mild to severe pneumonia. Pontiac fever has been associated with fever, chills, headache, and upper respiratory tract symptoms. Pneumonia occurs either sporadically or in small epidemics and is more likely to occur in immunocompromised hosts. After 2–8 days of incubation, headache, myalgia, high fever, and chills precede pneumonia by a few days. Initially, there is a nonproductive cough that may become productive of watery or even purulent sputum. Dyspnea, hemoptysis, and chest pain frequently occur. Extrapulmonary symptoms and signs are numerous and include abdominal pain, agitation, watery diarrhea, arthralgia, confusion, skin rash, headache, hematuria, hyponatremia, hypophosphatemia, myalgia, nausea, oliguria, proteinuria, renal failure, seizures, splenomegaly, and vomiting. Leukocytosis, neutropenia, lymphopenia, and hepatic inflammation may be observed. The chest radiograph shows consolidation, often unilateral and dense, initially localized and then spreading gradually. Pleural effusion is frequently present; cavitation is rare. The outcome depends on the early clinical recognition and treatment and on comorbidities. Mortality is increased in immunosuppressed patients and in those who have complications of the infection.

Gram-Negative Bacilli

Gram-negative bacilli include various Enterobacteriaceae and Pseudomonadaceae, in particular *Klebsiella pneumoniae*, *Escherichia coli*, *Pseudomonas aeruginosa*, and *Acinetobacter* species. Gram-negative bacilli are more often responsible for nosocomial pneumonia than for CAP, but CAP attributable to these agents may result from their colonization of the oropharynx followed by inhalation or microaspiration of the organisms. Comorbidity is usual in patients acquiring these pneumonias. The clinical presentation is that of a typical pneumonia. The prognosis is poor, particularly in cases of immunodepression, alcoholism, neutropenia, and old age.

Friedländer's pneumonia *(K. pneumoniae)* typically occurs in men older than 40 years; alcoholism, diabetes mellitus, and chronic lung disease are predisposing factors. Historically, patients were thought to produce particularly large volumes of thick and bloody sputum; they were likely to present with prostration and hypotension and to have multiple patches of consolidation, particularly in the upper lobes, with bulging fissures (Figure 27-3) and multicavitation on chest radiographs (i.e., an expanding pneumonia).

E. coli pneumonia and *P. aeruginosa* pneumonia usually occur in chronically ill patients; hemoptysis is rare, and pneumonia usually involves the lower lobes. Abscess and empyema occur frequently. *Acinetobacter* pneumonia progresses very quickly, leading to severe hypoxemia, shock, bilateral consolidation, empyema, and even death within a few days.

Pseudomonas pseudomallei, which causes melioidosis, is an aerobic, gram-negative bacillus found in soil, vegetation, and water in tropical regions. Infection of the lung occurs more commonly as a result of spread through the bloodstream after cutaneous infection than as a result of inhalation. The clinical presentation may be either acute or chronic. Acute melioidosis presents with high fever, dyspnea, chest pain, cough with purulent sputum, and hemoptysis. Local cellulitis and lymphangitis may be seen at the place of cutaneous inoculation. The chest radiograph shows diffuse miliary nodules, infiltrations, or cavitations. Chronic melioidosis may occur years after

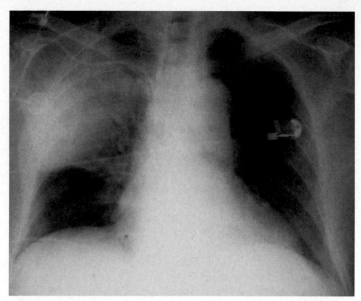

FIGURE 27-3 *Klebsiella* pneumonia. Chest radiograph showing a bulging fissure.

contracting the infection in the endemic area. Symptoms are either absent or may resemble those of pulmonary tuberculosis: asthenia, anorexia, weight loss, low-grade fever, productive cough, and hemoptysis. Chest radiographs show apical infiltrates, possibly with cavitations.

Anaerobic Bacteria

Anaerobic bacterial pneumonia results from aspiration; therefore, it typically occurs in situations involving alcoholism, coma, seizure, and general anesthesia. Chronic dental infection; head, neck, and lung cancer; and bronchiectasis are additional risk factors. Anaerobic pneumonia begins as a typical pneumonia with pleuritic pain; pulmonary infiltrations preferentially involve the lower lobes, particularly the right lower lobe. If patients aspirate while lying supine, the segments involved are typically the posterior segment of the right upper lobe and the apical segment of the right lower lobe. Necrosis and suppuration follow, and fever higher than 39°C (102.2°F), dyspnea, and pleuritic pain persist. Sputum is purulent and fetid, which is often obvious on entering the patient's room. Leukocytosis is high, and segmental infiltrations with small transparent areas of necrosis are seen. Abscess and empyema occur frequently. The outcome is closely related to treatment—delay in antibiotic treatment or inappropriate antibiotic choice will probably result in necrotizing pneumonia, abscess, and empyema, which increases the fatality rate.

Coxiella Burnetii

Coxiella burnetii is the causative agent of Q fever and is the most frequent pathogen responsible for pneumonia among the Rickettsiaceae. Ticks are vector agents, and various wild and domestic animals (cattle, sheep, goats) are infected with no evidence of disease; *C. burnetii* multiplies in the placenta of pregnant animals and spreads during parturition. Although *C. burnetii* is present in numerous species of ticks, the main route of transmission is by inhalation of infectious aerosols. *C. burnetii* is particularly resistant to chemical and physical agents. The clinical presentation is that of an atypical pneumonia. The onset occurs after a 2- to 4-week incubation period.

Patients present with high fever (40°C [104°F]), chills, myalgia, and headache, all of which appear abruptly; cough is usually nonproductive. Abdominal and thoracic pain, pharyngitis, and bradycardia may also occur. There is usually no rash, in contrast with other rickettsial infections. Hepatomegaly and splenomegaly may be found on physical examination. The chest radiograph shows dense nodular infiltrates; pleural effusion and linear atelectasis may be seen. There is no leukocytosis, and mild hepatitis may be found. The course is usually benign.

Nocardia Species

Nocardia asteroides and, to a lesser extent, *Nocardia brasiliensis* are responsible for most cases of *Nocardia* pneumonia. *Nocardia* are aerobic, gram-positive bacilli present mainly in soil. Approximately 50% of patients have no underlying disease. The others tend to have predisposing problems such as immunosuppression, malignancy, or long-term corticosteroid therapy. The onset of the infection is usually subacute, but it can be fulminant; in the latter case, there is a high fatality rate. Symptoms include fever, asthenia, anorexia, productive cough, and chest pain. Multiple subcutaneous abscesses may be present, as well as neurologic signs when there is central nervous system involvement. Chest radiograph abnormalities vary from infiltration to lobar consolidation; cavitation, nodules, abscesses, and pleural effusion may also be seen. The prognosis depends on whether the infection disseminates, but it is usually good in the case of isolated lung disease. Metastatic infection may occur anywhere but is particularly common in the central nervous system and the skin. Infection may also reach the pleura and the chest wall.

Actinomyces Israelii

Both *Actinomyces* species and *Arachnia* species can cause actinomycosis, but *Actinomyces israelii* is the main responsible organism. These are anaerobic, gram-positive, filamentous, branching bacilli (Figure 27-4) that were incorrectly thought to be fungi for many years. They normally reside in the oropharynx and become invasive pathogens when there is a defect in the anatomic barrier or when they are inhaled, at which time the infection may extend directly from one place to an adjacent area. Bad dentition, bronchiectasis, and COPD are risk factors for pulmonary infection. Men are far more frequently affected than women. The clinical presentation suggests tuberculosis, carcinoma, or chronic fungal infection; asthenia,

anorexia, weight loss, and low-grade fever may precede cough and chest pain by months. Cervicofacial and thoracic involvement coexists rarely. When infection progresses to the pleural space and chest wall, the opening of a sinus tract may disclose pus. Radiographic features are variable and include small cavitary nodules confined to one segment; cavitary infiltration; extension of infection to the interlobar fissure, chest wall, bone, or pleura; and empyema.

Pasteurella Multocida

Pasteurella multocida is a gram-negative coccobacillus present in the oropharynx of mammals. It causes cutaneous infection in humans after animal bites. Pneumonia has been reported in patients with chronic pulmonary diseases. The clinical presentation is nonspecific and includes fever, cough, purulent sputum, and dyspnea. Chest radiographs show lower lobe infiltrates; pleural effusion and empyema may occur.

Francisella Tularensis

Francisella tularensis is a gram-negative bacillus found in various mammals and insects of the northern hemisphere. Tularemia occurs after the bite of, or contact with, an infected animal. The onset of pneumonia is abrupt; fever, chills, and malaise precede dyspnea, cough, and chest pain. Painful ulceroglandular infection with adenopathy may be found at the site of bacterial inoculation. The chest radiograph shows signs of pneumonia, possibly with hilar adenopathy or pleural effusion.

Yersinia Pestis

Yersinia pestis or *Pasteurella pestis* is a short gram-negative rod that causes plague. It is a disease of rodents (squirrels, rabbits, rats) that is transmitted to humans by flea bites or by person-to-person contact through aerosol inhalation. Initial symptoms are chills, fever, prostration, delirium, headache, vomiting, and diarrhea. There are three forms of plague: bubonic, septicemic, and pneumonic. Bubonic plague consists of lymphadenopathy, with palpable masses forming in the cervical, axillary, femoral, and inguinal areas. Signs of septicemia are those of shock and petechial hemorrhages. Plague pneumonia results from either metastatic infection or inhalation of the pathogen. Pneumonia occurs within a week of initial exposure and is characterized by chest pain, productive cough, dyspnea, and hemoptysis. The chest radiograph shows lower lobe infiltrates, possibly nodules, lymphadenopathy, and pleural effusions.

Bacillus Anthracis

Bacillus anthracis is a large gram-positive rod that causes anthrax. *B. anthracis* is found in the soil, water, and vegetation and infects cows, sheep, and horses, which in turn infect humans after contact with contaminated materials. Fever and malaise usually appear progressively. Three forms of anthrax are found: cutaneous, intestinal, and pneumonic. Inoculation of *B. anthracis* into superficial wounds or skin abrasions causes cutaneous anthrax, which is characterized by a black-crusted pustule on a large area of edema. Intestinal anthrax results from ingestion of contaminated material, and it can be severe. Pneumonic anthrax is due to inhalation of the contaminated material. Nonproductive cough and chest pain precede dyspnea, stridor, tachypnea, cyanosis, and edema of the neck and anterior chest. Peribronchovascular edema, enlargement of the mediastinum, and pleural effusions are usually seen on the chest radiograph.

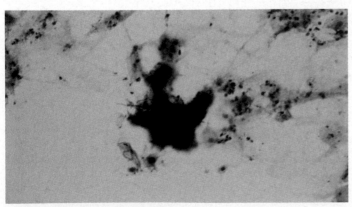

FIGURE 27-4 Sputum Gram stain showing actinomycetes (*center*).

Brucella Species

Brucella species are gram-negative coccobacilli found in the genitourinary tract of cows, pigs, goats, and dogs. Brucellosis results from contact with infected animals or from ingestion of unpasteurized milk products. The pathogen then spreads through the body by way of the bloodstream. General symptoms include fever, malaise, and headache. Hepatic enlargement and splenomegaly are common, as is lower back pain. Respiratory symptoms are less frequent than abnormalities on the chest radiograph, which include nodules, miliary infiltrates, and lymphadenopathy.

Moraxella Catarrhalis

Moraxella catarrhalis, formerly named *Branhamella catarrhalis*, is a gram-negative diplococcus that is commonly found in the oropharynx of normal subjects. *M. catarrhalis* pneumonia is seen in patients with underlying chronic diseases such as COPD, congestive heart disease, or malignancy. Symptoms and radiographic findings are nonspecific. Leukocytosis is common, and the course is usually favorable.

Diagnosis

History

The approach to the diagnosis of patients with CAP depends almost entirely on a careful history and physical examination that focus on the possibility that the infection may be the result of unusual pathogens (e.g., exposure to birds or parturient animals, recent foreign travel). The infection must also be considered in the context of the individual patient (e.g., recent influenza or varicella infection, oropharyngeal colonization with gram-negative rods in nursing home patients, occupations or hobbies involving animal exposures). Finally, the chest radiograph must be examined for findings that suggest other than common pathogens (e.g., abscess, effusion, adenopathy, cavitation). When the clinical presentation suggests an unusual pathogen, every attempt should be made to obtain a bacteriologic diagnosis. In the absence of this suspicion, the value of bacteriologic studies is unclear.

Bacteriology

There are various ways to obtain an etiologic diagnosis. Blood culture specimens (with more than two needle sticks performed at separate sites) should be obtained from patients who require hospital admission for acute pneumonia. If a pleural effusion is present, pleural fluid should be collected for examination and culture. The value of Gram staining of expectorated sputum is controversial, but it is recommended in consensus statements on inpatient care. A sputum specimen should be obtained by a deep cough before antibiotic therapy; it should then be rapidly transported and processed in the laboratory within a few hours of collection.

Routine laboratory tests should include Gram staining, cytologic screening, and aerobic culture of specimens that satisfy cytologic criteria. Cytologic criteria for judging the acceptability of specimens include the relative number of polymorphonuclear cells (PMN) and squamous epithelial cells (SEC) in patients with normal or elevated white blood cell counts, determined by a low-power field (LPF) examination; the acceptable values range from >25 PMN + <10 SEC/LPF–<25 SEC/LPF. Cultures should be performed rapidly. Interpretation of expectorated sputum cultures should include clinical correlations and semiquantitative results.

Numerous studies support the use of routine microscopic examination of Gram-stained sputum samples, with lancet-shaped, gram-positive diplococci suggestive of *S. pneumoniae*. Most show that the sensitivity of sputum Gram staining for patients with pneumococcal pneumonia is 50–60%, and the specificity is > 80%.

Routine cultures of expectorated sputum are neither sensitive nor specific when the common bacteriologic methods of many laboratories are used. The most likely explanation for unreliable microbiologic data is that the patient is unable to cough up a reliable specimen. Other reasons include prior administration of antibiotics, delays in processing the specimen, insufficient attention to separating sputum from saliva before smearing slides or culture plates, and difficulty with interpretation because of contamination by flora of the oral cavity and upper airways. In cases of bacteremic pneumococcal pneumonia, *S. pneumoniae* may be isolated in sputum culture in only 40–50% of cases when standard microbiologic techniques are used. The yield of *S. pneumoniae* is substantially higher from transtracheal aspirates, transthoracic needle aspirates, and quantitative cultures of BAL aspirates.

The usefulness of induced sputum specimens for detecting pulmonary pathogens other than *Pneumocystis jiroveci*, *L. pneumophila*, or *Mycobacterium tuberculosis* is poorly established.

Serologic tests are usually not helpful for the initial evaluation of patients with CAP but may provide useful data for epidemiologic surveillance. Management of patients on the basis of a single acute-phase titer is unreliable. Most laboratories request a follow-up (paired) serum sample 10–14 days later.

Cold agglutinins in a titer greater than 1:64 support the diagnosis of *M. pneumoniae* infection with a sensitivity of 30–60%, but this test has poor specificity. Immunoglobulin M antibodies to *M. pneumoniae* require up to 1 week to reach diagnostic titers; reported results for sensitivity are variable. The serologic responses to *Chlamydia* and *Legionella* species take even longer, and the acute antibody test for *Legionella* in Legionnaires' disease is usually negative or demonstrates a low titer only.

Antigen Tests

Urinary antigen tests are commercially available for detection of *S. pneumoniae* and *L. pneumophila* serogroup 1. The principal advantages of antigen tests are simplicity and rapidity (approximately 15 min). For pneumococcal pneumonia, urinary antigen testing studies in adults show a sensitivity of 50–80% and a specificity of more than 90%. False-positive results have been seen in children with chronic respiratory diseases who are colonized with *S. pneumoniae* and in patients with an episode of CAP within the previous 3 months. Urinary antigen testing seems to have a higher diagnostic yield in patients with more severe illness, but the ability to detect pneumococcal pneumonia after antibiotic therapy has been started.

For *Legionella*, several urinary antigen assays are available, but all detect only *L. pneumophila* serogroup 1. Although this serogroup accounts for most community-acquired cases of Legionnaires disease. Studies of culture-proven Legionnaires' disease indicate a sensitivity of 70–90% and a specificity of nearly 99% for detection of *L. pneumophila* serogroup1. The urine is positive for antigen on day 1 of illness and continues to be positive for weeks. The major issue with urinary bacterial antigen detection is whether the tests allow narrowing of empirical antibiotic therapy to a single specific agent.

Rapid antigen detection tests for influenza, which can also provide an etiologic diagnosis within 15–30 min, can lead to consideration of antiviral therapy. Test performance varies according to the test used, sample type, duration of illness, and patient age. Most show a sensitivity of 50–70% in adults and a specificity approaching 100%. Direct fluorescent antibody tests are available for influenza and RSV. For influenza virus, the sensitivity is better than with the point-of-care tests (85–95%). They will detect animal subtypes such as H5N1 and, thus, may be preferred for hospitalized patients. For RSV, direct fluorescent antibody tests have a very low sensitivity in adults (20–30%).

Recommendations for diagnostic testing remain controversial for the following reasons:

- Diagnostic testing is difficult to perform in the outpatient setting.
- Results are nonspecific and of questionable sensitivity.
- Antibiotic treatment, if needed, has to be started before the results are obtained, on the basis of the pathogens that are likely to be responsible for pneumonia in the community.

Therefore, diagnostic testing is not routinely performed for nonsevere CAP, but a specific clinical situation may justify more extensive diagnostic testing. These clinical situations are listed in Table 27-2.

In most studies, no microorganisms are found in up to 50% of outpatients investigated for CAP. Viruses are found in approximately 10%; *S. pneumoniae* in 25%; *H. influenzae* in 7%; *Mycoplasma*, *Legionella*, and *Chlamydia* species in 10%; and gram-negative bacteria and *S. aureus* in only 1%. In hospitalized patients with CAP, gram-negative bacteria and *S. aureus* strains are more frequent (Figure 27-5).

Specific Pathogens

Chest radiographs in patients with *H. influenzae* pneumonia often show a peribronchial distribution of infiltrates (e.g., bronchopneumonia) as opposed to the more peripheral lobar or segmental consolidations seen with *S. pneumoniae*. The sensitivity and specificity of this distinction are low, however.

In *M. pneumoniae* infections, the leukocyte count is usually normal, although mild to moderate leukocytosis can occur.

Cold agglutinins are frequently present. The diagnosis can be made by acute and convalescent blood serologic testing. Despite a favorable response to therapy, *M. pneumoniae* may persist in the oropharynx for 1–3 months, during which time it may be transmissible to others.

The diagnosis of *C. pneumoniae*, *C. psittaci*, and Q fever is on the basis of acute and convalescent blood serologies obtained 2–6 weeks apart.

Legionella pneumonia may be diagnosed within a few hours by direct immunofluorescence studies on respiratory tract specimens (e.g., sputum or tracheobronchial aspirates) or on urine for *Legionella pneumophila* serotype 1; respiratory tract specimens can be analyzed by a DNA probe and can be cultured. A fourfold increase in the antibody titers can be seen on two samples obtained within 2 months.

Bacteriologic diagnosis of anaerobic infections depends on the type of specimen and the quality of the anaerobic transport medium; various gram-negative and gram-positive agents are found, sometimes in conjunction with aerobic pathogens.

The pus in sinus tracts caused by *Actinomyces* contains sulfur granules made up of mineralized 2-mm yellow granules composed of *Actinomyces* or *Arachnia*. When examined by Gram stain, these appear as dense aggregates of the organism (Figure 27-6). Microbiologic diagnosis relies on the characterization of the pathogens in specimens from biopsy, exudate, or pus, by use of histopathologic evaluation and culture in anaerobic conditions.

Tularemia is diagnosed by serologic testing on paired serum specimens.

Microbiologic diagnosis of *Y. pestis* and *B. anthracis* is made on blood, sputum, or lymph node aspirate culture, by use of routine bacteriologic or fluorescent antibody staining techniques.

A titer of *Brucella* agglutinins equal to or greater than 1:160 indicates active brucellosis.

A diagnosis of *P. pseudomallei* is made when the organism is cultured from respiratory tract secretions, cutaneous lesions, or blood or when serologic tests are positive.

TREATMENT

Severity and Admission to Hospital

When a diagnosis of pneumonia is suspected, one of the important first steps is to evaluate severity and determine whether the patient needs hospital care (Figure 27-7).

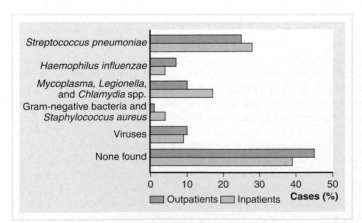

FIGURE 27-5 Community-acquired pneumonia. Cause in outpatients and in those requiring hospital admission.

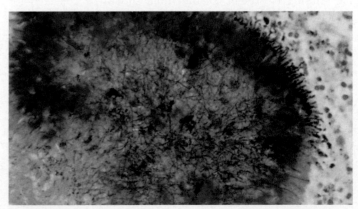

FIGURE 27-6 Sulfur granule seen in actinomycosis. Gram stain of sputum sample.

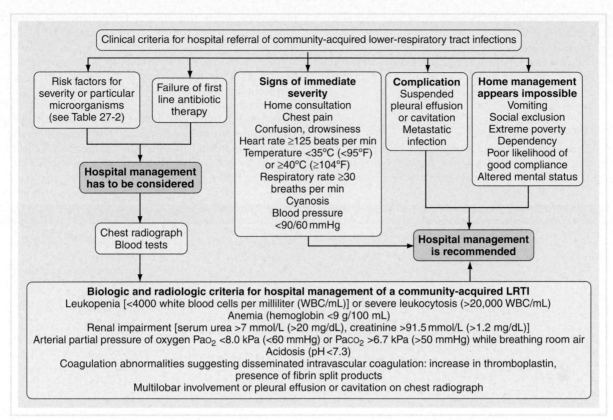

FIGURE 27-7 Criteria for admission to hospital. Biologic and radiologic investigations may be performed in patients referred to the hospital or in outpatients (depending, in part, on the local health care system and facilities), according to the criteria listed in Table 27-2. (Adapted from Huchon GJ, Woodhead MA, Gialdroni-Grassi G, et al: Guidelines for management of adult community-acquired lower respiratory tract infections. Eur Respir J 1998; 11:986–991.)

Severe CAP is defined as the presence of one of two major criteria, or the presence of two of three minor criteria. The major criteria are:

• Need for mechanical ventilation
• Septic shock

The minor criteria are:

• Systolic blood pressure 90 mmHg (12 kPa) or lower
• Multilobar disease
• PaO_2/FIO_2 ratio 250 or lower

Patients who have two of the four criteria from the 2001 British Thoracic Society (BTS) guidelines also have more severe illness and should be considered for admission to the intensive care unit. These criteria are:

• Respiratory rate 30 breaths/min or higher
• Diastolic blood pressure 60 mmHg (7.9 kPa) or lower
• Blood urea nitrogen 7.0 mM (19.1 mg/dL) or greater
• Confusion

Criteria for severe CAP suggested by the 2007 IDSA/ATS guidelines are shown in Box 27-1.

Empirical Antibiotic Therapy

The initial antibiotic choice for CAP is empirical for the following reasons:

• In at least half the cases, responsible organisms will not be isolated by use of even the most sophisticated methods.
• All the guidelines for the management of patients presenting with CAP suggest that antibiotic treatment should

be started as early as possible, without waiting for microbiologic results (if such investigations are performed). Delaying treatment increases the risk of complications and mortality, whereas correctly chosen empirical therapy improves outcome.

BOX 27-1 Criteria for Severe Community-Acquired Pneumonia (CAP)

Severe CAP is defined as the presence of one major criteria, or the presence of two minor criteria.

Minor criteria*

Respiratory rate = 30 breaths/min
Confusion/disorientation
Systolic blood pressure < 90 mmHg or diastolic blood pressure < 60 mmHg
PaO_2/FIO_2 ratio = 250
Multilobar infiltrates or bilateral involvement in chest radiograph
Uremia BUN level = 7 mmol/L (20 mg/dL) or serum creatinine ≥ 120 mmol/L (2 mg/dL)

Major criteria

Requirement for mechanical ventilation
Septic shock with the need for vasopressors

BUN, Blood urea nitrogen; PaO_2/FIO_2, arterial oxygen pressure/fraction of inspired oxygen; WBC, white blood cell.
Other criteria to consider include leukopenia (WBC count, <4000 cells/mm³), thrombocytopenia (platelet count, <100,000 cells/mm³), hypothermia = 36°C, hypoglycemia (in nondiabetic patients), acute alcoholism/alcoholic withdrawal, hyponatremia, unexplained metabolic acidosis or elevated lactate level, cirrhosis, and asplenia.

- Studies have shown that clinical data and radiologic findings, together with an assessment of comorbidity, risk factors for complications, and the severity of CAP, are sufficient for appropriate decisions regarding the choice of antibiotics and the necessity of hospital admission.

Antibiotic Selection

Table 27-4 summarizes antibiotic activity against bacteria that cause CAP. For patients with no risk factors who do not require hospitalization, an oral β-lactam antibiotic should be prescribed when the clinical presentation is consistent with *S. pneumoniae* or other bacteria associated with typical pneumonias. When the clinical presentation is consistent with an atypical pneumonia, a macrolide is recommended. Aminopenicillins have the advantage of being active against most extracellular bacteria, including *S. pneumoniae*, and against a few intracellular bacteria.

In patients with risk factors, an aminopenicillin associated with a β-lactamase inhibitor, or a second-generation cephalosporin, is indicated, possibly in conjunction with a macrolide or a fluoroquinolone (if there is a possibility of infection by intracellular agents). New quinolones are likely to be of

TABLE 27-4 Antibiotics Active Against Bacteria Responsible for Pneumonia

Bacteria	Antibiotics	Bacteria	Antibiotics
Acinetobacter spp.	Aminoglycosides and piperacillin Aminoglycosides and imipenem	*Moraxella catarrhalis*	Cephalosporins Aminopenicillin and penicillinase inhibitor Erythromycin Tetracyclines Quinolones Trimethoprim–sulfamethoxazole
Actinomyces spp.	Penicillins		
Anaerobes	Clindamycin Penicillin and metronidazole Cefoxitin Aminopenicillin and penicillinase inhibitor Impenem	*Mycoplasma pneumoniae*	Macrolides Tetracyclines Quinolones
		Neisseria meningitidis	Penicillin Cephalosporins (third generation) Chloramphenicol
Bacillus anthracis	Penicillins Chloramphenicol Erythromycin Tetracyclines	*Nocardia*	Trimethoprim-sulfamethoxazole Aminopenicillins Amikacin
Brucella	Streptomycin Trimethoprim–sulfamethoxazole	*Pasteurella multocida*	Penicillins Tetracyclines Chloramphenicol
Chlamydia burnetii	Tetracyclines Chloramphenicol	*Pseudomonas aeruginosa*	Aminoglycosides and piperacillin Aminoglycosides and ceftazidime Aminoglycosides and aztreonam Aminoglycosides and cefoperazone
Chlamydia pneumoniae	Tetracyclines Macrolides Quinolones		
Chlamydia psittaci	Tetracyclines Chloramphenicol	*Pseud. pseudomallei*	Tetracyclines Ceftazidime Sulfonamides Chloramphenicol Kanamycin
Chlamydia trachomatis	Macrolides Sulfisoxazole		
Coxiella burnetii	Tetracyclines Chloramphenicol	*Rhodococcus equi*	Vancomycin Erythromycin Chloramphenicol Rifampin (rifampicin)
Francisella tularensis	Aminoglycosides Tetracyclines Chloramphenicol		
Gram-negative enterobacteria, including *Klebsiella pneumoniae* and *Haemophilus influenzae*	Aminoglycosides and cephalosporins Aminoglycosides and aminopenicillins Cephalosporins (third generation) Clarithromycin Azithromycin Quinolones Aminopenicillin and penicillinase inhibitor Chloramphenicol Trimethoprim–sulfamethoxazole	*Staphylococcus aureus*	Oxacillin Cephalosporins (first generation) Methicillin Vancomycin and rifampin
		Streptococcus spp.	Penicillins Macrolides Cephalosporins (first generation) Vancomycin
		Streptococcus pneumoniae	Penicillins Macrolides Cephalosporins (first generation)
Legionella	Macrolides Trimethoprim–sulfamethoxazole Tetracyclines Quinolones	*Yersinia pestis*	Streptomycin

great benefit because they are active against *S. pneumoniae*, including penicillin-resistant strains and most intracellular and extracellular pathogens causing CAP.

Local resistance patterns of microorganisms to antibiotics obviously must be taken into account when choosing the appropriate medication, and studies document that patterns of resistance can vary markedly.

The incidence of drug-resistant *S. pneumoniae* (DRSP) seems to have stabilized somewhat in the past few years. Resistance to penicillin and cephalosporins may even be decreasing, whereas macrolide resistance continues to increase. However, the clinical relevance of DRSP for pneumonia is uncertain, and current levels of β-lactam resistance do not generally result in CAP treatment failures when appropriate agents (i.e., amoxicillin, ceftriaxone, or cefotaxime) and doses are used, even in the presence of bacteremia. Resistance to macrolides and older fluoroquinolones (ciprofloxacin and levofloxacin) results in clinical failure, but, to date, no failures have been reported for the newer fluoroquinolones (moxifloxacin and gemifloxacin).

Risk factors for infection with beta-lactam–resistant *S. Pneumoniae* include age <2 years or >65 years, β-lactam therapy within the previous 3 months, alcoholism, medical comorbidities, immunosuppressive illness or therapy, and exposure to a child in a daycare center. Although the relative predictive value of these risk factors is unclear, recent treatment with antimicrobials is likely the most significant. Recent therapy or repeated courses of therapy with β-lactams, macrolides, or fluoroquinolones are risk factors for pneumococcal resistance to the same class of antibiotic.

The recommended strategy for choosing first-line antibiotics is summarized in Table 27-5.

The recommended duration of antibiotic treatment for CAP is 1 week when the infection is due to extracellular organisms and 2 weeks when it is thought to be due to intracellular infection. Because they have a prolonged effect, macrolides such as azithromycin could be used for a shorter period; however, there is currently no definitive answer about the possible risk associated with shortening the duration of treatment.

Severe Bacterial Pneumonia

Bacterial pneumonia is also considered to be severe when it is accompanied by extension outside the lung parenchyma, when lung necrosis or septicemia develops, or when it occurs in patients with comorbid diseases. In these instances, it is much more important to establish a specific bacteriologic diagnosis. Antibiotic should initially be administered intravenously, and the choice of medication should include a consideration of the drug's diffusion into lung parenchyma, iatrogenic risks, and contraindications related to hepatic or renal function. Because *L. pneumophila* pneumonias may be severe and are frequently associated with diarrhea, they need to be treated with intravenous regimens that provide good intracellular penetration (e.g., erythromycin 3–4 g/24 h, pefloxacin 800 mg/24 h, and rifampicin 1200 mg/24 h).

Patients with *Actinomyces* infections should be treated for prolonged periods (up to 6 months). The choice of antibiotics to treat *Nocardia* should be based on *in vitro* susceptibility testing. Duration of treatment (usually not less than 6 weeks) and drainage of purulent collections are critical factors affecting outcome.

Mendelson's Syndrome (Aspiration of Gastric Contents)

The lower airways are suctioned as soon as possible after aspiration has occurred. When solid material is aspirated, fiberoptic bronchoscopy is useful in an attempt to remove as much of the material as possible by direct suctioning. The rigid bronchoscope may be more effective. Tracheobronchial lavage with buffering solutions has little effect on the course of the disease, because aspirated acids are rapidly neutralized by the outpouring of plasma that occurs in response to the chemical injury. Intravascular volume support may be needed. Fever, purulent secretions, leukocytosis, and new pulmonary infiltrates may develop in the absence of infection. Accordingly, prophylactic antibiotics are not generally used; they do not seem to modify the course of the disease and may predispose to resistant bacteria. The decision when to begin antibiotics is based on clinical suspicion that a secondary bacterial infection has developed. Trials of corticosteroids have been disappointing.

Aspiration Pneumonia

Antibiotics are selected for their activity against anaerobic bacteria. Choices include amoxicillin plus clavulanate (because up to 40% of anaerobic bacteria produce beta-lactamase), penicillin or amoxicillin plus metronidazole, or clindamycin. The increased risk of *Clostridium difficile* infection with clindamycin has led some investigators to suggest that it be given only to patients who have evidence of necrotizing pneumonia; in this group, the benefit of clindamycin over other treatments has been demonstrated.

When the areas of necrosis progress to involve the entire lobe, pulmonary gangrene must be considered. This condition is thought to result from thrombosis of the lobar pulmonary artery, such that the major blood supply to the lobe is lost. Older literature suggests that pulmonary gangrene should be treated with lobar resection or open drainage, because conservative treatment has been associated with increased mortality. There are, however, no studies to validate a surgical approach, which should probably only be recommended if sepsis and necrosis persists despite antibiotic therapy.

CLINICAL COURSE AND PREVENTION

The course of CAP is favorable in most cases. Fever declines over a few days, and the abnormalities seen on the chest radiograph generally begin to resolve in 1–3 weeks.

Nonresponding pneumonia to the initial antibiotic therapy, although difficult to define, may concern approximately 10% of hospitalized patients with CAP. Mortality among nonresponding patients is greatly increased. Nonresponding pneumonia may include failure to improve or deterioration or progression. Progressive pneumonia or rapid clinical deterioration, within the first 72 h of hospital admission, should lead to transfer of the patient to a higher level of care such as ICU in case of acute respiratory failure and/or septic shock. Persistence of fever should prompt concern about the presence of a resistant organism, a complication such as cavitation or empyema, the development of a nosocomial pneumonia caused by a resistant organism, or drug-related fever. An additional concern is that poor resolution may be caused by the presence of a coexistent problem such as lung cancer, bronchial foreign body, bronchiectasis, or chronic infection of the upper respiratory tract. Further diagnostic

TABLE 27-5 Recommended Empirical Antibiotics for Lower Respiratory Tract Infection (LRTI) and Community Acquired Pneumonia (CAP)

Setting	LRTI Type	Severity/Sub-Group	Preferred	Alternative*
Community	LRTI	All	Amoxicillin or tetracycline[†]	Co-amoxiclav Macrolide[‡] Levofloxacin Moxifloxacin
Hospital	COPD	Mild	Amoxicillin or tetracycline[†]	Co-amoxiclav Macrolide[‡] Levofloxacin Moxifloxacin
	COPD	Moderate/Severe	Co-amoxiclav	Levofloxacin Moxifloxacin
	COPD	+ risk factors for *P. aeruginosa*	Ciprofloxacin	
	CAP	Non-severe	Penicillin g ± macrolide[‡] • Aminopenicillin ± macrolide[‡] • Co-amoxiclav ± macrolide[‡] 2nd OR 3rd Cephalosporin ± macrolide[‡]	Levofloxacin Moxifloxacin
	CAP	Severe	3rd Cephalosporin + macrolide[‡]	3rd Cephalosporin + (levofloxacin or moxifloxacin)
	CAP	Severe + risk factors for *P. aeruginosa*	Anti-pseudomonal Cephalosporin + ciprofloxacin	Acylureidopenicillin/ β-lactamase inhibitor + ciprofloxacin or carbapenem + ciprofloxacin
	BRONCHIECT ASIS	No risk factors for *P. aeruginosa*	Amoxicillin clavulanate Moxifloxacin Levofloxacin	
	BRONCHIECT ASIS	Risk factors for *P. aeruginosa*	Ciprofloxacin	

(Adapted from Woodhead M, Blasi F, Ewig S, et al. ERS task force in collaboration with ESCMID. Guidelines for management of adult community-acquired lower respiratory tract infections. Eur Respir J 26:1138–1180, 2005).
Choice of a first-line strategy should depend on the local resistance of microorganisms, the patient's allergies, and the costs and side-effect profiles of antibiotics.
*Alternative choice of first-line strategy should depend on the local resistance of microorganisms, the patient's allergies, and side-effect profiles of antibiotics.
[†]High level of resistant pathogen in some areas (refer to local current epidemiological data).
[‡]High risk of resistant *Streptococcus pneumoniae* in some areas (refer to local current epidemiological data).

investigations, including extensive invasive and noninvasive microbiologic sampling and imaging procedures, are needed. Escalation or change in initial antibiotic treatment should also be considered. Etiologies of failure to respond are listed in Box 27-2.

Regarding gastric content aspiration, all the patients reported by Mendelson recovered rapidly, whereas subsequent studies demonstrated mortality rates as high as 60%. The discrepancy is probably because Mendelson's patients were healthy young women, whereas later reports included patients who were older and had numerous comorbid illnesses. There are three patterns of response to gastric aspiration:

1. Rapid recovery (62%).
2. Rapid deterioration into acute respiratory distress syndrome (ARDS), with death within 24 h (12%).
3. Initial recovery with subsequent development of fever and new infiltrates (26%), which suggests pulmonary superinfection, which may progress to ARDS.

When bacterial infection is demonstrated, the mortality increases by a factor of three.

BOX 27-2 Etiologies of Nonresponding Pneumonia

Resistant microorganism (uncovered or nonsensitive pathogen)
Parapneumonic effusion/empyema
Metastatic infection (pericarditis, endocarditis, meningitis, arthritis)
Nosocomial superinfection (nosocomial pneumonia or extrapulmonary nosocomial infection)
Noninfectious complication of pneumonia (ARDS, BOOP)
Inacurate diagnosis (PE, lung cancer, atelectasis, CHF, vasculitis)
Drug fever
Exacerbation of comorbid illness
Intercurrent noninfectious disease (PE, myocardial infarction, renal failure)
Abnormal host response (immunocompromized)

ARDS, Acute respiratory distress syndrome; *BOOP,* bronchiolitis obliterans organizing pneumonia; *CHF,* congestive heart failure; *PE,* pulmonary embolus.

COMPLICATIONS

Most cases of pneumonia resolve completely with appropriate antibiotic treatment and supportive care. However, a number of important complications may occur that require specific management. These include:

- Parapneumonic effusion
- Empyema
- Bronchopleural fistula
- Organizing pneumonia
- Bronchiectasis

Frequently, the diagnosis of these complications is delayed. Acute infective complications commonly present with a continuing pyrexia despite appropriate antibiotic therapy, but they may be more insidious, with or without a fever but with general ill health and continuing debility. The critical initial investigation is the chest radiograph. If an empyema or lung abscess is discovered, further imaging with CT or ultrasonography is often necessary.

Parapneumonic Effusion and Empyema

The symptoms suggestive of a parapneumonic collection are increased breathlessness, swinging pyrexia, and raised inflammatory markers. The chest radiograph usually demonstrates the collection of fluid. A lateral chest radiograph or ultrasonography is useful to confirm the presence of fluid.

All pleural fluid should undergo Gram stain and culture, because the identification of significant bacterial cultures confirms the diagnosis of infection and aids in antibiotic choice. Unfortunately, approximately 40% of infected pleural effusions are culture negative, and in this situation, biochemical pleural fluid markers (pH, lactate dehydrogenase [LDH], white cell count [WCC], and glucose) are central to establishing a diagnosis. Fluid drainage by means of a chest tube and prolonged antibiotic therapy is necessary in all cases of complicated parapneumonic pleural effusion and empyema.

Bronchopleural Fistula

A bronchopleural fistula is caused by a connection between the pleural space and the consolidated lung; it can complicate either an empyema or a lung abscess. The bronchopleural fistula causes a pyopneumothorax (i.e., air–fluid level in the pleural space), so that, on drainage of an empyema, not only pus but also air comes out through the chest drain. A bronchopleural fistula will not seal unless infection is controlled. Initial treatment is conservative, with antibiotics and tube drainage, to allow the fistula to seal. If this fails, surgery may be necessary to attempt primary closure of the fistula or closure of the potential space with other living tissues, such as muscle flaps. The management of bronchopleural fistulas that do not close with conservative treatment requires the surgical skills of a thoracic specialist.

Organizing Pneumonia

Organizing pneumonia, sometimes known as cryptogenic organizing pneumonia or bronchiolitis obliterans organizing pneumonia (BOOP), is a condition in which an organizing inflammatory exudate with fibroblast proliferation occurs after an episode of pneumonia. The consolidation is often patchy and may be fleeting. Organizing pneumonia after a bacterial infection is suggested when a residual consolidation (often fleeting) remains despite adequate antibiotic treatment.

Investigation includes examination of sputum or bronchial washings to exclude infection. CT may help to visualize the consolidation and exclude other causes. The definitive investigation is an open lung biopsy showing the typical histologic appearance. If suspicion is great enough and the physician is confident of the diagnosis, a course of steroids usually leads to resolution. When the steroids are stopped, however, there may be a relapse; in this case, treatment for several months may be necessary. (See Chapter 53.)

Bronchiectasis

Permanent dilatation of the bronchus can occur after severe pneumonia, causing localized bronchiectasis. CT scanning during or after an episode of acute pneumonia may show bronchial dilatation, so the diagnosis cannot be made with confidence until after the pneumonia has completely resolved. The presence of bronchiectasis is suggested by continual cough productive of sputum or recurrent infections in one part of the lung. Investigation consists of sputum examination, when organisms associated with bronchiectasis such as *H. influenzae* or *P. aeruginosa* may be isolated. The diagnostic test of choice is a thin-section, high-resolution CT scan. Management consists of postural drainage of the infected lobe and antibiotic treatment for any acute infection. In patients who have coexisting airflow obstruction, treatment with bronchodilators or inhaled steroids may be helpful.

RECURRENT PNEUMONIA

After clinical and radiologic improvement, a recurrent CAP episode is possible although not very frequent. The recurrence risk is higher in elderly patients, in smokers, and in those with chronic pulmonary diseases. Other underlying diseases may also be responsible for CAP recurrence. Local or general host defense impairment should be considered. Impairment of local host defense may be due to bronchial obstruction by foreign body, bronchial cancer, or localized or diffuse bronchiectasis. General causes of immune impairment include denutrition, intravenous drug abuse (Figure 27-8), alcoholism, cirrhosis, chronic renal failure and/or nephrotic syndrome, chronic heart failure, chronic humoral deficiency such as immunoglobulin quantitative or qualitative abnormalities, asplenia, sickle-cell disease, neutrophils, quantitative or qualitative abnormalities, underlying cancer or hematologic malignancy, HIV infections, and other T-cell deficiencies.

When possible, specific treatment of underlying disease may help to prevent recurrent bacterial pneumonia (e.g., immunoglobulin substitutive treatment in severe congenital immunoglobulin deficiency). In all cases, elimination of risk factors such as smoking and alcoholism and the use of vaccinations should be considered.

PREVENTION

There are various ways to prevent bacterial pneumonia, including the elimination of risk factors such as smoking and alcoholism and the use of vaccinations. Influenza vaccine is used in subjects older than 65 years, in those with chronic diseases, and in medical practitioners and nursing home employees. Pneumococcal vaccine is recommended in subjects older than 65 years and in younger patients with cardiovascular or pulmonary diseases, diabetes mellitus, alcoholism, cirrhosis,

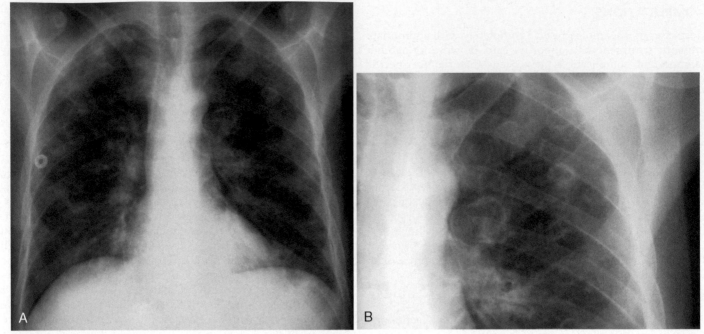

FIGURE 27-8 A, *Staphylococci aureus* pneumonia in an intravenous drug user, Chest radiograph showing multiple bilateral pulmonary abscesses related to hematogenous staphylococci spread. **B,** Pulmonary staphylococci related abscess (*detail*).

cerebrospinal fluid leak, and immunodepression (e.g., caused by HIV infection, chronic renal failure, organ transplantation, hematologic and lymphatic malignancies, asplenia, sickle-cell disease).

Steps for the prevention of aspiration pneumonia are summarized in Box 27-3 and should be applied in patients who have predisposing conditions. A number of surgical techniques have been advocated for patients who have anatomic abnormalities of the larynx or hypopharynx, including tracheostomy, cricopharyngeal myotomy, laryngeal suspension, cricoid resection, and vocal cord medialization. Aspiration of tube-fed patients can be detected by adding a food dye to the feeding formula and seeking evidence of its presence in tracheobronchial secretions or by measuring the glucose content of the secretions. Neither of these approaches seems to be cost-effective, however. Measuring the volume of residual gastric contents may help identify patients at risk (residual >100–200 mL).

PITFALLS AND CONTROVERSIES

Epidemiology

Antimicrobial resistance in community respiratory pathogens varies among countries and during time. Some countries have reported recent improvement in antimicrobial resistant; for example, a decrease in penicillin-resistant *S. pneumoniae* strains has been noted, but resistance to macrolide is still growing and several cases of levofloxacin-resistant *S. pneumoniae* have been reported. The clinical impact of antimicrobial resistance in CAP is debated. No clear increase in CAP-related mortality is reported with penicillin-resistant strains, but this is not the case with other drug-resistant *S. pneumoniae* (macrolides or levofloxacin-resistant *S. pneumoniae*).

Diagnosis

Recommendations for microbiologic diagnostic testing remain controversial, and there is no evidence that patients with CAP may have a better outcome when a microbiologic diagnosis is made. Fiberoptic bronchoscopy as a tool for microbiologic lung sampling of patients with severe CAP is a potentially invasive procedure and requires further assessment. Clinical value of commercially available new real-time PCR diagnostic tests are still under evaluation but could be useful in cases of atypical pathogens or viruses. New biomarkers of bacterial infection such as procalcitonin are probably useful to distinguish bacterial and nonbacterial LRTI and to limit antibiotic use but need further investigations.

BOX 27-3 Prevention of Aspiration Pneumonias

Position (elevation of the head of the bed)
Prefer jejunostomy to nasogastric tube for enteral feeding
Monitoring gastric residue
H_2 blockers, gastric acid pump inhibitors (avoid antacids, which may increase gastric fluid volume and cause pulmonary injury if aspirated)
Prokinetic agents? (no conclusive data)
Digestive decontamination in mechanically ventilated patients
Frequent upper airway suctioning in patients who have endotracheal tubes or tracheostomies
Gastric aspiration and awake endotracheal intubation for emergency general anesthetic?

(Data from Pachon J, Prados MD, Capote F, et al: Severe community-acquired pneumonia: aetiology, prognosis and treatment. Rev Respir Dis 142:369–373, 1990; Fine MJ, Smith DN, Singer DE: Hospitalization in patients with community-acquired pneumonia: a prospective cohort study. Am J Med 89:713–721, 1990.)

Assessment of Severity

Although assessment of severity is of crucial importance for the management of patients with CAP, there is no clear superiority of one score to another. Therefore, simple scores such as BTS CURB score are probably easier to use and efficient to decide where to treat the patient and to choose the initial empirical antibiotic therapy. CURB is a severity score for assessment of confusion, urea > 7 mmol/L, respiratory rate > 30 breaths per minute, systolic BP > 90 mmHg, or diastolic < 60 mmHg.

Antibiotic Treatment

Initial antibiotic therapy with coverage of atypical pathogens for inpatients with CAP could be associated with better outcome, but conflicting results have been reported. Pathogen-directed therapy could be a way to decrease antibiotic use and improve outcome but has not been demonstrated as more effective than empirical therapy. The use of most recent antibiotic therapy is probably not associated with a better outcome, because most clinical trials for antibiotic therapy of lower respiratory infections are designed to establish

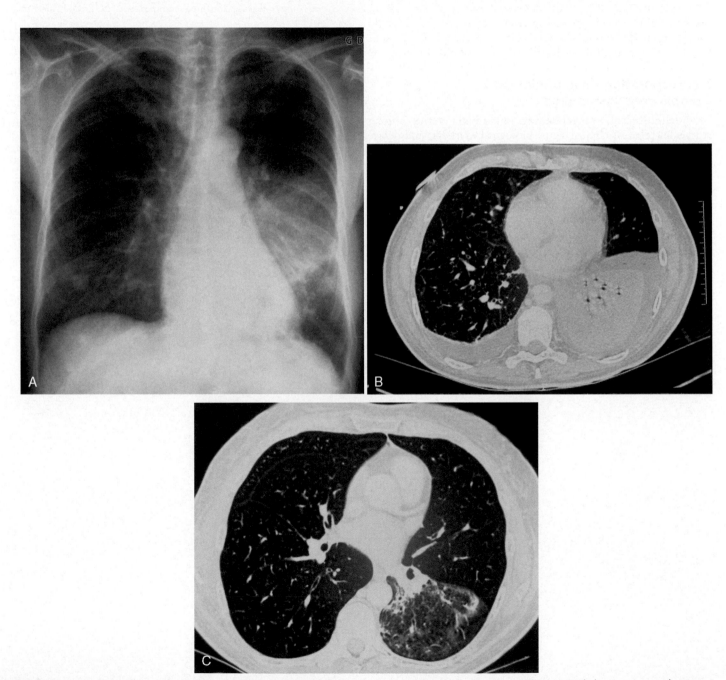

FIGURE 27-9 A, Legionellosis, initial chest radiograph showing left lower lobe consolidation. **B**, Legionellosis, initial chest computed tomography demonstrates left lower lobe alveolar infiltrate and pleural effusion. **C**, Legionellosis, chest computed tomography performed 6 weeks later (and after a 3-week course of macrolide) demonstrates partial resolution of left lower lobe alveolar infiltrate and disappearance of parapneumonic pleural effusion.

equivalency of newer agents rather than establish superiority of single or combined classes of agents. Duration of antibiotic treatment is largely empirical. Several studies even in severe CAP have reported no difference in outcome with shorter duration of treatment. Early oral switch for antibiotic treatment is recommended when clinical stability is achieved and the oral route available, but a clear definition of clinical stability is still necessary.

Adjuvant Therapy for Severe CAP

Because of their antiinflammatory properties, intravenous corticosteroid use has been suggested for patients with severe CAP admitted in ICU. The beneficial effect of steroids in severe CAP is largely debated. In case of severe sepsis or septic shock, patients should benefit from activated C protein therapy and or small doses of substitutive steroid therapy.

Nonresponding Pneumonia and Complicated Pneumonia

The definition of nonresponding pneumonia varies among studies in term of clinical signs, biological markers, and delay. Investigations for nonresponding CAP are not standardized. If chest X-rays and microbiologic investigations are recommended in non-responding or complicated CAP, many other diagnostic procedures are possible including chest CT scan (Figure 27-9), cardiac and thoracic echography, and flexible bronchoscopy. The respective indications and the clinical impact of these investigations are not well known. However, bronchoscopy is valuable for identifying an endobronchial tumor in a lobile pneumonia either not clearing or recurring. CT is also of value for identifying endobronchial disease, parapneumonic effusions that may be empyemas, and underlying bronchiectasis as a cause for poor response to treatment.

Outcome

Although several prospective and retrospective cohort studies showed a positive association between guideline adherence for initial antibiotic selection and short-term mortality, the best way to implement guidelines and improve adherence to these guidelines is unknown.

SUGGESTED READINGS

Bartlett JG: Diagnostic test for etiologic agents of community-acquired pneumonia. Infect Dis Clin North Am 2004; 18:809–827.

British Thoracic Society: Guidelines for the management of community acquired pneumonia in adults. Thorax 2001; 56(S4):1–64.

Fridkin SK, Hageman JC, Morrison M, et al: Methicillin-resistant *Staphylococcus aureus* disease in three communities. N Engl J Med 2005; 352:1436–1444.

Garau J, Gomez L: *Pseudomonas aeruginosa* pneumonia. Curr Opin Infect Dis 2003; 16:35–143.

Johnson JL, Hirsch CS: Aspiration pneumonia. Recognizing and managing a potentially growing disorder. Postgrad Med 2003; 113:99–102, 105–106, 111–112.

Mandell LA, Wunderink RG, Anzueto A, et al: Infectious Diseases Society of America/American Thoracic Society Consensus Guidelines on the management of community-acquired pneumonia in adults. Clin Infect Dis 2007; 44:S27–S72.

Moss PJ, Finch RG: The next generation: fluoroquinolones in the management of acute lower respiratory infection in adults. Thorax 2000; 55:83–85.

Murdoch DR: Diagnosis of *Legionella* infection. Clin Infect Dis 2003; 36:64–69.

Niederman MS, Ahmed OD: Community-acquired pneumonia in elderly patients. Clin Geriatr Med 2003; 19:101–120.

Niederman MS, Mandell LA, Anzueto A, et al: Guidelines for the management of adults with community-acquired pneumonia: diagnosis, assessment of severity, antimicrobial therapy, and prevention. Am J Respir Crit Care Med ; 163:1730–1754.

Woodhead M, Blasi F, Ewig S, et al: ERS task force in collaboration with ESCMID. Guidelines for management of adult community-acquired lower respiratory tract infections. Eur Respir J 2005; 26:1138–1180.

28 Nonbacterial Pneumonia

ANTOINE RABBAT • GÉRARD J. HUCHON

VIRAL PNEUMONIA

Although viral infections of the upper respiratory tract are common, viral pneumonia is rare in patients who are not immunocompromised, except for children and the elderly. Four major groups of viruses account for most viral pneumonias in immunocompetent children (Table 28-1).

Pneumonia accounts for 20–40% of viral lower respiratory tract infections in children. In adults, influenza is the most frequent cause of viral pneumonia, although respiratory syncytial virus (RSV) is also seen, and pneumonia may occur as part of systemic viral infections such as measles, chickenpox, and the hantaviruses. For each agent, epidemiology, risk factors, clinical features, diagnosis, treatment, clinical course, and prevention are considered.

Influenza Virus

Three types of influenza virus have been identified: A, B, and C. Type A is responsible for the most severe and widespread disease, and type C does not seem to be pathogenic. Major antigens of the virus envelope are hemagglutinin and neuraminidase (sialidase). In influenza A viruses, the former undergoes periodic changes, which may be major (resulting in antigenic shifts because of reassortments between strains, leading to an entirely new gene) or minor (resulting in antigenic drifts because of point mutations). Most of the host immune response is directed against hemagglutinin.

Influenza A and B viruses are responsible for at least 50% of the viral pneumonias encountered in immunocompetent adult subjects. Antigenic shifts are associated with pandemics when antigenic modifications lead to a decrease in the immunity of the community, whereas antigenic drifts are commonly associated with more limited epidemics. Outbreaks of severe disease occur every 10–30 years. During an outbreak, children are usually infected before adults (attack rates may reach 50–75%). The excess mortality caused by influenza may be as high as 10,000 patients per year, and the economic consequences of outbreaks are considerable.

The host immune response involves both cellular and humoral defenses, as well as local antibody responses caused by secretory immunoglobulin A (IgA). The result is mucosal inflammation that consists of hyperemia, edema, and, in severe cases, hemorrhage. Transmission is by respiratory secretions.

Pneumonia may occur directly after the acute illness (termed *primary pneumonia*, which is caused by the virus itself), or it may occur after a period of clinical improvement (*secondary pneumonia*, which results from bacterial superinfection, most commonly with *Streptococcus pneumoniae*, *Haemophilus influenzae*, or *Staphylococcus aureus*). Primary pneumonia seems to occur more commonly in association with conditions that result in increased left atrial pressure, whereas secondary pneumonia occurs mainly in older adults or in patients who have comorbid conditions, such as chronic cardiovascular or respiratory disease, diabetes mellitus, or chronic hepatic or renal failure.

A typical presentation includes the acute onset of cough, sore throat, conjunctival hyperemia, nasal discharge and congestion, fever, myalgia, headache, and malaise. Symptoms and findings of pneumonia are infrequent, and the disease is usually self-limited. Reappearance or worsening of respiratory symptoms and signs suggests pneumonia, but radiographic evidence of pneumonia may be found in the absence of such findings.

The typical radiographic findings of primary pneumonia are diffuse, interstitial, or patchy infiltrates. Secondary pneumonia may have a more segmental or lobar pattern. Primary and secondary pneumonia may occur in the same patient at the same time.

Indirect diagnosis is used primarily for epidemiologic purposes, because it requires two serologic assays performed 10–14 days apart. Direct diagnosis can be made by:

- Culture of respiratory secretions or lung tissue, a process that takes 2–5 days (less if antigen detection techniques are used).
- Immunofluorescence or enzyme-linked immunosorbent assay (ELISA) techniques on nasal or pharyngeal cells obtained by brushing or washing, a process that takes approximately 15 min.
- Antigen detection in respiratory secretions, a less sensitive but more rapid technique.

In addition to supportive care, treatment with specific antiviral therapy such as amantadine (100 mg/kg per day for 5 days) or rimantadine may be beneficial if administered early in the course of the disease (within 48 h of symptom onset). Zanamivir and oseltamivir are related antiviral drugs with a similar mechanism of action and a similar rate of effectiveness against both influenza A and B viruses, whereas the M2 inhibitors, amantadine, and rimantadine are active only against influenza A. Both are neuraminidase inhibitors; zanamivir is inhaled, and oseltamivir is given orally. Both drugs are approved for the treatment of influenza only in persons who have been symptomatic for less than 2 days. Clinical studies showed that the symptoms of influenza disappeared 1–1.5 days sooner in the drug-treated groups than in the placebo groups. Antibiotics active against *S. pneumoniae*, *H. influenzae*, and *S. aureus* are needed to treat patients who have secondary pneumonia.

The morbidity and mortality of influenza pneumonia are high, and patients can deteriorate to the point of acute respiratory distress syndrome (ARDS) developing. In such cases, the likelihood of a secondary pneumonia developing is high.

TABLE 28-1 Respiratory Viruses That Cause Pneumonias in Nonimmunocompromised Hosts

	Influenza	Parainfluenza	Respiratory Syncytial Virus	Adenovirus
Family	Orthomyxoviridae	Paramyxoviridae	Paramyxoviridae	Adenoviridae
Genome	Single-stranded RNA	Single-stranded RNA	Single-stranded RNA	Double-stranded DNA
Envelope antigens	Hemagglutinin Sialidase	Hemagglutinin Sialidase Fusion Glycoprotein	Fusion glycoprotein Glycoprotein	250 capsomeres
Serotypes	Three (pathogenic in humans: A and B)	Four (pathogenic in humans: 1, 2, and 3)	Two (A and B)	50
Infected cells	Epithelial cells	Epithelial cells	Epithelial cells	Epithelial cells Lymphoid cells
Frequency among lower respiratory tract infections	Type A: 1–13% Type B: 1–9%	4–41%	6–63%	2–35%

Inactivated influenza vaccines are modified each year to follow the antigenic modifications of influenza A strains. They provide 50–80% protection against influenza-related illnesses and 30–65% protection against influenza-related hospital admissions and deaths in the elderly. Accordingly, vaccination is recommended for all patients older than 65 years, all patients who have chronic comorbid conditions (regardless of age), patients who reside in chronic care facilities, and health care workers (because of their increased risk of contacting patients who have influenza and spreading it to other noninfected patients). Preventive administration of amantadine or rimantadine for 2 weeks after vaccination has been recommended in very high-risk patients to provide protection during the period required to develop an effective immunologic response.

Pandemic Influenza

Recent human infections caused by avian influenza A (H5N1) in Vietnam, Thailand, Cambodia, China, Indonesia, Egypt, and Turkey raise the possibility of a pandemic in the near future. The severity of H5N1 infection in humans distinguishes it from that caused by routine seasonal influenza. Respiratory failure requiring hospitalization and intensive care has been seen in most of the 1140 recognized cases, and mortality is as high as 50%.

Early clinical features of H5N1 infection include persistent fever, cough, and respiratory difficulty progressing over 3–5 days, as well as lymphopenia on admission to the hospital. Exposure to sick and dying poultry in an area with known or suspected H5N1 activity has been reported by most patients, although the recognition of poultry outbreaks has sometimes followed the recognition of human cases. In patients with suspected H5N1 infection, droplet precautions and careful routine infection control measures should be used until an H5N1 infection is ruled out.

Patients with an illness compatible with influenza and with known exposure to poultry in areas with previous H5N1 infection should be tested for H5N1 infection. Direct fluorescent antibody tests are available for influenza and require approximately 2 h. They will detect animal subtypes such as H5N1. Rapid bedside tests to detect influenza A have been used as screening tools for avian influenza in some settings. Throat swabs tested by reverse transcriptase–polymerase chain reaction (RT-PCR) have been the most sensitive for confirming H5N1 infection to date, but nasopharyngeal swabs, washes, and aspirates; bronchoalveolar lavage (BAL) fluid; lung and other tissues; and stool have yielded positive results by RT-PCR and viral culture with varying sensitivity. Convalescent-phase serum can be tested by microneutralization for antibodies to H5 antigen in a small number of international reference laboratories. Specimens from suspected cases of H5N1 infection should be sent to public health laboratories with appropriate biocontainment facilities; the case should be discussed with health department officials to arrange the transfer of specimens and to initiate an epidemiologic evaluation. Recommendations for such testing will evolve on the basis of the features of the pandemic, and guidance should be sought from the Centers for Disease Control and Prevention (CDC) and World Health Organization (WHO) Web sites (http://www.cdc.gov and http://www.who.int).

Patients with confirmed or suspected H5N1 influenza should be treated with oseltamivir. Most H5N1 isolates since 2004 have been susceptible to the neuraminidase inhibitors oseltamivir and zanamivir and resistant to the adamantines (amantadine and rimantadine). Patients with suspected H5N1 infection should be treated with oseltamivir and antibacterial agents targeting *S. pneumoniae* and *S. aureus*, the most common causes of secondary bacterial pneumonia in patients with influenza. The current recommendation is for a 5-day course of treatment at the standard dosage of 75 mg two times daily. Treatment recommendations may vary considerably with changes in the pandemic situation. More specific guidance can be found on the Infectious Disease Society of America (IDSA), American Thoracic Society (ATS), CDC, and WHO Web sites. In addition, droplet precautions should be used for patients with suspected H5N1 influenza, and they should be placed in respiratory isolation until that etiology is ruled out. Health care personnel should wear N-95 (or higher) respirators during medical procedures that have a high likelihood of generating infectious respiratory aerosols.

Parainfluenza Virus

Four serotypes have been identified, with types 1, 2, and 3 being responsible for most infections in humans. Parainfluenza viruses are responsible for up to 20% of the respiratory infections that occur in children but are found infrequently in immunocompetent adults. The epidemiologic and clinical characteristics depend on the serotype and are summarized in Table 28-2.

As with influenza, parainfluenza viruses are transmitted between humans by respiratory secretions. The incubation period

TABLE 28-2 Epidemiologic and Clinical Characteristics of Parainfluenza Infection Depending on the Serotype

	Serotypes	
	1 and 2	3
Epidemiology	Epidemics during the fall	Endemic with increases during fall, winter, or spring
Clinical features	Croup (laryngotracheobronchitis); less severe with type 2	Bronchiolitis Pneumonia

BOX 28-1 Preventive Measures Against Nosocomial Respiratory Syncytial Virus Infections

Isolation or cohorting of hospital-admitted infected infants in specific areas
Surface decontamination of objects and furniture
Isolation measures
 Handwashing
 Use of gowns, gloves, and eye–nose goggles

lasts 2–6 days, and humoral, local, and cellular immunities generate neutralizing circulating antibodies, local secretory IgA, and cytotoxic and helper T lymphocytes, respectively.

In adults, the disease may be completely asymptomatic or may present as a common upper respiratory tract infection with rhinitis and pharyngitis. Fever is unusual, as is the progression to pneumonia. When pneumonia does occur, the symptoms and signs are nonspecific, and the chest radiograph shows diffuse, interstitial infiltrates consistent with any type of atypical or viral pneumonia.

Although treatment with ribavirin (tribavirin) has some *in vitro* activity, it is only supportive. Corticosteroids have been reported anecdotally to accelerate recovery in patients who have severe involvement. No vaccine is yet available.

Respiratory Syncytial Virus

The leading cause of respiratory tract infection in young children, respiratory syncytial virus (RSV) is responsible for 25% of hospital admissions for pneumonia and 75% of bronchiolitis in children younger than 6 months old. The incubation period lasts 4–6 days; epidemics occur in the late fall and spring and usually last 1–5 months. Almost all children older than 5 years have anti-RSV antibodies.

Transmittal of RSV is by contaminated skin followed by autoinoculation in the conjunctiva or nose or by aerosols produced by coughing or sneezing.

Immunity involves mainly local and serum antibodies, but cell-mediated immunity also develops. Infection by RSV induces IgE production, the magnitude of which predicts the risk of subsequent wheezing episodes.

Usually, RSV infection begins in the upper respiratory tract with nasal congestion and pharyngitis and is associated with fever of variable intensity. The lower respiratory tract rapidly becomes involved in 25–40% of cases, which leads to worsening cough, dyspnea, wheezing, and rhonchi. Hypoxemia is common. Two types of lower respiratory tract involvement occur—pneumonia and bronchiolitis. Both are associated with interstitial infiltrates, the former from lung inflammation and the latter from peripheral atelectasis or hyperinflation. In older adults who have chronic cardiopulmonary disease, RSV may cause severe bronchitis, pneumonia, or both.

Serologic diagnosis can be made, but the tests may be less reliable in children younger than 4 months. Direct diagnosis requires cultures from respiratory secretions, nasopharyngeal washings, or throat swabs; virus detection is possible after 2–7 days. Immunofluorescence techniques are frequently used,

and they allow a reliable and more rapid detection in nasal scrapings or washings. The ELISA assay is less sensitive.

Treatment with aerosolized ribavirin improves the clinical course and should be administered for 12–18 hours/day for 2–5 days to patients who have severe disease. Systemic corticosteroids are also given to those who suffer the most severe involvement.

Because RSV may spread among hospitalized children and hospital staff, prevention of nosocomial infection is recommended (Box 28-1). No vaccine is available.

Adenovirus

Adenoviruses are responsible for up to 5% of respiratory infections in children but account for less than 2% of those in adults; an exception is military recruit populations, in which epidemics have been reported. Almost all adults have serum antibodies against adenoviruses (usually against several serotypes).

Adenovirus respiratory infection may be the consequence of airborne or of fecal-oral contamination. The incubation period lasts 4–7 days. Latent infection may develop and has even been implicated in the pathogenesis of chronic airway diseases such as asthma or chronic obstructive pulmonary disease. In children and military recruits, adenoviruses can cause bronchiolitis and pneumonia of variable severity.

Rapid diagnosis requires antigen detection or histopathologic examination of biopsy specimens (which show intranuclear basophilic inclusions). Virus isolation requires 3 days to several weeks, and serodiagnosis requires both acute and convalescent sera.

Treatment is supportive (e.g., analgesics, cough suppressants). Effective, enteric-coated live vaccines have been developed for military recruits, but they are not used in other settings.

Rubeola (Measles)

Measles virus belongs to the Paramyxoviridae family and is, therefore, similar to parainfluenza virus and RSV. Portals of entry are the respiratory tract and conjunctiva. Lower respiratory tract manifestations affect up to 50% of patients who have measles and include mainly bronchitis and pneumonia (which may be complicated by bacterial superinfection in up to 50% of cases). In the United States, pneumonia is the cause of 60% of measles-related deaths in children.

Patients who have measles show a typical viral prodrome that consists of fever, rhinitis, malaise, and anorexia and lasts for approximately 1 week before the onset of the rash. The maculopapular rash begins on the face and neck and progresses to the trunk and extremities. Leukopenia is seen early. Measles pneumonia can cause hilar lymphadenopathy and pleural effusions, in addition to reticulonodular parenchymal infiltrates. Secondary bacterial pneumonia also occurs.

Treatment is supportive, and antibiotics are required when bacterial secondary infection occurs. No consistent data are available on the effects of corticosteroids.

The measles vaccine has reduced the incidence of disease by 98% in developed countries and has shifted the median age of onset to the teenage years.

Varicella

Varicella causes pneumonia in adults, but this complication is unusual in immunocompetent children. Epidemics occur in the winter and spring, with infectivity rates that exceed 90% within the first 2–3 weeks after exposure.

Initially, a rash appears on the face and head, with subsequent spread to the thorax, abdomen, and extremities. The rash has a rather orderly progression, beginning with erythematous macules that progress to vesicles within hours to days. These subsequently become pustular and finally crust over. Lesions may also be found on mucosal surfaces (e.g., pharynx, vagina). When pneumonia occurs, it generally presents within the first 4–5 days after the onset of the rash. Cough is common, and pleuritic chest pain and hemoptysis may occur. Other organs such as the liver, kidney, heart, and brain may also be involved. Diffuse, small nodular infiltrates are the characteristic radiographic abnormality, and hilar adenopathy and effusions are common. With resolution, the nodules may calcify and persist for life (Figure 28-1).

Varicella infections can be diagnosed by a cytologic examination of scrapings from the lesions (e.g., the Tzanck smear, seeking multinucleated giant cells), although the sensitivity of this test is low. The virus may be cultured or found by polymerase chain reaction. A number of serologic tests are available, including the fluorescent antibody to membrane antigen test and ELISA.

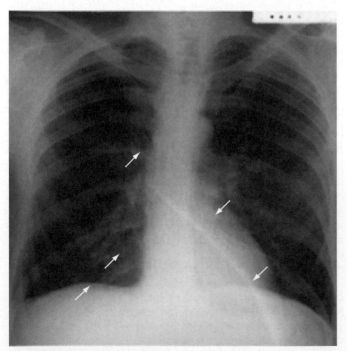

FIGURE 28-1 Calcific varicella nodules. Radiograph shows multiple 3- to 5-mm calcified nodules in the upper and lower lobes of a patient who had varicella pneumonia as a child.

Treatment with early administration of acyclovir (10–12.5 mg/kg intravenously every 8 h for 7 days) is recommended for immunocompromised hosts who have varicella and for immunocompetent patients who suffer pneumonia. Preventive administration of oral acyclovir in adults who have varicella may be prudent, especially in elderly subjects, pregnant women, or patients with chronic obstructive pulmonary disease. Zoster immune globulin is recommended to reduce the severity of illness in immunocompromised patients exposed to varicella.

The infection can spread readily in the hospital setting, so strict isolation must be instituted until all lesions have crusted over.

Hantavirus

The hantavirus pulmonary syndrome was first recognized in the United States in 1983, but the disease was retrospectively identified by use of serologic testing in patients who had a similar illness in 1959. The syndrome can result from several hantaviruses, such as Sin Nombre virus. Almost all cases have been reported in North and South America. Rodents (e.g., field mice, voles, chipmunks) serve as the reservoir, and transmission to humans results from aerosolization of viruses contained in their feces. Person-to-person spread rarely, if ever, occurs.

The initial presentation is that of a flulike syndrome of fever, myalgia, nausea, vomiting, and gastrointestinal pain suggestive of gastroenteritis. These are followed by a dry cough that portends diffuse noncardiogenic pulmonary edema (sometimes associated with bilateral pleural effusion), which may lead to ARDS and shock in severe cases. Hematologic examination usually demonstrates neutrophilic leukocytosis, hemoconcentration, thrombocytopenia, and circulating immunoblasts. Renal failure may occur but is uncommon.

The diagnosis can be made by serologic or immunohistochemical techniques.

Treatment is mainly supportive, but the results of controlled trials of intravenous ribavirin are pending. Although *in vitro* effects of ribavirin have been demonstrated, preliminary results from an open-label trial are not impressive.

Avoidance of areas in which infected rodents reside is the only recognized preventive measure.

Severe Acute Respiratory Syndrome (SARS)

An outbreak of SARS was recently reported, mainly in Asian countries and Canada. The origin of the epidemic was believed to be Guangdong province in China. None of the previously described respiratory pathogens was consistently identified, and a new coronavirus isolated from patients with SARS is thought to be the responsible pathogen.

The incubation period ranges from 2–11 days. The clinical presentation and radiologic features of SARS are those of atypical pneumonia.

No effective treatment is available, despite the use of antiviral therapy such as ribavirin or steroids in many cases.

SARS is a serious respiratory illness that can lead to significant morbidity, with 10–25% of patients requiring admission to an intensive care unit and a mortality rate of approximately 10%. Factors associated with a poor outcome are older than 60 years, significant comorbidities, diabetes mellitus, and initially elevated lactate dehydrogenase levels and elevated polymorphonuclear counts.

Because SARS is highly transmissible, it is recommended that patients be isolated in a single room (with negative pressure, if possible). Health care personnel should wear gloves, gown, mask, and eye protection and should wash their hands carefully after removing their gloves. The number of health care workers in contact with SARS patients should be limited. All suspected or confirmed cases should be reported to local health authorities and the World Health Organization.

FUNGAL PNEUMONIA

The most commonly encountered fungal and parasitic pulmonary infections are summarized in Table 28-3. The differential diagnosis in any given patient depends on his or her immunologic status, geographic locale, and travel history. A number of the fungal pneumonias occur almost exclusively in North America (e.g., histoplasmosis, blastomycosis, coccidioidomycosis). Although fungal and parasitic pulmonary infections are frequently self-limited, recurrent or severe disease is common when cell-mediated immunity is impaired. Infections in immunocompromised patients are covered in Chapter 29. Although amphotericin B remains the most effective medication for most fungal infections, treatment is now facilitated by a number of new agents that are easier to administer and better tolerated. Therapeutic options are summarized in Table 28-4.

Aspergillosis

Aspergillus species are ubiquitous saprophytic fungi that produce several toxic substances (e.g., endotoxin, proteases). Airway colonization by *Aspergillus* is usually seen in patients with chronic lung lesions, such as bronchiectatic cavities, pulmonary fibrosis, or tuberculosis sequelae, and local host defense

impairment. Invasive aspergillosis is an unusual finding in nonneutropenic patients but has been described in patients with chronic obstructive pulmonary disease on long-term steroid therapy.

In nonimmunocompromised patients, *Aspergillus* species cause hypersensitivity pneumonitis (generally from *Aspergillus fumigatus*) and Löffler's syndrome (discussed in Chapters 45 and 52, respectively), allergic bronchopulmonary aspergillosis (covered in Chapter 45), and aspergillomas. Chronic necrotizing pneumonia has been described in nonneutropenic patients with preexisting lung disease or on chronic steroid therapy.

Amphotericin B is the most effective medication for most fungal infections. Treatment is now facilitated, however, by a number of new agents that are easier to administer and better tolerated, such as itraconazole, voriconazole, and caspofungin.

Histoplasmosis

Histoplasma capsulatum is frequently isolated from soil that has been contaminated by bird or bat feces, which provide the organic nitrogen necessary for its growth. The disease occurs in the central United States (where the estimated prevalence and incidence of infection are $50/10^6$ and $500/10^3$, respectively), Mexico, and Puerto Rico. The disease was initially seen only in rural communities but is now found in patients who reside in urban settings as well, particularly in association with construction projects that involve moving contaminated soil. Numerous occupations have an increased risk of exposure.

The inhaled spores are contained in infective particles 2–5 μm in diameter, an ideal size to reach the airways and alveoli. After inhalation, multiplication converts the spores into yeasts, which are phagocytosed by macrophages in which they are able to survive, proliferate, and disseminate to

TABLE 28-3 Agents of Fungal and Parasitic Pneumonia, Classified According to the Immunologic Status of the Host

Type of Pathogen	Mainly in Normal Host	In Both Immunocompromised and Normal Host	Mainly in Immunocompromised Host
Fungi	Histoplasma capsulatum Blastomyces dermatitidis Coccidioides immitis Paracoccidioides braziliensis	Cryptococcus neoformans Aspergillus spp. Sporothrix schenckii Penicillium marneffei Geotrichum spp.	Zygomycetes Candida spp. Trichosporon spp. Fusarium spp. Penicillium spp. Hansenula spp. Mucor, Rhizopus, and Absidia genera (mucormycosis) Pseudoallescheria boydii Pneumocystis jiroveci
Parasites Protozoa	Plasmodium spp. (malaria) Entamoeba histolytica (amebiasis)	—	Toxoplasma gondii Cryptosporidium spp. Babesia spp.
Nematodes	Ascaris spp. Hookworm Toxocara canis (visceral larva migrans) Dirofilaria immitis Wuchereria bancrofti, Brugia malayi (tropical eosinophilia)	Strongyloides stercoralis	—
Platyhelminths	Paragonimus spp. Schistosoma spp. Echinococcus spp.	—	—

TABLE 28-4 Therapeutic Options in Fungal Pneumonias of the Nonimmunocompromised Host

Disease		First-Line Treatment	Alternatives
Allergic bronchopulmonary aspergillosis		Corticosteroids plus itraconazole	—
Aspergilloma		Surgical resection	Embolization Itraconazole Intracavitary instillation of amphotericin B
Histoplasmosis	Acute	No treatment	Itraconazole
	Chronic	Itraconazole	Ketoconazole Amphotericin B
	Disseminated	—	Amphotericin B
Blastomycosis	Acute	Itraconazole	—
	Chronic	Itraconazole	Amphotericin B
Coccidioidomycosis	Acute	Itraconazole	Ketoconazole
	Chronic	Itraconazole	Ketoconazole Amphotericin B
Paracoccidioidomycosis	Mild	Itraconazole	Itraconazole
	Chronic	Amphotericin B ± sulfadiazine	
Cryptococcosis		Fluconazole	Itraconazole Amphotericin B

TABLE 28-5 Clinical Presentations of Acute Histoplasmosis

	Mild Acute Pneumonitis	Pneumonic Histoplasmosis	Progressive Disseminating Primary Infection
Symptoms and physical signs	None or acute, influenza-like symptoms Arthralgia–erythema nodosum–erythema multiforme complex	Fever, chills, sweat, anorexia, weakness, cough with mucopurulent sputum, pleuritic chest pain Sometimes consolidation, rarely pleural effusion	Severe acute illness, often in immunocompromised patients Weight loss, low-grade fever, abdominal complaints, cough Sometimes mucosal ulcers, adrenal involvement
Chest radiography	Normal or consolidation 6 lymph node enlargement	Infiltrates of varying density, often with hilar lymph node enlargement, sometimes with pericarditis	Normal, or multiple nodules, linear opacities 6 lymph node involvement, or miliary aspect
Blood examination	—	—	In severe disease, leukopenia, thrombocytopenia, disseminated intravascular coagulation
Diagnosis	—	—	Few granulomas and many organisms in the most severe disease, the opposite in less severe forms
Clinical course	Spontaneous resolution; residual calcified nodules and lymph nodes	—	—

metastatic sites such as the liver and spleen. A lymphocyte-mediated, delayed-type hypersensitivity reaction occurs and results in the formation of granulomas that resemble those found in mycobacterial diseases; the necrotic material may become caseous and calcify. The granulomas may be found in the lung, as well as in a number of sites of metastatic infection. Patients affected by compromised cellular immunity (such as those who have AIDS or lymphoma) are more susceptible to histoplasmosis and may develop more severe disease.

Most patients who have acute primary infections are undiagnosed because histoplasmosis remains subclinical. Those who inhale larger numbers of spores (frequently as a result of exposure in a closed space) have a syndrome develop approximately 14 days later that has an abrupt onset and resembles influenza, bacterial pneumonia, or tuberculosis (Table 28-5).

When the inoculum is particularly large, patients may have ARDS develop.

The growth of *Histoplasma* species is slow, such that several weeks are needed for cultures to become positive. Giemsa staining of blood or bone marrow smears may be diagnostic when the fungus load is high, but this is unusual in immunocompetent patients. Tissue samples can demonstrate the organisms with silver or periodic acid–Schiff (PAS) staining. Indirect diagnosis may be provided by several serologic techniques, including complement fixation, immunodiffusion, or radioimmunoassay, all of which may require several weeks to become positive.

Treatment is needed only for patients who have chronic, progressive histoplasmosis or for those who have dissemination. The use of amphotericin B is limited by the need for intravenous administration and the frequent development of renal toxicity, febrile reactions, and phlebitis. Renal toxicity may be reduced by the coadministration of large volumes of intravenous fluids. Side effects may also be reduced by use of the newly developed, but considerably more expensive, liposomal form of amphotericin. Ketoconazole has frequent gastrointestinal and antitestosterone effects. Fluconazole and itraconazole (200–400 mg/day) are as effective as amphotericin or ketoconazole in patients who have mild illness. Thus, amphotericin B should be reserved for patients who have more severe or disseminated disease.

Most acute primary infections are self-limited, require no treatment, and do not come to medical attention. Recurrent infiltrates may occur in some patients in association with eosinophilia, mimicking Löffler's syndrome. Evidence of calcified granulomas may be present in the lung (Figure 28-2) and the spleen. On occasion, marked hilar lymphadenopathy or focal or diffuse mediastinal fibrosis may compress the central structures (e.g., airways, arteries, veins, esophagus).

Chronic, progressive disease occurs rarely, with symptoms of cough, hemoptysis, dyspnea, and fever. Chest radiographs usually show upper lobe or peripheral areas of consolidation, which evolve into cavities that mimic healed tuberculosis. Empyemas may occur, as may broncholithiasis, which has been associated with hemoptysis and bronchial obstruction. Chronic infection of the meninges, brain, or heart may occur rarely.

Blastomycosis

Blastomycosis is found in North America (in areas largely overlapping those where histoplasmosis occurs), Mexico, the Middle East, Africa, and India and results from inhalation of *Blastomyces dermatitidis*. The fungus grows in the soil, and the spores become airborne and are inhaled before converting to the yeast form in the lung. *B. dermatitidis* infection may occur sporadically or in epidemics. The initial defense mechanism involves polymorphonuclear cells, followed by macrophages and giant cells; epithelioid granulomas often develop.

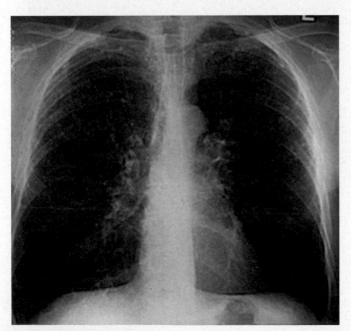

FIGURE 28-2 Calcified granulomas in the lung of a patient who has histoplasmosis.

Depending on the type of predominant inflammatory response (pyogenic or granulomatous), the histopathologic pattern can mimic that of a bacterial infection, sarcoidosis, or mycobacterial disease. After multiplication of the yeast in the lungs, it may spread to the skin, bones, brain, peripheral lymph nodes, or other organs, and extrapulmonary manifestations may occur many years after the initial infection.

The clinical manifestations of blastomycosis differ from one country to another. In North America, acute epidemic blastomycosis mimics bacterial pneumonia, with the abrupt onset of fever, chills, arthralgia and myalgia, cough with purulent sputum, and pleuritic chest pain. In milder cases, which are more frequent, the presentation is that of a more chronic disease, resembling tuberculosis; low-grade fever, cough, anorexia, and weight loss develop insidiously. Physical examination sometimes demonstrates erythema nodosum or findings of pulmonary consolidation, but it may be normal. The radiographic manifestations are nonspecific and include cavities, infiltrates, rounded densities, consolidation with air bronchograms, perihilar masses, or even a miliary pattern.

Mediastinal lymph node involvement is rare (<10% in most studies), and pleural effusions are quite uncommon. In the most severe cases, infection with *B. dermatitidis* can cause ARDS, even in immunocompetent hosts. Patients who have cutaneous blastomycosis frequently have a history of a self-limited pulmonary syndrome that occurred some years in the past.

The diagnosis of blastomycosis is made by microscopic examination of respiratory secretions digested by potassium hydroxide or by histopathologic examination of tissue samples after silver or PAS staining. In culture of respiratory samples, detectable growth takes up to 1 week.

Because blastomycosis is often self-limited, treatment is restricted to those who have chronic disease and those who have severe acute infections. Itraconazole has the best ratio of efficacy to side effects, but amphotericin B is preferred in the most severe cases. Ketoconazole is an alternative in slowly progressive disease.

Coccidioidomycosis

Coccidioidomycosis results from another soil-dwelling fungus, *Coccidioides immitis*. It is endemic in the southwestern United States and northern Mexico and occurs mainly during hot, dry summers. Inhalation of airborne spores leads to polymorphonuclear-mediated suppurative and cell-mediated granulomatous inflammatory responses. The incubation period is 10–16 days.

Patients who have coccidioidomycosis may complain of fever, chills, arthralgia, myalgia, and headache in addition to cough, pleuritic chest pain, dyspnea, and, on occasion, hemoptysis (which results from areas of lung necrosis manifested by cavitation). Physical examination may reveal a macular rash, erythema nodosum, or erythema multiforme, as well as rhonchi, wheezes, or signs of consolidation or pleural effusion. In many patients, the physical examination is normal. Chest radiographs initially show one or more areas of consolidation, which may cavitate. Hilar lymphadenopathy may be found. Cavities or multiple calcified nodules may persist for life. Occasionally, patients have progressive primary coccidioidomycosis develop, a condition in which the infiltrates and lymphadenopathy progress in association with fever, cough, and weight loss. Several months after the primary pulmonary infection, disseminated coccidioidomycosis may become manifest (affecting skin, bones, joints, genitourinary system, meninges), particularly but not exclusively in immunocompromised patients.

The diagnosis of coccidioidomycosis may be made by serologic or skin testing, both of which are most useful for epidemiologic purposes. Direct diagnosis can be made by microscopic examination of sputum or pus after potassium hydroxide digestion or Papanicolaou staining, by histopathologic examination of tissue biopsies after silver staining, or by cultures, which may demonstrate fungal growth after 5 days but pose an inhalation risk for laboratory personnel.

The treatment of coccidioidomycosis is similar to that of histoplasmosis and blastomycosis and relies on fluconazole and itraconazole, with amphotericin B and ketoconazole as alternatives. For most patients, no specific therapy is required.

Coccidioidomycosis is usually mild and self-limited, except in rare cases when it progresses or spreads hematogenously. Dissemination, which may be more common in dark-skinned races and in those who are immunocompromised, is associated with a high risk of meningitis and has a poor prognosis.

Paracoccidioidomycosis

Paracoccidioidomycosis results from inhalation of a soil fungus that is found mainly in South and Central America and in Mexico. In nonimmunocompromised patients, paracoccidioidomycosis presents as a chronic or subacute lung infection that is usually self-limited. In immunocompromised subjects, the clinical manifestations are those of an acute, severe disseminated infection.

The diagnosis of paracoccidioidomycosis relies on the same techniques used for coccidioidomycosis.

In severe or disseminated cases of paracoccidioidomycosis, treatment is similar to that of coccidioidomycosis but should be continued for up to 6 months.

Cryptococcosis

Cryptococcus neoformans is found throughout the world in bird guano. Cryptococcosis is a rare infection and is usually asymptomatic and self-limited in immunocompetent patients. In those who have impaired cell-mediated immunity, it may cause lung infection and meningitis. Symptoms of pulmonary infection include fever, malaise, cough, and chest pain. The chest radiograph may show large, nonspecific nodules (Figure 28-3) or infiltrates, sometimes associated with lymphadenopathy.

C. neoformans can colonize the airways of immunocompromised patients and those who have chronic bronchitis without causing illness. Accordingly, culture of fungus from sputum does not always indicate disease.

Because cryptococcosis resolves spontaneously in normal hosts, and because patients who have chronic mucopurulent pulmonary conditions may be colonized by *Cryptococcus* species, positive cultures do not, in and of themselves, denote a specific indication for treatment. For patients who have progressive disease, amphotericin B or ketoconazole, fluconazole, or itraconazole is recommended.

PARASITIC PNEUMONIA

Pulmonary infections that result from parasites are infrequent in immunocompetent hosts but must be included in the differential diagnosis when patients have lived in endemic areas.

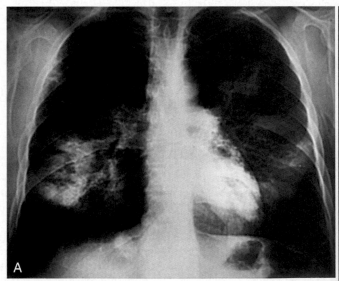

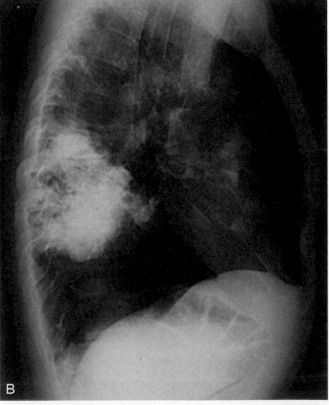

FIGURE 28-3 Cryptococcal lung infection. Chest radiographs (**A,** posteroanterior and, **B,** lateral view) of an immunocompetent patient show bilateral, large nodular densities.

Amebiasis

Entamoeba histolytica is endemic in West and South Africa, South and Southeast Asia, South America, and Mexico. The disease is transmitted by ingestion of contaminated food or water, and sexual transmission has been reported in homosexual men.

The parasite disseminates from the intestine to the liver or, much less frequently, to the lung (in <5% of those with intestinal infection) or brain. Pleuropulmonary complications occur in up to 50% of patients who have liver abscesses as a result of either direct spread from the liver or hematogenous dissemination.

The main features of the disease are intestinal, ranging from diarrhea and abdominal cramps to dysentery or even intestinal perforation because of mucosal ulcerations. Pleuropulmonary symptoms include cough, dyspnea, and pleuritic pain (usually right-sided) associated with fever and chills, diaphoresis, and weight loss. The chest radiograph may show elevation of the right hemidiaphragm, pleural effusion, atelectasis, lung consolidation (which usually affects the right lower lobe), or lung abscess. Hepatobronchial fistulas have been reported in 47% of patients who have pleuropulmonary complications of amebiasis; this finding is associated with the production of copious volumes of chocolate-colored sputum. Pericardial involvement may be observed in up to 10% of such patients.

The diagnosis can be made by microscopic examination of stool, which has a sensitivity of less than 30%, or by serologic techniques, which have sensitivities and specificities as high as 95% in invasive disease. Antigen may be detected on pleural fluid or respiratory secretions. Needle aspiration of lung or of liver abscesses is seldom necessary.

The drug of choice for treating invasive amebiasis is metronidazole (750 mg every 8 h for 10 days), in addition to agents that are active against intraluminal protozoa such as iodoquinol, diloxanide, or paromomycin.

Malarial Lung

Pleuropulmonary complications result from *Plasmodium falciparum*, the agent of the most severe form of malaria. Mild respiratory involvement is probably underdiagnosed and may affect up to 20% of patients who have falciparum malaria. Pulmonary involvement is commonly associated with cerebral disease and marked parasitemia. Histopathologic features include capillary congestion, pulmonary edema, alveolar hemorrhage, and endothelial cell injury.

The pulmonary manifestations of malaria include mild cough associated with pleural effusion, lung consolidation, or interstitial infiltrates. Severe respiratory involvement can occur as a result of lung edema and pleural effusions, and patients may present with ARDS.

The diagnosis is made by examination of thin or thick blood smears stained with Giemsa or Wright stain.

Besides supportive and respiratory care, treatment of severe disease requires intravenous quinidine and exchange transfusion in the most severe cases. Depending on the region of origin, drug-resistant strains must be considered, and alternative treatments offered. Despite these measures, prognosis for the malarial lung remains poor.

Pulmonary Ascariasis

The estimated worldwide prevalence of infection with the nematode *Ascaris lumbricoides* is 25%. The normal habitat of

the adult worm is the jejunum, and infection follows ingestion of embryonated eggs. Maturation occurs during pulmonary migration and may be responsible for ascaris pneumonia, a self-limited disease that occurs 4–16 days after ingestion and lasts for 10 days to several weeks.

Ascariasis is responsible for a Löffler-like syndrome in approximately 20% of cases. Symptoms are dominated by cough (sometimes with hemoptysis), wheezing, dyspnea, and high-grade fever. Abdominal pain, nausea and vomiting, and hepatomegaly may be present, as well as a variety of cutaneous reactions (e.g., urticaria, angioedema). The chest radiograph shows unilateral or bilateral patchy, migratory peribronchial infiltrates; eosinophilia may be present, and (on occasion) IgE elevation may be found.

Sputum analysis reveals eosinophils and Charcot–Leyden crystals. Stool examination may be negative at this early stage of ascariasis.

The pneumonia does not require any specific treatment, because it is usually self-limited. Bronchodilators and corticosteroids may be useful when bronchospasm is present. Antihelminthic therapy is necessary to eradicate intestinal adult worms (Table 28-6).

Strongyloidiasis and Ancylostomiasis

Although *Strongyloides stercoralis* is endemic in tropical and subtropical areas, strongyloidiasis is less frequent than ascariasis and ancylostomiasis. The life cycle of the parasite is the same as that of ascaris and hookworm. Ancylostomiasis, or hookworm infection, may be caused by two nematodes: *Ancylostoma duodenale* and *Necator americanus*. The prevalence and life cycles are similar to those of *Ascaris lumbricoides* and *Strongyloides stercoralis*.

Patients may be asymptomatic or experience a Löffler-like syndrome after transient urticaria in association with abdominal symptoms. In some cases, massive invasion (which is favored by abnormal cell-mediated immunity and malnutrition-related immunosuppression) leads to a much more severe disease, termed the hyperinfection syndrome, which develops from disseminated disease (Table 28-7).

The diagnosis can be made by sputum or stool examination or by duodenal or pleural aspiration. Serologic techniques may be of help in chronic cases.

The preferred treatment is thiabendazole 25 mg/kg every 12 h for 2 days (longer in disseminated disease), which may have to be repeated. Alternative agents are ivermectin and albendazole.

TABLE 28-6 First-Choice Antihelminthic Drugs Active Against *Ascaris lumbricoides* and Hookworms

Drug	Dose and Duration	Common Side Effects
Pyrantel pamoate	11 mg/kg, single dose	Anorexia, nausea, abdominal pain, diarrhea
Mebendazole	100 mg q12h for 3 days	Abdominal pain, diarrhea
Albendazole	400 mg, single dose	Abdominal discomfort, diarrhea

TABLE 28-7 Clinical Presentation of the Hyperinfection Syndrome or Disseminated Strongyloidiasis

Manifestation	Presentation
Abdominal	Anorexia, nausea, vomiting, diarrhea, abdominal pain ileus
Pulmonary	Cough, hemoptysis, wheezing, dyspnea Adult respiratory distress syndrome Bacterial superinfection
Other	Invasion of liver, skin, central nervous system Bacterial meningitidis Sepsis caused by secondary bacterial infection (usually gram-negative bacilli)

Visceral Larva Migrans

Human visceral larva migrans is caused by *Toxocara canis* or, less frequently, *Toxocara catis*. All canine species are hosts of the nematode, and the prevalence of the infection in dogs has been estimated at approximately 3%. Contamination of humans occurs after ingestion of eggs in contaminated food or soil. Larvae migrate to the liver and lungs through lymphatics and blood vessels and induce an IgE-mediated immune response. In rare cases, other organs may be involved, such as the heart or the central nervous system. Cells that infiltrate invaded tissues are mainly eosinophils and, to a lesser extent, lymphocytes.

Clinically apparent pulmonary involvement is common (20–85% of cases) and manifests as cough, wheezing, bronchiolitis, or pneumonia that may result in acute respiratory failure. Radiographic manifestations are usually mild migratory infiltrates, which are found in 50% of those who have respiratory symptoms. Systemic symptoms include weakness, malaise, anorexia, nausea, vomiting, weight loss, abdominal pain, or behavioral impairment. Overall, the severity of the clinical illness reflects the extent of the infestation.

Because *Toxocara* larvae do not mature in humans, the diagnosis can be made only by serologic or histologic examination of invaded tissues.

In mild cases, the disease is self-limited, so no treatment is required. In more severely affected patients, corticosteroids seem to improve the prognosis. Preventive measures are important to limit the spread of the disease (Table 28-8).

Dirofilariasis

Human dirofilariasis is the consequence of infestation by the nematode *Dirofilaria immitis*, which is a dog parasite transmitted by mosquitoes. In rare cases, larvae injected by mosquitoes into humans are transported by blood vessels to the pulmonary circulation, where they can cause thrombosis.

TABLE 28-8 Preventive Measures to Limit Visceral Larva Migrans in Humans

Behavioral Measures	Veterinary Measures	Environmental Measures
Avoid geophagia Limit close contact between children and canine species	Deworming of cats and dogs	Keep children's sandbox dry

Clinical signs of cough, hemoptysis, chest pain, and fever are present in half of affected patients. Chest radiographs may show peripheral nodules of 1–5 cm in diameter, which may calcify. A minority of patients exhibit peripheral eosinophilia.

The diagnosis can be made by serology or histologic examination of lung tissues. No treatment is required.

Tropical Pulmonary Eosinophilia

Tropical pulmonary eosinophilia results from infection with *Wuchereria bancrofti* or *Brugia malayi*, which are lymphatic-dwelling filariae found in tropical and subtropical areas. Pulmonary manifestations are the consequence of a hypersensitivity reaction after the discharge of microfilariae into the circulation by gravid female filariae. Transmission is by mosquitoes that ingest the microfilariae and inject larvae when they bite humans. Of the patients who have tropical eosinophilia, 80% are men, and the lungs are involved in more than 90% of cases.

Clinical manifestations include fever, weakness, anorexia, weight loss, cough, wheezing, and dyspnea. Chest radiographs usually show bilateral basal, interstitial infiltrates, and increased bronchovascular markings. Lymph node involvement and consolidation are infrequent.

The parasites may be found on histologic examination of affected organs, but the diagnosis is generally made by finding high levels of IgE and high titers of antibodies to filariae and by clinical improvement after treatment.

Standard treatment is diethylcarbamazine, 6–12 mg/kg body weight for up to 3 weeks. Alternatives are mebendazole and levamisole. New agents such as ivermectin are being evaluated. Corticosteroids or antihistamines may be used when patients exhibit allergic reactions to dying filariae. Some patients (10–20%) require repeated courses of treatment because the adult parasites may be relatively resistant. Response to treatment is inversely related to the duration of symptoms.

Paragonimiasis

Paragonimus species (most frequently *Paragonimus westermani*) are hermaphroditic flukes that are endemic in Southeast Asia, South America, and South Africa and are transmitted to humans by ingestion of insufficiently cooked crabs or crayfish that contain the encysted parasite. These go to the lung through the intestinal wall, peritoneal cavity, diaphragm, and pleura.

The illness may occur during the first weeks of infection, during the parasite's migration from the intestine to the lung. When this occurs, symptoms may include abdominal pain, diarrhea, hypersensitivity reactions (urticaria, eosinophilia, fever), chest pain, cough, and hemoptysis. In most cases, however, no symptoms appear until the adult parasite begins to produce eggs in the lung, which induces cough and hemoptysis. Chest radiographs usually show patchy infiltrates, which may progress to cavities surrounded by a rim of infiltration (ring cysts). Areas of fibrosis or pleural thickening are common. Pleural effusions are infrequent, except in some series of South Asian patients. The chest radiograph may be normal in up to 20% of cases.

The diagnosis is based on demonstrating eggs in bronchial secretions, pleural fluid, or feces. A number of serologic tests are also available.

The preferred treatment is praziquantel (25 mg/kg every 8 h for 3 days), which is effective in more than 90% of cases. Bithionol (40 mg/kg every other day for 2 weeks) is a less effective alternative.

Schistosomiasis

Several *Schistosoma* species may be pathogenic for humans. The most frequently encountered are described in Table 28-9. The parasite forms released by snails (in which asexual reproduction occurs) penetrate the skin and transform into immature parasites, which are transported in the blood, where they mature in venous plexuses (see Table 28-9) and reproduce. Eggs are deposited in the intestine or bladder, depending on the site of the infected venous plexus. The eggs, in turn, induce overwhelming granulomatous reactions; they may migrate to the liver and cause portal hypertension, with subsequent migration to the lung through portosystemic collaterals.

As shown in Table 28-10, symptoms depend on the stage of the disease. The most frequent pulmonary manifestation is pulmonary hypertension, which occurs in the chronic stages of infection with *Schistosoma mansoni* or *Schistosoma japonicum*. Nodular lesions can also develop, and this infestation should be included in the differential diagnosis of pulmonary nodules (Figure 28-4).

The direct diagnosis may be based on examination of the stool (Kato thick smear), urine, or rectal biopsies. Several serologic techniques have been developed.

The most effective treatment is praziquantel. Doses depend on the *Schistosoma* species (see Table 28-9).

Hydatidosis

Cystic hydatid disease (CHD) is caused by larvae of *Echinococcus granulosus*, and alveolar hydatid disease (AHD) is caused by *Echinococcus multilocularis*. Both are platyhelminths that infect humans through the ingestion of eggs. The parasite is transported by the blood or lymphatics to other sites, mainly the liver and lungs. Whereas CHD is the manifestation of the growth of larvae, which form spherical cysts, AHD results from persistent invasion by and destructive proliferation of the parasite. Of human hydatidosis cases, 90% of patients have CHD (with respiratory involvement in 25% of these), and 9% have AHD.

In CHD, symptoms occur in approximately 70% of cases and are related to compression of adjacent structures or to complications such as rupture or secondary infection. Accordingly, symptoms include chest pain, cough, expectoration of cyst contents (e.g., grape skins), dyspnea, hemoptysis, or even near drowning in cyst fluid. Rupture may also lead to dissemination of cysts within the lungs, hypersensitivity reactions, or pleural effusion. In rare instances (<10%), hydatid cysts may develop in the pleural space itself after the rupture of a pulmonary cyst. Chest radiographs typically show rounded opacities (called cannonballs), the borders of which can calcify. Sharply demarcated cysts, which may contain smaller daughter cysts, are shown by computed tomography scans. This finding allows CHD to be differentiated from AHD; in the latter, computed tomography shows less well-demarcated masses that have necrotic centers. Eosinophilia is frequent.

The diagnosis relies on the demonstration of associated hepatic cysts, serologic tests, and, in some cases, the presence

TABLE 28-9 Pathogenic *Schistosoma* Species

Species	Area	Predominant Venous Plexuses in Which Mature Parasites Develop	Treatment: Doses of Praziquantel
Schistosoma mansoni	Arabia, South America, Caribbean	Inferior mesenteric veins	20 mg/kg body weight × 2, for 1 day
Schist. japonicum	China, Japan, Philippines	Superior mesenteric plexus	20 mg/kg body weight × 3, for 1 day
Schist. haematobium	Africa, Middle East	Vesical plexus	20 mg/kg body weight × 2, for 1 day

TABLE 28-10 Clinical Presentations of Schistosomiasis

Stage of Disease	Involved Species	Clinical Signs
Skin penetration	All	Transient cutaneous symptoms ("swimming itch")
Tissue migration (immature parasite)	Mainly *Schistosoma japonicum*	Katayama fever: fever, chills, headache, myalgia, arthralgia, abdominal pain, diarrhea, weight loss, cough, wheezing, pulmonary infiltrates (sometimes with a miliary aspect), hepatosplenomegaly, lymphadenopathy, leukocytosis, eosinophilia, immune complexes
Chronic infection (mature reproducing parasites)	*Schistosoma mansoni* and *S. japonicum*	Abdominal pain, diarrhea, fatigue, portal hypertension, hepatic failure (presinusoidal hepatic fibrosis) Pulmonary hypertension Hypoxemia without pulmonary hypertension (intrapulmonary arteriovenous fistulas) Lung granulomas
	Schistosoma haematobium	Chronic bladder disease
Response to treatment	—	Transient and self-limited cough, wheezing, lung infiltrates, eosinophilia

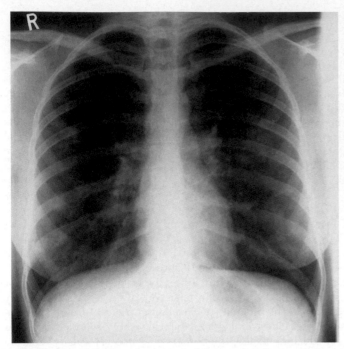

FIGURE 28-4 Multiple pulmonary nodules on the chest radiograph of a patient with schistosomiasis.

TABLE 28-11	Histopathologic Differences Between Exogenous and Endogenous Lipoid Pneumonias	
Characteristic	**Exogenous Lipids**	**Endogenous Lipids**
Fat	Large droplets	Small droplets
Foreign body granulomas	Present	Absent
Birefringence under polarized light	Absent	Present
Special stainings		
Periodic acid–Schiff	Negative	Positive
Sudan black	Light blue	Black
Sudan IV	Orange	Red
Oil red O	Orange	Red
Nile blue sulfate	Negative	Light violet
Osmium tetroxide	Negative	Positive

BOX 28-2   Findings in Exogenous Lipoid Pneumonia on Chest Radiography

Dense consolidation with air bronchograms
Ground glass infiltrates
Cavitation
Interstitial infiltrate
Fibrotic infiltrates
Nodules, masses
Atelectasis
Emphysema
Pleural effusion

---

of cyst material in sputum. Aspiration of the cyst should be avoided to limit the possibility of dissemination and hypersensitivity reactions.

The treatment of choice is surgical resection of the cysts. When surgery cannot be done, or when the cysts rupture and the parasite disseminates, the preferred treatment is albendazole 400 mg every 12 h (10–15 mg/kg per day) for 4 weeks. Treatment courses may be repeated.

LIPOID PNEUMONIA

Lipoid pneumonia results from the aspiration of exogenous lipids contained in orally administered laxatives or nasal decongestants. The histology is that of giant-cell inflammation with oil-containing vacuoles and phagocytes, type II cell metaplasia, degeneration of arteriolar or bronchial walls, necrosis, and fibrosis. Oil droplets or lipophages may be transported by lymphatics or through the blood to the liver, spleen, kidney, or other organs. Special stains allow exogenous lipoid pneumonia to be distinguished from conditions that arise from the accumulation of endogenous lipids, as occasionally occurs in the setting of chronic primary lung inflammation (Table 28-11).

Symptoms include cough, dyspnea, fever, chest pain, and hemoptysis. The onset may be acute, but more commonly it is chronic and is accompanied by weight loss. In 50% of cases, the disease is clinically silent and is discovered on a chest radiograph. A number of radiologic presentations may be found (Box 28-2; Figure 28-5). Computed tomography or magnetic resonance imaging scans may be useful when they demonstrate attenuation values of −30 to −150 Hounsfield units or high-intensity T1 signals with a slow decrease on T2-weighted images, respectively, as a result of the low density of fat. Sputum, bronchoalveolar lavage fluid, or transbronchial biopsies can be examined for fat-containing macrophages after the application of special stains.

The most important intervention is to stop the administration of the causative agent. Corticosteroids do not seem to be beneficial.

Exogenous lipoid pneumonia usually follows a benign course. The most frequently encountered complications are bacterial, fungal, or mycobacterial superinfections. Respiratory insufficiency occurs infrequently, unless the condition is far advanced (e.g., years of chronic aspiration), and neoplasm is uncommon. The use of oil-containing laxatives and decongestants should be discouraged.

SUGGESTED READINGS

American College of Physicians; Barnitz L, Berkwits M: The health care response to pandemic influenza. Ann Intern Med 2006; 145:135–137.

Batra P, Batra RS: Thoracic coccidioidomycosis. Semin Roentgenol 1996; 31:28–44.

Beigel JH, Farrar J, Han AM, et al; Writing Committee of the World Health Organization (WHO) Consultation on Human Influenza A/H5: Avian influenza A (H5N1) infection in humans. N Engl J Med 2005; 353:1374–1385.

Chapman SW, Bradsher RW Jr, Campbell GD Jr, et al: Infectious Diseases Society of America. Practice guidelines for the management of patients with blastomycosis. Clin Infect Dis 2000; 30:679–683.

Chitkara RK, Sarinas PS: Dirofilaria, visceral larva migrans, and tropical pulmonary eosinophilia. Semin Respir Infect 1997; 12:138–148.

Clancy CJ, Nguyen MH: Acute community-acquired pneumonia due to Aspergillus in presumably immunocompetent hosts: clues for recognition of a rare but fatal disease. Chest 1998; 114:629–634.

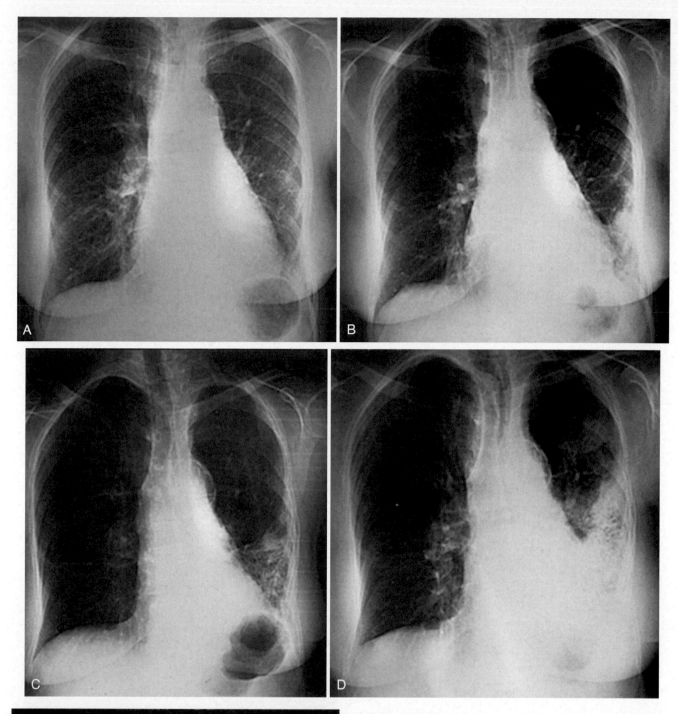

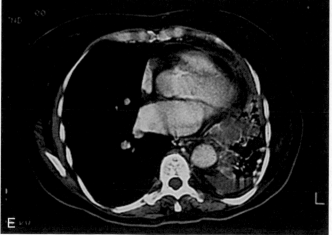

FIGURE 28-5 Lipoid pneumonia. This series of radiographs demonstrates infiltration of the left lower lobe that progressed slowly over 19 years—from 1974 **(A)** to 1993 **(D)**. The patient liberally applied a petrolatum-containing nasal grease each night before bed, and her husband documented that the patient routinely slept on her left side. The computed tomography scan shows low-density consolidation of the left lower lobe and a small left pleural effusion.

Couch RB: Drug therapy: prevention and treatment of influenza. N Engl J Med 2000; 343:1778–1787.

Ksiazek TG, Erdman D, Goldsmith CS, *et al*: A novel coronavirus associated with severe acute respiratory syndrome. N Engl J Med 2003; 348:1953–1966.

Lortholary O, Denning DW, Dupont B: Endemic mycosis: a treatment update. J Antimicrob Chemother 1999; 43:321–331.

Mandell LA, Wunderink RG, Anzueto A, *et al*: Infectious Diseases Society of America/American Thoracic Society Consensus Guidelines on the management of community-acquired pneumonia in adults. Clin Infect Dis 2007; 44:S27–S72.

Sarinas PS, Chitkara RK: Ascariasis and hookworm. Semin Respir Infect 1997; 32:130–137.

Spickard A 3rd, Hirschmann JV: Exogenous lipoid pneumonia. Arch Intern Med 1994; 154:686–692.

Wheat J, Sarosi G, McKinsey D, *et al*: Practice guidelines for the management of patients with histoplasmosis. Clin Infect Dis 2000; 30:688–695.

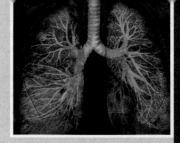

29 Pneumonia in the Non-HIV Immunocompromised Host

JEREMY BROWN

OVERVIEW

Lung infections are a common and frequently serious complication in patients with significant impairment of their immune system. For instance, pulmonary infiltrates occur in up to 25% of patients with neutropenia after chemotherapy, and up to 5% of patients undergoing hematopoietic cell transplantations will die from pneumonia. Compared with community-acquired pneumonia, the range of potential pathogens causing lung infections in immunocompromised patients is much broader and includes organisms such as *Aspergillus fumigatus* and human cytomegalovirus (CMV), the treatment of which is difficult and frequently toxic. As a consequence, management of lung infection in immunocompromised patients is considerably more complex than the management of community-acquired pneumonia, and the threshold for the use of invasive diagnostic tests such as bronchoscopy is low. This chapter will discuss the common causative pathogens and the clinical approach to pulmonary infections in severely immunocompromised patients because of chemotherapy, organ transplantation, or hematologic disease (Box 29-1) but excludes patients with HIV infection who are discussed in Chapter 34]. In addition to the effect of the immunodeficiency, these patients are also often at an increased risk of infection because of low-level microaspiration of oropharyngeal contents and because of damage to their mucosal surfaces by cytotoxic therapy, poor nutrition, or previous infection. Pneumonia in those patients with milder degrees of immunosuppression because of myeloma, low-dose cytotoxic therapy, or disease-modifying agents for rheumatology conditions generally should be managed as community- or hospital-acquired pneumonia, but with a low threshold for considering that the disease could be due to the opportunistic pathogens discussed in this chapter.

GENERAL PRINCIPLES OF THE CLINICAL APPROACH

The range of common potential pathogens causing lung infection in the immunocompromised host is given in Table 29-1. Given this intimidating range of potential pathogens that affect the immunocompromised patient and the potential toxicity of some antimicrobial therapies, blind empirical therapy against all possible pathogens is not feasible. Hence, the challenge in managing these patients is to (1) reduce the differential diagnosis to the most likely problems and so allow targeted empirical therapy, and (2) to identify when and which type of invasive diagnostic test(s) should be used to provide the most useful data. The likely potential causative pathogens can be defined by the following questions:

1. What is the clinical and radiologic presentation?
2. What is the speed of onset of the infection?
3. What is the type, duration, and severity of the patient's immune defect?
4. Has the patient had any positive microbiologic results?
5. Are there any other associated factors of importance? Important examples include recent local infective epidemics, the patient's prophylaxis regimen, and the patient's ethnic background and travel history.

Immune defects are generally predictable and caused by a combination of the disease and the treatment received and can be divided into two main groups, absolute or functional neutropenia and defects in cell-mediated immunity. Patients with neutropenia are mainly at risk of infection with extracellular pathogens such as pyogenic bacteria and filamentous fungi. Defects in cell-mediated immunity tend to predispose to intracellular pathogens such as viruses and mycobacteria, as well as some unusual extracellular infections such as *Pneumocystis* pneumonia (PCP) (see Table 29-2). In addition, a third less severe category of immune defect is deficiencies in antibody responses, which leads to a high incidence of infections caused by encapsulated bacteria like *Streptococcus pneumoniae* and by herpesviruses. Individual patients may have a combination of these immune defects; for example, hematopoietic cell transplantation initially causes severe neutropenia combined with impairment of cell-mediated immunity, but long term the patients have defects in cell-mediated immunity and often in antibody function.

By combining the clinical pattern of presentation with knowledge of the patient's immune defect, a differential diagnosis of likely pathogens can be suggested. For example, infections developing rapidly over 1–3 days with a marked rise in serum inflammatory markers such as C-reactive protein (CRP), pronounced fever, and focal radiologic changes are very likely to be due to infection with pyogenic bacteria. However, widespread ground glass infiltrations in both lungs developing over several days could be CMV pneumonitis or PCP, especially if the patient has a defect in cell-mediated immunity. In general, the more severe and prolonged the immune defect the greater the range of possible causative pathogens and the less usual the clinical presentation for a particular pathogen, prompting the need for early invasive investigation if the initial therapy is failing. Furthermore, the character of the disease can

TABLE 29-1 Range of Pathogens Commonly Associated with Pneumonia in the Non-HIV Immunocompromised Host

Pathogen	% Cases
Gram-negative pyogenic bacteria	
Escherichia coli	6
Proteus, Enterobacter, Serratia, and Citrobacter species	2
Haemophilus influenzae	<1
Klebsiella pneumoniae	<1
Pseudomonas aeruginosa	8
Acinetobacter species	2
Stenotrophomonas maltophilia	<1
Gram-positive pyogenic bacteria	
Streptococcus pneumoniae	2
Viridans streptococci	<1
Staphylococcus aureus	12
Enterococcus species	4
Other bacteria	
Anaerobes	<1
Legionella pneumophila	2
Chlamydia species	2
Mycoplasma pneumoniae	<1
Mycobacterium tuberculosis	4
Nontuberculous Mycobacteria	<1
Nocardia species	2
Fungi	
Pneumocystis jiroveciii	3
Candida species	9
Aspergillus species	24
Rarer molds (Mucor, Penicillium, Fusarium, etc.)	2
Endemic fungi (Histoplasma, Coccidiodes, etc.)	<1
Protozoa	
Toxoplasma gondii	<1
Helminths	
Strongyloides stercoralis	<1
Viruses	
CMV	6
Herpes simplex virus, varicella-zoster	2
Respiratory viruses (respiratory syncytial virus, Adenovirus, influenza, parainfluenza)	8

Adapted from Rañó et al: Thorax 2001; 56:379–387.

be dictated by the severity of the immune defect. For example, infections caused by filamentous fungi such as *Aspergillus* progress faster with increasing severity of neutropenia but may regress and become more focal when the neutrophil count recovers. Table 29-3 shows the common conditions that should be considered for different presentations of lung complications in immunocompromised patients.

Previous microbiologic results need to be reviewed, because these may provide a strong indication as to the cause of the present lung infection. For instance, infected indwelling vascular and urinary catheters can form foci of infection that can metastasize to the lungs, and previous *Aspergillus* infection may recur during new episodes of immunosuppression. Knowledge of previous and present CMV status identifies patients at risk of CMV pneumonitis, and positive sputum surveillance cultures for methicillin-resistant *Staphylococcus aureus* (MRSA) or *Pseudomonas aeruginosa* may indicate likely causes of a new pneumonia. In addition, positive samples from other patients may also be helpful, because local epidemics of respiratory virus infections are not uncommon in hospitals, and more rarely clusters of nosocomial *Aspergillus* (associated with building works on the hospital site) or *Legionella* infection can occur.

Other important factors that need to be taken into account include the patient's present antibiotic prophylaxis regimen and the travel history/ethnic background of the patient. A patient compliant with cotrimoxazole prophylaxis will rarely develop PCP, and fluconazole prophylaxis predisposes to non-albicans *Candida* infection. Patients with certain ethnic backgrounds or a pertinent travel history are more at risk of tuberculosis, endemic mycoses such as *Histoplasma*, or parasitic diseases such as disseminated *Strongyloides*. Finally, the patient's background lung structure and function need to be considered, because existing structural abnormalities may make certain pathogens more likely. For example, bronchiectasis could predispose to pneumonia caused by *P. aeruginosa* (Figure 29-1) and preexisting lung cavities to *Aspergillus* infection.

CLINICAL ASSESSMENT AND DIAGNOSTIC PROTOCOLS

Potential lung infections in immunocompromised patients are usually identified when a patient develops new respiratory symptoms or new radiologic findings with pyrexia. Occasionally, incidental radiologic or microbiologic results in an asymptomatic patient may suggest active lung infection. The initial assessment of an immunocompromised patient with potential lung infection requires a careful clinical assessment and review of the patient's previous laboratory and radiologic findings in

TABLE 29-2 Type of Immune Defect According to Disease/Treatment and Range of Pathogens Commonly Associated with Infections in Patients with This Type of Immune Defect

Immune Defect	Cause	Associated Pathogens
Neutropenia/functional neutrophil defects	Chemotherapy Early hematopoietic cell transplantation* Acute leukemia Chronic myelocytic leukemia Aplastic anemia Marrow infiltrations Azathioprine/mycophenolate[†] High-dose corticosteroids[†] Chronic granulomatous disease[†] Other inherited phagocyte defects[†]	Pyogenic bacteria and anaerobes Filamentous fungi (*Aspergillus*, rarer molds) *Candida* species
Cell-mediated immunity	Hematopoietic cell transplantation Chronic lymphocytic leukemia Lymphoma Tacrolimus/sirolimus Cyclosporin Azathioprine/mycophenolate High-dose corticosteroids Graft versus host disease Inherited disorders lymphocyte function	PCP Herpesviruses Respiratory viruses *L. pneumophila* Mycobacteria and *Nocardia* Endemic mycoses *T. gondii* *S. stercoralis*
Antibody deficiency	Hematopoietic cell transplantation Chronic lymphocytic leukemia Lymphoma Myeloma	Encapsulated bacteria (e.g., *Streptococcus pneumoniae*, *Haemophilus influenzae*) Herpesviruses

*Allograft up to 1 month, autografts usually <14 days.
[†]Usually have a normal neutrophil count but have functional defects in their function and/or a poor response to infection.

TABLE 29-3 Likely Differential Diagnosis Depending on CT Scan Appearances and the Rate of Development of the Clinical Problem

Predominate CT Scan Appearances	Rate of Progression		
	Acute (days)	Subacute (days to weeks)	Chronic (weeks)
Consolidation/focal ground glass infiltration	Bacterial pneumonia Aspiration Diffuse alveolar hemorrhage Adult respiratory distress syndrome (ARDS)*	Cryptogenic organizing pneumonia Aspiration *Mycobacteria*[†] *Nocardia*[†] Invasive filamentous fungi[†]	Cryptogenic organizing pneumonia Lymphoma *Mycobacteria*[†] *Nocardia*[†]
Diffuse ground glass infiltration	CMV pneumonia Viral pneumonia Diffuse alveolar hemorrhage ARDS*	CMV pneumonia PCP Idiopathic pneumonia syndrome (IPS) Drug reactions	Drug reaction
Nodules	Metastatic infection Invasive filamentous fungi	Metastatic infection Invasive filamentous fungi *Nocardia* *Mycobacteria*	Lymphoma Lymphoproliferative disease *Nocardia* *Mycobacteria*
Multiple nodules (> 10)	Metastatic infection	Metastatic infection *Mycobacteria*	Lymphoma Lymphoproliferative disease *Mycobacteria*
Bronchiolitis/tree and bud	Viral bronchiolitis *Chlamydia pneumoniae* *Mycoplasma pneumoniae*	Viral bronchiolitis *C. pneumoniae* *M. pneumoniae* Nontuberculous mycobacteria *Aspergillus* tracheobronchitis	Bronchiectasis Nontuberculous mycobacteria

*Extensive, patchy, mainly posterior.
[†]Usually focal patches.

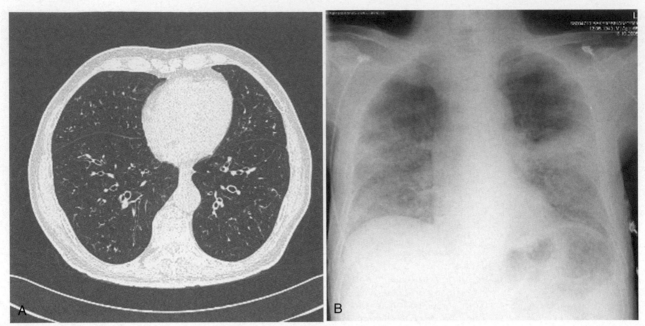

FIGURE 29-1 A, CT scan of a patient with a long history of chronic lymphatic leukemia and immunoglobulin deficiency showing dilated thick-walled bronchi caused by bronchiectasis. The patient produced purulent sputum daily, culture of which grew *P. aeruginosa*. **B,** A chest radiograph of the same patient presenting with a high fever, cough productive of purulent sputum, and marked hypoxia, showing consolidation (most marked in the left mid-zone) caused by *P. aeruginosa* pneumonia.

comparison to the new findings. Assessment of the patient's level of oxygenation is important for therapeutic considerations and may also aid diagnosis (severe hypoxia is more likely with a bacterial lobar pneumonia or extensive PCP or CMV infection). With the exception of bacterial pneumonia, chest radiographs are often not of sufficient sensitivity for an accurate assessment of lung shadowing, and a CT scan of the thorax will be required to fully evaluate the site and type of lung involvement. The high mortality associated with lung infections in immunocompromised patients requires that the clinical assessment and any necessary diagnostic tests be initiated rapidly.

All patients with suspected new lung infection will require blood and sputum cultures to be sent, as well as routine blood tests, and in many cases nasopharyngeal aspirates (NPA) for viruses and assessment of the CMV status. The main question for the respiratory physician is often when to use one of the three available invasive investigations: bronchoscopy (for BAL and possibly transbronchial biopsy), percutaneous radiologically guided biopsy, or surgical biopsy (usually performed with video-assisted thoracoscopy; VATs). Protocols based on the type of radiologic presentation (consolidation, diffuse ground glass, tree and bud changes, and nodules) to help guide this decision are described in Figures 29-2, 29-4, 29-5, and 29-6. These suggested protocols allow focused investigations, balancing the likelihood and necessity of a positive yield against the clinical probability that a particular disease will be identified and the potential complications of investigations. Because atypical presentations and dual pathology are not uncommon, the protocols should be used as guidance only, and individual cases may need a different approach. Although most cases of new lung infiltrates are caused by infection, immunocompromised patients are also at high risk of a range of noninfective causes of lung disease, including pulmonary edema, idiopathic pneumonia syndrome (IPS), and diffuse

alveolar hemorrhage (DAH) (see Chapter 63). These always have to be considered in the differential diagnosis and are included in the protocols. The protocols are discussed individually in the following.

Investigation of Consolidation (see Figure 29-2)

Rapidly developing unilateral consolidation is likely to be due to bacterial pneumonia and can be treated empirically with broad-spectrum antibiotics that are likely to be effective against gram-negative and gram-positive pathogens. If there is no improvement in the pyrexia or other clinical parameters of the patient's condition within 48–96 h, the most likely reason is infection with bacteria resistant to the first-line antibiotics. Second-line antibiotics likely to be effective against resistant organisms should be started. Alternatively, for patients at high risk of invasive fungal infection, or with nodular or widespread patchy consolidation, failure of first-line therapy should precipitate FOB for BAL and perhaps transbronchial biopsy. Patients with subacute or chronic consolidation in whom sputum is nondiagnostic or patients with rapidly developing consolidation not responding to second-line antibiotic therapy will need investigation by FOB for BAL and probably transbronchial biopsy. If FOB fails to achieve a diagnosis, percutaneous (mainly for dense consolidation adjacent to the pleura) or surgical biopsy should be considered.

Investigation of Diffuse Ground Glass Infiltration (Figures 29-3 and 29-4)

Diffuse ground glass changes on a CT scan have a wide differential diagnosis, including CMV and viral pneumonias, PCP, extensive bacterial infection and noninfective causes such as ARDS, drug toxicity, and IPS associated with hematopoietic cell transplantations (see Chapter 58). As a consequence, although these patients are often hypoxic and at risk of complications, unless an NPA identifies a respiratory viral infection, early

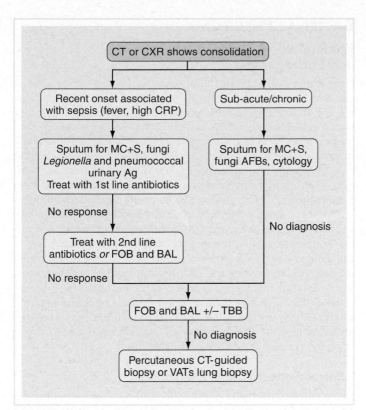

FIGURE 29-2 Investigation of consolidation in immunocompromised patients.

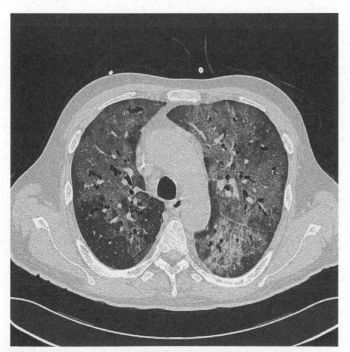

FIGURE 29-3 CT scan showing widespread bilateral ground glass infiltration in a hematopoietic cell transplant recipient. These appearances have a wide differential diagnosis, including CMV pneumonia, PCP, drug reactions, and IPS, and usually require early invasive investigation even though with such widespread lung disease the patient is likely to have significant hypoxia.

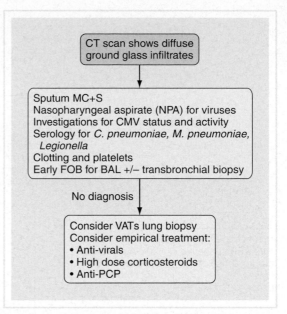

FIGURE 29-4 Investigation of diffuse ground glass pulmonary infiltrates in immunocompromised patients.

FOB with BAL and, if possible, transbronchial biopsy is usually necessary. Negative results from FOB do not exclude infective causes, and a decision then needs to be made about empirical treatment or proceeding to a VATs lung biopsy. CT-guided biopsy of diffuse lung disease will not be appropriate because of the high risk of complications and low diagnostic yield.

Investigation of "Tree and Bud" Changes
(Figure 29-5)

"Tree and bud" changes suggest small airways pathosis, which in immunocompromised patients is likely to be caused by respiratory virus infection, *Chlamydia pneumoniae* or *Mycoplasma pneumoniae*, or (especially if the changes are focal and associated with nodular changes) *Aspergillus* tracheobronchitis. Subacute or chronic changes could also reflect bronchiectasis or nontuberculous *Mycobacteria* infection. If an NPA is negative, early FOB for BAL and bronchial biopsies of macroscopically inflamed bronchial mucosa should be performed. *Aspergillus* tracheobronchitis is usually obvious macroscopically at FOB and is readily confirmed by culture and cytologic examination of bronchial washings and by bronchial biopsy, whereas viral, *C. pneumoniae* and *M. pneumoniae*, infections are often difficult to diagnose but are generally self-limiting illnesses. Hence, further investigation by surgical biopsy is usually not necessary.

Investigation of Pulmonary Nodules
(Figure 29-6)

The differential diagnosis of pulmonary nodules includes infection with *Aspergillus* (or other invasive filamentous fungi), *Nocardia*, or *Mycobacteria*. *Aspergillus* and *Nocardia* tend to cause a small number of nodules, whereas *Mycobacteria* can also cause large numbers of nodules. In addition, blood-borne spread of bacteria or *Candida* from infected indwelling devices can cause a variable number (often very numerous) of pulmonary nodules. Nodules caused by pyogenic bacterial and viral pneumonia tend to be associated with other radiologic findings such as ground glass infiltrates or consolidation. The other

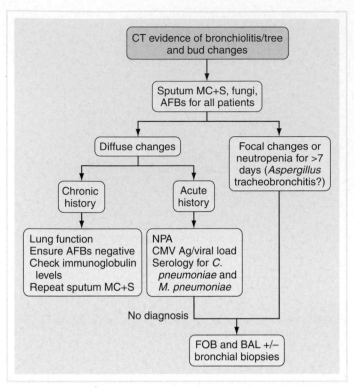

FIGURE 29-5 Investigation of "tree and bud"/bronchiolitis in immunocompromised patients.

major causes of nodules are underlying malignant disease or lymphoproliferative disorders caused by prolonged immunosuppression. In the absence of CT signs suggestive of invasive filamentous fungal infection (the halo and crescent signs), nodules in patients with line infections, or a positive blood culture could be treated empirically as metastatic infection. For most other patients with lung nodules, FOB for BAL is necessary, although for patients at high risk of invasive filamentous fungal infections with CT changes suggestive of *Aspergillus* infection, empirical antifungal therapy is a reasonable alternative strategy. If FOB is nondiagnostic, the patient should progress to percutaneous CT-guided or VATs lung biopsy, which is frequently diagnostic if invasive fungal infection is present because of specific histologic changes.

BRONCHOSCOPY

FOB with BAL of the affected part of the lung is the main invasive diagnostic test used in immunocompromised patients with pneumonia. Although many of these patients are hypoxic and have low platelet counts and/or abnormal clotting, FOB is generally safe and has a diagnostic yield of 30–50%. Even a negative result can be helpful, because exclusion of active infection is necessary to make a diagnosis of IPS after hematopoietic cell transplantation. In the authors experience, peroral FOB can be performed without significant bleeding in patients with a platelet count of 10,000/mL. Because BAL can commonly reduce PaO_2 by 2.5 kPa, BAL should only be performed in patients with marked hypoxia or severe tachypnea after careful consideration, because the procedure may precipitate the need for intubation and mechanical ventilation. Transbronchial biopsy improves the diagnostic yield of FOB but should be avoided unless the patient will be able to tolerate a pneumothorax and has a platelet count above 50,000/mL.

BACTERIAL PNEUMONIA

Epidemiology, Risk Factors, and Pathogenesis

Pneumonia caused by bacterial pathogens is the most common cause of lung infection in the immunocompromised host, causing approximately 40–50% of infective episodes. The main risk factor is neutropenia, but cell-mediated immune defects and functional defects in phagocyte responses because of cytotoxic or immunosuppressive therapy will also markedly increase the risk of pneumonia developing. Antibody deficiencies associated with lymphoproliferative disorders, myeloma, and after hematopoietic cell transplantation predispose to pneumonia with encapsulated organisms such as *Streptococcus pneumoniae* and *Haemophilus influenzae*. Many cases of bacterial pneumonia are nosocomial infections in patients who have been in the hospital for long periods and who have previously been treated with antibiotics and have had the normal oropharyngeal flora replaced mainly by gram-negative bacteria. As a consequence, the range of potential organisms causing bacterial pneumonia is very different to that seen in community-acquired pneumonia, with a high frequency of resistant organisms such as *P. aeruginosa* and MRSA (see Table 29-1).

Clinical Features and Diagnosis

Many cases of bacterial pneumonia will present with a similar clinical picture to that seen in immunocompetent hosts, with new-onset fever, cough, chest and radiologic signs of lobar consolidation and a rapid rise in inflammatory markers such as CRP (Figure 29-7). However, more insidious or diffuse disease is not uncommon and is harder to differentiate from other infective or noninfective causes. CT scanning of the thorax may be helpful in differentiating bacterial from fungal or viral pneumonia, with dense focal consolidation with a lobar distribution suggesting bacterial pneumonia. Blood culture will identify the causative organism in approximately 20% of cases (see Figure 29-7). Patients with an atypical clinical presentation or who do not respond to first- or second-line antibiotics should have an FOB and BAL, which has a high diagnostic yield for bacterial pneumonia. Protected specimen brush probably adds little information over and above directed BAL. Lung biopsy is unlikely to show specific features that confirm bacterial pneumonia and is mainly used to exclude other causes of lung infiltrates. Antigen testing of the urine may identify *Legionella pneumophila* or *S. pneumoniae* infections.

Treatment

Accurate assessment of the patient's level of oxygenation and oxygen therapy to maintain a normal PaO_2 is essential, and continuous positive airway pressure (CPAP) support may be necessary. Intubation of immunocompromised patients is associated with a poor prognosis (greater than 95% mortality in some series) but may be necessary if the patient's underlying disease does not preclude mechanical ventilation. Because of the range of bacteria that cause pneumonia in immunocompromised patients, initial therapy should be with antibiotics with good efficacy against the local pattern of hospital-acquired infections and is, therefore, likely to include extended-range β-lactams, aminoglycosides, or ciprofloxacin. If there is no response within 72–96 h and no organism has been isolated, the antibiotics should be switched to another broad-spectrum parenteral antibiotic (e.g., a carbapenem) in case the causative pathogen is resistant to the first-line therapy, and consideration

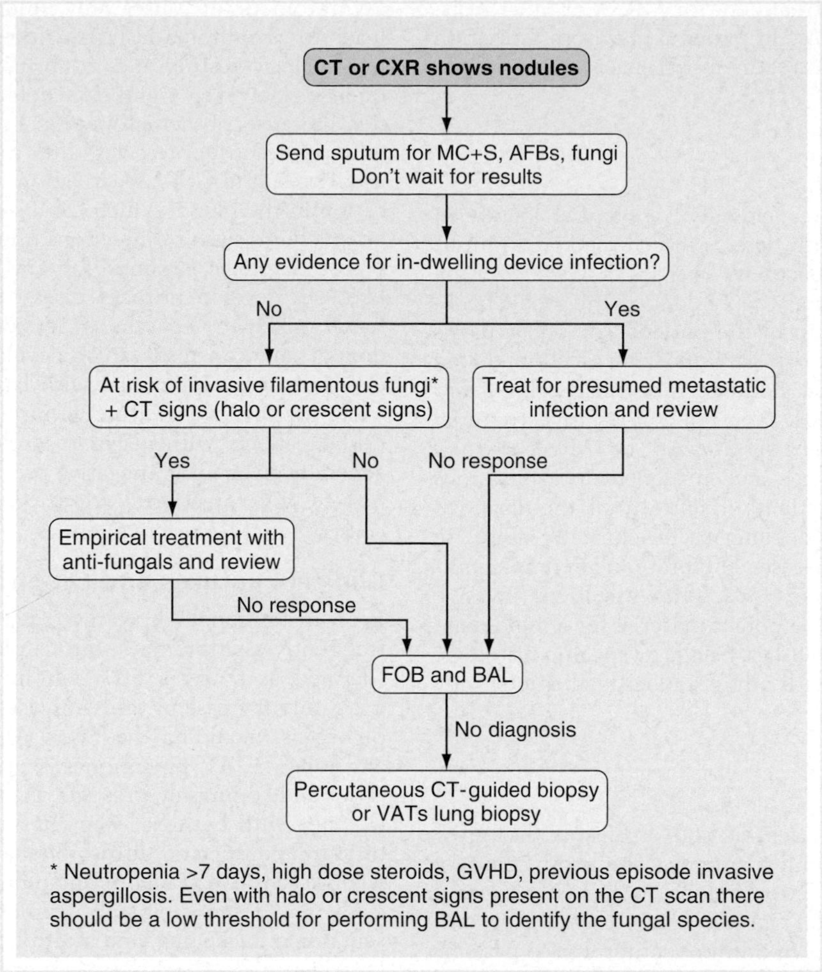

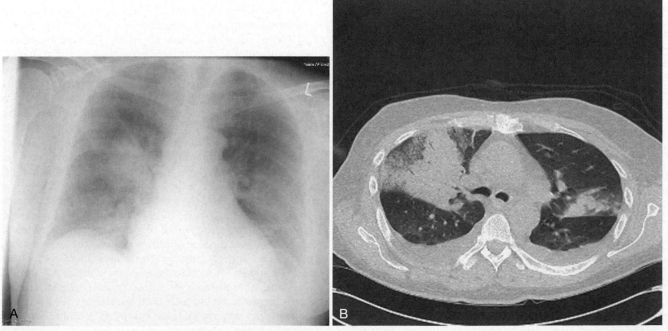

CT or CXR shows nodules

Send sputum for MC+S, AFBs, fungi
Don't wait for results

Any evidence for in-dwelling device infection?

No   Yes

At risk of invasive filamentous fungi*   Treat for presumed metastatic
+ CT signs (halo or crescent signs)   infection and review

Yes   No   No response

Empirical treatment with
anti-fungals and review

No response

FOB and BAL

No diagnosis

Percutaneous CT-guided biopsy
or VATs lung biopsy

* Neutropenia >7 days, high dose steroids, GVHD, previous episode invasive
aspergillosis. Even with halo or crescent signs present on the CT scan there
should be a low threshold for performing BAL to identify the fungal species.

FIGURE 29-6 Investigation of pulmonary nodules in the immunocompromised patient.

FIGURE 29-7 A, Chest radiograph showing a masslike consolidation in the right middle zone of a patient with acute myeloid leukemia recently treated with chemotherapy and presenting with a high temperature but no respiratory symptoms after 9 days of neutropenia. **B,** CT scan of the same patient, showing that the shadowing is due to dense consolidation in the right upper lobe, with a smaller area of consolidation in the left upper lobe. The blood cultures grew *E. coli,* and the patient improved rapidly on appropriate antibiotics, suggesting the consolidation was a hospital-acquired pneumonia caused by *E. coli.*

should be given to starting treatment for MRSA or other resistant gram-positive organisms. In patients in whom aspiration may have occurred, specific treatment for anaerobic organisms should be considered.

MYCOBACTERIA

Mycobacterial infections are generally a potential long-term complication of patients with defects in cell-mediated immunity and tend to develop subacutely. The risk of *Mycobacterium tuberculosis* infection is strongly dependent on the ethnic background and country of origin of the patient, and tuberculosis should be considered in at-risk patients with a cell-mediated immune defect, patchy or nodular lung shadowing from high-risk ethnic backgrounds. Nontuberculous mycobacterial infections (e.g., *Mycobacterium kansasii* or *Mycobacterium avium-intracellulare* complex) are infrequent complications in immunocompromised patients. Exclusion of the diagnosis by negative culture takes too long to be clinically useful in patients with progressive disease. Therefore, if there is significant clinical suspicion of mycobacterial infection, invasive investigations are necessary to obtain material for a rapid diagnosis by identification of acid-fast bacilli or specific histologic changes. Treatment is with the standard chemotherapy regimens.

NOCARDIA

Nocardia are gram-positive aerobic soil organisms that grow relatively slowly as branching filaments. The most common species causing human infection belong to the *N. asteroides* complex, but other *Nocardia* can also cause disease. Approximately 2% of lung infections in immunocompromised patients are due to *Nocardia* and, like mycobacterial infections, tend to affect patients with defects in cell-mediated immunity. Inhalation can result in lung infection, presenting as a relatively acute pneumonia or a more indolent disease similar to infection with *Mycobacteria* or *Aspergillus*. Radiologic changes include patches of consolidation, large nodules, and cavitation. Pleural involvement occurs in up to a third of cases. Hematogenous spread to other organs, mainly the brain, is common. The diagnosis is made by microscopy or histologic examination showing characteristic beaded branching gram-positive and weakly acid-fast filaments or by prolonged aerobic culture of respiratory samples. Blood cultures can also be positive. Most *Nocardia* are sensitive to cotrimoxazole, as well as carbapenems, amikacin, third-generation cephalosporins, tetracyclines, and co-amoxiclav, but treatment needs to be very prolonged, lasting up to 12 months in immunocompromised patients. In case series, the mortality associated with *Nocardia* infections is up to 70%.

CYTOMEGALOVIRUS

Epidemiology, Risk Factors, and Pathogenesis

CMV is the largest member of the Herpesviridae family of human double-stranded DNA viruses. It has a 230-kb genome that encodes more than 200 products, which are expressed in three overlapping phases termed immediate-early, early, and late. Infection in the general population is common, mainly occurring in children or young adults, but is usually asymptomatic or causes only mild disease. Previous infection leads to asymptomatic latent infection that can be identified by serologic testing and is normally of little clinical consequence. However, significant defects in cell-mediated immunity because of hematopoietic cell transplant or treatment with immunosuppressives after organ transplantation commonly result in CMV reactivation, characterized by viral replication in the blood, which can lead to CMV disease when an organ shows signs of infection. Immunocompromised patients whose serologic findings for CMV are negative are highly likely to develop primary disease when given transplants or blood products containing leukocytes from CMV-positive donors and can also rarely develop primary infection after exposure to an individual with latent CMV infection who is excreting the virus. Although rare now that immunocompromised patients with negative serologic findings for CMV are generally given CMV-negative products, disease caused by primary CMV infection tends to be more severe than disease caused by CMV reactivation.

Clinical Features and Diagnosis

Even in immunocompromised patients, CMV reactivation is frequently asymptomatic but can lead to the CMV syndrome (defined as fever, a 50% fall in the leukocyte count, and a 2.5-fold increase in transaminases) and infection in a variety of organs, including the liver, CNS, gastrointestinal system, and lungs. CMV pneumonia is usually relatively insidious in onset and commonly presents with fever, malaise, cough, and dyspnea with hypoxia. The chest radiograph may be normal or show nonspecific diffuse bilateral infiltrates. The CT scan is more sensitive at identifying pulmonary infiltrates and classically would show bibasal symmetric ground glass opacities, septal line thickening, and multiple small centrilobular nodules (see Figure 29-4). However, more asymmetric changes, consolidation, and effusions are not uncommon. The main clinical differential diagnoses are IPS, drug-induced pneumonitis, and (in patients not receiving effective prophylaxis) PCP.

To establish a diagnosis of CMV pneumonia first requires confirmation of CMV reactivation, usually by quantifying CMV copy number in the blood by PCR or by testing for the presence of CMV antigenemia. However, although CMV pneumonitis is unlikely in the absence of CMV reactivation, evidence of reactivation does not mean that new lung infiltrates are due to CMV. The greater the level of CMV in the blood, the greater the chance that CMV is causing disease, especially if the viral load is increasing rapidly. However, definitive confirmation that CMV is causing pneumonia requires identification of CMV in the respiratory tract, usually by FOB to obtain BAL and preferably a transbronchial biopsy, or possibly a VATs lung biopsy. Cytologic results can be obtained rapidly, and the presence of "owl's eyes" intranuclear inclusions is pathognomic for CMV infection. However, cytology is a relatively insensitive test for CMV pneumonia. CMV can be cultured from respiratory samples by use of fibroblast cell culture and looking for the appearance of a distinctive cytopathogenic effect. However, viral culture takes at least a week and, therefore, is of little clinical benefit. Hence, the main diagnostic techniques used to identify CMV in respiratory samples are rapid tests based on probing the samples directly for the presence of CMV antigens or by probing cell cultures inoculated with the samples after 24–48 h incubation (the shell vial or early antigen detection assays). These assays have good sensitivity compared with the "gold standard" of viral culture. However, the sensitivity of viral culture is questionable, and CMV pneumonia maybe difficult to prove in many potential cases. Tests for diagnosing CMV infections and their role in assessing patients with potential CMV pneumonia are described in Table 29-4.

Treatment

CMV pneumonia can be treated with ganciclovir, foscarnet, or cidofovir (see Table 29-5). The purine analog ganciclovir is the preferred treatment and, once phosphorylated within infected cells, competitively inhibits viral DNA polymerase.

TABLE 29-4 Types and Roles of Diagnostic Tests for Cytomegalovirus Infection

Test	Sample	Time Needed	Method	Role and General Comments
Serology	Blood	24–72 h	Enzyme-linked immunosorbent assay for CMV-specific IgM and IgG	Identifies latent infection. IgM unreliable as a marker for new infection
Antigenemia	Blood	6 h	Immunofluorescent staining of neutrophils with antibodies to pp65	Identifies CMV reactivation. Demanding on laboratory resources
Quantitative PCR	Blood, BAL	24 h	Uses PCR to amplify CMV DNA and calculate viral copy number in sample	Identifies CMV reactivation. Kinetics of copy number over time are important. PCR from BAL may identify CMV pneumonia
Culture	Blood, BAL	1–6 wk	Inoculate fibroblast cell culture and look for CMV cytopathic effect	Identifies CMV pneumonia, but low sensitivity and too slow to be useful
Immunocytochemistry	BAL, lung biopsy	6 h	Probe tissue samples with monoclonal antibodies to CMV	Identifies CMV pneumonia, but sensitivity with BAL probably poor
Shell vial assay or early antigen fluorescent foci test	BAL, blood	24–48 h	Probe with antibodies to CMV fibroblast cell culture 24+ hours after inoculation with sample	Identifies CMV pneumonia, sensitive and relatively rapid
Cytology	BAL	6 h	"Owl's eyes" intranuclear inclusions	Identifies CMV pneumonia, poor sensitivity
Histology	Lung biopsy	24–48 h	"Owl's eyes" intranuclear inclusions	Existing "gold standard" for diagnosis for CMV pneumonia

TABLE 29-5 Treatment Options for Viral Lung Infections

Treatment	Dose	Mode of Action	Viruses	Role and General Comments
Ganciclovir	2.5–5 mg/kg b.d./t.d.s. IV	Inhibitor of viral DNA polymerase	CMV, HSV, HHV6	First-line therapy; myelosuppressive; good efficacy
Foscarnet	60 mg/kg t.d.s. IV	Inhibitor of viral DNA polymerase	CMV	Second-line therapy; good efficacy; nephrotoxic
Acyclovir	10–15 mg/kg t.d.s. IV	Inhibitor of viral DNA polymerase	HSV, VZ, HHV6	Toxicity relatively uncommon
Cidofovir	1–5 mg/kg weekly IV	Inhibitor of viral DNA polymerase	CMV Adenovirus	Third-line agent for CMV infection; efficacy against adenovirus unclear; nephrotoxic
Ribavirin	0.8 mg/kg inh	Nucleoside analog	RSV, PIV, influenza, adenovirus	Questionable benefit; nebulizer requires a scavenger tent due to toxicity; given over 12–18 h
IVIG	e.g., 500 mg o.d.	Passive vaccination	CMV, RSV	Combination treatment with antiviral agent
Palivizumab	15 mg/kg IV	Humanized anti-RSV monoclonal antibody	RSV	Efficacy unclear; used in combination with ribavirin
Amantidine	100 mg b.d. orally	M2 inhibitor	Influenza A	Efficacy unclear; lowers incidence of progression to pneumonia?
Zanamivir	10 mg b.d. inh	Neuraminidase inhibitor	Influenza	Efficacy unclear; perhaps increased speed of recovery
Oseltamivir	75 mg b.d. orally	Neuraminidase inhibitor	Influenza	Efficacy unclear; perhaps increased speed of recovery

Ganciclovir has significant marrow-depressing effects and may be too toxic for patients with existing pancytopenia or who have had hematopoietic cell transplants. An oral formulation exists, and recently an oral prodrug formulation of ganciclovir called valganciclovir has been introduced. The second-line therapy foscarnet also inhibits the activity of viral DNA polymerase (by binding to the pyrophosphate binding site) and frequently causes significant renal abnormalities that limit treatment. Cidofovir has a broad spectrum of activity against DNA viruses, and like ganciclovir requires host cell phosphorylation before acting as a competitive inhibitor of viral DNA polymerases. Cidofovir causes both myelosuppression and renal toxicity, and patients should be prehydrated and given probenecid before starting treatment. Patients with CMV disease are also frequently given hyperimmune intravenous immunoglobulin (IVIG) as passive vaccination therapy. There are very few studies comparing the efficacy of these drugs in CMV pneumonia. Treatment lasts from 14–21 days. One popular treatment strategy is preemptive treatment of patients developing evidence of significant CMV reactivation before CMV disease develops, trading the increased numbers of patients requiring treatment for a better outcome in those developing disease because of earlier initiation of therapy. Mortality of CMV pneumonia is up to 50% in hematopoietic transplant recipients, but less in other types of immunocompromised patients.

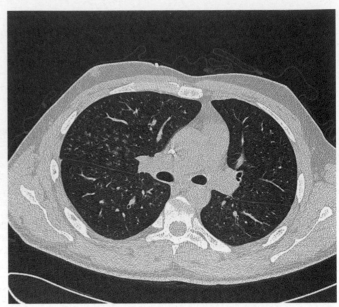

FIGURE 29-8 CT scan showing "tree and bud" changes (most obvious in the right upper lobe) caused by parainfluenza virus 3 bronchiolitis in a patient with relapsed acute myeloid leukemia who had had chemotherapy 25 days previously and presented with coryzal symptoms, cough, and a mild fever.

OTHER VIRAL INFECTIONS

Other Herpesviruses

Herpes simplex (HSV), varicella-zoster (VZ), and human herpesvirus 6 (HHV6) are rare causes of lung infection in immunocompromised patients, with a similar presentation to CMV pneumonia. HSV and VZ may have characteristic skin involvement. Microbiologic diagnosis relies on isolation of the virus from skin lesions or BAL, and treatment is with high-dose acyclovir.

Respiratory Viruses

Lower respiratory tract infections with respiratory viruses are relatively common in immunocompromised patients and are acquired by inhalation of infected respiratory droplets from other infected patients or mildly affected immunocompetent contacts. Respiratory viral infections are generally a late complication in transplant patients, reflecting continuing defects in cell-mediated immunity in hematopoietic cell transplant recipients and/or treatment with immunosuppressive therapy. The most common viruses identified are respiratory syncytial virus (RSV), influenza A, and parainfluenza virus (PIV). Infections with adenovirus and human metapneumovirus also occur, and recent studies have suggested that rhinovirus infection may be more common than previously thought. Respiratory virus infections often cause a bronchiolitis, presenting with cough, fever, wheeze, and inspiratory squeaks along with upper respiratory tract symptoms. The chest radiograph may be normal, but a CT scan will show evidence of small airways involvement, with widespread "tree and bud" changes (Figure 29-8). This clinical picture is highly suggestive of infection by a respiratory virus, with the main differential being *Chlamydia* or *Mycoplasma* infection or possibly *Aspergillus* tracheobronchitis. However, respiratory viruses may present with alveolar shadowing that has a much wider differential

diagnosis. The diagnosis can be rapidly confirmed by identifying viral antigen in a NPA or BAL sample (e.g., by use of a diffuse immunofluorescence test). Antigen testing is more sensitive in BAL than NPA, so a negative NPA should lead to FOB. Viral cultures from respiratory samples are the existing "gold standards" for the diagnosis of respiratory viruses but may be replaced by PCR because this probably has greater sensitivity. Treatment options depend on the underlying virus and are shown in Table 29-4. In general, the efficacy of antiviral treatments is not clear. In the absence of pneumonia, the mortality from respiratory virus infection in immunocompromised patients is relatively low, although infections can persist for weeks and might predispose to the development of obliterative bronchiolitis in hematopoietic cell transplant recipients. Patients with respiratory viral infection should be isolated, because these viruses can cause nosocomial epidemics.

INVASIVE ASPERGILLOSIS

Epidemiology, Risk Factors, and Pathogenesis

Invasive infections with *Aspergillus* are a common and important cause of lung infection in immunodeficient patients. *Aspergillus* species are saprophytic filamentous fungi that are found ubiquitously in the environment. They propagate by dispersal of airborne spores, which are 2–3 µm in diameter and, therefore, able to reach the distal airway. Exposure to airborne spores is essentially continuous, but this rarely causes a clinical problem unless the host's immune response is impaired. However, in a patient with impaired macrophage or neutrophil function, the spores can germinate and form a colony of branching multicellular hyphae that gradually expands and penetrates through host tissue, causing invasive pulmonary aspergillosis (IPA). The usual site of infection is the respiratory tract, including the sinuses, but blood-borne spread to internal organs (especially the CNS), bone, and skin is common. The most frequently isolated species causing infection are *A. fumigatus* (66% of cases), *A. flavus* (14%), *A. niger* (7%), and *A. terreus* (4%).

Clinical Features

Patients with significant neutropenia for longer than 10 days are most at risk of invasive aspergillosis, which means IPA is mainly a disease that affects patients with hematologic malignancies receiving chemotherapy, aplastic anemia, or in the early phase after hematogenous cell transplant. The risk of IPA is directly proportional to the depth and duration of neutropenia, developing in more than 50% of patients with neutropenia lasting for more than 4 weeks. Other patients at high risk include those who receive high-dose corticosteroids and/or have graft versus host disease (GVHD) (accounting for cases of IPA in the late phase after hematopoietic cell transplant), lung and liver transplant recipients, and patients with inherited disorders of phagocyte function such as chronic granulomatous disease (CGD), in which mutations in genes encoding the NADPH oxidase system impair the phagocyte oxidative burst.

Clinical presentation depends on the level of immunosuppression. Fever may be the only symptom of IPA, although cough, pleuritic chest pain, and hemoptysis are common. Chest radiographs show expanding patches of irregular consolidation or nodules that may cavitate. CT scans are very helpful, because they might identify the lung as the source of infection in patients with pyrexia and a normal chest radiograph and will define the nodular nature of infiltrates (with there being usually fewer than six nodules present in IPA) seen on chest radiograph and may show specific signs associated with IPA. These include the halo sign (an area of lower attenuation shadowing around a nodule or patch of consolidation), an early sign that usually occurs in the first week of infection (Figure 29-9), and the air crescent sign (a partial cavity formed by infarcted necrotic lung), a later sign that usually occurs around the third week of infection. If the patient's neutrophil count recovers, an intrapulmonary cavity containing a fungal ball may be created (see Figure 29-9). *Aspergillus* has a predilection for growing into blood vessels, and patients with IPA may have fatal massive hemorrhage. An unusual form of IPA is *Aspergillus* tracheobronchitis, in which infection is restricted to the tracheobronchial tree and presents with a severe unremitting cough and pyrexia. CT scans might show focal areas of bronchial wall thickening and "tree and bud" small airways disease (Figure 29-10). Milder degrees of immunosuppression associated with steroid and cytotoxic therapy lead to a more indolent form of invasive aspergillosis, called chronic necrotizing pulmonary aspergillosis (CNPA). CNPA presents as an indolent patch of consolidation with or without cavitation that progresses over weeks or months (Figure 29-11) and is associated with cough and marked systemic symptoms of malaise, fatigue, and weight loss.

Microbiologic Diagnosis (Table 29-6)

In high-risk patients with a compatible clinical syndrome and CT scan appearances highly suggestive of IPA (halo or crescent signs), the diagnosis can be made clinically and may not require confirmation by invasive investigations. However, some *Aspergillus* species (e.g., *A. terreus*) are resistant to amphotericin B, and a similar clinical presentation to IPA can be caused by rarer filamentous fungi that have different drug sensitivities to *Aspergillus*. Hence, microbiologic confirmation is reassuring, because it ensures that appropriate treatment is given. Microbiologic diagnosis of IPA can be achieved by culture, cytologic, or histologic appearances in BAL or lung biopsy specimens, or by the detection of fungal cell wall antigen (galactomannan or glucan) in blood or BAL. Compared with immunocompetent patients, isolation of *Aspergillus* from BAL in a high-risk immunodeficient patient is highly predictive of IPA. However, culture and microscopy for *Aspergillus* from BAL is relatively insensitive, identifying only 50% of

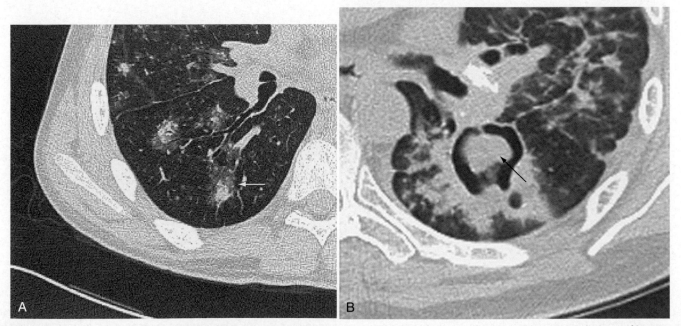

FIGURE 29-9 A, CT scan showing a nodule of invasive aspergillosis surrounded by an area of lower attenuation ground glass infiltration (the halo sign, indicated by the *white arrow*). **B,** CT scan showing an area of invasive aspergillosis that has cavitated, with the cavity containing a mycetoma (*arrow*).

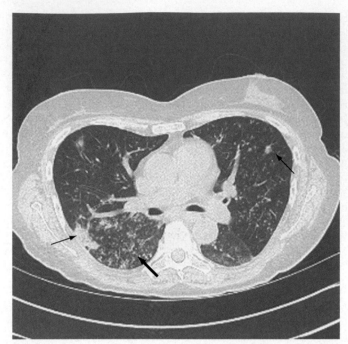

FIGURE 29-10 CT scan showing patchy "tree and bud" changes (*large arrow*) and occasional nodules (*smaller arrows*) caused by *Aspergillus* tracheobronchitis. The patient presented with a fever and a persistent cough and had had prolonged severe neutropenia caused by non-Hodgkin's lymphoma and recent chemotherapy.

cases of IPA. Culture from sputum and blood is even less sensitive. Biopsy of the affected area (either percutaneous under CT guidance or surgical by VATs) and histologic identification of fungal hyphae infiltrating through lung tissue is a highly sensitive and rapid method of diagnosing IPA. Hence, CT-guided or VATs biopsy should be considered in all patients with nodules not responding to conventional antibacterial antibiotics, especially if the BAL was nondiagnostic. Because invasive tests are most likely to be positive in patients with severe infection in whom mortality is high despite appropriate treatment, noninvasive tests have been developed to identify patients likely to have early IPA. These include detection of galactomannan or glucan cell wall antigen in the blood (or BAL if FOB has been performed) or PCR for *Aspergillus* DNA from the blood. These tests are highly sensitive, and, if performed routinely as surveillance of high-risk patients, could lead to preemptive antifungal therapy before clinically apparent disease has developed. However, galactomannan antigen frequently gives false-positive results (especially in patients treated with piperacillin-tazobactam) and as a consequence in many centers is not used routinely. FOB is usually diagnostic in *Aspergillus* tracheobronchitis, with distinctive macroscopic appearances of patchy highly inflamed mucosa with necrotic white slough, *Aspergillus* found in cultures and/or cytologic examination of bronchial washings, and evidence of fungal invasion of the respiratory mucosa in bronchial biopsy specimens. The diagnosis of CNPA is difficult, because the positive predictive value of isolation of *Aspergillus* from BAL in

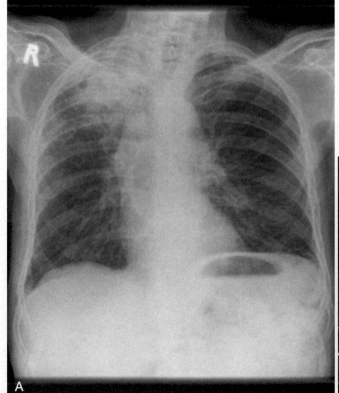

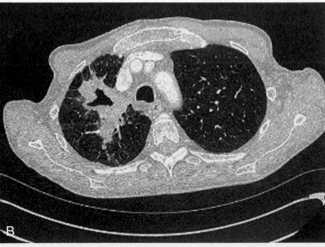

FIGURE 29-11 A, Chest radiograph showing a mass in the right upper lobe caused by CNPA in a patient treated for rheumatoid arthritis with a variety of immunosuppressive therapies. The diagnosis was confirmed by histologic identification of *Aspergillus* hyphae invading lung tissue in a VATs surgical biopsy sample. **B,** CT scan of the same patient, showing that the mass is caused by a thick-walled irregular cavity with no air–fluid level.

patients with lesser degrees of immunosuppression is poor, and surgical biopsy is frequently needed to exclude malignancy and confirm fungal invasion of lung tissue.

Treatment

The treatment options for invasive aspergillosis have been considerably improved by the introduction of a new azole, voriconazole, and a new class of antifungal agents, the echinocandins, the first example of which to reach clinical practice is caspofungin. Doses, modes of action, and common toxicities for the different treatment options are given in Table 29-7. Amphotericin B, voriconazole, and caspofungin seem to have similar efficacy, and which drug is used depends on the patient's tolerance of each drug and any preexisting medical conditions (e.g., amphotericin B should be avoided in patients with renal problems). Itraconazole is less efficacious and should be reserved for oral treatment of patients recovering from IPA after induction treatment with amphotericin B, caspofungin, or voriconazole or for the long-term treatment required for CNPA. Because voriconazole is more effective and can also be given orally, it is likely it will replace itraconazole as the oral preparation for treating cases of IPA. At present, the role of combination therapy is not clear, but is potentially attractive given that the three effective drugs have different mechanisms of action. Surgery should be urgently considered in patients with major hemoptysis to prevent future fatal bleeding and as a primary therapy for single lesions caused by IPA. In addition, the surgical removal of solitary areas of previous IPA that are causing persisting lung shadowing or contain an intracavitary mycetoma may prevent recurrence of IPA during subsequent immunosuppression. Treatment of IPA may have to be prolonged, and for CNPA is likely to last months. Mortality is high, at approximately 50% for IPA and 33% for CNPA, because of a combination of uncontrolled invasive aspergillosis and the underlying disease.

OTHER FUNGAL INFECTIONS

Non-*Aspergillus* Filamentous Fungi

Although *Aspergillus* species dominate infections caused by molds, other filamentous fungi can cause invasive pulmonary infections in immunocompromised patients including *Fusarium*, *Zygomycetes*, *Scedosporium*, and *Penicillium*. These infections are often clinically indistinguishable from invasive aspergillosis but have a different spectrum of susceptibilities to antifungal agents. Hence, non-*Aspergillus* filamentous fungal infection needs to be considered in patients with a clinical diagnosis of IPA who are not responding to antifungal therapy. Diagnosis is made by culture from respiratory samples or lung biopsy, and mortality is very high.

Candida Species

Candida species rarely cause pneumonia but may cause metastatic lung infection in patients with candidemia or colonization of an indwelling vascular catheter. Patients will present with pyrexia and radiologic evidence of lung nodules (sometimes very large). The frequent use of fluconazole as prophylaxis has led to increasing isolation of non-albicans species such as *Candida glabrata* and *Candida parapsilosis*.

Cryptococcus and Endemic Fungi

Cryptococcus neoformans infections are acquired by inhalation, and although respiratory infection is often asymptomatic, cryptococcal disease can cause multifocal consolidation and severe pneumonia in patients with defects in cell-mediated immunity. Diagnosis is by microscopic identification or culture of C. *neoformans* from respiratory tract samples, and suggested treatment is intravenous amphotericin B in combination with flucytosine followed by oral fluconazole. The mortality of cryptococcal pneumonia is 30%. Reactivation of latent infection with endemic fungi such as *Histoplasma* and *Coccidiodes* may occur in patients with defects in cell-mediated immunity and should be considered in patients who have lived in relevant geographical areas presenting with multifocal lung shadowing, especially if there is evidence of extrapulmonary involvement.

Pneumocystis jirovecii

Although PCP is particularly associated with HIV infection, PCP is also an important cause of pneumonia in non-HIV immunocompromised patients, causing 2–3% of lung infections in these patients. The clinical presentation can be fulminant or more insidious, and cough, dyspnea, and respiratory failure are common. The chest radiograph usually shows bilateral infiltrates but may be normal. CT scans of the thorax will show ground glass opacities with a predilection for the lung

TABLE 29-6 Types and Roles of Diagnostic Tests for Invasive Aspergillosis

Test	Sample	Time Needed	Method	Role and General Comments
Culture	Sputum, BAL, CSF, biopsy	2–4 days	Culture on fungal media	Low sensitivity (50% for BAL)
Cytology	BAL, biopsy	6 h	Microscopy for fungal elements	May not distinguish between fungal species
Histology	Biopsy	24–48 h	Visualization of dichotomous branching septate hyphae	Fungal stains necessary; may not distinguish between fungal species
Antigen testing	Serum, BAL	6 h	Galactomannan detection by ELISA	Cell wall antigen for *Aspergillus* and *Penicillium* species; sensitive; false positives occur
PCR	Blood, BAL	24 h	Amplification of target DNA	Technically challenging; role not yet established
CT appearances	—	Instant	Identification of halo or crescent signs	Specific for invasive filamentous fungal infection but does not identify fungal species

TABLE 29-7 Treatment Options for Invasive Aspergillosis

Treatment	Dose	Mode of Action	Role and General Comments	Toxicity
Amphotericin B	1–1.5 mg/kg per day IV	Binds to ergosterol in the fungal cell membrane	Effective; cheap; withdrawn in 1/3 of patients because of toxicity	Fever and chills; phlebitis; hypokalemia, hypomagnesaemia; uremia; bronchospasm; gastrointestinal disturbance; muscle pain
Lipid formulations of amphotericin B	1–5 mg/kg per day IV	As above	Expensive; much improved toxicity profile	As above (much lower incidence)
Itraconazole	200 mg o.d./ b.d./ t.d.s. IV/orally	Inhibits ergosterol biosynthesis	Poor efficacy versus acute IPA; poor absorbance (check levels)	Gastrointestinal disturbance; elevated hepatic transaminases; heart failure; neuropathy
Voriconazole	6 mg/kg ×2 then 4 mg/kg per day IV, 200 mg b.d. orally	Inhibits ergosterol biosynthesis	Effective; expensive; good absorption	Elevated hepatic transaminases; visual and CNS disturbances
Caspofungin	70 mg loading dose 50 mg per day IV	Inhibits fungal cell wall synthesis	Expensive; effective	Generally well tolerated; flushing; gastrointestinal disturbance
Surgery	—	—	For life-threatening hemoptysis or removal of single lesions	Pleural dissemination of *Aspergillus* as well as the usual postoperative complications

apices and thickening of the interlobular septa. The diagnosis is made by recognition of the clinical picture in an at-risk patient and should be confirmed by cytologic examination of BAL, identifying the characteristic *P. jirovecii* cysts. First-line treatment is with high-dose cotrimoxazole and adjuvant steroids according to the protocols used for PCP in HIV patients, but in hematology patients second-line therapy is often required because of myelosuppression by cotrimoxazole. Approximately 30% of non-HIV immunocompromised patients with PCP will need intubation and mechanical ventilation, and the mortality is also approximately 30%.

SUGGESTED READINGS

Doffman SR, Agrawal SG, Brown JS: Invasive pulmonary aspergillosis. Expert Rev Anti Infect Ther 2005; 3:613–627.

Herbrecht R, Denning DW, Patterson TF, et al: Voriconazole versus amphotericin B for primary therapy of invasive aspergillosis. N Engl J Med 2002; 347:408–415.

Hope WW, Walsh TJ, Denning DW: Laboratory diagnosis of invasive aspergillosis. Lancet Infect Dis 2005; 5:609–622.

de la Hoz RE, Stephens GS, Sherlock C: Diagnosis and treatment approaches to CMV infection in adult patients. J Clin Viral 2002; 25: S1–S12.

Ison M, Hayden FG: Viral infections in immunocompromised patients: what's new with respiratory viruses? Curr Opin Infect Dis 2002; 15:355–367.

Maschmeyer G, Beinert T, Buchheidt D, et al: Diagnosis and antimicrobial therapy of pulmonary infiltrates in febrile neutropenic patients. Ann Hematol 2003; 82(suppl 2):S118–S126.

O'Brien SN, Blijlevens NMA, Mahfouz TH, Anaissie EJ: Infections in patients with hematological cancer: recent developments. Hematology 2003; 438–472.

Patterson TF, Kirkpatrick WR, White M, et al: Invasive aspergillosis: disease spectrum, treatment practices and outcomes. Medicine 2000; 79:250–260.

Rañó A, Agusti C, Jimenez C, et al: Pulmonary infiltrates in non-HIV immunocompromised patients: a diagnostic approach using non-invasive and bronchoscopic procedures. Thorax 2001; 56:379–387.

Vogel MN, Brodoefel H, Hierl T, et al: Differences and similarities of cytomegalovirus and pneumocystis pneumonia in HIV-negative immunocompromised patients—thin-section CT-morphology in the early phase of the disease. Br J Radiol 2007; 80(955):516–523.

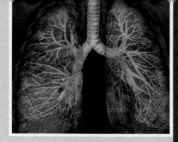

30 Nosocomial Pneumonia

MAURICIO VALENCIA • ANTONI TORRES

INTRODUCTION

Nosocomial pneumonia (NP) is one of the most important infections in hospitalized patients, and its mortality is not decreasing despite many advances in the field. A number of risk factors predispose patients to NP, some of which may be prevented or reduced. The diagnosis begins with clinical suspicion and requires that a respiratory sample be obtained by invasive or noninvasive means. Initial appropriate antimicrobial empiric treatment is the first objective of treatment. Treatment guidelines and knowledge of the bacteriology in each hospital and each intensive care unit will help determine which antibiotics to use. Then, deescalation of antibiotic therapy on the basis of the clinical response and results of respiratory cultures may help prevent development of bacterial resistance. Thirty percent of patients do not respond to antibiotic therapy, and these must be reevaluated with a new respiratory sample.

DEFINITIONS

NP is an inflammatory process resulting from infection of the pulmonary parenchyma by pathogenic microorganisms that develops in a patient who is hospitalized for more than 48 h. Ventilator-associated pneumonia (VAP) is a subcategory of NP defined by the additional requirement that patients have been intubated and received mechanical ventilation for at least 48 h. Ventilator-associated tracheobronchitis (VAT) has not been as widely studied as VAP and is characterized by the presence of signs of respiratory infection (e.g., an increase in the volume and purulence of respiratory secretions, fever, and leukocytosis in patients undergoing mechanical ventilation, who, in contrast to those with VAP, do not have consolidation on chest X-ray) (Figure 30-1).

Health-care–associated pneumonia (HCAP) has recently been defined in the latest American Thoracic Society guidelines for the diagnosis and treatment of NP. HCAP is found in patients who are *not* hospitalized at the time the infection develops. The epidemiologic characteristics of these patients (i.e., hospitalization for 2 days or more within the preceding 90 days, residence in a nursing home or extended care facility, home infusion therapy (including antibiotics, chronic dialysis within 30 days, home wound care, and family member with multidrug resistant pathogen colonization or infection) are similar to hospitalized patients in that they are also susceptible to colonization by potentially multiresistant bacteria.

Another classification system is based on the presence of microorganisms isolated in cultures of epidemiologic surveillance samples and includes (1) primary endogenous pneumonia: (with causative pathogenic microorganisms being found on admission surveillance cultures), and (2) secondary endogenous pneumonia (caused by nosocomial pathogens that were not present on admission colonizing the oropharynx, stomach, and/or the intestine, where they subsequently invade the lower respiratory tract).

Exogenous pneumonia is caused by microorganisms that are not isolated in surveillance cultures; that is, the patients are not previously carriers. Colonization of the artificial airway (e.g., ventilatory tubes, humidifiers), infection by invasive devices such as bronchoscopes, or infection by nebulization or inhalation plays an important role in this category.

Finally, the distinction of early (i.e., presenting within the first 4 days of hospital admission) versus late-onset (i.e., 5 days or more) NP has important implications with respect to etiology, empiric antimicrobial treatment, and outcome (although there are no well-designed trials supporting these specific time cutoffs). An interesting trial performed by Trouillet *et al* showed that according to logistic regression analysis, three variables predicted infection with multidrug-resistant VAP: duration of mechanical ventilation ≥ 7 days (odds ratio [OR] = 6.0), prior antibiotic use (OR = 13.5), and prior use of broad-spectrum drugs (third-generation cephalosporin, fluoroquinolone, and/or imipenem) (OR = 4.1).

EPIDEMIOLOGY, RISK FACTORS, AND PATHOGENESIS

After urinary tract infections, pneumonia is the second most common nosocomial infection, accounting for approximately 10–15% of all hospital-acquired infections. The incidence of NP is approximately 6.0–8.6 per 1000 admissions, but the risk is greatly increased for patients in intensive care units where the incidence ranges from 12–29%, making it the most frequent type of nosocomial infection encountered. The incidence in patients who receive mechanical ventilation ranges from 25–70%, depending on the population studied and the diagnostic criteria used.

Aerodigestive tract colonization and subsequent aspiration of contaminated secretions play a pivotal role in the pathogenesis of NP. Accordingly, risk factors include the duration of an artificial airway, nasal intubation, prior antibiotic treatment, medications altering gastric emptying and pH, nasogastric tube, reintubation, supine positioning, and host factors that may impair the mechanical, humoral, or cellular defense against lung infection.

The mortality of hospital-acquired pneumonia ranges from 25–50%. Up to 15% of all deaths that occur in hospitalized patients are directly related to NP. Patients with VAP may have a 2- to 10-fold greater risk of death than patients without this complication. Logistic regression analysis has suggest that

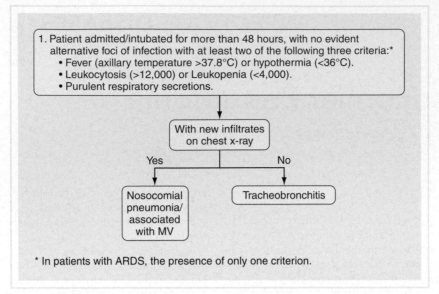

1. Patient admitted/intubated for more than 48 hours, with no evident
   alternative foci of infection with at least two of the following three criteria:*
   • Fever (axillary temperature >37.8°C) or hypothermia (<36°C).
   • Leukocytosis (>12,000) or Leukopenia (<4,000).
   • Purulent respiratory secretions.

With new infiltrates
on chest x-ray

Yes → Nosocomial pneumonia/associated with MV

No → Tracheobronchitis

* In patients with ARDS, the presence of only one criterion.

FIGURE 30-1 Clinical suspicion of nosocomial respiratory infection.

the following factors increase the mortality in patients with VAP: the identification of "high-risk" microorganisms (i.e., *Pseudomonas aeruginosa, Enterobacteriaceae*, and other gram-negative bacilli, *Enterococcus faecalis, Staphylococcus aureus, Candida* spp., *Aspergillus* spp., and episodes of polymicrobial pneumonia), bilateral involvement on chest X-ray, the presence of respiratory failure, inappropriate antibiotic therapy, age older than 60 years, and an ultimately or rapidly fatal underlying condition.

CLINICAL FEATURES

The clinical features leading to a suspicion of NP (see Figure 30-1) include the presence of new or persistent pulmonary infiltrates, a temperature greater than 38.3°C or less than 36°C, a white blood cell count greater than 12,000/mm^3 or less than 4000/mm^3, and purulent secretions. As a general rule, the presence of pulmonary infiltrates along with one of the remaining criteria should raise suspicion of NP. Although these criteria are well accepted for establishing a diagnosis in spontaneously breathing patients, a number of studies suggest that they are less reliable in diagnosing pneumonia in patients who require mechanical ventilation. Clinical criteria may result in a 29% false-positive diagnosis in patients with the acute respiratory distress syndrome (using autopsy findings as the "gold standard"). The incidence of a false-positive diagnosis using radiographic criteria alone is 32% in mechanically ventilated patients; other entities may result in pulmonary infiltrates and fever (e.g., atelectasis).

DIAGNOSIS

The first problem in the diagnosis of NP and VAP is the lack of a "gold standard" for comparing the different techniques used to confirm the suspicion of an infectious process. By use of histologic and microbiologic cultures from postmortem pulmonary biopsy samples, one study found that having radiologic abnormalities along with two or more clinical criteria still resulted in a sensitivity and specificity of only 69% and 75%, respectively.

In recent years, the Clinical Pulmonary Infection Score (CPIS), validated by Pugin and colleagues, has been widely used (Table 30-1). This score combines different clinical, radiologic, physiological, laboratory, and microbiologic parameters to increase the specificity of the clinical diagnostic approach. A score greater than 6 has been well correlated with the presence of pneumonia, but some studies show a sensitivity and specificity of only 77% and 42%, respectively. More recent studies have tried to improve these results by adding gram staining of lower airway secretions.

Blood cultures are obligatory when considering a diagnosis of NP. Unfortunately, the sensitivity is low (10–25%), and the specificity is reduced in critically ill patients who are at risk

TABLE 30-1 Clinical Pulmonary Infection Score

Variable	Criterion	Points
Temperature	≥36.5 to ≤38.4°C	0
	≥38.5 to ≤38.9°C	1
	≥39 to ≤36°C	2
Leukocyte count	≥4000 to ≤11,000	0
	<4000 to >11,000	1
	Band forms	1+
Tracheal secretions	<14+ aspirations	0
	≥14+ aspirations	1
	Purulent secretions	1+
Oxygenation (PaO$_2$/FiO$_2$ ratio)	>240 or acute respiratory distress syndrome	0
	≤240	2
Chest radiograph	No infiltrate	0
	Diffuse	1
	Localized	2
Semiquantitative tracheal aspirate cultures (0, 1, 2, or 3+)	Pathogenic bacteria ≤1+ or no growth	0
	Pathogenic bacteria >1+	1
	Same pathogenic bacteria on Gram's stain	1+

This score ranges from 0 to 12 and includes six variables. A clinical score higher than 6 has a good correlation with pulmonary infection.

of bacteremia from multiple infectious foci. Accordingly, microorganisms isolated in blood cultures can only be considered as the definitive etiologic cause of NP when they coincide with the microbiologic results of respiratory secretions.

NONINVASIVE APPROACHES

In patients breathing spontaneously, respiratory secretions can be obtained by expectoration. A valid sample for microbiologic processing requires more than 25 polymorphonuclear cells and less than 10 epithelial squamous cells per field. The operative values of Gram stain and cultures of sputum in hospital-acquired pneumonia are not well known.

In intubated patients, respiratory secretions can be obtained by tracheal aspirate. The sample may be cultured qualitatively or quantitatively with the former providing a good sensitivity (60–90%) but quite low specificity (0–33%) because of contaminates retrieved from the upper airway. The use of quantitative cultures with a cutoff of 10^6 cfu/mL increases the specificity of this noninvasive technique, and several studies have suggested that the diagnostic yield when done in this fashion may be comparable to secretions obtained by bronchoscopy. In the absence of prior antibiotic treatment, the negative predictive value of this techniques (i.e., negative cultures indicating absence of bacteria pneumonia) is high. Three Spanish studies found no significant differences comparing quantitive culture of tracheal aspiration versus more invasive techniques with respect to mortality or morbidity.

INVASIVE APPROACHES

Fiberoptic bronchoscopy provides direct access to the lower airways for sampling the bronchi and lung parenchyma. To reach the bronchial tree, however, the bronchoscope must traverse the endotracheal tube, where it can become contaminated by colonizing flora. Several devices have been developed to allow uncontaminated sampling of the lower airway and parenchyma, the most popular being the protected specimen brush (PSB). Bronchoscopy also has the disadvantage of requiring the presence of a physician trained to perform the procedure.

Protected Specimen Brush

The usefulness of the PSB was demonstrated nearly 25 years ago. This technique involves positioning the bronchoscope just above the orifice from which secretions are to be sampled and advancing the PSB catheter 3 cm from the end of the bronchoscope to avoid collecting secretions that may have accumulated on the bronchoscope tip. An inner cannula is extended, and this ejects a carbon-wax plug from the distal end of the catheter into the airway. The catheter is then advanced to the desired subsegment. If purulent secretions are visualized, the brush is rotated into them. After sampling, the brush is retracted into the inner cannula, the inner cannula is retracted into the outer cannula, and the catheter is removed from the bronchoscope. A small quantity of brushed secretions may be used for Gram stain. After wiping the cannula with 70% alcohol and cutting the catheter with sterile scissors, the brush is placed in 1 mL of diluent and immediately submitted for quantitative bacterial culture.

The volume of lower respiratory secretions retrieved is approximately 0.001 mL (range, 0.01–0.001), and, as a result of dilution in the holding medium, the colony count on the culture plate represents the result of a 100- to 1000-fold dilution.

Although a large body of work strongly supports the usefulness of performing quantitative cultures on the material retrieved by PSB to differentiate colonization from infection, questions persist regarding the true "gold standard" with which these data can be compared, as do concerns regarding the effects of antibiotics and the utility of the information obtained. The currently accepted threshold to separate "colonization" from "infection" is greater than 10^3 cfu/mL.

Bronchoalveolar Lavage

The BAL technique was developed to sample a larger portion of lung parenchyma (approximately 10^6 alveoli) than what is sampled by the PSB. Although the sensitivity of BAL is generally considered to be high (again with reservations about the true "gold standard" and the effects of antibiotics), the specificity has been limited, in part, by contamination with upper airway bacteria in up to one fourth of specimens. To perform BAL, 100–150 mL of saline is instilled in aliquots and the returned is pooled for analysis. Quantitative cultures showing greater than 10^4 colonies/mL correlate with the presence of pneumonia. Finding intracellular organisms in more than 2% of the polymorphonuclear cells or macrophages of centrifuged BAL fluid is also a sensitive and specific marker of pneumonia.

In the last few years, several devices have been developed that allow protected BAL to be performed with less fluid being instilled into the lower airways. These seem to be as accurate as a standard BAL.

Blind Methods

Several investigators have examined the usefulness of blindly sampling the lower airway secretions in mechanically ventilated patients (i.e., without the help of the fiberoptic bronchoscope). PSB performed in this fashion seems to have a similar accuracy as those done by bronchoscopy. Blind BAL has also been studied by a number of groups with mini-BAL protected catheters, Swan-Ganz catheters, or, more recently, protected catheters that can be directed to one or the other lung depending on the location of the infiltrate in question. In summary, when a blind system is used, the results obtained are similar to those obtained using guided, more invasive methods with the general advantage of having fewer side effects.

DIAGNOSIS

Two types of strategies may be used to diagnose NP. The clinical strategy is based on the previously mentioned clinical criteria in which the etiologic agent is defined by qualitative sputum cultures or tracheal aspirate. This strategy emphasizes the need for early initiation of empiric treatment in all patients suspected of having NP and may, therefore, result in a more frequent use of antibiotics than the bacteriologic strategy. The bacteriologic strategy uses the results of the quantitative cultures of lower respiratory secretions obtained by bronchoscopy or blindly to define the presence of pneumonia and the etiologic agent and has the advantage of being more specific, thereby reducing overtreatment with antibiotics.

With respect to studies aimed at determining which approach is associated with the lowest mortality, one found that patients treated according to the bacteriologic strategy had a lower mortality on day 14 but not on day 28 and also had more antibiotic-free days on day 28. A recent randomized study of patients thought to have NP on the basis of clinical indicators found no reduction in the use of antibiotics or in mortality when the patients subsequently underwent BAL and quantitative culture compared with tracheal aspirate and qualitative culture. This study included a group of patients with a low prevalence of *P. aeruginosa* and methicillin-resistant *S. aureus*.

TREATMENT

In patients suspected of having VAP, samples for microbiologic studies should be collected quickly (Figure 30-2). The initiation of antibiotic treatment should not, for any reason, be delayed by procedures for sample collection.

Several studies have demonstrated the importance of an early and appropriate initial empirical antibiotic treatment (at least one of the antibiotics selected should be active against the causal microorganism and administered in the correct doses, intervals, etc.) and initiated early. When the initial empiric treatment is inadequate and is subsequently adjusted on the basis of the quantitative cultures, mortality continues to exceed that of patients in whom the initial treatment is effective. To facilitate institution of effective empiric treatment that should be followed, taking microbiologic samples of each unit and each hospital into account.

The American Thoracic Society has recently published a guideline for the diagnosis and treatment of patients with NP. According to these guidelines the two most important factors determining the choice of antibiotics are (1) the presence of risk factors for infection by multiresistant microorganisms (Tables 30-2 and 30-3) and (2) the time of the onset of pneumonia (i.e., early or late). Recommendations for patients who

have NP of early onset but no risk factors for multiresistant microorganisms should be treated with monotherapy, with ceftriaxone, a respiratory fluoroquinolone, amoxicillin/clavulanic, or ertapenem. Patients with late-onset NP or those who have risk factors for having resistant microorganisms should have empiric treatment started with combined antibiotic that would be effective against drug-resistant *P. aeruginosa* such as an antipseudomonic beta-lactam (third- or fourth-generation cephalosporins, carbapenems, or penicillin associated with a beta-lactamase inhibitor such as piperacillin/tazobactam) and an aminoglycoside or a quinolone active against *Pseudomonas* (see Table 30-3). In those who seem to be responding to

TABLE 30-2 Initial Empiric Antibiotic Treatment in PN and VAP of Early Onset in Patients Without Risk Factors for Infection by MRMO and with any Degree of Severity

Probable Microorganism	Recommended Empiric Antibiotic
Streptococcus pneumonia *Haemophilus influenzae* Methicillin-resistant *Staphylococcus aureus*	Ceftriaxone *or*
Enteric gram-negative bacilli *Escherichia coli* *Klebsiella pneumoniae*	Levofloxacin *or*
Enterobacter spp. *Proteus* spp.	Ertapenem

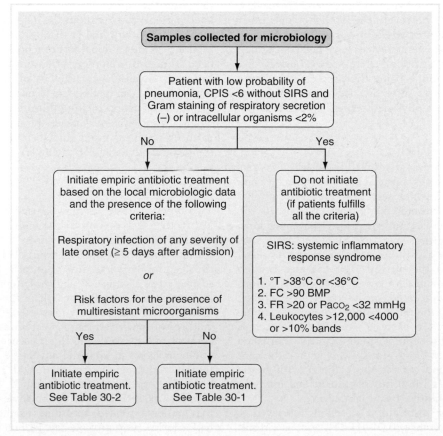

FIGURE 30-2 Algorithm for the treatment of patients with suspicion of nosocomial respiratory infection.

TABLE 30-3 Initial Empiric Antibiotic Treatment for PN and VAP of Late Onset or in Patients with Risk Factors for Infection by MRMO and with any Degree of Severity

Probable Microorganism	Combined Antibiotic Treatment
Microorganisms from Table 30-2 plus:	Antipseudomonic cephalosporin (ceftazidime or cefepime)
	or
Pseudomonas aeruginosa	Carbapenem (imipenem, meropenem)
	or
Klebsiella pneumoniae (ESBL+)	Betalactamic/betalactamase inhibitor (piperacillin/ tazobactam)
	+
Serratia marcescens	Antipseudomonic fluoroquinolone (ciprofloxacin, levofloxacin)
	or
Acinetobacter spp.	Aminoglycoside (amikacin)
	±
Methicillin-resistant *Staphylococcus aureus* (MRSA)	linezolid or vancomycin
Legionella pneumophila	
Other nonfermentative GNB	

treatment, the aminoglycoside or the quinolone may be discontinued after 5 days of combined treatment.

The tradition is for antibiotic treatment of patients with NP to be continued for 14–21 days. A randomized controlled trial has, however, shown that patients receiving treatment for 8 days had no greater mortality and no increased rate of recurrent infections (although patients with nonfermenting gram-negative bacilli such as *P. aeruginosa* showed a greater rate of recurrence of pulmonary infections).

A strategy currently used in clinical practice and which is being investigated in several ongoing studies is the so-called deescalation approach that involves narrowing the spectrum or the number of antimicrobial medications on day 3 of treatment on the basis of the results of microbial cultures performed. In several studies, this strategy has been shown to reduce the use of antimicrobials with no increase in either the rate of mortality or recurrence.

EVOLUTION

Most of the clinical and physiologic abnormalities resolve by day 6 after diagnosis is made in patients who receive adequate initial antibiotic therapy. Thirty percent of patients do not respond, however, and this figure may be as high as 50% in patients with VAP.

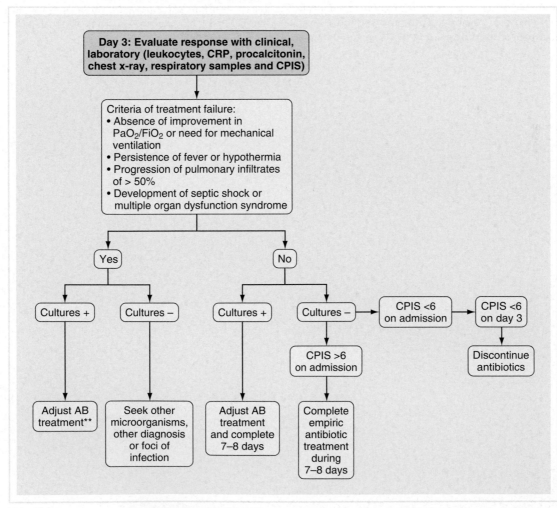

FIGURE 30-3 Follow-up of patients with nosocomial infection.

Oxygenation is the first variable to improve. There is a clear differentiation by day 3 between patients who are improving and those who are not. Other variables that may be useful include inflammatory markers such as C-reactive protein, procalcitonin, and some interleukins (especially IL-6). The Clinical Pulmonary Infection Score (CPIS) was originally described by Pugin and colleagues (see Table 30-1). When CPIS is <6 on the third and fifth day of evolution, the mortality is lower than if the score remained above this threshold.

When patients fail to improve, or when rapid deterioration occurs, reevaluation is needed, specifically considering the possibility that the process requiring treatment may not be pneumonia and that certain host, bacterial, or other therapeutic factors have not been overlooked. A number of noninfectious processes may be mistakenly labeled as NP, including atelectasis, congestive heart failure, pulmonary embolism with infarction, lung contusion (in trauma patients), chemical pneumonitis from aspiration, alveolar hemorrhage, and diffuse fibroproliferation in patients with acute respiratory distress syndrome. Host factors associated with failure to respond to appropriate treatment include the presence of other underlying diseases (e.g., endobronchial malignancy or foreign body), superinfections with organisms that are not sensitive to the antibiotics given, or any of a variety of types of immunosuppression. Bacterial factors associated with failure of initial therapy include primary or acquired resistance to the initial antibiotic(s) chosen. NP may be caused by pathogens that are not commonly included in the differential diagnosis (e.g., *Mycobacterium tuberculosis*, a variety of fungi, viruses). Although these may be more common in immunocompromised hosts, any of these can occur in apparently normal patients. Complications of the initial infection may also preclude a normal response to therapy (e.g., empyema, abscess formation).

Accordingly, patients with VAP must be reevaluated on day 3 (Figure 30-3). The following criteria indicate treatment failure: (1) failure to improve the PaO_2/FiO_2 ratio or need for MV 24 h after antibiotic initiation, (2) persistence of fever or hypothermia plus purulent respiratory secretions, (3) worsening of the pulmonary infiltrate by 50%, or (4) development of septic shock or multiple organ failure syndrome. The presence of any of these criteria together with the results of new respiratory sample cultures will determine the subsequent treatment.

SUGGESTED READINGS

Depuydt P, Myny D, Blot S: Nosocomial pneumonia: aetiology, diagnosis and treatment. Curr Opin Pulm Med 2006; 12:192–197.

Dominguez AA, Valencia M, Torres A: Treatment failure in patients with ventilator-associated pneumonia. Semin Respir Crit Care Med 2006; 27:104–113.

Niederman MS: De-escalation therapy in ventilator-associated pneumonia. Curr Opin Crit Care 2006; 12(5):452–457.

Niederman M, Craven D: Guidelines for the management of adults with hospital-acquired, ventilator-associated, and healthcare-associated pneumonia. Am J Respir Crit Care Med 2005; 171:388–416.

Ostendorf U, Ewig S, Torres A: Nosocomial pneumonia. Curr Opin Infect Dis 2006; 19(4):327–338.

Porzecanski I, Bowton DL: Diagnosis and treatment of ventilator-associated pneumonia. Chest 2006; 130:597–604.

Rello J: Bench-to-bedside review: Therapeutic options and issues in the management of ventilator-associated bacterial pneumonia. Crit Care 2005; 9:259–265.

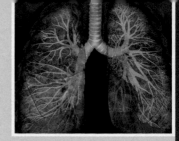

31 Tuberculosis and Nontuberculous Mycobacterial Infections

CHARLES L. DALEY

The genus *Mycobacterium* consists of slow-growing organisms that are widely disseminated throughout the world and range from organisms that cause no human disease to those like *Mycobacterium tuberculosis* and *Mycobacterium leprae* that cause enormous morbidity and mortality. *Mycobacteria* are aerobic bacilli with high concentrations of lipids in their cell wall, which make them impermeable to most common stains. However, because of their ability to retain carbolfuchsin dye despite decolorization attempts with acid alcohol, they are referred to as "acid-fast bacilli" (AFB). Although mycobacteria can produce disease in almost any site, two groups of mycobacteria have a propensity for causing pulmonary infections: some members of the *M. tuberculosis* complex and the nontuberculous mycobacteria (NTM).

Tuberculosis (TB) is the disease caused by bacteria of the *Mycobacterium tuberculosis* complex, which includes the clinically relevant species, *M. tuberculosis*, *M. bovis*, and *M. africanum*. Although *M. tuberculosis* is the most common cause of TB worldwide, both *M. bovis* and *M. africanum* can produce clinically indistinguishable forms of disease. The tubercle bacilli have been around for thousands of years with evidence of human infection dating back to Neolithic, pre-Columbian, and early Egyptian times. However, it was not until the Industrial Revolution that TB became a major cause of human disease and death. It is estimated that approximately 25% of all adults died from TB in Europe during the 17th and 18th centuries. Throughout this period, the etiology of TB was hotly debated, with some arguing for a hereditary cause, whereas others argued for a transmissible etiology. It was not until 1882 that Robert Koch presented his momentous discovery; the tubercle bacillus was the cause of TB. Early attempts at therapy, including the sanatorium movement, surgery, and collapse therapy, provided little relief from TB, and it was not until the discovery of paraaminosalicylate acid (PAS) and streptomycin in the 1940s that the age of antituberculosis chemotherapy had begun. Since that time, additional drugs have been developed, and most of the world treats TB with the same four-drug regimen administered for 6 months. However, HIV coinfection and the emergence of drug-resistant strains of *M. tuberculosis* have conspired to complicate the management of patients and create barriers for global TB control.

NTM refers to non-lepromatous organisms that are not members of the *M. tuberculosis* complex. The NTM have been referred to as mycobacteria other than tuberculosis (MOTT), atypical mycobacteria, and environmental mycobacteria. The latter designation refers to their ubiquitous presence in our environment. The NTM have several features that distinguish them from *M. tuberculosis*. They have a wide range of pathogenicity, are not always associated with disease, and, unlike *M. tuberculosis*, are not transmissible from human to human. However, the NTM are increasing in frequency in many areas of the world, and the cause for this increase is unknown. Unfortunately, the pathogenic NTM are relatively drug resistant compared with *M. tuberculosis* and, thus, difficult to treat. Because of our poor understanding of the transmission and pathogenesis of NTM infections, we have little insight in how to prevent these infections, and thus we have no public health strategy to control disease caused by these ubiquitous organisms.

TUBERCULOSIS

Epidemiology, Risk Factors, and Pathogenesis

Epidemiology

The World Health Organization (WHO) estimates that globally 30% of adults are infected with organisms in the *M. tuberculosis* complex. From this large reservoir of infected individuals, an estimated 8–9 million new cases of TB occurred in 2005, leading to approximately 2 millions deaths. TB is one of the leading causes of death from an infectious or parasitic disease worldwide, and it is the number one killer of HIV-infected individuals. High population growth rates and coinfection with HIV are expected to worsen the global morbidity and mortality caused by TB.

The burden of TB varies significantly throughout the world, with more than 90% of cases residing in developing countries (Figure 31-1). The highest incidence rates of TB are in sub-Saharan Africa, particularly in the southern region of the continent. Not surprisingly, the highest prevalence of HIV coinfection is also in this region. At present, approximately 23% of all TB cases have underlying HIV coinfection; however, in sub-Saharan Africa, an estimated 50% of TB cases have HIV/AIDS.

Recent reports of outbreaks of multidrug-resistant TB (MDR-TB) and extensively resistant TB (XDR-TB) have highlighted the importance of providing effective antituberculosis therapy to patients. MDR-TB refers to isolates of *M. tuberculosis* that are resistant to at least isoniazid and rifampin, whereas XDR-TB refers to MDR-TB isolates that are also resistant to fluoroquinolones and at least one injectable (amikacin, capreomycin, and kanamycin). Surveys have documented that approximately 2% of TB worldwide is due to MDR-TB, and 2% of these cases have XDR-TB. There are more cases of drug-resistant TB today than in recorded history, and this

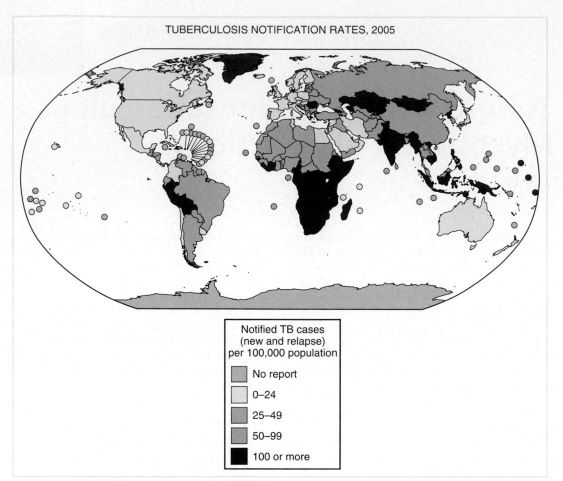

FIGURE 31-1 Tuberculosis notification rates, 2005. The legend depicts the number of notified tuberculosis cases, which includes both new and relapse cases per 100,000 population. (Source: World Health Organization.)

trend is likely to continue unless more effective TB control measures are implemented globally.

In the United States, the TB case rate declined 3–5% per year from 1953 to 1984. Between 1986 and 1992, the numbers of TB cases increased by approximately 20%. This increase in the number of cases was the result of at least three major factors: (1) inadequate public health measures; (2) immigration from countries where TB is prevalent; and (3) coinfection with HIV. Fortunately, since 1992, cases are again on the decline, but recent reports have described a decrease in the rate of decline. In 2006, a total of 13,767 cases of TB were reported, which is an incidence of 4.6/100,000 population. The average annual percentage decline has decreased from 7.3% per year during 1993–2000 to 3.8% during 2000–2006. Approximately 1% of new cases in the country have MDR-TB, but the frequency is higher in foreign-born patients. Of these MDR-TB cases, approximately 2% have XDR-TB.

Risk Factors

Certain individuals are at higher risk of TB developing simply because they are more likely to be exposed and, thus, infected with *M. tuberculosis* (Table 31-1). For example, approximately 50% of reported TB cases in the United States occur in foreign-born individuals who come from areas where the disease is endemic. Other populations with an increased prevalence of tuberculous infection include certain racial and ethnic groups, low-income populations, the homeless, and injection drug users.

Anyone infected with *M. tuberculosis* can have TB disease develop, but there are certain groups that have a higher-than-normal risk for progressing to active disease (see Table 31-1). Patients who have been recently infected with *M. tuberculosis* and those with medical conditions associated with significant immunosuppression are at particularly high risk of TB developing. HIV coinfection is the strongest known risk factor for the development of TB, but there are also other medical conditions associated with an increased risk of the disease developing.

Pathogenesis

TB is spread from person to person through the air by droplet nuclei: particles 1–5 μm in diameter that contain viable tubercle bacilli. Droplet nuclei are expelled into the air when patients with infectious TB create an aerosol by talking, coughing, or singing. Three factors determine the likelihood of transmitting TB: the number of bacilli being expelled into the air, the concentration of organisms in the air, and the length of time the contact breathes the infected air. Whether an inhaled tubercle bacillus establishes an infection in the contact's lung depends on both the bacterial virulence and the host's immune defenses.

The tubercle bacillus grows slowly, dividing approximately every 18–24 h until a cellular immune reaction develops after 2–8 weeks. However, before the development of cellular immunity, an inflammatory response appears and is associated with the spread of tubercle bacilli through the lymphatics to

TABLE 31-1 Criteria for a Positive Tuberculin Skin Test

Size of Reaction	Risk Groups
≥5 mm	HIV-infected persons Close contact to an infectious tuberculosis case Abnormal chest radiograph* consistent with prior tuberculosis Immunosuppressed patients receiving the equivalent of ≥15 mg/d of prednisone for at least 1 month
≥10 mm	Foreign-born persons recently arrived (<5 years) from high-prevalence countries Medical conditions† that increase the risk of tuberculosis Injection drug users Medically underserved, low-income populations (e.g., homeless persons) Residents and staff of long-term care facilities (e.g., nursing homes, correctional institutions, homeless shelters) Health care workers Children <4 years of age Tuberculin skin test converters (increase of ≥10-mm induration within a 2-year period)
≥15 mm	All others; these persons should not be screened in the absence of indication

*An abnormal chest radiograph consistent with prior tuberculosis refers to fibrotic lesions and does not mean pleural thickening or isolated calcified granulomas.
†Medical conditions that increase the risk of tuberculosis developing given latent tuberculosis infection include silicosis, end-stage renal disease, malnutrition, diabetes mellitus, carcinoma of the head or neck and lung, immunosuppressive therapy, lymphoma, leukemia, weight loss >10% ideal body weight, gastrectomy, and jejunoileal bypass.

the hilar lymph nodes or through the bloodstream. Small numbers of bacilli are deposited in other organs, which act as potential sites for extrapulmonary disease.

Once cell-mediated immunity develops, collections of activated T cells and macrophages form granulomas that wall off the mycobacterial organisms (Figure 31-2). For most persons with normal immune function, infection with *M. tuberculosis* seems to be arrested once cell-mediated immunity develops, even though small numbers of viable bacilli remain within the granuloma. Although a primary complex can sometimes be seen on chest radiograph, most tuberculous infections are asymptomatic and can only be detected with a tuberculin skin test (TST) or interferon-gamma release assay (IGRA). Persons with tuberculous infection who do not have active disease are not infectious and, thus, cannot spread the disease to others.

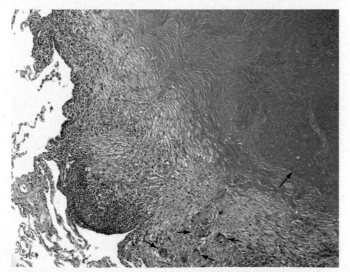

FIGURE 31-2 Caseating granuloma in lung tissue. The lung biopsy specimen depicts a caseating granuloma. The large arrow highlights the caseous center. The smaller arrows point out giant cells typical of granulomatous inflammation.

If cell-mediated immunity cannot contain the tubercle bacilli, the infected person progresses to active disease. Untreated, approximately 10% of infected persons have active TB develop, 5% within the first 1–2 years of infection (Figure 31-3). In contrast, persons who are coinfected with HIV have a 5–10% annual risk of active disease developing. When active TB develops soon after infection, the disease is referred to as primary TB. In contrast, when TB develops years or even decades after the initial tuberculous infection, the disease is referred to as postprimary or reactivation disease. Exogenous reinfection, because of acquisition of a second strain of *M. tuberculosis*, can also lead to disease and seems to be more common in HIV-infected individuals.

Genetics

Susceptibility and/or resistance to developing TB have long been thought to have a genetic component. Epidemiologic and genetic studies, including those in animal and human models, support this hypothesis. Recent investigations of specific candidate genes and genome-wide scans have identified individuals at increased risk for TB. Although polymorphisms in more than 10 genes have been associated with active TB, only polymorphisms in the HLA-DR molecules and in the genes for the Vitamin D_3 receptor, SCL11A-1, INF-γ promoter, and mannose-binding lectin have all been associated with increased susceptibility to *M. tuberculosis*. Because each association has been relatively modest at the individual level, the genetic susceptibility is likely to be polygenic in nature. Ultimately, whether an individual with TB infection progresses to disease will depend on the interplay between the host, organism, and environment.

Clinical Features

The clinical manifestations of TB may vary, depending on whether the disease is primary or reactivation in nature, the host's immune status, and possibly the strain of *M. tuberculosis*. It is important to note that the clinical features of active TB are the result of a balance between host defenses and

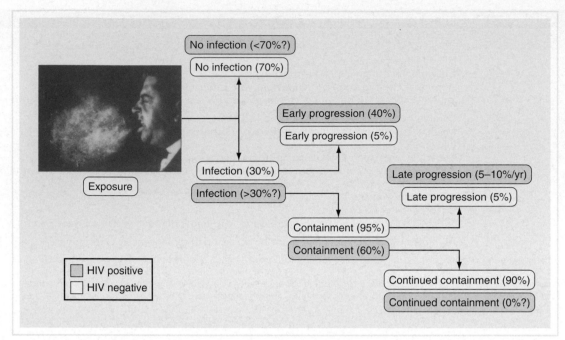

FIGURE 31-3 Pathogenesis of tuberculosis. After exposure to an infectious case of tuberculosis, approximately 30% of close contacts become infected with *Mycobacterium tuberculosis*. Of the contacts who become infected, approximately 5% will have active tuberculosis develop over the next year. Most infected individuals will not have tuberculosis develop. However, another 5% will have tuberculosis develop during their lifetime. When tuberculosis is introduced into an HIV-infected population, the pathogenesis of tuberculosis is altered. Although there are no scientific data that prove the point, it is likely that HIV-infected individuals are more likely to be infected than HIV-negative contacts. In outbreak settings, approximately 40% of contacts have tuberculosis develop within the first year. Coinfected individuals have tuberculosis develop at a rate of 5–10% per year.

bacterial virulence; therefore, there may be a continuum of disease, and the clinical presentation of disease may be altered in severely immunocompromised patients. Most patients are initially seen with pulmonary disease that is classically divided into primary disease or postprimary disease.

Pulmonary Tuberculosis

The initial infection in the lung, referred to as primary infection, causes an inflammatory infiltrate, which may be seen on a chest radiograph, often in the middle or lower lung zones. The draining lymph nodes may enlarge and compress adjacent bronchi, particularly in infants and children. Parenchymal disease usually clears as cell-mediated immunity develops, and it tends to clear more rapidly than nodal involvement. If the parenchymal disease persists beyond the development of cell-mediated immunity, cavitation may occur, although this is uncommon. Pleural effusions are a common manifestation of primary TB and presumably result when a peripheral, caseous focus ruptures into the pleural space (Figure 31-4). Pleuritis caused by TB may present as an acute illness characterized by cough, fever, and pleuritic chest pain.

During most initial infections with *M. tuberculosis*, small numbers of organisms are disseminated hematogenously, and some become seeded in the apices of the lung. The organisms seem to grow preferentially in this well-oxygenated environment and can progress to active disease months or years after the initial infection. This accounts for the characteristic radiographic location of reactivation disease, which in most cases occurs in the apical or posterior segments of the upper lobes (Figure 31-5). In areas of chronic infection or areas of caseation, fibrosis may occur. Fibrocaseous lesions may contain live

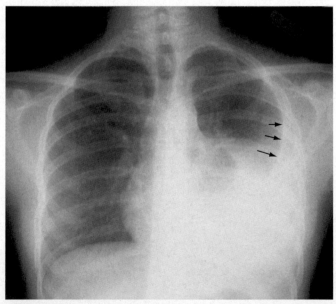

FIGURE 31-4 Chest radiograph of primary tuberculosis in a young adult. The radiograph demonstrates a large left-sided pleural effusion.

mycobacteria for many years, and these are the lesions that may reactivate years later.

Extrapulmonary Tuberculosis

As tubercle bacilli spread throughout the body during the initial infection, they can lodge in any organ and produce a focus

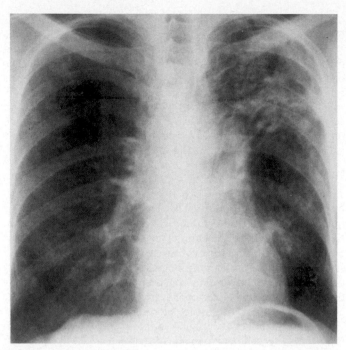

FIGURE 31-5 Chest radiograph of patient with postprimary tuberculosis. The patient with severe pulmonary tuberculosis has upper lobe airspace opacities with cavitation. There is evidence of bronchial spread of tuberculosis in the lower lung zones.

of disease. Approximately 17% of HIV-uninfected patients with TB have an extrapulmonary form of disease only. HIV-infected patients are more likely to have an extrapulmonary site of infection develop than HIV-seronegative persons, and the risk increases as the CD4 lymphocyte count decreases. The two most commonly involved extrapulmonary sites are peripheral lymph nodes and the pleura, but any site or organ can be involved. Other common sites for extrapulmonary TB are those in well-vascularized areas such as the kidney, the meninges, the spine, and the growing ends of long bones.

Tuberculous Lymphadenitis (*Scrofula*)

Lymphadenitis is the most common form of extrapulmonary TB, accounting for approximately 25% of extrapulmonary disease. Lymphadenitis usually presents with a painless, erythematous, firm mass most commonly involving the anterior and posterior cervical nodes or supraclavicular fossa. In HIV-uninfected individuals, the mass is usually unilateral, not associated with other sites, and systemic symptoms are absent. However, in HIV-infected patients, tuberculous lymphadenitis is often associated with multifocal disease and systemic symptoms. Without treatment, the mass will enlarge and a fistulous tract may develop.

Diagnosis of tuberculous lymphadenitis usually involves fine-needle aspiration or excisional biopsy with histopathologic examination, examination for acid-fast organisms, and culture for mycobacteria. Histologic evidence of mycobacterial infection, including caseating granulomas, are seen in nearly all cases, but the smear is positive in only approximately 25–50% of cases and the culture in approximately 70–80%.

Tuberculous Pleurisy

Pleurisy is usually a manifestation of primary TB and results when a subpleural caseous focus ruptures into the pleural space. The resulting delayed-type hypersensitivity reaction produces pleural liquid that has a high protein concentration. Most patients are initially seen with chest pain, fever, and a nonproductive cough. If left untreated, the pleural effusion will resolve spontaneously over 2–4 months. However, the incidence of reactivation is approximately 65% within the next 5 years.

Diagnosis of tuberculous pleural disease begins with sampling of the pleural fluid. Early in the course of disease, the fluid may have a polymorphonuclear predominance, but in almost all cases, mononuclear cells become the majority. Cell counts are typically in the 100–5000 cells/μL range, and the cells are almost all lymphocytes; the presence of mesothelial cells and/or eosinophils makes the diagnosis of tuberculosis extremely unlikely.

AFB smears are seldom positive, and pleural fluid cultures are only positive in approximately 20–40% of cases. *M. tuberculosis* can be isolated from 30% to 50% of induced sputum specimens and thus should be obtained in all patients. Pleural biopsy specimens provide the highest diagnostic yield, with positive culture results in up to 80–90% of cases when at least three specimens are obtained. Thoracoscopic biopsies are nearly always diagnostic, but the procedure is invasive, costly, and often not available.

Other tests that may be helpful in the diagnosis of pleuritis are adenosine deaminase (ADA) and interferon-γ (IFN-γ). ADA has been shown to have high sensitivity but variable specificity. IFN-γ has been reported to have high sensitivity and specificity in both HIV-infected and HIV-uninfected patients. Recently, stimulation of peripheral blood monocytes with ESAT-6 and measurement of IFN-γ production has been shown to be a potential diagnostic aid, but additional studies are needed.

When faced with a lymphocytic exudative pleural effusion in a patient with a positive TST or IGRA, the clinician should strongly consider TB. Whether to start treatment empirically or proceed with a pleural biopsy will depend on the certainty of the diagnosis and whether or not the patient is at risk for drug-resistant TB. In the later situation, pleural tissue should be obtained for smear and culture to obtain drug susceptibility results.

Genitourinary Tuberculosis

Genitourinary disease is responsible for approximately 15% of extrapulmonary cases and can affect either the kidneys or genitals. Renal disease may present with local symptoms that include dysuria, hematuria, urinary frequency, and flank discomfort. However, in many cases, the patient may be asymptomatic. Urine examination demonstrates sterile pyuria, hematuria, or both. *M. tuberculosis* can be isolated from urine in 80–95% of patients who have three morning urine specimens obtained for culture. In patients with pulmonary TB, urine cultures have been reported to be positive in approximately 5% of cases. An intravenous pyelogram may show evidence of destructive changes in the kidney or ureteral abnormalities like strictures and hydronephrosis. Computed tomography often demonstrates renal enlargement with abscess formation.

Genital involvement is common in patients with renal TB. Males usually present with a slowly enlarging mass in the seminal vesicles, prostate, or epididymis. TB is usually diagnosed with fine-needle aspiration or urine culture. In females, the fallopian tube is the primary site of involvement. Women tend to present with pelvic pain, abnormal uterine bleeding, irregular menses, amenorrhea, or infertility. Genital TB is diagnosed with urine culture and endometrial biopsy or curettage. Unfortunately, infertility is common even after successful treatment.

Bone and Joint Disease

Skeletal involvement is thought to arise from reactivation from foci that were seeded with the initial infection. The infection begins in the subchondral region of the bone and then spreads to cartilage, synovium, and joint space. Although weight-bearing bones are the most likely to be affected, any bone or joint may be involved. In most series, TB of the spine, or Pott's disease, makes up more than 50% of cases. In children, the upper thoracic spine is the most frequent site, whereas in adults, the lower thoracic and upper lumbar vertebrae are usually involved. After the spine, the hips or knee are the most common sites of skeletal TB.

Most patients are initially seen with pain in the involved joint. Systemic symptoms are usually absent, and delays in diagnosis are common. Tuberculous involvement of the joint is usually first suspected after a radiograph is obtained. Typical findings include metaphyseal erosion and cysts, loss of cartilage, and narrowing of the joint space. In Pott's disease, two vertebral bodies and the intervening joint space are usually involved. Computed tomography and/or MRI should be obtained to better define the pattern and extent of involvement. Confirmation of the diagnosis requires aspiration of joint fluid or periarticular abscesses or biopsy of affected bone or synovium. Acid-fast smears are positive in 20–25% of joint fluid aspirates, with mycobacteria being isolated in 60–80%. Histopathologic evidence of granulomatous inflammation is almost always present in bone and synovial biopsies.

Central Nervous Disease

Meningitis is the most common form of central nervous system TB, with tuberculomas occurring less commonly. Tuberculous meningitis, although less common than in the past, is still associated with the greatest morbidity and mortality of any form of tuberculosis with mortality of approximately 20%. Patients usually are initially seen with some combination of headache, abnormal behavior, confusion, fever, cranial nerve abnormalities, and occasionally seizures.

Computed tomography and magnetic residence imaging studies may provide evidence for a basilar meningitis, hydrocephalus, or demonstrate evidence of tuberculous abscesses. However, to confirm the diagnosis, cerebrospinal fluid (CSF) must be sampled for examination and culture. CSF protein is usually elevated, and glucose concentration decreased. Very high protein concentrations have been associated with a worse prognosis. White blood cell counts are elevated with values of 100–1000 cells/μL, most of which are lymphocytes. However, as with pleural effusions, there may be a polymorphonuclear predominance early in the disease. AFB smears are positive in only 10–25% of cases, and cultures are positive in approximately 55–80%.

Gastrointestinal Tuberculosis

Gastrointestinal disease is one of the most uncommon manifestations of extrapulmonary TB, although it is more common in HIV-infected patients. Classically, ileocecal involvement and tuberculous peritonitis are the most common forms. Patients with ileocecal involvement may be initially seen with abdominal pain simulating appendicitis or intestinal obstruction. Diagnosis of ileocecal TB can be difficult and is often made at the time of surgery.

Tuberculous peritonitis often presents with abdominal pain and swelling. Fever, weight loss, and anorexia are also common. Ascitic fluid is usually high in protein and contains 50–10,000 leukocytes, with most being lymphocytes. ABF smears are seldom positive, and cultures are positive in approximately 50–80% of cases; the higher yield has been reported when 1 L of fluid was cultured. Laparoscopic biopsy is usually required to make the diagnosis of peritoneal TB.

Tuberculous Pericarditis

Tuberculous pericarditis is a relatively uncommon manifestation of extrapulmonary TB. The clinical presentation is quite variable and determined by the stage of presentation. Early in the course of disease, fever and chest pain may occur. Some, because of a large volume of fluid, may present with signs and symptoms of tamponade. Although in others they present because of cardiac constriction. The fluid is usually serosanguineous and occasionally grossly bloody. It is typically an exudative fluid with white blood cell counts in the 5000–7000 cells/μL range, although counts up to 50,000 have been reported. The cells are usually mononuclear. AFB smears of the fluid are seldom positive, and cultures are positive in less than a third of cases. Often pericardial biopsy samples show histologic evidence consistent with a mycobacterial infection, but in some cases nonspecific inflammatory findings are described.

Miliary Tuberculosis

Miliary or disseminated TB occurs when tubercle bacilli spread throughout the body, through the bloodstream, resulting in small (approximately 1–2 mm) granulomatous lesions. Miliary TB is seen more commonly in infants, children less than 4 years old, and in immunocompromised individuals. Disease can result from early dissemination after infection or later after reactivation and dissemination. Disseminated TB usually develops insidiously with systemic symptoms such as fever, weakness, weight loss, fatigue, and anorexia. Cough and dyspnea may also be prominent symptoms. The mean duration of symptoms approaches 16 weeks, but some patients may go undiagnosed for more than 2 years. The chest radiograph typically shows the classic "miliary" pattern of diffuse small nodules (Figure 31-6). AFB smears are positive in the sputum of 20–25% of cases, whereas *M. tuberculosis* can be isolated in up to 65% of cases. Bronchoscopy should be considered in patients who are unable to produce sputum or who have produced negative sputum smears. Other potential sources include urine, which is positive in up to 25% of patients, liver and bone marrow in up to 25–40%.

Diagnosis of Tuberculosis

To diagnose TB, the disease must first be suspected. TB should be suspected in certain high-risk groups reviewed previously (see Table 31-1) and when the clinical and/or radiographic presentation is consistent with TB. The medical history should elicit whether or not the person suspected of having TB has been exposed to *M. tuberculosis* or has a previous history of tuberculous infection or disease. Symptoms at presentation will vary depending on the sites(s) of involvement and extent of disease as described previously. All persons with an unexplained cough lasting 2–3 weeks or more should be evaluated for TB. Of note, up to 20% of patients with pulmonary disease

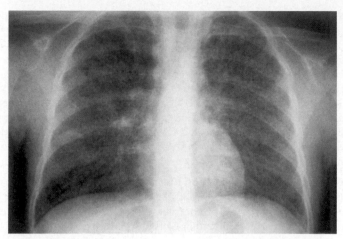

FIGURE 31-6 Chest radiograph of older child with miliary tuberculosis. The radiograph demonstrates diffuse small nodules 2–3 mm in diameter. The patient was diagnosed with disseminated tuberculosis with meningitis.

are asymptomatic. Findings at physical examination are rather nonspecific and vary depending on the site of involvement. Because patients coinfected with HIV are at increased risk of TB developing and the signs and symptoms of active disease may be atypical in this group, TB should be considered when any respiratory infection occurs in these patients or when there is a fever of unknown origin.

Tuberculin Skin Test and Interferon-Gamma Release Assays

The tuberculin skin test (TST) (see more detailed discussion later), which uses purified protein derivative (PPD), is the most common way to identify persons with latent tuberculosis infection (LTBI), but it should not be considered a diagnostic test for active TB. The sensitivity of the TST for active TB ranges from 65–94%. However, in critically ill patients with disseminated disease, the sensitivity decreases to only 50%. Thus, the diagnosis of TB should never be excluded because of a negative TST.

Tests are now available that measure the release of IFN-γ in whole blood in response to stimulation by various antigens. These assays are based on the quantification of IFN-γ that is released from sensitized lymphocytes in whole blood when it is incubated overnight with antigens found in *M. tuberculosis* (e.g., early secretory antigen target 6 [*ESAT-6*], culture filtrate protein 10 [*CFP10*]), and control antigens. IGRAs currently available include the QFT-TB Gold and QFT-TB Gold in tube that measure IFN-γ in the serum that uses enzyme-linked immunosorbent assay (ELISA) (Cellestis Limited, Carnegie, Victoria, Australia) and the T-Spot.*TB* Test that uses enzyme-linked immunospot (ELISPOT) (Oxford Immunotec, Oxford, UK) to identify INF-γ–producing cells.

The sensitivity of QFT-TB Gold in patients with active TB has varied from 55–88%, with a pooled sensitivity of 76%, whereas the T-Spot.*TB* test has a sensitivity that has ranged from 83–97%, with a pooled sensitivity of 88%. In contrast, the TST has a pooled sensitivity of 70% in patients with TB. The QFT-TB Gold in tube version may be more sensitive than QFT-TB Gold, but additional studies are needed. Although the IGRAs have improved sensitivity compared with the TST, the values are still too low to confidently rule out active TB, and neither test can differentiate latent from active TB.

Radiographic Examinations

The chest radiograph is a sensitive but nonspecific test to detect pulmonary TB. The radiographic manifestations may vary depending on when the initial infection occurred and whether or not the patient is coinfected with HIV. Patients who are initially seen with primary pulmonary TB may have radiographic opacities in the lower lung zones and an associated pleural effusion (see Figure 31-4). TB caused by reactivation typically involves the apical and posterior segments of the upper lobes or superior segment of the lower lobe (see Figure 31-5). Cavitation and volume loss are common in reactivation disease but not often seen in primary disease. The chest radiograph in patients coinfected with HIV differs, depending on the severity of immune suppression. Early in the course of HIV disease, the radiograph may look like typical reactivation pattern (Figure 31-7), but as the CD4 cell count declines, the radiographic appearance is more like the pattern seen in primary tuberculosis (Figure 31-8). Patients coinfected with HIV may sometimes have a normal chest radiograph but still be coughing up large numbers of tubercle bacilli.

Bacteriologic Examination

Sputum Microscopy. Diagnosis of pulmonary TB begins with obtaining three spontaneously expectorated sputum samples collected at 8- to 24-h intervals, with at least one being collected in early morning. Two methods are commonly used for acid-fast staining: the carbolfuchsin methods (Ziehl–Neelsen and Kinyoun methods) and a fluorochrome procedure that uses auramine-O or auramine-rhodamine dyes (Figure 31-9).

Approximately 5000–10,000 bacilli/mL are necessary to allow detection of bacilli in stained smears. The sensitivity of sputum AFB smears ranges from 50–80%, depending on the

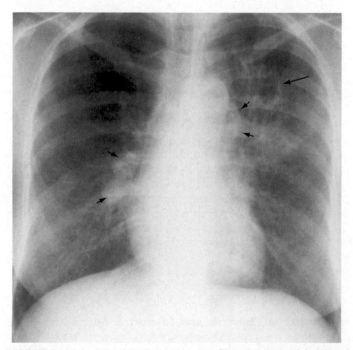

FIGURE 31-7 Chest radiograph of HIV-infected patient with tuberculosis. The radiograph demonstrates a left upper lobe cavitary process (*large arrow*). In addition, there is evidence of bilateral hilar adenopathy and aortopulmonary window adenopathy (*small arrows*).

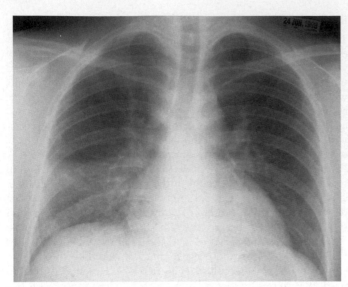

FIGURE 31-8 Chest radiograph of HIV-infected patient with primary-type presentation. The radiograph demonstrates right lower lobe and right middle lobe airspace consolidation with likely right hilar and paratracheal adenopathy.

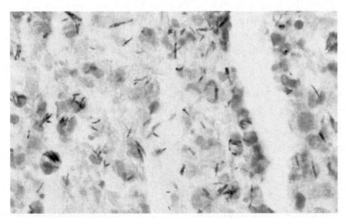

FIGURE 31-9 Acid-fast stain in tissue. Ziehl-Neelson stain of *Mycobacterium tuberculosis.*

extent of disease; patients with cavitary disease are more likely to expectorate tubercle bacilli than those without cavities. If patients are unable to produce sputum or have negative sputum smears, additional diagnostic tests may be indicated. In such circumstances, either sputum induction or fiberoptic bronchoscopy (FOB) may provide adequate specimens. Studies suggest that sputum induction with hypertonic saline and FOB with bronchoalveolar lavage produce similar yields in smear-negative cases. FOB can provide a rapid presumptive diagnosis of TB that can be particularly useful in smear-negative HIV-infected suspects. Because NTM are also acid-fast, staining with nucleic acid probes specific for MTB complex can be helpful.

Mycobacterial Cultures and Identification. Culture of *M. tuberculosis* remains the only way to confirm the diagnosis of TB, and thus all clinical specimens suspected of containing mycobacteria should be inoculated onto culture media. There are three different types of traditional culture media: egg based (Lowenstein–Jensen), agar based (Middlebrook 7H10 or 7H11),

and liquid (Middlebrook 7H12) media. Growth in the liquid media is faster than that in solid media, and automated commercial broth systems allow for growth detection within 1–3 weeks compared with solid media, where growth takes 3–8 weeks. However, solid media allow for observation of colony morphology and the ability to detect mixed infections. Because only 10–100 organisms are required to detect *M. tuberculosis*, cultures are more sensitive than smears, with sensitivities ranging from 80–93%. The tubercle bacilli can be identified from cultures and distinguished from other NTM by chemical means or with nucleic acid probes.

Nucleic Acid Amplification Assays. Nucleic acid amplification assays (NAA) that amplify *M. tuberculosis*–specific nucleic acid sequences by use of complementary probes allow for the direct and rapid identification of the organism in clinical specimens. There are two FDA-approved NAA assays available in the United States: the AMPLICOR M. tuberculosis (Roche Diagnostic Systems, Inc., Branchburg, NJ) and the Amplified Mycobacterium Tuberculosis Direct (MTD) Test (Gen-Probe, Inc., San Diego, CA). The enhanced MTD (E-MTD) assay is approved for use with both smear-negative and smear-positive specimen, but the AMPLICOR assay is approved for use with smear-positive specimens only. The assays show sensitivities of at least 80–90% in most studies, with specificities of approximately 98–99% in smear-positive specimens. The E-MTD assay has been shown to have a sensitivity and specificity close to 100% in smear-positive specimens, and in smear-negative specimens the sensitivity is 90% and specificity is 99%.

Studies have demonstrated that when NAA results are used in the context of clinical suspicion, they can be a useful adjunct for the diagnosis of TB. When the NAA assay and AFB smear are both positive, pulmonary TB is almost certain. If the smear is positive and the NAA negative, testing the sputum for inhibitors is advised and the assay repeated. If inhibitors are not detected and another sputum specimen is again NAA negative, the patient likely has an NTM infection. If smears are negative but the clinical suspicion is intermediate to high, an NAA should be ordered, and, if positive, TB is likely. NAA tests should not be performed on sputum specimens from patients at low risk for TB.

Use of NAA for testing extrapulmonary specimens has been systemically reviewed. The sensitivity of commercial assays for detecting *M. tuberculosis* in CSF and pleural fluid has been approximately 60% with a specificity of 98%. Therefore, NAA may be useful in confirming a diagnosis of CNS or pleural TB, but, because of the low sensitivity, they cannot be used to rule out disease.

Drug Susceptibility Testing. Drug susceptibility studies should be performed on all initial isolates and only by laboratories that have experience in culturing mycobacteria. Drug susceptibility testing should also be performed on patients whose treatment is failing or who have a recurrence. The agar proportion method and the liquid radiometric or chemoluminescence methods are the ones most commonly used in the Unites States. Automated radiometric procedures for drug susceptibility testing offer more rapid results but often require confirmation with solid media.

In the near future, nucleic amplification or other molecular techniques may allow for the rapid identification of drug resistance. Many of the mutations in the mycobacterial genome that confer resistance have been identified. Mutations in the rpoB region of *M. tuberculosis* account for approximately 98% of rifampin resistance, and thus this region can be targeted to identify underlying resistance producing mutations. Various methods of detecting these mutations have been developed and are beginning to make their way into clinical laboratories.

Treatment of Tuberculosis Disease

Identifying and treating patients with TB is the most effective way of preventing transmission in the community. TB must be treated with at least two drugs to which the organism is susceptible to prevent the emergence of drug resistance. Dosages of commonly used first-line and second-line drugs are shown in Tables 31-2 and 31-3, respectively. A regimen containing isoniazid (INH) and rifampin for 6 months, plus pyrazinamide for the initial 2 months is considered standard short-course therapy. Ethambutol should be added to the treatment regimen for the first 2 months of therapy, but once a drug-susceptible isolate has been demonstrated, ethambutol can be stopped (Table 31-4). After the first 2 months of treatment, one of several regimens can be chosen for the continuation phase of treatment. For HIV-negative patients who have a documented negative AFB smear after 2 months of therapy and have no evidence of cavitation on the initial chest radiograph, a once weekly regimen containing rifapentine and INH is effective. The total duration of therapy should be 6 months, but in patients whose 2-month culture remains positive and they have evidence of cavitation on a chest radiograph, the continuation phase should be extended by 3 months to complete a 9-month treatment course (Figure 31-10).

Some patients may be intolerant of a first-line drug or have underlying drug-resistant disease. In these cases, addition of a second-line drug may be necessary (see Table 31-3). These medications include the fluoroquinolones, paraaminosalicylic acid, ethionamide, cycloserine, clofazimine, and injectables like kanamycin, capreomycin, and amikacin. The duration of treatment for drug-resistant TB will be determined by the drugs used, the site, and the extent of the disease. Expert consultation should be obtained when treating drug-resistant TB.

To prevent acquired drug resistance, clinicians must prescribe an adequate regimen and ensure that patients adhere to therapy. Directly observed therapy (DOT) should be used whenever possible. If DOT is not available, combined preparations that include INH and rifampin, or INH, rifampin, and pyrazinamide, should be used.

Persons with active untreated pulmonary TB are infectious, particularly those who have AFB identified in a sputum specimen. Treatment of TB rapidly renders these patients noninfectious. According to the Centers for Disease Control and Prevention (CDC), patients are not considered infectious if they are on adequate therapy for 2 or more weeks, have a favorable clinical response to therapy, and have three consecutive negative sputum smear results from sputum collected on different days.

Special Circumstances

HIV Coinfection. Despite being immunocompromised, HIV-infected individuals with TB respond well to regimens containing INH and rifampin. Thus, the current recommendations are to begin the same antituberculosis regimens as used in HIV-seronegative cases. However, a recent study from San Francisco noted that the relapse rate among HIV-infected patients was 9.3/100 person-years versus 1.0 in HIV-uninfected/unknown patients. In addition, HIV-infected patients treated with a 6-month regimen were four times as likely to relapse as those treated longer. Studies have demonstrated that intermittent therapy is also associated with a higher rate of relapse and acquired rifampin resistance. Therefore, HIV-infected patients should not be treated with highly intermittent treatment regimens, particularly if they have advanced HIV disease.

The treatment of TB in HIV-infected individuals is more complicated because of the potential for drug interactions with the rifamycins and antiretroviral agents, such as the protease inhibitors (PIs) and nonnucleoside reverse transcriptase inhibitors (NNRTIs), the risk of an immune reconstitution syndrome, and the propensity to develop acquired drug resistance. The rifamycins (rifampin > rifapentine > rifabutin) are inducers of the cytochrome P450 pathway and thus can increase the metabolism of some antiretroviral drugs. Some combinations of these drugs are contraindicated, and for other combinations, dosages must be adjusted. Therefore, consultation with an expert in the field is necessary to determine the best treatment regimens for HIV-infected patients with TB. The optimal timing of antiretroviral therapy during TB treatment remains controversial; some experts recommend starting therapy within the first 2 weeks when the CD4 cell count is <100 cells/mm^3, whereas others recommend waiting until after 2 months of antituberculosis therapy before starting antiretroviral therapy.

Extrapulmonary Tuberculosis. In general, treatment of extrapulmonary TB follows the same principles as does pulmonary disease. However, both surgery and the use of corticosteroids may be needed more often in extrapulmonary TB. Corticosteroids should be considered in patients with confirmed CNS or pericardial TB. Corticosteroids have been demonstrated to improve the outcomes of tuberculous pericarditis in both acute and later phase disease. However, in neither setting is there a significant decrease in progression to constriction or need for pericardiectomy. In CNS TB, use of corticosteroids has been shown to decrease the frequency of neurologic sequelae in children. Treatment duration should be prolonged in patients with bone and joint disease to 6–9 months and for CNS disease 9–12 months.

Children. Children should be treated with the same regimens as those recommended for adults, but doses should be adjusted appropriately. Although some experts do not recommend the use of ethambutol in children, it seems to be safe and should be used whenever underlying drug resistance is suspected. In addition, some experts recommend increasing the duration of therapy to 9–12 months in children with disseminated and/or meningeal disease. HIV-infected children should receive at least 9 months of therapy.

Pregnancy and Breastfeeding. Pregnant and breastfeeding women with active TB must be treated, because the risk of untreated TB to the fetus or infant is always greater than any small risks of therapy. Pyrazinamide is not recommended currently in the United States in pregnant women because of a lack of data regarding teratogenicity, but the drug is recommended by the WHO and International Union Against Tuberculosis and Lung Disease (IUATLD).

TABLE 31-2 Doses of First-Line Antituberculosis Drugs for Adults and Children

Drug	Preparation	Adults/children	Daily	1×/wk	2×/wk	3×/wk
First-line drugs						
Isoniazid	Tablets (50 mg, 100 mg, 300 mg); elixir (50 mg/ 5 mL); aqueous solution (100 mg/mL) for intravenous or intramuscular injection	Adults (max)	5 mg/kg (300 mg)	15 mg/kg (900 mg)	15 mg/kg (900 mg)	15 mg/kg (900 mg)
		Children (max)	10–15 mg/kg (300 mg)	—	20–30 mg/kg (900 mg)	—
Rifampin	Capsule (150 mg, 300 mg); powder may be suspended for oral administration; aqueous solution for intravenous injection	Adults (max)	10 mg/kg (600 mg)	—	10 mg/kg (600 mg)	10 mg/kg (600 mg)
		Children (max)	10–20 mg/kg (600 mg)	—	10 mg/kg (600 mg)	—
Rifabutin	Capsule (150 mg)	Adults (max)	5 mg/kg (300 mg)	—	5 mg/kg (300 mg)	5 mg/kg (300 mg)
		Children (max)	Appropriate dosing for children is unknown	Appropriate dosing for children is unknown	Appropriate dosing for children is unknown	Appropriate dosing for children is unknown
Rifapentine	Tablet (150 mg film coated)	Adults	—	10 mg/kg (continuation phase) (600–900 mg)	—	—
		Children	Drug is not approved for children	Drug is not approved for children	Drug is not approved for children	Drug is not approved for children
Pyrazinamide	Tablet (500 mg scored)	Adults	20–25 mg/kg (2 g)	—	35–50 mg/kg (4 g)	30–40 mg/kg (3 g)
		Children	15–30 mg/kg (2 g)	—	50 mg/kg (4 g)	—
Ethambutol	Tablet (100 mg, 400 mg)	Adults	15–20 mg/kg (1.6 g)	—	35–50 mg/kg (4 g)	20–35 mg/kg (2.5)
		Children	15–20 mg/kg (1 g)	—	50 mg/kg (4 g)	—

(From Centers for Disease Control and Prevention. MMWR 52[No. RR-11]:1-80, 2003.)

TABLE 31-3 Doses of Second-Line Antituberculosis Drugs for Adults and Children

Drug	Preparation	Adults/children	Daily	1×/wk	2×/wk	3×/wk
Second-line drugs						
Cycloserine	Capsule (250 mg)	Adults (max)	10–15 mg/kg/d (1.0 g in two doses), usually 500–750 mg/d in two doses	There are no data to support intermittent administration		
		Children (max)	10–15 mg/kg (1 g)			
Ethionamide	Tablet (250 mg)	Adults (max)	15–20 mg/kg/d (10 g/d) usually 500–750 mg/d in a single daily dose or two divided doses	There are no data to support intermittent administration		
		Children (max)	10–20 mg/kg (1 g)			
Streptomycin	Aqueous solution (1-g vials) for intravenous or intramuscular administration	Adults (max)	15 mg/kg (1 g)	—	15–20 mg/kg (1.5)	15–20 mg/kg (1.5)
		Children (max)	20–40 mg/kg (1 g)	—	20 mg/kg	—
Amikacin/kanamycin	Aqueous solution (500-mg and 1-g vials) for intravenous or intramuscular administration	Adults (max)	15 mg/kg (1 g)	—	15–20 mg/kg (1.5)	15–20 mg/kg (1.5)
		Children (max)	15–30 mg/kg (1 g)	—	15–30 mg/kg	—
Capreomycin	Aqueous solution (1-g vials) for intravenous or intramuscular administration	Adults (max)	15 mg/kg (1 g)	—	15–20 mg/kg (1.5)	15–20 mg/kg (1.5)
		Children (max)	15–30 mg/kg (1 g)	—	15–30 mg/kg	—
p-Aminosalicyclic acid (PAS)	Granules (4-g packets) can be mixed with food; tablets (500 mg) are still available in some countries, but not in the United States; a solution for intravenous administration is available in Europe	Adults	8–12 g/d in two or three doses	There are no data to support intermittent administration		
		Children (max)	200–300 mg/kg in two to four divided doses			

Continued

Table 31-3 Doses of Second-Line Antituberculosis Drugs for Adults and Children—Cont'd

Drug	Preparation	Adults/children	Daily	Doses		
				1×/wk	2×/wk	3×/wk
Levofloxacin	Tablets (250 mg, 500 mg, 750 mg); aqueous solution (500-mg vials) for intravenous injection	Adults	500–1000 mg daily	There are no data to support intermittent administration	There are no data to support intermittent administration	There are no data to support intermittent administration
		Children (max)	Optimal dose not known			
Moxifloxacin	Tablets (400 mg); aqueous solution (400 mg/250 mL) for intravenous injection	Adults	400 mg daily	There are no data to support intermittent administration	There are no data to support intermittent administration	There are no data to support intermittent administration
		Children (max)	Optimal dose not known			

TABLE 31-4 Drug Regimens for Culture-Positive Pulmonary Tuberculosis Caused by Drug-Susceptible Organisms

Initial Phase			Continuation Phase		
Regimen	Drugs	Interval and Doses (minimal duration)	Regimen	Drugs	Interval and Doses (minimal duration)
1	INH RIF PZA EMB	Seven days per week for 56 doses (8 wk) or 5 d/wk for 40 doses (8 wk)	1a	INH/RIF	Seven days per week for 126 doses (18 wk) or 5 d/wk for 90 doses (18 wk)
			1b	INH/RIF*	Twice weekly for 36 doses (18 wk)
			1c	INH/RPT†	Once weekly for 18 doses (18 wk)
2	INH RIF PZA EMB	Seven days per week for 14 doses (2 wk), then twice weekly for 12 doses (6 wk) or 5 d/wk for 10 doses (2 wk), then twice weekly for 12 doses (6 wk)	2a	INH/RIF*	Twice weekly for 36 doses (18 wk)
			2b	INH/RPT†	Once weekly for 18 doses (18 wk)
3	INH RIF PZA EMB	Three times weekly for 24 doses (8 wk)	3a	INH/RIF	Three times weekly for 54 doses (18 wk)
4	INH RIF PZA EMB	Seven days per week for 56 doses (8 wk) or 5 d/wk for 40 doses (8 wk)	4a	INH/RIF	Seven days per week for 217 doses (31 wk) or 5 d/wk for 155 doses (31 wk)
			4b	INH/RIF	Twice weekly for 62 doses (31 wk)

(From Centers for Disease Control and Prevention. MMWR 52[No. RR-11]: 1-80, 2003.)
INH, Isoniazid; RIF, rifampin; RPT, rifapentine; PZA, pyrazinamide; EMB, ethambutol.
*Not recommended for HIV-infected patients with CD4 cell count <100 cells/μL.
†Should only be used in HIV-negative patients who have negative sputum smears at the time of completion of 2 months of therapy and who do not have cavitation on the initial chest radiograph.

Clinical Course and Prevention

Monitoring for Adverse Reactions and Response to Therapy

All patients receiving antituberculosis therapy must be educated about possible drug-related adverse reactions. The patients should be warned about insignificant side effects, such as the orange discoloration of urine from rifampin, as well as the symptoms of potentially serious side effects. Baseline measurements of hepatic enzymes, bilirubin, serum creatinine, and blood urea nitrogen, as well as a complete blood cell count including platelets, are obtained before beginning drug therapy. A serum uric acid level is obtained if pyrazinamide is included in the drug regimen. Visual acuity and red/green color discrimination are monitored in patients receiving ethambutol. Although routine laboratory monitoring for drug toxicity may not be necessary, many centers repeat liver function tests after 1 month of therapy and thereafter if symptoms develop or the liver function tests are elevated significantly.

Sputum examinations at monthly intervals are important to monitor response to therapy. Smears and cultures should be negative after 2–3 months of therapy. If the sputum remains positive after 3 months, the patient must be reevaluated; special attention is given to monitoring adherence and ruling out acquired drug resistance. Drug susceptibility tests are repeated, and the appropriateness of the drug regimen is reassessed.

Prevention of Tuberculosis

The best method of preventing TB is to identify active cases and treat them to cure, thus, preventing transmission to others.

Unfortunately, most transmission has occurred before diagnosis and initiation of therapy, so other methods are needed to prevent the development of TB. There are two methods that are used to do this. The first is to vaccinate individuals with the only available TB vaccine, Bacillus Calmette–Guérin (BCG). Although BCG is the most widely used vaccine in the world, there are serious shortcomings with this approach. The second is to diagnosis LTBI and treat those individuals with antituberculosis drugs to prevent progression to active disease.

Diagnosis of Latent Tuberculosis Infection

Most patients who are infected with M. tuberculosis are able to arrest the development of active disease with adequate cell-mediated immunity. However, as noted previously, approximately 10% of infected individuals have TB develop during their lifetime. One approach to TB control is to identify high-risk individuals with LTBI before they have TB develop and treat them (Figure 31-11). Until recently, the only method to detect LTBI was the TST. Recently, blood-based assays have been developed that provide an alternative to the TST. Whichever test is used, it is important to note that only those individuals or populations at increased risk of infection and/or disease should be tested and only after ruling out active TB.

Tuberculin Skin Test

The traditional test to diagnose LTBI for more than 100 years has been the TST. The reaction to intradermally injected tuberculin is a classic example of a delayed-type hypersensitivity

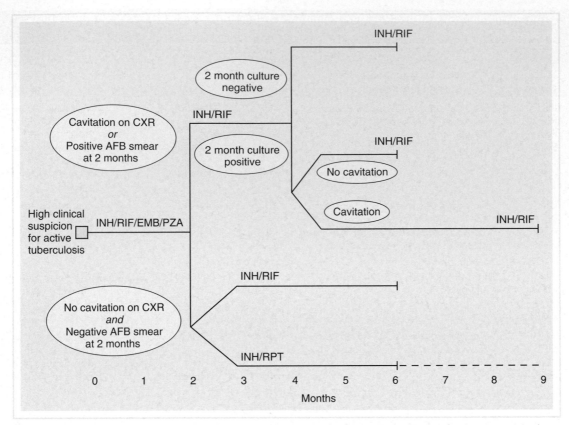

FIGURE 31-10 Treatment of pulmonary tuberculosis. Tuberculosis suspects who have no evidence of cavitation on a chest radiograph and who have negative AFB sputum smears after 2 months of therapy can be treated in the continuation phase with INH and rifampin to complete a 6-month duration of therapy. Alternately, they may be treated with INH and rifapentine administered once weekly. If cultures remain positive after 2 months of therapy, treatment duration should be extended by 3 months. TB suspects who have evidence of cavitation on the chest radiograph or who have a positive AFB smear after 2 months of therapy should be treated with INH and rifampin. If the 2-month culture is negative, they can be treated for a total of 6 months. If the 2-month culture is positive and there is no evidence of cavitation on the chest radiograph, they can be treated for 6 months. However, if cavitation is present, the continuation phase should be lengthened by 3 months. (From Centers for Disease Control and Prevention. MMWR 52[No. RR-11]:1-80, 2003.)

reaction, characterized by a peak reaction at 48–72 h marked by induration and, rarely, vesiculation and necrosis. The standard tuberculin test consists of 0.1 mL (5 tuberculin units) of purified protein derivative (PPD) administered intradermally, usually in the volar surface of the forearm. Sensitization is induced by infection with *M. tuberculosis* or other cross-reacting mycobacteria antigens. The TST should be read by trained readers 48–72 h after injection. The basis of the reading is the degree of induration present, not erythema.

Over time, delayed-type hypersensitivity resulting from mycobacterial infection may wane in some individuals, resulting in a nonreactive TST despite the fact that they are truly infected. The stimulus of this initial negative TST in these persons may "boost" or increase the size of the reaction to a second test administered later, resulting in a positive TST and incorrectly suggesting tuberculin conversion. This ability of the TST to recall the waned reactivity is known as the "booster" phenomenon.

Because of the difficulty in distinguishing boosting (indicating prior infection many years ago) from tuberculin conversion (indicating recent infection), it is recommended that persons who will undergo annual tuberculin skin testing and persons older than 55 years old receive two-step testing.

Because the TST is not entirely specific for the diagnosis of infection with *M. tuberculosis*, false-positive tests can occur from either infection with NTM or BCG vaccination. With respect to BCG vaccination, it can be difficult to distinguish between a TST reaction that is caused by LTBI and that caused by prior BCG vaccination. In 24 studies that involved almost 250,000 subjects BCG vaccinated as an infant, only 1% had a positive TST attributable after 10 years. BCG vaccination after infancy had a more significant and lasting impact on the TST reaction. In practice, most clinicians ignore prior BCG vaccination when interpreting the results of TSTs if it has been at least several years since the time of vaccination.

Three different thresholds (5, 10, and 15 mm) have been set for defining a positive tuberculin reaction, depending on the individual or population being tested (see Table 31-1). For persons at highest risk of TB developing, a cutoff of >5 mm is recommended. This group includes persons known or suspected of being HIV infected, close contacts of active TB cases, persons with an abnormal chest radiograph showing fibrosis consistent with prior TB (Figure 31-12), and other immunosuppressed patients. A cutoff of >10 mm is classified as positive for individuals at intermediate risk for TB. The remaining group consists of persons at low risk for TB who

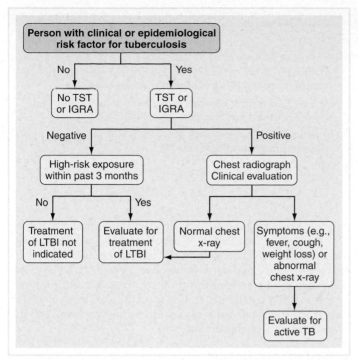

FIGURE 31-11 Flow diagram for screening for latent tuberculosis infection. In persons with clinical or epidemiologic risk factors for tuberculosis, a tuberculin skin test or interferon gamma release assay should be performed. If positive, a clinical evaluation and chest radiograph should be performed. If either is positive, the patient should be evaluated for the possibility of active tuberculosis. If the chest radiograph is normal, the patient is a candidate for treatment of LTBI. If the initial TST or IGRA is negative but there has been contact with infectious cases of tuberculosis, treatment may still be indicated.

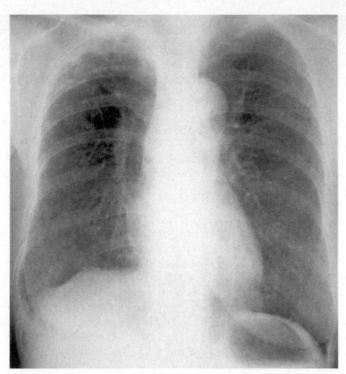

FIGURE 31-12 Chest radiograph of patient with previous tuberculosis. Note the right upper lobe linear and nodular opacities with pleural thickening. In addition, note the elevation of the right hemidiaphragm and superior retraction of the right hilum because of volume loss.

have no risk factors. These persons are classified as positive if the tuberculin reaction is >15 mm and, in general, should not be screened.

Recent TST converters are also at high risk of TB and have, therefore, been identified as a high-priority group for treatment of LTBI. Conversion is defined as an increase in induration of at least 10 mm within a 2-year period.

Interferon-γ Release Assays

As noted previously, there are two new T-cell–based tests for the diagnosis of LTBI, the QFT-TB Gold and T-Spot.*TB* test. The QFT-TB Gold uses an ELISA method to measure antigen-specific production of IFN-γ, whereas the T-Spot.*TB* test uses ELISPOT to measure the number of cells that produce IFN-γ. The CDC has recommended that these assays replace the TST, whereas the U.K. National Institute for Clinical Excellence has suggested that the IGRAs be used as adjuncts to the TST. Numerous studies have assessed the test characteristics of these assays by use of different versions of the tests, in different populations, and under different laboratory conditions. Overall, the specificity of QFT-TB Gold is approximately 97% and that of T-Spot.*TB* test approximately 92% when assessed in low-risk populations. On the other hand, as noted previously, the sensitivity of the

T-Spot.*TB* seems to be higher than that of the QFT-TB Gold when assessed in patients with active TB. It is important to note, however, that we do not have a "gold standard" for LTBI, so the true test characteristics of these assays is unknown. In studies assessing the correlation with degree of exposure, both IGRAs correlated with exposure better than the TST, and neither was affected by previous BCG vaccination.

The advantages of IGRAs compared with the standard TST are several: these blood-based tests have less cross-reactivity from vaccination with BCG and NTM, are less susceptible to reader variability that occurs with reading of the TST, require only one patient visit to obtain results, and may be more specific for identifying *M. tuberculosis* infection. However, longitudinal studies are needed to assess whether the results of IGRAs correlate with progression to disease.

Treatment of Latent Tuberculosis Infection

Persons who are infected with *M. tuberculosis* but do not have active disease should be considered for treatment of their LTBI. However, treatment is not recommended for all persons with LTBI, but instead, therapy should be provided to those persons at higher risk for tuberculous infection and/or TB. For persons who are at increased risk of progressing to disease, treatment of latent infection is indicated, regardless of age. Everyone being considered for therapy should receive a clinical and radiographic evaluation to exclude the possibility of active disease. The two most commonly used drugs for the treatment of LTBI are INH and rifampin (Table 31-5).

TABLE 31-5 Recommended Drug Regimens for Treatment of Latent Tuberculosis Infection in Adults

Drug	Duration (months)	Interval	Minimum No. of Doses	Comments
Isoniazid	9	Daily Twice weekly	270 76	9 months of isoniazid is preferred, but 6 months of isoniazid or 4 months of rifampin are acceptable alternatives.
Isoniazid	6	Daily Twice weekly	180 52	Not indicated for HIV-infected persons, those with fibrotic lesions on chest radiographs, or children.
Rifampin	4	Daily	120	For persons who are contacts of patients with isoniazid-resistant, rifampin-susceptible TB.

(From Centers for Disease Control and Prevention. MMWR 52[No. RR-11]:1-80, 2003.)

INH was evaluated in randomized controlled trials conducted by the United States Public Health Service that included more than 70,000 participants encompassing a variety of populations. In these studies, the effectiveness of the drug compared with placebo in reducing the incidence of active tuberculosis averaged approximately 60%, with a range of 25-92%, the higher values being associated with better adherence to the drug. On the basis of these studies, the American Thoracic Society and CDC recommend that INH be administered as a single daily dose or twice weekly. Completion of treatment is based on the total number of doses administered and not on duration of therapy alone.

Hepatitis is the most important adverse reaction related to INH. Although liver enzyme abnormalities are relatively common in persons taking INH, symptomatic hepatitis is uncommon. In fact, a recent study has estimated the rate of INH-related hepatitis to be 1/1000 persons. The most important cofactor for the development of INH hepatitis is alcohol consumption, so patients should be advised not to drink alcohol when they are taking INH. In addition, all persons taking INH should be educated about the symptoms of hepatitis, including nausea, vomiting, extreme fatigue, abdominal pain, dark urine, and jaundice, so that they can be evaluated before the hepatitis becomes severe.

The other potential side effect of INH is peripheral neuropathy that is caused by interference with the metabolism of pyridoxine. In persons predisposed to neuropathy (such as patients with diabetes, uremia, malnutrition, and HIV infection), in pregnant women, and persons with seizure disorders, pyridoxine (at a dose of 25 or 50 mg/day) should be given concurrently with isoniazid.

Rifampin alone for 4 months is the second option for treatment of LTBI. Rifampin for treatment of LTBI has not been well studied and, in the only large randomized trial evaluating its use, 10% of the patients taking rifampin alone for 3 months had active TB develop after completing therapy. In that study, rifampin taken daily for 3 months in persons with LTBI and silicosis had an efficacy equivalent to that of INH taken daily for 6 months. Rifampin should be used for patients who are intolerant of INH or who are presumed to have infection with INH-resistant strains of M. tuberculosis. Data regarding toxicity by use of rifampin alone for LTBI are limited, but in three published studies, rifampin alone seemed to be well tolerated and had a very low rate of hepatotoxicity.

Clinical Monitoring

Baseline laboratory testing of liver enzymes is not routinely indicated, except in the following instances: HIV-infected persons; pregnant women and those within 3 months postpartum; persons with a history of liver disease; and persons who use alcohol regularly. Follow-up laboratory testing of liver enzymes is indicated only if baseline liver enzyme tests are abnormal or when symptoms of hepatitis occur. Drugs should be withheld if a patient's serum transaminase level is greater than three times normal if associated with symptoms and five times normal if asymptomatic.

Special Circumstances

Coinfection with HIV. Because HIV-infected persons are clearly at highest risk for active TB developing once infected, they should be screened for TB and LTBI. HIV-infected individuals with LTBI should receive 9 months of INH once active TB has been ruled out. Rifampin should be used with caution in HIV-infected persons taking PIs or NNRTIs because of drug interactions described previously. In HIV-infected persons taking these antiretroviral drugs who have LTBI, rifabutin (often at an adjusted dose) can be substituted for rifampin in some circumstances.

Abnormal Chest Radiographs. In individuals with evidence of LTBI who have an abnormal chest radiograph with parenchymal fibrotic lesions (see Figure 31-12) who have not been previously treated, sputum should be collected to exclude active TB. Once active TB has been excluded, treatment options for LTBI include INH for 9 months and rifampin (with or without isoniazid) for 4 months.

Pregnancy and Lactating Women. Although INH can be given safely during pregnancy, most clinicians wait until after delivery to begin treatment for LTBI, unless the woman has HIV infection or has been in known contact with an infectious case.

Infants and Children. Infants and children younger than 5 years old are at high risk for progression to active TB once infected and should receive INH for 9 months.

Contacts to Drug-Resistant Cases. Contacts of patients with INH-resistant, rifampin-susceptible tuberculosis should be treated with rifampin for 4 months. The treatment of persons in recent contact with a MDR-TB case is challenging, however, and needs to be individualized on the basis of the susceptibility pattern of the source patient's organism, the probability that infection has occurred, and risk factors for progression to active TB. Treatment of contacts to MDR-TB often entails the administration of two drugs (to which the source case's isolate is susceptible) for 9-12 months.

Vaccination with Bacille Guérin Calmette (BCG)

BCG is a live attenuated vaccine derived from a strain of *Mycobacterium bovis*. BCG is used to vaccinate children, and in some cases adolescents and adults, throughout much of the world. Although the vaccine seems to be protective in children, it confers little protection in adults, who are the ones that usually transmit disease. Data suggest that BCG vaccination decreases the risk of disseminated disease in young children; that is the primary reason for its use today. In countries in which BCG vaccination was suspended, there was not a significant increase in TB rates reported.

As noted previously, BCG vaccination can influence the results of tuberculin skin testing because of cross-reaction with PPD. The effects of BCG vaccination on tuberculin reactivity vary, depending on the specific vaccine used, age of vaccination, and interval between vaccination and skin testing. Despite widespread use of BCG vaccination, it is difficult to demonstrate significant impact on TB control globally. New vaccines are greatly needed.

DISEASES CAUSED BY NONTUBERCULOUS MYCOBACTERIA

The NTM comprise more than 125 different species that are widely distributed throughout the environment and most of which have not been implicated as a cause of disease in humans. The rapidly growing list of mycobacterial species is primarily related to the availability of DNA sequencing, which has allowed identification of new species simply by detecting differences in the sequence of 1% or greater as new species.

The NTM were not widely recognized as a cause of human disease until the late 1950s. In 1959, Runyon reported a classification system that organized the NTM into four groups on the basis of microbiologic characteristics, including the formation of pigment and the speed of growth. This system has become less useful with the development of rapid molecular methods of diagnosis, but differentiating NTM on the basis of their rate of growth is still used today. NTM are typically divided into rapidly and slowly growing species (Table 31-6).

Epidemiology, Risk Factors, and Pathogenesis

Epidemiology

NTM have been isolated from soil and water sources, including both natural and treated water sources, from throughout the world. Because these organisms do not seem to be transmitted from human to human, the source of human infection is thought to be through environmental exposures. Skin test surveys of U.S. Navy recruits in the 1960s demonstrated higher rates of reactivity in those from the southeastern United States than from the northern states, suggesting higher rates of infection. Studies evaluating antibody to lipoarabinomannin (LAM) have demonstrated anti-LAM antibodies beginning early in life and rapidly rising through age 12.

Because NTM are usually not considered a reportable infection, there is a lack of surveillance data. The median rates of pulmonary NTM isolation have been approximately 6.2/

TABLE 31-6 Nontuberculous Mycobacteria by Rate of Growth	
Slowly growing (>7 days of incubation for mature growth)	Rapidly growing (≤7 days of incubation for mature growth)
M. avium	M. fortuitum group
M. intracellulare	M. fortuitum
M. kansasii	M. peregrinum
M. xenopi	M. fortuitum third biovariant
M. simiae	complex
M. szulgai	M. chelonei/abscessus group
M. scrofulaceum	M. abscessus
M. malmoense	M. chelonae
M. haemophilum	M. immunogenum
M. genavense	M. smegmatis
M. marinum*	
M. gordonae*	

*These organisms often grow within 7–10 days.

100,000 in North America, 8.3/100,000 in Europe, 15/100,000 in Asia, and 7.2/100,000 in Australia. Recent data support the view that the incidence of NTM infections is increasing. In a retrospective cohort review from 1997–2003 in Ontario, Canada, 222,247 pulmonary isolates from 10,231 patients were identified. The prevalence was 9.1/100,000 in 1997 and increased to 14.1/100,000 by 2003 ($P < .0001$), with an average annual increase of 8.4%. Increases were noted among *M. avium* complex, *M. xenopi*, rapidly growing mycobacteria, and *M. kansasii*. Of note, the rate of TB declined 4.0% over the study period. Two hundred patients were evaluated in more detail, and 33% fulfilled the clinical, radiologic, and bacteriologic ATS criteria.

The most common NTM pathogens vary geographically. *M. avium* complex has been reported as the most common cause of NTM-related pulmonary disease in almost all studies. However, the next most common NTM vary. For example, in the United States, *M. kansasii* is the second most common cause of pulmonary disease followed by *M. abscessus*. In Canada, and some parts of Europe, *M. xenopi* is the second most common, whereas in northern Europe and Scandinavia, *M. malmoense* is second.

Risk Factors

Patients who have pulmonary infections caused by NTM often have structural lung disease such as chronic obstructive pulmonary disease, bronchiectasis, cystic fibrosis, pneumoconiosis, prior TB, alveolar proteinosis, and chronic aspiration. A study from France noted more than 50% of the patients who met ATS disease criteria (except for those with *M. kansasii*) had underlying predisposing factors such as preexisting pulmonary or immune deficiency. HIV-infected patients and those with abnormalities in the IFN-γ or interleukin-12 (IL-12) pathways are predisposed to severe NTM infections.

Of note, many women with NTM infection have nodular bronchiectasis and similar body types: scoliosis, pectus excavatum, mitral valve prolapse, and joint hypermobility. The reason for this association has not been definitively determined.

Pathogenesis

Although little is known about the pathogenesis of NTM infections, several observations have provided some insight into this disease. First, in patients with HIV infection, disseminated NTM infections typically occur only after the CD4 lymphocyte count falls below 50 cells/μL, suggesting that specific T-cell products or activities are required for mycobacterial resistance. Second, in HIV-uninfected patients, certain genetic syndromes have been identified that are associated with disseminated NTM infections. These syndromes have been traced to mutations in IFN-γ and IL-12 synthesis and response pathways. Third, there is a striking association between bronchiectasis, nodular pulmonary NTM infections, and a particular body habitus, predominantly in postmenopausal women. In the latter instance, it remains to be seen whether or not these women have some sort of subtle immune deficiency that predisposes them to NTM pulmonary infections or their predisposition is related to ineffective mucociliary clearance or poor tracheobronchial secretion drainage.

NTM do not seem to live in a state of dormancy like *M. tuberculosis.* Moreover, unlike with TB, simply isolating an NTM from a respiratory specimen does not mean that the patient has NTM-related disease. For years the term "colonization" has been used to differentiate those who have a single or small number of positive cultures over time and in whom progressive disease cannot be demonstrated. However, with longer follow-up, many of these patients do, in fact, demonstrate clinical and/or radiographic progression of disease, so it may be more appropriate to think of these patients as having indolent infection.

Genetics

The genetics of NTM infection are not well understood. In a study from Japan, 170 patients with *Mycobacterium avium* complex (MAC) lung infection were studied and of 622 siblings of these patients, 3 also had MAC lung disease. The authors concluded that the rate of infection among the siblings was higher than previously estimated among the general population.

Clinical Features

The most common clinical manifestation of NTM infection is lung disease. However, lymphatic, skin/soft tissue, bone/joint involvement, as well as disseminated disease are also important. The propensity for a specific manifestation varies with the NTM species and certain host factors. For example, HIV-infected patients typically are seen with disseminated disease caused by *M. avium,* whereas elderly white women usually have pulmonary disease caused by *M. intracellulare.*

Pulmonary Disease

Chronic pulmonary disease is the most common clinical presentation of NTM disease, and patients usually are seen with chronic cough, fatigue, malaise, dyspnea, fever, hemoptysis, chest pain, and weight loss. Patients with pulmonary disease because of rapidly growing mycobacteria are typically white, female nonsmokers, older than 60 years of age with no obvious predisposing conditions. Most patients present with cough and easy fatigability. These patients should be evaluated for possible gastroesophageal disorders that lead to aspiration, lipoid pneumonia, cystic fibrosis, and α$_1$-antitrypsin anomalies. Physical examination may identify certain morphologic characteristics in postmenopausal women, and occasionally men, that include thin body habitus, scoliosis, pectus excavatum, and mitral valve prolapse.

Radiographic features will depend on whether the patient has primarily fibrocavitary disease or nodular bronchiectatic disease. Patients who are seen with primarily fibrocavitary disease are typically diagnosed because they are being evaluated for possible TB. The abnormalities consist of upper lobe opacities with evidence of cavitation and volume loss. Classically, this pattern of disease was recognized in older men with underlying lung disease (Figure 31-13). Patients with predominantly noncavitary nodular bronchiectatic disease have opacities in the mid and lower lung fields. High-resolution computed tomography scans demonstrate bronchiectasis often

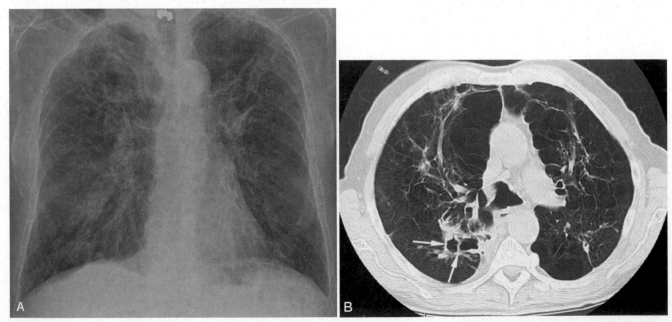

FIGURE 31-13 A, Chest radiograph of patient with upper lobe emphysema and severe lung disease caused by *M. avium* complex. **B,** Chest computed tomography demonstrates severe emphysema with cavitation posteriorly (*arrows*) in the right lower lobe.

in the middle lobe and lingula with evidence of small nodules, centrilobular in location (Figure 31-14). It is important to recognize that there is a great deal of overlap between the two classic radiographic presentations and between the patterns of disease produced by the various NTM species.

Patients with *M. kansasii* infection usually are seen with upper lobe cavitary opacities, and the cavities are typically thin walled (Figure 31-15). The chest radiograph in patients with rapidly growing mycobacterial infections usually shows multilobar, patchy, reticulonodular or mixed interstitial alveolar opacities, with an upper lobe predominance (Figure 31-16). Cavitation is reported to occur in 15%. High-resolution CT will show bronchiectasis and small nodules similar to MAC.

Lymphadenitis

In children, the most common form of NTM disease is cervical lymphadenitis. *M. avium* is the most common etiology, accounting for 80% of culture-proven cases. *M. scrofulaceum*

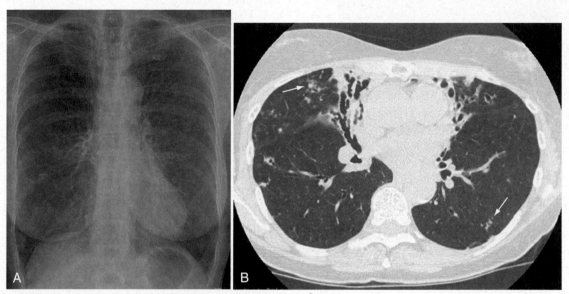

FIGURE 31-14 A, Chest radiograph with right middle lobe and lingular bronchiectasis in a patient with *M. avium* complex and *M. simiae.* **B,** Chest computed tomography demonstrating bronchiectasis in the right middle lobe and lingula. Note also the nodular opacities and tree-in-bud opacities (*arrows*).

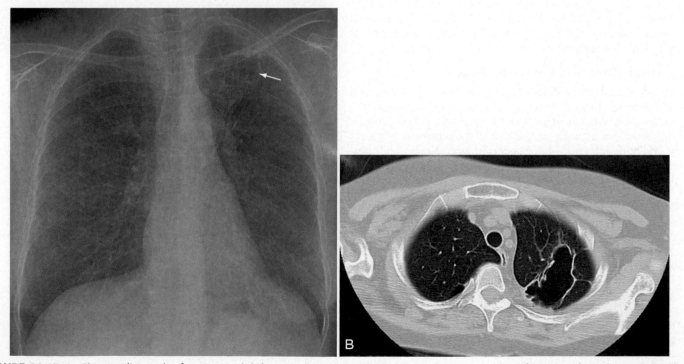

FIGURE 31-15 A, Chest radiograph of patient with left upper lobe thin walled cavity (*arrow*) caused by infection with *M. kansasii.* **B,** Chest computed tomography demonstrating a thin-walled left upper lobe cavity.

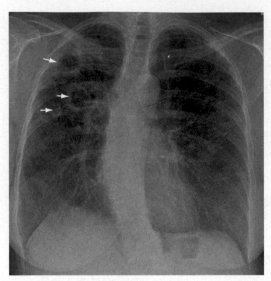

FIGURE 31-16 Chest radiograph of a patient with infection caused by *M. abscessus*. Note the multiple cavities, diffuse nodular opacities, and kyphoscoliosis.

is the second most common cause of lymphadenitis in the United States and Australia, whereas *M. malmoense* and *M. haemophilum* are in Scandinavia, the United Kingdom, and other areas of northern Europe. *M. tuberculosis* is isolated in only 10% of culture-proven mycobacterial cervical lymphadenitis in the United States, but in adults 90% are due to TB.

Infection usually involves the submandibular, submaxillary, cervical, and preauricular lymph nodes in children between 1 and 5 years of age. The disease occurs insidiously and is rarely associated with systemic symptoms. Involvement of the lymph nodes is usually unilateral and nontender. The lymph nodes may enlarge and eventually rupture, producing sinus tracts just like tuberculous lymphadenitis. Diagnosis is usually made by fine-needle aspiration or surgical excision of the involved lymph nodes. Only 50–82% of excised nodes will be culture positive. Treatment for most NTM-related cervical lymphadenitis is surgical excision.

Soft Tissue, Skin, and Bone Infections

Although virtually any NTM can cause skin, soft tissue, and bony infection, the most common species to do so are the rapid growers, *M. marinum* and *M. ulcerans*. Rapid growers often produce infections at the site of punctures or surgery. Joint and bone infections have occurred after surgery and traumatic injuries. Tissue biopsy is the most sensitive way to diagnose these infections.

Disseminated Infections

Disseminated infections are most commonly associated with HIV infection and other forms of severe immunosuppression. More than 90% of reported disseminated infection in HIV-infected patients are due to MAC, and almost all of these are due to *M. avium*. The next most common cause of disseminated NTM disease in HIV patients is *M. kansasii*, but a number of other species have also been implicated. Most patients are seen with advanced HIV disease and complain of fever, night sweats, and weight loss. Abdominal pain and diarrhea may also be reported. In non-HIV–infected patients, fever of unknown origin is a common presentation. Diagnosis is usually through detection of the causative organism in the blood.

In HIV-infected patients *M. avium* can be isolated in more than 90% of cases.

Diagnosis

Patients suspected of having a NTM infection should be evaluated with a chest radiograph and/or high-resolution computed tomography, particularly when there is no evidence of cavitation on the radiograph. If there is evidence of radiographic abnormalities consistent with an NTM infection, at least three sputum specimens should be obtained for AFB examination and mycobacterial culture. TB, as well as other disorders, should be excluded.

To diagnose NTM infection, the clinician must weigh clinical, bacteriologic, and radiographic information (Box 31-1). NTM pulmonary infections should be suspected when a patient is seen with a compatible clinical picture and has nodular or cavitary opacities on the chest radiograph or an HRCT scan that shows multifocal bronchiectasis with multiple small nodules. In addition to these clinical criteria, the patient should have at least two positive cultures from separate sputum specimens or a positive culture from at least one bronchial wash or lavage. Additional diagnostic criteria include transbronchial or other lung biopsy with mycobacterial histopathologic features and positive culture for NTM or biopsy showing mycobacterial histopathologic features and one or more sputum or bronchial washings that are culture positive. In patients who do not meet the preceding definition for disease, close follow-up should occur, because many of the patients will demonstrate progression over time.

The same methods that are used to stain and grow *M. tuberculosis* are used for NTM. Both solid and liquid culture media support growth of the NTM, and both are recommended for use in the clinical laboratory. Although cultures in broth media have a higher yield and provide a more rapid result, they do

---

BOX 31-1 Clinical and Microbiologic Criteria for Diagnosing Nontuberculous Mycobacterial Lung Disease

Clinical (both required)

1. Pulmonary symptoms, nodular or cavitary opacities on chest radiograph, or a high-resolution computed tomography scan that shows multifocal bronchiectasis with multiple small nodules
   and
2. Appropriate exclusion for other diagnoses

Microbiologic

1. Positive culture results from at least two separate expectorated sputum samples. If results are nondiagnostic, consider repeat sputum AFB smears and cultures.
   or
2. Positive culture result from at least one bronchial wash or lavage.
   or
3. Transbronchial or other lung biopsy with mycobacterial histopathologic features (granulomatous inflammation or AFB) and positive culture for NTM or biopsy showing mycobacterial histopathologic features (granulomatous inflammation or AFB) and one or more sputum or bronchial washings that are culture positive for NTM.

(From Griffith DE, Aksamit T, Brown-Elliott BA, *et al.* Am J Respir Crit Care Med 175:367–416, 2007.)

not allow for observation of colony morphology, growth rates, and recognition of mixed cultures as do solid media. For most mycobacteria, the optimum temperature for growth is 28°–37°C, and most clinically significant NTM grow at 35°–37°C. However, some NTM (*M. marinum*, *M. chelonae*, *M. ulcerans*, and *M. haemophilum*) require lower temperatures for optimum growth. Others, like *M. xenopi*, grow best at higher temperatures. Some species require special media such as iron or heme for *M. haemophilum* and mycobactin J for *M. genavense*. Most NTM grow within 2–3 weeks on subculture, but it may take up to 8–12 weeks to grow *M. ulcerans* and *M. genavense*. Rapidly growing mycobacteria usually grow within 7 days.

Species identification can be performed biochemically or more commonly with high-performance liquid chromatography (HPLC), genetic probes, and/or 16S ribosomal DNA sequencing. Genetic probes are commercially available only for *M. tuberculosis*, *M. kansasii*, *M. avium*, *M. intracellulare*, and *M. gordonae*. These probes have a sensitivity of between 85 and 100%, with a specificity of 100%. HPLC is a practical and rapid way to detect differences in mycolic acid content between NTM species, although this method cannot differentiate some species of NTM. DNA sequence analysis is able to differentiate strains on the basis of two hypervariable sequences.

The role of *in vitro* susceptibility testing for managing patients with NTM disease remains controversial. Unlike with *M. tuberculosis*, the *in vitro* susceptibility results and clinical outcome do not always correlate, and this is particularly true of infections caused by *M. avium* complex, *M. xenopi*, and *M. simiae*. On the other hand, there seems to be better correlation with *M. marinum*, *M. kansasii*, and the rapid growers. Drug susceptibility testing can be performed through a variety of methods, and the following drugs are usually tested: clarithromycin, ciprofloxacin, doxycycline, a sulfonamide, amikacin, cefoxitin, imipenem, and tobramycin.

For slowly growing mycobacteria, no single method is recommended for all species. For isolates of MAC, a broth-based method with both microdilution or macrodilution methods is acceptable. For other slowly growing NTM, broth and solid media may be used, but they must be validated within each laboratory performing the tests. Clarithromycin testing is currently recommended for new, previously untreated MAC isolates, those who fail macrolide-based treatment regimens, or prophylaxis regimens. Previously untreated *M. kansasii* isolates should be tested *in vitro* against rifampin. Isolates resistant to rifampin should also be tested against rifabutin, ethambutol, isoniazid, clarithromycin, fluoroquinolones, amikacin, and sulfonamides.

Treatment

When a patient grows *M. tuberculosis*, treatment is always indicated, assuming that the isolate was not due to laboratory cross contamination. However, with NTM, isolation should not always lead to treatment. The decision to treat is based on the potential risks and benefits for the individual patient. Thus, management of patients with NTM infections is complicated and requires a great deal of individualization of therapy. In addition, *in vitro* susceptibility results for many NTM do not correlate well with clinical response to antimicrobial therapy, thus clinicians should use such data with a clear understanding of the limitations.

Pulmonary Infections

Mycobacterium avium Complex

Before the availability of the newer macrolides, the long-term treatment outcomes for patients treated with antituberculosis regimens was approximately 50%. Small, noncomparative studies of azithromycin- and clarithromycin-containing regimens have been associated with higher bacteriologic response rates, but long-term follow-up is often lacking. The ATS currently recommends that the treatment regimen be based on the presence or absence of cavitary disease and whether or not the patient has been treated previously (Table 31-7). For patients with noncavitary nodular bronchiectasis disease, a three times a week regimen should be considered. For patients with cavitary and/or advanced disease and in those who have been treated previously, daily therapy is recommended. An aminoglycoside should be considered in patients, at least for the first 2–3 months of therapy, if they have cavitary disease or have been treated previously and treatment has failed. Surgery should be considered in patients who have a macrolide-resistant strain of MAC, have had treatment fail, or who have primarily focal cavitary disease.

M. kansasii

Patients with lung disease caused by *M. kansasii* should be treated with isoniazid, rifampin, and ethambutol (see Table 31-7). On the basis of *in vitro* activity, the newer macrolides could probably be substituted for INH. In one study, no relapses were seen after 46 months of follow-up in patients who received clarithromycin, rifampin, and ethambutol. The treatment duration should include 12 months of negative sputum cultures. For patients whose isolate is resistant to the rifamycins, a three-drug regimen is recommended on the basis of *in vitro* susceptibility data to clarithromycin or azithromycin, moxifloxacin, ethambutol, sulfamethoxazole, or streptomycin. Surgical resection is almost never necessary in patients infected with *M. kansasii*.

Rapidly Growing Mycobacteria

M. abscessus is the third most frequently encountered NTM respiratory pathogen in the United States and accounts for 80% of rapidly growing mycobacteria (RGM) lung disease. Treatment outcomes with *M. abscessus* are generally poor, in part because the organism is resistant to almost all of the standard antituberculosis drugs. *In vitro* susceptibility testing is recommended for selection of a treatment regimen; however, *M. abscessus* is susceptible to only a few antimicrobials, including the macrolides, imipenem, cefoxitin, amikacin, tigecycline, and occasionally linezolid. Moreover, no antibiotic regimen has demonstrated long-term sputum conversion in patients with pulmonary disease. Current recommendations are to provide periodic drug administration of multidrug therapy, including a macrolide, and one or more parenteral agents such as amikacin, cefoxitin, or imipenem for 4–6 months to help control symptoms and prevent progression (see Table 31-7). For patients who are good candidates, surgical resection should be considered but only if done by an experienced surgeon and after a period of intensive antimicrobial therapy.

M. chelonae is typically susceptible to tobramycin, macrolides, linezolid, imipenem, and amikacin and may demonstrate susceptibility to fluoroquinolones and doxycycline. Isolates are usually resistant to cefoxitin. Treatment should consist of at least two drugs to which there has been demonstrated

TABLE 31-7 Diseases Caused by the Nontuberculous _Mycobacteria_ and Recommended Therapy

Clinical Disease	Common Etiologies	Recommended Antimicrobial Therapy	Other Etiologies
Pulmonary disease	1. _M. avium_ complex 　a. _Nodular bronchiectasis_	Clarithromycin 1000 mg tiw or azithromycin 500–600 mg tiw, rifampin 600 mg tiw, ethambutol 25 mg/kg tiw	1. _M. simiae_ 2. _M. malmoense_ 3. _M. szulgai_
	b. _Cavitary disease_	Clarithromycin 1000 mg daily or azithromycin 250 mg daily; rifampin 450–600 mg daily, ethambutol 15 mg/kg daily and consider amikacin 15 mg/kg (for the first 2–3 mo) tiw	4. _M. celatum_ 5. _M. asiaticum_ 6. _M. haemophilum_
	c. _Previously treated_	Clarithromycin 1000 mg daily or azithromycin 250 mg daily, rifampin 450–600 mg daily or rifabutin 150–300 mg daily, amikacin 15 mg/kg (for the first 2–3 months) tiw	7. _M. smegmatis_ 8. _M. chelonae_ 9. _M. fortuitum_
	2. _M. kansasii_	Isoniazid 300 mg/day, rifampin 600 mg/day, ethambutol 15 mg/kg/day with at least 12 mo of negative sputum cultures. Can add aminoglycoside in severe disease.	10. _M. scrofulaceum_ 11. _M. shimodei_
	3. _M. abscessus_	Clarithromycin 1000 mg/daily or azithromycin 250 mg/daily, amikacin 15 mg/kg and cefoxitin max 12 g/day divided in 3–4 doses/day or imipenem 500–1000 mg q 8–12 h/day plus amikacin 15 mg/kg tiw	
	4. _M. xenopi_	See treatment for MAC	
Lymphadenitis	1. _M. avium_ complex 2. _M. haemophilum_	Surgical excision of infected lymph nodes Surgical excision of infected lymph nodes if immunocompetent	1. _M. fortuitum_ 2. _M. chelonae_ 3. _M. abscessus_ 4. _M. kansasii_ 5. _M. haemophilum_ 6. _M. genavense_ 7. _M. szulgai_
Skin, soft tissue, and bone disease	1. _M. marinum_	Ethambutol 15 mg/kg/day and any of the following for at least 4 mo; clarithromycin 500 mg bid, minocycline or doxycycline 100 mg bid, TM/SM 160/800 bid, or rifampin 600 mg/day	1. _M. avium_ complex 2. _M. kansasii_ 3. _M. nonchromogenicum_
	2. _M. fortuitum_	At least two drugs with _in vitro_ susceptibility for 4 mo. Six months if bone infection. Surgery required for extensive disease.	4. _M. smegmatis_ 5. _M. haemophilum_ 6. _M. immunogenum_
	3. _M. chelonae_	At least two drugs with _in vitro_ susceptibility for at least 4 mo. Six months if bone infection. Surgery for extensive disease.	7. _M. malmoense_ 8. _M. smegmatis_ 9. _M. szulgai_
	4. _M. abscessus_	Clarithromycin 1000 mg/day or azithromycin 250 mg/day plus one or more parenteral drugs (imipenem, cefoxitin, and amikacin) may be effective. Surgery required for more extensive disease.	10. _M. terrae_ complex
Disseminated disease	1. _M. avium_ complex	Three drugs are recommended: clarithromycin 500 mg bid or azithromycin, ethambutol 15 mg/kg/day, and a rifamycin. Consider adding amikacin or streptomycin in severe disease.	1. _M. abscessus_ 2. _M. xenopi_ 3. _M. malmoense_ 4. _M. genavense_
	2. _M. kansasii_	See _M. kansasii_ in the pulmonary disease section.	5. _M. simiae_ 6. _M. conspicuum_ 7. _M. marinum_
	3. _M. haemophilum_	Suggested drugs: ciprofloxacin, clarithromycin, and rifampin	8. _M. fortuitum_ 9. _M. celatum_ 10. _M. cimmunogenum_ 11. _M. mucogenicum_ 12. _M. scrofulaceum_ 13. _M. szulgai_

in vitro drug susceptibility. The duration should be for at least 12 months of culture negativity.

M. fortuitum isolates are typically susceptible to newer macrolides, fluoroquinolones, doxycycline, minocycline, sulfonamides, cefoxitin, and imipenem. Therapy should be with at least two agents with _in vitro_ activity for at least 12 months of culture negativity.

Lymphadenitis

Cervical lymphadenitis is usually caused by _M. avium_ complex or _M. scrofulaceum_ infection. Surgical excision of the involved lymph nodes without chemotherapy is usually curative, with success rates of approximately 95%. In patients who have surgical excision fail, a macrolide-based treatment regimen with or without repeat excision is usually successful.

Skin, Soft Tissue, and Bone/Joint Infections

For most patients with MAC infection, a combination of surgical excision plus multidrug chemotherapy is usually successful. The optimal duration of therapy is not known but should probably be 6–12 months in duration. For serious infections caused by rapidly growing mycobacteria, a newer macrolide should be combined with a parenteral medication (amikacin, cefoxitin, or imipenem) or perhaps another oral agent in the case of *M. fortuitum* infection. Therapy should continue for a minimum of 4 months for skin infections and at least 6 months for bone infections. Surgery is generally indicated for extensive disease, and removal of foreign objects such as breast implants, percutaneous catheters, and joint prostheses is necessary.

Disseminated Infections

Treatment of disseminated MAC infection in HIV-infected patients should include clarithromycin, 500 bid, and ethambutol, 15 mg/kg daily with or without rifabutin 300 mg daily. Azithromycin, 500 mg daily, could be used as an alternative to clarithromycin. Treatment should be considered lifelong, unless immune restoration is achieved by antiretroviral therapy. MAC treatment can be stopped for patients who are asymptomatic and have achieved a CD4 lymphocyte count of more than 100 cells/µL for at least 12 months. Prophylaxis should be reintroduced if the count falls below 100 cells/µL.

The treatment for disseminated disease caused by *M. kansasii* is the same as for pulmonary disease. Unlike with MAC, there is no known prophylactic regimen.

Clinical Course and Prevention

The clinical course will depend on the specific species of NTM that is being treated, the extent of disease, and the treatment regimen used. Untreated *M. kansasii* is usually progressive, much like TB. However, with appropriate treatment, almost all patients respond well, and both treatment failure and relapse are uncommon. Untreated *M. avium* pulmonary disease is quite variable in its progression. In some patients progression can be seen over a matter of months, and in others it may take years to demonstrate progressive disease. Treatment responses are also variable with cure rates ranging from 60–85%. Genotyping data suggest that reinfection is common in women with nodular bronchiectasis, so a patient in whom cure is achieved may become infected again. The clinical course of untreated *M. abscessus* is generally slow and progressive, but more rapidly progressive presentations have been described, particularly in patients with CF or esophageal disorders associated with aspiration.

Treatment is complicated and cure extremely rare. The mortality rate with *M. xenopi* infection has been reported to be as high as 57%, but this probably reflects the severity of the underlying lung disease.

Prevention

Strategies for preventing NTM infections are difficult to formulate because of our poor understanding of the transmission and pathogenesis of these infections. There are at least two to three areas in which there are potential ways to prevent NTM disease. The first is in HIV-infected patients with advanced disease. Preventive therapy for disseminated MAC is recommended for HIV-infected patients with fewer than 50 CD4 lymphocytes/µL. Azithromycin given as 1200 mg once weekly is the preferred agent. Alternate regimens include clarithromycin, 500 mg, twice daily or rifabutin, 300 mg daily. Primary prophylaxis should be discontinued when patients who have responded to HAART with an increase in CD4 cell count to more than 100 cells/µL for more than 3 months. Prophylaxis should be reintroduced if the cell count falls to less than 50–100 cells/µL.

The second way to prevent NTM infections is in health care settings, where contamination of water sources, biologicals, and multidose vials have been implicated in postsurgical infections. In these settings, specific steps can be taken to prevent the use of tap water to wash wounds or equipment, and multidose vials should be avoided for injections.

Prevention of community-acquired pulmonary infections remains elusive. The organisms have been isolated in tap water and water distribution systems, survive well at water temperatures of 45°C, and are resistant to our typical decontamination methods. Therefore, it is not clear how to best decrease our environmental exposure.

PITFALLS AND CONTROVERSIES

TB remains one of the most important public health problems in the world. Despite effective treatment and preventive regimens, TB continues to spread, particularly in resource-poor countries, where both HIV coinfection and drug-resistant *M. tuberculosis* create additional barriers to control. Delays in the diagnosis and initiation of effective antituberculosis chemotherapy lead to higher morbidity and mortality in the individual and continued transmission to others. The first step in preventing these scenarios is the timely diagnosis and initiation of therapy, which begins by suspecting that TB could be the cause of a patient's illness. Because of the increased frequency of drug-resistant TB, more rapid diagnostics are greatly needed particularly in areas where HIV coinfection is common. Current treatment regimens require that multiple drugs be administered over a prolonged treatment course. Poor adherence to therapy, which has resulted in poor outcomes including the development of drug-resistant disease, remains a barrier to completion of therapy. New drugs that would allow for shorter treatment regimens, ideally administered intermittently, could improve our ability to treat patients to cure.

As the United States and other industrialized countries move toward the goal of elimination, they will need improved diagnostics for detecting LTBI and ideally for identifying those at increased risk of progression to active disease. It remains to be seen whether the new IGRAs will provide us with such tools. Once diagnosed with LTBI, we face a similar problem as with the treatment of TB, a long duration of treatment. To overcome this barrier, shorter treatment regimens are needed. Finally, BCG has failed as a significant TB control measure, because it does not prevent infection from occurring and it does not prevent the development of active TB in adults, thereby allowing continuation of the cycle of transmission. New vaccines are greatly needed if we truly wish to eliminate TB on a global scale.

As TB declines in many countries, NTM infections are increasing to fill the ecologic void. The reasons for this and just how much NTM exists is not really known because of the lack of epidemiologic and surveillance data. We need better data on the natural history of NTM infections and how and where individuals become infected. Because of the difficulty in determining colonization from disease, it is important to develop better diagnostic tests and to develop new drugs and better treatment regimens for these resistant and difficult-to-treat infections. It is remarkable what we do not know about the treatment of these infections. Which macrolide is superior? Which rifamycin is superior? Does addition of an aminoglycoside improve outcomes? What is the role of the fluoroquinones? Importantly, how do we prevent these infections?

Only better epidemiologic data and clinical trials can answer these questions.

WEB RESOURCES FOR GUIDELINES/PROTOCOLS

American Thoracic Society (www.thoracic.org)
Centers for Disease Control and Prevention (www.cdc.org)
World Health Organization, Stop TB Partnership (www.stoptb.org)
International Union Against Tuberculosis and Lung Disease (www.iuatld.org)
Francis J. Curry National Tuberculosis Center (www.nationaltbcenter.org)
Heartland National Tuberculosis Center (www.heartlandntbc.org)
Southeastern National Tuberculosis Center (sntc.medicine.ufl.edu)
Northeastern Regional Training and Medical Consultation Consortium (www.umdnj.edu/globaltb/home.htm)

SUGGESTED READINGS

American Thoracic Society/Centers for Disease Control and Prevention/Infectious Diseases Society of America: Controlling tuberculosis in the United States. Am J Respir Crit Care Med 2005; 172:1169–1227.
Brodie D, Schluger NW: The diagnosis of tuberculosis. Clin Chest Med 2005; 26:247–271.
Centers for Disease Control and Prevention: Update: Nucleic acid amplification tests for tuberculosis. MMWR 2000; 49(No. 26):593–594.
Centers for Disease Control and Prevention. Treatment of Tuberculosis, American Thoracic Society, CDC, and Infectious Diseases Society of America. MMWR 2003; 52(No. RR–11):1–80.
Centers for Disease Control and Prevention: Guidelines for preventing the transmission of Mycobacterium tuberculosis in health-care settings. MMWR 2005; 54(No.RR-17).
Diagnostic Standards and Classification of Tuberculosis in Adults and Children. Am J Respir Crit Care Med. 2000; 161:1376–1395.
Griffith DE, Aksamit T, Brown-Elliott BA, et al: ATS Mycobacterial Diseases Subcommittee; American Thoracic Society; Infectious Diseases Society of America. An official ATS/IDSA statement: diagnosis, treatment, and prevention of nontuberculous mycobacterial diseases. Am J Respir Crit Care Med 2007; 175(4):367–416.
Hopewell PC, Pai M, Maher D, Uplekar M, Raviglione MC: International standards for tuberculosis care. Lancet Infect Dis 2006; 6:710–725.
Menzies D, Pai M, Comstock G: Meta-analysis: new tests for the diagnosis of latent tuberculosis infection: Areas of uncertainty and recommendations for research. Ann Intern Med 2007; 146:340–354.
Targeted tuberculin testing and treatment of latent tuberculosis infection. Am J Respir Crit Care Med 2000; 161:S221–S247.

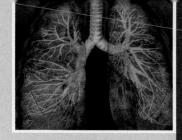

32 Rhinitis and Sinusitis

GLENIS K. SCADDING

EPIDEMIOLOGY, RISK FACTORS, AND PATHOPHYSIOLOGY

Rhinitis and sinusitis are terms that refer to inflammatory conditions of the nose and paranasal sinuses characterized by symptoms of:

- Rhinorrhea (anterior or posterior)
- Itching
- Sneezing
- Nasal obstruction

Secondary symptoms include:

- Headache
- Cough
- Facial pain
- Poor olfaction
- Disturbed sleep
- Pharyngitis
- Poor concentration
- Exacerbation of lower respiratory tract problems

In practice, inflammatory changes are usually continuous from nasal to sinus mucosa (Figure 32-1); therefore, the terminology *rhinosinusitis* is more accurate, but cumbersome—the two will be used interchangeably in this chapter.

The condition has marked effects on quality of life and is responsible for reduced school and workplace attendance (by 3–4%) and performance (by 30–40%). The resulting economic burden is high, and rhinosinusitis and related conditions occupy approximately one third of primary care consultations.

The causes of rhinitis can be simply considered as:

- Allergy
- Infections
- Other causes or unknown

The recent classification of rhinitis taken from the ARIA (Allergic Rhinitis and its Impact on Asthma) guidelines is shown in Table 32-1, with the differential diagnoses shown in Table 32-2.

Considerable overlap between causes occurs; for example, allergic rhinitis characterized by sneezing, itching, and watery discharge results in considerable mucosal swelling, which may result in reduced sinus drainage and allow secondary infection to occur. Both allergic and infective inflammatory rhinosinusitis may be exacerbated by the presence of anatomic and mechanical defects, such as a deviated nasal septum or enlarged turbinates.

It is also important to consider the possibility of serious underlying conditions and their early recognition, which may be necessary to prevent later damage (e.g., defects of immunity, defects of cilial motility, vasculitic and granulomatous disease).

Rhinosinusitis is frequently associated with lower respiratory disease; for example, approximately one third of patients who have bronchiectasis also have chronic sinusitis, and patients who have cystic fibrosis invariably have sinusitis and frequently have nasal polyps develop. Rhinitis is practically ubiquitous in asthmatics, with 10% of adults with late-onset asthma exhibiting aspirin hypersensitivity, often with nasal polyps (Samter's triad). Most asthma exacerbations begin with rhinitis, either infective, allergic, or both.

Rhinitis is a global problem with increasing prevalence. It is common in Westernized societies, with up to one third of the population affected (Figure 32-2).

Genetics

Risk factors for allergic rhinitis are both genetic—with an affected parent or sibling being associated with increased risk—and environmental. Westernization seems to be associated with an increased prevalence of allergic disorders (asthma, eczema, rhinitis); the mechanisms involved are still under investigation, but several lines of evidence exist for a deviation of the immune response away from Th1 (protective immunoglobulin IgG immunity and delayed hypersensitivity) toward Th2 (atopy with IgE production) by decreased bacterial contact. As in asthma, multiple genes are involved, many of these code for epithelial molecules concerned with innate immunity. Nasal polyposis also demonstrates a strong heritable component with a relative risk of 18 times the normal rate and 6 times the normal rate with an affected father and mother, respectively. There are a number of genes associated with aspirin-exacerbated respiratory disease—e.g., leukotriene C4 synthase promoter region—which vary among different populations. HLA-DQB1 is associated with allergic fungal sinusitis. The genetics of cystic fibrosis are discussed in Chapter 46; heterozygotes for cystic fibrosis are overrepresented in the chronic rhinosinusitis population. Primary ciliary dyskinesia is also genetic, with an incidence of approximately 1 in 20,000. Various structural ciliary defects have been described, but one common defect—a lack of inducible nitric oxide synthase in nasal mucosa—has recently been found.

Allergy
Allergic Rhinosinusitis

Apart from viral colds, allergic rhinosinusitis is the most common cause of nasal symptoms; it results from IgE-mediated immediate hypersensitivity reactions that occur in the mucous membranes of the nasal airways. Allergic rhinitis occurs in atopic individuals who have the genetic predisposition to produce IgE antibody responses to allergens, which are innocuous to normal individuals. The allergens responsible are usually

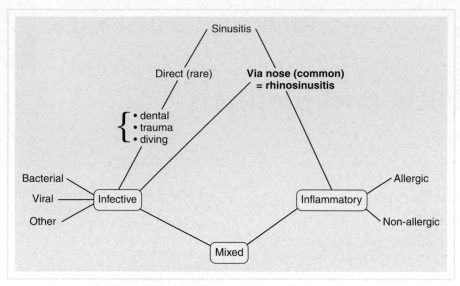

FIGURE 32-1 Causes of sinusitis.

TABLE 32-1 **Classification of Rhinitis**	
Infectious	Viral
	Bacterial
	Other infectious agents
Allergic	Intermittent
	Persistent
Occupational (allergic and non-allergic)	Intermittent
	Persistent
Drug-induced	Aspirin
	Other medications
Hormonal	
Other causes	NARES
	Irritants
	Food
	Emotional
	Atrophic
	Gastroesophageal reflux
Idiopathic	

NARES, Nonallergic rhinitis with eosinophilia syndrome.

TABLE 32-2 **Differential Diagnosis of Rhinitis**	
Polyps	
Mechanical factors	Deviated septum
	Adenoidal hypertrophy
	Foreign bodies
	Choanal atresia
Tumors	Benign
	Malignant
Granulomas	Wegener's granulomatosis
	Sarcoid
	Infectious
	Malignant-midline destructive granulomas
Ciliary defects	
Cerebrospinal rhinorrhea	

airborne, so-called aeroallergens, and consist of plant pollen, fungal spores, house dust mite and cockroach aeroallergens, and dander from domestic pets. Allergic rhinitis was formerly categorized as seasonal, perennial, and occupational; however, the recent World Health Organization ARIA guidelines suggest that intermittent and persistent are better divisions, because they are globally applicable and influence treatment.

In the United Kingdom and other North European countries, symptoms in the spring are frequently caused by allergy to tree pollens such as birch, plane, ash, and hazel. In late spring and early summer—the classic hay fever season—allergic rhinitis results from allergy to grasses such as rye, timothy, and cocksfoot. In late summer, weed pollens, such as nettle and mugwort, are responsible, whereas in autumn the fungi *Cladosporium* spp, *Alternaria* spp, and *Aspergillus* spp provoke symptoms. In the United States, ragweed pollen allergy is a common cause of rhinitic symptoms, usually from mid-August to mid-September.

Allergy to grass pollen is probably the most common in the United Kingdom, and symptoms correlate with the presence of high airborne pollen counts. Perennial rhinitis—in which symptoms occur throughout the year—in the United Kingdom is most commonly caused by allergy to the fecal pellets of the house dust mite (*Dermatophagoides pteronyssinus*), which flourishes in warm, humid environments and lives in bedding and soft furnishings.

Allergy to dander from domestic pets (such as cats, dogs, rabbits, and hamsters) can account for perennial rhinitis, whereas allergens encountered in the workplace are responsible for occupational rhinitis. Examples include sensitization to latex, flour, and grain (bakers); allergies to small mammals among laboratory workers; and allergy to wood dust, biologic products (such as antibiotic powder and enzyme-enhanced detergents), and rosin (colophony) from solder flux.

Allergic rhinitis is caused by a specific, immediate hypersensitivity reaction in the nasal mucosa that arises from IgE production to allergens. The allergic reaction can exhibit two phases: immediate and late (Figure 32-3). Mast cell degranulation with release of mediators such as histamine, leukotrienes,

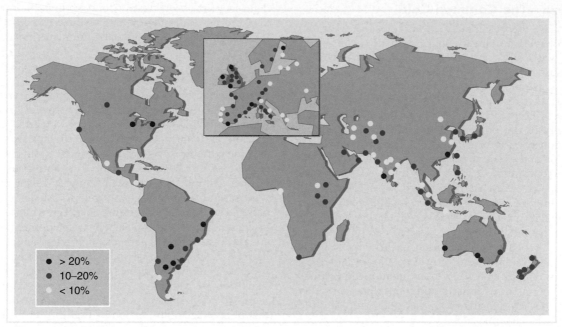

FIGURE 32-2 Global prevalence of hay fever in 13- to 14-year-olds. (From Strachan D, Sibbald B, Weiland S, et al: Worldwide variations in prevalence of symptoms of allergic rhinoconjunctivitis in children: the International Study of Asthma and Allergies in Childhood [ISAAC]. Pediatr Allergy Immunol 1997; 8[4]:161–176.)

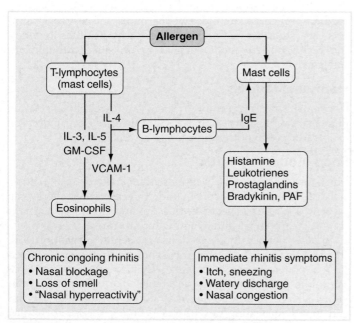

FIGURE 32-3 Immediate and late phases of the allergic rhinitis reaction. Mast cell degranulation leads to immediate symptoms, which are easily recognized. The late reaction, seen predominantly in persistent rhinitis, involves inflammation and produces nasal congestion and hyperreactivity, often unrecognized as allergic. (Courtesy of Professor Stephen Durham.)

TABLE 32-3 Pathophysiology of Rhinitis and Asthma

Rhinitis	Asthma
Epithelium intact	Epithelium disrupted
Basement membrane normal	Basement membrane abnormal
No airway smooth muscle	Bronchial smooth muscle hypertrophy
Venous sinusoids	None
Submucosal glands	Less prominent
Antihistamine effective	Ineffective
β_2-agonists ineffective	Effective

decreased olfaction, and mucosal irritability—changes similar to those seen in chronic asthma. Similar, but more marked, inflammatory changes occur in aspirin-sensitive disease, without the involvement of interleukin-4 and systemic IgE. Constant allergen contact or very high levels produce such symptoms, the allergic nature of which may not be recognized. Symptoms produced by consequent hyperreactivity to nonspecific irritants, such as inhaled fumes, dusts, and cold air, may lead to an erroneous diagnosis of "vasomotor" rhinitis.

True food allergy is rarely the cause of isolated rhinitis but may be relevant in small children with multisystem allergies.

Table 32-3 shows the similarities and differences between the pathophysiology of asthma and rhinitis.

Nonallergic Rhinosinusitis

Infectious Rhinosinusitis

The nasal and sinus mucosa can be infected by all types of organisms: viruses, bacteria, fungi, and protozoa. Of these, viral infections are the most frequent.

prostaglandins, bradykinin, and other mediators (platelet-activating factor, substance P, tachykinins) causes immediate symptoms of sneezing, itching, and running, typically seen where allergen contact is intermittent—for example, hay fever.

The late phase response involves ingress of inflammatory cells, particularly eosinophils, and is characterized by obstruction,

Acute Coryza—The Common Cold

Most people have approximately three colds per year, but small children have from six to eight. Humans spend 2 years of their lives with colds, of which 50% result from rhinoviruses, a further 20% from coronaviruses, and a further 20% from influenza, parainfluenza, adenoviruses, and respiratory syncytial virus; the remainder are caused by other viruses, including enteroviruses. Viral invasion occurs at the point of infection usually in the posterior nasopharynx and results in transient vasoconstriction of the mucous membrane followed by vasodilatation and edema with mucus production. A leukocytic inflammatory infiltrate develops, followed by desquamation of mucous epithelial cells. Initially, a clear watery secretion is produced, but it is followed by epithelial desquamation with opacification of secretions, which does not necessarily indicate bacterial infection, which complicates only approximately 2% of colds. Resolution occurs in a few days in uncomplicated viral infections; however, allergic individuals have more colds of greater severity than no atopic individuals. Rhinovirus infections in asthmatic children exposed to allergens to which they are sensitized give an odds ratio of 20 for hospitalization with asthma.

Acute Sinusitis

Although the nose harbors bacteria, the sinuses are normally largely sterile, possibly because of the nitric oxide concentrations therein and continuous mucociliary clearance. Acute sinusitis rarely occurs directly after trauma, dental infections, and diving into polluted water but usually arises from the secondary bacterial infection of a common cold. The mucous membranes of the nose and sinuses become swollen, which leads to blockage of the ostiomeatal complex and bacterial infection of the sinuses, particularly with *Haemophilus influenzae* and *Streptococcus pneumoniae*, with other causative bacteria being *Staphylococcus aureus*, *Moraxella catarrhalis*, *Streptococcus pyogenes*, and gram-negative bacteria such as *Klebsiella* spp and *Pseudomonas* spp. Anaerobic organisms may also be involved.

Chronic Rhinosinusitis

This, with or without nasal polyps, is defined clinically in the EPOS (European Position Paper on Chronic Rhinosinusitis and Nasal Polyposis) document as:

1. Two or more of the major symptoms:
   - Blockage/congestion
   - Reduced olfaction
   - Discharge anterior/postnasal drip
   - Facial pain/pressure
   and either
2. Endoscopic signs of
   - Polyps
   - Mucopurulent discharge from middle meatus
   - Edema/mucosal obstruction primarily in middle meatus
   or
3. CT changes
   - Mucosal changes within ostiomeatal complex and/or sinuses
   Cough is a predominant symptom in children, leading to a possible misdiagnosis of asthma.

Chronic sinusitis can occur after failure of resolution of acute sinusitis after weeks with the same bacterial pathogens involved. However, there are often other factors present such as eosinophilic inflammation (allergic or nonallergic rhinosinusitis), immune deficiency (innate or adaptive), or structural abnormalities; the role of pathogens is disputed. One possibility is persistence of organisms as a biofilm that continually stimulates a damaging immune response.

Drug-Induced Rhinitis

Antihypertensives, particularly β-blockers, can cause nasal obstruction by abrogation of the normal sympathetic tone, which maintains nasal patency. Exogenous estrogens in oral contraceptives or hormone replacement therapy also invoke rhinitis in some patients. Overuse of α-agonists results in rhinitis medicamentosa: a tachyphylaxis of α-receptors to extrinsic and intrinsic stimuli. The mucosa becomes swollen and reddened.

Aspirin hypersensitivity develops usually in adult life in patients with rhinitis (often nonallergic rhinitis with eosinophilia syndrome) with subsequent development of nasal polyps and asthma. Mast cell and eosinophil degranulation are seen in biopsies, and polyclonal local IgE production stimulated by superantigens from staphylococci has been described. Cox I inhibition by aspirin or nonsteroidal antiinflammatory drugs seems to promote leukotriene production, whereas inhibiting that of prostaglandins, including PGE-2, a bronchodilator. Leukotrienes cause bronchoconstriction, mucosal swelling, and excess mucus production, and sensitivity to their effects is high in aspirin sensitivity, probably because of increased numbers of specific receptors. The clinical picture is often one of aggressive polyposis, severe asthma with life-threatening reactions to aspirin, nonsteroidal antiinflammatory drugs, and frequent need for oral corticosteroids. A subgroup reacts also to E numbers (i.e., additives and preservatives, such as sulfites in wine), and high-salicylate foods such as herbs, spices, dried fruit, and jams.

Hormonal Rhinitis

Hormonal rhinitis is seen in pregnancy, occasionally in relation to menstruation, and at puberty. Chronic nasal obstruction can be a feature of hypothyroidism and acromegaly.

Food-Induced Rhinitis

Much rarer than popularly supposed, food allergy rarely causes isolated rhinitis, but in small children, milk or egg allergy can cause it as part of a spectrum that can include atopic dermatitis, gut symptoms, asthma, and failure to thrive.

In older people, food reactions are seen in association with rhinitis as part of the oral allergy syndrome in which sensitization to pollen results in cross-reactivity to components such as profilin in fresh fruit and vegetables. For example, an individual allergic to tree pollen may notice irritation of the lips and mouth on eating raw apples. These give rise to itching of mouth and lips, sometimes with swelling, rarely severe enough to compromise the airway, and provision of an EpiPen is usually unnecessary. Profilin is heat labile, so cooked fruits and vegetables are usually tolerated. Cross-reacting foods are shown in Table 32-4. An individual will react to only one or two of the fruits and vegetables on the list and, therefore, does not need to avoid all of them.

Allergy to food may be confused with food intolerance (in which IgE-mediated mechanisms are not involved). Some foods are rich in histamines (cheese, some fish, and some wines) that may result in flushing, headache, and rhinitis, and the same may occur with tyramine-rich foods (bananas). Food additives and coloring agents (such as sulfites, benzoates, and tartrazine) may also provoke reactions, especially in

TABLE 32-4 Oral Allergy Syndrome—Cross-Reacting Foods

Plant Material	Cross-Reacting Foods	
Silver birch pollen	Almond	Mango
	Anise seed	Nectarine
	Apple (raw)	Onion (raw)
	Apricot	Orange
	Caraway	Parsley
	Carrot (raw)	Peach
	Celery (raw)	Pepper (capsicum)
	Cherry	Plum
	Coriander	Potato (raw)
	Hazelnut	Tomato (raw)
	Kiwi	Walnut
	Lychee	
Grass pollen	Kiwi	Tomato (raw)
	Melon	Watermelon
	Peanut	Wheat
Daisy family pollens	Lychee	Sunflower seeds
Mugwort (weed) pollen	Aniseed	Fennel
	Carrot (raw)	Parsley
	Celery (raw)	Spices (some)
	Celery salt	
Latex (contact and/or inhaled allergy)	Avocado	Papaya
	Banana	Peach
	Chestnut	Peppers
	Kiwi	Pineapple
	Mango	Plum
	Melon	Tomato (raw)
	Orange	

Animal material	Cross-reacting foods	
House dust mite	Shellfish	Snails

aspirin-sensitive subjects. Finally, alcohol or spicy, hot food containing capsaicin may irritate c fibers and nonspecifically provoke rhinitic symptoms.

Atrophic Rhinitis

Atrophic rhinitis is characterized by atrophy of mucosa plus the bone beneath. The nose is widely patent, but there is crusting and an unpleasant smell. *Klebsiella ozaenae* has been found in many patients, and cure with long courses of ciprofloxacin has been reported. However, it is uncertain whether this condition is primarily infective. It may follow extensive surgery, radiation, chronic granulomatous disease, or trauma. Possibly, the primary problem is failure of normal mucociliary clearance mechanisms.

Other Causes

Emotional stimuli such as sexual arousal and stress have powerful effects on the nasal mucosa through the autonomic system. Gastroesophageal reflux is thought to be a cause of rhinitis, especially in small children. Chronic exposure to dry air or occupational irritants—for example, those found in the shipbuilding industry—can lead to nasal mucosal changes, often with squamous cell abnormalities.

Nonallergic, Noninfectious Rhinitis

Patients with none of the aforementioned causes are usually divided according to the presence or absence of nasal eosinophilia.

Nonallergic Rhinitis with Eosinophilia Syndrome

The presence of eosinophils in nasal smears (more than 5–25% according to different authorities) characterizes a condition that is probably the counterpart of intrinsic asthma and may precede nasal polyposis and aspirin sensitivity. It is usually responsive to topical nasal corticosteroids.

Noneosinophilic Nonallergic Rhinitis

Autonomic Rhinitis. In autonomic rhinitis, there is no evidence of nasal inflammation, but of autonomic dysfunction. Nasal and, in some patients, cardiovascular reflexes are abnormal, and there may be associated chronic fatigue syndrome. Topical ipratropium is useful in decreasing watery rhinorrhea; capsaicin applications may also relieve symptoms for several months after a few weeks of treatment.

The nasal mucosa receives a rich innervation from both the sympathetic and parasympathetic nervous system. Adrenaline and other sympathomimetics lead to vasoconstriction of the nasal mucosa, with increased nasal patency. Both α- and β-adrenergic blockers increase nasal resistance and can produce symptoms of nasal stuffiness. Stimulation of the parasympathetic system leads to an increase in nasal secretions. However, patients who have this condition also have increased responsiveness to both histamine and methacholine, which results in nasal blockage and rhinorrhea. It is also associated with hypertrophy of the inferior turbinates, and nasal polyps are sometimes present. Certain stimuli such as cold air, exercise, mechanical or thermal, and humidity changes result in rhinorrhea and other symptoms of rhinitis, and a period of nasal hyperresponsiveness often follows viral infection.

Idiopathic or Intrinsic Rhinitis

Idiopathic or intrinsic rhinitis is a diagnosis of exclusion with no evidence for any of the aforementioned causes. Symptoms tend to be perennial, and local allergy has been suggested as a cause, on the basis of histologic findings of mast cells and eosinophils in resected turbinates and on positive responses to local nasal allergen challenge in a subgroup.

Direct release of mediators from mast cells or neurogenic mechanisms may be involved here.

Finally, emotional factors may play a part, ranging from stress that compounds nasal blockage and discharge to the patient emphatically or consistently complaining of gross nasal symptoms, yet with no abnormal findings on examination.

Structural Causes

Variant anatomy was thought to predispose to rhinosinusitis as a result of interference with normal drainage and aeration of the paranasal sinuses (Figure 32-4) at the ostiomeatal complex, the crucial point at which the maxillary, frontal, and anterior ethmoid sinuses drain into the nose. However, in three recent studies, patients with chronic rhinosinusitis showed no greater prevalence of structural abnormalities than did normal controls.

Neoplasms, foreign bodies, and trauma can all produce symptoms of obstruction, pain, purulent discharge, and epistaxis. In adults, the possibility of neoplasm is always considered in patients who have persistent symptoms, particularly if these are unilateral. In children, the presence of foreign bodies should be considered if nasal discharge is unilateral and foul smelling. Local disease in the pharynx and larynx may also have an impact on the nose and paranasal sinuses (e.g., enlarged adenoids),

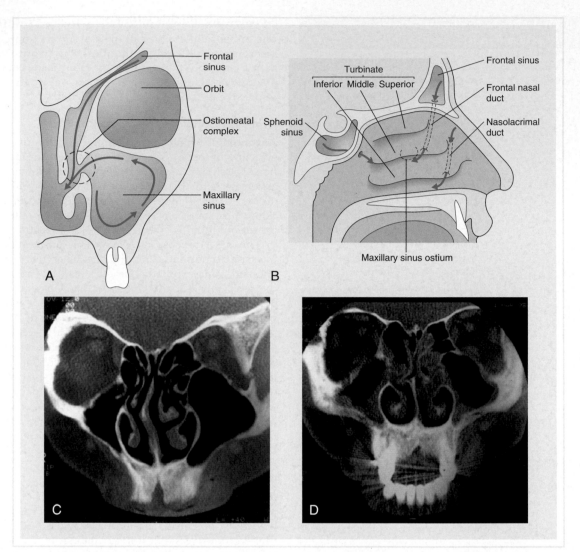

FIGURE 32-4 The top diagrams show sinus drainage pathways. **A,** In the left coronal diagram, the ostiomeatal complex is seen to drain the frontal, anterior ethmoid, and maxillary sinuses. **B,** The right diagram demonstrates these from the lateral view. **C,** The left coronal computed tomography (CT) scan shows clear paranasal sinuses in a patient with a deviated nasal septum. **D,** In the right scan, significant thickening of the mucosal lining is seen. CT changes do not correlate well with nasal symptoms but do relate to eosinophil counts in blood and sputum and to pulmonary function in accompanying asthma. (CT scans courtesy of Mr. Ian Mackay.)

as may dental disease (e.g., maxillary dental root infection), which may spread to the maxillary sinus.

Immune Defects

Panhypogammaglobulinemia is a severe condition with variable absence of all classes of immunoglobulin; it presents with bacterial and other infections at many sites. Initial presentation may be to the otorhinolaryngologist with symptoms of recurrent acute or chronic rhinosinusitis. It is important to make the diagnosis early before irreversible damage occurs at other sites (the lungs) and so that appropriate immunoglobulin therapy can be instituted. Total or relative absence of IgA may be present in the absence of any obvious clinical disease. However, IgA deficiency is now known to be associated in some patients with IgG_2 subclass deficiency, and such individuals may be more prone to episodes of sinusitis caused by capsulated bacteria such as *H. influenzae* and *S. pneumoniae*. Acute, chronic, and recurrent sinusitis are common in individuals who have human immunodeficiency virus infection, the most common organisms being *S. pneumoniae* and *H. influenzae*. A tendency to chronicity and to relapse is found, and in addition, fungal (*Cryptococcus* spp, *Alternaria* spp, and *Aspergillus* spp) and viral (cytomegalovirus) sinusitis may occur.

Mucus Clearance Defects

The nose and paranasal sinuses are lined with ciliated epithelium, which in a coordinated fashion moves a mucus blanket toward the nasopharynx. This mucus is important for the entrapment and removal of particulate material and toxic substances, which include bacteria and allergens. The integrity of the mucociliary clearance pathway is vital to the appropriate drainage and ventilation of the paranasal sinuses and the nose (see Figure 32-4). Primary ciliary dyskinesia is inherited as an autosomal-recessive trait and is characterized by the presence of sinusitis, bronchiectasis, situs inversus (Kartagener's syndrome, present in 50% of these patients), and male infertility that results from dyskinetic sperm. Various ciliary structural defects have been described (e.g., absence of inner or outer dynein arms or both), but some cilia appear normal (Young's syndrome). Recent work suggests that deficiency of iNOS (inducible nitric oxide synthase) may be the common underlying abnormality. Presentation is with chronic sinusitis, bronchiectasis or bronchitis, and obstructive azoospermia.

Secondary ciliary defects may arise after viral or bacterial infections; a number of mechanisms are involved:

- Mucous membranes become swollen and inflamed, which may result in blockage of the sinus ostia and thus prevent clearance (this is particularly critical at the ostiomeatal complex).
- If viruses or bacteria damage the epithelial cell layer, the integrity of cilial clearance is destroyed.
- Some bacteria produce toxins that inhibit cilial clearance mechanisms.
- Mucus during infection becomes thick and difficult to clear.

Granulomas/Vasculitis

A number of granulomatous diseases may involve the nose and sinuses as part of the generalized disease, or nasal symptoms may be the first manifestation. These include Wegener's granulomatosis, Churg–Strauss syndrome, and sarcoidosis, particularly in Afro-Caribbean individuals. Mucous membrane infiltration and thickening with granulomas may be present and may involve the septum, inferior turbinates, and occasionally the sinuses. Nasal congestion is a prominent symptom, sometimes with epistaxis and marked crusting. Sufferers feel unwell, with fatigue and malaise. Infective granulomatous disease may involve the nose and sinuses; examples are tuberculosis, leprosy, syphilis, blastomycosis, histoplasmosis, and aspergillosis.

Nasal Polyps

Nasal polyps (Figure 32-5) result from prolapse of the mucous membrane that lines the nose and present as pale, grapelike protuberances arising predominantly from the middle meatus. They are insensitive to pain but produce symptoms of nasal blockage and loss of sense of smell and may be associated with aspirin hypersensitivity and asthma. Nasal polyps may also be related to infection and are common in patients who have cystic fibrosis. Nasal polyps are rare in children, but when they do occur, they are often associated with cystic fibrosis. Classification of nasal polyps is similar to that of rhinitis (Table 32-5).

Occupational Rhinitis

Occupational rhinitis can be allergic or nonallergic, with the former nearly always preceding or developing concurrently with occupational asthma.

CLINICAL FEATURES

Allergy

Allergic Rhinitis

This presents in two forms.

Runners/Sneezers/Itchers. Symptoms tend to be intermittent and changeable and are often closely related to allergen exposure during the day. Severity varies from trivial to extremely disabling. In addition, itching and injection of the conjunctivae may occur, with watery discharge and conjunctival swelling, and itching in the mouth, oropharynx, and ears.

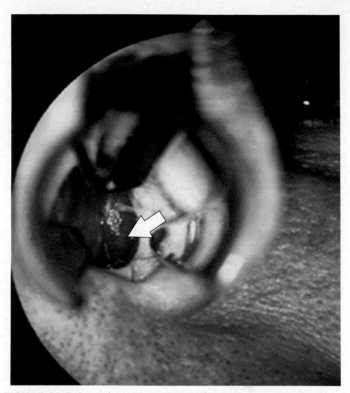

FIGURE 32-5 Speculum examination of nostril shows a pale watery polyp (*arrow*). Polyps are insensate and grayish, unlike turbinates, which are sensitive and bluish pink. (Courtesy of St. Mary's Hospital Audio-Visual Department.)

TABLE 32-5 Classification of Nasal Polyps	
Allergic	Eosinophil rich
	Skin prick tests may be negative
	Allergic fungal
	Sinusitis
	Aspirin sensitive
	Churg-Strauss
Infective	Neutrophil-rich
	Cystic fibrosis
	Immune deficiency
Structural	Antrochoanal
Other	Malignancy

This form of allergic rhinitis tends to be a disorder of children and young adults, and up to one third have associated asthma.

Blockers. The nose is chronically obstructed, with little in the way of immediate allergic symptoms.

Facial ache, headache, nasal hyperreactivity, and loss of sense of smell may also be present. Examination of the nose reveals pale or bluish mucosa, which is boggy and swollen, and a watery discharge may be present. Examination of the nose is important to exclude the concomitant presence of polyps, septal deviation, prominent turbinates, and evidence of other systemic disease and tumors.

Nonallergic Rhinosinusitis

Infections

Acute Coryza (The Common Cold). The prodrome normally consists of a feeling of dryness, itching, and heat in the nose, which may last for a few hours and is often followed by a dry, sore throat; sneezing; watery discharge; and constitutional symptoms of feverishness and malaise. This phase is followed in a day or so with symptoms of nasal obstruction and mucopurulent discharge, feverishness, and malaise, which may continue until resolution after 5–10 days. Initially, the symptoms of allergic rhinitis and coryza may be difficult to distinguish.

Acute Sinusitis. Acute maxillary sinusitis is characterized by facial pain, localized to the cheek, but also in the frontal area or the teeth, that is made worse by stooping down or straining. The pain can be unilateral or bilateral, and tenderness may overlie the sinus. Acute frontoethmoidal sinusitis may cause pain around the eye and in the frontal region, with overlying tenderness and erythema of the skin. There is usually fever, and toxemia may occur. Differential diagnosis of facial pain is wide and includes dental disease and the numerous causes of headache. Recently, all the accepted clinical signs and symptoms noted here have been shown to be unreliable as diagnostic aids to acute sinusitis, with the combination of erythrocyte sedimentation rate (ESR) and C-reactive protein (CRP) giving the best guide.

Chronic sinusitis is frequently pain free and presents with a sensation of congestion, poor concentration, tiredness, and malaise. Other symptoms of chronic sinusitis include purulent nasal discharge (often postnasal), sore throat, and a productive cough, especially in children in whom misdiagnosis of asthma is not uncommon. Loss of smell and halitosis are additional features.

Noninfective Rhinosinusitis

Symptoms are similar to those of blockers, as mentioned previously. The differential diagnosis from allergic rhinitis depends on skin prick or other allergy testing.

Clinical Presentations that Need Physician Referral

Unilateral symptoms, bloody discharge, polyps presenting for the first time, and systemically ill patients should be seen by an otorhinolaryngologic surgeon. Orbital cellulitis and sinusitis with severe headache or vomiting demand urgent referral.

DIAGNOSIS, EVALUATION, AND TESTS

Examination

It is frequently possible to arrive at a diagnosis of rhinosinusitis on the basis of a good detailed history. Physical examination should never be omitted, and it is vitally important that chronic symptoms are appropriately investigated.

Observation of the patient's face may reveal an allergic crease or salute, a deviated nose, or more sinister collapse of the nasal bridge.

Anterior rhinoscopy with a bright light or head mirror by use of a Thudicum speculum allows simple examination of the anterior nasal cavity; also, the mucous membrane can be viewed, and the presence of nasal polyps and disorders of the anterior part of the nasal septum can be seen.

Nasal endoscopy by use of either a rigid or fiberoptic flexible endoscope allows more detailed examination and assessment. Congenital defects, such as cleft palate and atresia, septal deviation and perforation, abnormalities of the turbinates, state of the mucous membranes, presence of purulent secretions, polyps, neoplasms, and foreign bodies can be determined.

Diagnosis of Coryza

Coryza is normally diagnosed on the basis of a patient's history, and further investigations are rarely required. Viral culture or immunofluorescent techniques can identify specific viruses.

Diagnosis of Acute Sinusitis

On examination, red, swollen nasal mucous membranes are present, and pus may be seen in the middle meatus. Endoscopy, together with imaging techniques, allows assessment of the severity and extent of involvement (diagnostic antral puncture and lavage are now rarely required). Middle meatal swabs provide material for bacteriologic culture. Immunoglobulin classes and subclasses are checked in cases of recurrent or chronic sinusitis.

Imaging Techniques

Radiography is rarely needed for diagnosis, unless a tumor is suspected. There is a high incidence of abnormalities in the general population: one third of unselected adults and 45% of children have abnormal scans. After a cold, computed tomography (CT) scans show changes for at least 6 weeks. The role of imaging is largely to provide a road map for the surgeon after failure of medical treatment.

Since the advent of computed tomography, plain sinus radiographs now have only a very limited role in acute rather than chronic sinusitis, because opacification or a fluid level may be seen in a sinus or gross soft tissue swelling may be evident. The imaging investigation of choice is CT, which is the best technique to demonstrate mucosal disease and underlying anatomic abnormalities (see Figure 32-4). The detailed anatomy of both bone and soft tissue is provided, and axial and coronal sections can be obtained. The coronal cuts provide views of the ostiomeatal complex, important for planning surgery for acute and chronic sinusitis (Figure 32-6). Preoperatively, coronal sections at 3–4 mm give maximal anatomic detail, whereas axial views provide vital information regarding the relation of the optic nerve to the posterior ethmoidal and sphenoid sinuses. Magnetic resonance imaging is of very limited value, because bone is not well imaged. It is useful

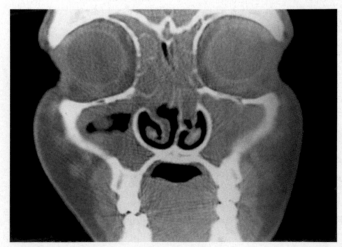

FIGURE 32-6 Coronal computed tomography scan of paranasal sinuses showing almost complete opacification of maxillary and ethmoid sinuses with polyps that obstruct the ostiomeatal complex. (Courtesy of Mr. Ian Mackay.)

in distinguishing one soft tissue from another and has the advantage of avoiding irradiation.

Mucociliary Function Tests

Saccharin Clearance

One quarter of a grain of saccharin is placed on the lateral nasal wall, 1 cm behind the anterior end of the inferior turbinate. A sweet taste is detected within 20 min if cilial function is normal—that is, the mucociliary mechanism is able to transport the particle to the nasopharynx and the pharynx, where taste is detected. If abnormal, more sophisticated tests of cilial activity by use of cells detached by brushings taken from the turbinate undertaken by use of phase contrast microscopy. Significant abnormalities on this test lead to electron microscopic examination of cilia.

Confirmation of observations of very low nasal nitric oxide (NO) in primary ciliary dyskinesia means that a nasal NO of greater than 250 ppb excludes this diagnosis with 95% sensitivity.

Nasal Airway Tests

Dynamic tests include nasal inspiratory peak flow (by use of a mask attached to a peak flow meter, the patient sniffs hard with a closed mouth) and rhinomanometry. The technique is used to assess nasal airway resistance by measuring airflow across a pressure gradient with a pneumotachograph and facemask. Acoustic rhinometry uses a sound pulse to measure the nasal cross-sectional area.

Nasal resistance can change very dramatically within a few minutes. Congestion is produced by engorgement of venous erectile tissue within the nose; the mucous membrane receives dense, autonomic innervation. Nasal resistance falls with adrenaline and other sympathomimetic drugs, but also with exercise, rebreathing, and adoption of the erect posture. Nasal resistance increases in rhinitis and, in some individuals, with alcohol, aspirin, and other drugs, as well as when the supine posture is adopted.

Evaluation of Allergic Rhinitis

The diagnosis is usually obvious from a careful history and examination but can easily be missed in chronic blockers; thus, skin prick tests should be performed in all rhinitis clinic patients. Skin tests that use allergen extracts to elicit IgE-mediated immediate hypersensitivity responses can be used to confirm or exclude atopy. If all the skin tests are negative, it is unlikely that the rhinitis is allergic. However, positive tests do not confirm the diagnosis, because many asymptomatic individuals have positive skin tests to common allergens. Correlation between skin prick tests and history should be sought, because occasionally it is possible to identify an allergen that can be avoided. Measurement of total IgE is not helpful; however, measurement of specific IgE levels to common aeroallergens by means of radioallergosorbent testing may be useful, and the results show a good correlation with skin test results. Occasionally, particularly where occupational rhinitis may be a possibility, nasal challenge and provocation tests (with the offending allergen, histamine, aspirin, or methacholine) may be required.

Nasal Cytology

It may be of value to determine the presence or absence of eosinophils in patients who have perennial rhinitis, negative skin tests, and who are not atopic. A subset of these patients have nasal secretion eosinophilia and are more likely to have allergic features such as sneezing and congestion; they may also respond to topical corticosteroids.

TREATMENT

Allergic Rhinitis

The basis of treatment for allergic rhinitis is:

1. Allergen avoidance
2. Pharmacotherapy
3. Immunotherapy
4. Rarely surgery
5. Patient education (vital)

Identify and Avoid Allergens

In practice, the identification and avoidance of allergens may be extremely difficult. House dust mites are responsible for much perennial allergic rhinitis. Mites flourish at temperatures of approximately 15°C and 60–70% relative humidity, conditions present in many homes that contain central heating. They flourish particularly in soft furnishings, mattresses, pillows, and bed covers, as well as in carpets. Allergen avoidance and measures to reduce the load (i.e., wooden floors rather than carpets, regular vacuum cleaning, and barrier covers for mattresses and pillows) effectively reduce rhinitic symptoms. Acaricides that kill the mites do not eliminate the antigen, which is present in the fecal pellets. Removal of a pet may not remove symptoms, because allergens may persist in rooms for many months, if not years. Avoidance of pollen is difficult, but vacationing or, failing that, staying indoors when the pollen count is high, closing windows, shutting car windows, and avoiding open grassy spaces may help.

Medical Suppressive Therapy

The treatment plan for allergic rhinitis according to ARIA is shown in Figures 32-7 and 32-8.

Topical Corticosteroids. Meta-analysis has shown that these are the most effective treatment for allergic rhinitis. Regular use is needed and preseasonal dosing reduces development of seasonal rhinitis symptoms. For polyps or marked nasal

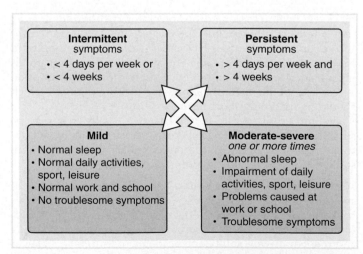

FIGURE 32-7 Division of rhinitis according to frequency and severity. (From Bousquet J, Van Cauwenberge P, Khaltaev N: J Allergy Clin Immunol 2001; 108[Suppl]:5147–5276.)

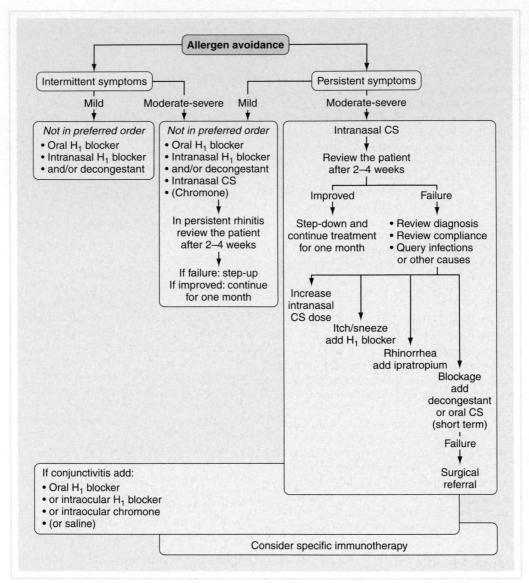

FIGURE 32-8 Rhinitis treatment on the basis of the subdivision in Figure 32-6. (From Bousquet J, Van Cauwenberge P, Khaltaev N: J Allergy Clin Immunol 2001; 108[Suppl]:5147–5276.)

blockage, betamethasone drops or oral corticosteroids for the first 2 weeks of therapy may be needed, followed by a nonabsorbed drop formulation, Flixonase nasules, in the long term for polyps (Figure 32-9). Side effects of topical corticosteroids include local irritation and minor epistaxis. Steroid absorption is low except for betamethasone and dexamethasone, which should be used only short term.

Sodium cromoglycate is less effective nasally, but may be suitable for small children, whereas severe conjunctival symptoms are best treated with sodium cromoglicate or nedocromil sodium. Corticosteroid eye drops are avoided.

Antihistamines. Antihistamines provide excellent relief of sneezing, itching, and rhinorrhea, but not congestion; oral ones have the advantage of being effective for mouth and eye symptoms. Chlorpheniramine is best avoided, because it is sedating and reduces driving ability and academic performance. Newer H_1-antagonists are largely nonsedating. Certain molecules (terfenadine, astemizole, and diphenhydramine in particular) can produce QT prolongation and fatal cardiac arrhythmias,

especially if blood levels are high because of overdosing or combining with other hepatically metabolized drugs. Fexofenadine cetirizine, levocetirizine, and desloratadine seem safe in this respect and possess some measurable nasal unblocking activity. Azelastine and levocabastine are useful topical antihistamines.

Other Agents. Vasoconstrictors are useful in the short term for marked congestion, but long-term use must be avoided because of the risk of rhinitis medicamentosa. Anticholinergics such as ipratropium bromide may be useful if extensive, watery secretion is a major problem.

Antileukotrienes are of similar efficacy to antihistamines in allergic rhinitis, with no major benefits from a combination of the two. However, in some patients with polyps, they can reduce symptoms and polyp size when used with a topical steroid.

Douching the nose with isotonic saline can reduce symptoms of allergic rhinitis and improve endoscopic appearances and quality of life in chronic rhinosinusitis.

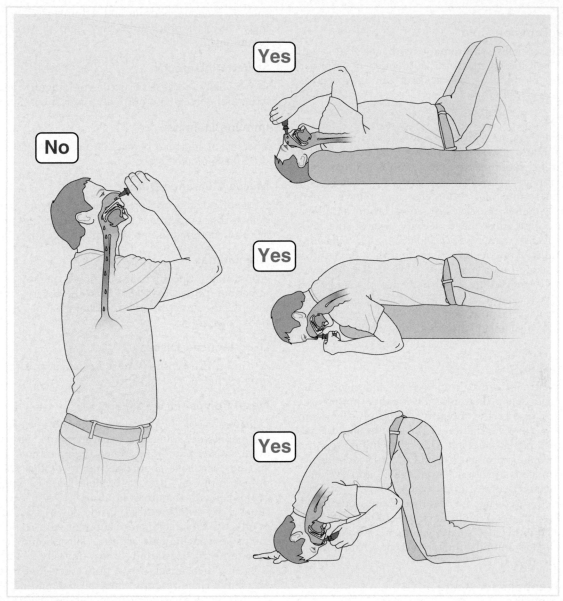

FIGURE 32-9 Correct instillation of nasal drops. (Adapted from BSACI Rhinitis Management Guidelines.)

Immunotherapy

This is the only treatment that has been shown to influence the course of disease. Three years treatment reduces symptoms for several years thereafter. In children with rhinitis, subcutaneous immunotherapy reduces progression to asthma at 3, 5, and 10 years afterwards. There is also a reduction in new allergic sensitization.

Desensitization involves the administration of increasing doses of relevant allergen extract by subcutaneous injection over a period of months and has been shown to effectively diminish symptoms of allergic seasonal rhinitis to grass pollen, ragweed, and birch pollen. Some studies also suggest efficacy to house dust mite and some animal danders. Desensitization has largely been superseded by the success of effective medical therapy in the suppression of allergic inflammation and so is reserved for nonresponders with severe disease. It is not always effective, and concerns have been raised regarding occasional anaphylactic reactions and deaths after the procedure, so it must be undertaken by well-trained individuals in a hospital setting with cardiorespiratory resuscitation facilities at hand.

Safer sublingual approaches have now been demonstrated to be effective, and grass pollen tablets will become available in the United Kingdom in 2007. The first sublingual dose needs to be under medical supervision; after this, each dose is taken every day at home. Eight weeks preseasonal therapy followed by continuation throughout the pollen season is suggested. Trials are in progress to assess the long-term effects of 3 years regular treatment.

Surgical Intervention

When medical treatment is only partially successful, a full otorhinolaryngologic assessment is performed because correction of a deviated nasal septum or reduction of hypertrophied mucosa may improve the symptoms. With coexistent chronic sinus infection, functional endoscopic sinus surgical techniques (FESS) may be necessary to facilitate sinus drainage, aeration, and access for medications, although a recent study showed that medical therapy with corticosteroid and long-term macrolide use was equally effective. Both improved concomitant asthma.

Infections

Coryza—The Common Cold

Treatment is essentially symptomatic with analgesics, antipyretics, rest, and broad-spectrum antibiotics if secondary infection is present. Oral or topical nasal zinc may decrease symptoms and their duration.

Acute Sinusitis

Most cases resolve spontaneously. Analgesics and antipyretics provide symptomatic relief, but aspirin must be avoided in those who may be hypersensitive. Acetaminophen (paracetamol) and codeine are satisfactory alternatives. Decongestants such as oxymetazoline and xylometazoline reduce edema and may improve sinus drainage. Broad-spectrum antibiotics are appropriate but must have activity against the most common pathogens, namely *S. pneumoniae*, *H. influenzae*, and *M. catarrhalis*. Amoxicillin, trimethoprim-sulfamethoxazole (co-trimoxazole), or a macrolide such as clarithromycin are appropriate. Amoxicillin-clavulanate has the added advantage of activity against *S. aureus* and penicillin-resistant *H. influenzae*. If anaerobic infection is suspected, a combination of amoxicillin-clavulanate and metronidazole or clindamycin is appropriate.

Chronic Rhinosinusitis

The aims of treatment are to remedy any underlying cause (e.g., immunologic defect, anatomic abnormality that prevents drainage) and to restore the integrity of the mucous membranes to allow normal ventilation of the sinuses and drainage (see Figure 32-3). Nasal douching with saline improves symptoms and endoscopic appearances. Topical corticosteroids may help to reduce mucous membrane swelling and improve drainage. Initially, betamethasone drops taken in the head-down position are briefly used, but no absorbed Fluticasone nasules are safer in long-term use. Prolonged courses of macrolide antibiotics produced improvements equivalent to FESS surgery, possibly because of their antiinflammatory activity. Amphotericin douching is ineffective.

Surgical Interventions for Acute and Chronic Sinusitis

Major changes have occurred in recent years as a result of the advent of high-resolution CT scans and FESS. Better demonstration of the nasal and sinus anatomy is achieved with CT scans, as well as of the important ostiomeatal complex, the vital region where sinus drainage by mucociliary clearance occurs. Obstruction in this zone is very important in the generation of chronic sinus disease. The main aim of FESS is to restore adequate drainage for the frontal, maxillary, and ethmoidal sinuses (see Figure 32-4). When this fails, more radical sinus surgery may be needed, but complete investigation for underlying medical factors (e.g., immune deficiency) should be undertaken first.

Noninfectious Causes

Intrinsic Rhinitis (Figure 32-10)

Anticholinergics (ipratropium bromide) are useful for troublesome rhinorrhea, particularly when eosinophils are absent from nasal secretions. When eosinophilia is present, a response to topical corticosteroid therapy is usual. α-Agonist decongestants, such as pseudoephedrine and xylometazoline, are used sparingly. Surgical procedures may help if nasal obstruction is predominant.

Structural Defects

Occasionally, topical corticosteroid therapy may ameliorate structural defects, but normally surgical correction is required.

Immune Defects

Therapy of immune defects is directed toward correction of the immunologic defect.

Mucus Clearance Defect

It is not possible to correct the underlying mucus clearance defect, so therapy relies on regular douching, improved drainage and aeration, and prevention of secondary infection.

Granulomas

Appropriate, specific antimicrobial therapy is required for infectious causes of granulomatous disease. Sarcoidosis that involves the nose responds to either local or systemic glucocorticoid therapy.

Drug-Induced Disease

A careful drug history must be taken and the incriminated drug excluded.

Nasal Polyps (Figure 32-11)

Unilateral nasal polyps must be referred to exclude transitional cell papilloma, squamous cell carcinoma, encephalocoele, or other sinister pathology. When there are no contraindications and no suspicions about the nature of the polyp, a medical polypectomy by use of prednisolone (0.5 mg/kg, enteric-coated) plus betamethasone drops (two in each nostril three times a day with the head upside down) for 5 days can prove as effective as surgery and is superior with respect to improvements in concomitant asthma. This should be followed by long-term corticosteroid drops—initially betamethasone for 2 weeks, then nonabsorbed fluticasone. Subsequently, a trial of a leukotriene receptor antagonist should be undertaken for 2–4 weeks, with continuation if beneficial. Other measures being evaluated include regular saline douching and topical lysine aspirin in patients sensitive to this on nasal challenge. Failure of medical treatment is an indication for surgery.

Patients with aspirin-exacerbated respiratory disease should be warned to avoid all Cox-1 inhibitors and to watch for exacerbation by similar substances: E numbers, preservatives, high-salicylate foods. Most can tolerate 500 mg paracetamol or Cox-2 inhibitors.

CLINICAL COURSE AND PREVENTION

Allergic Rhinosinusitis

The clinical course is variable. With good compliance, allergen avoidance, and regular pharmacotherapy, symptoms are usually minimal. Understandably, patients want a cure. Immunotherapy remains of limited value, but with development in understanding of the mechanism of generation of IgE responses and of ways in which this can be modulated, it may become more useful.

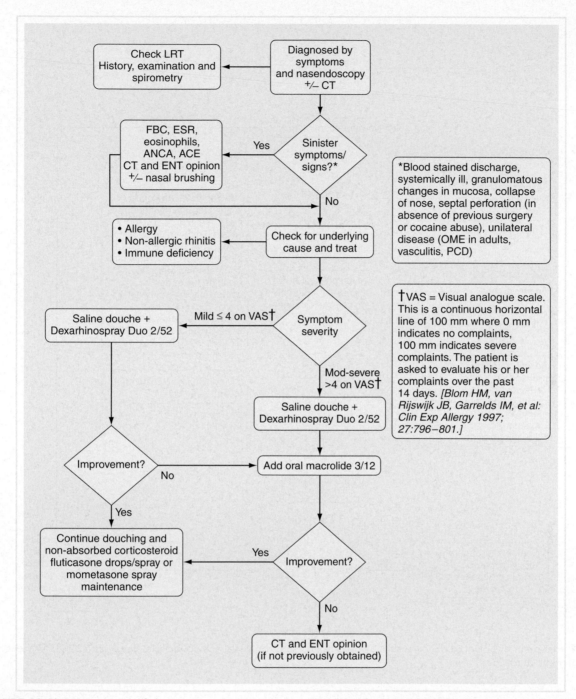

FIGURE 32-10 Management of chronic nonpolyp rhinosinusitis. (Adapted from BSACI Rhinitis Management Guidelines.)

Infections

Coryza—The Common Cold

Unfortunately, avoidance of the common cold is virtually impossible, and prevention by immunization has so far been a failure. However, colds are self-limiting and normally last approximately 5 days. Clinical trial data support the value of zinc in reducing the duration and severity of symptoms of the common cold when administered within 24 h of the onset of common cold symptoms.

Most asthma exacerbations (80% in children and 60% in adults) start with a viral upper respiratory tract infection. Synergy between allergen sensitization, exposure, and rhinoviral infection leads to an almost 20-fold likelihood of an asthmatic child needing hospital admission. Other complications include acute sinusitis, pharyngitis, otitis media, mastoiditis, and tonsillitis. The common cold frequently leads to lower respiratory infection, including laryngotracheitis, bronchitis, and occasionally pneumonia. Those who have other cardiorespiratory diseases may also experience exacerbations.

Acute Bacterial Sinusitis

Before the antibiotic era, acute sinusitis had a significant morbidity and mortality because of spread of bacterial sepsis beyond the sinuses. Osteolysis of the sinus wall occurred often,

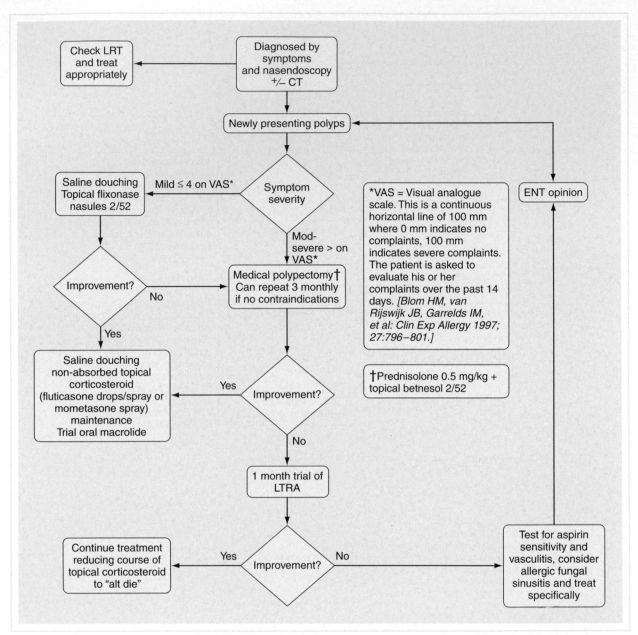

FIGURE 32-11 Treatment of polypoid rhinosinusitis. Symptoms and signs on visual analogue scale. See Figure 32-10. (Adapted from BSACI Rhinitis Management Guidelines.)

with abscess formation and direct spread to neighboring structures, in addition to local spread and thrombophlebitis. These local complications include orbital cellulitis with or without abscess formation, cavernous sinus thrombosis, sagittal sinus thrombosis, intracranial abscess, meningitis and encephalitis, osteomyelitis, and septicemia.

Complications are now rarely seen, because most patients are prescribed broad-spectrum antibiotics.

Intrinsic Rhinitis

Intrinsic rhinitis often has an onset in middle age or later and is often refractory to treatment. Combinations of therapy may prove helpful.

PITFALLS AND CONTROVERSIES

Points to consider in patients with rhinitis and sinusitis:

- Not all patients who have nasal symptoms have allergic rhinitis—neoplasm or foreign body could be present.
- Unilateral discharge in children is probably a foreign body, but in adults it may be carcinoma.
- Unilateral lesions must be biopsied to exclude malignancy.
- Nasal decongestants must be used sparingly, if at all.
- Most medical treatment failures result from poor compliance—once daily treatment is best, if possible.
- Common cold, a cause of widespread morbidity, remains a major research challenge.

...rinsic rhinitis can be troublesome to treat, and further ...earch is required.

...urbinates and polyps are difficult to distinguish—turbi...ates are rigid and pain-sensitive, polyps are mobile and ...nsensitive to pain.

...acial pain in the absence of nasal symptoms is rarely ...aused by sinus disease, so other causes such as migraine, dental problems, and temporomandibular joint syndrome are considered.

Chronic refractory sinusitis stimulates investigation for underlying immune or other defects.

- CT scan is the investigation of choice—plain radiographs or magnetic resonance imaging has a limited role.
- Treatment of rhinosinusitis benefits asthma.

SUGGESTED READINGS

Bousquet J, Van Cauwenberge P, Khaltaev N: The Aria Workshop Panel—Allergic rhinitis and its impact on asthma. J Allergy Clin Immunol 2001; 108(Suppl):5147–5276.

British Society of Clinical Immunology and Allergy Rhinitis Management Guidelines, 2007. Clin Exp Allergy (in press).

Fokkens WF, Lund VJ, Bechert C: EAACI Position Paper on rhinosinusitis and nasal polyps. Allergy 2005; 60:583–601.

Pharmacologic and anti-IgE treatment of allergic rhinitis ARIA update (in collaboration with GA2LEN): Allergy 2006; 61(9):1086–1096.

Ragab S, Scadding GK, Lund VJ, Saleh H: Treatment of chronic rhinosinusitis and its effects on asthma. Eur Respir J 2006; 28(1):68–74. Epub 2006 Mar 1.

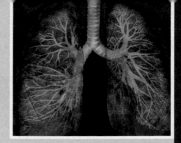

33 Bronchiectasis

ALAN F. BARKER

DEFINITION

Bronchiectasis is a chronic respiratory disease involving repeated infection and inflammation of large and small airways. Bronchiectasis has been defined as permanent dilatation of bronchi. Clinical features include frequent cough, the daily production of mucopurulent phlegm, often accompanied by recurrent sinopulmonary infections, and chest imaging that demonstrates dilated and thickened airways.

EPIDEMIOLOGY

There are no reliable estimates of the frequency of the disease, but prevalence varies by country and region. Susceptible populations include those with relatively poor access to health care and delayed treatment of respiratory infections. An increased prevalence has been reported in Native Americans from remote areas of Alaska, Maori in New Zealand, and impoverished tribes from Nigeria and perhaps other sub-Saharan areas of Africa. An estimated 110,000 individuals have bronchiectasis in the United States on the basis of review of the ICD codes from a large insurance database. The prevalence of bronchiectasis increases with age, and, in contrast to COPD, bronchiectasis is more common in women than men.

ETIOLOGY AND RISK FACTORS

Although 50% of individuals with bronchiectasis have no proven etiology, there are broad and specific categories of associations that merit attention (Table 33-1). Several of these associations warrant closer scrutiny.

Individuals with humoral immunodeficiencies of IgG, IgM, and IgA are at risk for suppurative sinopulmonary infections, including recurrent sinusitis, otitis media, and bronchiectasis. Immune globulin replacement reduces the frequency of acute infectious exacerbations and probably reduces airway mucosal damage. Selective IgG subclass deficiency may also contribute to bronchiectasis.

The respiratory complications (bronchiectasis) of cystic fibrosis may not become apparent until adulthood. The clinical paradigm is sputum cultures growing *Pseudomonas aeruginosa* and/or *Staphylococcus aureus* and upper lobe infiltration on chest radiograph. Confirmatory testing includes sweat chloride levels greater than 50–60 mmol. Genetic testing with identification of an abnormal allele can also provide confirmation.

Primary ciliary dyskinesia (PCD) is inherited as an autosomal-recession abnormality, affecting 1 in 15,000–30,000 individuals. PCD is a condition in which poorly functioning cilia contribute to reduced clearance of airway secretions, foreign particles, and bacteria, leading to recurrent infections and bronchiectasis. Approximately half of patients with PCD have classic Kartagener's syndrome (bronchiectasis, sinusitis, situs inversus). The most common ciliary defect is an absence or shortening of the outer (dynein) arms that are responsible for propelling or moving mucus out of the respiratory tract (Figure 33-1). Low levels of nasal and exhaled nitric oxide (NO) are suggestive of PCD.

Regarding infectious contributions and their sequelae, whooping cough and measles have been reduced, if not eliminated, in most parts of the world. Endemic tuberculosis is reduced and effectively treated in most developed nations. Primary *Mycobacterium avium* complex (MAC) can cause an indolent respiratory syndrome in immunocompetent individuals. White, usually slender, women older than the ages of 50–60 are particularly recognized with unrelenting cough. The middle lobe and/or lingula on chest imaging shows changes of bronchiectasis. MAC can also be cultured in patients with cystic fibrosis (CF) and other patients with bronchiectasis. A major component of allergic bronchopulmonary aspergillosis (ABPA) is bronchiectasis. Individuals with asthma may have cough productive of mucus plugs. The *Aspergillus* organism causes an allergic and, perhaps, infectious airway damage. An emerging concern or contributing cause is esophageal reflux. Whether this is a primary cause or frequent, paroxysmal, or violent coughing promotes reflux is uncertain.

PATHOGENESIS

The induction of bronchiectasis requires an infectious insult, airway obstruction, and/or a defect in host defense. Some specific infectious insults were discussed in the preceding paragraph. Episodes of acute bronchitis with bacterial pathogens such as *Pseudomonas* will perpetuate and worsen mucosal injury. This tissue injury is mediated by neutrophilic cellular infiltration and both host and organism inflammatory mediators including proteases, reactive oxygen intermediates, and cytokines such as interleukin-8. An impairment in host defense may be mainly confined to the respiratory tract such as in CF or ciliary dyskinesia or systemic with hypogammaglobulinemia or AIDS. Airway obstruction can be caused by a foreign body aspiration such as popcorn or a peanut in children or food particulate, crown, or fragmented tooth in an adult. Inebriation or altered mental status secondary to a stroke may delay recognition of the initial aspiration event. An intraluminal (partially) obstructing tumor such as carcinoid or fibroma or extrinsic compression of an airway (enlarged lymph node) may interfere with proper drainage and lead to recurrent infections and bronchiectasis. Figure 33-2 is a chest CT image of bronchiectasis caused by middle lobe syndrome.

TABLE 33-1 Conditions Associated with Bronchiectasis

Focal bronchiectasis	Foreign body aspiration Benign tumors (fibroma, lipoma) Lymph node encroachment (middle lobe syndrome)
Diffuse bronchiectasis	**Post-infectious** Bacteria (pertussis) Virus (adenovirus, measles, human immunodeficiency) Fungi (*Aspergillus fumigatus, Coccidoides imitis, Histoplasma capsulatum*) *Mycobacterium tuberculosis* or *avium complex* **Immunodeficiency** Primary humoral (hypogammaglobulinemia) Secondary (CLL) **Congenital** Primary ciliary dyskinesia Alpha-one antitrypsin deficiency Cystic fibrosis Cartilage deficiency (Williams-Campbell syndrome) Tracheobronchomegaly (Mounier-Kuhn syndrome) Marfan syndrome **Rheumatic and other** Rheumatoid arthritis Inflammatory bowel disease

GENETICS

Two associated diseases have genetic bases, both transmitted as autosomal recessive. Cystic fibrosis involves a defect in the cystic fibrosis transmembrane conductance regulatory protein. Most common is the delta F508 mutation, but many other abnormal alleles have been identified. In PCD, genetic abnormalities of heavy (DNAH5) and intermediate (DNAIl) chains have been identified in 30–40% of PCD patients. These genetic defects are present in the outer dynein arms and contribute to the discoordinated ciliary propelling of mucus.

CLINICAL FEATURES

Daily cough and mucopurulent sputum production are cardinal features of almost every patient. More than half of affected patients will exhibit chronic and intermittent dyspnea, pleuritic chest pain, and hemoptysis. The hemoptysis can vary from blood streaking to massive volume (greater than 300 mL in a day) during an acute exacerbation caused by erosion of a mucosal neovascular arteriole. Physical findings noted on chest auscultation include crackles and rhonchi. Airway obstruction can produce wheezes that mimic findings in asthma. Layering of sputum in a container has distinctive features that yield a clue to the diagnosis (Figure 33-3). The older literature described a frequent finding of digital clubbing, but this probably occurs in less than 5% of patients currently seen. Pulmonary function tests provide a guide to impairment. Spirometry shows a normal or reduced forced vital capacity (FVC), reduced forced expiratory volume in 1 second (FEV_1), and reduced FEV_1/FVC consistent with obstructive impairment. Many patients will have an improved FEV_1 and/or FVC after aerosol

bronchodilator. Key confirmatory testing includes chest imaging. The chest X-ray is abnormal in most patients with bronchiectasis. Suspicious findings include linear atelectasis, dilated and thickened airways noted as ring shadows on cross section, and tram or parallel lines when seen in a longitudinal plane. Old granulomatous disease and cystic fibrosis have an upper lobe predominance of findings. A central distribution is typical of ABPA (Figure 33-4), and a middle lobe or lingular lobe distribution suggests MAI as the genesis (Figure 33-5). Most other associations and idiopathic bronchiectasis present a lower lobe distribution of radiographic findings.

The high-resolution chest CT (HRCT) has become the defining tool if not the "gold standard" for confirmation of the diagnosis of bronchiectasis. Noncontrast studies are adequate with 1.0–1.5 mm sections and images obtained every 1 cm by use of a high spatial algorithm. The major HRCT findings are mentioned in Box 33-1 and Figure 33-6 and illustrated in the accompanying HRCTs. Controversy and confounding diagnoses occur when some of these radiographic findings are seen in other diseases. During acute pneumonia and the resolution phase, airways may be seen as dilated and even thickened. Those findings would resolve. Individuals with asthma and even chronic bronchitis may have a few dilated areas and inspissated secretions that could be interpreted as bronchiectasis. Other diseases associated with parenchymal destruction can distort airways that mimic bronchiectasis. In pulmonary fibrosis, parenchymal scars contract and pull airways open, leading to so-called traction bronchiectasis. In emphysema, small bullae may simulate the dilated airways of bronchiectasis, but the walls are thin-walled and often not complete.

The HRCT is complementary when the diagnosis is in doubt, location of changes may give a clue to an underlying association, bleeding needs to be localized, or a map is needed when surgical resection is considered.

DIAGNOSIS

Symptoms or a history of repeated lower respiratory tract infections and sometimes chest findings would usually suggest the diagnosis. Chest imaging is required to confirm the diagnosis. Sinus CT will be helpful and usually abnormal when there are upper respiratory complaints or host defense are impaired affecting the entire respiratory system such as ciliary dyskinesia, humoral immunodeficiency, or cystic fibrosis. A complete blood cell count (CBC) will not show specific changes, but eosinophilia may point to ABPA. Immunoglobulin (IgG, IgM, IgA) quantitation should be performed because of therapeutic implications. If the IgG is borderline low or there is a history of repeated otitis media, IgG subclasses can be analyzed. In addition, vaccination with a common humoral antigen such as polyvalent *Haemophilus* or pneumococcal vaccine followed by measurement of the antibody response 2–4 weeks later can be useful. Failure to produce *Haemophilus* or pneumococcal antibodies suggests humoral subclass deficiency and consideration of IVIG replacement. Other blood tests such as rheumatoid factor, α_1-antitrypsin level, or precipitins for aspergillus are guided by clinical suspicion. Performance of sweat chloride iontophoresis and/or genetic testing will also depend on a suspicion of cystic fibrosis. Bronchoscopy is warranted when focal obstruction from a foreign body or tumor is suspected. Confirmation of ciliary dyskinesia requires a respiratory tract biopsy of the nasal mucosa or lower airway with examination of cilia by electron microscopy. Bacterial sputum cultures are not routinely helpful but can

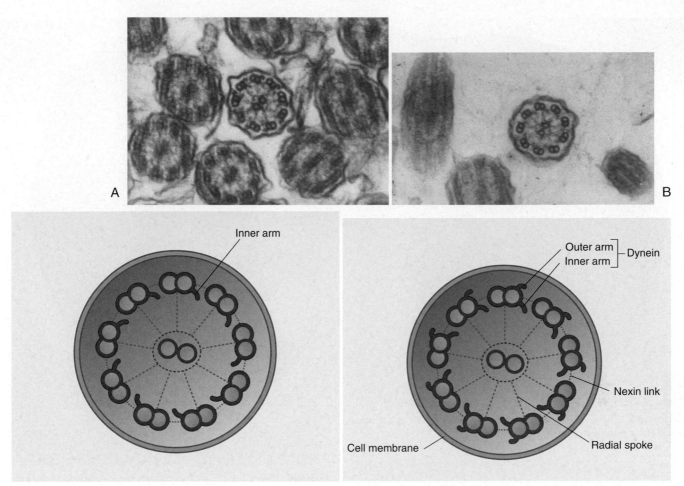

FIGURE 33-1 A, Electron micrograph of normal cilia and a stylized diagram noting inner and outer dynein arms. **B,** Electron micrograph of cilia of patient with the most common dyskinetic abnormality. The diagram illustrates the presence of inner arms and lack of outer arms.

point to a single or potentially resistant pathogen such as *Moraxella* or *Pseudomonas*. Cultures for fungus and mycobacteria can highlight problematic pathogens.

TREATMENT

Treatment of bronchiectasis includes attention to eight principles:

1. Antibiotic therapy of acute exacerbations
2. Prevention of acute exacerbations by reducing the burden of microbial pathogens with antibiotics
3. Treatment of resistant or problematic pathogens
4. Reduction of inflammation with antiinflammatory agents
5. Enhance secretion removal with bronchial hygiene
6. Surgical removal of affected parts of the lung
7. Control of hemoptysis
8. Protection against gastric acid reflux

ANTIBIOTIC THERAPY OF ACUTE EXACERBATIONS

Because cough and phlegm production are present most days for individuals with bronchiectasis, deciding when an acute exacerbation occurs is problematic. The sputum often increases in amount (although may be harder to expectorate), becomes more tenacious, and is darker in color. Hemoptysis may be an accompanying complaint. Other features include worsening dyspnea and pleuritic chest pain. Fatigue is usually present, but fever and chills are lacking. Leukocytosis and new chest radiographic findings do not occur or are minimal.

The genesis of acute exacerbations must be suspected bacterial bronchitis. Prompt antibacterial therapy is warranted. For ambulatory patients, choosing an antibiotic involves an educated guess unless recent sputum culture data are available. For individuals with no or few recent exacerbations, the colonizing flora can be presumed similar to individuals with chronic bronchitis. Coverage against *Streptococcus pneumoniae*, *Haemophilus influenzae*, and perhaps *Moraxella* is satisfactory. Choices are shown in Table 33-2. For individuals with a longer duration of illness or failed previous antibiotic courses, *Pseudomonas aeruginosa* has to be a suspected pathogen. Therapy with a quinolone provides the only effective oral regimen. A choice would be ciprofloxacin, 500–750 mg, twice daily. Other quinolones such as levofloxacin, 500 mg daily, or moxifloxacin, 400 mg daily are reasonable alternatives. The duration of therapy should probably extend to 10–14 days. In any individual who has a first course of antibiotics fail, sputum culture and sensitivity provide information to make an informed decision about subsequent therapy. Decisions about the need for hospitalization involve systemic findings, including hemodynamic or respiratory compromise, comorbid disease, or presence of a highly resistant organism that requires initiation of parenteral antibiotics.

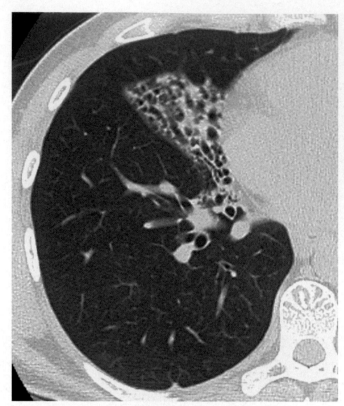

FIGURE 33-2 Chest CT of a patient with extensive cystic or saccular bronchiectasis confined to the middle lobe.

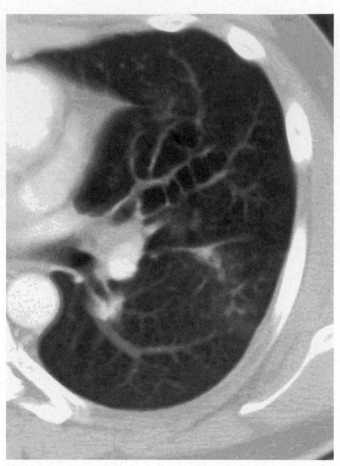

FIGURE 33-4 Chest CT of a patient with ABPA and very dilated airways extending centrally to the periphery.

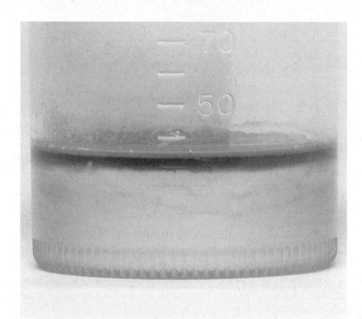

FIGURE 33-3 Sputum (in a cup) from a patient with bronchiectasis. The heavier cells, pigments, and debris sink to the bottom; there is a clear watery middle layer; airway mucus will foam or layer at the top.

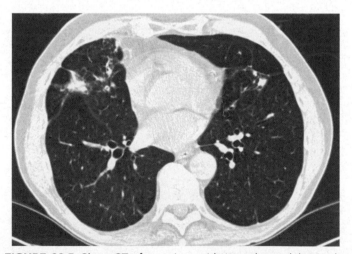

FIGURE 33-5 Chest CT of a patient with irregular nodules in the middle lobe and lingula consistent with *Mycobacterium avium* complex.

PREVENTION OF ACUTE EXACERBATIONS AND REDUCTION OF BACTERIAL BURDEN

The strategy of reducing the bacterial load makes sense in patients with bronchiectasis but is not proven. The easiest strategy for patient administration involves an oral antibiotic on an intermittent basis. Table 33-3 lists several such strategies. Pilot studies with tobramycin delivered by aerosol have shown dramatic microbiologic reductions in *Pseudomonas* burden. One double-blind placebo-controlled trial of 74 patients showed a 10,000-fold reduction in *Pseudomonas* density but no change in FEV$_1$ in the tobramycin group. The use of a macrolide is attractive when *Pseudomonas* is a pathogen, because there is evidence that it may reduce surrounding biofilms or inflammatory burden.

TREATMENT OF RESISTANT OR PROBLEMATIC PATHOGENS

Expectorated (sometimes induced) sputum cultures or cultures obtained at bronchoscopy and lavage will be required to identify resistant pathogens. *Pseudomonas aeruginosa* is almost impossible to eradicate from patients with bronchiectasis. Strategies for suppression are noted in the previous paragraph. Treatment of ABPA includes augmentation or introduction of systemic steroids. Itraconazole, 400 mg daily, may reduce the burden of *Aspergillus* but is less effective in individuals with bronchiectasis (see Chapter 52). Decisions about the diagnosis and therapy of *Mycobacterium avium* complex (MAC) are discussed in a Statement of the American Thoracic Society. Therapy with a macrolide, rifampin or rifabutin, and ethambutol is required for many months (see Chapter 31).

TREATMENT WITH ANTIINFLAMMATORY AGENTS

The neutrophilic influx into airways accompanying infection is presumed to be injurious and destructive. Systemic steroids at the time of an acute exacerbation (particularly with respiratory compromise) is a reasonable approach but has not been tested in a clinical trial. Clinical trials have demonstrated the usefulness of aerosol steroids to reduce inflammatory mediators and symptoms. Two agents that have been studied include beclomethasone and fluticasone.

ENHANCE SECRETION REMOVAL WITH BRONCHIAL HYGIENE

Because viscous secretions are part of the disease process, attention to bronchial hygiene is important. Strategies include hydration (systemic and airway), mucolytic agent administration, chest physiotherapy, and bronchodilator administration.

Oral liquids will usually maintain airway hydration, but nebulization of hypertonic (7%) saline solutions will also reduce viscosity of tenacious secretions. Acetyl cysteine administered as a 20% solution by nebulizer is an effective mucolytic agent, with its role mainly confined to patients in whom saline nebulization is not effective. Acetyl cysteine may provoke bronchospasm and a bronchodilator can be delivered as adjunctive therapy. Recombinant DNAse is not effective in bronchiectasis.

Chest physiotherapy involves a variety of mechanical measures to loosen tenacious secretions and enhance their removal from the airways. Chest clapping is effective for some individuals, but is time intensive and requires an assistant. Mechanical percussors or vibrating vests applied to the chest, positive expiratory pressure valves, or flutter devices producing oscillatory positive airway pressures are modern approaches that are sometimes more comfortable and can be used or applied without an assistant. Postural chest drainage requires an individual to lie in multiple positions (to drain various affected lobes) on a bed, table, or couch and is often used in conjunction with chest clapping or mechanical percussors. Many patients find such positioning uncomfortable and time intensive.

Between 30% and 50% of patients with bronchiectasis have a response to bronchodilators when tested in the pulmonary function laboratory. Bronchodilators such as beta-agonists or anticholinergics administered on an acute or chronic basis are probably effective.

SURGICAL REMOVAL OF AFFECTED LUNG

The role of surgery has certainly declined over the past 3–4 decades. Because most individuals now have multiple affected areas of lung, total cure is not usually possible. There are several indications for which surgery should be considered: Removal of a lobe or segment obstructed by a tumor or foreign

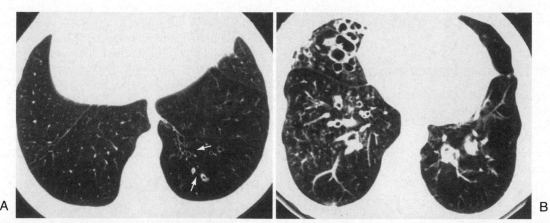

FIGURE 33-6 A, HRCT of patient with bronchiectasis. Upper arrow shows six or more very dilated airways. Lower arrow shows both dilated and thickened airways. **B,** HRCT of a patient with advanced bronchiectasis caused by Kartagener's and ciliary dyskinesia. There are multiple areas dilated and thickened airways and peripheral small airways filled with mucus ("tree-in-bud"). At the top on the right are hugely dilated cystic areas (grapelike clusters).

TABLE 33-2 Oral Antibiotics for Acute Exacerbations of Bronchiectasis

Category	Agents	Organisms
Penicillins	Amoxicillin 500 mg, q8h Amoxicillin-clavulanate 875 mg, q12h	S. pneumoniae, H. influenzae S. pneumoniae, H. influenzae M. catarrhalis
Cephalosporins	Cefaclor 500 mg, q8h or Cefuroxime 500 mg, q12h	S. pneumoniae, H. influenzae M. catarrhalis same
Macrolides	Azithromycin 500 mg 1st day, then 250 mg daily or Clarithromycin 500 mg, q12h	S. pneumoniae, H. influenzae
Quinolones	Ciprofloxacin 500–700 mg, bid or Levofloxacin 500 mg, qd or Moxifloxacin 400 mg, qd	P. aeruginosa S. pneumoniae, H. influenzae
Other	Trimethoprim-sulfa 160–180 mg, bid	S. maltophilia

TABLE 33-3 Prevention Strategies for Bronchiectasis

Strategy	Example
Intermittent or daily oral antibiotic	Ciprofloxacin 500–700 mg, bid or Azithromycin 250 mg
High-dose oral	Amoxicillin 3 gm, sache qd*
Aerosol antibiotic (alternate months)	Tobramycin 300 mg, bid*
Intermittent IV antibiotics (10–21 days)	Depends on bacterial flora in sputum

*Not approved in the United States.

body, reduction of an area of lung thought to be contributing to massive suppurative and tenacious secretions contributing to dyspnea or acute exacerbations, removal of an airway subject to massive or recurrent hemorrhage, elimination of necrotic lung tissue thought to harbor resistant organisms such as MAC, and multidrug resistant *Mycobacterium tuberculosis*, or *Aspergillus*. Bilateral lung transplantation has been performed on some individuals with extensive bronchiectasis. Recurrence of bronchiectasis has been seen.

CONTROL OF MASSIVE HEMORRHAGE

Hemoptysis in bronchiectasis can be blood-streaked or massive, causing respiratory compromise. Prompt identification of the location of hemorrhage with chest CT and bronchoscopy is warranted. Positioning of the patient in bed with the affected side down and opiate cough suppression may temporize. Intubation with a divided endotracheal tube to protect the unaffected side is also a temporizing strategy. Definitive therapy includes aortography with bronchial or intercostal artery selective catheterization and potential embolization of a previously identified bleeding area or one with neovascularization (see Chapter 24). Thoracotomy and resection may be necessary when such efforts fail or proximal airways and vessels are involved.

TREATMENT OF GASTRIC ACID REFLUX

Because this is an evolving consideration, there is uncertainty whether all patients should have diagnostic testing for acid reflux or whether gastric acid suppression is warranted and diagnostic testing saved for more refractory patients.

CLINICAL COURSE AND PREVENTION

Although it is difficult to generalize about the course of patients with bronchiectasis, the number of acute exacerbations requiring antibiotics averages 2–3/patient/year. The number of hospitalizations varies widely, depending on severity of respiratory compromise, comorbid diseases, and practice patterns. In some locales, hospitalization is necessary for intravenous antibiotics for most exacerbations. In other areas, intravenous antibiotics can be administered in an ambulatory setting. Repeated exacerbations may lead to airway and parenchymal destruction, accelerated decline in pulmonary function, hypoxemia, and cor pulmonale. As noted previously, hemoptysis may be life threatening. Concerning mortality, there are data from a Hospital Registry in Finland. Patients with bronchiectasis, asthma, and COPD were age matched (ages 35–74) and followed for 8–13 years. Twenty-eight percent of bronchiectasis patients, 20% of asthma patients, and 38% of COPD patients died. The underlying disease was the primary cause of death in the bronchiectasis and COPD patients. Cardiac disease was the primary cause of death in the asthma patients. Retrospective analysis of 48 patients (ages 35–88) admitted to an ICU in France for the first time between 1990 and 2000 revealed a 19% mortality in the ICU and a 40% mortality at 1 year. Age older than 65 and previous use of supplemental oxygen were associated with reduced survival.

PITFALLS AND CONTROVERSIES

Bronchiectasis is an important chronic respiratory disease that uses frequent medical resources. The increased use of HRCT has helped identify many unrecognized patients. The meaning or role of bronchiectasis on chest imaging when there are scant clinical findings needs clarification. Most studies of etiology come from retrospective reviews or tertiary centers. A registry with testing for key associated conditions such as CF, ABPA, MAC might help our understanding. Treatment strategies are most often based on experiences at single institutions and referral centers. Their experiences may not reflect practice or disease conditions in a general pulmonary or even internal or family medicine practice. Larger clinical trials with aerosolized antibiotics would provide better credence to their utility. There is a great need for antibiotics against the emerging resistant pathogens. Virtually all treatment strategies have been adopted from practices and multicenter clinical trials in patients with cystic fibrosis. Because bronchiectasis is the main respiratory disease in cystic fibrosis, it would seem logical that CF treatment strategies should be effective in non-CF bronchiectasis. Such generalities are not always correct. Aerosolized DNAse is a proven effective mucolytic agent in CF. In the largest multicenter trial of a therapy in non-CF bronchiectasis, DNAse was found ineffective and may cause decline in pulmonary function.

SUGGESTED READINGS

Angrill J, Aguisti C, de Celis R, et al: Bacterial colonization in patients with bronchiectasis: microbiologic pattern and risk factors. Thorax 2002; 57:15–19.

Barker AF: Medical progress: Bronchiectasis. N Engl J Med 2002; 346:1383–1393.

Cohen M, Sahn SA: Bronchiectasis in systemic diseases. Chest 1999; 116:1063–1074.

Dupont M, Gacouin A, Lena H, et al: Survival of patients with bronchiectasis after the first ICU stay for respiratory failure. Chest 2004; 125:1815.

King PT, Holdsworth SR, Freezer NJ, et al: Characterization of the onset and presenting clinical features of adult bronchiectasis. Respir Med 2006; 100:2183.

McCool FD, Rosen MJ: Nonpharmacologic airway clearance therapies: ACCP evidence-based clinical practice guidelines. Chest 2006; 129:250S.

Pasteur MC, Helliwell SM, Houghton SJ, et al: An investigation into causative factors in patients with bronchiectasis. Am J Resp Crit Care Med 2000; 162:1277–1284.

O'Donnell AE, Barker AF, Ilowite JS, Fick RB: Treatment of idiopathic bronchiectasis with aerosolized recombinant DNAse I. Chest 1998; 113:1329–1334.

Schneiter D, Meyer N, Lardinois D, et al: Surgery for non-localized bronchiectasis. Br J Surg 2005; 92:836.

Weycker D, Edelsberg J, Oster G, et al: Prevalence and economic burden of bronchiectasis. Clin Pulm Med 2005; 12:205.

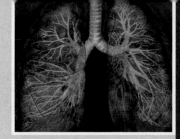

SECTION VIII

ACQUIRED IMMUNODEFICIENCY SYNDROME AND THE LUNG

34 Pulmonary Infections

ROBERT F. MILLER • MARC C.I. LIPMAN

EPIDEMIOLOGY, RISK FACTORS, AND PATHOPHYSIOLOGY

Human Immunodeficiency Virus Infection—Background

It is hard to believe that the first consistent reports of acquired immunodeficiency syndrome (AIDS) were only 25 years ago. Since then, respiratory and general physicians have become accustomed to dealing with an extraordinary range of esoteric and previously unheard of conditions. *Pneumocystis carinii* (now known as *Pneumocystis jirovecii*) pneumonia is frequently part of the differential diagnosis of treatment-nonresponsive pneumonic illness. Human immunodeficiency virus (HIV) testing is almost routinely offered as a "rule out" test in clinical cases that defy simple diagnosis. In many parts of the developing world, advanced HIV disease is unfortunately the likeliest reason for seeking medical care. The change this has wrought on people, countries and their economies is huge and depressing.

The isolation of HIV from patients with AIDS in the mid 1980s paved the way for intensive research with the ultimate development of drugs directed against this chronic infection. However, despite such advances, the methods by which HIV infection leads to severe immune dysregulation and clinical disease are still not fully defined.

The introduction in 1996, in the developed world, of highly active antiretroviral therapy, also known as combination antiretroviral therapy (cART) hereto referred to as HAART, has altered the natural history of this extraordinary condition. Before HAART, defined as a combination of medications that usually includes at least three potent anti-HIV agents, treatment largely consisted of specific opportunistic infection management and less effective antiretroviral therapy. The clinical consequences of this change are enormous. The relative hazard for development of *Pneumocystis* pneumonia (PCP) in an HIV-infected individual has fallen by more than 80%. Drug therapy does have a down side. It has significant unwanted effects, as well as major interactions with other medication (e.g., rifamycins used in treating tuberculosis). The profound change in immunity induced by HAART may also lead to disease (the immune reconstitution inflammatory syndrome [IRIS]).

Notwithstanding HAART, respiratory disease remains an important cause of morbidity and mortality. Much of the world cannot afford such medication, and more than two thirds of HIV-infected individuals have at least one respiratory episode during the course of their illness. In the early stages of HIV infection, when patients have relatively preserved immune responses, individuals have the same infections found in the general population, although at a greater incidence.

With progressive HIV disease, subjects are at an increased risk of opportunistic disease. For example, the North American Prospective Study of Pulmonary Complications of HIV Infection (PSPC), a multicenter cohort drawn from all HIV risk groups at various stages of immunosuppression, revealed over an 18-month study period that of approximately 1000 subjects who were not using HAART:

- 33% reported an upper respiratory tract infection
- 16% had an episode of acute bronchitis
- 5% had acute sinusitis
- 5% had bacterial pneumonia
- 4% had PCP develop

The immune dysregulation that arises from HIV infection means that bacteria, mycobacteria, fungi, viruses, and protozoa can all cause disease in subjects with advanced infection. Table 34-1 shows the organisms that typically infect the lung in HIV disease. Of these, bacterial infections, tuberculosis, and PCP are the most important. In the West, 40% of AIDS diagnoses are due to PCP. This chapter provides a brief general overview of the epidemiology and pathogenesis of HIV infection before concentrating on HIV and its infectious pulmonary complications.

It is reported that by the end of 2006, 39.5 million individuals worldwide had acquired HIV infection (Figure 34-1). Of these, more than 40% are thought to have had AIDS develop (for definition of AIDS, see Tables 34-2 and 34-3, and Box 34-1). Globally, 4.3 million individuals acquired HIV infection in 2006, and over this time 2.9 million died of AIDS. The developing world has been most affected. Sub-Saharan Africa is the current epicenter of the pandemic (two thirds of all infections); here, one in five adults is HIV infected. South and Southeast Asia are responsible for almost a fifth of the estimated HIV global burden. In Central-Eastern Europe and Central Asia, there are currently 1.7 million HIV-infected individuals. In the developed world, North America and Western Europe account for approximately 1.4 million and 740,000 infections, respectively. Most of these are spread through sexual contact, although vertical (mother-to-child) and bloodborne infections are also common. In the developing world, heterosexual transmission is the norm; however, in North America and Europe, homosexual and bisexual men constitute the largest group of infected individuals.

Virology and Immunology of the Human Immunodeficiency Virus

HIV was first isolated in 1983 from patients with symptoms and signs of immune dysfunction. Two subtypes (HIV-1 and HIV-2) have subsequently been identified. HIV-1 (hereafter

TABLE 34-1 Common Etiologies of HIV-Related Pulmonary Infections

Bacteria	Fungi	Parasites	Viruses
Streptococcus pneumoniae	Pneumocystis jirovecii	Toxoplasma gondii	Cytomegalovirus
Haemophilus influenzae	Cryptococcus neoformans	Cryptosporidium spp.	
Staphylococcus aureus	Histoplasma capsulatum	Microsporidium spp.	
Pseudomonas aeruginosa	Candida albicans	Leishmania spp.	
Nocardia asteroides	Aspergillus spp.	Strongyloides stercoralis	
Rochalimaea henselae	Penicillium marneffei		
Mycobacterium tuberculosis			
Mycobacterium avium-intracellulare			
Mycobacterium kansasii			

referred to as HIV) is responsible for most infections, has a more aggressive clinical course, and is the focus of this chapter.

HIV is a human retrovirus belonging to the lentivirus family. Cell-free or cell-associated HIV infects through attachment of its viral envelope protein (gp120) to the CD4 antigen complex on host cells. The CD4 receptor is found on several cell types, although the T-helper lymphocyte is the main site of HIV infection in the body. HIV gp120 must also bind to a cell surface protein coreceptor called chemokine receptor 5 (CCR5) or to other co-receptors, including CXCR4, depending on the host cell type. Polymorphisms in genes for CCR5 may affect disease progression by reducing the ability of HIV to enter and infect cells. However, at a population level, this effect is small.

Once HIV is inside the cell, it can, by use of the enzyme reverse transcriptase (RNA-dependent DNA polymerase), transcribe its HIV RNA into a DNA copy that can translocate to the nucleus and integrate with host cell DNA by use of its viral integrase. The virus (as proviral DNA) remains latent in many cells until the cell itself becomes activated. This may arise from cytokine or antigen stimulation. The viral genetic material is then transcribed into new RNA, which, in the form of a newly created virion, buds from the cell surface and is free to infect other CD4-bearing cells.

HIV infection directly attacks the immune system and in particular the T-helper cells that are central to a coordinated immune response. This leads to progressive immune dysfunction and an inability to resist opportunistic disease. The pathogenic process is not well defined, although it is thought that at the time of primary infection, HIV spreads to the lymph nodes, circulating immune cells, and thymus. This is a massive viral infection of the human host; and although there seems to be a relatively potent immune response, in fact, this initial onslaught is so devastating (targeting as it does specific memory T cells responsible for sustaining long-term protective immunity) that the scene is set for progressive immune failure. This occurs through a combination of direct cell killing by HIV replicating within cells, as well as the negative effects of chronic immune activation. Ultimately, these lead in most individuals to immune system destruction and dysfunction.

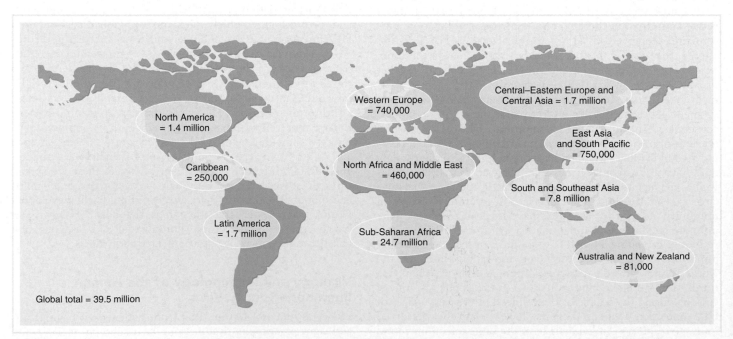

FIGURE 34-1 Estimated number of adults and children with human immunodeficiency virus (HIV) infection (to December 2006) by regions of the world. (Source: UNAIDS/WHO AIDS epidemic update: December 2006.)

TABLE 34-2 Centers for Disease Control and Prevention Classification

Group	Infection
I	Acute primary
II	Asymptomatic
III	Persistent generalized lymphadenopathy
IV	Other disease
Subgroup A	Constitutional disease (e.g., weight loss >10% of body weight or >4.5 kg; fevers >38.5°C lasting >1 month; diarrhea lasting >1 month)
Subgroup B	Neurologic disease (e.g., HIV encephalopathy, myelopathy, peripheral neuropathy)
Subgroup C	Secondary infectious diseases
Subgroup C1	AIDS-defining secondary diseases (e.g., Pneumocystis jirovecii pneumonia, cerebral toxoplasmosis, cytomegalovirus retinitis)
Subgroup C2	Other specified secondary infectious diseases (e.g., oral candida, multidermatomal varicella zoster)
Subgroup D	Secondary cancers (e.g., Kaposi sarcoma, non-Hodgkin lymphoma)
Subgroup E	Other conditions (e.g., lymphoid interstitial pneumonitis)

BOX 34-1 Adult AIDS Indicator Diseases (1993)

Candidiasis of esophagus, trachea, bronchi, or lungs
Cervical carcinoma, invasive
Coccidioidomycosis, disseminated or extrapulmonary
Cryptococcosis, extrapulmonary
Cryptosporidiosis, with diarrhea for >1 month
Cytomegalovirus diseases (not in liver, spleen, or lymph nodes)
Encephalopathy caused by HIV (AIDS-dementia complex)
Herpes simplex: ulcers for >1 month, or pneumonitis, esophagitis
Histoplasmosis, disseminated or extrapulmonary
Isosporiasis, with diarrhea for >1 month
Kaposi sarcoma
Lymphoma: Burkitt or immunoblastic or primary in CNS
Mycobacteriosis (including pulmonary tuberculosis)
Pneumocystis jirovecii pneumonia
Pneumonia recurrent within a 12-month period
Progressive multifocal leukoencephalopathy
Salmonellal (nontyphoidal) septicemia, recurrent
Toxoplasmosis of brain
Wasting syndrome caused by HIV

This is reflected not only by clinical disease indicating profound immunosuppression but also by a measurable reduction in the circulating absolute CD4 cell count, the percentage of T cells expressing CD4 markers, and in the progressive reduction in CD4/CD8 T-cell ratio.

Natural History of Human Immunodeficiency Virus Infection

The use of HAART, as well as preventative (prophylactic) therapies for opportunistic infections, has changed the clinical picture of HIV disease in countries where these interventions are available. Death rates have fallen to one sixth of their previous levels. However, in the absence of such treatments, the median interval between HIV seroconversion and progression to AIDS in the developed world has been estimated to be 10 years, although rather less in resource-poor countries. Almost all individuals have AIDS develop if untreated, and without HAART, 95% of these will die within 5 years. In many parts of the world, the main causes of death in patients with HIV infection include bacterial pneumonia, tuberculosis, and PCP.

The course of HIV infection can be divided clinically into several distinct periods:

- Acquisition of the virus
- Seroconversion, with or without a clinical illness (primary HIV infection)
- Clinically silent period, lasting several months to years
- Development of symptoms and signs indicating some degree of immunosuppression
- AIDS (where the subject has opportunistic disease implying profound immunosuppression [e.g., PCP])

Acute Primary Human Immunodeficiency Virus Infection

The time from acquisition of HIV infection to development of detectable antibodies (the "window" period) is usually approximately 6–8 weeks. Between 30 and 70% of individuals who become infected will have a seroconversion illness. HIV antibody is normally present within 2–3 weeks of these symptoms, although this can take longer. HIV RNA in peripheral blood is detectable before this and is often used to confirm infection.

The nonspecific features of primary HIV infection are almost always self-limiting, and typically seroconversion mimics a "flulike" illness or glandular fever. Most individuals with primary HIV infection recover from the acute symptoms within 4 weeks. A proportion may have persistent symmetric

TABLE 34-3 Revised (1993) CDC Classification System for HIV Infection—Clinical Categories

CD4 T-cell Categories (cells/mL)	A: Acute (primary) HIV, Asymptomatic or Persistent Generalized Lymphadenopathy	B: Symptomatic (not A or C)	C: AIDS Indicator Conditions
≥500	A1	B1	C1
200–499	A2	B2	C2
<200	A3	B3	C3

Patients are stratified clinically (A–C) and immunologically (1–3). Category B consists of symptomatic conditions that are not included within AIDS indicator diseases (category C) but can either be attributed to, or are complicated by, HIV infection. Examples include persistent candidiasis, thrombocytopenia, and peripheral neuropathy.

generalized lymphadenopathy. There is no difference in prognosis in this group compared with asymptomatic HIV-positive individuals.

Chronic Human Immunodeficiency Virus Infection

Although a proportion of individuals remain completely well without any treatment for an extended period (approximately 20% after 10 years), many HIV-infected individuals have minor symptoms and signs suggesting immune dysfunction. Examples of these include new or worsening rashes (including herpes simplex), tiredness, cough, and low-grade anemia. Certain clinical symptoms and signs provide important prognostic information. Most studies have shown that oral candidiasis and constitutional symptoms (e.g., malaise, idiopathic fever, night sweats, diarrhea, and weight loss) are the strongest clinical predictors of progression to AIDS.

The term AIDS was created as an epidemiologic tool to capture those conditions that early in the HIV epidemic seemed to suggest significant immune destruction. Over time, it has been modified to incorporate the expanding spectrum of recognized diseases affecting immunosuppressed individuals, such as cervical carcinoma and recurrent bacterial pneumonia (see Box 34-1). The 1993 Centers for Disease Control and Prevention (CDC) classification included an immunologic criterion for AIDS (CD4 count <200 cells/µL or CD4 percentage <14% of total lymphocytes) regardless of clinical symptoms (see Table 34-3). These data are used to define a point at which the risk of severe opportunistic infection rises dramatically. An example of this can be seen in the Multicenter AIDS Cohort Study (MACS) of homosexual and bisexual men without AIDS, which found that the incidence of PCP in subjects who did not use prophylaxis rose from 0.5% at 6 months in men with a baseline CD4 count >200 cells/µL to 8.4% in those with a CD4 count <200 cells/µL.

Apart from cervical carcinoma, AIDS indicator diseases differ little between men and women. Injecting drug users have a high incidence of wasting syndrome, recurrent bacterial pneumonia, and tuberculosis. Geographic differences in diseases occur that reflect the opportunistic pathogens present in the local environment (e.g., histoplasmosis or visceral leishmaniasis usually occur only in patients from endemic areas). In the developed world, sexual, racial, and HIV risk factor survival differences after an AIDS diagnosis mainly arise from variation in ease of access to medical care. It is certainly the case, however, that better treatment outcomes are associated with genuine specialist care provided by people with extensive experience in the field.

In countries where HAART is available, the spectrum of HIV-related disease has changed. In the EuroSIDA cohort (a pan-European prospective study of HIV infection), between 1994 and 2002, opportunistic infections associated with very low CD4 counts (e.g., cytomegalovirus [CMV] retinitis and *Mycobacterium avium-intracellulare* complex [MAC] infection) were observed less frequently over time. Malignant disease, such as non-Hodgkin lymphoma, increased as an AIDS-defining event between 1994 and 2004.

Although death rates have fallen in HAART-treated populations, there has been a rise in the proportion of non-AIDS deaths. In some series, this accounts for most events. Causes include liver disease (often caused by viral hepatitis) and cancer, as well as cardiovascular disease and drug-related toxicity. In such circumstances, AIDS deaths usually occur among patients who have not accessed medical care regularly and who are initially seen with advanced HIV disease.

A new manifestation of opportunistic infection has been described in patients commencing HAART. The immune reconstitution disease, IRIS, may cause severe, if temporary, clinical illness as the individual's immunity recovers. Patients will appear to develop a relapse of their original (and partially treated) disease. This is often seen in MAC infection, tuberculosis, hepatitis B, CMV retinitis, and herpesviral infection. Metabolic complications of HAART, such as ischemic heart disease and diabetes, are a potential problem in HIV practice in the developed world. A significant number of individuals taking HAART also experience drug toxicity. An increasing number of patients are also surviving to manifest symptoms associated with chronic hepatitis B and C infection. HIV-associated nephropathy (often with chronic kidney disease) is common in black Africans and is a significant cause of long-term morbidity.

Prognostic Markers

Laboratory markers and clinical symptoms (e.g., oral thrush) can independently reflect the immune changes that lead to serious disease. Staging systems have been developed that can predict the risk of progression to severe opportunistic disease (AIDS). The fall in absolute blood CD4 T-lymphocyte count is the most widely used prognostic marker, although CD4 counts may be affected by a number of factors apart from HIV, including intercurrent infection, cigarette smoking, exercise, time of day, and laboratory variation. The percentage of CD4 cells and ratio of CD4/CD8 cells are more stable measures and may be used if the CD4 absolute counts seem to vary widely from visit to visit.

Measurement of plasma HIV RNA "viral load" provides important prognostic information that can both guide therapy and suggest long-term outcome. It has a particular value in subjects who are clinically well and have high CD4 counts, because it can give some indication of the expected speed of clinical progression.

Pulmonary Immune Response During Human Immunodeficiency Virus Infection

It is clear from the frequency with which HIV-related respiratory disease occurs that the pulmonary immune response is profoundly dysregulated. However, the mechanism underlying this has not been fully explained. In part, this is because the alterations that arise reflect the complex interplay between systemically derived HIV and other circulating antigens trafficking through the pulmonary vasculature, local immune cells, and airborne antigen. Most studies investigating the pulmonary immune response have used *in vitro* cell culture systems that seek to mimic the pulmonary environment or in some cases bronchoscopy and bronchoalveolar lavage (BAL) to recover lung cells from infected individuals. Until recently, these have been performed on symptomatic patients who required bronchoscopy as a diagnostic procedure. Such subjects generally have advanced HIV infection, are often taking a number of different drugs (including antiretrovirals), and may have any number of different pathogens causing their pulmonary disease—which by themselves can influence the immune findings. Finally, the question of whether BAL fluid truly represents the site of the immune response (the lung parenchyma) remains unclear. For all these reasons, reported data should be interpreted with some care.

Risk Factors for Respiratory Disease

An individual's risk for respiratory disease is determined by his or her medical history (e.g., receipt of effective preventative or antiretroviral therapy), place of residence and travel history (e.g., the influence of geography on mycobacterial and fungal disease), and state of host immunity. Falling blood CD4 counts or high plasma RNA "viral loads" increase the chance of respiratory infection, with an increased spectrum of potential organisms responsible for infection in the more immunosuppressed individual. For example, HIV-infected individuals with a CD4 count <200 cells/μL are four times more likely to have one episode of bacterial pneumonia per year than those with higher CD4 cell counts. More exotic organisms are found in subjects with very low CD4 counts. These include bacteria such as *Rhodococcus equi* and *Nocardia asteroides* and fungi such as *Aspergillus* species and *Penicillium marneffei*. Just as with *P. jirovecii*, this reflects the importance of T-cell depletion and macrophage dysfunction in the loss of host immunity (a process that has been confirmed by animal experiments).

Among HIV-infected patients, injecting drug users are at greatest risk for development of bacterial pneumonia and tuberculosis. Individuals who have had previous respiratory episodes (PCP or bacterial pneumonia) seem to be at increased risk of further disease. Whether this relates to host or environmental factors is not certain, although it seems likely that structural lung damage and abnormal pulmonary physiology would, in part, contribute to this. This argument is supported by the increased rates of pneumonia in HIV-infected smokers compared with nonsmokers. Recent work has shown chronic obstructive pulmonary disease (COPD) and lung cancer occur more frequently among HIV-infected individuals compared with the general population. Given that a large number of HIV-infected individuals smoke heavily, there is a pressing need to target this population for smoking cessation. This is reinforced by the association demonstrated in some (but not all) studies between smoking and a more rapid progression to first AIDS illness and death.

CLINICAL FEATURES

Bacterial Infection

Bronchitis

The presentation mimics bacterial exacerbations of chronic obstructive lung disease; most patients have a productive cough and fever. The pathogens commonly identified are similar to those in the general population (i.e., *Streptococcus pneumoniae* and *Haemophilus influenzae*). However, patients with advanced disease may be infected with *Pseudomonas aeruginosa* or *Staphylococcus aureus*. Response to appropriate antibiotic therapy in conventional doses is good, although relapses frequently occur.

Bronchiectasis

Bronchiectasis is increasingly recognized in HIV-infected patients with advanced HIV disease and low CD4 lymphocyte counts. It probably arises secondary to recurrent bacterial or *P. jirovecii* infections. The diagnosis is most often made by high-resolution/fine-cut computed tomography (CT) scanning. Its prevalence has not been accurately determined, although with improved survival from both opportunistic infections and HIV disease, it is likely that it will be increasingly common in clinical practice. The pathogens isolated in patients with bronchiectasis are those seen in bronchitis. In addition, *Pseudomonas cepacia* and *Moraxella catarrhalis* have been described.

Pneumonia

Community-acquired bacterial pneumonia occurs more frequently in HIV-infected patients than in the general population. It is especially common in HIV-infected injecting drug users. The spectrum of bacterial pathogens is similar to that in non-HIV–infected individuals (see Table 34-1). *S. pneumoniae* is the most common cause, followed by *H. influenzae*. HIV-infected individuals with *S. pneumoniae* pneumonia are frequently bacteremic. In one study, the rate of pneumococcal bacteremia in HIV-infected individuals was 100 times that of an HIV-negative population. More recent work has confirmed this to be the case for all causes of HIV-related bacterial pneumonia. Typically, blood cultures have a 40-fold increased pickup rate in HIV-positive patients. The widespread use of HAART has led to some decrease in rates of bacterial pneumonia and bacteremia, although they are still considerably higher than those seen in a non-HIV–infected population.

Bacterial pneumonia has a similar presentation in HIV-infected and uninfected individuals. Chest radiographs are frequently atypical, mimicking PCP in up to 50% of cases (Figure 34-2). By contrast, radiographic lobar or segmental consolidation may also be seen in a wide range of bacterial organisms (Figure 34-3); these include *S. pneumoniae*, *P. aeruginosa*, *H. influenzae*, and *Mycobacterium tuberculosis*. PCP may also present with lobar or segmental consolidation.

In subjects with more advanced HIV disease and low CD4 lymphocyte counts, *P. aeruginosa* and *S. aureus* also cause pneumonia.

Complications of bacterial pneumonia frequently occur, and pleural effusions are twice as likely in HIV infection (often occurring with *S. aureus* infection); empyema and intrapulmonary abscess formation are present in up to 10% of patients. Inevitably, the mortality rate is high (approximately 10%).

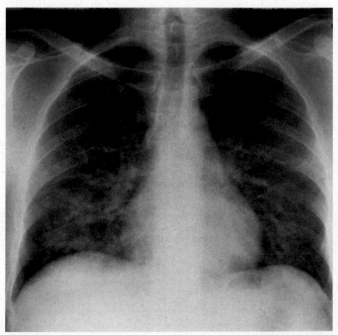

FIGURE 34-2 Chest radiograph showing bilateral, diffuse, interstitial infiltrates mimicking *Pneumocystis jirovecii* pneumonia. Etiology is *Streptococcus pneumoniae*.

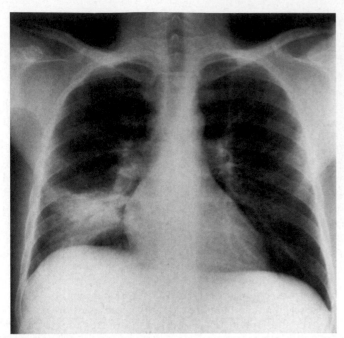

FIGURE 34-3 Chest radiograph showing lobar consolidation. Etiology is *Salmonella cholera-suis*.

Other Bacteria

***Nocardia Asteroides* Infection.** This has been reported in patients with advanced HIV disease and low CD4 lymphocyte counts. The widespread use of trimethoprim/sulfamethoxazole (TMP/SMX) for prophylaxis of PCP may have reduced the incidence of infection. The clinical presentation is often indistinguishable from that of other bacterial infections. Chest radiographic appearances may mimic tuberculosis (see later), with upper lobe consolidation, cavitation, interstitial infiltrates, pleural effusion, and hilar lymphadenopathy. The diagnosis is made by identification of the organism in sputum/BAL fluid or lung tissue.

Rhodococcus equi. *R. equi* usually produces pneumonia in patients who have advanced HIV infection and have been in contact with farm animals or with soil from fields or barns where animals are housed. The presentation is subacute, with 2–3 weeks of cough, dyspnea, fever, and pleuritic chest pain. The chest radiograph typically shows consolidation with cavitation.

Pleural effusions are common. The diagnosis is usually made by culture of sputum or blood; bronchoscopy with BAL or pleural aspiration may be necessary in some cases.

Bartonella henselae. *B. henselae* is a gram-negative bacillus that causes bacillary angiomatosis in HIV-infected patients. Clinically, the cutaneous lesions may mimic Kaposi sarcoma, from which they may be distinguished by demonstration of organisms in tissue with Warthin–Starry silver stain. Bacillary angiomatosis may also infect the lungs, where it produces endobronchial red or violet polypoid angiomatous lesions, which may resemble Kaposi sarcoma. Biopsy is necessary to confirm a diagnosis.

Mycobacterial Infections

Tuberculosis

HIV infection is associated with at least a 40-fold increased risk of an individual having active tuberculosis develop compared with noninfected subjects. Taken together with its ability to infect both the immunosuppressed and immunocompetent, tuberculosis is perhaps, therefore, the single most important disease associated with HIV infection. It is estimated that there are at least 13 million individuals with HIV-tuberculosis coinfection. As such, tuberculosis is a major cause of HIV-related morbidity and mortality. It is also a major driver in both resource-rich and resource-poor countries for the current overall increase in tuberculosis rates. Where HIV infection is endemic, tuberculosis control at a population level is almost impossible if treatment for both infections is not available.

In the United Kingdom, many centers routinely offer HIV antibody testing to all patients with tuberculosis, regardless of risk factors for HIV infection. In the United States, the CDC now recommends HIV testing as a routine part of health care for all patients aged 13–64 accessing medical services. The advantage of this is that individuals who are found to be HIV infected can be given HAART. Furthermore, strategies to modify high-risk behavior and reduce ongoing HIV transmission may be offered.

Active tuberculosis can occur at any stage of HIV infection, and unlike almost every other HIV-related infection, may do so despite effective antiretroviral therapy. In the United States, United Kingdom, and most European countries, reporting of tuberculosis in both HIV-infected and non-HIV–infected individuals is mandatory.

Clinical disease in HIV-infected patients may arise in several different ways: by reactivation of latent tuberculosis, by rapid progression of pulmonary infection, and by reinfection from an exogenous source.

Pulmonary disease is the most common presentation; and clinical manifestations are related to the level of an individual's cell-mediated immunity. For example, subjects with early HIV disease have clinical features similar to "normal" adult postprimary disease (Table 34-4). Symptoms typically include

TABLE 34-4 Tuberculosis and HIV Infection		
	Stage of HIV Disease	
	Early	**Late**
Chest radiograph	Upper lobe infiltrates and cavities (c.f. postprimary infection)	Lymphadenopathy, effusions, miliary or diffuse infiltrates (c.f. primary infection) Normal
Sputum or bronchoalveolar lavage "smear positive"	Frequently	Less commonly
Tuberculin test positive	Frequently	Less commonly

weight loss, fever with sweats, cough, sputum, dyspnea, hemoptysis, and chest pain. These patients may have no clinical features to suggest associated HIV infection. The chest radiograph frequently shows upper lobe consolidation, and cavitary change is common (Figure 34-4). The tuberculin skin test (purified protein derivative [PPD]) is usually positive, and the likelihood of spontaneously expectorated sputum or BAL fluid being smear positive for acid-fast bacilli is high.

In individuals with advanced HIV disease (i.e., low CD4 lymphocyte counts and clinically apparent immunosuppression), it may be difficult to diagnose tuberculosis. The clinical presentation here is often with nonspecific symptoms. Fever, weight loss, fatigue, and malaise may be mistakenly ascribed to HIV infection itself. In this context, pulmonary tuberculosis is often similar to primary infection, with the chest radiograph showing diffuse or military-type shadowing (Figure 34-5), hilar or mediastinal lymphadenopathy, or pleural effusion; cavitation is unusual. In up to 10% of patients the chest radiograph may appear normal; in others, the pulmonary infiltrate can be bilateral, diffuse, and interstitial in pattern, thus mimicking PCP. Hilar lymphadenopathy and pleural effusion may also be produced by pulmonary Kaposi sarcoma or lymphoma, with which *M. tuberculosis* may coexist. The tuberculin skin test is usually negative, and spontaneously expectorated sputum and BAL fluid are often smear negative (but culture positive).

In addition to pulmonary tuberculosis, extrapulmonary disease occurs in a high proportion of HIV-infected individuals with low CD4 lymphocyte counts (<150 cells/µL). Mycobacteremia and lymph node infection (Figure 34-6) are common, but involvement of bone marrow, liver, pericardium, meninges, and brain also occurs.

Evidence of extrapulmonary tuberculosis should be sought in any HIV-infected patient with suspected or confirmed pulmonary tuberculosis, by culture of stool, urine, and blood or bone marrow. Traditional solid phase culture and speciation techniques may take 6–10 weeks. Liquid culture methods (e.g., BACTEC, Becton Dickinson) that detect early growth may provide a diagnosis in only 2–3 weeks. Molecular diagnostic tests that use *M. tuberculosis* genome detection (e.g., by polymerase chain reaction [PCR]) offer the possibility of yet more rapid diagnosis (within hours), but are not yet in routine clinical use. They are also less useful in primary samples with low bacterial load (e.g., smear negative sputum)—which is often when they will be most needed in HIV-coinfected patients. The recent description of simple, but highly sensitive

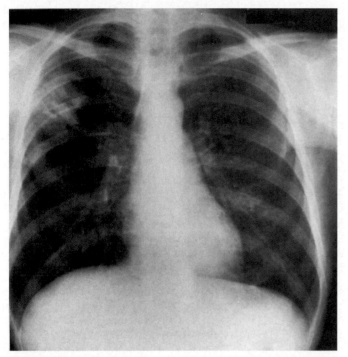

FIGURE 34-4 Chest radiograph of pulmonary tuberculosis in early-stage human immunodeficiency virus infection. Upper lobe infiltrates and cavities are shown.

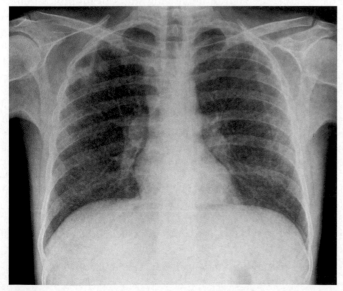

FIGURE 34-5 Chest radiograph showing miliary tuberculosis. Patient's CD4 count was 80 cells/µL.

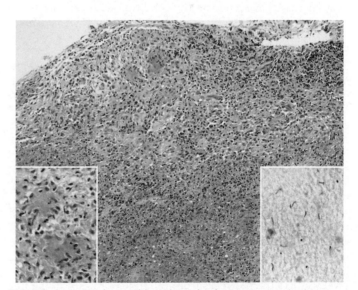

FIGURE 34-6 Mediastinal lymph node showing necrotic tissue surrounded by poorly developed granulomatous inflammation (*left insert*). A Ziehl Neelsen stain showed numerous acid-fast bacilli (*right insert*). (Reproduced with permission from Miller RF, Shahmanesh M, Talbot MD, Wiselka MJ, Shaw PJ, Bacon C, Robertson CM: Progressive symptoms and signs after institution of highly active antiretroviral therapy and subsequent antituberculosis therapy: Immune reconstitution syndrome or infection? Sexually Transmitted Infections 2006; 82: 111–116, BMJ Publishing Group.)

and specific, methods that use the inoculation of large quantities of, for example, sputum onto microscopic plates with subsequent rapid detection (in days) of both mycobacterial growth and resistance patterns (MODS) is of great potential significance.

Until the results of culture and speciation are known, acid-fast bacilli identified in respiratory samples, biopsy tissue, an aspirate, or blood in an HIV-infected individual, regardless of the CD4 lymphocyte count, should be regarded as being *M. tuberculosis*, and conventional antituberculosis therapy should be commenced. If culture fails to demonstrate *M. tuberculosis* and instead another mycobacterium (see later) is identified, treatment can be modified.

Drug-Resistant Tuberculosis

Multiple drug-resistant (MDR) tuberculosis—that is, *M. tuberculosis* that is resistant to isoniazid and rifampicin (rifampin), with or without other drugs, is now an important clinical problem in HIV-infected individuals in the United States, where it is responsible for approximately 3% of all tuberculosis in HIV-infected patients. Outbreaks of MDR tuberculosis have occurred in both HIV-infected and non-HIV–infected individuals in the United States in prison facilities, hostels, and hospitals. Similar outbreaks have also been documented among HIV-infected patients in Europe. Inadequate treatment (including case management and supervision of medication) of tuberculosis and poor patient compliance with antituberculosis therapy are the most important risk factors for development of MDR tuberculosis. Other cases have arisen because of exogenous reinfection of profoundly immunosuppressed HIV-infected patients who are already receiving treatment for drug-sensitive disease.

Despite antituberculosis therapy, the median survival in HIV-infected individuals with MDR-tuberculosis was initially only 2–3 months. Recently this has improved, largely because of an increased awareness of the condition with early initiation of suitable therapy as determined by drug sensitivity testing.

Extensively Drug-Resistant Tuberculosis

Extensively drug-resistant (XDR) tuberculosis—that is, *M. tuberculosis* resistant to isoniazid and rifampicin (rifampin), plus any fluoroquinolone and one or more of the three injectable second-line drugs (capreomycin, kanamycin and amikacin)—is an increasingly important clinical problem. Originally described in South Africa in association with HIV infection, XDR tuberculosis has also been identified in most parts of the world. As of March 2007, 35 countries had reported at least one case; although in many places, testing for fluoroquinolone sensitivity is not standard practice; this number may be, in fact, a huge underestimate. What is of concern about XDR tuberculosis is that, despite specific therapy, mortality is high among HIV-infected individuals. The current picture seems to mirror early reports of MDR tuberculosis in HIV infection: in the original South African study from KwaZulu Natal, survival was less than 3 weeks from the time of receipt of the first sputum sample.

Mycobacteria Other Than Tuberculosis

***Mycobacterium avium-intracellulare* Complex.** Before the widespread availability of HAART, disseminated MAC infection developed in up to 50% of HIV-infected patients. It remains a problem in patients with advanced HIV disease not receiving antiretroviral therapy and who have CD4 lymphocyte counts <50 cells/µL. Clinical presentation is nonspecific and may be confused with the effects of HIV itself. Fever, night sweats, weight loss, anorexia, and malaise are common. Anemia, hepatosplenomegaly, abdominal pain, and chronic diarrhea are frequent findings. The diagnosis of disseminated MAC infection is based on culture of the organism from blood, bone marrow, lymph node, or liver biopsy specimens. Also, MAC is frequently identified in BAL fluid, sputum, stool, and urine, but detection of the organism at these sites is not diagnostic of disseminated infection. Evidence of pulmonary MAC infection is not usually obtained from a chest radiograph, which may be negative or show nonspecific infiltrates. Rarely, focal consolidation, nodular infiltrates, and apical cavitation (resembling *M. tuberculosis*) have been reported.

Mycobacterium kansasii. *Mycobacterium kansasii* is the second most common nontuberculous opportunistic mycobacterial infection in HIV-infected individuals and usually appears late in the course of HIV infection in patients with CD4 lymphocyte counts <100 cells/µL. The most frequent presentation is with fever, cough, and dyspnea. In approximately two thirds of those who have *M. kansasii* infection, the disease is localized to the lungs; the remainder have disseminated disease that affects bone marrow, lymph node, skin, and lungs. The diagnosis is made by culture of the organism from respiratory secretions or from bone marrow, lymph node aspirate, or skin biopsy. Focal upper lobe infiltrates with diffuse interstitial infiltrates are the most common radiographic abnormalities; thin-walled cavitary lesions and hilar adenopathy have also been reported.

Mycobacterium xenopi. *Mycobacterium xenopi* may occasionally be isolated from sputum or BAL fluid samples, but its significance is uncertain. Patients have low CD4 counts, and *M. xenopi* is usually accompanied by isolation of a co-pathogen, such as *P. jirovecii*. Treatment of the latter condition is associated in most cases with resolution of symptoms. There is some evidence that starting HAART prevents disease recurrence, provided there is an adequate immune response.

***Pneumocystis jirovecii* Pneumonia.** The development of PCP is largely related to underlying states of immunosuppression induced by malignancy or treatment thereof, organ transplantation, or HIV infection. In 2007 in the United States, United Kingdom, Europe, and Australasia, PCP is largely seen only in HIV-infected individuals unaware of their serostatus or in those who are intolerant of, or noncompliant with, anti–*P. jirovecii* prophylaxis and HAART.

Until recently, *P. jirovecii* was regarded taxonomically as a protozoan, on the basis of its morphology and the lack of response to antifungal agents such as amphotericin B. The organism has now been ascribed to the fungal kingdom. The demonstration of antibodies against *P. jirovecii* in most healthy children/adults suggests that organisms are acquired in childhood and persist in the lungs in a dormant phase. Subsequent immunosuppression (e.g., as a result of HIV infection) allows the fungus to propagate in the lung and cause clinical disease. However, this "latency" hypothesis is challenged by several observations:

- *P. jirovecii* cannot be identified in the lungs of immunocompetent individuals.
- "Case clusters" of PCP in health care facilities suggest recent transmission.

- Different genotypes of *P. jirovecii* are identified in each episode in HIV-infected patients who have recurrent PCP.
- Genotypes of *P. jirovecii* in patients who have PCP correlate with place of diagnosis and not with their place of birth—suggesting infection has been recently acquired.

Taken together, these data suggest that PCP arises by reinfection from an exogenous source.

The clinical presentation of PCP is nonspecific, with an onset of progressive exertional dyspnea over days or weeks, together with a dry cough with or without expectoration of minimal quantities of mucoid sputum. Patients often complain of an inability to take a deep breath, which is not due to pleurisy (Table 34-5). Fever is common, yet patients rarely complain of temperatures or sweats. In HIV-infected patients, the presentation is usually more insidious than in patients receiving immunosuppressive therapy, with a median time to diagnosis from onset of symptoms of more than 3 weeks in those with HIV compared with less than 1 week in non-HIV–infected patients. In a small proportion of HIV-positive individuals, the disease course of PCP is fulminant, with an interval of only 5–7 days between onset of symptoms and progression to development of respiratory failure. In others, it may be much more indolent, with respiratory symptoms that worsen almost imperceptibly over several months. Rarely, PCP may present without respiratory symptoms as a fever of undetermined origin.

Clinical examination is usually remarkable only for the absence of physical signs; occasionally, fine, basal, end-inspiratory crackles are audible. Features that would suggest an alternative diagnosis include a cough productive of purulent sputum or hemoptysis, chest pain (particularly pleural pain), and signs of focal consolidation or pleural effusion (see Table 34-5). It should be noted that infection with more than one pathogen occurs in almost one fifth of individuals, and thus symptoms may be the product of several agents.

The chest radiograph in PCP is typically unremarkable initially. Later, diffuse reticular shadowing, especially in the perihilar regions, is seen and may progress to diffuse alveolar consolidation that resembles pulmonary edema if untreated or if the patient is seen late in disease. At this stage, the lung may be massively consolidated and almost airless (Figure 34-7). Up to 20% of chest radiographs are atypical, showing lobar consolidation, honeycomb lung, multiple thin-walled cystic air space formation (pneumatoceles), intrapulmonary nodules, cavitary lesions, pneumothorax, and hilar and mediastinal lymphadenopathy. Predominantly apical changes, resembling tuberculosis, may occur in patients who have PCP develop having received anti-*P. jirovecii* prophylaxis with nebulized pentamidine (Figure 34-8). All these radiographic changes

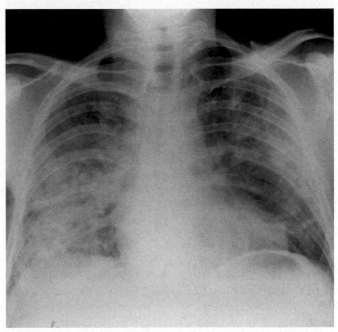

FIGURE 34-7 Chest radiograph of severe *Pneumocystis jirovecii* pneumonia. Diffuse bilateral interstitial infiltrates are shown.

TABLE 34-5 Presentation of *Pneumocystis jirovecii* Pneumonia		
Examination	**Typical Presentation**	**Atypical Presentation**
Symptoms	Progressive exertional dyspnea over days or weeks	Sudden onset of dyspnea over hours or days
	Dry cough ± mucoid sputum	Cough productive of purulent sputum Hemoptysis
	Difficulty in taking in a deep breath not because of pleuritic pain	Chest pain (pleuritic or "crushing")
	Fever ± sweats	
	Tachypnea	
Signs	Normal breath sounds or fine end-inspiratory basal crackles	Wheeze, signs of focal consolidation or pleural effusion
Chest radiograph	Early: perihilar "haze" or bilateral interstitial shadowing	
	Late: alveolar-interstitial changes or "white out" (marked alveolar consolidation with sparing of apices and costophrenic angles)	
Arterial blood gases	Pao$_2$: early, normal: late, low	
	Paco$_2$: early, normal or low; late, normal or high	

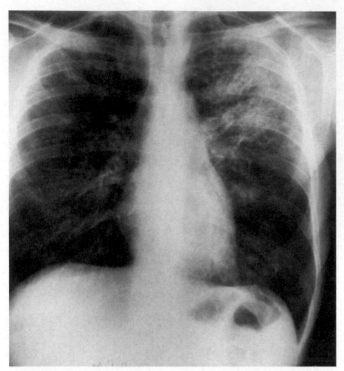

FIGURE 34-8 Chest radiograph of *Pneumocystis jirovecii* pneumonia. Upper lobe infiltrates are seen in this patient who had received nebulized pentamidine.

are nonspecific, and similar changes occur with other pulmonary pathogens, including pyogenic bacterial, mycobacterial, and fungal infection, as well as Kaposi sarcoma and nonspecific interstitial pneumonitis. Respiratory symptoms in an immunosuppressed, HIV-infected individual with a negative chest radiograph should not be discounted, because over an interval of 2–3 days radiographic abnormalities may appear.

The diagnosis of PCP is made by demonstration of the organism in induced sputum, BAL fluid, or lung biopsy material by use of histochemical or immunofluorescence techniques. The early promise of molecular diagnostic techniques has not been borne out.

Fungal Infections

Many fungal infections of the lung are confined to specific geographic regions, although with widespread travel, they may present in patients outside these areas. *Candida*, *Aspergillus*, and *Cryptococcus* species are ubiquitous and occur worldwide.

Candidal Infection

In contrast to infections of the oropharynx and esophagus, candidal infection of the trachea, bronchi, and lungs is rare in HIV-infected patients, as are candidemia, disseminated candidiasis, and deep focal candidiasis. The clinical presentation of pulmonary candidal infection has no specific features. Chest radiography is equally nonspecific—it may be negative or show patchy infiltrates. Isolation of *Candida* from sputum may simply represent colonization and does not mean the patient has candidal pneumonia. Indirect evidence may be obtained from positive cultures or rising antibody titers. However, in HIV-infected patients, a high antibody titer alone is a less reliable indicator, and antibodies may be absent in proven cases of invasive candidal infection. Some correlation occurs between

identification of large quantities of *Candida* species in BAL fluid and *Candida* species as the cause of pneumonia. Definitive diagnosis is made by lung biopsy.

Aspergillus *Infection*

By contrast with patients immunosuppressed and rendered neutropenic by systemic chemotherapy, infection with *Aspergillus* species is relatively rare in HIV-positive individuals. Risk factors for aspergillosis are neutropenia, which is commonly drug induced (zidovudine or ganciclovir), or patient's receipt of corticosteroids. Fever, cough, and dyspnea are the most common presenting symptoms, but pleuritic chest pain and hemoptysis are found in approximately one third of patients.

Patterns of pulmonary disease include cavitating upper lobe disease, focal radiographic opacities resembling bacterial pneumonia, bilateral diffuse and patchy opacities (nodular or reticular-nodular in pattern), pseudomembranous aspergillosis, which may obstruct the lumen of airways, and tracheobronchitis. Diagnosis of pulmonary aspergillosis is made by the identification of fungus in sputum, sputum casts, or BAL fluid associated with respiratory tract tissue invasion (Figure 34-9). The role of antigen testing (such as galactomannan assays), which is commonplace in hematology patients at risk of invasive aspergillus, has not been clearly defined in HIV-infected individuals.

Cryptococcal Infection

Infection may present in one of two ways: either as primary cryptococcosis or complicating cryptococcal meningitis as part of disseminated infection with cryptococcemia, pneumonia, and cutaneous disease (umbilicated papules mimicking molluscum contagiosum; Figure 34-10). Primary pulmonary cryptococcosis presents in a very nonspecific way and is frequently indistinguishable from other pulmonary infections. In disseminated infection, the presentation is frequently overshadowed by headache, fever, and malaise (caused by meningitis). The duration of onset may range from only a few days to several weeks. Examination may reveal skin lesions, lymphadenopathy, and meningism. In the chest, signs may be absent or crackles may be audible. Arterial blood gas tensions may be normal or show hypoxemia. The most common abnormality on the chest radiograph is focal or diffuse interstitial infiltrates.

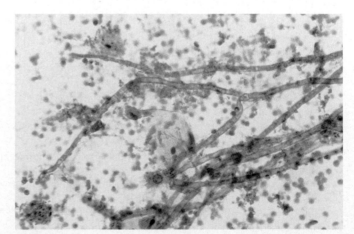

FIGURE 34-9 Bronchoalveolar lavage fluid containing *Aspergillus fumigatus*.

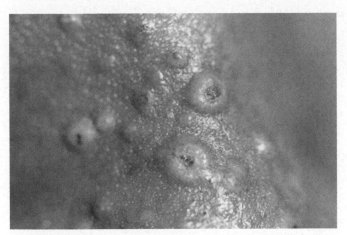

FIGURE 34-10 Skin in disseminated cryptococcosis. The multiple, umbilicated lesions resemble molluscum contagiosum.

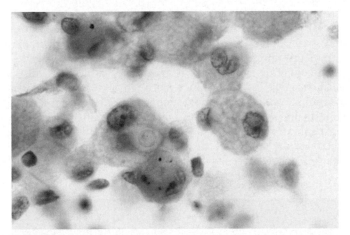

FIGURE 34-11 Bronchoalveolar lavage fluid containing *Cryptococcus neoformans*.

Less frequently, masses, mediastinal or hilar lymphadenopathy, nodules, and effusion are noted.

The diagnosis of cryptococcal pulmonary infection (Figure 34-11) is made by identification of *Cryptococcus neoformans* (by staining with India ink or mucicarmine, and by culture) in sputum, BAL fluid, pleural fluid, or lung biopsy. Cryptococcal antigen may be detected in serum by use of the cryptococcal latex agglutination (CrAg) test. Titers are usually high but may be negative in primary pulmonary cryptococcosis, in which case BAL fluid (CrAg) is positive. In patients with disseminated infection, *C. neoformans* may also be cultured from blood and cerebrospinal fluid. The mortality rate is high in this disseminated form (up to 80%).

Endemic Mycoses

The endemic mycoses caused by *Histoplasma capsulatum*, *Coccidioides immitis*, and *Blastomyces dermatitidis* are found in HIV-infected patients living in North America (especially the Mississippi and Ohio River valleys). Histoplasmosis is also found in Southeast Asia, the Caribbean Islands, and South America. Coccidioidomycosis is endemic in the southwest United States (southern California), northern Mexico, and in parts of Argentina and Brazil. Blastomycosis has a similar distribution, with an extension north into Canada.

Histoplasmosis

Progressive, disseminated histoplasmosis in patients with HIV typically presents with a subacute onset of fever and weight loss; approximately 50% of patients have mild respiratory symptoms with a nonproductive cough and dyspnea. Hepatosplenomegaly is frequently found on examination, and a rash (similar to that produced by *Cryptococcus* species) may be seen. Rarely, the presentation may be rapidly fulminant, with clinical features of the sepsis syndrome, including anemia or disseminated intravascular coagulation. The chest radiograph may be unremarkable (in up to one third of patients), although characteristic abnormalities are bilateral, widespread nodules 2–4 mm in size. Other radiographic features are nonspecific and include interstitial infiltrates, reticular nodular shadowing, and alveolar consolidation. Histoplasmosis may disseminate to the central nervous system and produce meningoencephalitis or mass lesions. The diagnosis is made reliably by identification of the organism in Wright-stained peripheral blood or by Giemsa staining of bone marrow, lymph node, skin, sputum, BAL fluid, or lung tissue. It is important that identification is confirmed by detection of *H. capsulatum* var. *capsulatum* polysaccharide antigen by radioimmunoassay, which has a high sensitivity. False-positive results may occur in patients infected with *Blastomycosis* and *Coccidioides* species. Tests for *Histoplasma* antibodies by complement fixation or immunodiffusion may be negative in immunosuppressed, HIV-positive patients.

Coccidioidomycosis

The clinical presentation of coccidioidomycosis is variable. The chest radiograph may show focal pulmonary disease with focal alveolar infiltrates, adenopathy, and intrapulmonary cavities or, alternately, diffuse reticular infiltrates. Diagnosis is made by isolation of the organism in sputum or BAL fluid. Disseminated disease is identified by isolating the fungus in blood, urine, or cerebrospinal fluid. Serologic tests may also be used for diagnosis.

Blastomycosis

Blastomycosis presents in patients who have advanced HIV infection, when CD4 lymphocyte counts are usually less than 200 cells/μL. Clinical symptoms include cough, fever, dyspnea, and weight loss. Patients may present late in respiratory failure. Disseminated disease can occur with both pulmonary and extrapulmonary features. There is frequently multiple involvement of the skin, liver, brain, and meninges. Chest radiographic abnormalities include focal pneumonic change, miliary shadowing, or diffuse interstitial infiltrates. Diagnosis is made by culture from BAL fluid, skin, and blood. In this infection, cytologic or histologic diagnosis is important for early diagnosis, because culture of the organism may take 2–4 weeks. The mortality rate is high in patients with disseminated infection.

PENICILLIUM MARNEFFEI INFECTION

P. marneffei infection is particularly common in Southeast Asia. Most HIV-infected patients present with disseminated infection and solitary skin or oral mucosal lesions, or with multiple infiltrates in the liver or spleen, or bone marrow (leading to presentation with pancytopenia). Pulmonary infection has no specific clinical features, and chest radiographs may be negative or show diffuse, small nodular infiltrates. Diagnosis is made by identifying the organism in bone marrow, skin biopsy samples, blood films, or BAL fluid. The differential diagnosis of *P. marneffei* infection includes both PCP and tuberculosis.

Viral Infections
Community-Based Respiratory Viral Infections

These occur with equal frequency in HIV-infected and non-HIV–infected patients; however, respiratory complications after influenza infection are increased in patients affected with underlying conditions such as cardiac or pulmonary disease and immunosuppression. In prospective studies of HIV-infected patients undergoing bronchoscopy for evaluation of suspected lower respiratory tract disease, the community-acquired respiratory viral infections (i.e., influenza, parainfluenza, respiratory syncytial virus, rhinovirus, coronavirus and adenovirus) are found only rarely, if at all.

Cytomegalovirus

CMV chronically infects most HIV-infected individuals, and up to 90% of homosexual HIV-infected men shed CMV intermittently in urine, semen, and saliva. Clinical disease may be caused by CMV in patients who have advanced HIV infection and CD4 counts <100 cells/μL. Chorioretinitis is most frequently encountered, but encephalitis, adrenalitis, esophagitis, and colitis are also seen. Frequently, CMV is isolated from BAL fluid, being found in 40% of samples from patients with CD4 counts <100 cells/μL. However, the role of CMV in causing disease in this context is unclear (see later).

In patients who have CMV as the sole identified pathogen, clinical presentation and chest radiographic abnormalities (usually diffuse interstitial infiltrates) are nonspecific. Diagnosis of CMV pneumonitis is made by identifying characteristic intranuclear and intracytoplasmic inclusions, not only in cells in BAL fluid but also in lung biopsy specimens (Figure 34-12).

Protozoal Infections
Leishmaniasis

Pulmonary involvement with *Leishmania* species may rarely occur as part of the syndrome of visceral leishmaniasis in HIV-infected patients. Patients usually have advanced HIV disease with CD4 lymphocyte counts less than 300 cells/μL and present with unexplained fever, splenomegaly, and leukopenia. Respiratory symptoms are often absent. Diagnosis of visceral leishmaniasis is most often made by staining a splenic or bone marrow aspirate and subsequent culture. Occasionally, the parasite is found by chance in a skin or rectal biopsy or BAL fluid taken for other purposes. The chest radiograph may be negative or show reticular-nodular infiltrates.

Toxoplasmosis

Toxoplasma gondii infection in patients who have AIDS usually occurs as a result of reactivation of latent, intracellular protozoa acquired in a primary infection. Patients are invariably systemically unwell, with malaise and pyrexia. Clinical disease in association with HIV infection is most commonly seen in the central nervous system, where it produces single or multiple abscesses. Multisystem infection with *T. gondii* is uncommon in patients who have HIV infection.

Toxoplasmic pneumonia is frequently difficult to distinguish from PCP. Nonproductive cough and dyspnea are the symptoms most commonly reported. Chest radiographic abnormalities include diffuse interstitial infiltrates indistinguishable from those of PCP (Figure 34-13), as well as micronodular infiltrates, a coarse nodular infiltrate, cavitary change, and lobar consolidation. The diagnosis is made by

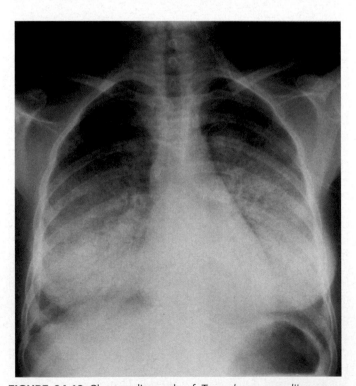

FIGURE 34-13 Chest radiograph of *Toxoplasma gondii* pneumonia. The diffuse bilateral infiltrates resemble *P. jirovecii* pneumonia. (Reproduced with permission from Miller RF, Lucas SB, Bateman NT: Disseminated *Toxoplasma gondii* infection presenting with a fulminant pneumonia. Genitourinary Med 1996; 72:139–143, BMJ Publishing Group.)

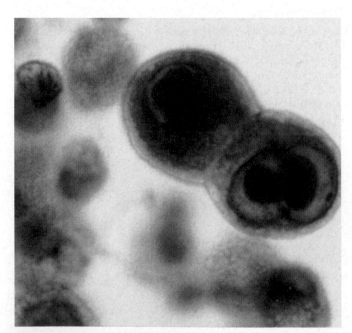

FIGURE 34-12 Bronchoalveolar lavage fluid containing cytomegalovirus inclusions.

hematoxylin–eosin or Giemsa staining of BAL fluid that reveals cysts and trophozoites of *T. gondii*. Staining of BAL fluid is not always positive; the diagnostic yield is increased either by staining of transbronchial biopsy material or by performing nucleic acid amplification procedures such as PCR to detect *T. gondii* DNA in BAL fluid.

Cryptosporidiosis

The most frequent manifestation of infection with *Cryptosporidium* species in HIV infection is a noninflammatory diarrhea that may be of high volume, intractable, and life threatening. *Cryptosporidium* species may colonize epithelial surfaces, including the trachea and lungs, occasionally resulting in pulmonary infection. Most cases of pulmonary cryptosporidiosis have co-pathology such as PCP or bacterial pneumonia; ascertaining the exact role of cryptosporidiosis as the cause of respiratory symptoms may be difficult. Diagnosis is made by Ziehl–Neelsen or auramine-rhodamine staining of BAL fluid or transbronchial biopsy specimens.

Microsporidiosis

Pulmonary *Microsporidia* infection may occur as part of systemic dissemination from gastrointestinal infection with *Septata intestinalis* or *Encephalitozoon hellem*. The organism may be identified by conventional staining in BAL fluid. Electron microscopy is necessary to distinguish the two species.

Strongyloidiasis

The nematode *Strongyloides stercoralis* is endemic in warm countries worldwide. In immunosuppressed patients, the organism has an increased ability to reproduce parthenogenetically in the gastrointestinal tract without the need for repeated exposure to new infection—so-called autoinfection. This results in a great increase in worm load and a hyperinfective state ensues; massive acute dissemination with *S. stercoralis* may occur in the lungs, kidneys, pancreas, and brain. Although infection with *S. stercoralis* is more severe in immunocompromised patients, it is no more common in patients who have HIV infection. Presentation with hyperinfection may be with fever, hypotension secondary to bacterial sepsis, or disseminated intravascular coagulation. The clinical features of respiratory *S. stercoralis* infection are nonspecific. *S. stercoralis* in sputum or BAL fluid (Figure 34-14) may be identified in HIV-positive patients in the absence of symptoms elsewhere;

this can predate disseminated infection and, as such, requires prompt treatment.

DIAGNOSIS

It is apparent from the foregoing discussion that HIV-related pneumonia of any cause may present in a similar manner. A wide range of investigations is available to aid diagnosis. These are listed in Table 34-6. If the subject is producing sputum, it is important to obtain samples for bacterial and mycobacterial detection. In up to one third of cases, these will assist in diagnosis. Three samples on consecutive days (preferably either with overnight or early morning production) is the critical first step in the diagnosis of pulmonary tuberculosis. This is considerably easier and safer for health care personnel than obtaining hypertonic saline-induced sputum or BAL fluid. Blood cultures are also important, because very high rates of bacteremia have been reported in both bacterial and mycobacterial disease (see earlier).

A patient who is initially seen with symptoms and signs consistent with pneumonia should have chest radiography and arterial oxygen assessments performed at his or her first consultation. The question at this stage is usually whether this infectious episode is due to bacterial infection, tuberculosis, or PCP. In general, alveolar and interstitial shadowing is taken as evidence for PCP, although important caveats apply.

Arterial Oxygen Assessments

Transcutaneous pulse oximetry and arterial blood gas analysis are useful tests for hypoxemia. They can be used to distinguish an alveolar condition (i.e., PCP) from bacterial pneumonia. The alveolitis produces a greater impairment of oxygen transfer (especially during exercise), such that for a given clinical situation there will be more hypoxemia and a wider alveolar-arterial oxygen gradient (A-aO_2) in those with PCP. With pulse oximetry, this manifests as low oxygen saturations at rest that decrease further with exercise. In general, more information

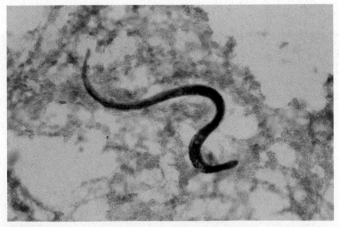

FIGURE 34-14 Bronchoalveolar lavage fluid containing *Strongyloides stercoralis*.

TABLE 34-6	Tests Available to Aid Diagnosis of HIV-Related Pneumonia
Type	**Test**
Physiologic	Transcutaneous pulse oximetry
	Arterial blood gas analysis
	Lung function
Radiologic	Chest radiography
	Computed tomography of thorax
Pathologic	Serology (antigen or antibody testing)
	Serum lactate dehydrogenase enzyme measurement
	Microscopy and culture of body fluid/tissue (e.g., sputum, blood, bronchoalveolar lavage fluid, lung tissue) obtained by:
	Sputum induction
	Bronchoscopy and bronchoalveolar lavage fluid
	Bronchoscopy and transbronchial biopsy
	Thorascopic biopsy
	Open-lung biopsy
	Nucleic acid detection of specific organisms (e.g., polymerase chain reaction for *Pneumocystis jirovecii* in bronchoalveolar lavage fluid or sputum)

can be obtained from arterial blood gas analysis, although this advantage is offset by the need for direct arterial puncture.

Of patients with PCP, fewer than 10% have a normal Pa_{O_2} and a normal $A\text{-}a_{O_2}$. These measures are sensitive, although not particularly specific for PCP, and similar results may occur with bacterial pneumonia, pulmonary Kaposi sarcoma, and *M. tuberculosis* infection. The diagnostic value of identifying exercise-induced desaturation, measured by transcutaneous oximetry, has been validated only in HIV-infected patients who have PCP and a normal or "near normal" appearance on chest radiographs. The test's value has not been confirmed in patients with abnormal chest radiographs because of PCP or other pathogens. Exercise-induced desaturation may persist for many weeks after treatment and recovery from PCP, even in the absence of active pulmonary disease.

Lung Function Testing

Abnormalities of lung function are well documented with HIV infection. The most common of these relate to tests measuring gas exchange, rather than the size of the conducting airways. In general, an overall reduction in diffusing capacity for carbon monoxide (DL_{CO}) occurs at all stages of HIV infection, with the largest changes found in HIV-infected patients with PCP. Thus, to some extent, patients who have probable PCP can be differentiated and treatment guided. A normal DL_{CO} in an individual who has symptoms but a negative or unchanged chest radiograph makes the diagnosis of PCP extremely unlikely. Data from the North American PSPC cohort study suggest that individuals with rapid rates of decline in DL_{CO} are at an increased risk for development of PCP. Recent work suggests that HIV-infected smokers are at increased risk of early-onset emphysema. Smoking history must, therefore, be taken into account when assessing a patient's lung function results in the context of possible PCP.

Computed Tomography Scanning

High-resolution (fine-cut) CT scanning of the chest may be helpful when the chest radiograph is normal, unchanged, or equivocal. The characteristic appearance of an alveolitis (i.e., areas of ground-glass attenuation through which the pulmonary vessels can be clearly identified) may be present, which indicates active pulmonary disease (Figure 34-15). This feature, however, is neither sensitive nor specific for PCP, although its sensitivity can be improved if evidence for reticulation and/or small cystic lesions is added to this. Hence, a negative test result implies an alternative diagnosis.

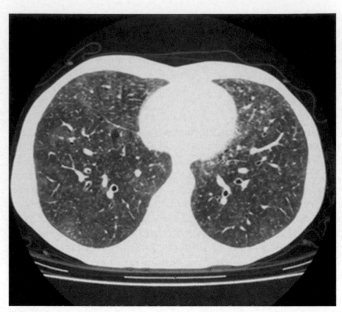

FIGURE 34-15 CT scan of thorax showing diffuse bilateral ground-glass shadowing typical of PCP.

Lactate Dehydrogenase Enzyme

In the context of an HIV-infected patient who is seen with an acute or subacute pneumonitis, an elevated serum lactate dehydrogenase (LDH) enzyme level is strongly suggestive of PCP. When interpreting such results, it is important to remember that other pulmonary disease processes (e.g., pulmonary embolism, nonspecific pneumonitis, and bacterial and mycobacterial pneumonia) and extrapulmonary disease (Castleman disease and lymphoma) may also cause elevations of LDH and may need to be considered in the correct clinical context.

From the previous information, it is evident that noninvasive tests cannot reliably distinguish the different infecting agents from each other but may be useful in excluding acute opportunistic disease. Thus, the clinician is left with either proceeding to diagnostic lung fluid or tissue sampling (by either induced sputum collection or bronchoscopy and BAL with or without transbronchial biopsy Table 34-7) or treating an unknown condition empirically. HAART has also altered the investigation of respiratory disease. The numbers of invasive procedures performed are falling and tend to be in patients

TABLE 34-7 Induced Sputum, Bronchoalveolar Lavage, and Surgical Biopsy in Diagnosis of *Pneumocystis jirovecii* Pneumonia

Technique	Ease of Procedure	Diagnostic Sensitivity (%)	Cost	Notes
Induced sputum	Simple once technique established	50–90	Low	Requires dedicated health care worker(s) and facility Risk to health care workers from expectorated aerosol
Bronchoalveolar lavage	Moderate	90–>95	Moderate	Risk of deterioration post procedure Risk to health care workers from coughed secretions Sensitivity may be increased by two-lobe lavage
Surgical biopsy	Complex	>95	High	Requires health care workers with surgical expertise

not taking antiretroviral drugs (usually to exclude PCP) or where there has been no response to empiric antibiotic therapy (regardless of the CD4 count).

Induced Sputum

Spontaneously expectorated sputum is inadequate for diagnosis of PCP. Sputum induction by inhalation of ultrasonically nebulized hypertonic saline may provide a suitable specimen (see Table 34-7). The technique requires close attention to detail and is much less useful when samples are purulent. Sputum induction must be carried out away from other immunosuppressed patients and health care workers, ideally in a room with separate negative-pressure ventilation, to reduce the risk of nosocomial transmission of tuberculosis. Although very specific (>95%), the sensitivity of induced sputum varies widely (55–90%), and therefore a negative result for *P. jirovecii* prompts further diagnostic studies. The use of immunofluorescence staining enhances the yield of induced sputum compared with standard cytochemistry.

Bronchoscopy

Fiberoptic bronchoscopy with BAL is commonly used to diagnose HIV-related pulmonary disease. When a good "wedged" sample is obtained, the test has a sensitivity of more than 90% for detection of *P. jirovecii* (Figure 34-16). Just as with induced sputum, fluorescent staining methods increase the diagnostic yield, which makes it the procedure of choice in most centers. More technically demanding (both of the patient and the operator) than induced sputum collection, bronchoscopy and BAL have the advantage that direct inspection of the upper airway and bronchial tree can be performed and, if necessary, biopsies taken. Transbronchial biopsies may marginally increase the diagnostic yield of the procedure. This is relevant for the diagnosis of mycobacterial disease, although the relatively high complication rate in HIV-infected individuals (pneumothorax and the possibility of significant pulmonary hemorrhage in up to 10%) outweighs the advantages of the technique for routine purposes.

Samples of BAL fluid are examined for bacteria, mycobacteria, viruses, fungi, and protozoa. Inspection of the cellular component may also provide etiologic clues—cooperation of a pathology department with experience in opportunistic infection diagnosis is vital. The drug interactions associated with antiretroviral protease inhibitor (PI) therapy mean that special care should be exercised when sedation is used with either benzodiazepine or opiate drugs. Prolonged sedation and life-threatening arrhythmias have been reported.

A diagnostic strategy, therefore, includes sputum induction and, if results are nondiagnostic or if the test is unavailable, bronchoscopy and BAL. If this does not yield a result, consideration is given to either a repeat bronchoscopy and BAL with transbronchial biopsies or surgical biopsy. The latter can be performed as either an open lung or thoracoscopic procedure. Surgical biopsy has a high sensitivity.

Empirical Diagnosis and Therapy

Although empirical therapy is usually reserved for the management of presumed bacterial pneumonias, and at first sight may seem unwise when dealing with possible opportunistic infection, in reality PCP is almost invariably a diagnosis of exclusion, and certain clinical and laboratory features may guide the assessment of an HIV-infected individual's risk for this condition. The likelihood that *P. jirovecii* is the causative organism increases if the subject is not taking effective anti-*Pneumocystis* drug prophylaxis or has a previous medical history with clinical or laboratory features that suggest systemic immunosuppression (i.e., recurrent oral thrush, longstanding fever of unknown cause, clinical AIDS, or blood CD4 count <200 cells/μL). Hence, some centers advocate use of empirical therapy for HIV-infected patients who are seen with symptoms and chest radiographic and blood gas abnormalities typical of mild PCP, without the need for bronchoscopy. Invasive measures are reserved for those with an atypical radiographic presentation, those who fail to respond to empirical therapy by day 5, and those who deteriorate at any stage.

Most clinicians in North America and the United Kingdom would seek to obtain a confirmed diagnosis in every case of suspected PCP. In practice, both strategies seem to be equally effective, although a number of caveats should be borne in mind when empirical treatment is given for PCP. Patients who have PCP typically take 4–7 days to show clinical signs of improvement, so a bronchoscopically proven diagnosis ensures that the treatment being given is correct, particularly in the first few days of therapy, when it may not be well tolerated. In addition, the diagnosis of PCP has implications for the infected individual, because it may influence the decision to start either HAART or anti-*Pneumocystis* prophylaxis. Finally, empirical therapy requires the patient to be maximally adherent to treatment, because nonresolution of symptoms may be seen as failure of therapy rather than of compliance.

Nucleic Acid Detection

Molecular biologic techniques (such as PCR) are increasingly used in the diagnosis of respiratory disease. Two examples of this are DNA amplification of loci of the *P. jirovecii* and *M. tuberculosis* genomes. The advantages of molecular methods are that the diagnosis may be made by use of samples that are more readily obtained than BAL fluid (i.e., expectorated sputum or nasopharyngeal secretions) and also that these methods are rapid (the answer may be available within a working day, compared with conventional mycobacterial culture, which may take weeks). Despite encouraging results in the research setting (sensitivity and specificity have been reported as 60–100% and 70–100%, respectively), problems persist when these techniques are applied to routine diagnostic samples. These include extraction of nucleic acid from clinical material, cross-contamination with the products of previous assays, and clinical interpretation of a test result. Currently,

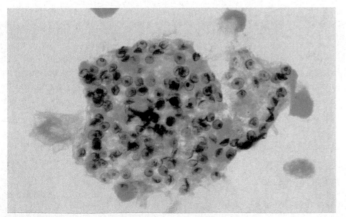

FIGURE 34-16 Bronchoalveolar lavage fluid containing *Pneumocystis jirovecii* (Grocott silver staining).

molecular methods are not part of the standard diagnostic workup.

TREATMENT

Individuals infected with HIV, compared with the non-HIV–infected general population, have an increased likelihood of adverse reactions to therapy. This includes TMP/SMX (see later) and other antibacterial and antimycobacterial agents. In addition, there are complex drug interactions with other medications, particularly components of HAART. Before instituting therapy for any infectious complication in an HIV-infected individual, it is important to consult with a physician experienced in the care of patients with HIV infection and to seek advice from a specialist pharmacist.

Bacterial Pneumonia

The main organisms causing pneumonia in HIV-infected individuals are similar to those found in the general population with community-acquired pneumonia. Thus, bacterial pneumonia in HIV-infected patients should be treated in a similar manner to that in HIV-negative individuals, by use of the published American Thoracic Society (ATS) and British Thoracic Society (BTS) guidelines. In addition, expert advice on local antibiotic resistance patterns should be sought from infectious disease or microbiology colleagues, because treatment is usually begun on an empirical basis before the causative organism is identified and antibiotic sensitivities known. The same clinical and laboratory prognostic indices that are described for the general population apply to HIV-infected patients and should be documented on presentation.

Response to appropriate antibiotic therapy is usually rapid and is similar to that seen in the non-HIV–infected individual. Early relapse of infection after successful treatment is well described. Those HIV-infected patients who have presumed PCP and are being treated empirically with high-dose TMP/SMX, and who have infection with either *S. pneumoniae* or *H. influenzae* rather than *P. jirovecii*, may also improve. In addition, in those patients who are treated with benzylpenicillin for proven *S. pneumoniae* pneumonia but do not respond, and penicillin resistance can be discounted as the cause, it is important to consider whether there is a second pathologic process, such as PCP. Co-pathogens are reported in up to 20% of cases of pneumonia.

Pneumocystis jirovecii Pneumonia

Before instituting treatment, assessment of the severity of PCP should be performed on the basis of history, findings on examination, arterial blood gas estimations, and chest radiographic abnormalities. Patients can then be stratified into those with mild, moderate, or severe disease (Table 34-8). This is important, because some drugs are of unproven benefit and others are known to be ineffective for the treatment of severe disease. In addition, adjuvant glucocorticoid therapy may be given to patients with moderate or severe pneumonia. Patients with glucose-6-phosphate dehydrogenase deficiency should not receive TMP/SMX, dapsone, or primaquine, because these drugs increase the risk of hemolysis.

Trimethoprim-Sulfamethoxazole

Several drugs are effective in the treatment of PCP. TMP/SMX is the drug of first choice (Tables 34-9 and 34-10). Overall it is effective in 70–80% of individuals when used as first-line therapy. Adverse reactions to TMP/SMX are common and usually become apparent between days 6 and 14 of treatment. Neutropenia and anemia (in up to 40% of patients), rash and fever (up to 30%), and biochemical abnormalities of liver function (up to 15%) are the most frequent adverse reactions. Hematologic toxicity induced by TMP/SMX is neither attenuated nor prevented by coadministration of folic or folinic acid. Furthermore, the use of these agents may be associated with reduced therapeutic success. During treatment with TMP/SMX, full blood count, liver function, and urea and electrolytes should be monitored at least twice weekly.

It is not known why HIV-infected individuals, especially those with higher CD4 counts, have such a high frequency of adverse reactions to TMP/SMX. The optimum strategy for an HIV-infected patient who has PCP and who becomes intolerant of high-dose TMP/SMX has not been established. Many physicians "treat through" minor rash, often adding an antihistamine and a short course of oral prednisolone (30 mg every 24 h, reducing to zero over 5 days).

Other Therapy

If treatment with TMP/SMX fails, or is not tolerated by the patient, several alternative therapies are available (see Tables 34-9 and 34-10).

TABLE 34-8 Grading of Severity of *Pneumocystis Jirovecii* Pneumonia			
	Mild	**Moderate**	**Severe**
Symptoms and signs	Dyspnea on exertion with or without cough and sweats	Dyspnea on minimal exertion and occasionally at rest; cough and fever	Dyspnea and tachypnea at rest; persistent fever and cough
Oxygenation PaO_2 room air, at rest (kPa; mmHg)	>11.0; >83	8.1–11.0; 61–83	≤8.0; ≤60
SaO_2, room air	>96	91–96	<91
SaO_2, on exercise	>90	<90	<90
$A-aO_2$ (kPa; mmHg)	<4.7; <35	4.7–6.0; 35–45	>6.0: >45
Chest radiograph	Normal or minor perihilar shadowing	Diffuse interstitial shadowing	Extensive interstitial shadowing with or without diffuse alveolar shadowing

TABLE 34-9 Treatment of *Pneumocystis jirovecii* Pneumonia According to Disease Severity

	Mild	Moderate	Severe
First choice	Trimethoprim-sulfamethoxazole	Trimethoprim-sulfamethoxazole	Trimethoprim-sulfamethoxazole
Second choice	Clindamycin-primaquine Trimethoprim-dapsone	Clindamycin-primaquine Trimethoprim-dapsone	Clindamycin-primaquine Intravenous pentamidine
Third choice	Atovaquone	Trimetrexate-folinic acid	Trimetrexate-folinic acid
Fourth choice	Trimetrexate-folinic acid Intravenous pentamidine	Atovaquone Intravenous pentamidine	
Adjuvant corticosteroids	Benefit not proven	Benefit proven	Benefit proven

TABLE 34-10 Treatment Schedules for *Pneumocystis jirovecii* Pneumonia

Drug	Dosage	Notes
Trimethoprim-sulfamethoxazole	Trimethoprim 20 mg/kg iv q24h and sulfamethoxazole 100 mg/kg iv q24h in 2–3 divided doses for 3 days then reduced to trimethoprim 15 mg/kg iv q24h and sulfamethoxazole 75 mg/kg iv. q24h in 2–3 divided doses for 18 further days Same daily doses of trimethoprim-sulfamethoxazole po q24h, in 3 divided doses for 21 days 1920 mg (2 trimethoprim-sulfamethoxazole double strength tablets) po q8h for 21 days	Dilute 1:25 in 0.9% saline infused over 90–120 min
Clindamycin-primaquine	Clindamycin 600–900 mg iv q6h or q8h iv and primaquine 15–30 mg po q24h for 21 days Clindamycin 300–450 mg po q6h to q8h and primaquine 15–30 mg po q24h for 21 days	Methemoglobinemia Less likely if dose of 15 mg po q24h of primaquine is used
Pentamidine	4 mg/kg iv q24h for 21 days	Dilute in 250 mL 5% dextrose in water and infuse over 60 min
Trimethoprim-dapsone	Trimethoprim 20 mg/kg po q24h in 3 divided doses and dapsone 100 mg po q24h for 21 days	
Trimetrexate-folinic acid	45 mg/m^2 or 1.2 g/kg iv q24h for 21 days with folinic acid 20 mg/m^2 or 0.5 mg/kg q6h for 24 days	Folinic acid must be continued for 3 days after last dose of trimetrexate
Atovaquone	750 mg po q12h for 21 days	Give with food to increase absorption
Glucocorticoids Prednisolone	40 g po q12h, days 1–5 40 g po q24h, days 6–10 20 g po q24h, days 11–21	Regimen recommended by CDC/NIH/IDSA, widely used in USA
Methylprednisolone	iv at 75% of dose given above for prednisolone	
Methylprednisolone Prednisolone	1 iv q24h, days 1–3 0.5 iv days 4–6 then 40 g po q24h reducing to 0, days 7–16	Regimen widely used in United Kingdom

NB, None of these regimens for adjuvant glucocorticoid therapy have been compared in prospective clinical trials.

Clindamycin-Primaquine

The combination of clindamycin and primaquine is widely used for treatment of PCP whatever the severity, although there is no license in the United Kingdom or United States for this indication. The combination is as effective as oral TMP/SMX and oral trimethoprim-dapsone for the treatment of mild and moderate-severity disease. As a second-line treatment it is effective in up to 90% of patients. Methemoglobinemia caused by primaquine occurs in up to 40% of patients. If 15 mg four times daily of primaquine is used, rather than 30 mg four times daily, the likelihood of methemoglobinemia is reduced. Diarrhea develops in up to 33% of patients receiving clindamycin. If this occurs, stool samples should be analyzed for the presence of *Clostridium difficile* toxin.

Trimethoprim-Dapsone

This oral combination is as effective as oral TMP/SMX and oral clindamycin plus primaquine (see earlier) for treatment of mild and moderate-severity PCP. The combination has not been shown to be effective in patients who have severe PCP. Most patients experience methemoglobinemia (caused by dapsone), which is usually asymptomatic. Up to one half of patients have mild hyperkalemia (<6.1 mmol/L) caused by trimethoprim.

Trimetrexate

A methotrexate analog, trimetrexate, is given intravenously together with folinic acid "rescue" to protect human cells from trimetrexate-induced toxicity. In patients who have moderate to severe disease, trimetrexate-folinic acid is less effective than high-dose TMP/SMX, but serious treatment-limiting hematologic toxicity occurs less frequently with trimetrexate-folinic acid.

Atovaquone

Atovaquone is licensed for the treatment of mild and moderate-severity PCP in patients who are intolerant of TMP/SMX. In tablet formulation (no longer available), this drug was less effective but was better tolerated than TMP/SMX or intravenous pentamidine for treatment of mild or moderate-severity PCP (see Tables 34-9 and 34-10). There are no data from prospective studies that compare the liquid formulation (which has better bioavailability) with other treatment regimens. Common adverse reactions include rash, fever, nausea and vomiting, and constipation. Absorption of atovaquone is increased if it is taken with food.

Intravenous Pentamidine

Intravenous pentamidine is now seldom used for the treatment of mild or moderate-severity PCP because of its toxicity. Intravenous pentamidine may be used in patients who have severe PCP, despite its toxicity, if other agents have failed (see Tables 34-9 and 34-10). Nephrotoxicity develops in almost 60% of patients given intravenous pentamidine (indicated by elevation in serum creatinine), leukopenia develops in approximately half, and up to 25% have symptomatic hypotension or nausea and vomiting. Hypoglycemia occurs in approximately 20% of patients. Given the long half-life of the drug, this may occur up to several days after the discontinuation of treatment. Pancreatitis is also a recognized side effect.

Adjuvant Glucocorticoids

For patients who have moderate and severe PCP, adjuvant glucocorticoid therapy reduces the risk of respiratory failure by up to half and the risk of death by up to one third (see Tables 34-9 and 34-10). Glucocorticoids are given to HIV-infected patients with confirmed or suspected PCP who have a PaO_2 <9.3 kPa (<70 mmHg) or an A-aO_2 of >4.7 kPa (<33 mmHg). Oral or intravenous adjunctive therapy is given at the same time as (or within 72 h of starting) specific anti–P. jirovecii therapy. Clearly, in some patients treatment is commenced on a presumptive basis, pending confirmation of the diagnosis. In prospective studies, adjuvant glucocorticoids have not been shown to be of benefit in patients with mild PCP. However, it would be difficult to demonstrate this, given that survival in such cases approaches 95% with standard treatment.

General Management of Pneumocystis jirovecii Pneumonia

Patients with mild PCP may be treated with oral TMP/SMX as outpatients if they are able to manage at home, willing to attend the outpatient clinic for regular review, and that there is clinical and radiographic evidence of recovery. If the patient is intolerant of oral TMP/SMX despite clinical recovery, either the treatment is given intravenously or treatment may be changed to oral clindamycin plus primaquine. All patients with moderate and severe PCP should be hospitalized and given intravenous TMP/SMX or intravenous clindamycin and oral primaquine (plus adjuvant steroids). Patients with moderate or severe disease who show clinical and radiographic response by day 7–10 of therapy may be switched to oral

TMP/SMX to complete the remaining 14 days of treatment. If the patient has failed to respond within 7–10 days or deteriorates before this time while receiving TMP/SMX, then treatment should be changed to clindamycin and primaquine or trimetrexate plus folinic acid.

Deterioration in the Patient with Pneumocystis jirovecii Pneumonia

Deterioration in a patient who is receiving anti–P. jirovecii therapy may occur for several reasons (Table 34-11). Before ascribing deterioration to treatment failure and considering a change in therapy, these alternatives should be evaluated carefully. It is also important to consider treating any co-pathogens present in BAL fluid, to perform bronchoscopy if the diagnosis was made empirically, to repeat the procedure, or to carry out open lung biopsy to confirm that the diagnosis is correct.

Intensive Care

Most centers advocate admission to the ICU for PCP with respiratory failure and for acute severe deterioration after bronchoscopy. The prognosis for severe PCP in such circumstances has improved over the past decade. This is likely because of a greater understanding of successful general ICU management of respiratory failure and acute respiratory distress syndrome (ARDS) rather than specific improvements in PCP care. Factors associated with poor outcome include increasing patient age, need for mechanical ventilation, and development of a pneumothorax. The latter reflects both the association between this complication and PCP, as well as the subsequent difficulty in successful mechanical ventilation of such individuals.

Treatment of Mycobacterial Diseases
Treatment of Tuberculosis

The treatment of HIV-related mycobacterial disease is complex. Not only do individuals have to take prolonged courses of relatively toxic agents, but also these antimycobacterial drugs have side effects similar to those of other prescribed

TABLE 34-11 Causes of Deterioration in an HIV-Infected Individual who has Pneumocystis jirovecii Pneumonia

Cause	Notes
Severe progressive pneumonia	
Side effects of therapy	Drug-induced anemia Drug-induced methemoglobinemia
Iatrogenic	Pulmonary edema caused by fluid overload
Postbronchoscopy	Sedation Pneumothorax
Pneumothorax	Spontaneous
Copathology in lung	Bacterial infection CMV infection Intercurrent pulmonary embolism
Wrong diagnosis	When diagnosis of PCP is empiric and is in fact bacterial pneumonia
Inadequate therapy	Wrong dose or route of administration Adjuvant glucocorticoids omitted in moderate or severe disease

medications, especially HAART. Drug–drug interactions are also extremely common.

Overlapping Toxicity

In the developed world, isoniazid-related peripheral neuropathy is rare in HIV-negative subjects taking pyridoxine. The nucleoside reverse transcriptase inhibitors (RTI) didanosine and stavudine, which are now less frequently used in the United States and the United Kingdom but which remain a mainstay of HAART in the developing world, can also cause a painful peripheral neuropathy. This complication develops in up to 30% of patients if stavudine and isoniazid are co-administered. Rash, fever, and biochemical hepatitis are common adverse events with rifamycins, pyrazinamide, and isoniazid (occurring more frequently in patients with tuberculosis who have HIV infection with hepatitis C coinfection). The nonnucleoside RTI drugs (e.g., nevirapine) have a similar toxicity profile. If treatment for both HIV and tuberculosis is co-administered, ascribing a cause may be problematic.

Drug–Drug Interactions

Drug–drug interactions between medications used to treat tuberculosis and HIV infection occur because of their common pathway of metabolism through the hepatic cytochrome P-450 enzyme system. Rifampin is a potent inducer of this enzyme (rifabutin less so), which may result in subtherapeutic levels of nonnucleoside RTI and PI antiretroviral drugs, with the potential for inadequate suppression of HIV replication and the development of resistance to HIV. In addition, the PI class of antiretroviral drugs inhibits the metabolism of rifamycins, which leads to increases in their plasma concentration and is associated with increased drug toxicity. The nonnucleoside RTI drugs are inducers of this enzyme pathway. Coadministration of rifabutin with efavirenz requires an increase in the dose of rifabutin to compensate for the increase in its metabolism induced by efavirenz (see later).

Type and Duration of Therapy for Tuberculosis

The optimal duration of treatment of tuberculosis, by use of a rifamycin-based regimen, in a patient who has HIV infection is unknown. Current recommendations (Joint Tuberculosis Committee of the BTS and the ATS/CDC/Infectious Disease Society of North America [IDSA]) are to treat tuberculosis in HIV-infected patients in the same way as for the general population (i.e., for 6 months for drug-sensitive pulmonary TB). In addition, ATS/CDC/IDSA guidelines recommend that treatment be extended to 9 months in those who have cavitation on the original radiograph, continuing signs, or a positive culture after 2 months of therapy.

Recent work has highlighted the increased risk for development of rifampin monoresistance in HIV-infected individuals on treatment. This is especially so if intermittent regimens are used and may arise from a lack of efficacy of the other drugs present in the combination (e.g., intermittent isoniazid). Hence, daily medication regimens are recommended and should be closely supervised in all HIV-positive patients. It should be remembered that although rifabutin is usually given three times a week with ritonavir-boosted protease inhibitors, this seems to achieve adequate rifamycin levels; there have been no reports of this leading to rifamycin resistance in patients who are appropriately adherent. Directly observed therapy (DOT) is an important, although fairly labor-intensive, strategy that has the support of the World Health Organization.

When to Start Antiretroviral Therapy in a Patient with Tuberculosis

The best time to start therapy in patients being treated for tuberculosis is unknown. Decision analyses show that early treatment with antiretroviral therapy leads to a marked reduction in further opportunistic disease. Against this is balanced the risk of needing to discontinue antituberculosis therapy or HIV therapy because of drug toxicity or drug–drug interactions. IRIS is reported to be more likely if the treatments are started at the same time as each other.

Pragmatically, delaying the start of antiretroviral therapy simplifies patient management and may reduce or prevent adverse drug reactions and drug–drug interactions and may also reduce the risk of IRIS. On the basis of current evidence, patients with CD4 counts >200 cells/μL have a low risk of HIV disease progression or death during 6 months of treatment for tuberculosis. In these patients, the CD4 count should be closely monitored, and antiretroviral therapy may be deferred until treatment for tuberculosis is completed. In patients who have CD4 counts from 199–100 cells/μL, many centers currently delay starting antiretroviral therapy until after the first 2 months of treatment for tuberculosis have been completed; patients are given concomitant PCP prophylaxis. In patients who have CD4 counts of <99 cells/μL, antiretroviral therapy is started as soon as possible after beginning treatment for tuberculosis. This is based on evidence that shows a significant short-term risk of HIV disease progression and death in this patient group if antiretroviral therapy is delayed.

Two options exist for starting antiretroviral therapy in a patient already being treated for tuberculosis. First, the rifampin-based regimen is continued, and antiretroviral therapy is commenced, for example, with a combination of two nucleoside RTIs and a non-nucleoside RTI, such as efavirenz (if the patient weighs <50 kg, the efavirenz dose is often increased to 800 mg once daily to compensate for rifampin-induced metabolism of efavirenz). Alternately, the rifampin is stopped and rifabutin is started: Antiretroviral therapy is given, with a combination of two nucleoside RTI drugs and either a single ritonavir-boosted PI or a nonnucleoside RTI. Here the dose of rifabutin is adjusted to take into account the pharmacokinetic effect of the co-administered drug. With a boosted PI, it is usually prescribed at a dose of 150 mg three times weekly and with efavirenz it is increased to 450 mg once a day.

Immune Reconstitution Inflammatory Syndrome

Before the advent of antiretroviral therapy, it was recognized by tuberculosis physicians that patients who were apparently responding to their antimycobacterial treatment would sometimes have a short period of clinical deterioration develop. This "paradoxical reaction" (in the face of overall treatment response) was seen as an interesting and probable immune-based phenomenon of generally little consequence. The widespread introduction of HAART has led to an increased awareness by clinicians of similar, but generally more severe, events in HIV-infected individuals. In the context of HIV, these are termed IRIS, or immune reconstitution disease.

They can present in a number of ways and with a range of opportunistic conditions. Perhaps the most common of these is similar to a paradoxical reaction. Here, after initiation of antiretroviral therapy in a patient being treated for tuberculosis, for example, there arises the return of the original or the development of new symptoms and signs. These are often of a systemic nature and may be associated with marked radiographic changes. Examples of this include fever, dyspnea, lymphadenopathy, effusions, parenchymal pulmonary infiltrates, or expansion of cerebral tuberculomas. This form of IRIS is seen most frequently with mycobacteria (commonly tuberculosis or MAC), fungi (notably, *Cryptococcus*), and viruses (hepatitis and herpes viridae).

IRIS develops in up to one third of HIV-infected patients being treated for tuberculosis when antiretroviral therapy is started. The median onset of tuberculosis-related IRIS is approximately 4 weeks from beginning antituberculosis treatment or 2 weeks from commencing HAART. It seems to be more likely in patients who have disseminated tuberculosis (and hence presumably more antigen present as well as more potential for significant inflammatory reactions) and a lower baseline blood CD4 count. A rapid fall in HIV load, as well as a large increase in CD4 counts in response to HAART, may also predict IRIS. The relationship between early use of HAART and low blood CD4 counts suggests that care must be taken when starting antiretrovirals in patients with TB at sites where rapid expansion of an inflammatory mass could be life threatening. Examples of this would include cerebral, pericardial, or peritracheal disease (Figure 34-17).

It is important to note that IRIS is currently a diagnosis of exclusion. There is no laboratory test available to assist with this; it should be made only after progressive or (multi) drug-resistant tuberculosis, poor drug adherence (to either antituberculosis or antiretroviral agents) and drug absorption, or an alternative pathologic process have been excluded as an explanation for the presentation. Criteria have been drawn up that seek to provide clinical diagnostic criteria (Table 34-12).

The mechanism leading to IRIS is unclear. It is not due to failure of treatment of tuberculosis or to another disease process; if anything, it is most likely to represent an exuberant and uncontrolled response to mycobacterial antigens (from both dead and live organisms).

Current treatments include nonsteroidal antiinflammatory drugs or glucocorticoids. The latter are undoubtedly effective, although they can lead to hyperglycemia and hypertension. Recent preliminary data suggest that the leukotriene receptor antagonist montelukast may be of benefit in IRIS (this drug is unlicensed for this indication). Recurrent aspiration of lymph nodes or effusion may also be needed. Although IRIS is often self-limiting, it may persist for several months. Rarely, temporary discontinuation of antiretroviral therapy is required. In this situation there may be precipitous falls in CD4 counts; patients are at risk of other opportunistic infections.

Attention has also focused on what is possibly more of a concern—the form of IRIS referred to as "unmasking phenomenon." Here, individuals with presumably latent tuberculosis infection who start HAART have systemic active (and often infectious) tuberculosis develop within a 3-month period. Although it is likely that the patient's disease would have presented in time anyway and that some of the reported cases may, in fact, represent ascertainment bias, the current view is that this is real and represents an adverse effect of HAART. Given that the people most at risk live in countries with limited facilities for pre-HAART screening, this has major implications for antiretroviral therapy roll-out programs in resource-poor areas.

Treatment of Disseminated *Mycobacterium avium-intracellulare* Complex Infection

Combination antimycobacterial therapy by itself does not cure MAC infection. A commonly used regimen is oral rifabutin, 300 mg once daily, with oral ethambutol, 15 mg/kg once daily,

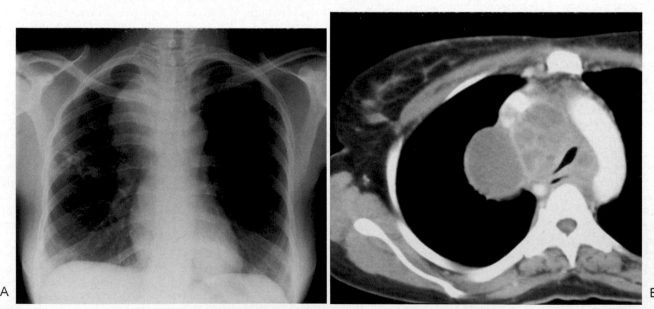

FIGURE 34-17 A, Chest radiograph. **B,** CT scan showing massive mediastinal lymphadenopathy in a patient with IRIS caused by *M. tuberculosis.* (Reproduced with permission from Buckingham SJ, Haddow LJ, Shaw PJ, Miller RF: Immune reconstitution inflammatory syndrome in HIV-infected patients with mycobacterial infections starting highly active antiretroviral therapy. *Clin Radiol* 2004; 59:505–513, Elsevier Ltd.)

TABLE 34-12 Immune Reconstitution Inflammatory Syndrome in HIV-Infected Individuals with Tuberculosis

Evidence supporting diagnosis	A. Initial diagnosis of tuberculosis confirmed by laboratory methods or by appropriate response to treatment
	B. Development of new clinical phenomena temporally associated with starting HAART. This includes, but is not limited to:
	  1. New or enlarging lymphadenopathy, cold abscesses, or other focal tissue involvement
	  2. New or worsening central nervous system disease
	  3. New or worsening radiological features of tuberculosis
	  4. New or worsening serositis (pleural effusion, ascites, pericardial effusion, or arthritis.
	  5. New or worsening constitutional symptoms such as fever, night sweats, and/or weight loss
	  6. Retrospective review indicating that a clinical or radiologic deterioration occurred with no change having been made to tuberculosis treatment
	C. Immune restoration, e.g., a rise in CD4 lymphocyte count in response to HAART
	D. A fall in HIV "viral load" in response to HAART

Alternative diagnoses to be excluded	Progressive underlying infection Treatment failure due to drug resistance (MDR or XDR) Treatment failure from poor adherence Adverse drug reaction Another diagnosis coexisting (e.g., non-Hodgkin lymphoma)

and oral clarithromycin, 500 mg once daily or every 12 h. If clarithromycin is not used, oral rifabutin, 600 mg once daily, is given—the lower dose adjusting for yet more drug–drug interactions. Use of three drugs has no impact on overall outcome, although it reduces the risk of resistance and possibly enhances early mycobacterial killing. In patients severely compromised by symptoms, intravenous amikacin, 7.5 mg/kg once daily for 2–4 weeks, is also given. Trough blood levels must be measured to ensure toxic accumulation of amikacin does not occur. Fluoroquinolones such as moxifloxacin or levofloxacin may be extremely useful, because they have good antimycobacterial activity with limited side effects. At present, many of these agents are not licensed for this indication. Given the concerns over XDR tuberculosis, it is important to ensure that patients are adherent to such treatments, and hence reduce the risk of fluoroquinolone resistance developing.

Mycobacterium kansasii Infection

A frequently used regimen includes rifampin, isoniazid, and ethambutol in conventional doses; all drugs are given by mouth.

Treatment of Fungal Infections

The treatment regimens for fungal infections complicating HIV infection are shown in Table 34-13.

Cryptococcosis

After initial treatment of cryptococcal infection, there is a high likelihood of relapse of infection; hence, lifelong secondary preventative therapy is needed unless antiretroviral therapy is commenced and results in sustained improvements in CD4 counts (>250 cells/µL) and suppression of HIV load in peripheral blood. Secondary prophylaxis is most often oral fluconazole 200–400 mg four times daily. Just as with mycobacterial disease, "late" IRIS events can occur after months or even years. These should be investigated to exclude active disease and other conditions.

Histoplasmosis

Oral itraconazole, 200 mg twice daily, is the current treatment of choice. The dose is adjusted to achieve blood trough drug levels that are above the standard lowest effective concentration. There are no data on the impact of antiretroviral therapy on which to base decisions about discontinuation of secondary prophylaxis.

Coccidioidomycosis

Treatment of this infection is difficult. After initial treatment with amphotericin B, itraconazole or fluconazole may be given for long-term suppression. The overall prognosis is poor, with a 40% mortality rate despite therapy. There are no data on the impact of antiretroviral therapy on which to base decisions about discontinuation of secondary prophylaxis.

PENICILLIUM MARNEFFEI INFECTION

Oral itraconazole has now replaced amphotericin B as the treatment of choice for *P. marneffei* infection, apart from the subgroup who are acutely unwell. Fluconazole is less effective than itraconazole. After initial treatment, lifelong suppressive therapy with itraconazole is needed. There are no data on the impact of antiretroviral therapy on which to base decisions about discontinuation of secondary prophylaxis.

Treatment of Parasitic Infections

The treatment regimens are shown in Table 34-14.

Toxoplasmosis

A combination of sulfadiazine and pyrimethamine is the regimen of choice for *T. gondii* infection. The most frequent dose-limiting side effects are rash and fever. Adequate hydration must be maintained to avoid the risk of sulfadiazine crystalluria and obstructive uropathy. Alternate regimens are given in Table 34-14. Once treatment is completed, lifelong maintenance is necessary to prevent relapse, unless antiretroviral therapy achieves adequate immune restoration (blood CD4 count >250 cells/µL and undetectable HIV load).

Visceral Leishmaniasis

Visceral leishmaniasis is usually treated with liposomal amphotericin B, although this is still associated with a high rate of relapse. Second-line therapy (or first-line in resource-poor environments) is to use sodium stibogluconate (see Table 34-14).

TABLE 34-13 Treatment of Fungal Pulmonary Infection in HIV-Infected Individuals

Infectious Cause	Drug	Notes
Candida spp.	Amphotericin B IV for 2–20 weeks	Continue until clinical/mycologic response is achieved
Aspergillus spp.	Amphotericin B 1 mg/kg or liposomal amphotericin 3 mg/kg IV q24h or itraconazole 200 mg PO q12h or voriconazole 6 mg/kg q12h	Use for severely ill patients Monitor renal function Adjust dose to measured trough levels
Cryptococcus neoformans	Amphotericin B 0.8–1.0 mg/kg or liposomal amphotericin 3 mg/kg IV q24h for 2–4 weeks and flucytosine 25–50 mg/kg IV q6h or fluconazole 300–400 mg PO q12h for 2–4 weeks	Monitor renal function Monitor blood count, liver and renal function
Histoplasma capsulatum	Itraconazole 200 mg PO q8h for 3 days, then 200 mg PO q12h for 6–12 weeks Amphotericin B 0.7 mg/kg or liposomal amphotericin 4 mg/kg IV q24h for 2–4 weeks	Adjust dose to measured trough levels Use for severely ill patients Monitor renal function
Coccidioides immitis	Amphotericin B 0.5–1 mg/kg or liposomal amphotericin 4 mg/kg IV q24h for 2–4 weeks	Monitor renal function
Penicillium marneffei	Itraconazole 400 mg PO q24h for 4–6 weeks Amphotericin B 0.6–1.0 mg/kg or liposomal amphotericin 3 mg/kg IV q24h for 2–4 weeks	Adjust dose to measured trough levels Use for severely ill patients Monitor renal function

TABLE 34-14 Treatment of Parasitic Infections in HIV-Infected Individuals

Infectious Cause	Drug	Notes
Toxoplasma gondii First choice	Sulfadiazine 2 g PO q8h and pyrimethamine 50 mg PO q24h and folinic acid 15 mg PO q24h for 14–28 days	Rash and fever are common
Second choice	Clindamycin 450–600 mg PO q6h and pyrimethamine 50 mg PO q24h and folinic acid 15 mg PO q24h for 14–28 days	If diarrhea develops, analyze stool for *Clostridium difficile*
Leishmania spp. First choice	Liposomal amphotericin B 2–5 mg/kg IV q24h for 10 days	
Second choice	Sodium stibogluconate (equivalent to pentavalent antimony 10 g/mL) 10–20 mg/kg IV q24h for 3–4 weeks	
Strongyloides stercoralis	Ivermectin 200 µg/kg PO q24h × 4 doses over 16 days	

STRONGYLOIDES STERCORALIS INFECTION

The treatment of choice is ivermectin. Risk of treatment failure with thiabendazole in HIV-infected individuals is higher than that in non-HIV–infected patients.

Treatment of Viral Infections

Cytomegalovirus pneumonitis is treated with intravenous ganciclovir, 5 mg/kg every 12 h, for 14 days. Drug-induced neutropenia is managed with granulocyte colony-stimulating factor. Some centers use valganciclovir, an oral formulation of ganciclovir, at a dose of 900 mg orally every 12 h, to treat CMV pneumonitis. Side effects and their management are as for ganciclovir. There are no data that demonstrate efficacy for cidofovir for treatment of CMV pneumonitis, but this agent is used as second-line therapy in many centers. Phosphonoformate (foscarnet) can be used for treatment of CMV end-organ disease (e.g., pneumonitis), although it has an extensive toxicity profile. It is also a moderately effective antiretroviral agent. This effect is occasionally used as an adjunct in controlling nonresponsive viral infections.

CLINICAL COURSE AND PREVENTION

Within the past few years, drug therapy has radically altered the depressingly predictable nature of progressive HIV infection. Combinations of specific opportunistic infection prophylaxis and antiretroviral therapy can reduce both the incidence and the mortality associated with common conditions. The observational North American MACS cohort demonstrated that the risk of PCP in individuals with blood CD4 counts of <100 cells/µL can be reduced almost fourfold if both specific prophylaxis and HAART are taken (from 47% to 13%). However, as common conditions are prevented, so other less treatable illnesses may arise.

The initial impact of *P. jirovecii* prophylaxis was a reduction in the incidence of PCP at the expense of an increase in cases of disseminated MAC infection, CMV infection, esophageal candidiasis, and wasting syndrome. New prophylactic therapies targeting those conditions associated with high morbidity and mortality (in particular MAC) have further improved survival. It has become apparent that specific infection prophylaxis may also confer protection against other agents. This "cross-prophylaxis" is particularly seen with the use of TMP/SMX for *Pneumocystis*, which also provides cover against cerebral toxoplasmosis and several common bacterial infections (although not *S. pneumoniae*) and with macrolides for MAC infection, which further reduce the incidence of bacterial disease and also PCP. Use of large amounts of antibiotic raises the possibility of future widespread drug resistance. This is clearly of concern, and recent reports suggest that, indeed, in some parts of the world the incidence of pneumococcal TMP/SMX resistance is rising. Current preventive therapies pertinent to lung disease focus on *P. jirovecii*, MAC, *M. tuberculosis*, and certain bacteria (Table 34-15).

Pneumocystis jirovecii Prophylaxis

Numerous studies have demonstrated the greatly increased risk in subjects who do not take adequate drug therapy with blood CD4 counts <200 cells/μL. Clinical symptoms are also an independent risk factor for PCP, and hence the current guidelines recommend lifelong prophylaxis against *P. jirovecii* in HIV-infected adults who have had prior PCP, CD4 counts <200 cells/μL, constitutional symptoms (documented oral thrush or fever of unknown cause of <37.8°C that persists for more than 2 weeks), or clinical AIDS. The importance of secondary prophylaxis (i.e., used after an episode of PCP) becomes clear from historical data, which indicate a 60% risk of relapse in the first 12 months after infection.

The increase in systemic and local immunity that occurs with HAART has led to several studies evaluating the need for prolonged prophylaxis in individuals with sustained elevations in blood CD4 counts and low HIV RNA load. In summary, it seems that both primary and secondary PCP prophylaxis can be discontinued once CD4 counts are >200 cells/μL for more than 3 months. A caveat to this is that the patient should have a low or undetectable HIV RNA load, that the CD4 percentage is stable or rising and is >14%, and that the individual plans to continue HAART long term with good adherence.

The risk of PCP recurrence is real if the CD4 count falls below 200 cells/μL. If this does happen, PCP prophylaxis should be restarted. Similar algorithms have been successfully used for all the major infections except tuberculosis. They all rely on an estimation of the general blood CD4 count above which clinical disease is highly unlikely. For example, secondary prophylaxis of MAC may be discontinued once the blood CD4 count is consistently >100 cells/μL. This is a general guideline, however, and patients must be assessed on an individual basis.

Trimethoprim-Sulfamethoxazole

As with treatment strategies, TMP/SMX is the drug of choice for prophylaxis (Table 34-16). It has the advantages of being highly effective for both primary and secondary prophylaxis (with 1-year risk of PCP while on the drug being 1.5 and 3.5%, respectively). It is cheap, can be taken orally, acts systemically, and provides some cross-prophylaxis against other infections, such as toxoplasmosis, *Salmonella* species, *Staphylococcus* species, and *H. influenzae*. Its main disadvantage is that adverse reactions are common (see earlier), occurring in up to 50% of individuals taking the prophylactic dose.

The standard dose of TMP/SMX is one double-strength tablet (160 mg trimethoprim, 800 mg sulfamethoxazole) per day. Other regimens have been tried; these include one "double-strength" tablet three times weekly and one single-strength tablet per day. In general, when used for primary prophylaxis, these regimens are tolerated well (if not better than the standard) and seem as efficacious as one double-strength tablet per day. The data are less clear on secondary prophylaxis, in which subjects are at a much higher risk of recurrent PCP. Attempts to desensitize patients who are intolerant of TMP/SMX have met with some success.

Dapsone

In patients who cannot tolerate TMP/SMX, dapsone is a safe and inexpensive alternative. It has been studied in a number of trials as both primary and secondary prophylaxis and is effective at an oral dose of 100 mg/day. When combined with pyrimethamine (25 mg three times weekly), it provides a degree of cross-prophylaxis against toxoplasmosis. Before starting dapsone, patients are tested for glucose-6-phosphate dehydrogenase deficiency.

TABLE 34-15 Prevention of Respiratory Infections in HIV-Infected Adults

Organism	Preventive Method	Specific Agent	Indications	Cost	Notes
Pneumocystis jirovecii	Regular drug	Trimethoprim-sulfamethoxazole (daily)	Persistent thrush, fever, AIDS; CD4 count <200 cells/μL	Cheap	Provides cross-protection; May lead to resistance
Mycobacterium tuberculosis	Regular drug	Isoniazid (6–12 months)	Purified protein derivative positive; Close contact with active case	Cheap	Compliance a potential problem, therefore resistance possible
Mycobacterium avium-intracellulare complex	Regular drug	Clarithromycin (daily) or azithromycin (weekly)	CD4 count <50 cells/μL	Expensive	Provides cross-protection; May lead to resistance
Streptococcus pneumoniae	Immunization	23-valent capsular polysaccharide (single dose)	All subjects at diagnosis and at 5 years	Cheap	Uncertain protection; Transient increase in HIV "load"
Influenza virus	Immunization	Whole or split virus (yearly)	All subjects	Cheap	Uncertain protection; Transient increase in HIV "load"

TABLE 34-16 Primary and Secondary Prophylaxis Regimens for *Pneumocystis jirovecii*

Drug	Dose	Notes
Trimethoprim-sulfamethoxazole	1 Double-strength* tablet PO q24h	Other options for primary prophylaxis: 1 double-strength* tablet PO q24h three times a week or 1 single-strength† tablet PO q24h Protects against toxoplasmosis and certain bacteria
Dapsone	100 mg PO q24h	With pyrimethamine (25 mg PO q24h three times a week) protects against toxoplasmosis
Pentamidine	300 mg via *Respirgard II* (jet) nebulizer every 4 weeks	Less effective in subjects with CD4 <100 cells/μL Provides no cross-prophylaxis
Atovaquone	750 mg PO q12h	Absorption increased if administered with food Protects against toxoplasmosis
Azithromycin	1250 mg PO once weekly	Protects against *Mycobacterium avium-intracellulare* complex and certain bacteria

*160 mg trimethoprim, 800 mg sulfamethoxazole.
†80 mg trimethoprim, 400 mg sulfamethoxazole.

Pentamidine

Nebulized pentamidine has largely fallen from use as a prophylactic agent. This is despite it being better tolerated and having a similar efficacy to TMP/SMX for primary preventive therapy. However, its breakthrough rate is higher in subjects who have lower CD4 counts (i.e., <100 cells/μL) and in those who take it as secondary prophylaxis. Other disadvantages include equipment costs and complexity (alveolar deposition is crucial, and hence the nebulizer system used is important), the risk of transmission of respiratory disease (e.g., tuberculosis) to other patients and staff during the nebulization procedure, an alteration in the clinical presentation of PCP while on pentamidine (increased frequency of radiographic upper zone shadowing, increased incidence of pneumothorax), and a lack of systemic protection against *Pneumocystis* and other infectious agents. There is also an acute bronchoconstriction effect during nebulization. Long-term follow-up studies have not demonstrated any significant negative effect on lung function.

Atovaquone

Atovaquone oral suspension is used as a second-line prophylactic agent in subjects intolerant of TMP/SMX. It seems to have similar efficacy to dapsone (given together with weekly pyrimethamine), with a reduced incidence of side effects, of which the most frequent are rash, fever, and gastrointestinal disturbance.

Azithromycin

Azithromycin is used in many centers as a third-line prophylactic agent. It is given at a dose of 1250 mg once weekly, and may provide protection against some bacterial infections, as well as MAC.

Predictors of *Pneumocystis* Prophylaxis Failure

A low blood CD4 count (<50 cells/μL) is the current best laboratory predictor of prophylaxis failure. This is not particularly surprising given that the median blood CD4 count of subjects not on prophylaxis who have PCP develop is below 50 cells/μL. Persistent fever of unknown cause is an important clinical risk factor for PCP. Used as preventive therapy, TMP/SMX significantly reduces the chance for development of *Pneumocystis*. It is, therefore, vital that subjects who are most vulnerable be encouraged to use this drug on a regular basis. The PSPC cohort study revealed that 21% of subjects with a CD4 count <200 cells/μL were not receiving any form of PCP prophylaxis.

Bacterial Infection Prophylaxis

The effective and safe (i.e., replication incompetent) bacterial vaccines that are available would be expected to be widely used to prevent HIV-related disease. In fact, uptake of both pneumococcal and the *H. influenzae* type b (Hib) vaccines is poor (current estimates for the former are at most only 40% of the infected population with the recommended 23-valent vaccine). One reason for this may be that the protection conferred by vaccination (90%) in the general population is not seen in immunosuppressed HIV-infected individuals, reflecting their inability to generate adequate memory B-cell responses (especially those subjects with CD4 counts <200 cells/μL). However, in North America, CDC/IDSA recommend the pneumococcal vaccine as a single dose as soon as HIV infection is diagnosed, with a booster at 5 years, or if an individual's blood CD4 count was <200 cells/μL and subsequently increased on HAART. Several studies show pneumococcal immunization reduces the risk of invasive pneumococcal infection in this population. This does not seem to be the case in a developing world setting, where not only is the 23-valent vaccine ineffective against both invasive and noninvasive pneumococcal disease, but the overall incidence of pneumonia is increased.

Infection with *H. influenzae* type b is much less common in HIV-infected adults and, therefore, immunization with Hib vaccine is not routinely recommended.

There is little evidence to suggest that the high frequency of bacterial infections in the HIV population is related to bacterial colonization. Therefore, continuous antibiotics are rarely indicated, although both TMP/SMX and the macrolides (clarithromycin and azithromycin) given as long-term prophylaxis for opportunistic infections have been shown to reduce the incidence of bacterial pneumonia, sinusitis/otitis media, and infectious diarrhea. The use of TMP/SMX also confers a survival advantage in many studies performed in resource-poor settings. There is little evidence, however, that TMP/SMX protects against pneumococcal infection.

Mycobacterium tuberculosis Prophylaxis

The interaction between HIV and tuberculosis is of fundamental importance, because the annual risk for the development of clinical tuberculosis in a given individual is estimated to be 5–15% (i.e., similar to a non-HIV–infected subject's *lifetime* risk). HIV-infected individuals with pulmonary tuberculosis are less likely to be smear positive than their HIV-negative counterparts, although they can still transmit tuberculosis. Thus, within a community, tuberculosis prevention involves case finding and treatment of active disease, as well as specific prophylactic drug therapies for those exposed. If possible, HIV-positive subjects should make every effort to avoid encountering tuberculosis (e.g., at work, homeless shelter, health care facility).

One of the problems with standard methods of tuberculosis contact tracing in HIV infection is that both tuberculin skin test results and chest radiology may be unreliable. However, in the absence of bacillus Calmette–Guérin (BCG) immunization, a positive PPD (e.g., <5 mm induration with 5 tuberculin units) indicates a greatly increased risk (6- to 23-fold compared with nonanergic, PPD-negative, HIV-infected subjects) of future active disease. The chance that HIV-infected subjects may contract disseminated infection if given BCG means that (having excluded active infection) the only option in these circumstances is to use a preventative drug regimen. Options include at least 6 months of isoniazid (together with pyridoxine to prevent peripheral neuropathy). This is safe and well tolerated, although compliance is a problem (especially with regimens longer than 6 months), and DOT may need to be instituted (e.g., 900 mg isoniazid twice weekly). There is little evidence to suggest that this single-agent regimen leads to isoniazid resistance, which probably reflects the low mycobacterial load present in such individuals.

Attempts to shorten the length of treatment for latent infection have produced variable results. Recent studies used rifampin and pyrazinamide for short-course prophylaxis (2 months). This was as effective as 12 months of isoniazid in HIV-coinfected individuals, although it was associated with fatal hepatotoxicity (almost exclusively in the HIV-negative population). Hence, it is currently out of favor. If used, liver function should be closely monitored, and it is recommended that this regimen not be given to patients with preexisting liver disease (e.g., because of alcohol or viral hepatitis). Because rifampin should not be used by subjects taking PIs, this may also limit widespread application of the two-drug regimen. The same applies to combinations of isoniazid and rifampin taken for at least 3 months, which are also effective in HIV-negative individuals. Alternate protocols also exist for subjects thought to be resistant to first-line prophylactic agents. These have not been widely clinically evaluated. It is recommended that HIV-infected subjects who have had close contact with an active case of tuberculosis should also receive prophylaxis. There is little evidence to suggest that anergy confers an increased risk for development of clinical disease. However, patients who have not had BCG, have a negative skin test, and have started HAART may benefit from regular skin tests, because some studies suggest that cutaneous responses may return with increasing CD4 counts, and that this may help in identifying newly infected individuals requiring prophylaxis.

In populations where the prevalence of tuberculosis is low and BCG may be given during childhood or adolescence (e.g., the United Kingdom), the value of PPD testing is more limited. Here, an arbitrary cutoff of 10 mm for tuberculin reactions is used to define who should receive preventive therapy. The introduction of immune-based blood tests that can accurately distinguish between BCG vaccination and tuberculosis infection may be helpful when screening for evidence of latent tuberculosis. The two currently available commercial tests use fairly specific CD4-directed mycobacterial antigen responses with consequent production of detectable interferon-γ. The need for reasonably intact CD4 function means that they may, in fact, be less useful in HIV infection, especially in those subjects with very low blood CD4 counts, who are possibly at greatest risk of developing active tuberculosis.

Secondary tuberculosis prophylaxis may be important, because studies indicate a high rate of relapse in endemic areas. Here, no specific guidelines exist, although 6 months of isoniazid and rifampin after a full treatment course shows a greatly reduced risk of relapse within the subsequent 2 years. Whether this is enough to prevent clinical disease (which may also arise from reinfection in areas of high tuberculosis prevalence) without concomitant antiretroviral therapy is unclear. In the developed world, secondary prophylaxis is usually not recommended.

The use of HAART also can reduce the risk of tuberculosis in endemic areas. Work in South Africa indicates that this is most beneficial in patients with advanced disease and leads to a reduction in RR of at least 80%.

Mycobacterium avium-intracellulare Complex Prophylaxis

Data from North America indicate that the prevention of disseminated MAC infection has an effect on survival (25% reduction in mortality rate in subjects taking clarithromycin). The US guidelines advise prophylaxis with a macrolide (either clarithromycin, 500 mg orally twice per day, or azithromycin, 1250 mg orally, once a week) in all HIV-infected individuals with blood CD4 counts >50 cells/μL. In Europe, where the prevalence of disseminated MAC infection is probably lower (perhaps because of previous BCG vaccination), this may be less relevant. Here, surveillance cultures of blood may be more cost-effective in the at-risk HIV population with low CD4 counts. Routine stool and sputum cultures probably do not add much to this strategy, because disseminated MAC is much more common than isolated organ disease.

Single-agent prophylaxis may lead to antibiotic resistance. This does not seem to be reduced by the addition of a second drug (rifabutin) to the prophylactic regimen. The latter is now a second-line prophylactic agent, largely as a result of its rather worse protective effect and its adverse interaction profile with PIs. As mentioned earlier, if an individual sustains a rise in CD4 count >100 cells/μL for >6 months, it is safe to discontinue prophylaxis.

PROGNOSIS

Pneumocystis jirovecii

Several clinical and laboratory features have prognostic significance in HIV-infected individuals with PCP (Box 34-2). A severity score on the basis of the serum LDH levels, the A-aO$_2$, and the percentage of neutrophils in the BAL fluid can predict survival reasonably accurately, with the highest scores indicating the worst outcome. Other workers have shown that increased age (<50 years) leads to an increased

BOX 34-2 Prognostic Factors Associated with Poor Outcome in *Pneumocystis jirovecii* Pneumonia

On admission	Patient's age
	No previous knowledge of HIV status
	Tachypnea (respiratory rate >30/min)
	Second or subsequent episode of *Pneumocystis jirovecii* pneumonia
	Poor oxygenation – PaO_2 <7.0 kPa (<53 mmHg) or $A-aO_2$ >4.0 kPa (>30 mmHg)
	Low serum albumin (<35 g/dL)
	Low hemoglobin (<12.0 g/dL)
	Peripheral blood leukocytosis ($>10.8 \times 10^9$/L)
	Elevated serum lactate dehydrogenase levels (>300 IU/L)
	CD4 count <50 cells/µL
	Marked chest radiographic abnormalities-diffuse bilateral interstitial infiltrates with or without alveolar consolidation
	Medical comorbidity (e.g., pregnancy)
Following admission	At bronchoscopy
	1. In bronchoalveolar lavage fluid detection of
	a. Copathology CMV bacteria
	b. Neutrophilia (>5%)
	2. Detection of pulmonary Kaposi sarcoma
	Serum lactate dehydrogenase levels that remain elevated
	Development of pneumothorax
	High APACHE II score on admission to the ICU
	Need for mechanical ventilation

mortality rate—in part as a result of late, "unsuspected" diagnosis. The overall mortality rate from an episode of PCP is approximately 14% and has not changed since the advent of HAART.

Among individuals with access to HAART, post-PCP survival has improved. In 1981, the median survival after PCP was 9 months. By 1995, this had risen to 20 months. The introduction of HAART has led to a further improvement, with survival in the period up to year 2000 of 40 months. In those without access to HAART and/or prophylaxis, survival post-PCP, unfortunately, remains poor.

Bacterial Infection

In general, mortality from bacterial respiratory infection in HIV-infected individuals is similar to that seen in the general population. Clinical and laboratory markers of disease severity that have been defined in the adult general population (e.g., those described in the ATS or the BTS Guidelines for the management of community-acquired pneumonia in adults) apply to HIV-infected patients. These are confusion, raised respiratory rate, abnormal renal function, and low blood pressure. Recurrent pneumonia is common (reported in up to 55% of cases) and may lead to chronic pulmonary disease (see earlier).

Mycobacterium Tuberculosis

Although tuberculosis normally responds to standard multiple-drug therapy, work from Africa has highlighted the increased mortality rate in HIV-infected compared with non-HIV–infected individuals. A relationship has also been described between mortality and declining blood CD4 count: HIV-infected patients with CD4 counts <200 cells/µL have a mortality rate of 10% compared with 4% in those with CD4 counts from 200–499 cells/µL. Compared with HIV-infected individuals without tuberculosis, the main effect on mortality is seen in patients with higher CD4 counts (>200 cells/µL), where the relative risk of death is three times that of the non-tuberculous population.

Mycobacterium avium-intracellulare Complex

Several case-controlled studies have indicated that in the absence of effective treatments, MAC-infected patients have a reduced survival compared with blood CD4 level-matched control subjects (approximately 4 months vs 9 months, respectively). Currently available treatment regimens may reduce this difference, although severe anemia seems to be an independent predictor of mortality.

Cytomegalovirus

The presence of CMV in BAL fluid also containing *P. jirovecii* has been related to outcome (see earlier). The mortality rate at 3 and 6 months after bronchoscopy is greater in those with CMV detected at bronchoscopy. However, CMV recovered as a sole pathogen does not impact on survival.

PITFALLS AND CONTROVERSIES

The Effect of Antiretroviral Therapy on Opportunistic Infections

The introduction of HAART, together with the wide availability of accurate methods of determining plasma RNA viral load, has led to profound changes in both clinical practice and HIV outcome. Although it is still the case that respiratory disease remains above non-HIV infected background levels, in particular, bacterial pneumonia, TB, and lung cancer are more common, despite apparently effective HAART, in HIV-infected subjects. Overall data indicate that clinical progression is rare in subjects who are able to adhere rigorously to at least 95% of their antiretroviral drug regimen. Mortality rates have fallen by 80% for almost all conditions, and it seems that a damaged immune system can, to a clinically significant extent, be reconstituted for a period of at least several years. Hence, clinicians need to consider not only opportunistic infection or malignancy within their diagnostic workup but also the effects of drug therapy itself. The side effect profile of HAART (e.g., metabolic and mitochondrial toxicities, liver damage, and neuropsychiatric disorders), as well as the large number of drug–drug interactions, makes this a very complex area of management. The best example of this is HIV-related tuberculosis. Here, not only is there overlapping toxicity and pharmacologic interaction, but IRIS is common. Research is needed to address this area. Studies should inform the decision on when to start HAART in patients already on antituberculosis medication. Other work needs to focus on understanding why full pulmonary immunity is not restored. This may reflect abnormalities in the innate immune response, which is currently poorly described in HIV infection.

Predictors of Disease

Despite the benefits of HAART, it is likely that in the long term many patients will progress to severe disease. There is currently little research in this area. Research should focus on correlating clinical and laboratory findings. An example of this would be assessing the risk of an individual for development of active tuberculosis. It is clear that much of the excess mortality in HIV-tuberculosis coinfection occurs early in HIV infection. Thus, if tests can be devised that indicate who has latent tuberculosis infection (and who is, therefore, most likely to have clinical disease develop), steps can be taken to prevent illness.

As discussed previously, immune-based tests have shown promise in immunocompetent individuals with tuberculosis infection. If these can be refined to work consistently in patients with HIV infection at a reasonable cost, there is the possibility of targeting those at risk of future tuberculosis, or of tuberculosis "unmasking" after starting HAART.

The other role for a test such as this would be in rapid diagnosis of active tuberculosis. It is common to be faced with a patient who has nonspecific symptoms and a wide differential diagnosis. Often treatment is multiple and empirical. A quantitative test would help resolve some of these dilemmas by indicating the chance of the condition being caused by a particular disease. An example would be the patient from an endemic tuberculosis area, with low CD4 counts, who has both pulmonary and central nervous system disease. Is this tuberculosis, toxoplasmosis, cryptococcosis, or viral or bacterial infection? Any such test for tuberculosis would also have to distinguish between the different states of old (treated), old (inactive), old (latent), and active. Although not insurmountable, at present, this is not possible.

Rapid diagnostic assays that assess organism viability are also important. If a clinician can receive early feedback on whether treatment is producing a suitable killing effect, therapy can be tailored to the individual. This enables regimens to be "dose adjusted" as needed and removes the element of concern that is often present when patients are slow to respond. Examples of this would be in the treatment of PCP or mycobacterial disease.

Bacterial Infections

The frequency of bacterial infection (often recurrent) with its attendant sequelae makes effective strategies for vaccination an important priority. It is uncertain why there is a differential response to vaccination; even in the United States, African Americans do not seem to derive the same benefit as whites. This needs further research, together with more emphasis on identifying the local immune response present in the lung in such individuals.

Bacterial infections may be clinically indistinguishable from other pathogens, and only two thirds of all respiratory infections are formally diagnosed. There is a need for improved methods to assist with this. The use of rapid antigen tests may be one way forward. This is especially so given the high incidence of (potentially fatal) bacteremia present in such populations. For maximum benefit, this needs to use a system that is simple and cheap, and hence suitable to both resource-rich and resource-poor countries.

Mycobacterial Diseases

M. tuberculosis is globally the most important HIV-related pathogen. Strategies of control and prevention are vital to ensure that millions of people do not become coinfected and that those who are do not go on to have clinical disease develop. Rapid diagnostics are critical. The encouraging reports of the simple and cheap method of MODS to both diagnose tuberculosis and then provide resistance data in field settings (see earlier) argues for large-scale roll out and evaluation.

Beyond public health measures, such as DOT, fixed-dose combination drugs, case management, and education, research needs to improve on current drug therapy. Long-acting preparations such as rifapentine show promise but, as the problem with rifampicin monoresistance demonstrates, there is still much work to be done. For the first time in many years, there are several antimycobacterial drugs that are in various stages of clinical trials. All are promising, and several have novel mechanisms of action. The Global Alliance and the WHO "Stop TB" campaigns have been crucial in this regard. The fluoroquinolones, moxifloxacin and gatifloxacin, are closest to the market. They are potent drugs with considerable ability both to kill and also sterilize mycobacteria-infected sites. Trials of treatment-shortening regimens are ongoing worldwide.

Vaccination against *M. tuberculosis* with BCG has understandably not been widely used in an immunosuppressed HIV-infected population. However, a safe vaccine may be the only affordable way of protecting large parts of the world from tuberculosis. So far there seems to be more success in vaccines to either enhance or replace the primary protective effects of BCG. The use of immunotherapy (e.g., with heat-killed *Mycobacterium vaccae*) in combination with chemotherapy has been disappointing in clinical trials.

Pneumocystis jirovecii

Newer methods of diagnosis (e.g., PCR tests on saliva) may prove invaluable for quick and easy disease confirmation, although their applicability to routine samples needs further evaluation.

P. jirovecii prophylaxis was the first important HIV treatment widely available. However, despite the efficacy of TMP/SMX, compliance remains a problem. Regimens that use a gradual increase in dosage when starting prophylaxis may help. One concern with widespread use of prophylaxis is that resistance will start to occur to TMP/SMX. Reports have indicated that there are mutations in the *P. jirovecii* dihydropteroate synthase gene that confer resistance. These seem to be increasing over time, although they do not seem to be present in many patients who fail treatment for PCP with TMP/SMX. The implications of this are uncertain but could include a greater likelihood of treatment failure and the possibility of worsening patterns of global bacterial drug resistance.

Smoking-Related Diseases

HIV-infected populations in the developed world have high rates of smoking. The evidence that this is harmful above those effects seen in the general population continues to accrue. The accelerated course of both obstructive lung disease and cancer, together with the increased risk of respiratory infection in smokers, persuasively argues the case for targeted smoking cessation. That HIV infection and HAART have profound (and probably negative) effects on blood lipids and insulin resistance further support the need to reduce smoking rates in this population. It seems that we are starting to see increased rates of cardiovascular disease in this now aging population.

The natural history of HIV-related respiratory disease continues to evolve. HAART and newer therapeutic strategies have made a significant impact on morbidity and mortality. Yet individuals continue to become HIV infected, progress, and die from an ever-expanding range of conditions. *P. jirovecii* remains the most common AIDS-defining event in the developed world, whereas *M. tuberculosis* is globally the most common cause of death. Bacterial respiratory infection is not far behind. Given the huge number of individuals with HIV infection, the only effective way to manage this disease is to find simple ways of treating HIV itself, and thus contain the worst ravages of this illness.

SUGGESTED READINGS

Benson CA, Kaplan JE, Masur H, *et al*: Treating opportunistic infections among HIV-infected adults and adolescents. MMWR 2004; 53(RR15): 1–112.

Branson BM, Handsfield HH, Lampe M, *et al*: Revised recommendations for HIV testing of adults, adolescents, and pregnant women in health-care settings. MMWR 2006; 55(RR14):1–47.

Burman WJ, Jones BE: Treatment of HIV-related tuberculosis in the era of effective antiretroviral therapy. Am J Respir Crit Care Med 2001; 164: 7–12.

Castro M: Treatment and prophylaxis of *Pneumocystis carinii* pneumonia. Semin Respir Infect 1998; 13:296–303.

Lawn SD, Bekker LG, Miller RF: Immune reconstitution disease associated with mycobacterial infections in HIV-infected individuals starting anti-retroviral therapy. Lancet Infectious Diseases 2005; 5:361–373.

Lipman MCI, Breen RA: Immune reconstitution inflammatory syndrome in HIV. Curr Opin Infect Dis 2006; 19:20–25.

Masur H, Kaplan JE, Holmes K: Guidelines for preventing opportunistic infections among HIV-infected persons—2002. Ann Intern Med 2002; 137:435–478.

Pozniak AL, Miller RF, Lipman MCI, *et al*, on behalf of the BHIVA Guidelines Writing Committee. HIV Medicine 2005; 6(Suppl 2): 62–83.

Redhead SA, Cushion MT, Frenkel JK, Stinger JR: *Pneumocystis* and *Trypanosoma cruzi*: nomenclature and typifications. J Eukaryot Microbiol 2006; 53:2–11.

Semple SJG Miller RF, eds: AIDS and the lung. Oxford: Blackwell Scientific; 1997.

Zumla A, Johnson MA, Miller R, eds: AIDS and respiratory medicine. London: Chapman & Hall; 1997.

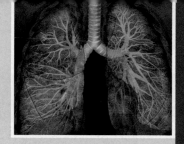

35 Noninfectious Conditions

THOMAS BENFIELD

INTRODUCTION

Although most complications affecting the lungs during the course of HIV arise from infection, especially early in the epidemic HIV-infected patients may present with, or develop, complications related to alterations in their immune regulation. A marked CD8 T-cell infiltration in the lung may be caused by HIV in both symptomatic and nonsymptomatic patients. The effects of HIV on the pulmonary microenvironment include a progressive decline in local immunocompetence that results in failure to mount a protective immune response against opportunist infections. The spectrum of noninfectious complications associated with HIV infection encompasses other idiopathic conditions and pulmonary malignancies, which include Kaposi sarcoma (KS), Hodgkin's and non-Hodgkin's lymphoma, and solid tumors.

NEOPLASTIC DISEASES

Cancer incidence is higher in persons with immunodeficiency of all causes. In HIV-1 infection, cancers that are uncommon in the general population predominate and include mainly lymphoma and Kaposi's sarcoma. However, other more common cancers are now seen with increasing frequency with HIV-1 infection (Table 35-1).

Kaposi's Sarcoma

Epidemiology, Risk Factors, and Pathogenesis

In the general population, Kaposi's sarcoma is a rare benign skin tumor that develops in the skin of the lower extremities in elderly men from the Mediterranean area. The disease was originally described in 1872 by the Hungarian physician, Moricz Kaposi. KS is up to 1000 times more frequent in persons with HIV-1 infection than in the general population and is associated with an aggressive course. The incidence of AIDS-associated KS has, however, declined substantially over the past two decades. Before combination antiretroviral therapy (cART), the incidence of KS ranged from 25–50 cases per 1000 person-years of follow-up (PYFU) but has steadily declined so that the incidence in a cART-treated population is less than 5 per 1000 PYFU. Approximately 5–10% of all AIDS diagnoses are based on the presentation of KS. HIV-1 infected men who have sex with men have a 20-fold higher risk of KS developing than other transmission groups. Development of KS increases with lower CD4 T-cell counts but can occur at all levels of immunodeficiency (Table 35-2). Thus, when KS is the AIDS-defining illness, it may have occurred at a relatively higher CD4 T-cell count than other AIDS-defining illnesses.

KS is an angioproliferative inflammatory condition that is associated with infection with human herpesvirus 8 (HHV-8). Gene expression profiling shows that KS consists of aberrant endothelial and inflammatory cells of lymphatic origin. HHV-8, a γ-2 herpesvirus of the rhadinovirus genus, has been demonstrated in all forms of KS, and in situ hybridization has demonstrated the presence of HHV-8 RNA and DNA in spindle cells, endothelium, and mononuclear cells of KS. HHV-8 DNA is detectable in peripheral blood before the development of KS, and increased viral replication is evident before symptomatic KS. More than 80% of individuals with AIDS-associated KS have antibodies toward HHV-8. HHV-8 may exert its oncogenic potential in several ways. The HHV-8 genome contains several genes that are homologs to human genes. Among these is a latent nuclear antigen that binds to p53 and associates viral DNA to human DNA during mitosis; a viral cyclin that activates cyclin-dependent kinases that prevent human cells from remaining in a G_1 phase; a constitutively expressed receptor (viral interleukin-8 receptor) that may be involved in angiogenesis; a Bcl-2–like protein that prevents apoptosis; and viral cytokines (vMIP and viral interleukin [IL]-6) that may explain some of the constitutive symptoms associated with KS. Cytokines are required for HHV-8–infected endothelial cells to acquire their phenotype and for continued growth of KS. The HIV-1 Tat protein upregulates cytokines and metalloproteinases, which further promotes the oncogenic potential of KS cells.

Genetics

Genetic polymorphisms of the Fc-γ receptor IIIA, the IL-6 and IL-8 promoter regions, have been associated with an increased risk of developing KS. Some human leukocyte antigen (HLA) types have also been associated with KS.

Clinical Features

Cutaneous and mucocutaneous manifestations of AIDS-associated KS are the more common and usually precede visceral disease by months to years. Skin and visceral lesions appear as red or violet macules, papules, or nodules that may coalesce to form plaque-like lesions. Lesions may affect any area of the skin and involve any organ system. Lymphadenopathy is frequent.

Pulmonary KS may cause nonproductive cough, hemoptysis, shortness of breath, chest pain, and fever. In rare instances, involvement of the larynx or trachea may cause airway obstruction. Extrapulmonary involvement is frequent, but 15% of KS occurs without skin lesions. CD4 cell counts are low (0–100/µL) at the time of diagnosis. Examination of the lungs is usually normal. Chest radiograph may be

TABLE 35-1 Noninfectious Pulmonary Complications Associated with HIV-1 Infection

Neoplastic disease	Kaposi's sarcoma
	Castleman's disease
	Non-Hodgkin's lymphoma
	Primary effusion lymphoma
	Lung cancer
Inflammatory disease	Non-specific interstitial pneumonitis
	Lymphocytic interstitial pneumonitis
Airway disease	Chronic obstructive pulmonary disease
Pulmonary vascular disease	Pulmonary hypertension
Miscellaneous	Antiretroviral treatment–induced respiratory disease

TABLE 35-2 Association with Degree of Immunodeficiency

Degree of Immunodeficiency	Noninfectious Pulmonary Complication
Severe (CD4 cell count < 50/μL)	Kaposi's sarcoma
	Castleman's disease
	Non-Hodgkin's lymphoma
	Primary effusion lymphoma
	Lung cancer
	Non-specific interstitial pneumonitis
	Lymphocytic interstitial pneumonitis
	Chronic obstructive pulmonary disease
	Pulmonary hypertension
	Antiretroviral treatment–induced respiratory disease
Moderate to severe (CD4 cell count 50–200/μL)	Kaposi's sarcoma
	Non-Hodgkin's lymphoma
	Lung cancer
	Non-specific interstitial pneumonitis
	Lymphocytic interstitial pneumonitis
	Chronic obstructive pulmonary disease
	Pulmonary hypertension
	Antiretroviral treatment–induced respiratory disease
Moderate (CD4 cell count 200–350/μL)	Non-Hodgkin's lymphoma
	Lung cancer
	Chronic obstructive pulmonary disease
	Pulmonary hypertension
	Antiretroviral treatment–induced respiratory disease
Normal (CD4 cell count > 350/μL)	Lung cancer
	Chronic obstructive pulmonary disease
	Pulmonary hypertension

normal but commonly shows single or multiple peribronchovascular nodules (Figure 35-1, *A*). Diffuse infiltration and air space consolidation may also be present. Pleural effusion is common. Hilar and mediastinal lymphadenopathy may be visible on chest films but are better visualized with CT scan.

In pulmonary KS, CT scans typically reveal peribronchovascular thickening and nodules that are larger than 1 cm in diameter (see Figure 35-1, *B*). The role of magnetic resonance imaging or positron emission tomography in the diagnosis and management of pulmonary KS is not clear.

Diagnosis

Pulmonary KS is highly likely in an HIV-1–infected person with a CD4 cell count of < 100/μL, with cutaneous or mucocutaneous KS and with pulmonary symptoms and bronchoscopy is useful to visualize typical endobronchial lesions (see Figure 35-1, *C*). These are flat or slightly raised and occur throughout the tracheobronchial tree but are most frequent at airway bifurcations. Pleural effusions are usually exudative and may be serous or serosanguineous. Serum lactate dehydrogenase may be elevated. Histologic verification is usually not required for a diagnosis of KS. Endobronchial biopsy may confer a substantial risk of severe bleeding, but biopsy may be necessary in cases where there is no bronchial involvement. In these cases, transbronchial or percutaneous needle biopsy are useful to establish the diagnosis. In cases of pleural KS, video-assisted thorascopy can be used to visualize pleural KS lesions and to perform biopsy. Open lung biopsies are obsolete because of the complications associated with the procedure. Lung biopsies show typical features of KS that include a tumor-like infiltrate with a peribronchovascular distribution of spindle cells. Slitlike spaces without endothelium contain extravasated erythrocytes (see Figure 35-1, *D*). *In situ* hybridization and immunostaining is usually positive for HHV-8. HHV-8 DNA is detectable in bronchoalveolar lavage cells.

Treatment

All patients with KS should be treated with cART, but immune reconstitution may induce an inflammatory reaction and flare of KS within 2–8 weeks of cART. Cutaneous and mucocutaneous AIDS-associated KS usually regresses with cART without chemotherapy but may require additional local radiotherapy. Visceral KS, however, will require chemotherapy. Concomitant use of cART increases the response rate to chemotherapy. All patients should be offered *Pneumocystis jirovecii* prophylaxis regardless of their CD4 cell count. The most widely used regimen for the treatment of pulmonary KS has been adriamycin (20 mg/m^2), bleomycin (10 mg/m^2), and vincristine (1.4 mg/m^2) (ABV) combination chemotherapy. Vincristine may be replaced with vinblastine in patients with polyneuropathy. The combination is given every 2 weeks. Response is evaluated after four to six courses of chemotherapy. Response rates are 30–50%. Adverse side effects include anemia, neutropenia, thrombopenia, neuropathy, mucositis, and alopecia. There are potential drug–drug interactions between vincristine/vinblastine and antiretroviral agents.

Alternative regimens to ABV are liposomal anthracyclines and paclitaxel. Liposomal daunorubicin (40–60 mg/m^2) or doxorubicin (20 mg/m^2) given every 2 weeks is associated with comparable response rates and less severe adverse effects than ABV. Therefore, liposomal anthracyclines are considered to be first-line chemotherapeutic agents for visceral KS by many clinicians. The risk of drug–drug interactions with antiretroviral agents is low with anthracyclines. Paclitaxel (100 mg/m^2) every 2 weeks in combination with granulocyte-colony stimulating factor (G-CSF) is approved for second-line treatment of KS. Experience with paclitaxel and

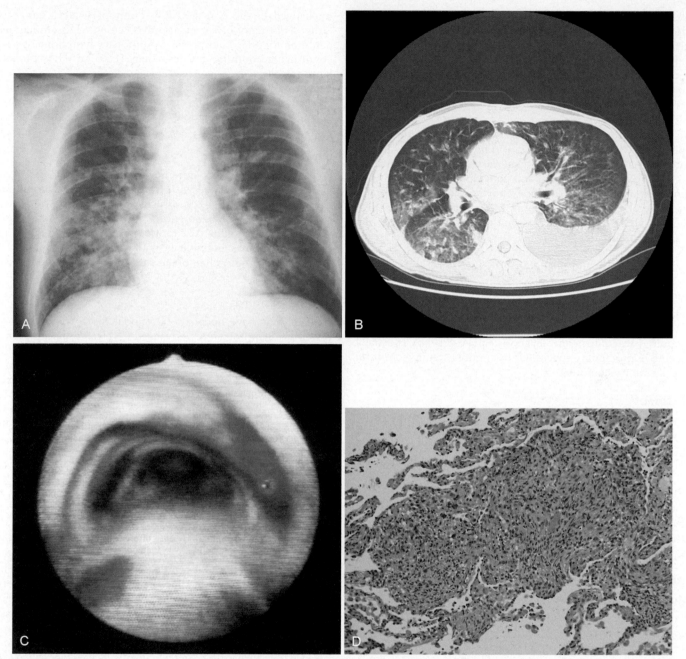

FIGURE 35-1 Pulmonary Kaposi's sarcoma. **A** and **B**, Chest radiograph and CT scan of multiple peribronchovascular nodules. **C**, Typical violet-red endobronchial nodule visualized through a fiber bronchoscope. **D**, Transbronchial biopsy of pulmonary Kaposi's sarcoma lesion. (**C**, Courtesy of Dr. L. Huang. **D**, Courtesy of Dr. J. Junge.)

pulmonary KS is limited, and the use of paclitaxel is associated with more severe adverse effects than anthracyclines, and paclitaxel has potential serious drug–drug interactions with antiretroviral drugs. Investigational agents include thalidomide, imatinib, IL-12, and fumagillin.

Clinical Course and Prevention

Untreated pulmonary KS is associated with a median survival of less than 6 months. cART is associated with improved survival in HIV-1–infected patients with pulmonary KS receiving chemotherapy, and the 5-year overall survival has improved to 50% and above. Severe immunodeficiency (CD4 cell count <100/µL), pleural effusion, and/or hypoxia are associated with a particularly rapid course of KS. KS is best prevented through

treatment of the underlying HIV-1–related immunodeficiency with cART.

Multicentric Castleman's Disease

Epidemiology, Risk Factors, and Pathogenesis

Castleman's disease is a rare lymphoproliferative disease characterized by angiofollicular proliferation. Three histologic variants (hyaline vascular, plasma-cell, and mixed) and two clinical types (localized and multicentric) of Castleman's disease have been described. The incidence of Castleman's disease increases with HIV-1 infection. Multicentric disease is associated with concomitant AIDS-associated Kaposi's sarcoma. One study found HHV-8 DNA in all 14 cases of HIV-1–associated multicentric Castleman's disease but only in 7 of 17 non-HIV-1–infected cases. HHV-8 DNA was only detected in 1 of 34 lymph node biopsy samples of HIV-1–uninfected individuals with localized disease. Multicentric Castleman's disease frequently transforms to non-Hodgkin's lymphoma. Pulmonary involvement of Castleman's in HIV1 infection is exceedingly rare but probably also is underdiagnosed.

Clinical Features

The localized form usually presents as mediastinal lymph node hyperplasia without systemic symptoms. Symptoms of multi-centric disease include fever, generalized lymphadenopathy, fatigue, hepatosplenomegaly, and pancytopenia. Symptoms of pulmonary involvement include shortness of breath, cough, and bilateral crackles. Worsening of symptoms is often pre-ceded by HHV-8 viremia. CD4 cell counts vary from normal to severe immunodeficiency. Chest radiographs and CT scans may show noduloreticular interstitial infiltration, mediastinal lymphadenopathy, and pleural effusions.

Diagnosis

Bronchoscopy is usually normal. Analysis of BAL cells may show hypercellularity and lymphocytosis. A pulmonary biopsy is required to confirm the diagnosis. HHV-8 DNA is usually detected in pulmonary specimens by immunostaining or *in situ* hybridization techniques.

Treatment

Localized disease is cured by surgical resection. Multicentric disease requires chemotherapy with vinblastine or etoposide. Etoposide effectively prevents the onset of multicentric Castleman's disease. Anti-CD20 therapy is under investigation.

Clinical Course and Prevention

Survival rates are poor but have improved in the era of cART, with a 5-year overall survival of approximately 50%. Patients with multicentric Castleman's diseases often have non-Hodgkin's lymphoma (NHL) develop.

Non-Hodgkin's Lymphoma
Epidemiology, Risk Factors, and Pathogenesis

In the pre-cART era, NHL represented the second most common HIV-1–associated cancer after KS. With the intro-duction of cART, rates of NHL have declined by 40–70% for most histologic types. Despite the decline in incidence, NHL is now one of the most common initial AIDS-defining illnesses. Compared with non-HIV-1–infected individuals, the risk of low-grade lymphoma (although not AIDS defining) is increased fourfold, the risk of high-grade lymphoma is increased 600-fold, and the risk of primary brain lymphoma is increased 3600-fold with HIV-1 infection. The increased risk is associated with concomitant infection with Epstein–Barr virus (EBV) and/or HHV-8. Male sex, increased age, and immunodeficiency are other risk factors for NHL. A prior AIDS diagnosis usually precedes primary pulmonary lym-phoma. Most AIDS-related NHLs belong to one of three cate-gories of high-grade B-cell lymphomas: Burkitt's lymphoma, centroblastic lymphoma, and immunoblastic lymphoma. Bur-kitt and Burkitt-like lymphoma tend to occur in patients with relative high CD4 cell counts compared with centroblastic large cell and immunoblastic lymphoma that occur at low CD4 cell counts. The incidence of Burkitt lymphoma remains unchanged in the era of cART. Pulmonary NHL can occur either as primary or secondary involvement. Dissemination is common for NHL, but primary pulmonary lymphoma is a rare condition accounting for less than 0.5% of HIV-1–related lymphomas.

The pathogenesis of NHL is complex and involves immune dysfunction together with dysregulation of cytokine responses, chronic antigen stimulation, and coinfection with EBV and HHV-8.

Genetics

Somatic mutations of immunoglobulin, c-MYC, bcl-6, and p53 genes are associated with transformation into lymphoma. Overexpression of bcl-2 is associated with resistance to che-motherapy and a poor prognosis. Individuals heterozygous of the CCR-5 chemokine $\Delta 32$ mutation may have a reduced risk of NHL, whereas individuals with the stromal cell–derived factor 1 (SDF1)-3′A chemokine variant may be associated with an increased risk of NHL.

Clinical Features

Patients may have nodal or extranodal disease with systemic systems. Symptoms of advanced NHL with pulmonary involvement include fever, night sweats, and weight loss (B symptoms). Symptoms of primary pulmonary involvement include shortness of breath, cough, and chest pain. Primary pulmonary lymphoma is associated with CD4 cell counts less than $50/\mu L$. Anemia, thrombocytopenia, and leukopenia are frequent. Serum lactate dehydrogenase is commonly elevated with secondary, but not primary, pulmonary involvement. Chest radiographs and CT scans commonly show isolated or multiple central or peripheral nodules (Figure 35-2, *A*). Mediastinal lymphadenopathy and pleural effusion are less common.

Diagnosis

Fiberoptic bronchoscopy is usually normal. Bronchoalveolar lavage cytology may reveal lymphoma cells, but a biopsy is required to establish a histologic diagnosis. Transbronchial biopsy has a reasonable diagnostic yield for secondary, but not primary, pulmonary lymphoma. Percutaneous thoracic core needle biopsy is the most used method to obtain tissue for diagnosis. In rare cases, video-assisted thorascopic or open lung biopsy may be necessary. Histologically, the lymphoma invades the alveolar septa and vascular walls (see Figure 35-2, *B*). Necrosis is frequent. Most are high-grade centroblastic or immunoblastic large B-cell lymphoma that are EBV positive and overexpress bcl-2.

Treatment

There is no evidence to indicate that primary or secondary pulmonary NHL should be treated differently than NHL in general. Chemotherapy regimens that include cyclophospha-mide, doxorubicin, vincristine, and prednisolone (CHOP), or CHOP-rituximab (CHOP-R), or etoposide, prednisone, vincristine, cyclophosphamide, and doxorubicin (EPOCH) are used in conjunction with cART. CHOP-R may be benefi-cial in primary pulmonary lymphoma, because these often overexpress bcl-2. There are no significant drug–drug interac-tions between commonly used cART regimens and CHOP. Use of cART is associated with less anemia, thrombocytopenia, and other adverse effects of chemotherapy.

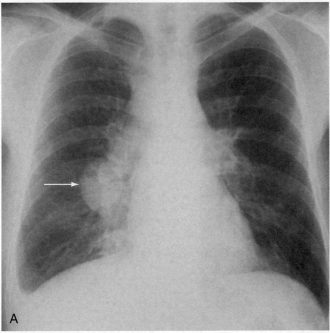
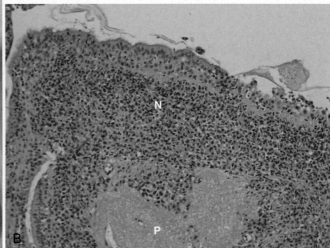

FIGURE 35-2 Primary pulmonary non-Hodgkin's lymphoma (NHL). **A,** Chest radiograph showing a single, large central nodule. **B,** Transbronchial biopsy of pulmonary NHL and *Pneumocystis jirovecii* pneumonia. *N,* Lymphoma cell infiltration; *P,* characteristic foamy, eosinophilic exudate of *P. jirovecii* trophozoites and cysts. (Courtesy of Dr. J. Junge.)

Clinical Course and Prevention

The median survival from primary pulmonary lymphoma is less than 4 months with chemotherapy alone. Survival from lymphoma in general has greatly improved in the cART era.

Primary Effusion Lymphoma (Body-Cavity–Associated Lymphoma)

Epidemiology, Risk Factors, and Pathogenesis

Primary effusion lymphoma (PEL) is a rare type of non-Hodgkin's lymphoma that almost exclusively occurs with HIV-1 infection. PEL grow mainly in the body cavities (pleural, pericardial, and peritoneal) as lymphomatous effusions without an identifiable contiguous tumor mass. PEL predominantly occurs in men who have sex with men and who are seropositive for HHV-8. In contrast to NHL, PEL lacks c-myc gene rearrangements. PEL contains HHV-8, Epstein–Barr virus, expresses CD45, exhibits clonal immunoglobulin gene rearrangements, and lacks *bcl-2*, *bcl-6*, *ras*, and p53 gene alterations.

Clinical Features

PEL is associated with progressive immunodeficiency and consequently low CD4 cell counts. Patients usually have a prior diagnosis of KS. Symptoms include fever, generalized lymphadenopathy, and fatigue. Symptoms of pleural involvement include shortness of breath and cough. Chest radiographs show unilateral or bilateral effusions. CT scans are useful to identify localized masses representing NHL, KS, or other neoplastic disease. PEL usually remains localized to the body cavity of origin.

Diagnosis

The diagnosis is based on the demonstration of morphologic, immunophenotypical, immunogenotypical, viral, and molecular characteristics of pleural fluid. Demonstration of HHV-8 is often essential.

Treatment

Treatment follows guidelines for treatment of NHL and should include chemotherapy together with cART.

Clinical Course and Prevention

PEL has an aggressive clinical course and is associated with a high mortality rate. The 1-year overall survival rate is 40%.

Lung Cancer

Epidemiology, Risk Factors, and Pathogenesis

The risk of small cell carcinoma, non-small cell carcinoma, and bronchioalveolar carcinoma is twofold to fivefold greater among persons with HIV-1 infection compared with the general population. Adenocarcinoma accounts for most cases. Men have a higher risk than women. Pulmonary neoplastic diseases develop at a younger age. The risk is increased with a CD4 cell count less than 300/μL but not at higher CD4 cell counts. Between 60% and 80% of HIV-1–infected individuals smoke, and this contributes significantly to the excess risk. However, epidemiologic modeling shows that smoking alone cannot account for the excess risk, suggesting that other cofactors are at play. It is possible that smoking may additively or synergistically together with HIV-1 infection affect the lung more severely than in non-HIV-1–infected individuals. HIV-1 may enhance lung damage and lead to increased oxidative stress.

Clinical Features

These do not differ from lung cancer in general, but HIV-1–infected individuals tend to be younger at presentation. Symptoms of localized disease may be subtle but may include persistent cough, shortness of breath, chest pain, and weight loss as the disease develops. Chest radiographs and CT scans may show nodular or diffuse infiltrates, hilar or mediastinal lymphadenopathy, and pleural effusion.

Diagnosis

Fiberoptic bronchoscopy may reveal bronchial invasion. Biopsy is required to establish a histologic diagnosis and can be obtained by transbronchial, percutaneous thoracic, open lung, or video-assisted thorascopic biopsy.

Treatment

Treatment of HIV-1–associated lung cancer follows current guidelines for treatment of non-HIV-1–associated lung cancer as described in Chapter 47.

Clinical Course and Prevention

Individuals with HIV-1 infection tend to present with more advanced disease. Studies indicate that overall survival is shortened for individuals with HIV-1 and lung cancer compared with the general population.

INFLAMMATORY PULMONARY DISORDERS

Nonspecific Interstitial Pneumonitis
Epidemiology, Risk Factors, and Pathogenesis

Nonspecific interstitial pneumonitis (NIP), also known as chronic interstitial pneumonitis, is a common cause of pulmonary disease in adults with advanced, untreated HIV-1 infection. Half of HIV-1–infected adults without pulmonary symptoms and with less than 200 CD4 T lymphocytes per μL show histopathologic changes characteristic of NIP. The incidence of NIP at different CD4 strata is unknown. NIP is rare in children. The etiology of NIP is unknown. There is evidence of HIV-1 RNA expression in pulmonary CD4 T lymphocytes and macrophages. Cytotoxic CD8 T lymphocytes are the predominant lymphocyte, and it is speculated that these cells induce pulmonary inflammation. Other mechanisms of lung damage include increased levels of inflammatory mediators (e.g., cytokines and leukotrienes) and release of superoxide anion from activated alveolar macrophages.

Clinical Features

The symptoms of NIP are nonspecific and resemble many symptoms of the infectious complications of HIV-1 such as cough, shortness of breath, and fever. Extrapulmonary involvement is rare. Examination of the lungs is usually normal. There may be discreet hypoxia that further increases on exercise. Chest radiographs and CT scans may be normal or show diffuse alveolar, nodular, or interstitial infiltrates that are indistinguishable from other common HIV-1–associated infections (Figure 35-3, A and B). Pleural effusion is less common.

Diagnosis

Suspicion of NIP should arise when standard histocytology, microbiological staining and culture, and molecular techniques do not yield a pathogen. Thus, NIP is an exclusion diagnosis. Tissue specimens are required to establish the diagnosis and may be obtained by bronchoscopy, fine-needle aspiration, or open lung procedures. Transbronchial biopsy specimens characteristically show varying degrees of perivascular, peribronchial, and pleural lymphocyte and plasma cell infiltration, edema, fibrin deposition, pneumocyte hyperplasia, and thickening of alveolar septa. Alveolar septal infiltration is uncommon (see Figure 35-3, C). Lymphoid aggregates are common. Bronchoalveolar fluid analysis shows lymphocytosis and a decrease in relative and absolute numbers of alveolar macrophages. Because of

the risks involved with biopsy procedures, some clinicians make a presumptive diagnosis after ruling out an infectious cause of the patient's pulmonary symptoms.

Treatment

Symptoms may resolve without therapy. However, given the association of NIP with severe immunodeficiency, initiation of combination antiretroviral therapy is almost always indicated. Several case series indicate that cART leads to resolution of symptoms and pathosis.

Clinical Course and Prevention

The natural course of NIP without cART is chronic and rarely leads to respiratory failure. Some individuals may be asymptomatic. NIP is best prevented by initiating cART before the development of moderate to severe immunodeficiency.

Bronchiolitis Obliterans Organizing Pneumonia

The presenting clinical features of bronchiolitis obliterans organizing pneumonia (BOOP) in HIV-infected patients may be dramatic, with the development of a flulike illness with acute or subacute symptoms (fever, malaise, anorexia, weight loss, nonproductive cough, and dyspnea). Usually this syndrome develops in immunocompromised patients who have infections or malignancy. Physical examination often reveals bibasal crackles, and the chest radiograph shows multiple, bilateral, alveolar opacities. Linear or nodular opacities may also be present. In those with typical BOOP, alveolar lavage may demonstrate an alveolitis characterized by $CD8^+$ lymphocytes; foamy macrophages; and a small increase in neutrophils, eosinophils, and mast cells.

Treatment with glucocorticosteroids causes a remission or stabilization of the disease. However, relapse is common if the steroids are withdrawn.

Lymphocytic Interstitial Pneumonitis
Epidemiology, Risk Factors, and Pathogenesis

Lymphocytic interstitial pneumonitis (LIP) is a disease of unknown etiology associated with HIV-1 infection and autoimmune disease. LIP occurs predominantly, and not infrequently, among untreated infants and children where LIP is an AIDS-defining illness. LIP is rare among adults. There seems to be an association between LIP and advanced HIV-1 disease. Similar to NIP, there is evidence of HIV-1 RNA expression in pulmonary CD4 T lymphocytes and macrophages.

Clinical Features

As with NIP, the symptoms of LIP are nonspecific and include nonproductive cough, shortness of breath, and fever. Extrapulmonary involvement of lymph nodes is common, and generalized lymphadenopathy is frequent. Peripheral CD8 T lymphocytosis is characteristic. Clubbing has been reported among children. Chest radiographs may be normal but commonly show diffuse alveolar, nodular, or interstitial infiltration. Pleural effusion is common. CT scans may reveal peribronchial nodules or a diffuse ground-glass appearance.

Diagnosis

Again, as with NIP, LIP is a diagnosis of exclusion that requires tissue samples to establish the diagnosis. Transbronchial biopsy is characterized by peribronchial, perivascular, and pleural infiltration of lymphocytic and plasma cells. These findings

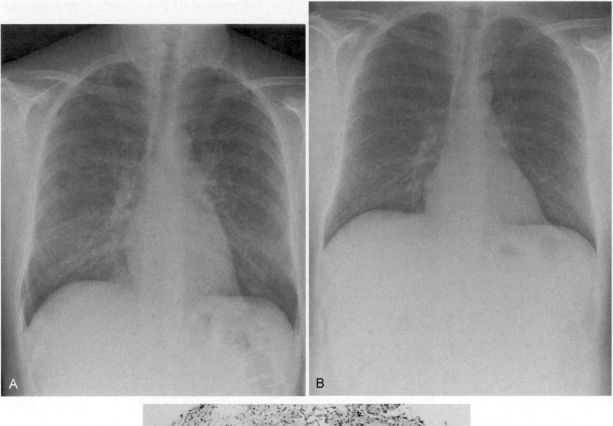

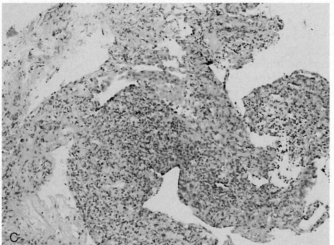

FIGURE 35-3 Nonspecific interstitial pneumonitis. **A,** Chest radiograph showing bilateral diffuse infiltration before start of combination antiretroviral therapy. **B,** Chest radiograph 1 year after start of combination antiretroviral therapy. **C,** Transbronchial biopsy showing nonspecific inflammation. The alveolar septae are thickened due to alveolar epithelial proliferation, edema, and a cellular infiltration of lymphocytes and plasma cells. (Courtesy of Dr. J. Junge.)

are also characteristic of NIP. However, septal infiltration differentiates LIP from NIP. Lymphoid aggregates are common.

Treatment

Treatment of LIP is directed at the underlying immunodeficiency caused by HIV-1, and initiation of cART is associated with resolution of pulmonary symptoms.

Clinical Course and Prevention

The natural course of LIP is variable and ranges from spontaneous remission to respiratory failure. LIP is best prevented by initiating cART before the development of moderate to severe immunodeficiency.

Chronic Airway Disease and Emphysema
Epidemiology, Risk Factors, and Pathogenesis

HIV-1–infected smokers are twice as likely to have chronic obstructive pulmonary disease (COPD) as smokers without HIV-1 infection. Several factors that increase the risk of COPD developing are frequent among HIV-1–infected individuals, including a high prevalence of tobacco smoking, intravenous drug use, and recurrent bacterial and opportunistic infections. COPD develops at younger age and is more prevalent among African-Americans. Currently, it is unknown whether HIV-1 infection per se, the increased life expectancy associated with combination antiretroviral therapy, or both account for the increased prevalence of COPD. Evidence seems to support all three possibilities. Ongoing viral replication and activation of pulmonary cytotoxic T lymphocytes may lead to parenchymal destruction similar to the effects of tobacco smoking. Advanced HIV-1 disease is associated with impaired lung function tests. Some studies suggest a synergistic effect of HIV-1 and smoking, and this may explain why HIV-1 individuals may have COPD develop at a younger age. HIV-1–infected intravenous drug users have reduced FEV_1, FVC, and diffusing capacity of carbon monoxide (DLco) compared with other transmission categories. This may, in part, be explained by the fact that they more frequently are heavy smokers and have recurrent lower respiratory tract infections. Pulmonary bacterial and opportunistic infections (e.g., *Pneumocystis jirovecii* pneumonia) are associated with permanent reductions in FEV_1, FVC, FEV_1/FVC, and DLco after infection. Chapter 38 deals with COPD in detail.

Genetics

Mutations in the α_1-antitrypsin gene predispose to emphysema.

Clinical Features

Signs and symptoms of COPD do not differ between individuals with and without HIV-1 infection and include cough, sputum production, shortness of breath, wheezing, and chest tightness. HIV-1–infected patients may be younger.

Diagnosis

Spirometry is central to the diagnosis. Reductions in FEV_1, FVC, and FEV_1/FVC will confirm the diagnosis and establish the severity of the condition. A radiograph is useful to distinguish between other lung and heart conditions with similar symptoms. Arterial blood gas tension analysis is performed to confirm hypercapnia and/or establish the need for oxygen treatment.

Treatment

Treatment does not differ from COPD treatment in general. Therapy includes bronchodilators, inhaled glucocorticosteroids, and pulmonary rehabilitation. Influenza and pneumococcal vaccination is recommended and does not confer any increased risk of HIV-1 disease progression. Oxygen treatment follows general guidelines.

There are no important drug interactions between antiretrovirals and bronchodilators, except between some protease inhibitors and theophylline. There is the potential of drug interactions between protease inhibitors and inhaled glucocorticosteroids, but not with nucleoside and nonnucleoside analogs. Nicotine can be used to treat tobacco dependency together with antiretrovirals. There is a potential drug interaction with bupropion and protease inhibitors and nonnucleoside analogs. Similar interactions may occur with varenicline.

Clinical Course and Prevention

The clinical course is usually not any different from COPD among non-HIV-1–infected individuals. Smoking cessation is central to successfully preventing further disease progression. Care should also be taken to avoid secondary smoke. Avoidance of lung irritants is important. COPD is not believed to affect HIV-1 disease progression. Antiretroviral management of HIV-1 should follow national and international guidelines and should not be delayed.

HIV-1–Associated Pulmonary Hypertension

Non-HIV-1–associated pulmonary hypertension is described in detail in Chapter 62.

Epidemiology, Risk Factors, and Pathogenesis

Pulmonary hypertension (PH) is an infrequent cause of pulmonary disease among HIV-1–infected individuals. However, the incidence (<0.5%) is greater than for non-HIV-1–infected individuals (~0.02%). A careful examination is required to distinguish between primary and secondary pulmonary hypertension. HIV-1 per se is assumed to induce vascular changes associated with primary PH, whereas drug use (foreign particle microembolism), COPD, interstitial pulmonary disease, essential hypertension, ischemic heart disease, chronic thromboembolism, and valvular heart disease contribute to secondary PH. Some reports have implicated concurrent infection with HHV-8 in the pathogenesis of PH.

The pathogenesis remains unclear. Remodeling of the media and adventitia of the arterial pulmonary tree, the extracellular matrix, and plexiform lesion characterize HIV-1–related and non-HIV-1–related sporadic forms. The increase in pulmonary vascular resistance may be caused by vascular growth factors, mechanical obstruction of the pulmonary arteries, hypoxia, or other stimuli. Chronic changes may remain even after the initiating insult factor is removed. Pulmonary vascular resistance increases right ventricular systolic pressure, leading to dilatation and dysfunction ultimately leading to right ventricular failure.

Genetics

Familial primary pulmonal hypertension (PPH) is characterized by autosomal-dominant inheritance and incomplete penetrance. A mutation in the type II bone morphogenetic protein receptor (BMPR II) has been associated with familial PPH.

Clinical Features

The predominant symptom is dyspnea, particular exertional dyspnea. This symptom is nonspecific and, therefore, the diagnosis is often made late in its course. Other common symptoms may include other nonspecific symptoms such as fatigue, angina, syncope, near syncope, and peripheral edema. PH may occur at any CD4 cell count.

Diagnosis

A full diagnostic evaluation is crucial to rule out non-HIV-1–related causes, because they may require other specific therapy. The chest radiograph shows cardiomegaly and enlarged central pulmonary arteries, or signs of emphysema suggestive of chronic obstructive pulmonary disease, or interstitial infiltration suggestive of parenchymal disease. Echocardiogram usually confirms right axis deviation and right ventricular hypertrophy (P pulmonale). Echocardiography provides imaging of right atrial and ventricle enlargement, tricuspidal regurgitation, and reduced left ventricular size. Arterial blood gases commonly demonstrate hypoxia. Pulmonary function tests are helpful to distinguish between obstructive or restrictive underlying pulmonary pathology. Perfusion lung scans or computed tomography with intravenous contrast can rule out central and peripherally located thrombi. In addition, the lung parenchymal CT images may establish alternative diagnoses. Magnetic resonance pulmonary angiography is promising, because it also provides assessment of right ventricular function. Eventually, cardiac catheterization is necessary to measure pulmonary artery pressure, cardiac output, and left ventricular filling pressure.

Treatment

HIV-1–associated PH has been treated with epoprostenol, inhaled prostacyclin, inhaled iloprost, bosentan (an endothelin receptor antagonist), and sildenafil. The effect of each agent is variable but generally improves dyspnea and exercise tolerance. However, the effect is temporary, and there are concerns related to adverse effects. cART is associated with improved hemodynamics and survival. Use of anticoagulation is not supported by evidence.

Clinical Course and Prevention

PH progresses to heart failure within 1–2 years despite therapy and is associated with a poor survival rate. Higher CD4 cells have been associated with better survival.

MISCELLANEOUS

Antiretroviral Therapy and Respiratory Symptoms

Antiretroviral treatment may cause unexpected respiratory symptoms. Lactic acidosis and hepatic steatosis with hepatic failure are rare, but severe complications associated with nucleoside reverse transcriptase inhibitor therapy (NRTI), particularly the thymidine analogues, stavudine, and zidovudine, may occur after a few to several months of treatment. Lactic acidosis has a high mortality rate. Patients with elevated serum lactate levels may be asymptomatic, critically ill, or may have nonspecific symptoms such as dyspnea, tachypnea, fatigue, nausea, diarrhea, vomiting, and abdominal pain.

Another NRTI, abacavir, can produce a hypersensitivity reaction with fever, rash, and myalgias. Respiratory symptoms, including cough, dyspnea, and pharyngitis, frequently accompany the hypersensitivity reaction.

Third, in HIV-1–infected individuals with severe immunodeficiency at the time of institution of combination antiretroviral therapy, an inflammatory reaction to asymptomatic or residual opportunistic pathogens may arise and cause serious clinical conditions or aggravation of symptoms. Typically, such reactions have been observed within the first few weeks or months of therapy. Pulmonary examples are HIV-1 per se, *Mycobacterium avium* complex, *M. tuberculosis*, *Pneumocystis jirovecii* pneumonia, sarcoidosis, vasculitis, and other autoimmune disease. Any inflammatory symptoms should be evaluated and treatment instituted when necessary. Optimal therapy has not been determined. Antiinflammatory therapy may attenuate symptoms but many cases may resolve spontaneously.

PITFALLS AND CONTROVERSIES

Noninfectious pulmonary complications of HIV-1 infection are very often an exclusion diagnosis, because pulmonary infectious complications are many times more frequent than noninfectious complications. Therefore, extensive microbiologic and histopathologic workup is often required to rule out, for example, PCP.

Given the extended life expectancy with cART and high prevalence of smoking, non-AIDS pulmonary malignancy are expected to increase in frequency. Many clinicians have been reluctant to refer HIV-1–infected individuals to oncology services because of the dismal prognosis associated with HIV-1 infection, pulmonary cancer, and the adverse effects of aggressive chemotherapy. However, recent studies indicate that chemotherapy is better tolerated and that response rates are higher with concomitant cART.

Some controversy exists as to whether to initiate cART for nonspecific pulmonary inflammatory disease, COPD, PH, and other non-AIDS pulmonary disease. In cases of immunodeficiency (CD4 cell count $< 300/\mu L$) or constitutional symptoms, cART should always be offered according to national and international guidelines. In other cases, I believe that initiation of cART is prudent if the underlying condition leading to pulmonary inflammatory disease, COPD, PH, or other is believed to be HIV-1 per se. Most adverse effects to cART, interactions, and compliance issues are easily managed today with the introduction of less toxic compounds and once-daily dosing regimens.

WEB RESOURCES

AIDS Malignancy Program of the National Cancer Institute: www.cancer.gov/dctd/aids

Antiretroviral treatment guidelines: www.aidsinfo.nih.gov

HIV Drug Interactions: www.hiv-druginteractions.org

SUGGESTED READINGS

Aboulafia DM: The epidemiologic, pathologic, and clinical features of AIDS-associated pulmonary Kaposi's sarcoma. Chest 2000; 117(4): 1128–1145.

Chaturvedi AK, Pfeiffer RM, Chang L, et al: Elevated risk of lung cancer among people with AIDS. AIDS 2007; 21(2):207–213.

Crothers K, Butt AA, Gibert CL, et al: Increased COPD among HIV-positive compared with HIV-negative veterans. Chest 2006; 130(5): 1326–1333.

Grubb JR, Moorman AC, Baker RK, Masur H: The changing spectrum of pulmonary disease in patients with HIV infection on antiretroviral therapy. AIDS 2006; 20(8):1095–1107.

Guihot A, Couderc LJ, Agbalika F, et al: Pulmonary manifestations of multicentric Castleman's disease in HIV infection: a clinical, biological and radiological study. Eur Respir J 2005; 26(1):118–125.

Nador RG, Cesarman E, Chadburn A, et al: Primary effusion lymphoma: a distinct clinicopathologic entity associated with the Kaposi's sarcoma-associated herpes virus. Blood 1996; 88(2):645–656.

Ray P, Antoine M, Mary-Krause M, et al: AIDS-related primary pulmonary lymphoma. Am J Respir Crit Care Med 1998; 158(4):1221–1229.

Rosen MJ, Beck JM: Human immunodeficiency virus and the lung. New York, NY: Marcel Dekker; 1998.

Sparano JA: Human immunodeficiency virus associated lymphoma. Curr Opin Oncol 2003; 5(5):372–378.

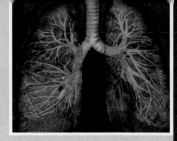

SECTION IX

AIRWAY DISEASES

36   β₂-Agonists, Anticholinergics, and Other Nonsteroid Drugs

PETER J. BARNES

INTRODUCTION

Asthma therapy can be classified into two main types—bronchodilators (or relievers) that give rapid relief of asthma symptoms, and controllers that give long-term control of asthma symptoms by suppression of the chronic inflammatory process (antiinflammatory drugs), by inhibition of the release of bronchoconstrictors, or by some other mechanism that does not involve a direct relaxant effect on airway smooth muscle (Table 36-1). Chronic obstructive pulmonary disease (COPD) is treated predominantly by bronchodilators, because there is no evidence yet that controllers influence progression of the disease. In this chapter, the mode of action and the clinical use of the main classes of drugs used in asthma therapy are reviewed, apart from corticosteroids (see Chapter 37). Although drugs are traditionally classified as controllers and relievers, some drugs, such as theophylline and antileukotrienes, seem to have bronchodilator and antiinflammatory properties.

β₂-AGONISTS

Inhaled β₂-agonists are the most effective bronchodilators and have minimal side effects when used correctly, and so they are the treatment of choice. Nonselective β-agonists, such as isoproterenol (isoprenaline) and orciprenaline, have no place.

Mode of Action

β₂-Agonists produce bronchodilatation by directly stimulating β₂-receptors in airway smooth muscle, which leads to relaxation. This can be demonstrated *in vitro* by the relaxant effect of β-agonists on human bronchi and small airways and *in vivo* by a rapid decrease in airway resistance. β-Receptors have been demonstrated in airway smooth muscle by direct receptor-binding techniques, and autoradiographic studies indicate that β-receptors are localized to smooth muscle of all airways from the trachea to the terminal bronchioles.

Activation of β₂-receptors results in activation of adenylate cyclase and an increase of intracellular cyclic adenosine-3′,5′-monophosphate (cAMP) (Figure 36-1). This leads to activation of a specific kinase (protein kinase A) that phosphorylates several target proteins within the cell, resulting in:

- Lowering of intracellular calcium ion (Ca^{2+}) concentration by active removal of Ca^{2+} from the cell into intracellular stores
- Inhibitory effect on phosphoinositide hydrolysis
- Direct inhibition of myosin light-chain kinase

- Opening of large-conductance, calcium-activated potassium channels (K_{Ca}) that repolarize the smooth muscle cell and may stimulate the sequestration of Ca^{2+} into intracellular stores (β-agonists may be directly coupled to K_{Ca} and relaxation of airway smooth muscle may, therefore, occur independently of an increase in cAMP).

β₂-Agonists act as functional antagonists and reverse bronchoconstriction, irrespective of the contractile agent. This is an important property, because multiple bronchoconstrictor mediators (inflammatory mediators and neurotransmitters) are released in asthma.

β₂-Agonists may have additional effects on airways, and β₂-receptors are localized to several different airway cells (Table 36-2 and Figure 36-2):

- Inhibition of mediator release from mast cells and other inflammatory cells
- Inhibitory effects on neutrophil migration and activation
- Reduction and prevention of microvascular leakage and thus the development of bronchial mucosal edema after exposure to mediators such as histamine and leukotrienes
- Increased mucus secretion from submucosal glands and ion transport across airway epithelium (effects that may enhance mucociliary clearance and, therefore, reverse the defect in clearance found in asthma)
- Reduction in neurotransmitter release from airway cholinergic nerves, thus reducing cholinergic reflex bronchocon-striction
- Inhibition of the release of bronchoconstrictor and inflammatory peptides, such as substance P, from sensory nerves.

Although these additional effects of β-agonists may be relevant to the prophylactic use of the drugs against various challenges, their rapid bronchodilator action is probably caused by a direct effect on airway smooth muscle.

Antiinflammatory Effects?

The inhibitory effects of β-agonists on the release of mast-cell mediators and microvascular leakage are clearly antiinflammatory effects, which suggests that β-agonists may modify acute inflammation. However, β-agonists do not have a significant inhibitory effect on the chronic inflammation of asthmatic airways, which is suppressed by corticosteroids or in COPD airways. Bronchial biopsy specimens in asthmatic patients who regularly take β-agonists show no significant reduction in the number of or activation in inflammatory cells in the airways in contrast to suppression of inflammation that occurs with inhaled corticosteroids. This is probably explained by the fact

471

TABLE 36-1 Current Therapy for Asthma

Relievers (Bronchodilators)	Controllers (Antiinflammatory Treatments)
β₂-Agonists	Corticosteroids
Theophylline	Cromones
Anticholinergics	Antileukotrienes
	Corticosteroid-sparing therapies: Methotrexate Gold Cyclosporin A

TABLE 36-2 Localization and Function of Airway β-Adrenoreceptors

Cell Type	Subtype	Function
Smooth muscle	β₂	Relaxation (proximal = distal) Inhibition of proliferation
Epithelium	β₂	Increased ion transport Secretion of inhibitory factor Increased ciliary beating Increased mucociliary clearance
Submucosal glands	β₁/β₂	Increased secretion (mucus cells)
Clara cells	β₂	Increased secretion
Cholinergic nerves	β₂	Reduced acetylcholine release
Sensory nerves	β₂/β₃	Reduced neuropeptide release Reduced activation?
Bronchial vessels	β₂	Vasodilation Reduced plasma extravasation
Inflammatory cells:		
Mast cells	β₂	Reduced mediator release
Macrophages	β₂	No effect?
Eosinophils	β₂	Reduced mediator release?
T-lymphocytes	β₂	Reduced cytokine release?

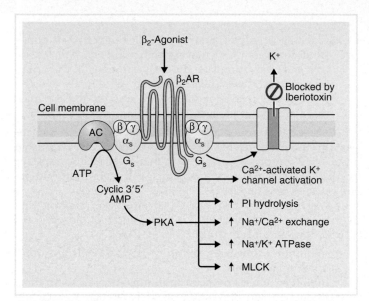

FIGURE 36-1 Molecular mechanisms involved in bronchodilator response to β₂-agonists. Activation of β₂-adrenoceptors on airway smooth muscle cells is coupled by means of a G-protein to adenylyl cyclase, which results in increased intracellular cyclic adenosine monophosphate formation. This activates protein kinase A, which phosphorylates a number of substrates, including large, conductance calcium-activated potassium channels (K_{Ca}), which can also be directly coupled to β₂-receptors.

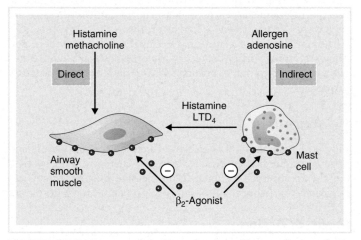

FIGURE 36-2 Direct and indirect bronchodilator effects of β₂-agonists. β₂-Agonists may cause bronchodilatation directly by means of activation of β₂-receptors on airway smooth muscle and also indirectly by inhibition of mediator release from mast cells.

that β-agonists do not have a long-term inhibitory effect on macrophages, eosinophils, or T lymphocytes, the cells involved in chronic inflammation and airway hyperresponsiveness because of downregulation of β₂-receptors.

Clinical Use

Short-acting inhaled β₂-agonists (SABA), such as albuterol (salbutamol) and terbutaline, are the most widely used and effective relievers for the treatment of asthma. When inhaled from metered-dose inhalers (MDIs) or dry powder inhalers, they are convenient, easy to use, rapid in onset, and without significant side effects. In addition to an acute bronchodilator effect, they effectively protect against various challenges, such as exercise, cold air, and allergen. They are the bronchodilators of choice for the treatment of acute severe asthma, for which the nebulized route of administration is as effective as intravenous use. The inhaled route of administration is preferable to the oral route because side effects are less common and also because it may be more effective (better access to surface cells such as mast cells). Short-acting, inhaled β₂-agonists should

not be used on a regular basis for the treatment of mild asthma and should be used only as required by symptoms. Increased use is an indication for the need for more antiinflammatory therapy. Oral β-agonists are very occasionally indicated as an additional bronchodilator in patients who cannot use inhalers properly. Slow-release preparations (such as slow-release albuterol and bambuterol) may be indicated in nocturnal asthma but are less useful than inhaled β-agonists because of an increased risk of side effects.

Choice of SABA

Several SABA are available (Figure 36-3). These drugs are as effective as nonselective agonists in their bronchodilator action, because airway effects are mediated only by β₂-receptors.

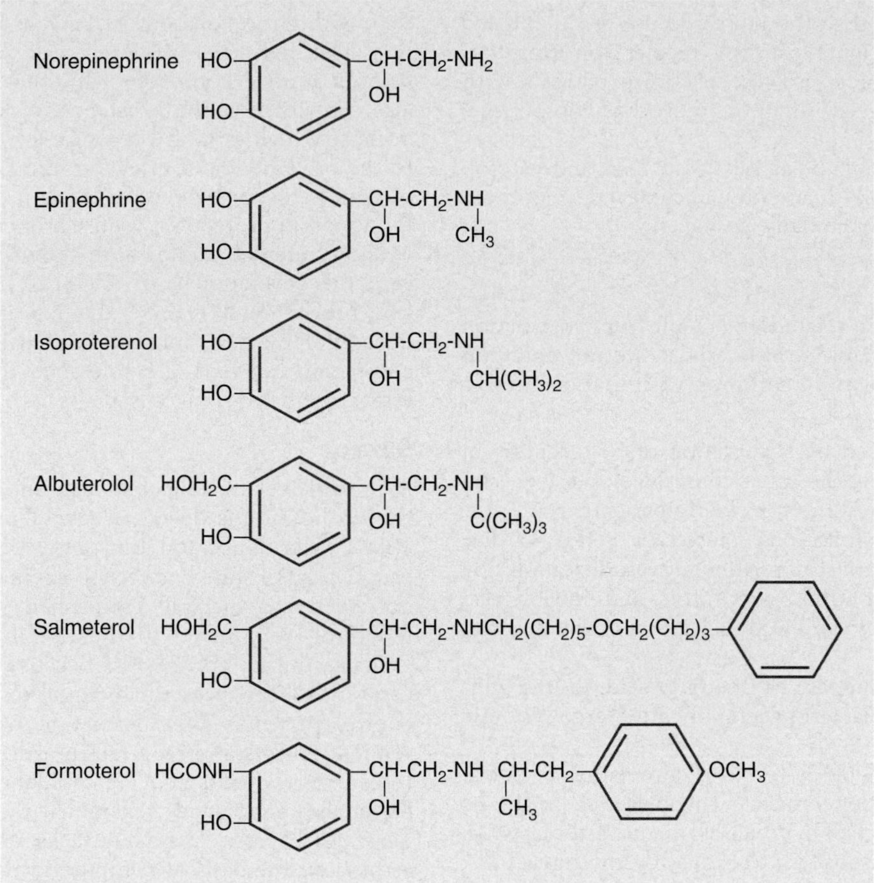

FIGURE 36-3 Structures of catecholamines showing the development of short- and long-acting selective β₂-agonists.

However, they are less likely to produce cardiac stimulation than isoproterenol, because β₁-receptors are stimulated relatively less. With the exception of rimiterol (which retains the catechol ring structure and is, therefore, susceptible to rapid metabolism), their duration of action is longer, because they are resistant to uptake and enzymatic degradation. There is little to choose between the various SABAs currently available; all are usable by inhalation and orally and have similar duration of action (usually 3–4 h, but less in severe asthma) and side effects. Differences in β₂-selectivity have been claimed but are not clinically important. Drugs in clinical use include albuterol, terbutaline, fenoterol, tulobuterol, rimiterol, and pirbuterol. It has been claimed that fenoterol is less β₂-selective than albuterol and terbutaline, which results in increased cardiovascular side effects, but this evidence is controversial, because all of these effects are mediated by β₂-receptors. The increased incidence of cardiovascular effects is more likely to be related to the greater effective dose of fenoterol used and perhaps to more rapid absorption into the circulation.

Long-Acting Inhaled β₂-Agonists

Long-acting inhaled β₂-agonists (LABA) include salmeterol and formoterol, which have a bronchodilator action of >12 h and also protect against bronchoconstriction for a similar period. Both are used as an add-on therapy in asthma patients not controlled on low doses of inhaled corticosteroids (beclomethasone dipropionate 400 μg daily or equivalent). Both improve asthma control (when given twice daily) compared with regular treatment with short-acting β₂-agonists four times daily. Salmeterol and formoterol are also used as a maintenance bronchodilator therapy in COPD. Both drugs are well tolerated. Tolerance to the bronchodilator effect of formoterol and the bronchoprotective effects of formoterol and salmeterol have been demonstrated, but a loss of protection does not occur, the tolerance does not seem to be progressive, and is of doubtful clinical significance.

Although both drugs have a similar duration of effect in clinical studies, there are some differences. Formoterol has a more rapid onset of action and is a fuller agonist than salmeterol but also does not have cumulative side effects when repeated doses are given. This means that formoterol, but not salmeterol, may be used as a reliever, and studies have shown it to be more effective than conventional SABA.

It is recommended that LABA should be used only in patients who are also prescribed inhaled corticosteroids (see later). Fixed-combination inhalers (fluticasone propionate/salmeterol or budesonide/formoterol) are now widely used and not only improve compliance and guard against discontinuation of the inhaled corticosteroids but may also give better control of asthma, because the two drugs are delivered to the same areas of the lung to allow positive molecular interactions between these two classes of drug. Recently, budesonide/formoterol has also been used as a reliever as well as for maintenance therapy twice daily in asthma patients. This single inhaler approach has been shown to be more effective in controlling asthma and particularly in reducing exacerbations. Its efficacy may be related to the increased use of the inhaled corticosteroid when patients use the inhaler for symptom relief. Combination inhalers are also useful in patients with COPD and are more effective than the individual components used alone.

Several ultra-long-acting β_2-agonists, such as indacaterol, which last for more than 24 h, are now in clinical development and may be suitable for once daily dosing.

Side Effects

Unwanted effects are dose related and result from stimulation of extrapulmonary β-receptors. Side effects are not common with inhaled therapy but more common with oral or intravenous administration:

- Muscle tremor caused by stimulation of β_2-receptors in the skeletal muscle is the most common side effect, and may be more troublesome for elderly patients.
- Tachycardia and palpitations caused by reflex cardiac stimulation secondary to peripheral vasodilatation, by direct stimulation of atrial β_2-receptors, and possibly also by stimulation of myocardial β_1-receptors as the doses of β_2-agonist increase.
- Metabolic effects (increase in free fatty acid, insulin, glucose, pyruvate, and lactate) seen only after large systemic doses.
- Hypokalemia caused by β_2-receptor stimulation of potassium entry into skeletal muscle (hypokalemia might be serious in the presence of hypoxia, as in acute asthma, when there may be a predisposition to cardiac dysrhythmias).
- Increased ventilation-perfusion ($\dot{V}/\dot{Q}$) mismatching by causing pulmonary vasodilatation in blood vessels previously constricted by hypoxia, which results in the shunting of blood to poorly ventilated areas and a fall in arterial oxygen tension—although, in practice, the effect of β-agonists on PaO_2 is usually very small, a fall of <0.7 kPa (<5 mmHg), occasionally in severe chronic airways obstruction it is large, but it may be prevented by giving additional inspired oxygen.

Tolerance

Continuous treatment with an agonist often leads to tolerance (subsensitivity, desensitization), which may be caused by uncoupling and/or downregulation of the receptor. Many studies of bronchial β-receptor function after prolonged therapy with β-agonists have been conducted. Tolerance of nonairway β-receptor responses, such as tremor, cardiovascular, and metabolic, is readily induced in normal and asthmatic subjects. Tolerance of human airway smooth muscle to β-agonists *in vitro* has been demonstrated, although the concentration of agonist necessary is high and the degree of desensitization is variable. Animal studies suggest that airway smooth muscle β-receptors may be more resistant to desensitization than β-receptors elsewhere because of a high receptor reserve; it is necessary to reduce β-receptor number by 95% before the maximal bronchodilator response is reduced. In normal subjects, bronchodilator tolerance has been demonstrated in some studies after high-dose, inhaled albuterol, but not in others. In asthmatic patients, tolerance to the bronchodilator effects of β-agonists has not usually been found. However, tolerance develops to the bronchoprotective effects of β_2-agonists, which is more marked with indirect constrictors, such as adenosine, allergen, and exercise (which activate mast cells), than with direct constrictors, such as histamine and methacholine. The high level of β_2-receptor gene expression in airway smooth muscle compared with that of peripheral lung may also contribute to the resistance to development of tolerance, because a high rate of β-receptor synthesis is likely. Tolerance to the bronchodilator effects of the LABA formoterol but not to salmeterol has been reported, but both LABA cause a small reduction in protection against bronchoconstrictors.

Experimental studies have shown that corticosteroids prevent the development of tolerance in airway smooth muscle and prevent and reverse the fall in pulmonary β-receptor density. However, inhaled corticosteroids do not seem to completely prevent the tolerance to the bronchoprotective effect of inhaled β_2-agonists.

Safety

A possible relationship between adrenergic drug therapy and the rise in asthma deaths in several countries during the early 1960s casts doubts on the safety of β-agonists. However, a causal relationship between β-agonist use and mortality has not been convincingly established. A particular β_2-agonist, fenoterol, was linked to the rise in asthma deaths in New Zealand during the 1980s, because significantly more fatal cases had been prescribed fenoterol than the case-matched control patients. This association was strengthened by subsequent studies and by a fall in asthma mortality when fenoterol was withdrawn. An epidemiologic study based in Saskatchewan, Canada, examined the links between death or near death from asthma attacks and drugs prescribed for asthma on the basis of computerized records of prescriptions. A marked increase in the risk of death was associated with high doses of all inhaled β-agonists. The risk was greater for fenoterol, but when the dose was adjusted to the equivalent dose of albuterol, no significant difference in the risk for these two drugs was found. The link between high β-agonist use and increased asthma mortality does not prove a causal association, because patients with more severe and poorly controlled asthma, and who are, therefore, more likely to have an increased risk of fatal attacks, are more likely to be using higher doses of β-agonist inhalers, and less likely to be using effective antiinflammatory treatment. Indeed, in patients who regularly used inhaled corticosteroids, there was no significant increase in the risk of death.

Regular use of inhaled β-agonists was also suggested to increase asthma morbidity. In a study carried out in New Zealand, the regular use of fenoterol was associated with worse control and an increase in airway hyperresponsiveness compared with patients who use fenoterol "on demand" for symptom control over a 6-month period. However, this was not found in several subsequent careful studies that used albuterol. Some evidence suggests that regularly inhaled albuterol may increase exercise-induced asthma and inflammation in asthmatic airways.

Recently, concerns have been raised about the safety of LABA in the management of asthma, and this is particularly relevant to the use of an LABA in treating exacerbations. A controlled trial of salmeterol versus placebo in more than 26,000 patients with asthma showed a small but significant excess of asthma mortality and life-threatening events in the LABA-treated patients, raising concerns that this treatment may be causally related to the increased deaths. Subgroup analysis showed that most of these deaths occurred in inner-city African-Americans, and it is very likely that this can be explained by failure to use concomitant inhaled corticosteroids as recommended in clinical practice. It is also possible that this could be explained by genetic differences in β₂-receptors in this group. A meta-analysis that included this study with other smaller studies, including studies with formoterol treatment, concluded that LABA may increase severe exacerbations and mortality but did not analyze whether this effect was not seen if patients were treated with concomitant inhaled corticosteroids.

Patients on high doses of β-agonists (>1 canister per month) and all patients on LABA should be treated with inhaled corticosteroids, and attempts should be made to reduce the daily dose of inhaled β-agonist. The use of LABA in a fixed combination with inhaled corticosteroids (ICS) ensures that LABA are not taken alone.

β₂-Receptor Polymorphisms

Several polymorphisms of the β₂-receptor have now been identified, and some affect the amino acid sequence of the receptor. Arg-Arg homozygosity at position 16 that occurs in approximately 15% of the Caucasian population is associated with a reduced bronchodilator response to β₂-agonists compared with the normal Arg-Gly variant. However, this is a small effect and unlikely to be of major clinical importance. It is possible that it could be relevant is some patients, however.

THEOPHYLLINE

Methylxanthines related to caffeine, such as theophylline, have been used in the treatment of asthma since 1930. Indeed, theophylline is still widely used in developing countries because it is inexpensive. Theophylline became more useful with the availability of rapid plasma assays and the introduction of reliable slow-release preparations. However, the frequency of side effects and the relative low efficacy of theophylline have recently led to reduced use, because β-agonists are far more effective as bronchodilators, and inhaled corticosteroids have a greater antiinflammatory effect. In patients who have severe asthma and COPD, it still remains a very useful drug, however. Evidence is increasing that theophylline has an antiinflammatory or immunomodulatory effect and may be effective in combination with inhaled corticosteroids.

Mode of Action

Although theophylline has been in clinical use for more than 70 years, its mechanism of action is uncertain and several modes of action have been proposed (Table 36-3):

- Inhibition of phosphodiesterases, which break down cAMP in the cell, leads to an increase in intracellular cAMP concentrations (Figure 36-4)—theophylline is a

TABLE 36-3 Mechanisms of Action of Theophylline

Phosphodiesterase inhibition

Adenosine receptor antagonism

Stimulation of catecholamine release

Mediator inhibition

Inhibition of intracellular calcium release

Increased histone deacetylase activity

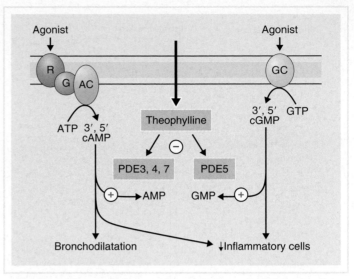

FIGURE 36-4 Theophylline as an inhibitor of phosphodiesterases. Theophylline is a weak phosphodiesterase (PDE) inhibitor and increases the concentrations of cyclic adenosine monophosphate and cyclic guanosine monophosphate in airway cells, which results in bronchodilatation and inhibition of inflammatory cells.

nonselective phosphodiesterase inhibitor, but the degree of inhibition is minor at the concentrations of theophylline within the new "therapeutic range." This is likely to account for the bronchodilator action of theophylline, however. Phosphodiesterase (PDE) inhibition may account for the most common side effects of theophylline, namely nausea and headaches.

- Adenosine receptor antagonism, because adenosine is a bronchoconstrictor in asthmatic patients through activation of mast cells—adenosine antagonism may account for some of the dangerous side effects of theophylline, such as central nervous system stimulation, cardiac arrhythmias, and diuresis.
- Increased secretion of adrenaline from the adrenal medulla, but the increase in plasma concentration is small and insufficient to account for any significant bronchodilator effect.

Recently a novel mechanism of action has been proposed to account for the antiinflammatory actions of theophylline at low plasma concentrations; this involves activation of histone deacetylases, nuclear enzymes that are recruited by corticosteroids to switch off inflammatory gene expression. This mechanism also accounts for the synergistic interaction with the antiinflammatory effect of corticosteroids and may lead to reversal of corticosteroid resistance in severe asthma and in COPD.

It is possible that any beneficial effect in asthma is related to its action on other cells (such as T lymphocytes or macrophages) or on airway microvascular leak and edema (Figure 36-5). Theophylline is a relatively ineffective bronchodilator, and its antiasthma effect is more likely to be explained by an antiinflammatory action, particularly at low plasma concentrations now used clinically. Theophylline is ineffective when given by inhalation until a therapeutic plasma concentration is reached. A placebo-controlled theophylline withdrawal study indicates that it seems to have an immunomodulatory effect and decreases the number of activated T lymphocytes in the airways, probably by blocking their trafficking from

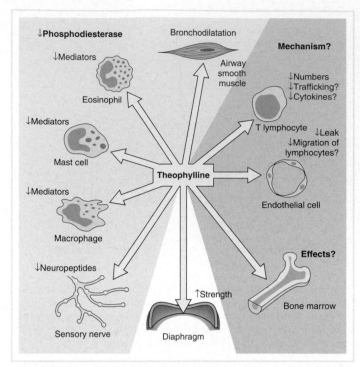

FIGURE 36-5 The multiple actions of theophylline in asthma. Some of these effects are probably mediated by phosphodiesterase inhibition, but others are so far unexplained.

TABLE 36-4 Factors That Affect Clearance of Theophylline	
Increased Clearance	**Decreased Clearance**
Enzyme induction—rifampin (rifampicin), phenobarbital (phenobarbitone), ethanol	Enzyme inhibition—cimetidine, erythromycin, ciprofloxacin, allopurinol, zileuton
Smoking—tobacco, marijuana	Congestive heart failure
High-protein, low-carbohydrate diet	Liver disease
	Pneumonia
Barbecued meat	Viral infection and vaccination
Childhood	High-carbohydrate diet
	Old age

the circulation. Theophylline also reduces eosinophils in bronchial biopsy specimens and induced sputum at low plasma concentrations. Theophylline reduces neutrophils in the sputum of COPD patients, whereas inhaled corticosteroids are ineffective in this respect. Theophylline withdrawal leads to a clinical deterioration in COPD patients, as in asthma.

Clinical Use

In patients who have acute asthma, intravenous aminophylline is less effective than nebulized β-agonists and is, therefore, reserved for the few patients who fail to respond to β-agonists. Theophylline should not be added routinely to nebulized β-agonists, because it does not increase the bronchodilator response and may only increase their side effects. There is no evidence that theophylline is useful in exacerbations of COPD.

Theophylline has little or no effect on bronchomotor tone in normal airways but reverses bronchoconstriction in asthmatic patients, although it is less effective than inhaled β-agonists and is more likely to have unwanted effects. Theophylline and β-agonists have additive effects, even if true synergy is not seen, and evidence exists that theophylline may provide an additional bronchodilator effect even when maximally effective doses of β-agonist have been given. Thus, if adequate bronchodilatation is not achieved with a β-agonist alone, theophylline may be added to the maintenance therapy with benefit. Theophylline may be useful in some patients who have nocturnal asthma, because slow-release preparations can provide therapeutic concentrations overnight and are more effective than slow-release β-agonists. Although theophylline is less effective than a β-agonist and corticosteroids, some asthmatic patients seem to derive particular benefit. Even patients on high-dose inhaled corticosteroids and oral corticosteroids may show deterioration in lung function when theophylline is withdrawn. Addition of low-dose theophylline is as or more effective than doubling the dose of inhaled corticosteroids in patients not controlled on low doses of inhaled corticosteroids. However, it is less effective as an add-on therapy than an LABA, although it is less expensive and so may be a preferred option in countries where medication costs are limited.

Theophylline is readily and reliably absorbed from the gastrointestinal tract, but many factors affect plasma clearance and, therefore, plasma concentration, so the drug is relatively difficult to use (Table 36-4).

Many different formulations of slow-release theophylline or aminophylline are available and differ in their pharmacokinetic profile. Several preparations are available for twice-daily administration, and also once-daily preparations. Twice-daily administration may be preferable with a higher dose given at night to prevent nocturnal bronchoconstriction, whereas a lower dose is needed in the day, because inhaled β-agonists may be used as additional bronchodilators. The frequency of side effects may be reduced. Caution must be observed when switching from one slow-release preparation to another.

Recent studies suggest that low-dose theophylline (which give plasma concentrations of 5–10 mg/L) effectively controls asthma, and such doses are below the previously recommended doses for theophylline on the basis of plasma concentrations needed for bronchodilatation (10–20 mg/L).

Side Effects

Unwanted effects of theophylline are usually related to plasma concentration and tend to occur when plasma levels exceed 20 mg/L. However, some patients develop side effects even at low plasma concentrations. To some extent, side effects may be reduced by gradually increasing the dose until therapeutic concentrations are achieved. The most common side effects are headache, nausea and vomiting, abdominal discomfort, and restlessness (Table 36-5). Increased acid secretion and diuresis may also occur. Concern that theophylline, even at therapeutic concentrations, may lead to behavioral disturbance and learning difficulties in school children is not supported by convincing evidence. At high concentrations, convulsions, cardiac arrhythmias, and death may occur.

ANTICHOLINERGICS

Atropine is a naturally occurring compound that was introduced for the treatment of asthma but, because of side effects (particularly drying of secretions), less soluble quaternary compounds (e.g., ipratropium bromide, tiotropium bromide) were

TABLE 36-5 Side Effects of Theophylline
Nausea and vomiting
Headaches
Gastric discomfort
Diuresis
Behavioral disturbance (?)
Cardiac arrhythmias
Epileptic seizures

developed. These compounds are topically active and are not significantly absorbed from the respiratory tract or from the gastrointestinal tract.

Mode of Action

Anticholinergics are specific antagonists of muscarinic receptors and inhibit cholinergic nerve–induced bronchoconstriction. A small degree of resting bronchomotor tone is caused by tonic cholinergic nerve impulses, which release acetylcholine in the vicinity of airway smooth muscle, and cholinergic reflex bronchoconstriction may be initiated by irritants, cold air, and stress. Although anticholinergics afford protection against acute challenge by sulfur dioxide, inert dusts, cold air, and emotional factors, they are less effective against antigen challenge, exercise, and fog. This is not surprising, because anticholinergic drugs only inhibit reflex cholinergic bronchoconstriction and have no significant blocking effect on the direct effects of inflammatory mediators, such as histamine

and leukotrienes, on bronchial smooth muscle (Figure 36-6). Furthermore, cholinergic antagonists probably have little or no effect on mast cells, microvascular leak, or the chronic inflammatory response. For these reasons, in patients who have asthma, anticholinergics are less effective as bronchodilators than β₂-agonists. By contrast, anticholinergics are the bronchodilators of choice in COPD.

Clinical Use

In asthmatic subjects, anticholinergic drugs are less effective as bronchodilators than β₂-agonists and offer less-efficient protection against various bronchial challenges, although their duration of action is longer. These drugs may be more effective in older patients who have asthma and in whom an element of fixed airway obstruction is present. Nebulized anticholinergic drugs are effective in acute severe asthma, although they are less effective than β-agonists in this situation. Nevertheless, in the acute and chronic treatment of asthma, anticholinergic drugs may have an additive effect with β-agonists and should, therefore, be considered when control of asthma is not adequate with β-agonists, particularly if there are problems with theophylline or inhaled β-agonists give troublesome tremor in elderly patients. The time course of bronchodilatation with anticholinergic drugs is slower than with β-agonists, reaching a peak only 1 h after inhalation but persists for more than 6 h.

In COPD, anticholinergic drugs are even more effective than β-agonists. Their relatively greater effect in chronic obstructive airways disease than in asthma may be explained by an inhibitory effect on vagal tone, which, although not necessarily being increased in COPD, may be the only reversible

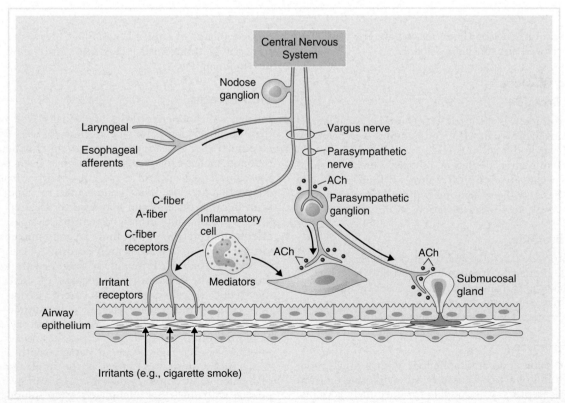

FIGURE 36-6 Cholinergic control of airway smooth muscle. Preganglionic and postganglionic parasympathetic nerves release acetylcholine (ACh) and can be activated by airway and extrapulmonary afferent nerves. Note that mediators released from inflammatory cells directly activate airway smooth muscle cells, as well as a cholinergic reflex, so that anticholinergics are less effective than β₂-agonists as bronchodilators in asthma, because the latter counteract the effect of all bronchoconstrictors.

FIGURE 36-7 Cholinergic control of airways in patients who have chronic obstructive pulmonary disease (COPD). The normal airway has a certain degree of vagal cholinergic tone caused by tonic release of acetylcholine, which is blocked by muscarinic antagonists. This effect may be exaggerated in patients who have COPD, because of fixed narrowing of the airways as a result of geometric factors. Thus, anticholinergic drugs have a greater bronchodilator effect in COPD than in normal airways.

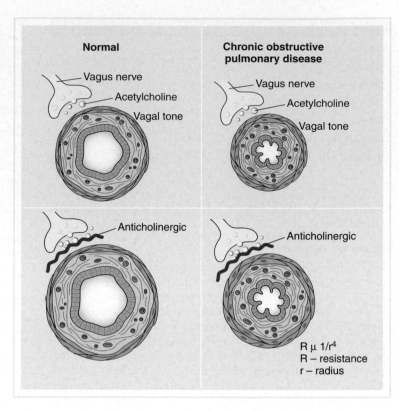

element of airway obstruction that is exaggerated by geometric factors in a narrowed airway (Figure 36-7).

Therapeutic Choices

Ipratropium Bromide

Ipratropium bromide was the most widely used anticholinergic inhaler and is available as an MDI and nebulized preparation. The onset of bronchodilatation is relatively slow and is usually maximal 30–60 min after inhalation, but may persist for more than 6 h. It is usually given by MDI three to four times daily on a regular basis, rather than intermittently for symptom relief, in view of its slow onset of action.

Oxitropium Bromide

Oxitropium bromide is a quaternary, anticholinergic bronchodilator that is similar to ipratropium bromide in terms of receptor blockade. It is available in higher doses by inhalation, and its effect may, therefore, be more prolonged, so it may be useful in some patients who have nocturnal asthma.

Tiotropium Bromide

Tiotropium bromide is an anticholinergic with a much more prolonged duration of action caused by slow dissociation from muscarinic M₃ receptors. It is suitable for once-daily administration and is superior to four times daily ipratropium bromide. It reduces gas trapping in COPD, reduces exertional dyspnea, and improves exercise performance. It is now the

bronchodilator of choice in COPD. Several other long-acting muscarinic antagonists (LAMA) are now in clinical development.

Side Effects

Inhaled anticholinergic drugs are usually well tolerated, and there is no evidence for any decline in responsiveness with continued use. On stopping inhaled anticholinergics, a small, rebound increase in responsiveness has been described, but the clinical relevance of this is uncertain. Atropine has side effects that are dose related and caused by cholinergic antagonism in other systems and may lead to dryness of the mouth, blurred vision, and urinary retention. Systemic side effects after taking ipratropium bromide are very uncommon, because virtually no systemic absorption occurs.

Several studies of mucus secretion with anticholinergic drugs have been carried out because of concern that they may reduce secretion and lead to more viscous mucus. Atropine reduces mucociliary clearance in normal subjects and in patients who have asthma and chronic bronchitis, but ipratropium bromide, even in high doses, has no detectable effect in either normal subjects or in patients with airway disease. A significant, unwanted effect is the unpleasant bitter taste of inhaled ipratropium, which may contribute to poor compliance with this drug. Nebulized ipratropium bromide may precipitate glaucoma in elderly patients, a direct effect of the nebulized drug on the eye, which is prevented by nebulization with a mouthpiece rather than a facemask.

Reports of paradoxical bronchoconstriction with ipratropium bromide, particularly when given by nebulizer, were largely explained by the hypotonicity of the nebulizer solution and by antibacterial additives, such as benzalkonium chloride. Nebulizer solutions free of these problems are less likely to cause bronchoconstriction. Occasionally, bronchoconstriction may occur with ipratropium bromide given by MDI. It is possible that this results from blockade of prejunctional M_2-receptors on airway cholinergic nerves, which normally inhibit acetylcholine release. The most common side effect with tiotropium bromide is dryness of the mouth, which occurs in ~10% of patients.

CROMONES

Cromones include cromolyn sodium (sodium cromoglycate) and nedocromil sodium. Cromolyn sodium is a derivative of khellin, an Egyptian herbal remedy that was found to protect against allergen challenge without bronchodilator effect. Nedocromil sodium is structurally related and has very similar clinical effects, although some evidence indicates that it is more potent.

Mode of Action

Initial investigations indicated that cromolyn sodium inhibited the release of mediators by allergen in passively sensitized human and animal lungs and inhibited passive cutaneous anaphylaxis in the rat, although it had no effect in guinea pig. This activity was attributed to stabilization of the mast-cell membrane, and thus cromolyn sodium was classified as a mast-cell stabilizer. However, cromolyn sodium has a rather low potency in stabilizing mast cells of the human lung, and other drugs more potent in this respect have little or no effect in clinical asthma. This has raised doubts that mast-cell stabilization is the major mode of action of cromolyn sodium.

Cromones potently inhibit bronchoconstriction induced by sulfur dioxide, metabisulfite, and bradykinin, which are believed to activate sensory nerves in the airways. In dogs, cromones suppress firing of unmyelinated C-fiber nerve endings, which reinforces the view that they might suppress sensory nerve activation and thus neurogenic inflammation. Cromones have variable inhibitory actions on other inflammatory cells that may participate in allergic inflammation, including macrophages and eosinophils. *In vivo* cromolyn sodium can block the early response to allergen (which is mediated by mast cells) but also the late response and airway hyperresponsiveness, which are more likely to be mediated by macrophage and eosinophil interactions.

The molecular mechanism of action of cromones is not understood, but recent evidence suggests that they may block a particular type of chloride channel that may be expressed in sensory nerves, mast cells, and other inflammatory cells. It remains unclear why cromones are effective only in allergic inflammation.

Current Use

Cromolyn sodium is a prophylactic treatment and needs to be given regularly. It protects against various indirect bronchoconstrictor stimuli, such as exercise and fog. It is only effective in mild asthma but does not seem to be effective in all patients, and no sure way of predicting the patients likely to respond has been established. Indeed, a systematic review

of clinical studies of cromolyn in children concluded that it provided little benefit. One reason for the discrepancy between its beneficial effects in various indirect challenges and its poor efficacy in clinical practice is likely to be its short duration of action (~2 h), and it needs to be given at least 4 times daily. Because of its poor efficacy and high cost, it is now used less and less, particularly as low doses of inhaled corticosteroids have been shown to be much more effective and just as safe in children with mild asthma.

In clinical practice, nedocromil has a similar efficacy to cromolyn sodium and is, therefore, indicated in patients who have mild asthma, but the unpleasant taste makes cromolyn sodium preferable to many patients. Cromones are far less effective than inhaled corticosteroids and are not now routinely recommended in guidelines. No place exists for cromones in the management of COPD.

Side Effects

Cromolyn sodium is one of the safest drugs available, and side effects are extremely rare. The dry powder inhaler may cause throat irritation, coughing, and (occasionally) wheezing, but this is usually prevented by prior administration of a β-agonist inhaler. Very rarely, a transient rash and urticaria are seen, and a few cases of pulmonary eosinophilia have been reported, all of which arise from hypersensitivity. Side effects with nedocromil are not usually a problem, although some patients have noticed a sensation of flushing after the use of the inhaler. Many patients find the bitter taste unpleasant, but a menthol-flavored version is now available and seems to overcome this problem.

ANTILEUKOTRIENES

Antileukotrienes are a relatively new class of antiasthma agent.

Mode of Action

Elevated levels of cysteinyl leukotrienes (cys-LTs: LTC_4, LTD_4, LTE_4) are detected in bronchoalveolar lavage fluid and elevated LTE_4 levels in the urine of asthmatic subjects. Cys-LTs are generated from arachidonic acid by the rate-limiting enzyme 5'-lipoxygenase (5-LO; Figure 36-8). Cys-LTs are potent constrictors of human airways *in vitro* and *in vivo*, cause airway microvascular leakage in animals, and stimulate airway mucus secretion (Figure 36-9). These effects are all mediated in human airways by cys-LT_1 receptors, and potent cys-LT_1 antagonists (montelukast, zafirlukast, pranlukast) are now available. Antileukotrienes reduce allergen-induced, exercise-induced, and cold air–induced asthma by approximately 50–70%, and inhibit aspirin-induced responses in aspirin-sensitive patients with asthma almost completely. The only 5-lipoxygenase inhibitor tested clinically is zileuton, which is not currently available. Antileukotrienes have also been shown to have weak antiinflammatory effects and may reduce eosinophilic inflammation, which may be provoked by cys-LTs.

Clinical Use

Antileukotrienes may have a small and variable bronchodilator effect, indicating that leukotrienes may contribute to baseline bronchoconstriction in asthma. Long-term administration reduces asthma symptoms and the need for rescue β₂-agonists and improves lung function. The effects are significantly less than with inhaled corticosteroids in terms of symptom control,

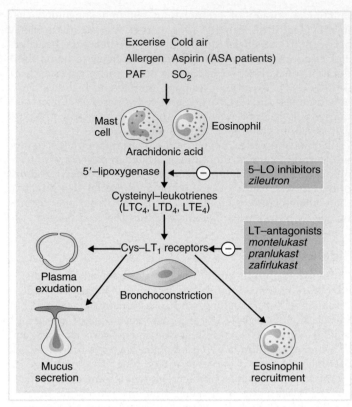

FIGURE 36-8 Cellular origin and effects of cysteinyl leukotrienes.

improvement in lung function, and reduction in exacerbations. Antileukotrienes may be useful in patients whose asthma is not controlled on inhaled corticosteroids and are as effective as doubling the dose of inhaled corticosteroids. They are effective in some, but not all, patients with aspirin-sensitive asthma. Patients differ in their response to antileukotrienes, but it is impossible to predict which patients will respond best.

A major advantage of antileukotrienes is that they are orally active, and this is likely to improve compliance with long-term therapy. However, they are expensive, and a trial of therapy is indicated to determine which patients will benefit most. Antileukotrienes have no place in the management of COPD.

Side Effects

Side effects are uncommon. Some drugs produce mild liver dysfunction, so liver function tests are important. Several cases of Churg–Strauss syndrome (systemic vasculitis with eosinophilia and asthma) have been observed in patients taking antileukotrienes, but this is very likely to be explained by a concomitant reduction in oral corticosteroids (made possible by the antileukotriene), which allows the vasculitis to flare up.

KETOTIFEN

Ketotifen is described as a prophylactic antiasthma compound. Its predominant effect is histamine H_1-receptor antagonism, which accounts for its sedative effect. Ketotifen has little effect in clinical asthma—in acute challenge, on airway hyperresponsiveness, or on clinical symptoms. A long-term placebo-controlled trial of oral ketotifen in children who had mild asthma showed no significant clinical benefit. It is claimed that ketotifen has disease-modifying effects if started early in asthma in children and that it may even prevent the development of asthma in atopic children. More carefully controlled studies are needed to assess the validity of these claims.

IMMUNOSUPPRESSIVE OR CORTICOSTEROID-SPARING THERAPY

Immunosuppressive therapy has been considered in asthma when other treatments have been unsuccessful or to reduce the dose of oral corticosteroids required. Immunosuppressives are, therefore, indicated in only a very small proportion of asthmatic patients (<1%) at present.

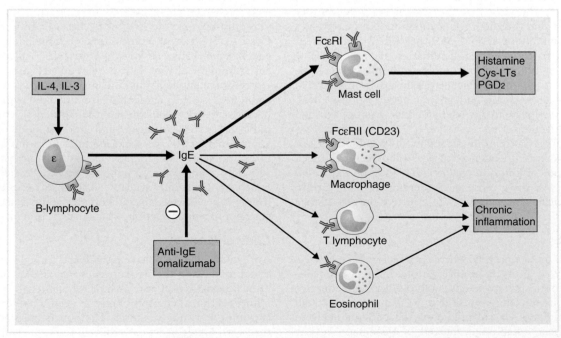

FIGURE 36-9 Inhibition of IgE by omalizumab.

Methotrexate

Low-dose methotrexate (15 mg weekly) has a corticosteroid-sparing effect in asthma and may be indicated when oral corticosteroids are contraindicated because of unacceptable side effects (e.g., in postmenopausal women when osteoporosis is a problem). Some patients show better responses than others, but whether a patient will have a useful corticosteroid-sparing effect is unpredictable. In some studies, no useful beneficial effect is reported. Side effects of methotrexate are relatively common and include nausea (reduced if methotrexate is given as a weekly injection), blood dyscrasias, and hepatic damage. Careful monitoring of such patients (monthly blood counts and liver enzymes) is essential. Methotrexate has been disappointing in the clinical experience of most physicians.

Gold

Gold has long been used in the treatment of chronic arthritis. Anecdotal evidence suggests that it may also be useful in asthma, and it has been used in Japan for many years. A controlled trial of an oral gold preparation (auranofin) demonstrated some corticosteroid-sparing effect in chronic asthmatic patients maintained on oral corticosteroids. Side effects such as skin rashes and nephropathy are a limiting factor.

Cyclosporin A

Cyclosporin A is active against $CD4^+$ lymphocytes and is, therefore, potentially useful in asthma, in which these cells are implicated. A trial of low-dose oral cyclosporin A in patients who had corticosteroid-dependent asthma indicated that it can improve control of symptoms in patients who have severe asthma and are taking oral corticosteroids, but other trials have been unimpressive, and a systematic review has concluded that its poor and unpredictable efficacy is outweighed by the risk of side effects. Its use is limited by severe side effects, such as nephrotoxicity and hypertension, which are common. In clinical practice, it is very disappointing as a corticosteroid-sparing agent and has largely been abandoned.

Intravenous Immunoglobulin

When high doses were used (2 g/kg), intravenous immunoglobulin was reported to have corticosteroid-sparing effects in corticosteroid-dependent asthma, although in controlled trials at lower doses it is ineffective. This is an extremely expensive treatment that cannot be recommended.

Anti-IgE

Omalizumab is a blocking antibody that neutralizes circulating IgE without binding to cell-bound IgE and, thus, inhibits IgE-mediated reactions. This also inhibits the production of IgE from B-lymphocytes, resulting in a marked downregulation of high-affinity IgE receptors on mast cells. This treatment has been shown to significantly reduce the number of exacerbations (by up to 50%) in patients with severe asthma and may improve asthma control and reduce the need for corticosteroids while having little effect on airway hyperresponsiveness and lung function. However, the treatment is very expensive and is only suitable for highly selected patients who are not controlled on maximal doses of inhaled therapy and have a circulating IgE within a specified range. Patients should be given a 3–4 month trial of therapy to show objective benefit. The treatment is only likely to be cost-effective in patients who have frequent hospitalization for acute severe asthma. Omalizumab is usually given as a subcutaneous injection every 2–4 weeks and seems to have no significant side effects.

Specific Immunotherapy

Specific immunotherapy that uses injected extracts of pollens or house dust mite has not been very effective in controlling asthma and may cause anaphylaxis. A meta-analysis of immunotherapy in asthma compared with placebo shows modest clinical efficacy. One problem is that most asthma patients are sensitized to several environmental allergens, but immunotherapy against multiple allergens has not been successful. Side effects may be reduced by sublingual dosing, but sublingual immunotherapy is rather poorly effective in asthma for the same reason. Specific immunotherapy is not recommended in most asthma treatment guidelines because of lack of evidence of clinical efficacy and lack of studies comparing it with traditional therapy, particularly inhaled corticosteroids.

FUTURE TRENDS IN THERAPY

Asthma

Currently available therapy for asthma is highly effective if used correctly, but there are some unmet needs. For example, there is a need for more effective oral controllers in the treatment of mild asthma, particularly in children, and for more effective add-on therapies in patients with severe asthma who are not controlled by maximal inhaled therapy. Many new therapeutic approaches to the treatment of asthma based on a better understanding of the disease may be possible, yet there have been few new drugs to reach the clinic. β₂-Agonists are by far the most effective bronchodilator drugs, and it is unlikely that more effective bronchodilators could be discovered. For many patients, a fixed combination inhaler of LABA and corticosteroid inhaler is a convenient and effective way to control asthma, particularly when used as a reliever, as well as a controller. Several new fixed combination inhalers with formoterol and different corticosteroids are now in development, so there is likely to be a wide choice of brands available. Once-daily β₂-agonists and corticosteroids are also in clinical development.

The ideal drug for asthma is probably a tablet that could be administered once daily to improve compliance. It should have no side effects, which means that it should be specific for the abnormality of asthma (or allergy). So far, inhibitors of specific cytokines have proved to be ineffective, and a more generalized antiinflammatory treatment is needed. Phopshodiesterase-4 inhibitors may be useful, but so far orally administered drugs have been limited by side effects, so that inhaled preparations are now in development. Vaccines or bacterial products to stimulate protective (TH1) immunity are also in development, but so far clinical results have proved to be disappointing. The possibility of developing a "cure" for asthma seems remote, but when more is known about the genetic abnormalities of asthma, a search for such a therapy may be feasible.

Chronic Obstructive Pulmonary Disease

No current available therapy alters the progression of COPD, and there is no evidence that corticosteroids are effective. Future approaches may include drugs that inhibit the characteristic neutrophilic inflammation of COPD (LTB₄ antagonists, interleukin-8 antagonists, phosphodiesterase-4 inhibitors), more potent antioxidants (glutathione analogs), and drugs that inhibit proteases (neutrophil elastase inhibitors, matrix metalloproteinase inhibitors). The molecular mechanisms of corticosteroid resistance in COPD are now better understood, and an alternative approach is to develop drugs that reverse this resistance. The testing of these new drugs is difficult, because long-term studies will be necessary to demonstrate a reduction in the progressive decline in lung function.

SUGGESTED READINGS

Barnes PJ: New drugs for asthma. Nat Rev Drug Discov 2004; 3:831–844.

Barnes PJ: Theophylline: new perspectives on an old drug. Am J Respir Crit Care Med 2003; 167:813–818.

Barnes PJ, Hansel TT: Prospects for new drugs for chronic obstructive pulmonary disease. Lancet 2004; 364:985–996.

Capra V, Ambrosio M, Riccioni G, Rovati GE: Cysteinyl-leukotriene receptor antagonists: present situation and future opportunities. Curr Med Chem 2006; 13:3213–3226.

Global Initiative for Asthma: Global strategy for asthma management and prevention. NHLBI/WHO Workshop Report. 2006; *www.ginasthma. com*

GOLD. Global Initiative for Chronic Obstructive Lung Disease (GOLD): Global strategy for the diagnosis, management and prevention of COPD. GOLD, 2006; www.goldcopd.com

Kips JC, Pauwels RA: Long-acting inhaled β_2-agonist therapy in asthma. Am J Respir Crit Care Med 2001; 164:923–932.

Mundy C, Kirkpatrick P: Tiotropium bromide. Nat Rev Drug Discov 2004; 3:643–644.

Nelson HS, Dorinsky PM: Safety of long-acting beta-agonists. Ann Intern Med 2006; 145:706–710.

O'Byrne PM, Parameswaran K: Pharmacological management of mild or moderate persistent asthma. Lancet 2006; 368:794–803.

Rennard SI: Treatment of stable chronic obstructive pulmonary disease. Lancet 2004; 364:791–802.

Walker S, Monteil M, Phelan K, *et al*: Anti-IgE for chronic asthma in adults and children. Cochrane Database Syst Rev 2006; 19:CD003559.

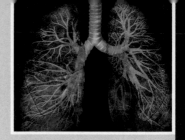

37 Corticosteroids

RYAN M. MCGHAN

INTRODUCTION

Corticosteroids (CS, also known as glucocorticoids) are the foundation of antiinflammatory therapy in modern medicine. They are used to treat inflammatory diseases throughout the body. The remarkable therapeutic potential of CS was acknowledged with the 1950 Nobel Prize for Medicine and Physiology, awarded only 2 years after the description of their efficacy in treating rheumatoid arthritis. CS were applied to the treatment of inflammatory diseases of the lungs as early as 1949. The development of inhaled CS (ICS), providing local antiinflammatory properties while minimizing systemic side effects, has revolutionized the care of patients with asthma, and this mode of therapy has recently been shown to reduce acute exacerbations of selected patients with chronic obstructive pulmonary disease (COPD).

This chapter will review the mechanisms underlying the therapeutic antiinflammatory properties of CS and the pharmacokinetics of these drugs and their toxicities. Some of the most commonly used systemic and inhaled CS will be compared, with particular attention to dosing equivalence.

PHARMACODYNAMICS

Cellular, Tissue, and Systemic Effects

The primary therapeutic effects of CS result from their action on white blood cells, although they also affect other cells in inflamed tissues and throughout the body. CS inhibit the recruitment of inflammatory cells by reducing chemotaxis and adhesion, decrease phagocytosis and respiratory burst activity, and decrease the production of inflammatory mediators such as cytokines and eicosanoids. In circulating blood, CS induce lymphopenia through lytic effects on lymphocytes and neutrophilia through decreased adhesion and demargination of polymorphonuclear cells.

CS also influence blood flow through their effects on endothelial and smooth muscle cells, generally promoting vasoconstriction by potentiating the action of catecholamines and decreasing the release of nitric oxide. In airway epithelium, CS may reduce shedding of epithelial cells and the production of mucus and of cytokines such as TGF-β. They may also interfere with airway remodeling in chronic inflammatory states by reducing fibroblast activity, collagen production, basement membrane thickness, and smooth muscle cell proliferation, although some of these findings are controversial.

CS decrease both pulmonary and systemic inflammation in both asthma and COPD; ICS, particularly in combination with a long-acting β_2-agonists (LABA) reduce airway inflammation detected by endobronchial biopsy (Figure 37-1). In addition, both inhaled and systemic CS reduce systemic inflammation as reflected by C-reactive protein levels in patients with COPD (Figure 37-2).

Molecular Mechanisms

CS act primarily by binding to intracellular glucocorticoid receptors that, in turn, regulate gene expression through glucocorticoid response elements (GREs). Glucocorticoids diffuse across the cell membrane, where they bind to glucocorticoid receptor-α. Binding of glucocorticoid to the glucocorticoid receptor causes dissociation of the receptor from chaperone proteins and promotes translocation of the receptor to the nucleus. Once inside the nucleus, glucocorticoid receptors dimerize and bind to GREs in the promoter regions of steroid-responsive genes, altering gene transcription (Figure 37-3).

The number of genes directly regulated by GREs is small and may not explain the entire spectrum of biologic activity of CS. Clearly, direct regulation of gene expression through GREs may initiate a cascade of events resulting in downstream effects on the expression of genes without GREs. Other non-genomic mechanisms of corticosteroid activity have been described, including direct interaction between glucocorticoid receptors and transcription factors, coactivators, and signal transduction pathways, including AP-1 and the p-65 subunit of NF-κ-B (see Figure 37-3). CS can also decrease protein synthesis by decreasing the stability of mRNA.

Recent work has focused on the role of CS in regulating gene expression through their effect on histone acetylation and chromatin compaction. Inflammatory signals cause chromatin unwinding by histone acetyl-transferase activity. CS can directly inhibit histone acetyl-transferases and recruit histone deacetylases (HDACs) to their site of action seemingly independent of glucocorticoid receptor binding to GREs. CS interact with specific HDACs (such as HDAC2) that target specific histone proteins (e.g., histone H4), regulating expression of particular regions of the genome. The net effect of CS is to decrease histone acetylation, promoting chromatin compaction and downregulation of inflammatory gene expression (Figure 37-4).

Many of the antiinflammatory properties of CS are independent of receptor dimerization and binding to GREs. A transgenic mouse model has been developed with mutant glucocorticoid receptors that bind CS without dimerizing; in these mice, CS still inhibit inflammation *in vivo* and *in vitro*. If the antiinflammatory properties of CS can be produced by glucocorticoid receptor monomers, but their side effects are regulated by dimer binding to GREs, drugs might be developed with greater antiinflammatory activity and reduced toxicity. Such "dissociated" CS are under development.

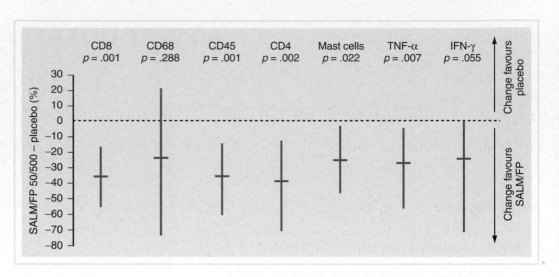

FIGURE 37-1 Inhaled corticosteroid and long-acting beta-agonist reduces airway inflammation in COPD. Endobronchial biopsies were obtained before and after 12 weeks of treatment. This figure demonstrates the reduction in inflammatory cells and cytokines with combination therapy compared with placebo. (Reproduced with permission from Barnes NC, Qiu Y, Pavord ID, et al: Antiinflammatory effects of salmeterol/fluticasone propionate in chronic obstructive lung disease. Am J Respir Crit Care Med 2006; 173[7]:736–743.)

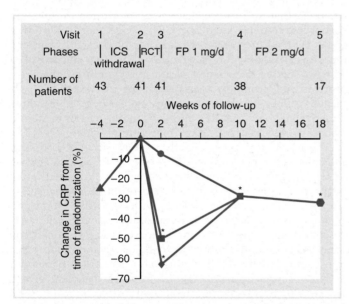

FIGURE 37-2 Inhaled and systemic corticosteroids reduce markers of systemic inflammation in COPD. Patients stopped inhaled corticosteroids (time, 4 weeks) and were then randomly assigned to 2 weeks of inhaled fluticasone (1000 μg/day, *square*), oral prednisone (30 mg/day, *diamond*), or placebo (*circle*). Both oral and inhaled corticosteroids significantly reduced ($P < .05$) C-reactive protein (CRP); this reduction was sustained after an additional 16 weeks of open-labeled fluticasone (1000 μg/day weeks 2–10, and 2000 μg/day weeks 10–18). (Reproduced with permission from Sin DD, Lacy P, York E, Man SF: Effects of fluticasone on systemic markers of inflammation in chronic obstructive pulmonary disease. Am J Respir Crit Care Med 2004; 170[7]:760–765.)

Nongenomic Effects

When used to treat acute inflammatory states of the lung (e.g., acute exacerbations of asthma), the time-course of clinical improvement is 4–24 h after administration, consistent with alterations occurring in gene transcription and protein synthesis. However, inhaled CS seem to have biologic activity within minutes of administration, raising the possibility that they may work through nongenomic effects. The most striking acute effect of topical CS is decrease in mucosal blood flow. Additional effects include anesthesia and alterations in smooth muscle tone. The exact mechanisms underpinning these

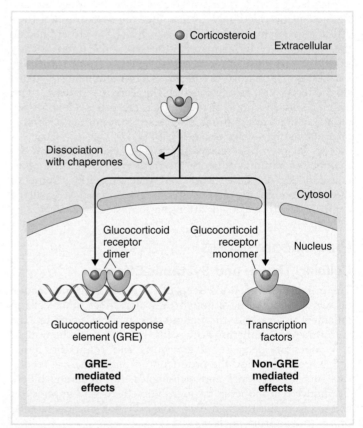

FIGURE 37-3 Molecular mechanisms of corticosteroid action. Corticosteroids diffuse readily across the cell membrane, where they bind glucocorticoid receptors. Corticosteroid binding causes dissociation of chaperone proteins (such as heat shock protein 90); this allows translocation of the glucocorticoid receptor to the nucleus. Once in the nucleus, the glucocorticoid receptor can dimerize and bind to glucocorticoid response elements (*GREs*), or it can bind to other transcription factors (such as activator protein 1 and nuclear factor κ-B) as a monomer.

nongenomic effects are not clear, but may include interaction with membrane-bound or cytoplasmic receptors, as well as nonspecific interactions with cell membranes. These acute, nongenomic effects may have clinical relevance. Although systemic CS are the mainstay of therapy in acute exacerbations of

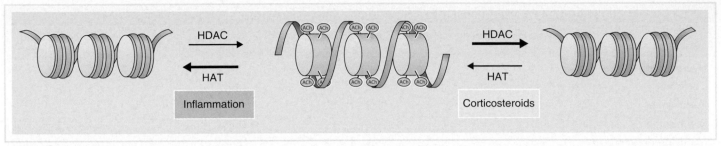

FIGURE 37-4 Effects of inflammation and corticosteroids on chromatin compaction. Inflammation promotes acetylation of histones by increasing histone acetyltransferase *(HAT)* activity; in addition, histone deacetylase *(HDAC)* activity is decreased in inflammatory lung diseases, including asthma and COPD. Corticosteroids promote chromatin compaction and silencing of gene transcription by inhibiting HAT activity and by increasing HDAC activity.

asthma, recent articles suggest that frequent, high-dose administration of inhaled CS might provide additional benefit, potentially through nongenomic mechanisms.

Synergy with Bronchodilators

Molecular biology provides a rationale for administrating combinations of inhaled CS and bronchodilators. CS upregulate β_2-adrenoreceptors and prevent downregulation of β_2-adrenoreceptors in response to agonists (i.e., tachyphylaxis). β_2-Agonists, in turn, increase translocation of glucocorticoid receptors from the cytoplasm to their site of action in the nucleus. CS may also be effective in combination with theophylline, because theophylline activates HDAC and may accentuate CS action through chromatin compaction.

Steroid Resistance

Although CS have potent antiinflammatory effects in a number of different tissues and disease states, some patients may be relatively resistant to the therapeutic effects of these drugs while remaining sensitive to their toxic side effects.

Several mechanisms of corticosteroid resistance have been described. Inactivating mutations in the glucocorticoid receptor occur in rare cases of familial corticosteroid resistance. These patients will typically have no evidence of corticosteroid side effects. In patients who are corticosteroid resistant but who lack evidence of corticosteroid side effects, one should also consider nonadherence to the medication.

More commonly, corticosteroid resistance is acquired during the course of inflammatory diseases and may, in fact, be induced selectively in inflamed tissues through the action of inflammatory cytokines. Alternative splicing of the glucocorticoid receptor may result in accumulation of β-glucocorticoid receptors that do not bind CS and that decrease the activity of steroid-bound α-glucocorticoid receptors through formation of heterodimers and through competitive binding to GREs. Additional mechanisms may include phosphorylation of glucocorticoid receptors that alter their biologic activity and acquired HDAC deficiency, resulting in decreased corticosteroid-induced chromatin compaction.

PHARMACOKINETICS

Systemic

Oral CS are readily absorbed by the gastrointestinal tract. The degree of first-pass hepatic elimination varies, with oral bioavailability ranging from 60–90%. Cortisone and prednisone are pro-drugs and require hydroxylation in the liver for

activation. After absorption, CS are bound to proteins such as albumin and corticosteroid binding globulin and circulate systemically. The rate-limiting step in the elimination of CS is reduction and conjugation in the liver, although the final fate of these water-soluble metabolic end products is excretion in the urine. The metabolism of parenteral steroids is similar, except without first-pass elimination.

The route of administration for systemic CS depends, to some degree, on the indication. Very high doses of CS given for acute conditions generally require parenteral administration. When the dose of corticosteroid can be achieved by oral administration (e.g., prednisone 1 mg/kg daily), there is no clear benefit to parenteral therapy. For chronic corticosteroid therapy, the preferred route is enteral, although intramuscular injection is also an alternative.

The biologic activity of systemic CS depends on both pharmacokinetic and pharmacodynamic properties of the drug. Dosing equivalence is based on the biologic activity of a given dose, as measured by antiinflammatory activity and sodium-retaining activity. Table 37-1 lists commonly used systemic CS and their dosing equivalence.

Inhaled

The minority of an inhaled dose of CS is deposited in the lungs (10–40%). Once deposited in the lung, the drug will eventually be released into the systemic circulation and cleared through the liver. The remainder of the dose is deposited in the pharynx. Typically, some of this dose is swallowed and undergoes absorption into the portal circulation and first-pass elimination, as for oral steroids, earlier.

The route of administration for inhaled drugs is, by definition, inhalation, but there are a number of methods for delivering ICS, most commonly a metered-dose inhaler (MDI). Historically, the propellants used in MDIs were chlorofluorocarbon. Recognition that these agents depleted atmospheric ozone led to the development of MDIs that use hydrofluoroalkanes as the propellant. Dry-powdered inhalers have also been developed. Finally, a formulation of budesonide is now available for use with a nebulizer. These methods of delivering ICS differ with respect to the particle size generated and velocity of delivered drug, resulting in small differences in equivalent dosing, but the efficiency of drug delivery is similar for each (8–15%).

The pharmacokinetic characteristics of ICS are more complex than those of systemic CS. These drugs have undergone extensive development to improve activity in the lungs while decreasing systemic activity. The factors that promote this

TABLE 37-1 Relative Potency and Equivalent Dosing of Systemic Corticosteroids

Name	Relative Glucocorticoid Activity	Relative Mineralocorticoid Activity	Biologic Half-Life (h)	Equivalent Glucocorticoid Dose (mg)
Hydrocortisone	1	1	8–12	20
Cortisone	0.8	0.6	8–12	25
Prednisone	4	0.6	18–36	5
Prednisolone	4	0.8	18–36	5
Methylprednisolone	5	0.5	18–36	4
Triamcinolone	5	0	18–36	4
Dexamethasone	20–30	0	36–54	0.75
Betamethasone	20–30	0	36–54	0.6

Adapted from Harris E: Kelley's Textbook of Rheumatology, 7th ed. Philadelphia, 2005, Saunders.

TABLE 37-2 Receptor Affinity and Pharmacokinetic Properties of Inhaled Corticosteroids

Corticosteroid	Relative Receptor Affinity*	Half-Life (h)	Oral Bioavailability (%)	Protein Binding (%)	Lipid Conjugation	Prodrug
Beclomethasone[†]	0.5/13	0.1/2.7	15/26	87/NA		Yes
Budesonide	9.4	2–3	11	88	Yes	
Flunisolide	1.8	1.6	21	80		
Fluticasone	18	4–14	<1	90		
Triamcinolone	3.6	1.5	23	71	Yes	
Mometasone	2200	4.5	<1	NA		
Ciclesonide[†]	0.1/12	0.4/3.6–5.1	<1/<1	99/99	Yes	Yes

*Affinity relative to dexamethasone.
[†]Values are given for the prodrug before the slash, and active compound after the slash.

TABLE 37-3 Adult Dosing for Inhaled Corticosteroids*

Corticosteroid	Delivery	Dose Per Actuation (µg)	Low Dose (µg)	Medium Dose (µg)	High Dose (µg)
Beclomethasone	CFC	42 or 84	168–504	504–840	>840
	HFA	40 or 80	80–240	240–480	>480
Budesonide	DPI	200	200–600	600–1200	>1200
Flunisolide	MDI	250	500–1000	1000–2000	>2000
Fluticasone	MDI	44, 110, 220	88–264	264–660	>660
	DPI	50, 100, 250	100–300	300–600	>600
Triamcinolone	MDI	100	400–1000	1000–2000	>2000
Mometasone	MDI	220	220–440	440–660	>660
Ciclesonide	MDI	80,160	80–160	160–320	>320

*Modified from the NAEPP Expert Panel Report and the GINA Global Strategy for Asthma Management and Prevention. For dosing in children, please reference package inserts.

"ideal" profile include low oral bioavailability, long residence in the lung (through slow absorption and/or lipid conjugation), delivery of a pro-drug that is activated in the lung, high receptor affinity, and avid binding to protein in circulating blood. Table 37-2 reviews many of these properties for seven commercially available inhaled CS (ciclesonide is not yet available in the United States but is available in Canada and in Europe).

As with systemic CS, the biologic activity of ICS depends on the integration of numerous pharmacokinetic and pharmacodynamic properties. Direct comparison of the biologic activity of various inhaled agents is difficult, but important, because management of airway diseases requires the ability to titrate the potency of delivered drug to achieve the desired clinical effect. The National Asthma Education and Prevention Program Expert Panel Report, the Global Initiative for Asthma, and the Global Strategy for Asthma Management and Prevention integrated a large amount of clinical and pharmacokinetic data to classify equivalent doses of a variety of different inhaled steroids (Table 37-3). In general, the low to medium doses were the range across which there seems to be a dose-response relationship without increased systemic effect, and the high doses were the threshold beyond which there is significant suppression of the hypothalamic-pituitary axis.

TOXICITIES

Upper Airway

Oropharyngeal candidiasis (thrush) may occur with either systemic or inhaled corticosteroid therapy, but thrush and dysphonia are particularly problematic with ICS.

Musculoskeletal

A major concern in pediatric patients is the impact of corticosteroid therapy on growth. Systemic CS commonly retard growth, and this effect can be permanent. Growth retardation has also been described with ICS, but it is thought to be transient and without long-term significance. The Childhood Asthma Management Program study followed 1041 children treated with budesonide, nedocromil, or placebo for 4–6 years and found a 1.1-cm lag in height gained in patients taking budesonide compared with placebo. This lag was experienced primarily during the first year of the study, because growth velocity toward the end of the study was similar. Projections of adult height were also similar.

CS adversely affect bone health, with osteoporosis, osteoporotic fractures, and avascular osteonecrosis being relatively common and severe toxicities resulting from systemic administration. The incidence of osteoporosis seems related to daily use, duration of use, and cumulative lifetime dose. Osteoporosis has been seen with doses as low as 5–7.5 mg/day of prednisone. There is less risk with ICS, although they have been associated with decreased bone mineral density in at least one randomized controlled trial. The risk of fractures associated with ICS is unclear, although some observational studies suggest an increased risk, particularly with long-term use of very high doses.

In addition to their effects on bone health, systemic CS are also associated with steroid-induced myopathy. Although myopathy has also been described with ICS, it seems to be exceedingly rare.

Adrenal Suppression

Adrenal insufficiency is a well-described consequence of systemic corticosteroid use. The risk seems minimal with ICS. Although suppression of morning cortisol levels does occur in response to ICS, the risk of clinically apparent adrenal insufficiency is small (although case reports of this do exist).

Ocular

CS are used to treat many inflammatory conditions of the eye but can also result in ocular toxicity. Ocular toxicity seems to be a greater problem in patients with exogenous CS administration than in those with endogenous CS excess. The most common ocular toxicity is posterior subcapsular cataract formation. Increased ocular pressure is also common after CS and may result in clinically significant glaucoma. Risk factors for developing glaucoma in the setting of CS therapy include a personal or family history of glaucoma, older age, race, hypertension, migraine headaches, and vasospastic disorders. Less common ocular toxicities include exophthalmos and central serous chorioretinopathy.

There are case reports of cataracts and glaucoma in association with use of high doses of ICS, but these seem to be uncommon. A potential source of confounding, however, is the use of systemic CS in patients receiving the medication by the inhaled route.

Skin and Soft Tissues

The most common cutaneous side effects are ecchymoses and atrophy. Others include acne, alopecia or hypertrichosis, striae, and impaired wound healing. There is some evidence that systemic CS may increase the risk of nonmelanoma skin cancer. The physiognomy of Cushing's syndrome (i.e., buffalo hump, moon facies, and truncal obesity) results from weight gain and maldistribution of adipose tissue. The cutaneous manifestations of inhaled steroids are milder than those with systemic CS and consist primarily of atrophy and easy bruising (Figure 37-5).

Infection

Systemic CS are potent immunosuppressors, particularly when prescribed in higher doses and for prolonged periods of

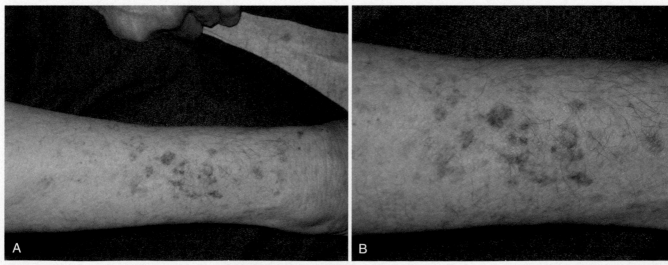

FIGURE 37-5 A and **B**, Steroid-inducted purpura.

time. Courses of 2–8 weeks of systemic CS used to treat acute exacerbations of COPD do not seem to be associated with increased rates of infection. Chronic CS use does pose a risk for *Pseudomonas*, *Pneumocystis*, tuberculosis, and herpes zoster.

Until recently, ICS were not thought to increase the risk of lung infections. The recently published TORCH trial, however, found an increase in the proportion of patients who have pneumonia develop in the two groups of patients treated with fluticasone propionate compared with the groups not receiving ICS. This result was also seen in a second recent trial. The increase in pneumonia could be a result of local immunosuppression in the lungs.

Central Nervous System

Euphoria is a commonly described side effect of systemic CS. More concerning, central nervous system (CNS) complications include hypomania, depression, psychosis, memory loss,

akathisia, and sleep disturbances. Pseudotumor cerebri is a rare complication of CS; CNS toxicity has been rarely associated with ICS.

Cardiovascular

In observational studies, systemic CS have been associated with increased risk of cardiovascular disease, including heart failure, ischemic heart disease, and cerebrovascular disease, as well as all-cause mortality. This may be mediated, in part, by salt retention and hypertension, insulin resistance, hyperglycemia, and/or adverse alteration of lipid profiles. ICS seem safe in patients with cardiovascular disease; indeed, there is some suggestion that these drugs may reduce the risk of cardiovascular events in patients with COPD by reducing systemic inflammation.

Gastrointestinal

Systemic CS have been associated with upper gastrointestinal bleeding from peptic ulcer disease, but this seems to be

TABLE 37-4 Adverse Effects of Inhaled and Systemic Corticosteroids

System	Inhaled	Systemic	Prevention
Upper airway	Thrush Dysphonia	Thrush	Wash out mouth after using inhaled steroids Use a spacer device
Musculoskeletal	Growth delay Decreased bone mineral density Possible increase in fractures	Decreased adult height Osteoporosis Fractures Avascular osteonecrosis Myopathy	Follow bone mineral density Calcium/vitamin D Bisphosphonates Weight-bearing exercise HCTZ
HPA axis	Suppression of cortisol secretion Case reports of clinical adrenal insufficiency	Adrenal insufficiency well described	Avoid abrupt discontinuation of chronic steroids Stress dosing when appropriate
Ocular	Possible increase in posterior subcapsular cataracts, glaucoma	Posterior subcapsular cataracts Glaucoma	Serial ophthalmologic examination
Skin and soft tissues	Ecchymosis Atrophy	Ecchymosis Atrophy Acne Impaired wound healing Striae Buffalo hump Moon facies Weight gain	Face washing after use of nebulized drug in children
Immunologic	Increased pneumonias	Increased infection Opportunistic infection	TB screening and prophylaxis where appropriate Pneumocystis prophylaxis
Central nervous system	Case reports of psychiatric disturbance	Euphoria Depression Psychosis Memory loss Hypomania Sleep disturbance	
Gastrointestinal	None	GI bleeding in conjunction with NSAIDs Visceral perforation Steatohepatitis	Avoid NSAIDs
Cardiovascular	None	Increased cardiovascular events Hypertension Hyperlipidemia Hyperglycemia	Treat modifiable risk factors (lipids, blood pressure, glucose)

HCTZ, Hydrochlorothiazide.

attributable to the patients also being on nonsteroidal anti-inflammatory drugs. CS may also predispose to diverticular or other visceral rupture (with the antiinflammatory effects masking presentation of the rupture) and to fatty liver.

Prevention and Management of Corticosteroid Toxicity

The most important principle with respect to the use of either systemic or ICS is to minimize the dose and duration of treatment.

Patients on ICS should be educated on proper inhaler technique and on washing out their mouth after use, and those who use MDIs should be given a spacer. If symptoms occur with an MDI, they may be reduced or eliminated by switching to a dry-powder inhaler. Children who use nebulized CS should wash their face after the use of the medication.

In patients on pharmacologic doses of systemic CS, periodic ophthalmologic examination can detect the development of cataracts and glaucoma, which may respond to reduction of corticosteroid dose or, if CS cannot be reduced, other treatments. The role of ophthalmologic assessment in patients on ICS is less clear, but these patients should certainly be referred for any ophthalmologic symptoms and for routine, age-appropriate care.

Screening for and management of cardiovascular risk factors, including hypertension, hyperglycemia, and hyperlipidemia, is warranted in patients receiving chronic systemic CS.

Patients receiving chronic systemic or ICS should have routine bone mineral density measurements (particularly in high-risk groups), and they should be encouraged to perform weight-bearing exercise and to use calcium and vitamin D (unless there is a contraindication). Hormone replacement, bisphosphonates, calcitonin, and hydrochlorothiazide (HCTZ) can be considered in patients with established osteoporosis.

Avoidance of NSAIDs is appropriate in patients receiving systemic CS.

Vigilance for psychiatric symptoms is prudent and, if present, can be managed by reducing the dose of CS and/or by pharmacotherapy targeting the psychiatric symptoms.

Patients receiving chronic CS should be alerted to the increased risk of infection and should be encouraged to seek prompt evaluation at the earliest sign of infection. If possible, PPD status should be established before initiation of therapy, and any vaccinations that are appropriate should be administered. If long-term administration of moderate to high doses of systemic CS is anticipated, prophylaxis for *Pneumocystis* may be appropriate (trimethoprim sulfate/sulfamethoxazole 1 DS daily or 3×/week).

Patients receiving chronic systemic CS should be alerted to the symptoms of adrenal insufficiency and should be encouraged not to skip doses. If the patient experiences major illness or surgery, stress-doses of steroids may be indicated.

CONCLUSION

CS remain an essential treatment for many inflammatory diseases of the lung. Their clinical benefits must be weighed against the risk of adverse effects (Table 37-4). Inhaled CS offer many of the benefits of systemic CS while minimizing toxicity. New insights into the pharmacokinetics and pharmacodynamics of these medications may lead to the development of new drugs that maximize the antiinflammatory effects that minimize the side effects and to increased synergy between CS and other medications such as bronchodilators.

SUGGESTED READINGS

Allen DB, Bielory L, Derendorf H, et al: Inhaled corticosteroids: Past lessons and future issues. J Allergy Clin Immunol 2003; 112(3 Suppl): S1–S40.

Barnes PJ: How corticosteroids control inflammation: Quintiles Prize Lecture 2005. Br J Phamacol 2006; 148:245–254.

Derendorf H, Nave R, Drollman A, et al: Relevance of pharmacokinetics and pharmacodynamics of inhaled corticosteroids to asthma. Eur Respir J 2006; 28(5):1042–1050.

Leung DY, Bloom JW: Update on glucocorticoid action and resistance. J Allergy Clin Immunol 2003; 111:3–22.

Rodrigo GJ: Rapid effects of inhaled corticosteroids in acute asthma: An evidence-based evaluation. Chest 2006; 130:1301–1311.

Sin DD, Man SF: Corticosteroids and adrenoceptor agonists: The compliments for combination therapy in chronic airways diseases. Eur J Pharmacol 2006; 533:28–35.

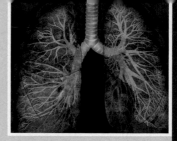

38 Chronic Obstructive Pulmonary Disease: Epidemiology, Physiology, and Clinical Evaluation

WILLIAM MACNEE

Chronic obstructive pulmonary disease (COPD) is a preventable and treatable condition that is characterized by airflow limitation that is not fully reversible and is progressive. Although hidden by the generic term "COPD," it is a collection of syndromes that result from pathologic changes in the large and small airways and in the lung parenchyma that are variably expressed in individual patients resulting in heterogeneity of the condition.

Our understanding of the pathogenesis, physiology, clinical features, and management of COPD has increased substantially in recent years. The condition is thought to arise from an abnormal inflammatory response in the lungs to inhaled particles and gases. Although cigarette smoking is a major risk factor, COPD occurs in nonsmokers, and individuals vary greatly in their susceptibility to the effects of tobacco smoke. Although primarily a disease of the lungs, it is now recognized that COPD has important systemic consequences that influence morbidity and mortality and comorbidities that affect the severity of the disease.

In 1990, COPD was the 12th leading cause of morbidity and the 6th leading cause of death worldwide. Of all the major chronic diseases, COPD is the one whose burden is rising fastest, and it is projected that it will be the 5th leading cause of disability and the 3rd leading cause of death by 2020 (Figure 38-1).

Patients frequently attribute their symptoms of breathlessness, cough, and sputum production to aging or to their cigarette smoking. In addition, many health care providers consider the condition to be irreversible and that treatment offers very little. Accordingly, COPD is markedly underdiagnosed, despite the fact that it is a relatively easy diagnosis to make and is also frequently undermanaged.

It is now well recognized that treatment of COPD can result in clinically significant improvement. Whereas treatment was previously considered for patients at the severe, end stage of the disease, it is now recognized that diagnosis and treatment at an earlier stage can offer important benefits for patients. Although current treatments are unable to cure COPD, they can be of considerable benefit in reducing symptoms, improving function and health-related quality of life and acute exacerbations, and may decrease the enormous health care costs associated with COPD.

DEFINITIONS

Chronic obstructive pulmonary disease is not truly a disease but a group of diseases—chronic bronchitis, small airways disease (obstructive bronchiolitis), and destruction of the lung parenchyma (emphysema). Although these conditions comprise the syndrome, the terms describe clinical or pathologic findings rather than pertaining to airflow limitation.

Chronic bronchitis is defined clinically as the presence of a chronic productive cough on most days for 3 months, in each of two consecutive years, in patients in whom other causes of chronic cough have been excluded. Cough and sputum production may precede the development of airflow limitation. Some patients, however, have airflow limitation develop without cough and sputum production.

Emphysema is defined as abnormal, permanent enlargement of airspaces distal to terminal bronchioles, accompanied by the destruction of airspace walls without obvious fibrosis. As with the definition of chronic bronchitis, the definition of emphysema does not require the presence of airflow limitation.

Obstructive bronchiolitis, or *small airways disease*, results from inflammation, squamous metaplasia, and/or fibrosis in airways less than 2 mm in diameter. These changes are among the earliest to appear in cigarette smokers, but they are difficult to detect by physiologic measurements. Although relatively little is known of the natural history of this condition, it is thought to progresses to the airflow limitation that is in COPD.

It is difficult to determine the relative contributions to the airflow limitation in individual patients by airway abnormalities versus distal air space enlargement. Thus, the term COPD was introduced in the 1960s to describe patients with incompletely reversible airflow limitation resulting from a combination of airways disease and emphysema, without defining the contribution of these conditions to the airflow limitation.

In their statement on the standards for diagnosis and care of patients with COPD, the American Thoracic Society and European Respiratory Society defined the syndrome as "a preventable and treatable disease state characterized by air flow limitation that is not fully reversible. The airflow limitation is usually progressive and is associated with an abnormal inflammatory response in the lungs to noxious particles or gases, primarily caused by cigarette smoking. Although COPD affects the lungs, it also produces significant systemic consequences." The recent update of the Global Initiative for Chronic Obstructive Pulmonary Disease (GOLD) has a very similar working definition, emphasizing again that the pulmonary component, airflow limitation, is associated with an abnormal inflammatory response of the lungs to particles or

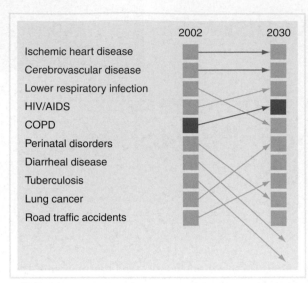

FIGURE 38-1 Predicted changes in global causes of mortality.

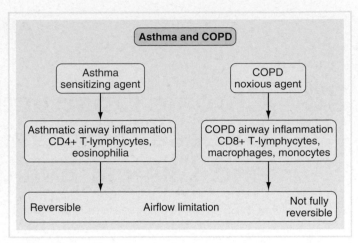

FIGURE 38-2 Differences in pathophysiology between asthma and COPD.

gases and that there are extrapulmonary events and comorbidities that may contribute to the severity of the disease in individual patients.

In clinical practice diagnosis of COPD should be considered in individuals over the age of 35 with:

- History of chronic progressive symptoms (cough, wheeze, and/or breathlessness)
- Exposure to risk factors such as cigarette smoke, occupational or environmental dust, or gases

The diagnosis of COPD requires objective evidence of airflow limitation determined by spirometry. A postbronchodilator forced expiratory volume in the first second (FEV_1)/forced vital capacity (FVC) <0.7 confirms the presence of airflow limitation that is not fully reversible.

A number of specific causes of airways obstruction such as cystic fibrosis, bronchiectasis, and bronchiolitis obliterans are not included in the definition of COPD and should be considered in its differential diagnosis.

COPD AND ASTHMA

A major problem in defining COPD is the difficulty in differentiating this condition from asthma, particularly the chronic persistent or poorly reversible airways obstruction that occurs in older patients with chronic asthma that is often difficult or even impossible to distinguish from COPD. An additional difficulty is the considerable overlap between the physiologic mechanisms that underlie chronic asthma and the syndromes that comprise COPD. A large proportion of patients with COPD show some reversibility of their airflow obstruction with bronchodilators. Furthermore, COPD can coexist with asthma, and individuals with asthma who are exposed to noxious particles and gases, such as cigarette smoke, can also have fixed airflow limitation develop. Epidemiologic studies also show that long-standing chronic asthma can itself lead to fixed airflow limitation.

Chronic airway inflammation underlies both of these conditions but is different in type between these two diseases (Figure 38-2). However, some patients with COPD demonstrate an airway inflammatory pattern similar to that in asthmatic subjects such as increased eosinophils in the airways. Thus, although asthma can usually be distinguished from COPD, in some individuals with chronic symptoms and a degree of fixed airflow limitation, it is difficult to differentiate these two diseases.

In such cases, a history of heavy cigarette smoking, evidence of emphysema by imaging techniques, decreased diffusing capacity for carbon monoxide, and chronic hypoxemia in more severe disease favor a diagnosis of COPD.

Population studies suggest that chronic airflow limitation can occur in up to 10% of individuals who are lifelong nonsmokers aged 40 years or older. The cause of the airflow limitation in these cases is not apparent.

COPD AND COMORBIDITIES

COPD is associated with a number of comorbid diseases that are related to several factors, including smoking, extrapulmonary effects of COPD, and/or aging. Weight loss and skeletal muscle dysfunction are recognized extrapulmonary effects of COPD. Whether these changes represent pathologic or compensatory changes in response to worsening COPD is debated, however. Patients with COPD are also at increased risk of a number of other conditions (Box 38-1). These comorbidities can add to the severity of the disease, and, furthermore, in managing COPD, attention should be paid to the comorbidities and their effects on patients.

BOX 38-1 Comorbidities in COPD

Weight loss
Skeletal muscle dysfunction
Ischemic heart disease
Osteoporosis
Diabetes
Sleep disorders
Depression
Anemia
Glaucoma
Peptic ulceration

PATHOLOGY

The pathologic changes in COPD are complex and occur in the central conducting airways, the peripheral airways, the lung parenchyma, and the pulmonary vasculature. The relative contribution of pathologic changes in the airways versus those of emphysema to the observed airflow limitation is still debated. In general, pathologic changes correlate rather poorly with both clinical and functional patterns of disease. Indeed, there is still no clear consensus on whether the fixed airways obstruction in COPD results from inflammation and scarring in the small airways producing narrowing of the airway lumen or to loss of support for the airways because of the loss of alveolar walls as in emphysema. The clinicopathologic picture is complicated by the fact that these three entities may coexist singly or in any combination in an individual patient.

Inflammation initiated by exposure to particles or gases is thought to underlie most of the pathologic changes associated with COPD. There is good evidence that all smokers have inflammation in their lungs as a result of the innate and adaptive immune response to long-term exposure to noxious particles and gases. There is, however, individual susceptibility in the inflammatory response to tobacco smoking such that people who have COPD develop are also thought to have an enhanced or abnormal response to the inhaled toxins. This amplified response may result in abnormal mucus hypersecretion (chronic bronchitis), tissue destruction (emphysema), and destruction of normal repair and defense mechanisms, causing small airway inflammation and eventual fibrosis (bronchiolitis). These pathologic changes result in increased resistance to airflow in the small conducting airways, increased compliance of the lungs, leading to increasing air trapping, and progressive airflow obstruction that are characteristic features of COPD.

Some believe that chronic asthma should be included as part of the spectrum of COPD. Although the clinical and physiologic presentation of asthma can be indistinguishable from that of COPD, the pathologic changes are distinct from those in most cases.

The pathologic features of COPD in the 10% of COPD patients who are nonsmokers have not yet been studied in detail.

Chronic Bronchitis

Chronic hypersecretion of mucus results from changes in the central airways (i.e., the trachea, bronchi, and bronchioles >2–4 mm in diameter). Mucus is produced by mucus glands in the larger airways and by goblet cells in the airway epithelium (Figure 38-3). In healthy subjects who have never smoked, goblet cells are predominantly seen in the proximal

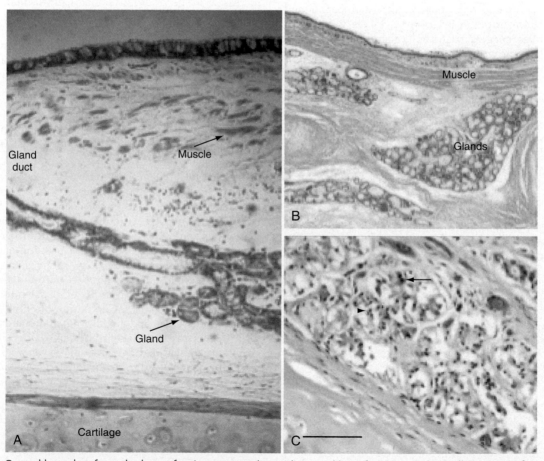

FIGURE 38-3 A, Central bronchus from the lung of a cigarette smoker with normal lung function. Only small amounts of muscle are present, and the epithelial glands are small. This contrasts sharply with a diseased bronchus **(B),** where the muscle appears as a thick bundle and the glands are enlarged. **C,** Enlarged glands at a higher magnification. There is evidence of a chronic inflammatory process involving polymorphonuclear *(arrowhead)* and mononuclear cells, including plasma cells *(arrow).* (Permission of Dr. J. C. Hogg and Dr. S. Greene.)

airways, and they decrease in number in more distal airways, normally being absent in the terminal or respiratory bronchioles. By contrast, in smokers and in patients with COPD, goblet cells increase in number and extend more peripherally. Thus, mucus is produced in greater quantity in peripheral airways where the mucociliary escalator is less developed. The function of the mucociliary escalator is also decreased in smokers. The volume of sputum produced correlates with mucus gland area or volume and with the degree of inflammation in the airway wall. Neutrophils are present, particularly in the mucus glands, and become more prominent as the disease progresses. Squamous metaplasia of the airway epithelium occurs. Bronchial biopsy and studies of resected lung material show bronchial wall inflammation in chronic bronchitis (Box 38-2). As in asthma, activated T lymphocytes are prominent in the proximal airway walls. In contrast to asthma, however, macrophages are also prominent, and the CD8 suppressor T-lymphocyte subset predominates, rather than the CD4 subset, as occurs in asthma.

Several studies of bronchoalveolar lavage (BAL) and spontaneous or induced sputum demonstrate intraluminal inflammation in the airspaces of patients with chronic bronchitis, with or without airflow obstruction. In stable chronic bronchitis, the high percentage of intraluminal neutrophils is associated with the presence of neutrophil chemotactic factors, including interleukin (IL)-8 and leukotriene B4. There is evidence that the airspace inflammation in patients with chronic bronchitis persists after smoking cessation, particularly if the production of sputum persists, although cough and sputum production improve in most smokers who quit. Preliminary studies suggest that the inflammatory changes present in the large airways may reflect those present in the small airways and in the alveolar walls.

Airway wall changes include squamous metaplasma of the airway epithelium, loss of cilia and ciliary function, and increased smooth muscle and connective tissue. Bronchial biopsy samples taken from patients during mild exacerbations of chronic bronchitis indicate increased numbers of eosinophils in the bronchial wall, although far fewer than are present in exacerbations of asthma. Increased numbers of neutrophils are also observed. Eosinophils may not be predominant in severe exacerbations.

Emphysema

Pulmonary emphysema is defined as "abnormal permanent enlargement of airspaces distal to the terminal bronchioles accompanied by destruction of their walls." The major types of emphysema distinguished by the distribution of enlarged airspaces within the acinar unit (the acinar unit being that part of the lung parenchyma supplied by a single terminal bronchiole):

- Centriacinar (centrilobular emphysema), in which large airspaces are initially clustered around the terminal bronchiole
- Panacinar (or panlobular) emphysema, where the large airspaces are distributed throughout the acinar unit (Figure 38-4)

In the early stages of the disease, emphysematous lesions are microscopic (<1 mm in diameter) (Figure 38-5). Airspace enlargement can be identified macroscopically when the enlarged airspace reaches 1 mm. These may progress to become macroscopic lesions or bullae. A bulla represents a localized area of emphysema that has locally overdistended, conventionally greater than 1 cm in size. Bullous disease can also occur in the absence of COPD.

Although obvious fibrosis is, by definition, not present emphysema, in the region of the terminal respiratory bronchioles, fibrosis has been recognized as part of a respiratory bronchiolitis that occurs in smokers, and lung collagen content is increased in mild emphysema. Centriacinar and panacinar emphysema can occur alone or in combination. The association with cigarette smoking is greater for centriacinar than panacinar emphysema, whereas smokers can have both types develop. Those with centriacinar emphysema seem to have more abnormalities in the small airways than those with panacinar emphysema. Panacinar emphysema seems to be more severe in the lower lobes, whereas centriacinar emphysema usually predominates in the upper lobes. Panacinar emphysema is associated with alpha$_1$-antitrypsin deficiency but can also be found in patients in whom no genetic abnormality has been identified.

Other types of emphysema exist such as periacinar (paraseptal or distal acinar) emphysema, which describes enlarged airspaces along the edge of the acinar unit, but only where it abuts against a fixed structure such as the pleura or a vessel. This is usually of little clinical significance except when it occurs extensively in a subpleural position and may be associated with pneumothorax. Scar or irregular emphysema is used to describe enlarged airspaces around the margins of a scar unrelated to the structure of the acinus. This lesion is excluded from the current definition of emphysema.

The bronchioles and small bronchi are supported by outer attachments to the adjacent alveolar walls. This arrangement maintains the tubular integrity of the airways. Loss of these attachments may lead to distortion and irregularities of the airways because of loss of lung elastic recoil that results in airflow limitation.

The inflammatory cell profile in the alveolar walls is similar to that described in the airways and persists throughout the course of the disease.

Small Airways Disease/Bronchiolitis

The smaller bronchi and bronchioles <2 mm in diameter are a major site of airflow obstruction in COPD. Small airway

---

BOX 38-2   Inflammation, Inflammatory Cells, and Mediators in COPD

- Neutrophils increase in sputum and distal airspaces in smokers with a further increase in COPD related to disease severity. Important in secretion and the release of proteases.
- Macrophages increased in number in airways, lung parenchyma, and in bronchoalveolar lavage fluid. Produce increased inflammatory mediators and proteases.
- T lymphocytes. Both CD4 and CD8 cells increase in airways and in lung parenchyma with an increase in CD8/CD4 ratio. Increase in TH1 and TC1 cells that produce interferon gamma. CD8$^+$ cells may be cytotoxic, causing alveolar wall destruction.
- T lymphocytes increase in the peripheral airways and within lymphoid follicles, possibly as a response to chronic infection of the airways. Eosinophil proteins in sputum and increased eosinophils in airway walls occur in some exacerbations of the disease.

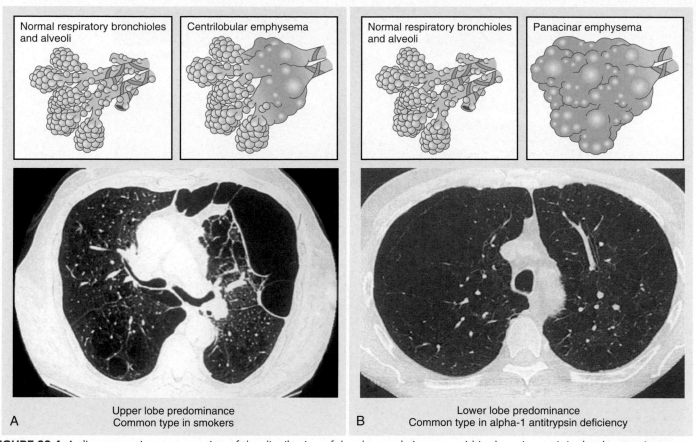

FIGURE 38-4 A diagrammatic representation of the distribution of the abnormal airspaces within the acinar unit in the three major types of emphysema. **A**, Acinar unit in a normal lung (*left top*) and in centriacinar emphysema (*left bottom*): focal enlargement of the airspaces around the respiratory bronchiole. A CT scan showing patchy centrilobular emphysema with bullous disease (*right*) is also shown. **B**, Panacinar (panlobular) emphysema: confluent even involvement of the acinar unit. A CT scan with diffuse low attenuation areas of panlobular emphysema is shown (*right*).

inflammation is one of the earliest changes to occur, and there is evidence of small airway inflammation in asymptomatic cigarette smokers. Considerable inflammatory change can occur in absence of symptoms or in absence of abnormal spirometry. The inflammatory cell changes in the small airways are similar to those in larger airways, including the predominance of CD8$^+$ lymphocytes and the increase in the CD8/CD4 ratio. The increased peripheral airway resistance is a result of several processes:

1. Destruction of the alveolar support
2. Loss of elastic recoil in the parenchyma that provides this support consequent on a narrowing of the airways
3. Occlusion of the lumen by mucus and cells

Mucosal ulceration, goblet cell hyperplasia, and squamous cell metaplasia may be present. In addition, there may be mesenchymal cell accumulation and fibrosis. As the condition progresses, structural remodeling may occur, characterized by increased collagen content and scar tissue formation that narrows the airways and produces fixed airway obstruction (Figure 38-6).

Bronchiolitis is present in the peripheral airways at an early stage of disease. Recent studies that used resected lung specimens and those obtained from lung volume reduction surgery have shown the changes in inflammatory response as the disease progresses (Figure 38-7). An increase in T lymphocytes,

B lymphocytes, and lymphoid follicles around the bronchioles has been shown to occur in the later stages of the disease. The cause(s) of these changes is not known, and autoimmune and adaptive immune responses to chronic lower respiratory infection are two possibilities currently being investigated.

Pulmonary Vasculature

Changes in the pulmonary arteries occur early in the course of COPD, the first of these being thickening of the intima, followed by increase in smooth muscle and infiltration of the vessel wall with inflammatory cells such as macrophages and CD8$^+$ T lymphocytes. As the disease progresses, greater amounts of smooth muscle, proteoglycans, and collagen accumulate in the arterial wall and cause it to thicken. The development of chronic alveolar hypoxia in patients with COPD results in hypoxic vasoconstriction and contributes to structural changes in the pulmonary vasculature, pulmonary hypertension, and right ventricular dilatation and hypertrophy.

ETIOLOGY AND RISK FACTORS

The risk of COPD developing is thought to result from an interaction between genes and the environment. Thus, cigarette smoking results in COPD as a function of genetic predisposition, infection, or failure of lung growth and development.

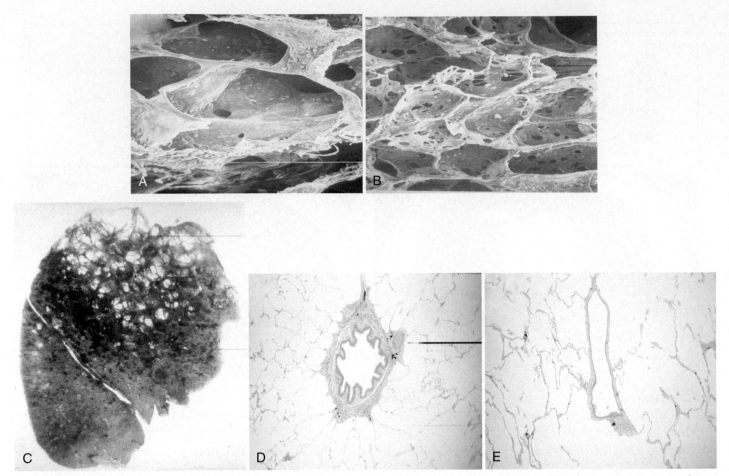

FIGURE 38-5 Scanning electron micrograph of the alveoli in a normal **(A)** and in microscopic emphysema **(B)**. **C**, Entire lung section from a lung with severe macroscopic centrilobular emphysema (note that the centrilobular form is more extensive in the upper regions of the lung). **D**, Histologic section of normal small airway and surrounding alveoli connecting with attached alveolar walls. **E**, Histologic section showing emphysema, with enlarged alveolar spaces, loss of alveolar wall, and attachments and collapsed airways.

Cigarette Smoking

Cigarette smoking is the single most important identifiable etiologic factor in COPD. In general, there is a correlative dose effect, with smokers having lower lung function the more and longer they smoke. There is, however, considerable variation (Figure 38-8). Some nonsmokers have impaired lung function, and as many as 20% of patients with COPD are lifelong nonsmokers. Conversely, some heavy smokers are able to maintain normal lung function. The frequently quoted 10–20% of smokers in whom clinically significant COPD is thought to develop is now known to be an underestimate.

Cigarette smokers have a higher prevalence of respiratory symptoms and lung function abnormalities, a greater annual rate of decline in FEV_1, and a greater mortality rate than nonsmokers. Morbidity and mortality rates are greater in pipe and cigar smokers than in nonsmokers, although their rates are lower than those for cigarette smokers.

There is a trend toward an increased relative risk of chronic airflow limitation from passive smoking, but the effect is not powerful enough to demonstrate clinical significance. Exposure to environmental tobacco smoke during childhood, however, is associated with a lower FEV_1 in adulthood. Furthermore, maternal smoking is associated with low birth weight, and smoking by either parent is associated with an increased frequency of respiratory illness in the first 3 years of life, and this may also result in airflow limitation in later life.

Air Pollution

Air pollution has been recognized as a risk factor in chronic respiratory disease as a result of various air pollution episodes, such as the London smog of December 1952 in which 4000 excess deaths from cardiorespiratory disease occurred. Indoor air pollution from the combustion of biomass fuel in fires and stoves is an important etiologic factor in the development of COPD, particularly in women from developing countries in which open fires are used for heating and cooking in housing offering limited venting to the resulting smoke.

The introduction of air quality standards in many countries in the 1950–1960s led to a decrease in smoke and sulfur dioxide levels, which resulted in less discernible associations between peaks of pollution and respiratory morbidity and mortality. More recent studies, however, show an association between respiratory symptoms, general practitioner consultations, and hospital admissions in patients with airways diseases, including COPD, at levels of particulate air pollution that are currently experienced in many urban areas (i.e., levels below 100 $\mu g/m^3$). Furthermore, increased levels of particulate

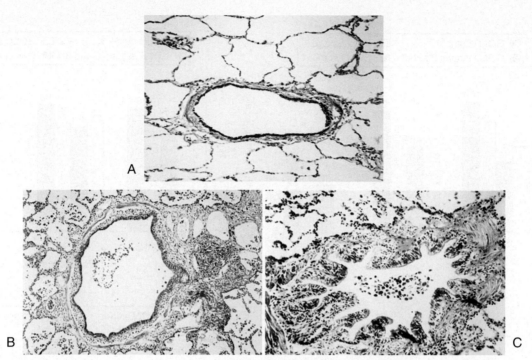

FIGURE 38-6 Histologic sections of peripheral airways. **A,** Section from a cigarette smoker with normal lung function, showing a nearly normal airway. **B,** Section from a patient with small airways disease, showing inflammatory exudates in the wall and the lumen of the airway. **C,** A more advanced case of small airways disease, with reduced lumen, structural reorganization of the airway wall, increased smooth muscle, and deposition of peribronchiolar connective tissue. (Reproduced with permission from Dr. J. C. Hogg.)

air pollution are associated with deaths from all causes, particularly cardiorespiratory deaths. There are also clear associations between the levels of outdoor air pollution, especially particulate air pollution, and exacerbations of COPD. The role of long-term exposure to outdoor air pollution as a risk factor for the development of COPD is still debated. Air pollution does seem to be a risk factor for mucus hypersecretion, although the association with airflow limitation and accelerated decline in FEV_1 is less clear. Air pollution may affect the growth of lung function in childhood, which may influence the risk of COPD in adulthood

Occupation

There is a causal link between occupational exposure to organic and inorganic dusts and the development of mucus hypersecretion. In addition, longitudinal studies in workers exposed to dust show an association between the exposure and a more rapid decline in FEV_1. It has been estimated that occupational exposures account for 10–20% of either symptoms or lung function impairment consistent with COPD. Exposure to welding fumes or cadmium is also associated with a small, but significant, risk of COPD or emphysema developing, respectively.

Genetic Factors

The increased risk of siblings of patients with severe COPD having airflow limitation develop suggests the presence of genetic susceptibility. A number of candidate genes have been associated with the development of COPD, including microsomal epoxide hydrolase-1, tumor necrosis factor, and transforming growth factor-beta. However, the associations are not consistent across different populations. The only proven association is with α_1-antitrypsin (α_1-proteinase inhibitor) deficiency (see later).

Chronic Mucus Hypersecretion: Chronic Bronchopulmonary Infection

Population studies indicate a higher prevalence of cough and sputum among smokers than nonsmokers. Cessation of smoking is associated with cessation of sputum production in 90% of patients. In studies of working men in London, Fletcher and Peto showed that smoking accelerated the decline in FEV_1, but they failed to show a correlation between the degree of mucus hypersecretion and an accelerated decline in FEV_1 or mortality. By contrast, mortality was strongly related to the development of a low FEV_1. More recent data from a more general population study in Copenhagen between 1976 and 1994, however, suggested that mucus hypersecretion was associated with increased risk of hospital admission and accelerated decline in FEV_1. Moreover, as the FEV_1 decreases, the association between mucus hypersecretion and mortality becomes stronger. Differences in the degree of airflow obstruction between the populations in these two studies may explain the different findings

Studies by Fletcher and Peto in the 1960s and 1970s in men with chronic bronchitis did not show a relationship between recurrent infective exacerbations of bronchitis and the decline in lung function. This has been challenged recently in the Lung Health Study, which showed an association in continued smokers between lower respiratory tract infection and a faster rate of decline in lung function. This is supported by newer population studies of patients with COPD.

Cough and sputum production in adulthood are more commonly reported in those with a history of chest illness in childhood. The association between childhood respiratory illness and ventilatory impairment in adulthood is probably multifactorial. Several factors, such as low economic status, greater exposure to passive smoking, poor diet and housing, and

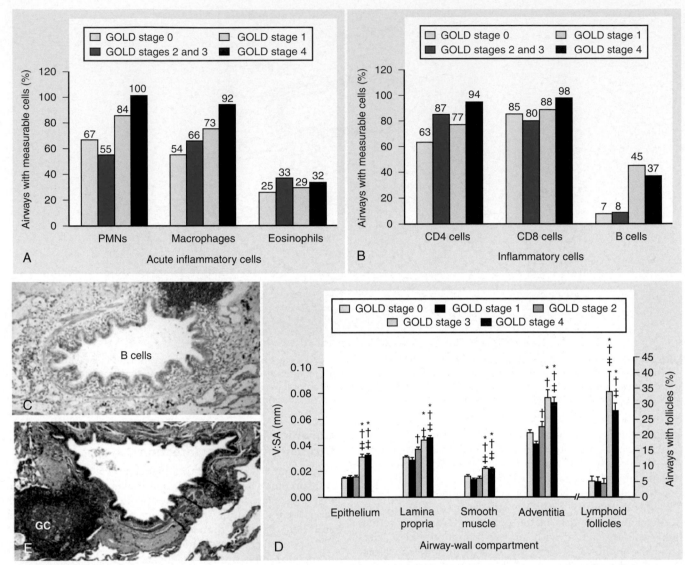

FIGURE 38-7 Changes in inflammatory cells in the small airway walls in different disease severity according to GOLD staging. **A,** Enhanced innate immune response as the disease progresses **(B)** increases in CD4- and CD8-positive T lymphocytes and **(C)** B cells and **(D and E)** increased lymphoid follicles represents an enhanced acquired immune response. (Reproduced from Hogg JC: N Engl J Med 2004; 24:2645.)

residence in areas of high pollution, may contribute to this finding.

Socioeconomic Factors

The risk of COPD developing is inversely related to socioeconomic status. This may reflect exposures to indoor/outdoor air pollutants, poor housing or poor diet, and other factors related to low socioeconomic status.

Growth and Nutrition

Several studies indicate that mortality from chronic respiratory diseases and adult ventilatory function correlates inversely with birth weight and weight at 1 year of age. Thus, it seems that impaired growth *in utero* may be a risk factor for the development of chronic respiratory diseases, including COPD. Any factor that adversely affects lung growth during gestation will potentially increase an individual's risk of COPD developing.

Diet may have an influence on the development of COPD. One study of British adults showed a correlation between consumption of fresh fruit and ventilatory function, a relationship that held both in smokers and in subjects who had never smoked. Dietary factors, particularly a low intake of vitamin C and low plasma levels of ascorbic acid, were related to a diagnosis of bronchitis in the US National Health and Nutrition Examination Survey (NHANES).

Gender

The role of gender as a risk factor in COPD remains unclear. Historical studies showed that COPD prevalence and mortality was greater among men than among women. More recent studies, however, now show that in developed countries, the prevalence of COPD is now almost equal in men and women, which probably reflects the changing patterns of tobacco smoking. There are some studies that suggest that women are more susceptible to the effects of tobacco smoke than men.

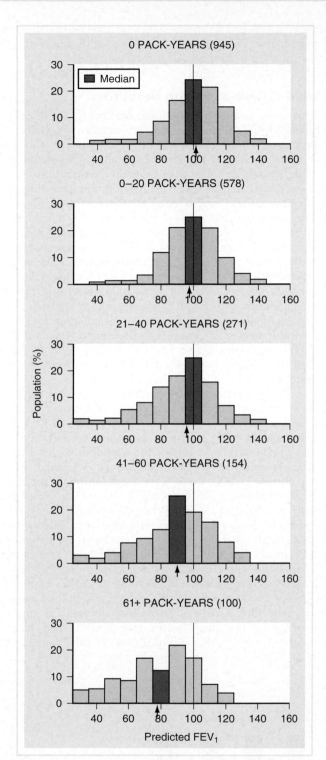

FIGURE 38-8 Distribution of FEV$_1$ values as a percentage of predicted value for groups with differing smoking histories. (From Traver GA, Cline MG, Burrows B: Am Rev Respir Dis 1979; 119:895.)

However, the question of gender as a risk factor for COPD remains unresolved.

Atopy and Airway Hyperresponsiveness

A hypothesis was proposed in the 1960s that smokers with chronic, largely irreversible airways obstruction and subjects with asthma shared a common constitutional predisposition to allergy, airway hyperresponsiveness, and eosinophilia—the "Dutch hypothesis." Smokers tend to have higher levels of immunoglobulin E and higher eosinophil counts in blood than nonsmokers, but not as high as those found in patients with asthma. Studies in middle-aged smokers with an airflow limitation show a positive correlation between accelerated decline in FEV$_1$ and increased airway responsiveness to either methacholine or histamine, but there is no increase in atopy in cigarette smokers (defined by positive skin tests). Whether airway hyperresponsiveness is a cause or consequence of COPD remains a subject of debate.

EPIDEMIOLOGY

The prevalence of COPD, its morbidity, and mortality vary across countries, but it is a leading cause of morbidity and mortality worldwide. The imprecise and variable definitions of COPD and the lack of spirometry to confirm the diagnosis have made it difficult to quantify the true morbidity and mortality of this disease. In addition, prevalence data underestimate the total disease burden, because COPD is not usually diagnosed until it is clinically recognized, usually when it has already progressed to at least a moderately advanced stage. The mortality from this condition is also likely to be underestimated, because it is often cited as a contributory, rather than a primary, cause of death.

Prevalence

Existing data on the burden of COPD vary depending on the method of survey, diagnostic criteria, and analysis of the data. The methods that have been used in surveys include:

- Spirometry with or without bronchodilator
- Questionnaires of the prevalence of respiratory symptoms
- Self-reported doctor diagnosis for COPD or equivalent condition

Prevalence estimates on the basis of self-reporting of a doctor diagnosis of COPD produce the lowest estimates of prevalence. Such data show that <6% of the population has a diagnosis of COPD, which is likely to reflect underrecognition/underdiagnosis of the condition. By contrast, prevalence surveys that have used spirometry have estimated that up to 25% of adults aged 40 and older may have airflow limitation.

Older studies reported a prevalence of cough and excessive sputum production of between 15 and 50% in middle-aged men with a lower prevalence of between 8% and 22% in women. A study in the late 1980s showed a decline in the prevalence of chronic cough and phlegm in middle-aged men to 15–20%, with little change in women.

Prevalence studies of COPD on the basis of spirometry have produced different prevalence data, depending on the spirometric criteria used to define COPD.

Defining irreversible airflow limitation on the basis of a fixed postbronchodilator FEV$_1$/FVC ratio of less than 0.70 can lead to an underdiagnosis of COPD in younger adults and an overdiagnosis in those older than 50. In a population survey in the United Kingdom in 1987 of a representative sample of 2484 men and 3063 women, in the age range 18–64 years, 10% of men and 11% of women had an FEV$_1$ that was greater than 2 standard deviations below their predicted values, with the percentage of affected patients increasing with age, particularly in smokers. In current smokers in the age range 40–65 years, 18% of men compared with 14% of women had an FEV$_1$ greater than 2 standard deviations below normal compared with 7% of male and 5% of female nonsmokers. A further study in the Manchester area of England found nonreversible airflow limitation in 11% of adults >45 years of whom 65% had not had a diagnosis of COPD.

Approximately 14 million people in the United States have COPD, and the number has increased by 42% since 1982. The best data available come from the third NHANES study, a large national survey conducted between 1988 and 1994. The prevalence of mild COPD (defined as FEV_1/FVC <70% predicted and FEV_1 >80% predicted) was 6%, and of moderate COPD (defined as FEV_1/FVC <70% and FEV_1 ≤80% predicted) was 6% for subjects 25–75 years of age. The prevalence of both mild and moderate COPD was higher in men than women and in whites than in blacks, and it increased steeply with age in all groups. Airflow limitation was estimated to be present in 14% of current white male smokers, 7% of ex-smokers, and 3% of never-smokers. In white female subjects, airflow limitation occurred in 14% of smokers, 7% of ex-smokers, and 3% in never-smokers. Interestingly, fewer than 50% of individuals with COPD on the basis of the presence of airflow limitation had a physician's diagnosis of COPD.

In England and Wales, some 900,000 people have a diagnosis of COPD—although because of underdiagnosis, the true number is likely to be closer to 1.5 million. The mean age at diagnosis in the United Kingdom is 67 years, and the prevalence increases with age. COPD is more common in men than in women and is associated with low socioeconomic state.

The prevalence of diagnosed COPD has increased in the United Kingdom in women from 0.8% in 1990 to 1.4% in 1997, but it did not change over the same period in men (Figure 38-9). Similar trends are found in the United States and probably reflect changes in smoking habits over time in men and women. National surveys of consultations in British general practices have shown a modest decline in the number of middle-aged men consulting their doctor with symptoms suggestive of COPD and a slight increase among middle-aged women. These trends are confounded by changes over the years in the application of the diagnostic labels for this condition, particularly the overlap between COPD and asthma.

Studies from the Latin American Project for the Investigation of Obstructive Lung Disease (PLATINO) found in five major Latin American cities, each in a different country,

that the prevalence of mild COPD, as assessed by the post-bronchodilator FEV_1, increased steeply with age, with the highest prevalence in those older than the age of 60 years, with a wide variation between these five Latin American cities.

Morbidity/Use of Health Resources

COPD places an enormous burden on health care resources, including physician visits, emergency department visits, and hospitalizations. The economic costs of COPD are more than twice those of asthma. The effect on quality of life is considerable, particularly in those with frequent exacerbations. It has been calculated that airways diseases (chronic bronchitis and emphysema, COPD, and asthma) account for 24.4 million lost working days per year in the United Kingdom, which represents 9% of all certified sickness absence among men and 3.5% of the total among women. Respiratory diseases in the United Kingdom rank as the third most common cause of days of certified incapacity; COPD accounts for 56% of these days lost in men and 24% in women. In 2002–2003, there were 110,000 hospital admissions for COPD exacerbations in England, representing 8% of all emergency admissions. The burden in primary care is even greater. Direct costs to the United Kingdom NHS for COPD are estimated to be £819 million (1208 M Euros, 1625 M U.S. dollars), with 54% of these costs caused by hospital admissions and 19% caused by drug treatment.

The European Respiratory Society White Book provides data on the mean number of consultations for major respiratory diseases across 19 countries of the European Economic Community. In most of these countries, consultations for COPD equate with the number for consultations for asthma, pneumonia, lung cancer, and tuberculosis combined. In the United States in 2000, there were 8 million physician office/hospital outpatient visits for COPD, 1.5 million emergency department visits, and 673,000 hospitalizations. The morbidity burden of disease can also be estimated by calculating years of living with disability (yld). It has been estimated that COPD results in 1.68 yld/1000 population, representing 1.8% of all yld with a greater burden in men than in women.

In developed countries, exacerbations of COPD account for the greatest burden on the health care system. In the European Union, total direct costs of respiratory diseases are approximately 6% of the total health care budget, with COPD accounting for 56% (38.6 billion Euros) of this figure. In the United States in 2002, direct costs of COPD were

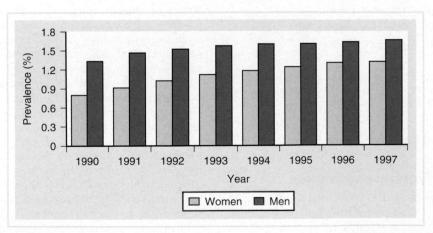

FIGURE 38-9 Prevalence of diagnosed COPD in UK men and women during 1990–1997.

approximately $18 billion and indirect costs approximately $14 billion. There is a direct relationship between the cost of care for COPD and the severity of the condition. Diagnoses related to COPD accounted for 461,000 hospital discharges in the United States in 2004, the fourth most common reason for hospitalization.

Morbidity data in patients with COPD are less available and less reliable than mortality data, but the prevalence of physician visits, emergency department visits, and hospitalizations in COPD increase with age, are greater in men than women, and are likely to increase in the future with the aging of populations.

Mortality

The Global Burden of Disease study undertaken by the World Bank and the World Health Organization concluded that COPD will become the third leading cause of death worldwide by 2020 and will increase its ranking relative to the number of disability-adjusted life years lost from 12th to 5th, largely because of the increase in smoking in the developing world. There are large international variations in the death rate for COPD that cannot be entirely explained by differences in diagnostic patterns, diagnostic labels, or smoking habits. Figures from death certificates underestimate the mortality from COPD, because COPD is often cited as a contributory, rather than as a primary, cause of death. COPD death rates are very low under the age of 45 years and increase steeply with age. Although the mortality from COPD in men has been falling slightly, the mortality in women has increased. COPD accounted for 120,000 deaths in the United States in 2001. Although the death rate is low in patients <45 years old, the mortality increases with age, and for patients >45 years, COPD is the fourth leading cause of death. Worldwide, COPD is the sixth leading cause of death and is the only condition in the top 10 causes of death that has an increasing prevalence and mortality

In the United Kingdom in 2003, 26,000 (14,000 men and 12,000 women) people died of COPD, which represents 4.9% of all deaths, 5.4% of all male deaths, and 4.2% of all female deaths. Within the United Kingdom, age-adjusted death rates from chronic respiratory diseases vary by a factor of 5–10 in different geographic locations. Mortality rates tend to be higher in urban areas than in rural areas.

Mortality from COPD in the United Kingdom has fallen in men but risen in women over the past 25 years, except in the group older than 75 years of age. In American women, the decline in mortality that was recorded until 1975 has reversed and has increased substantially, between 1980 and 2000 from 20.1–56.7/100,000, whereas the increase in men has been more modest from 73.0–82.6/100,000. These trends presumably relate to the later time of the peak prevalence of cigarette smoking in women than men.

Trends in death rates for COPD seem to be rising in the United States but falling in Europe, and the reason for the difference in trends in North America and Europe are, as yet, unexplained.

Natural History and Prognosis

COPD is generally a progressive disease, particularly if the patient's exposure to noxious agents continues. However, the natural history of COPD is variable, not all individuals following the same course. Stopping exposure to noxious agents,

such as cigarette smoke, may result in some improvement in lung function and may slow or halt progression of the disease.

The airways obstruction in susceptible smokers develops slowly as a result of an accelerated rate of decline in FEV_1 that continues for years. As noted previously, impaired growth of lung function during childhood and adolescence as a result of recurrent infections or exposure to tobacco smoke may lead to lower maximally attained lung function in adulthood. This failure in lung growth, often combined with a shortened plateau phase in teenage smokers, increases the risk of COPD. In never-smokers, the FEV_1 declines at a rate of 20–30 mL/year (Figure 38-10). Smokers as a population have a faster rate of decline, and reported changes in FEV_1 in patients with COPD are >50 mL/year. There is a relationship between the initial level of FEV_1 and the annual rate of decline in FEV_1, and individuals in the highest or lowest FEV_1 percentiles remain in the same percentiles over subsequent years. This suggests that susceptible cigarette smokers can be identified in early middle age by a reduction in FEV_1.

Longitudinal data from the Lung Health Study in the United States show that stopping smoking, even after significant airflow limitation is present, can result in some improvement in function and will slow or even stop the progression of airflow limitation. Men who quit smoking at the beginning of the study had an FEV_1 decline of 30.2 mL/year, whereas in those who continued to smoke throughout the study, the decline was 66.1 mL/year. Similar findings were seen in women.

FEV_1 is a strong predictor of survival. Fewer than 50% of patients whose FEV_1 has fallen to 30% of the predicted values are alive 5 years later. The best association between FEV_1 and survival is the postbronchodilator, rather than prebronchodilator, FEV_1. Other clinical parameters have also been shown to be important prognostic indicators independent of FEV_1, such as weight loss, which is a bad prognostic sign. A recently described index that combined the FEV_1, dyspnea, body weight, and the results of a 6-min walk more accurately described prognosis than the FEV_1 alone (Figure 38-11).

Other unfavorable prognostic factors include severe hypoxemia, raised pulmonary arterial pressure, and low carbon monoxide transfer, which become apparent in patients with severe disease.

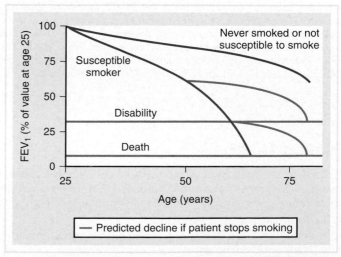

FIGURE 38-10 FEV_1 decline in smokers and non-smokers.

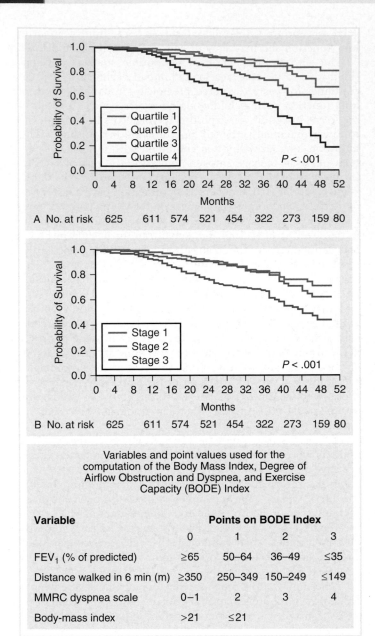

Variables and point values used for the computation of the Body Mass Index, Degree of Airflow Obstruction and Dyspnea, and Exercise Capacity (BODE) Index

Variable	Points on BODE Index			
	0	1	2	3
FEV$_1$ (% of predicted)	≥65	50–64	36–49	≤35
Distance walked in 6 min (m)	≥350	250–349	150–249	≤149
MMRC dyspnea scale	0–1	2	3	4
Body-mass index	>21	≤21		

FIGURE 38-11 The body mass index, degree of airflow obstruction and dyspnea, and exercise capacity (**BODE**) Index in COPD. The variables used for computation of the BODE index are show on the left. The relationship between different quartiles of body mass index on survival in a population of patients with COPD seem to be the stage of COPD as assessed by the level of FEV$_1$. The BODE index indicates survival better than the FEV$_1$. (Adapted from Celli BR, Cote CG, Marin JM, *et al*: N Engl J Med 2004; 350:1005.)

PATHOGENESIS

Central to the pathogenesis seems to be an enhanced inflammatory response to inhaled particles or gases. Several pathogenic processes are involved in this inflammatory response.

- Increased airspace inflammation
- Increased protease burden/decreased antiprotease function
- Oxidant/antioxidant imbalance—oxidative stress
- Defective lung repair

Airway Inflammation

Inflammation is present in the lungs of all smokers. This inflammatory response is thought to be a normal protective innate immune response to inhaled toxins but is amplified in patients who have COPD develop. The mechanism(s) by which this amplification occurs is not understood. COPD does develop in some patients who do not smoke, but the inflammatory response in these patients is not well characterized. The abnormal inflammatory response in COPD leads to tissue destruction, impairment of defense mechanisms that limit such destruction, and impairment of the repair mechanisms. In general, the inflammatory and structural changes in the airways increase with disease severity and persist even after smoking cessation.

Both central and peripheral airways are inflamed in smokers with COPD. Smokers with chronic bronchitis have greater inflammation around gland ducts. Recent studies characterizing the inflammation show increased infiltration of mast cells, macrophages, and neutrophils in smokers with chronic bronchitis (see Box 38-2; see also Figure 38-7). An increase in T lymphocytes, mainly because of an increase in the CD8-positive subset, is present, in contrast to the predominance of the CD4 T-cell subset in asthma. CD8 lymphocytes may have a role in apoptosis and destruction of alveolar-wall epithelial cells through the release of perforins and TNF-α. Excessive recruitment of CD8 T lymphocytes may occur in response to repeated viral infections damaging the lungs in susceptible smokers.

Although several studies have shown that smoking cessation has beneficial effects on pulmonary function, the few studies that have performed a direct assessment of airway inflammation after smoking cessation show persistence of the inflammatory response in the airways, suggesting that there are perpetuating mechanisms that maintain the chronic inflammatory process once it has become established despite the absence of direct smoke exposure.

In addition to inflammatory cells, several inflammatory mediators are involved in the inflammation in the lungs of patients with COPD (Box 38-3).

Proteinase/Antiproteinases Imbalance

The observation of an association between α$_1$-antitrypsin deficiency and the development of early-onset emphysema was important for the pathogenesis of COPD. From these studies

---

BOX 38-3 Inflammatory Mediators

Many inflammatory mediators are increased in COPD, including leukotriene B$_4$, a neutrophil, and T-cell chemoattractant, which is produced by macrophages, neutrophils, and epithelial cells.

Chemotactic factors such as the CXC chemokines interleukin-8 and growth-related oncogene α, which are produced by macrophages and epithelial cells. These attract cells from the circulation and amplify proinflammatory responses.

Proinflammatory cytokines such as tumor necrosis factor-α and interleukins-1β and 6.

Growth factors such as transforming growth factor β, which may cause fibrosis in the airways either directly or through release of another cytokine, connective tissue growth factor.

a hypothesis was developed that, under normal circumstances, the release of proteolytic enzymes from inflammatory cells that migrate to the lungs to fight infection or after cigarette smoke inhalation does not cause damage because of inactivation of these proteolytic enzymes by an excess of inhibitors. In conditions of excessive enzyme load, however, or where there is an absolute or a functional deficiency of antiproteinases, such as may occur during cigarette smoking, an imbalance develops between proteinases and antiproteinases in favor of proteinases, leading to uncontrolled enzyme activity and degradation of lung connective tissue in alveolar walls, resulting in emphysema

This simplified proteinase/antiproteinase theory is complicated by the presence of other antiproteases such as antileukoprotease and other proteases such as metalloproteases released from macrophages (Table 38-1).

α_1-Antitrypsin is the major inhibitor of serine proteases, including neutrophil elastase, and has greatest affinity for the enzyme neutrophil elastase. It is synthesized in the liver and increases from its usual plasma concentration of approximately 2 g/L as part of the acute-phase response. The activity of the protein is critically dependent on the methionine-serine sequence at its active site.

A deficiency in antitrypsin levels, particularly the inability to increase levels in the acute response, leads to unrestrained proteolytic damage to lung tissue leading to emphysema, which develops at an earlier age than in the common variety of emphysema in COPD. Cigarette smoking is a cofactor in the development of emphysema in α_1-antitrypsin–deficient patients, probably as a result of oxidation and, hence, inactivation of the remaining functional α_1-antitrypsin by oxidants in cigarette smoke.

More than 75 biochemical variants of α_1-antitrypsin have been described in relation to their electrophoretic properties, giving rise to the phase inhibitor (Pi) nomenclature. The most common allele in all populations is PiM, and the most common genotype is PiMM, which occurs in 86% of the population in the United Kingdom (Table 38-2). PiMZ and PiS are the two next most common genotypes and are associated with α_1-antitrypsin levels of between 15 and 75% of the mean levels of PiMM subjects. Similar levels occur in the much less common PiSS type. In the PiSZ genotype, basal α_1-proteinase inhibitor levels are 35–50% of normal values. The threshold point for increased risk of emphysema is a level of approximately 80 mg/dL, which is approximately 30% of normal. The homozygous PiZZ type, in which serum levels are

TABLE 38-2 Alpha$_1$-Antitrypsin Phenotypes: Frequency in UK Population, Concentration of Serum Alpha$_1$-Protease Inhibitor, and the Risk for Emphysema

Phenotype	Frequency (%)	Average Concentration (g/L)	Risk Factor for Emphysema
MM	86	2	No
MS	9	1.6	No
MZ	3	1.2	No
SS	0.25	1.2	No
SZ	0.2	0.8	Yes
ZZ	0.03	0.4	Yes

10–20% of the average normal value, is the strongest genetic risk factor for the development of emphysema.

The average α_1-antitrypsin plasma levels for the more common phenotypes are shown in Table 38-2. Although the liver and mononuclear cells from PiZ patients can manufacture normal amounts of mRNA, and the protein can be translated, there is little secretion of the protein. The Z α_1-antitrypsin gene is normal apart from a single point mutation, resulting from substitution of a glycine nucleotide for adenine in the DNA sequence that codes for the amino acid at position 342 on the molecule. This results in spontaneous polymerization of the protein such that these large polymers are unable to pass through the endoplasmic reticulum and accumulate in the liver accounting for the periodic acid–Schiff (PAS)–positive inclusion bodies seen on histologic examination. These polymers may also be chemotactic for inflammatory cells, thereby contributing to the increased elastase burden. It is postulated that a deficiency in α_1-proteinase inhibitor results in excess activity of neutrophil elastase and, therefore, tissue destruction and emphysema.

A-1AT occurs with a prevalence of 1 in 2700 in the United States as determined by screening of adult blood donors (most of whom had normal spirometry). Approximately 1 in 5000 children in the United Kingdom are born with a homozygous PiZZ abnormality. However, the number of subjects affected with the disease is much less than predicted from the known prevalence of the deficiency, and a few PiZZ individuals live beyond their sixth decade and escape the development of airways obstruction. Follow-up of PiZZ subjects has shown an accelerated decline in FEV_1 but with large variations among individuals. There is a clear interaction with cigarette smoking, but this cannot entirely account for the variation observed in the decline in FEV_1. Individuals with PiZZ have predominantly panacinar, basal emphysema develop.

Elastase Synthesis and Repair

An abnormality of elastin synthesis and repair may be involved in the pathogenesis of emphysema. Severe starvation has been reported to cause COPD both in humans and animals; in addition, starvation can exacerbate proteinase-induced emphysema in animal models. Whether the milder malnutrition that occurs in emphysematous patients has a role in the pathogenesis is unknown.

Certain disorders of connective tissues, including Ehlers–Danlos syndrome and cutis laxa, have been associated with

TABLE 38-1 Proteinases and Antiproteinases Involved in COPD

Proteinases	Anti-Proteinases
Serine proteinases	α_1-Antitrypsin
Neutrophil elastase	α_1-Antitrypsin
Cathepsin G	Secretory leukoprotease inhibitor
Proteinase 3	Elafin
Cysteine proteinases	Cystatins
Cathepsins B, K, L, S	
Matrix metalloproteinases	Tissue inhibitor of MMP (TIMP1–4)
MMP-8, MMP-9, MMP-12	

the development of emphysema. Emphysema also develops in some animal models with genetic defects in tissue metabolism.

Oxidant/Antioxidant Imbalance

There is considerable evidence supporting the presence of increased oxidative stress in patients with COPD as a result of an imbalance in the ratio of oxidants to antioxidants. Cigarette smoke itself produces a huge oxidant burden in the airspaces, and oxidants are released in increased amounts from the activated inflammatory cells that migrate into the airspaces in response to smoking. Important antioxidants such as glutathione may also be affected by cigarette smoke. Smoking initially depletes glutathione, but a subsequent rebound occurs, presumably as a protective mechanism.

There is evidence of increased oxidative stress in BAL fluid, sputum, exhaled breath, and breath condensate and also systemically in peripheral blood and skeletal muscle in patients with COPD. There is also evidence that oxidative modification of target molecules occurs to a greater extent in the lungs of patients with COPD compared with smokers in whom the disease has not developed, supporting a role for oxidative stress in the pathogenesis of this condition. Oxidative stress can directly damage cells, increase airspace epithelial permeability, inactivate antiproteases, and, importantly, trigger an enhanced inflammatory response by activating redox-sensitive transcription factors such as Nf-κB and AP1. Oxidative stress may also result in decreased histone deacetylase activity in the lungs of patients with COPD, which would enhance the gene expression of proinflammatory genes such as IL-8.

Other Mechanisms

Both oxidants and proteases such as elastase are important secretagogues for mucous and may, therefore, contribute to the hypersecretion of mucus in chronic bronchitis. Recent studies have shown that airway mucus synthesis is regulated by the epidermal growth factor receptor (EGFR) system. Cigarette smoke upregulates EGFR expression and activates EGFR tyrosine phosphorylation, causing mucus synthesis in epithelial cells by a mechanism that probably involves oxidative stress.

Recent studies have also suggested that apoptosis may be a central feature in the development of emphysema as a result of apoptotic loss of epithelial and endothelial cells in the alveolar walls. This may occur as a result of downregulation of the important maintenance factor vascular endothelial growth factor (VEGF). Oxidative stress may also have a role in both the downregulation of VEGF and in apoptosis. More recently, it has been suggested that enhanced inflammatory response, particularly that which occurs in the later stages of the disease, may result from an upregulation of acquired immunity as the result of an autoimmune inflammatory response or as a result of reaction to respiratory infection.

PATHOPHYSIOLOGY

Mucus Hypersecretion and Ciliary Dysfunction

Mucus hypersecretion results in a chronic productive cough (i.e., chronic bronchitis). Chronic bronchitis is not necessarily associated with airflow limitation, and, conversely, not all patients with COPD have chronic productive cough. Mucus hypersecretion is due to squamous metaplasia and increased numbers of goblet cells and increased size of bronchial submucosal glands in response to chronic irritation by noxious particles and gases. Ciliary dysfunction results from squamous metaplasia of the epithelial cells and produces abnormal function of the mucociliary escalator and thus difficulty expectorating sputum.

Airflow Limitation and Hyperinflation

The characteristic physiologic abnormality in COPD is a decrease in maximum expiratory flow resulting from loss of lung elasticity and an increase in small and/or large airways resistance.

In healthy young subjects, significant airway closure occurs only below functional residual capacity (FRC). However, enhanced airway closure occurs in the early stages of COPD as demonstrated by the single-breath nitrogen test. The "closing volume" so derived measures the lung volume at which some lung units close their airways and, hence, stop emptying, as manifested by abrupt increases in expired nitrogen concentrations. In healthy young nonsmokers, the closing volume is approximately 5–10% of vital capacity (VC), increasing to 25–35% of VC in old age. Compared with nonsmokers, young, asymptomatic adult smokers have an increase in closing volume. As the airways disease progresses, the ability to define a closing volume decreases, and, therefore, the test is not useful in established disease.

The main site of airflow limitation in COPD occurs in the conducting airways, less than 2 mm in diameter, as a result of inflammation, narrowing (airway remodeling), and inflammatory exudates in the small airways, features that correlate with the reduction in FEV_1. Other factors contributing to the airflow obstruction include loss of the lung elastic recoil (because of the destruction of alveolar walls) and the destruction of alveolar support (from alveolar attachments). The consequent airway obstruction results in progressive air trapping during expiration, resulting in hyperinflation at rest and dynamic hyperinflation during exercise. Lung hyperinflation reduces the inspiratory capacity and thus FRC increases, particularly during exercise (Figure 38-12). These features are thought to occur early in the course of the disease and result in breathlessness and limited exercise capacity typical of COPD. Bronchodilators reduce air trapping and thus decrease lung volumes, thereby improving symptoms and exercise capacity (Figure 38-13). Tests of overall lung mechanics, such as the FEV_1 and airways resistance, are usually abnormal in patients with COPD when breathlessness develops.

Residual volume, FRC, and (in some cases) TLC increase. Maximum expiratory flow-volume curves show a characteristic convexity toward the volume axis, with preservation of peak expiratory flow initially (Figure 38-14).

The uneven distribution of ventilation in advanced COPD causes a reduction in "ventilated" lung volume, and thus the carbon monoxide transfer factor is almost always reduced, although the lung diffusing capacity for carbon monoxide (DL_{CO}), normalized to ventilated alveolar volume ($DL_{CO}/V_A/K_{CO}$), may remain relatively well preserved in those without emphysema.

The ability to draw air through the conducting airways during inspiration depends on the strength of the respiratory muscles (which in turn depends on their resting length), the compliance of the respiratory system (i.e., lung and chest wall), and the resistance of the airways. Exhalation is normally passive and is a result of the elastic recoil of the lungs.

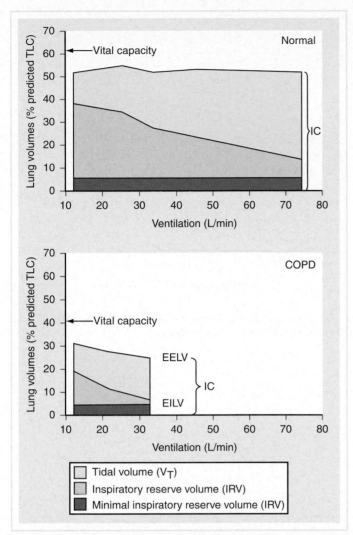

FIGURE 38-12 In good health, the body meets the increased oxygen demand produced by exercise by use of some of the inspiratory reserve volume of the lungs to increase tidal volume. The vertical axes here are presented inverted from the pulmonologic convention for clarity. *EELV,* End expiratory lung volume; *EILV,* end inspiratory lung volume; *IC,* inspiratory capacity; *IRV,* inspiratory reserve volume; *TLC,* total lung capacity. (Data from O'Donnell DE, Revill SM, Webb KA: AJRCCM 2001; 164:770.)

The characteristic changes in the static pressure-volume curve of the lungs in COPD are an increase in static compliance and a reduction in static transpulmonary pressure at any given lung volume (Figure 38-15). These changes are generally thought to indicate emphysema.

The resistance to airflow depends on the length and diameter of the airways and the physical properties of the respirable gas. At a constant airway diameter, flow during inhalation is proportional to the difference between the pressures of atmospheric gas and that in the alveolus. During exhalation, it depends on the difference between alveolar and atmospheric pressures. Throughout inhalation and during the initial portion of exhalation, this relationship is constant. However, at a certain point during exhalation, flow cannot increase despite further increases in alveolar pressure. This is a result of dynamic compression of the airways, which limits flow as illustrated

in the flow-volume curve (Figure 38-16). During exhalation from TLC, flow increases to a point beyond which additional expiratory effort has no effect. During tidal breathing, expiratory flow is well below that attainable during maximum expiration. In COPD, however, the flow-volume curve is markedly different. The major site of the fixed airway narrowing is in the peripheral airways. Dynamic expiratory compression of the airways is enhanced by loss of lung recoil and by atrophic changes in the airways and loss of support from the surrounding alveolar walls, allowing flow limitation at lower driving pressures and flows.

In addition to a decrease in peak expiratory flow, the later expiratory portion of the flow-volume curve is markedly concave relative to the volume axis in patients with COPD. In severe disease, the flow that is generated during tidal breathing may actually reach the maximum possible flow. Such patients, in response to the increased metabolic demands of exercise, for example, are unable to increase ventilation. Increases in respiratory rate result in gas trapping from incomplete alveolar emptying—so-called dynamic overinflation. This increased lung volume increases the elastic recoil and is associated with an increase in the end-expiratory alveolar pressure. The result is an increase in the work of breathing, because pleural pressure has to drop below alveolar pressure before inspiration of air can occur.

VENTILATORY CONTROL

The respiratory center, which controls ventilation, is situated in the upper part of the medulla and integrates a variety of sensory inputs (e.g., mechanical from stretch receptors; neural factors from the resultant dyspnea; chemical factors related to blood gases and pH; and other sensory inputs such as the work of breathing). Output is through the peripheral nervous system to the respiratory muscles, which shorten to deform the rib cage and abdomen and generate intrathoracic pressures. Coupling is the term used to describe the relationship between respiratory drive and respiratory pressure or volume. In normal subjects, breathing is perceived as effortless. In circumstances when breathing requires an increased effort that is perceived as work, the resulting symptom is breathlessness. The relationship between central drive (i.e., control of output) and final output (i.e., ventilation) is complex. Accordingly, it has been difficult to ascribe breathlessness to any given individual component of the system.

Ventilation ($\dot{V}_E$, $\dot{V}$) represents the final effectiveness of the ventilatory drive. $\dot{V}_E$ has two components, the tidal volume (V_T) and respiratory frequency. In COPD, as the disease progresses, adverse lung mechanics and changes in ventilation perfusion ($\dot{V}/\dot{Q}$) relationships occur, and $\dot{V}_E$ increases as a response. The increase in $\dot{V}_E$ is affected initially by an increase in V_T, but as airflow limitation worsens and the consequent work increases, V_T decreases. The respiratory rate increases as the airflow limitation worsens.

$\dot{V}_E$ can be expressed in terms of the ratio of inspiratory time (T_I) and the total volume of inspiration (T_{TOT}) (T_I/T_{TOT}) and V_T. V_T/T_I reflects the respiratory drive; T_I/T_{TOT} reflects respiratory timing. In COPD, T_I/T_{TOT} is reduced from the normal value of 0.38 by the increase in V_T, whereas V_T/T_I increases.

It is apparent from these measurements that as the degree of airflow limitation progresses, the central drive to breathing increases and is maximum in patients who have respiratory failure. In the early stages of the disease, respiratory drive is

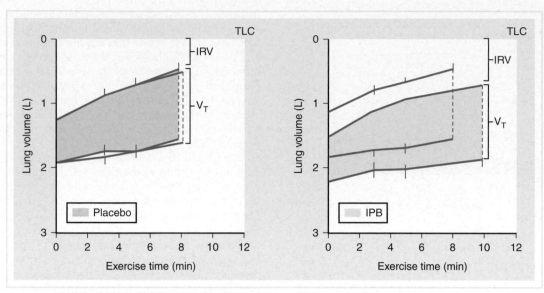

FIGURE 38-13 Operational lung values before and after a bronchodilator (*IPB*, ipratropium bromide) that results in a decrease in operational lung volumes and an increase in inspiratory reserve volume (*IRV*). V_T, Tidal volume; *TLC*, total lung capacity.

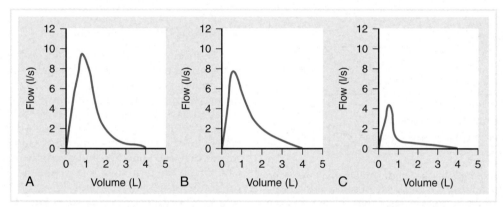

FIGURE 38-14 Examples of flow-volume curves. **A**, Mild obstruction; **B**, moderate obstruction; and **C**, severe obstruction.

effectively coupled to the increase in V_T. As the work of breathing increases, V_T drops, and when this occurs, the only way to increase V_E is to increase the respiratory rate. However, the ability to increase respiratory rate to increase V_E is limited by a reduction in the elastic recoil, which limits expiratory flow and results in air trapping. Increases in lung volume may help dilate the airways, but this benefit is offset by a concurrent reduction in respiratory muscle strength and the development of autopositive end-expiratory pressure.

Pulmonary Gas Exchange

$\dot{V}/\dot{Q}$ mismatching (as a result of decreased alveolar ventilation without a corresponding reduction in perfusion) is the most important cause of impaired pulmonary gas exchange in COPD. Other causes, such as impaired alveolar-capillary diffusion of oxygen and increased shunt, are of much less importance. In general, gas exchange worsens as the disease progresses but is not likely to be abnormal until the FEV_1 drops at least below 50% predicted. The distribution of ventilation is very uneven in patients with COPD. A reduction of blood flow is produced by several mechanisms, including local destruction of vessels in alveolar walls as a result of emphysema, hypoxic vasoconstriction in areas of severe alveolar hypoxemia, and passive vascular obstruction as a result of increased alveolar pressure and distention (if cardiac output is reduced).

Respiratory Muscles

In patients with severe COPD, lung overinflation, compensatory or pathologic loss of muscle mass, and perhaps malnutrition result in muscle weakness reducing the capacity of the respiratory muscles to generate pressure over the range of tidal breathing. In addition, the load against which the respiratory muscles need to act is increased because of the increase in airways resistance. Overinflation leads to shortening and flattening of the diaphragm, impairing its ability to generate inspiratory force. During quiet tidal breathing in normal subjects, expiration is largely passive and depends on the elastic recoil of the lungs and the chest wall. Patients with COPD increasingly need to use their rib cage muscles and inspiratory accessory muscles, such as the sternocleidomastoids, even during quiet breathing. During exercise, this pattern may be even

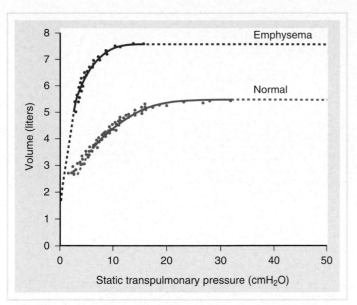

FIGURE 38-15 Representative static expiratory pressure-volume curves of lungs in a subject with severe emphysema compared with a normal subject. Lung volume measured by body plethysmography. Solid lines through experimental points were derived by exponential curve-fitting procedure. Broken lines, extrapolation of curve to infinite pressure and to volume axis at zero pressure. Values of k (cm H_2O^{-1}): for emphysema, 0.325: normal, 0.143. (Adapted from Gibson GJ, Pride NB, Davis J, Schroter RC: Am Rev Respir Dis 1979; 120:799.)

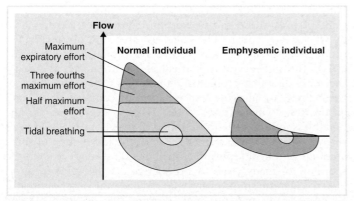

FIGURE 38-16 Flow-volume loop of a normal individual and a patient who has chronic obstructive pulmonary disease (COPD). Patients who have COPD may reach airflow limitation even during tidal breathing. (From Celli B: In Albert R, Spiro SG, Jett JR [eds]: Comprehensive Respiratory Medicine. St Louis: Mosby, 1999.)

more distorted and may result in paradoxical motion of the rib cage.

Patients with COPD have impaired values of global function of the respiratory muscles such as maximum inspiratory mouth pressures (Pe_{max}), although these measurements are very effort dependent. Diaphragmatic function can be assessed during inspiration by measurement of transdiaphragmatic pressure (Pdi) by use of balloon-tipped catheters with small transducers placed in the esophagus and stomach. Measurements of Pdi are reduced in patients with COPD.

BREATHLESSNESS

Breathlessness limits exercise in patients with COPD. The symptom arises from increases in lung volume producing secondary respiratory muscle activation and parallels the increased sensation of respiratory effort. The sensation of breathlessness increases as the ratio of the pressure needed to ventilate to the maximum possible inspiratory pressure increases, and it also worsens in proportion to the duration of inspiration (i.e., Ti/Ttot) and to the respiratory frequency. The respiratory muscles of patients with severe COPD function at a level that approaches the threshold of fatigue. Electromyographic evidence of fatigue has been shown during acute exacerbations of COPD. Respiratory muscle weakness or fatigue may also contribute to the carbon dioxide retention that occurs in some patients with COPD as the disease progresses. Because these circumstances also result in acute gas trapping, with the resulting increase in lung volume, it is difficult to distinguish decreased respiratory strength occurring as a result of fatigue from that attributable to weakness from the muscles having to work at their maximum length.

There is a good relationship between the sensation of breathlessness and the end-expiratory lung volume or the change in end-expiratory lung volume that occurs during exercise. Reducing the degree of overinflation by bronchodilators can reduce breathlessness at rest in more severe cases.

The changes in chest wall geometry that accompany these altered lung volumes reduce the capacity of the inspiratory muscles to develop pressure. Indeed, reduced maximum inspiratory pressure predicts those patients with COPD complaining of breathlessness. The importance of lung mechanical abnormalities, particularly elastic loading secondary to overinflation, has been confirmed by the effect of lung volume reduction surgery in reducing resting and exercise breathlessness. Reductions in lung volumes are accompanied by an increased ability to develop inspiratory pressure and a decreased tension-time index of the respiratory muscles. Thus, changes in lung mechanics seem to be the critical factor in generating breathlessness in COPD.

The role of blood gases in producing breathlessness has been difficult to establish. Patients with COPD do increase their perceived effort as the Pa_{CO_2} rises, but hypoxia seems to be less important in producing breathlessness. Oxygen desaturation during exercise, for example, does not relate to subsequent intensity of breathlessness.

Cor Pulmonale

Pulmonary arterial hypertension occurs late in the course of COPD, concurrent with the development of hypoxemia and usually hypercapnia. Cor pulmonale is a major cardiovascular complication of COPD, is associated with the development of right ventricular hypertrophy, and carries a poor prognosis. Peripheral edema results from a combination of increased venous pressure and cardiac and renal hormonal changes, leading to increased salt and water retention (Figure 38-17).

Systemic Effects

Although primarily a disease of the lungs, it is increasingly recognized that, as in many chronic diseases, COPD is associated with a number of important systemic features that may affect morbidity and mortality and may result in comorbid diseases (see Box 38-1). The effects are more commonly seen in more severe disease. Systemic effects are associated with

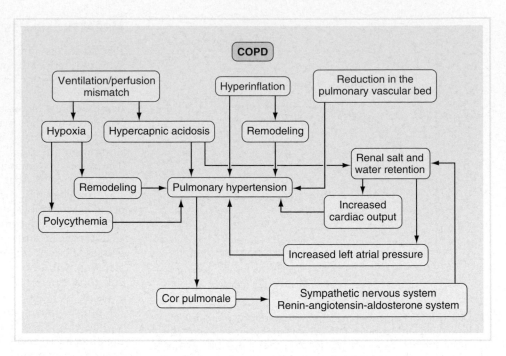

loss of skeletal muscle mass and dysfunction of the skeletal muscles. Weight loss is associated with a poor prognosis in COPD patients. Weight loss and loss of muscle mass may result from a number of factors, including the effects of systemic inflammation, muscle apoptosis, and muscle disuse. Increased systemic inflammatory mediators such as TNFα, IL-6, and oxygen free radicals may mediate some of these systemic effects. Other systemic effects of COPD include osteoporosis, depression, anemia, and an increased risk of cardiovascular disease.

Pathophysiology of Exacerbations

Exacerbations of COPD are associated with a further increase in the inflammatory response in the lungs with an increase predominantly neutrophils and in some mild exacerbations, an increased number of eosinophils.

This increased inflammatory response can be triggered by infection with bacterial viruses or by environmental pollutants. Exacerbations are associated with increased concentrations of mediators such as TNFα, LTB$_4$, and IL-8 in the airways and increased markers of oxidative stress.

In mild exacerbations, airflow limitation is unchanged or only slightly increased. Severe exacerbations are associated with worsening of pulmonary gas exchange because of increased inequality between ventilation and perfusion and respiratory muscle fatigue. The worsening ventilation/perfusion mismatch results from airway inflammation, edema, mucus hypersecretion, and bronchial constriction. These effects also reduce ventilation and cause hypoxic vasoconstriction of pulmonary arterioles, which, in turn, impairs perfusion.

Respiratory muscle fatigue and alveolar hypoventilation can contribute to the hypoxemia, hypercapnia, and respiratory acidosis, and lead to severe respiratory failure and death. Hypoxia and respiratory acidosis can induce pulmonary vasoconstriction that increases the load on the right ventricle, which, together with renal and hormonal changes, can result in peripheral edema.

CLINICAL FEATURES

A summary of the clinical evaluation of patients with COPD is given in Box 38-2.

Symptoms

Patients with COPD characteristically complain of the symptoms of breathlessness on exertion, sometimes accompanied by wheeze and cough. The cough is often, but not invariably, productive. Breathlessness is the symptom that commonly causes the patient to seek medical attention and is usually the most disabling problem. Patients often date the onset of their illness to an acute exacerbation of cough with sputum production, which leaves them with a degree of chronic breathlessness. Close questioning, however, usually reveals many years of a "smokers cough" with the production of small amounts of mucoid sputum (usually <60 mL/day) often in the morning for many years. A productive cough occurs in up to 50% of cigarette smokers and may precede the onset of breathlessness. Many patients may dismiss this as simply being related to their smoking. The frequency of nocturnal cough does not seem to be increased in stable COPD. Paroxysms of coughing in the presence of severe airway obstruction generate high intrathoracic pressures, which can produce syncope and "cough fractures" of the ribs.

Breathlessness is usually first noticed on climbing hills or stairs or hurrying on level ground. It usually heralds the existence of at least moderate impairment of expiratory flow.

Patients may adapt their breathing pattern and their behavior to minimize the sensation of breathlessness. The perception of breathlessness varies greatly between individuals with the same impairment of ventilatory capacity. However, when the FEV$_1$ has fallen to 35% or less of the predicted value, breathlessness is usually present on minimal exertion. Severe breathlessness is often affected by changes in environmental temperature or occupational exposure to dust and fumes. Some patients have severe orthopnea, relieved by leaning forward, whereas others find greatest ease when lying flat. Breathlessness can be assessed on the Medical Research Council (MRC) Dyspnea Scale, the Borg Scale, and visual analog scales (Table 38-3 and Box 38-4).

Wheeze is common, but not specific, to COPD, because it is due to turbulent airflow in large airways from any cause.

Substernal chest pain is common in patients with COPD. It may be a result of the COPD itself or may result from underlying ischemic heart disease or gastroesophageal reflux. Chest tightness is a common complaint during periods of worsening breathlessness, particularly during exercise, and this is sometimes difficult to distinguish from ischemic cardiac pain. Pleuritic chest pain may suggest an intercurrent pneumothorax, pneumonia, or pulmonary infarction. Hemoptysis can be associated with purulent sputum and may be due to inflammation or infection. However, this symptom should also prompt consideration of the possibility of bronchial carcinoma.

Weight loss and anorexia are features of severe COPD and are thought to result from decreased calorie intake, hypermetabolism, or perhaps as a compensatory mechanism for the reduced alveolar ventilation and accompanying decrease in the ability to take up oxygen and excrete carbon dioxide.

Psychiatric morbidity, particularly depression, is common in patients with severe COPD. Sleep quality and sexual function are impaired, which may be contributing factors.

Exposure History

Patients should be questioned about previous and present occupations, particularly exposure to dust and chemicals. Occupational exposure to dust has an additive effect with smoking on the decline in lung function, as has been shown in coal miners, where both smoking and years of dust exposure contribute to the decline in FEV_1, although the contribution of smoking was three times as great as that of the dust exposure.

Differential Diagnosis of COPD

Several conditions should be considered in the differential diagnosis in COPD. Asthma can be particularly difficult as a differential diagnosis (Table 38-4).

The history in COPD should also include:

- History of asthma, allergy, respiratory infections in childhood, or any other respiratory diseases such as tuberculosis
- Family history of COPD or other respiratory diseases
- Number of exacerbations or hospitalizations
- Comorbidities, particularly those that have the same risk factor (smoking) such as ischemia, heart disease, osteoporosis, peptic ulceration, or peripheral vascular disease
- Current drug treatment
- Social support

Clinical Signs

Patients typically are seen in the fifth decade of life. The physical examination may be completely normal early in the course of COPD. The physical signs are not specific and depend on the degree of airflow limitation and pulmonary overinflation. Because of the heterogeneity of COPD, patients may show a range of phenotypic clinical presentations. The sensitivity of

TABLE 38-3 The Modified Borg Scale for Assessing Breathlessness	
Scale	**Severity Experienced by Patient**
0	Nothing at all
0.5	Very, very slight (just noticeable)
1	Very slight
2	Slight (light)
3	Moderate
4	Somewhat severe
5	Severe (heavy
6	Very severe Very, very severe (almost maximal) Maximal

BOX 38-4 The Modified MRC Dyspnea Scale for Assessing Breathlessness

Grade degree of breathlessness related to activities:
0 Not troubled by breathlessness except on strenuous exercise
1 Short of breath when hurrying or walking up a slight hill
2 Walks slower than contemporaries on the level because of breathlessness, or has to stop for breath when walking at own pace
3 Stops for breath after walking about 100 m or after a few minutes on the level
4 Too breathless to leave the house, or breathless when dressing or undressing
5 Breathless at rest

TABLE 38-4 Differences Between COPD and Asthma		
	COPD	**Asthma**
Age	>35 years	Any age
Cough	Persistent and productive	Intermittent and nonproductive
Smoking	Almost invariable	Possible
Breathlessness	Progressive and persistent	Intermittent and variable
Nocturnal symptoms	Uncommon unless in severe disease	Common
Family history	Uncommon unless family members also smoke	Common
Concomitant eczema or allergic rhinitis	Possible	Common

physical examination to detect or exclude moderately severe COPD is rather poor.

General Examination

The respiratory rate may be increased. A forced expiratory time greater than 5 sec strongly suggests the presence of airflow limitation. A breathing pattern with a prolonged expiratory phase, with or without pursing of the lips, is characteristic of patients with COPD. Use of accessory muscles of respiration, particularly the sternocleidomastoids, is often seen in advanced disease, and these patients often adopt a posture in which they lean forward, supporting themselves with their arms to fix the shoulder girdle. This allows use of the pectorals and the latissimus dorsi to increase chest wall movement.

Tar-stained fingers indicate the smoking habit in many patients. In advanced disease, cyanosis may be present, indicating hypoxemia, but it may be diminished by anemia or accentuated by polycythemica and is a fairly subjective sign. The asterixis associated with hypercapnia is neither sensitive nor specific, and papilledema associated with severe hypercapnia is rare.

Weight loss may also be apparent in advanced disease, as well as a reduction in muscle mass. Finger clubbing is not a feature of COPD and should suggest the possibility of complicating bronchial neoplasm or bronchiectasis.

Examination of the Chest

In the later stages of COPD, the chest is often barrel-shaped with a kyphosis, resulting in an increased anteroposterior chest diameter, horizontal ribs, prominence of the sternal angle, and a wide subcostal angle. The distance between the suprasternal notch and the cricoid cartilage (normally 3 finger breadths) may be reduced because of the elevation of the sternum. These are all signs of overinflation. An inspiratory tracheal tug may be detected, attributed to contraction of the low, flat diaphragm. The horizontal position of the diaphragm also acts to pull the lower ribs in during inspiration (i.e., Hoover's sign). Widening of the xiphosternal angle and abdominal protuberance occur, the latter because of forward displacement of the abdominal contents, giving the appearance of apparent weight gain. Increased intrathoracic pressure swings may result in indrawing of the suprasternal and supraclavicular fossae and of the intercostal muscles.

There is decreased hepatic and cardiac dullness on percussion, indicating overinflation. A useful sign of gross overinflation is the absence of a dull percussion note, normally because of the underlying heart, over the lower end of the sternum. Breath sounds may have a prolonged expiratory phase or may be uniformly diminished, particularly in the advanced stages of the disease. Wheeze may be present both on inspiration and expiration, but is not an invariable sign. Crackles may be heard, particularly at the lung bases, but are usually scant and vary with coughing.

Cardiovascular Examination

Air trapping decreases venous return and compresses the heart. Accordingly, tachycardia is common. The presence of positive alveolar pressure at the end of exhalation (i.e., auto- or intrinsic positive end-expiratory pressure) results in the need to create a more negative pleural pressure than usual, manifested by the presence of a paradoxical pulse. Overinflation makes it difficult to localize the apex beat and reduces

the cardiac dullness. The characteristic signs that indicate the presence or consequences of pulmonary arterial hypertension may be detected in advanced cases. The heave of right ventricular hypertrophy may be palpable at the lower left sternal edge or in the subxiphoid regions. Heart sounds are usually soft, although the pulmonary component of the second heart sound may be exaggerated in the second left intercostal space. A right ventricular gallop rhythm may be detected (disappearing on exhalation) in the fourth intercostal space to the left of the sternum. The jugular venous pressure can be difficult to see in patients with COPD, because it swings widely with respiration and is difficult to discern if there is prominent accessory muscle activity. There may be evidence of functional tricuspid incompetence, producing a pansystolic murmur at the left sternal edge. The liver may be tender and pulsatile, and a prominent "v" wave may be visible in the jugular venous pulse. The liver may also be palpable below the right costal margin as a result of overinflation of the lungs.

Peripheral vasodilatation accompanies hypercapnia, producing warm peripheries with a high-volume pulse. Pitting peripheral edema may also be present as a result of fluid retention.

INVESTIGATIONS

Physiologic Assessment

The degree of airflow obstruction cannot be predicted from the symptoms and signs noted on clinical evaluation. Accordingly, the degree of airflow limitation should be assessed in every patient. At an early stage of the disease, conventional spirometry may reveal no abnormality. Results of tests of small airway function, such as the frequency dependency of compliance and closing volume, may be abnormal; however, these tests are difficult to perform, have high coefficients of variation, and are valid only when lung elastic recoil is normal and there is no increase in airways resistance. They are, therefore, not recommended in normal clinical practice.

Spirometry

Spirometry is the most robust test of airflow limitation in patients with COPD. Spirometric measurements have a well-defined range of normal values. A low FEV_1 with an FEV_1/VC ratio below the normal range is a diagnostic criterion for COPD. The rate of decline of the FEV_1 can be used to assess susceptibility in cigarette smokers and progression of the disease.

It is important that a volume plateau is reached when performing the FEV_1, which can take 15 sec or more in patients with severe airways obstruction. If this maneuver is not carried out, the VC can be underestimated. The FEV_1 as a percentage of the predicted value can be used as part of the assessment of severity of the disease (Table 38-5). FEV_1 values within ±20% of the predicted value are considered to be within the normal range. Thus, an FEV_1 of 80% or more of the predicted value is considered to be normal. Under normal circumstances, 70–80% of the total volume of the air in the lungs (FVC) should be exhaled in the first second. When the FEV_1/FVC ratio falls below 70%, airflow limitation is present. The reproducibility the FEV_1 varies by less than 170 mL between maneuvers. To avoid the effect of airway collapse in patients with COPD during forced expiration, it is suggested that a slow or relaxed vital capacity (VC) measurement, which

TABLE 38-5	Spirometric Classification of COPD Severity
Stage	**Characteristics**
0: At risk	Normal spirometry Chronic symptoms (cough, sputum production)
I: Mild COPD	$FEV_1/FVC < 70\%$ $FEV_1 \geq 80\%$ predicted With or without chronic symptoms (cough, sputum production)
II: Moderate COPD	$FEV_1/FVC < 70\%$ $50\% \leq FEV_1 < 80\%$ predicted With or without chronic symptoms (cough, sputum production)
III: Severe COPD	$FEV_1/FVC < 70\%$ $30\% \leq FEV_1 < 50\%$ predicted With or without chronic symptoms (cough, sputum production)
IV: Very severe COPD	$FEV_1/FVC < 70\%$ $FEV_1 < 30\%$ predicted or FEV_1, 50% predicted plus chronic respiratory failure

allows patients to exhale at their own pace, be used. The slow VC is often 0.5 L greater than the FVC.

Spirometry measurements are evaluated by comparing results with appropriate reference values on the basis of age, height, gender, and race. The presence of a postbronchodilator FEV_1 <80% predicted, together with an FEV_1/FVC ratio <0.7, confirms the presence of airflow limitation that is not fully reversible (Figure 38-18).

The FEV_1 as a percentage of the predicted value can be used to assess the severity of the disease, but other measurements, in addition to spirometry, are required to fully assess the effect of COPD on patient's functional ability. Breathlessness can be gauged by the MRC Scale (see Box 38-4). Exercise capacity can be objectively measured by a reduction in self-paced walking distance, which is a strong predictor of health status impairment and prognosis.

Reversibility Testing

Assessment of reversibility to bronchodilators should be performed in patients with COPD to help distinguish those patients with underlying asthma (i.e., those with marked reversibility) and to establish the postbronchodilator FEV_1, which is the best predictor of long-term prognosis.

There is no agreement on a standardized method of assessing reversibility, but this is usually quantified on the basis of a change in the FEV_1. There may be changes in other lung volumes after bronchodilators (e.g., inspiratory capacity, residual volume), which may explain why some symptoms improve in some patients after a bronchodilator without a change in spirometry results. An improvement in FEV_1 in response to a bronchodilator does not necessarily predict a symptomatic response.

Bronchodilator reversibility can vary from day to day, depending on the degree of bronchomotor tone. A change in FEV_1 that exceeds 200 mL is considered to be greater than random variation. Therefore, changes should be reported as significant only if they exceed 200 mL. In addition to this absolute change in FEV_1, a percentage change of 12% over baseline as an absolute change has been suggested as significant by the European Respiratory/American Thoracic Society and GOLD Guidelines, whereas an improvement of 15% over baseline FEV_1 and 200 mL absolute change has been suggested by the British Thoracic Society Guidelines. A suggested protocol is shown in Box 38-5.

It is usually recommended that reversibility be assessed by use of a large bronchodilator dose, either by use of repeated

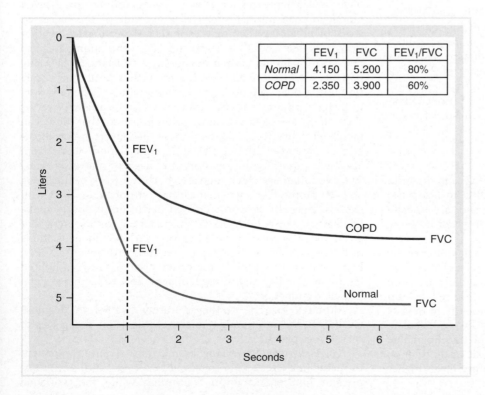

	FEV_1	FVC	FEV_1/FVC
Normal	4.150	5.200	80%
COPD	2.350	3.900	60%

FIGURE 38-18 Static expiratory pressure-volume curves of lungs in a subject with severe emphysema compared with a normal subject. The broken lines represent extrapolation of the curve to infinite pressure and to the volume axis at zero pressure.

doses from a metered dose inhaler or by the nebulization, because this produces a larger number of patients with a significant response. In some cases, the addition of a second drug, such as an anticholinergic drug, to a β-agonist produces a further increase in FEV_1.

Reversibility testing with a bronchodilator is usually indicated only at the time of diagnosis. Approximately 30% of patients with COPD show significant reversibility of their airflow obstruction in response to a bronchodilator.

Reversibility to Corticosteroids

Whether all patients with symptomatic COPD should have a formal assessment of steroid reversibility remains controversial, but this practice is not included in the most recent guidelines for assessment and management of the disease. The most common method for doing this is to administer of 30 mg of prednisolone for a period of 2 weeks. Although patients who have previously shown a response to nebulized bronchodilators are more likely to show a response to steroids, it is not possible to predict an individual patient.

Lung Volumes

Static lung volumes such as TLC, RV, and FRC, and the ratio RV/TLC are measured in patients with COPD to assess the degree of overinflation and gas trapping and are usually increased. These measurements are not necessary in every patient.

The standard method of measuring static lung volumes, by use of the helium dilution technique during rebreathing, may underestimate lung volumes in COPD, particularly in those patients with bullous disease, because the inspired helium may not have sufficient time to equilibrate properly in the airspaces. Body plethysmography uses Boyle's law to calculate lung volumes from changes in mouth and plethysmographic pressures. This technique measures trapped air in the thorax, including poorly ventilated areas, and, therefore, gives higher readings than the helium dilution technique.

Gas Transfer for Carbon Monoxide (DLco)

A low DLco is present in many patients with COPD. Although there is a relationship between the DLco and the extent of microscopic emphysema, the severity of the emphysema in an individual patient cannot be predicted from the DLco, nor is a low DLco specific for emphysema. The commonly used method is the single-breath technique, which uses alveolar volume calculated from the helium dilution during a single breath test. This method underestimates alveolar volume in patients with severe COPD, producing a lower value for the DLco. This test can be useful to distinguish patients with COPD from those with asthma, because a low DLco excludes asthma.

Arterial Blood Gases

Arterial blood gases are needed to confirm the degree of hypoxemia and hypercapnia that develops in patients with COPD. Hypoxemia and hypercapnia are not usually observed until the FEV_1 falls below 50% of predicted. It is essential to record the inspired oxygen concentration when reporting blood gases. It is also important to note that it may take at least 30 min for a change in inspired oxygen concentration to have its full effect on the PaO_2, because of long time constants for alveolar gas equilibration in COPD, particularly during exacerbations. Pulse oximetry is increasingly used to measure the level of oxygenation, but it should not replace an assessment of blood gas tensions in patients with FEV_1s below 50% predicted or in those with elevations of their serum bicarbonate concentrations, because measurements of $PaCO_2$ are often required.

Blood gas abnormalities may worsen during exercise and sleep and during exacerbations.

Exercise Tests

Exercise increases oxygen consumption and carbon dioxide production from skeletal muscle. Patients with COPD may have considerably higher oxygen consumptions for a given workload than normal subjects as a result of the increased work of breathing they may experience. Dead space ventilation is higher and thus larger minute ventilations are also needed to maintain carbon dioxide at a constant level. Many patients with COPD have expiratory airflow limitation occurring in the tidal volume range. In these patients, the only way to increase minute ventilation is to increase inspiratory flow or shift the end-expiratory lung volume up so that flow can increase (Figure 38-12). Both of these maneuvers are problematic in patients with COPD and require more work from already compromised inspiratory muscles or result in progressive overinflation, which increases both the work of breathing and symptoms. The increased cardiac output that occurs with exercise may also lead to increased perfusion of poorly ventilated areas, worsening the V̇/Q̇ mismatching to the extent that arterial oxygenation may fall. Moreover, metabolic acidosis develops at lower work rates in patients with severe COPD. In patients with COPD, progressive cycle exercise is limited by dyspnea in 40% and by leg fatigue in 25% reflecting skeletal muscle dysfunction.

Although exercise testing is rarely needed to diagnose COPD, useful information might accrue from doing any of three types of tests:

Progressive symptom limited exercise tests require the patient to maintain exercise on a treadmill or a cycle until symptoms prevent him or her from continuing while the workload applied is continuously increased. A maximum test is usually defined as a heart rate of greater than 85% of predicted or ventilation greater than 90% predicted. The results are particularly useful when simultaneous electrocardiography and blood pressure monitoring are performed to assess whether coexisting cardiac or psychologic factors contribute to exercise limitation.

Self-paced exercise tests are simple to perform and give information on sustained exercise that may be more relevant to problems in daily life. The commonly used test is the 6-min walk, which has a coefficient of variation of approximately 8%. A learning effect, however, may influence the result of repeated tests. This test is useful only in patients with moderately severe COPD (FEV_1, <1.5 L), who would be expected to have an exercise tolerance of less than 600 m in 6 min. There is a weak relationship between 6-min walking distance and FEV_1, although walking distance is a predictor of survival in patients with severe disease.

An alternative test is the shuttle walking test, in which the patient performs a paced walk between two points 10 m apart (the shuttle). The pace of the walk is increased at regular intervals dictated by bleeps on a tape recording until the patient is forced to stop because of breathlessness. The number of completed shuttles is recorded.

Steady-state exercise tests involve exercise at a sustainable percentage of maximum capacity for 3-6 min during which blood gases are measured, enabling calculation of dead space/tidal volume ratio (V_D/V_T) and shunt. This assessment is seldom required in patients with COPD.

OTHER TESTS

Lung pressure volume curves are difficult to measure, requiring assessment of esophageal pressure with an esophageal balloon and are not part of the routine assessment of patients with COPD. They may be necessary in special circumstances.

Measurements of small airway function with nitrogen washout test, helium flow flow-volume loops, or frequency dependence of compliance have poor reproducibility in patients with COPD. Although they can differentiate smokers from nonsmokers, they are not useful for predicting in which smokers COPD will develop and thus are not used in routine practice.

Respiratory Muscle Function Tests

The usual tests of respiratory muscle function in COPD are maximum inspiratory and expiratory mouth pressures. These tests can be useful in cases in which breathlessness or hypercapnia is not fully explained by other lung function testing following suspected peripheral muscle weakness.

Sleep Studies

Selected patients should be assessed for the presence of nocturnal hypoxemia. Finding nocturnal hypoxemia does not, however, provide any further prognostic or clinically useful information in the assessment of patients with COPD, unless coexisting sleep apnea syndrome is suspected.

Assessment of Breathlessness

Symptomatic improvement, particularly in breathlessness, is one of the important goals of treatment in COPD. Breathlessness is a subjective feature but can be quantified. The appearance of breathlessness heralds moderate to severe impairment of airway function. By the time patients seek medical advice, the FEV_1 has usually fallen to approximately 1–1.5 L in an average man (30–45% of the predicted value). The perception of breathlessness varies greatly between individuals with the same degree of ventilatory capacity. It can be assessed by use of a modified Borg Scale (see Table 38-3), a visual analog scale (see Figure 38-13), or the MRC Dyspnea Scale (see Box 38-4). The oxygen-cost diagram is more sensitive to change than the MRC scale and allows the patient to mark a 10-cm line to represent the point beyond which he or she becomes breathless (Figure 38-19). The distance in centimeters from the zero point can be used to obtain a score.

Health Status

Health-related quality of life is a measure of the impact of disease on daily life and well-being. Several questionnaires are available to assess health status. The Chronic Respiratory Disease Index Questionnaire is sensitive to change but is very time-consuming and requires training to administer properly. The St. George's Respiratory Questionnaire is a self-completed questionnaire with three components: symptoms, which measures distress because of respiratory symptoms; activity, which measures disturbance of daily activities; and impact, which measures psychosocial function. The three components are summed to give a total score of overall health status. The Breathing Problems Questionnaire is a self-completed questionnaire that is easy to complete but relatively insensitive to change. The St. George's Respiratory Questionnaire is the most validated in COPD.

There is a rather poor relationship between the St. George's Respiratory Questionnaire and FEV_1. It is clear from various studies that there can be improvement in health status without

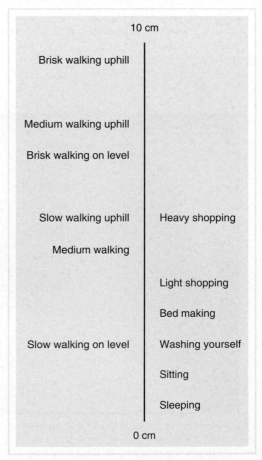

FIGURE 38-19 Oxygen-cost diagram.

any improvement in FEV_1 in response to drugs. The threshold of clinical improvement is a change of four units in the St. George's Respiratory questionnaire. Exacerbations of COPD have a clear detrimental effect on health status.

Other Measurements

Erythrocythemia/polycythemia is important to identify in patients with COPD, because it predisposes to peripheral vascular, cardiovascular, and cerebrovascular events. Erythrocythemia does not develop until there is clinically important hypoxemia (PaO_2 <7.2 kPa, 55 mmHg) and is not an inevitable occurrence even at this level. Polycythemica should be suspected when the hematocrit is greater than 47% in women and 52% in men and/or the hemoglobin is greater than 16 g/dL in women or 18 g/dL in men, provided other causes of spurious polycythemica, because of decreased plasma volume, such as caused by dehydration or diuretics, can be excluded.

A full blood count may reveal the anemia of chronic disease that occurs in COPD.

Alpha$_1$-antitrypsin deficiency screening with measurements of the level and determination of allelic phenotype is indicated for patients with an early onset of emphysema (<45 years of age) and in those with a family history of premature emphysema. Because of the potential importance for other family members, some experts recommend that all patients with COPD be screened.

Electrocardiography is not routinely required in the assessment of patients with COPD except when coexisting cardiac morbidity is suspected. It is an insensitive technique for the diagnosis of cor pulmonale. Overinflation of the chest increases the retrosternal air space, which transmits sound waves poorly, making echocardiography difficult in patients with COPD. Thus, an adequate examination can be achieved in only 65–85% of patients with COPD.

Two-dimensional echocardiography has been used in the investigation of right ventricular dimensions. Pulsed-wave Doppler echocardiography is used to assess ejection flow dynamics of the right ventricle in patients with pulmonary hypertension. The tricuspid gradient can be used to calculate the right ventricular systolic pressure. The technique estimates the pressure gradient across the tricuspid regurgitant jet recorded by Doppler ultrasound. The maximum velocity of the regurgitant jet is measured from the continuous-wave Doppler recordings, and the simplified Bernoulli equation is used to calculate the maximum pressure gradient between the right ventricle and the right atrium as: $P_{RV} - P_{RA} = 4v^2$; where P_{RV} and P_{RA} are the right ventricular and right atrial pressures and v is the maximum velocity. The right atrial pressure is estimated from clinical examination of the jugular venous pressure.

Imaging

Plain Chest Radiography

COPD does not produce any specific features on a plain chest radiograph unless features of emphysema are present. There may be no abnormalities, however, even in patients with very severe disability. The most reliable radiographic signs of emphysema can be divided into those caused by overinflation, vascular changes, and bullae.

The following radiologic features are indicative of overinflation.

- A low, flattened diaphragm (i.e., the border of the diaphragm in the midclavicular line on the posteroanterior film is at or below the anterior end of the seventh rib, and is flattened if the perpendicular height from a line drawn between the costal and cardiophrenic angles to the border of the diaphragm is < 1.5 cm [Figure 38-20]).
- Increased retrosternal airspace, visible on the lateral film at a point 3 cm below the manubrium, is present when the horizontal distance from the posterior surface of the aorta to the sternum exceeds 4.5 cm (see Figure 38-20).

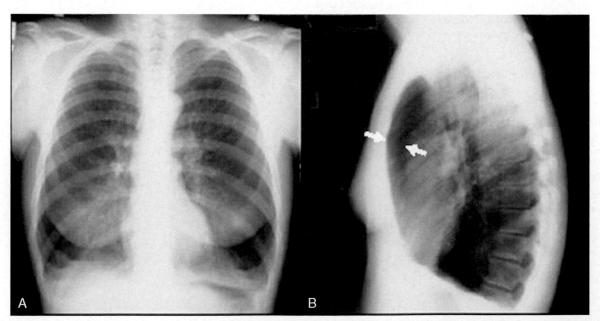

FIGURE 38-20 Plain chest radiographs of generalized emphysema particularly affecting the lower zones. **A,** Posteroanterior radiograph showing a low, flat diaphragm (below the anterior ends of the seventh ribs), obtuse costophrenic angles, and reduced vessel markings in lower zones, which are transradiant. **B,** Lateral radiograph showing a low, flat, and inverted diaphragm and widened retrosternal transradiancy (*white arrows*) that approaches the diaphragm inferiorly (*black arrows*).

- An obtuse costophrenic angle on the posteroanterior or lateral chest radiograph
- An inferior margin of the retrosternal airspace 3 cm or less from the anterior aspect of the diaphragm.

The vascular changes associated with emphysema result from loss of alveolar walls and are shown on the plain chest radiograph by:

- A reduction in the number and size of pulmonary vessels, particularly at the periphery of the lung
- Vessel distortion, producing increased branching angles and excess straightening or bowing of vessels
- Areas of increased lucency

Critical to the assessment of vascular loss in emphysema is the quality of the chest radiograph, because increased lucency may simply be due to overexposure.

The accuracy of diagnosing emphysema on a plain chest radiograph increases with severity of the disease and has been reported as being 50–80% in patients with moderate to severe disease. However, the sensitivity has been reported as being as low as 24% in patients with mild to moderate disease.

Right ventricular hypertrophy or enlargement produces nonspecific cardiac enlargement on the plain chest radiograph. The plain chest radiograph can be used as a screening tool to assess pulmonary hypertension. The width of the right descending pulmonary artery, measured just below the right hilum, where the borders of the artery are delineated against air in the lungs laterally and the right main stem bronchus medially, is normally up to 16 mm in men and 15 mm in women. Measurements greater than this can predict the presence, but not the level, of the pulmonary arterial hypertension.

Computed Tomography (CT)

Computed tomography (CT) scanning has been used to detect and quantify emphysema. Techniques can be divided into those that provide a visual assessment of low-density areas on the CT scan, which can be either semiquantitative or quantitative, or those that use CT lung density to quantify areas of low X-ray attenuation. These techniques are used to measure macroscopic or microscopic emphysema, respectively.

A visual assessment of emphysema on CT scanning shows:

- Areas of low attenuation without obvious margins or walls
- Attenuation and pruning of the vascular tree
- Abnormal vascular configurations.

Areas of low attenuation correlate best with areas of macroscopic emphysema. Visual inspection of the CT scan can be used to locate macroscopic emphysema, although assessing the extent is insensitive and subject to high intraobserver and interobserver variability. The CT scan can be used to assess different types of emphysema—centrilobular emphysema produces patchy areas of low attenuation prominent in the upper zones, whereas those of panlobular emphysema are diffuse throughout the lung zones (see Figure 38-4).

A more quantitative approach of assessing macroscopic emphysema is by highlighting picture elements (pixels) in the lung fields in a predetermined low-density range, between −910 and −1000 Hounsfield units, the so-called density mask technique.

Although the choice of the density range is fairly arbitrary, there is a good correlation between pathologic emphysema score and the CT density score. This technique may still miss areas of mild emphysema.

Microscopic emphysema can be quantified by measuring CT lung density. CT density is measured on a linear scale in Hounsfield Units (water = 0; air = −1000). CT lung density is a direct measure of physical density, and, thus, as emphysema develops, a decrease in alveolar surface area occurs as alveolar walls are lost, associated with an increase in distal airspace size, which would decrease lung CT density.

More studies are required before CT lung density can be used as a standardized technique to quantify microscopic emphysema.

A bulla is defined arbitrarily as an emphysematous space greater than 1 cm in diameter. On the plain chest radiograph, a bulla appears as a localized avascular area of increased lucency, usually separated from the rest of the lung by a thin, curvilinear wall. Marked compression of the surrounding lung may be seen, and bullae may also depress the diaphragm.

CT scanning is much more sensitive than plain chest radiography at detecting bullae and can be used to determine the number, size, and position.

CT scanning has been used to quantify the extent and distribution of emphysema as part of the assessment for surgery in bullous disease and for lung volume reduction surgery.

PITFALLS AND CONTROVERSIES

Differentiation of COPD from asthma has been difficult because of the overlap in pathophysiology, clinical presentation, pulmonary function test results, and treatment. This differentiation is important, however, because treatment options now differ for both conditions (e.g., importance of anticholinergics vs β-agonist therapy, use of corticosteroids, use of pulmonary rehabilitation).

The pathogenesis of emphysema is thought to result from an abnormal inflammatory response in the lungs to inhaled particles and gases, usually cigarette smoking. The enhanced inflammatory response involves both an increase in the innate and acquired immune responses. Other pathogenic mechanisms such as antioxidant imbalance, protease/antiprotease imbalance, and abnormal lung repair are also thought to be involved.

Spirometry is essential in the diagnosis of COPD, but the FEV_1 may not be the best measure of functional status in COPD. It is, therefore, necessary to make other assessments of exercise tolerance, breathlessness, and weight loss to assess the severity of the disease and its impact in COPD patients fully.

SUGGESTED READINGS

Anto JM, Vermeire P, Vestbo J, Sunyer J: Epidemiology of chronic obstructive pulmonary disease. Eur Respir J 2001; 17:982–994.

Barnes PJ: Chronic obstructive pulmonary disease. N Engl J Med 2000; 343:269–280.

Calverley PMA, MacNee W, Pride NB, Rennard SI, eds: Chronic Obstructive Pulmonary Disease, 2nd ed. London: Chapman & Hall; 2003.

Celli BR, MacNee W: Standards for the diagnosis and treatment of patients with COPD. Eur Respir J 2004; 23:841–845.

European Respiratory Monograph: 2006 Management of chronic obstructive pulmonary disease, Issue 38. (*www.ersnet.org*)

Glenny R, Wagner PD, Roca J, *et al*: Gas exchange in health: rest, exercise, and aging. In Roca J, Rodriguez-Roisin R, Wagner PD, eds: Pulmonary and Peripheral Gas Exchange in Health and Disease. New York: Marcel Dekker; 2000:121–148.

Global Initiative for Chronic Obstructive Pulmonary Disease Workshop Report: www.goldcopd.com (accessed June 2005).

Hogg JC, Chu F, Utokaparch S, *et al*: The nature of small-airway obstruction in chronic obstructive pulmonary disease. N Engl J Med 2004; 350:2645–2653.

Hogg JC, Senior RM: Chronic obstructive pulmonary disease. II. Pathology and biochemistry of emphysema. Thorax 2002; 57:830–834.

MacNee W: Pathogenesis of chronic obstructive pulmonary disease. Proc Am Thorac Soc 2005; 2:258–266.

MacNee W, Calverley PMA: Chronic obstructive pulmonary disease 7: Management of COPD. Thorax 2003; 58:261–265.

Saetta M, Turato G, Maestrelli P, *et al*: Cellular and structural bases of chronic obstructive pulmonary disease. Am J Respir Crit Care Med 2001; 163:1304–1309.

Schols AMWJ, Soeters PB, Dingemans AMC, *et al*: Prevalence and characteristics of nutritional depletion in patients with stable COPD eligible for pulmonary rehabilitation. Am Rev Respir Dis 1993; 147:1151–1156.

Voelkel NF, MacNee W, eds: Chronic obstructive lung disease. London: BC Decker; 2002.

Wouters EFM: Muscle weakness in chronic obstructive pulmonary disease. Eur Respir Rev 2000; 10:349–353.

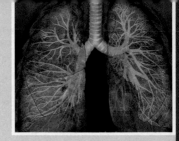

39 Management of Acute Exacerbations of Chronic Obstructive Pulmonary Disease

JOHN R. HURST • JADWIGA A. WEDZICHA

EPIDEMIOLOGY

Chronic obstructive pulmonary disease (COPD) is the fifth most common cause of death in the world, has an increasing mortality rate, and much of the morbidity and mortality relate to episodes of symptom deterioration (i.e., acute exacerbations [AEs]) that punctuate the course of disease. AEs of COPD account for approximately one in ten emergency medical admissions to hospital, and the in-hospital mortality is 10%. AEs are responsible for 70% of the direct costs attributable to COPD.

AEs generally become both more frequent and more severe as the severity of the underlying COPD progresses. On average, patients with moderate to severe COPD, typical of those attending secondary care, will have between one and two AEs requiring additional treatment annually. There are, however, large differences in the annual AE incidence rates of individual patients, and those prone to more frequent AEs experience a particular burden of disease as outlined in Figure 39-1. The factors predisposing some patients to frequent AEs are poorly understood but may include daily bronchitic symptoms, greater severity of underlying disease, greater airway inflammation in the stable state, a predisposition to acquiring respiratory viral infection, and/or the presence of lower airway bacterial colonization (described later).

PATHOPHYSIOLOGY

COPD has been defined by the World Health Organization as a disease state characterized by airflow limitation that is progressive, not fully reversible, and associated with an abnormal inflammatory response to noxious particles or gases. Airway inflammation is even greater at the time of AE, and the assumption has been made that this additional inflammation provokes symptoms such as worsening dyspnea and sputum production by mechanisms relating to airway tone, airway wall edema, and mucus production. The resultant airtrapping increases the work of breathing and causes additional impairment to respiratory muscle function. Triggers of increased airway inflammation are, therefore, considered to be the most common causes of AEs, predominantly tracheobronchial infection and with a lesser role for pollutants. The effects of increased inflammation at AE require further clarification, however, because a direct relationship between the clinical severity of the AE and the degree of airway inflammation has never been conclusively demonstrated.

Defining the role of airway infection in causing AEs is not a simple task. Recent advances in molecular biology have enabled the isolation of respiratory viruses and potentially pathogenic bacteria from the airways of many patients during exacerbations. The most common organisms identified are listed in Table 39-1. Patients with more severe underlying disease, however, are also colonized with bacteria when in their stable state. The presence of an organism at AE does not, therefore, imply a role in causing that exacerbation. More recently, it has been suggested that a change in the colonizing bacterial strain may be the precipitating event. However, not all strain changes are associated with an AE, and not all AEs are associated with strain change. Reflecting this, and as discussed later, antibiotics may not be of universal benefit during AEs. Rhinovirus is the most commonly identified viral pathogen, and consequently, AEs are more common during the winter months when viral circulation in the community is higher. The role of atypical organisms such as *Chlamydia* and *Mycoplasma* species remains unclear.

Large epidemiologic studies link increases in pollutant levels with increases in hospital admission for respiratory disease. PM_{10} (particulate matter less than 10 μm in size) appear particularly important. It is possible that pollutants and microorganisms may interact to amplify the risk of exacerbation.

It has recently been recognized that COPD is associated with systemic inflammation, and there is now ample evidence to demonstrate that systemic inflammation increases during AEs. This may be important given the associations between cardiovascular death and raised systemic inflammatory markers and the finding that many patients with COPD die from cardiovascular disease. This systemic inflammation is thought to represent "spill over" from the lung.

Understanding the pathophysiology of AEs promotes an appreciation of the rationale for the various therapies used: bronchodilators may be helpful for increased bronchoconstriction and hyperinflation; corticosteroids may reduce airway inflammation; and antibiotics may be appropriate in those AEs caused by bacteria (although making this distinction is difficult). This concept is illustrated in Figure 39-2, and the various therapeutic strategies are described in further detail in the following sections.

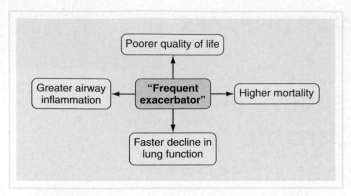

FIGURE 39-1 Consequences of exacerbations in COPD.

TABLE 39-1 Commonly Isolated Organisms at Exacerbation of COPD	
Bacteria	**Respiratory Viruses**
Haemophilus influenzae	Rhinovirus
Moraxella catarrhalis	Influenza
Streptococcus pneumoniae	Parainfluenza
*Pseudomonas aeruginosa**	Coronavirus
	Respiratory syncytial virus
	Adenovirus

*In patients with more severe underlying COPD.

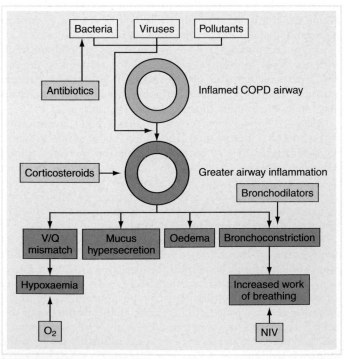

FIGURE 39-2 The pathophysiology of exacerbation provides a rationale for understanding exacerbation therapy. *NIV*, Noninvasive ventilation; $\dot{V}/\dot{Q}$, ventilation-perfusion.

CLINICAL FEATURES

The cardinal feature of an AE is an increase in respiratory symptoms beyond that which is usual for the patient. Typically, such symptoms include dyspnea, sputum production, sputum purulence, cough, and wheeze, perhaps accompanied by upper respiratory tract symptoms (such as rhinorrhea), peripheral edema, and/or confusion. Clinical signs are nonspecific but may include tachycardia, tachypnea, cyanosis, the use of accessory respiratory muscles, polyphonic expiratory wheeze or crackles on auscultation, an abnormal mental status, elevated jugular venous pressure, edema, and other manifestations of cor pulmonale.

AEs are very heterogeneous events, and the clinical features vary widely. Patients with mild underlying disease may experience no more than a troublesome worsening of symptoms, whereas those with more severe COPD are at significant risk of respiratory failure. Furthermore, other conditions occurring in patients with underlying COPD may mimic or complicate exacerbations. Proper assessment, as described below, is therefore important.

DIAGNOSIS

An AE of COPD is a clinical syndrome, and, as such, there is no confirmatory diagnostic test. Although there has been controversy about the exact definition of AE, and although such differences may be important when interpreting the results of various studies, it is now widely accepted that an AE may be defined as a sustained worsening of a patient's symptoms that is acute in onset, beyond day-to-day variation, and that may necessitate a change in therapy.

Although laboratory investigations are not helpful in the diagnosis of AEs, diagnostic tests are of value in assessing the severity of the event and in excluding other conditions that may mimic or complicate the syndrome. Such diagnoses include pneumonia, pneumothorax, pulmonary embolus, and cardiac failure, and appropriate investigations would, therefore, include a chest radiograph, electrocardiogram, oxygen saturations and/or arterial blood gas analysis, and simple venous blood tests, including full blood count, urea and electrolytes, and C-reactive protein. Spirometry is not generally helpful, because absolute values may be misleading, changes at exacerbation are small, and patients who are acutely dyspneic may have difficulty performing the maneuvers accurately. Sputum microscopy and culture may help to refine empiric antibiotic therapy in those not improving or in those with resistant *Pseudomonas* infection, but the role of microbiologic studies in the initial evaluation has not been clarified. For those mild exacerbations that respond to an increase in inhaled bronchodilators alone, further investigation may not be warranted.

There is no accepted method of assessing exacerbation severity. Quantifying changes in symptoms or lung function is not generally helpful and is difficult to achieve, because it requires knowledge of the patient at baseline. Consequently, the degree of health care utilization has been used as a surrogate assessment of severity: mild exacerbations are defined as those that require no more than an increase in inhaled bronchodilators, moderate exacerbations as those requiring antibiotics and or corticosteroids in the community, and severe exacerbations as those requiring hospital admission. pH is the best indicator of an acute change in alveolar ventilation, and most exacerbations associated with respiratory failure will require hospital assessment. The decision to admit a patient to the hospital is, however, dependent on more than the severity of the exacerbation itself and would include, for example, the patient's social circumstances and the support available to the patient at home.

TREATMENT

The principles of therapy at the time of an AE are twofold: to modify the course of the event and to support respiratory function while such disease-modifying therapies are able to act. Treatment is given in proportion to the clinical severity of the event, and the sequential approach is illustrated in Figure 39-3. Many published guidelines exist to guide appropriate therapy, including recent evidence-based statements from the UK National Institute of Clinical Evidence (NICE). Attention to comorbidities is also important, and in the recovery phase, one should consider interventions that may reduce the risk of subsequent exacerbations.

Inhaled Bronchodilator Therapy

An increase in the dose or frequency of inhaled short-acting bronchodilators is the mainstay of therapy. There is little to choose from in terms of bronchodilator effect between the β_2-agonist salbutamol (albuterol) and the anticholinergic drug ipratropium bromide. Although often used in combination, there is little evidence to suggest an additive benefit. There is also no evidence that administering the medications by nebulization is any more effective than by a metered-dose inhaler and large-volume spacer. However, nebulizers are often preferred in dyspneic patients. Nebulizers for COPD should be driven on compressed air rather than oxygen because of concern for the effect of high alveolar oxygen tensions on ventilation-perfusion relationships. Patients prescribed long-acting bronchodilators could continue this therapy, but there is little evidence to support introducing long-acting agents during an AE, and short-acting drugs are preferred. The recommended approach is, therefore, to increase the dose and or frequency of either a short-acting β_2-agonist or an anticholinergic, with both drugs used together in the event of inadequate clinical response.

Corticosteroids

Systemic corticosteroids are indicated in all but the mildest of exacerbations that respond to an increase in inhaled

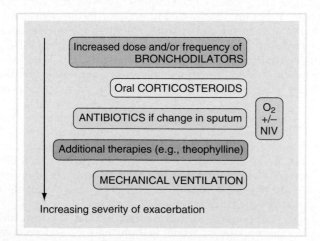

FIGURE 39-3 A summary of the stepwise therapeutic approach to COPD exacerbation. *NIV,* Noninvasive ventilation.

bronchodilators alone. A number of randomized trials, now summarized in systematic reviews, demonstrate a more rapid improvement in FEV_1 after administration of steroids, although effects on outcomes such as oxygenation, hospitalization, and length of hospital stay are more variable, and an effect on mortality has not been documented. Guidelines vary in their specific recommendations, generally suggesting oral prednisone at a dose between 30 and 40 mg for between 10 and 14 days. Prolonged courses are not of additional benefit (and increase the risk of side effects), and there is no evidence to suggest that tapering the dose is advantageous. Many physicians choose to give the first dose intravenously. Nebulized budesonide results in similar improvements in lung function to oral dosing but is more expensive. Intriguingly, the use of systemic steroids may delay the time to subsequent exacerbation, and although there is no role for the initiation of inhaled steroids at exacerbation, inhaled corticosteroids also have an important role in exacerbation prevention as discussed further in the following.

Antibiotics

The seminal work on antibiotics at exacerbation, by Anthonisen and colleagues, demonstrated benefit only when patients had an increase in at least two of the following three symptoms: breathlessness, sputum volume, and sputum purulence. Sputum purulence reliably indicates the presence of bacteria at exacerbation. A meta-analysis of the six sufficiently well-designed randomized trials by Saint and colleagues confirmed a small, but statistically significant, benefit in favor of antibiotics. Local resistance patterns and antibiotic policies will dictate the choice of drug, but coverage should include the common pathogens *Haemophilus influenzae, Moraxella catarrhalis,* and *Streptococcus pneumoniae.* An oral aminopenicillin, macrolide, or tetracycline is, therefore, an appropriate empiric choice. Comparative data across drug classes are sparse. Intravenous antibiotics are rarely required. There are little data on the optimal duration of therapy.

Oxygen Therapy

Oxygen is indicated to correct the hypoxemic respiratory failure that may occur with AEs. Hypoxemia is due to a combination of increased ventilation-perfusion mismatch and alveolar hypoventilation. Oxygen should be administered in a controlled manner with monitoring of arterial blood gas tensions or saturations to avoid CO_2 retention and the development of hypercapnic respiratory failure that may occur in a portion of patients. Studies have shown little risk of hypercapnia if oxygen is titrated to a maximum saturation of 90–92%. Failure to correct hypoxemia to $> 90\%$ with $FiO_2 > 40\%$ suggests the presence of additional pathology such as pulmonary embolus. Achieving adequate oxygenation only at the expense of rising $PaCO_2$ or falling pH is an indication for ventilatory support. Venturi masks provide a more reliable FiO_2 than nasal cannulae, but the latter may be better tolerated.

Noninvasive Ventilation

Noninvasive ventilation (NIV) refers to the provision of ventilatory support by means of a nasal or full-face mask in the absence of an endotracheal tube. There is now considerable evidence supporting the use of NIV for patients with hypercapnic respiratory failure caused by AEs. The benefit in mortality with additional reduction in hospital stay, complications, and cost may largely be attributed to the reduced need for sedation, intubation, and invasive ventilation. In addition, and in contrast to invasive ventilation, NIV may be used earlier and intermittently, which, therefore, facilitates communication, nutrition, and physiotherapy. NIV is usually administered as pressure-cycled bilevel positive airway pressure in which the inspiratory and expiratory pressures may be independently varied. NIV is not, however, a substitute for invasive ventilation when the latter is required. Therefore, a plan of management should be made with regard to suitability for invasive ventilation should NIV fail. In addition, some patients may have relative contraindications to NIV or respiratory failure of such severity that they should be immediately assessed for invasive ventilation. The indications and relative contraindications for NIV are provided in Table 39-2. Most, but not all, patients suitable for NIV are able to tolerate the treatment. The application of a nasal mask for NIV at exacerbation is illustrated in Figure 39-4.

Invasive Ventilation

The primary indications for invasive ventilation at exacerbation of COPD are severe hypoxia or respiratory acidemia

TABLE 39-2	Indications and Relative Contraindications for Noninvasive Ventilation (NIV) at Exacerbation of COPD	
Indications	**Relative Contraindications**
Exacerbation with hypercapnic respiratory failure ($Paco_2 > 6$ kPa) and pH < 7.35 but > 7.25	More severe acidemia Life-threatening hypoxemia Inability to protect the airway Hemodyanmic instability Inability to clear secretions Undrained pneumothorax Impaired consciousness or agitation

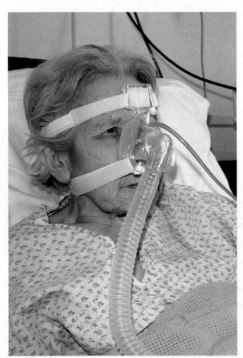

FIGURE 39-4 Application of noninvasive ventilation (NIV) by a nasal mask in a patient with exacerbation of COPD. Note the addition of entrained oxygen. Reproduced with written patient consent.

(pH < 7.26) in a patient unsuitable for, or failing, NIV. However, although data suggest that patients with COPD have similar outcomes after invasive ventilation to that seen in patients with respiratory failure from other causes, the decision to institute invasive ventilation should consider the prior functional status of the patient, the severity of the current and underlying illness, the degree of reversibility of the present deterioration, the presence and severity of comorbidities, and the wishes of the patient and their families or other caregivers. Mortality after invasive ventilation is approximately 20%, and weaning from the ventilator can be challenging. This is a further setting in which NIV may be valuable. The aim of ventilation is to support gas exchange and respiratory muscle function until other therapies have had sufficient time to be effective. In such circumstances, corticosteroids and antibiotics are usually given parenterally, and bronchodilator drugs may be added to the ventilator circuit from an inhaler and spacer.

Other Therapies

Methylxanthine drugs such as theophylline have a variety of potentially beneficial effects on respiratory and cardiac function, yet, randomized, controlled trials have failed to show any benefit in lung function or symptoms during exacerbations. Despite this, and in addition to well-recognized problems with drug interactions, side effects, and a narrow therapeutic range necessitating the monitoring of drug levels, theophyllines are still sometimes used in patients who are not demonstrating sufficient progress on otherwise maximal therapy. One action of theophyllines is as phosphodiesterase (PDE) inhibitors, and newer, selective PDE_4 inhibitors are currently being tried (although initial results have been disappointing).

There are no data to support the use of intravenous salbutamol for exacerbation of COPD. Side effects are more common than with the inhaled route, and routine use is not recommended.

Although exacerbations are often associated with an increased volume or tenacity of sputum, there is currently no firm evidence supporting the use of mucolytic drugs to treat AEs of COPD. There is also no evidence to support strategies aimed at facilitating expectoration such as physiotherapy or saline nebulization (although this largely reflects an absence of evidence rather than evidence supporting the absence of benefit). Cough suppressants are contraindicated.

Central respiratory stimulants such as intravenous doxapram have now been all but superseded with the availability of NIV, a therapy that is clearly superior in the management of hypercapnic respiratory failure. A limited role for doxapram may remain if NIV is not appropriate, as a bridge to NIV, or (with specialist advice) in conjunction with NIV. The use of doxapram is often limited by side effects, especially agitation, and any potential benefits do not appear to persist beyond 48 h.

Although intravenous magnesium may be an effective bronchodilator in exacerbations of asthma, there are no convincing data supporting its effectiveness in AE of COPD, and its routine use is not recommended. Heliox (a mixture of helium and oxygen) has a lower viscosity than air and may, therefore, reduce the work of breathing. However, there remains no evidence of benefit in treating AEs of COPD.

Other supportive measures that should be instituted include appropriate attention to fluid balance and consideration of prophylaxis against venous thromboembolism. Finally, for patients not responding to maximal therapy or for those in whom escalation is inappropriate, a range of palliative approaches to achieve symptom control should be considered.

CLINICAL COURSE AND PREVENTION

By use of analysis of symptoms and lung function changes, the median length of an exacerbation is approximately 7–10 days, although there is wide variability, and a proportion of exacerbations take considerably longer to improve. Some patients appear never to fully recover to their preexacerbation lung function. Those patients admitted to the hospital have an in-hospital mortality of approximately 10%, and for patients with hypercapnic respiratory failure, the mortality approaches 50% at 2 years. Some patients may be suitable for early supported discharge schemes. Although these are associated with similar outcomes, they appear no more cost-effective than standard care.

Given the importance of AEs and having managed the acute event, it is important to consider instituting a range of preventative measures to reduce the risk of future AEs. There is accumulating evidence to suggest that a number of classes of medications reduce the incidence of AEs. These include the long-acting β_2-agonists, long-acting anticholinergics, and inhaled corticosteroids (at least for those with moderately severe underlying disease). Combination therapy with long-acting β_2-agonists and inhaled corticosteroids appears superior to the use of either component alone, and this combination may also have a mortality benefit. Oral corticosteroids are ineffective at preventing exacerbations, and because they also have no effect on other outcomes measures, they are not indicated in stable COPD. Ongoing trials are reexamining the role of antibiotics in reducing exacerbation frequency; there is some existing evidence that these drugs may be effective, but many existing trials included patients with simple chronic bronchitis, the drugs used were older, and any benefit must be balanced against the possibility of promoting drug resistance. Macrolides hold particular promise given their recognized antiinflammatory action. Vaccinations against influenza and *S. pneumoniae* are recommended. Pulmonary rehabilitation has also been shown to reduce hospitalization in patients with COPD. Furthermore, early treatment has been shown to reduce exacerbation length, and this might be included in a patient education program. There are, therefore, a variety of measures that may be instituted to reduce the number and consequences of exacerbations. For this reason and for further assessment of patients who presented in respiratory failure, it is usually appropriate to review patients in an ambulatory care setting after an admission with acute exacerbation.

PITFALLS AND CONTROVERSIES

Recently, there has been increasing research focusing on AEs of COPD, but we still understand little about the relationships between AEs and bacterial type and load or how bacterial and viral pathogens might interact. More effective antiinflammatory agents are required, and the role of antibiotics in preventing exacerbations is unclear. We currently have no effective interventions targeting viral pathogens, especially rhinovirus. Finally, it is now recognized that COPD is associated with systemic inflammation that may cause considerable cardiovascular comorbidity, and ways to assess and manage this may also lead to a reduction in the number or impact of exacerbations.

WEB RESOURCES AND GUIDELINES/PROTOCOLS

World Health Organization (WHO) Global Initiative for Obstructive Lung Disease (GOLD) resources. www.goldcopd.com

American Thoracic Society (ATS)/European Respiratory Society (ERS) standards for the diagnosis and treatment of COPD. www.ersnet.org

United Kingdom National Institute for Clinical Excellence (NICE) COPD guidelines. www.nice.org.uk

Cochrane Airways Group (up-to-date, accurate systematic reviews and meta-analyses). www.cochrane-airways.ac.uk

SUGGESTED READINGS

Anthonisen NR, Manfreda J, Warren CP, *et al:* Antibiotic therapy in exacerbations of chronic obstructive pulmonary disease. Ann Intern Med 1987; 106:196–204.

Connors AF, Dawson NV, Thomas C, *et al:* Outcomes following acute exacerbations of severe chronic obstructive pulmonary disease. Am J Respir Crit Care Med 1996; 154:959–967.

Lightowler JV, Wedzicha JA, Elliott MW, *et al:* Non-invasive positive pressure ventilation to treat respiratory failure resulting from exacerbations of chronic obstructive pulmonary disease. Cochrane systematic review and meta-analysis. BMJ 2003; 326:185–187.

Niewoehner DE, Erbland ML, Deupree RH, *et al:* Effect of systemic glucocorticoids on exacerbations of chronic obstructive pulmonary disease. N Engl J Med 1999; 340:1941–1947.

Saint S, Bent S, Vittinghoff E, *et al:* Antibiotics in chronic obstructive pulmonary disease exacerbations. A meta-analysis. JAMA 1995; 273: 957–960.

Seemungal TAR, Donaldson GC, Bhowmik A, *et al:* Time course and recovery of exacerbations in chronic obstructive pulmonary disease. Am J Respir Crit Care Med 2000; 161:1608–1613.

Sethi S, Evans N, Grant BJB, *et al:* New strains of bacteria and exacerbations of chronic obstructive pulmonary disease. N Engl J Med 2002; 347:465–471.

Siafakas NM, Anthonisen NR, Georgopoulos D, Eds: Lung Biology in Health and Disease. Volume 183: Acute exacerbations of chronic obstructive pulmonary disease. New York: Marcel Dekker; 2003.

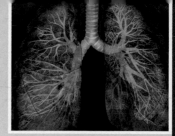

SECTION IX

AIRWAY DISEASES

40 Chronic Obstructive Pulmonary Disease: Management of Chronic Disease

PRESCOTT G. WOODRUFF • REBECCA E. SCHANE

Chronic obstructive pulmonary disease (COPD) is an irreversible and progressive disorder that causes severe physiologic and functional impairment in patients with advanced disease. Although COPD is not curable, available therapies do reduce the effect of the disease on patients. Beneficial outcomes can be obtained with appropriate use of medications, ambulatory oxygen, pulmonary rehabilitation, and selected surgical interventions. Management of COPD requires a multifaceted, multidisciplinary approach as described in the Global Initiative for Chronic Lung Disease or GOLD guidelines:

1. Establish a correct diagnosis and assess severity of disease with spirometry.
2. Reduce the risk for progression by encouraging smoking cessation and avoidance of other causative agents.
3. Reduce dyspnea by appropriate administration of bronchodilators.
4. Prevent and treat complications such as hypoxia and acute exacerbations.

REDUCE RISK WITH SMOKING CESSATION

COPD is the fourth leading cause of death in the United States, and the World Health Organization (WHO) predicts it will become the fourth leading cause of death worldwide by 2030. The most effective way to decrease the risk of disease progression is smoking cessation. All patients who are current or former smokers and/or have occupational or other risk factors for the development of COPD should be strongly and repeatedly encouraged to discontinue smoking. A clear, concise smoking cessation message should be provided during *every visit* with any health care provider. *Smoking cessation is the most effective tool* to preserve lung function and functional capacity. Current smokers have an increased risk of all cause mortality from COPD, cardiovascular disease, cerebrovascular disease, and/or lung cancer.

Patients who are susceptible to the adverse effects of cigarettes have a more rapid decline in lung function than nonsmokers (Figure 40-1). The Lung Health Study showed that smoking cessation reduces the rate of decline in FEV_1, essentially to that of a nonsmoker or nonsusceptible smoker, but it does not *reverse* the damage that has already occurred (although pulmonary function improves slightly in the year after smoking cessation [Figure 40-2]).

The key features of a successful smoking cessation program are vigilance in inquiring about smoking status of patients who smoke and assessing their preparedness or motivation to quit. Direct physician inquiry and advice to discontinue smoking can lead to a 10–20% cessation rate at 1 year. Many smokers require repeated attempts at smoking cessation before they are successful.

A useful approach to smoking cessation is the "five As" set forth in the GOLD Guidelines (Box 40-1):

Ask if the patient is still smoking every visit.
Advise the patient about the advantages and reasons to quit.
Assess the patient's willingness to quit.
Assist in quitting by educating the patient about nicotine withdrawal and addictive behavior, providing follow-up counseling and support, and prescribing nicotine replacement therapy (NRT) and bupropion as needed.
Arrange for regularly scheduled follow-up contact, either in person or by telephone, to check on status.

Who is likely to be a sustained quitter? From the Lung Health Study, patients who were able to achieve and maintain smoking cessation tended to have a significant other present at counseling sessions, were married, and/or had made previous long-term quit attempts. Those who were more likely to fail tended to have had more frequent cessation attempts, greater life stressors, and were still actively using nicotine replacement therapy 1 year after quitting.

Methods to facilitate smoking cessation include counseling and pharmacotherapy. At present, NRT is the treatment standard, because it results in twice the quit rate observed in patients receiving placebo. NRT is available as skin patches, gum, inhalers, and nasal sprays. Physicians should understand the method for the use of each of these formulations and educate patients on the appropriate technique of administration. The combination of (1) nicotine replacement therapy, (2) bupropion, and (3) behavioral counseling provides the highest smoking cessation rates.

Patients smoking less than 10 cigarettes per day should be put on NRT with caution and should be monitored for signs of nicotine toxicity. Pregnant/breastfeeding women, adolescents, and patients with unstable coronary artery disease, recent myocardial infarction, or untreated peptic ulcer disease should be considered for NRT only with caution and reservation.

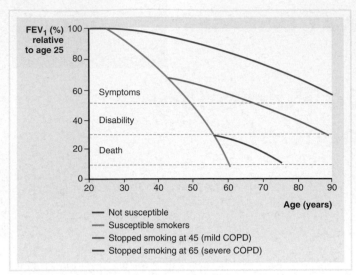

FIGURE 40-1 Graphic depiction of decline in lung function in cigarette smokers and the effects of smoking cessation. Lung function declines more rapidly in smokers who are susceptible to the adverse effects of cigarettes compared with nonsmokers. Discontinuing smoking in both a 45-year-old patient with mild disease and in a 65-year-old with more severe disease reduces the accelerated decline in lung function and delays progression of symptoms. *COPD,* Chronic obstructive pulmonary disease. (Modified from Fletcher C, Peto R: The natural history of chronic airflow obstruction. BMJ 1977; 1:1645–1648.)

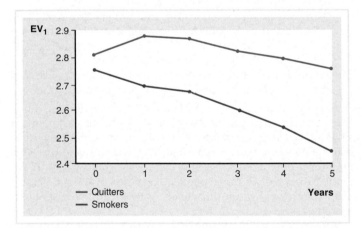

FIGURE 40-2 Effect of smoking cessation on lung function. In this study, the forced expired volume in 1 sec (FEV_1) improved in the year after smoking cessation. The decline in lung function in later years was less in former smokers compared with continuing cigarette smokers. (From Anthonisen N, Connett JE, Kiley JP, et al: Effects of smoking intervention and the use of an inhaled anticholinergic bronchodilator on the rate of decline of FEV_1: The Lung Health Study. JAMA 1994; 272:1497–1505.)

Varenicline is a new agent recently released by the FDA (2006) as an alternative to nicotine replacement therapy. It is a partial agonist of nicotinic acetylcholine receptors and should be administered at a dose of 1 mg twice daily for 12 weeks. Varenicline has been studied in two randomized control trials, with results showing higher abstinence rates when compared with bupropion or placebo. Adverse events (nausea) were similar for all treatment groups. Varenicline has not yet been studied in a randomized control trial against the current standard of NRT.

Other agents such as clonidine, the tricyclic antidepressant nortriptyline, and buspirone show no benefit compared with bupropion and/or nicotine replacement therapy.

REDUCE SYMPTOMS WITH BRONCHODILATORS

No pharmacologic interventions have been shown to alter disease progression. Bronchodilators remain the mainstay of pharmacologic therapy for most patients, however, because they provide symptomatic relief and improve exercise capacity by reducing gas trapping and hyperinflation, increasing airflow, and improving inspiratory capacity. These effects can be achieved without necessarily increasing FEV_1. Thus, relying on FEV_1 alone to monitor response to therapy may result in physiologic and clinical benefits being missed.

Inhaled bronchodilators are the first line of treatment. Current recommendations are based in part on disease severity as defined in the GOLD guidelines (Figure 40-3). Therapy begins with the use of short-acting bronchodilators for symptomatic treatment of mild COPD (GOLD stage I). Options for short-acting bronchodilators include β_2-agonists, anticholinergics, or both drugs in combination. For patients with persistent symptoms, and those with GOLD stage II–IV COPD, a long-acting bronchodilator should be added (either a β_2-agonist or an anticholinergic). The subsequent choices for third-line therapy include addition of a second long-acting inhaled bronchodilator (chosen from the alternate class of drug), an inhaled corticosteroid, or theophylline. Factors influencing the choice of third-line therapy include frequency of COPD exacerbations, risk of adverse effects, cost, and patient preference. Additional clinical studies relevant to the choice of third-line therapy will be published in the near future and may provide further guidance.

Anticholinergic Bronchodilators

Ipratropium bromide is a quaternary ammonium derivative of atropine sulfate that blocks muscarinic (M) receptors on airway smooth muscle and submucosal gland cells in a relatively nonselective fashion (Figure 40-4). Preganglionic blockade of M_2 receptors can actually *increase* acetylcholine release, because cholinergic stimulation of the M_2 receptors leads to inhibition of the release of acetylcholine (negative feedback). This seems to be of less importance in terms of the actions of ipratropium bromide compared with M_3 stimulation on airway smooth muscle, which is the primary site of action leading to reductions in bronchomotor tone.

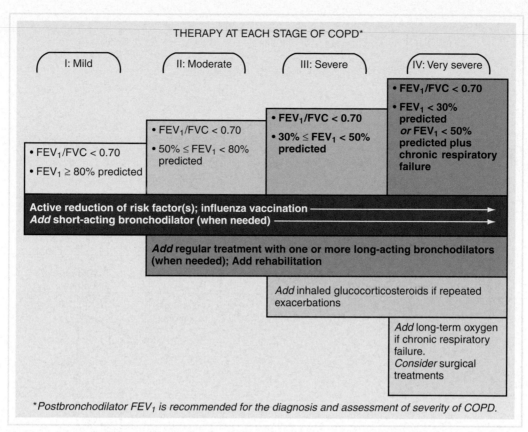

THERAPY AT EACH STAGE OF COPD*

I: Mild	II: Moderate	III: Severe	IV: Very severe
• $FEV_1/FVC < 0.70$ • $FEV_1 \geq 80\%$ predicted	• $FEV_1/FVC < 0.70$ • $50\% \leq FEV_1 < 80\%$ predicted	• $FEV_1/FVC < 0.70$ • $30\% \leq FEV_1 < 50\%$ predicted	• $FEV_1/FVC < 0.70$ • $FEV_1 < 30\%$ predicted *or* $FEV_1 < 50\%$ predicted plus chronic respiratory failure

Active reduction of risk factor(s); influenza vaccination ————————→
Add short-acting bronchodilator (when needed) ————————————→

Add regular treatment with one or more long-acting bronchodilators (when needed); Add rehabilitation

Add inhaled glucocorticosteroids if repeated exacerbations

Add long-term oxygen if chronic respiratory failure.
Consider surgical treatments

Postbronchodilator FEV_1 is recommended for the diagnosis and assessment of severity of COPD.

FIGURE 40-3 Therapeutic recommendations at each stage of COPD as defined by the GOLD Guidelines. (From Global Initiative for Chronic Obstructive Lung Disease: Global strategy for the diagnosis, management and prevention of COPD, 2006.)

Cholinergic stimulation of the muscarinic receptors causes bronchoconstriction and mucus secretion. Although Ipratropium bromide leads to a decrease in bronchomotor tone, no significant changes in mucus secretion occur with the use of anticholinergic bronchodilators. The duration of action of short-acting anti-cholinergics is 4–6 h, similar to that of the short-acting β_2-agonists. Ipratropium bromide is available in the United States in a metered-dose inhaler (MDI) dispensing 21 μg/dose or in an MDI in combination with albuterol (dispensing 18 μg/dose of ipratropium and 90 μg/dose of albuterol). Typical dosing is two puffs four times per day (maximum recommended daily dose, 12 puffs), but higher doses are recommended in patients with more severe disease. Increased doses can cause clinically important adverse effects, but these are uncommon. Ipratropium bromide is also available as a nebulized 0.02% solution (500 μg/2.5-mL unit dose), and patients typically receive a unit dose of 500 μg three or four times daily. Atropine-like side effects of the anticholinergics are relatively few, because they are not systemically absorbed but include hypertension, skin rashes, urinary retention, constipation, and headache. Dry mouth is the most common side effect. There is no evidence that individuals have tachyphylaxis to ipratropium bromide.

The bronchodilator effects of ipratropium bromide are equal, if not superior, to those of β_2-agonists in COPD. Regular use of ipratropium bromide reduces symptoms and improves health status.

Oxitropium bromide is similar to ipratropium bromide, with the same duration of action and side-effect profile. It is available in MDI form (100 μg) and as a nebulized solution of 1.5 mg/mL. It is reported to have a slightly longer duration

of action than ipratropium. This drug is not available in the United States.

Tiotropium is a long-acting anticholinergic bronchodilator that requires only once-daily dosing, because its effects last more than 24 h. Tiotropium binds with equal avidity to M_1, M_2, and M_3 receptors but dissociates fairly rapidly from the M_2 receptors but more slowly from M_1 and M_3 receptors. It is available as an 18-μg/dose dry powder inhaler (DPI) formulation. Reports of side effects indicate they are no greater than those seen with the short-acting anticholinergics (with the primary adverse effect being dry mouth). Tiotropium's onset of peak bronchodilation is between 1 and 3 h. In clinical studies, tiotropium is more effective than regularly scheduled ipratropium (or placebo) in terms of improving lung function, symptoms, quality of life, and decreasing acute exacerbations (Figures 40-5 and 40-6). In addition, studies to date suggest that tiotropium produces better bronchodilation and improvements in dyspnea than salmeterol (a long-acting β_2-agonist described later) in patients with COPD.

β_2-Agonist Bronchodilators

Short-acting β_2-specific agonists (SABAs) cause smooth muscle relaxation by directly stimulating β_2 receptors, mimicking endogenous adrenergic neurotransmitters. β_2 stimulation activates adenylate cyclase and increases concentrations of intracellular cyclic adenosine monophosphate. SABAs preferentially bind to the hydrophilic site of the β_2 receptor and have minimal binding to the β_1 receptors of the heart. Nonetheless, controlled clinical studies have shown that SABAs can produce tachycardia, hypertension, electrocardiographic changes, and cardiac symptoms in some patients.

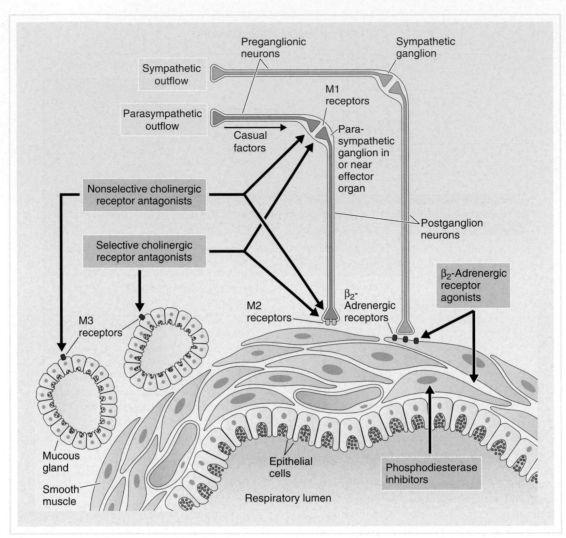

FIGURE 40-4 Sites of action of β-agonist and anticholinergic bronchodilators. (From Manda W, Rennard SI: COPD: New treatments. Consultant 2003; 43:953–965.)

SABAs have a rapid onset of action, reaching peak bronchodilation within 5–15 min and abating within 4–6 h, thus requiring redosing at least four times per day. Dose-response relationships for SABAs are relatively flat for many patients with COPD, with only modest changes in FEV_1 with increasing doses of medication. Albuterol (or salbutamol) is a SABA that is available for inhalation in the United States as an MDI, 90 μg/dose, and as a solution for nebulization (at concentrations ranging from 0.5–0.021%). Typical dosing with a nebulized solution is 2.5 mg (e.g., a 3-mL unit dose of the 0.083% solution). It is also available orally as a long-acting pill and as a syrup (0.024% 2 mg/5 mL). Dosing of the MDI devices is typically two puffs four times per day when used on a regular basis or as a "rescue" medication for intermittent dyspnea.

SABAs, however, can downregulate the $β_2$ receptors, leading to tachyphylaxis. Accordingly, overzealous rescue use (more than six times total per day) should be discouraged. Toxicity of SABAs is somewhat greater than with ipratropium bromide, because they are systemically absorbed. Side effects include tachycardia, palpitations, nervousness, gastrointestinal (GI) upset, esophageal reflux, and hypokalemia.

Levalbuterol tartrate is the R-enantiomer of albuterol (i.e., a racemic mixture of R- and S-enantiomers). The bronchodilatory effects of racemic albuterol are attributable to the R-enantiomer. The motivation for development of the R-enantiomer in a pure preparation is that the S-enantiomer, which is found in the racemic mixture, could have adverse effects. However, direct administration of the S-enantiomer has not revealed specific effects in clinical studies and, like other β-adrenergic agonists, levalbuterol can produce cardiovascular side effects. Levalbuterol is available as an MDI, 45 μg/dose, and as a solution for nebulization (at concentrations ranging from 0.01–0.25%).

There are two long-acting β-agonists (LABA) available for use. Salmeterol preferentially binds to the lipophilic site of the β receptor, takes 30–60 min to reach maximum bronchodilation, and lasts for up to 12 h. Formoterol is amphiphilic and binds with equal avidity to the hydrophilic and lipophilic sites on the β receptors. This provides a relatively rapid onset of action, from 5–15 min, and a 12-h duration of action. The LABAs share the same properties of the SABAs, causing smooth muscle relaxation by direct stimulation of adrenergic receptors. Salmeterol is available as a 50-μg/dose DPI preparation that is

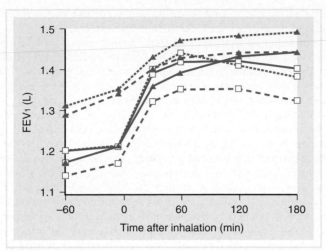

FIGURE 40-5 Effect of short-acting versus long-acting anticholinergic on lung function in COPD. Tiotropium improves trough peak forced expired volume in 1 sec (FEV$_1$) compared with ipratropium with long-term use. Mean FEV$_1$ before and during the 3 h after inhalation of tiotropium (*solid triangles*) or ipratropium (*open squares*) at baseline (*solid lines*) and after 8 days (*dotted lines*) and 364 days (*dashed lines*). (From Vincken W, van Noord JA, Greefhorst AP, et al: Dutch/Belgian Tiotropium Study Group: Improved health outcomes in patients with COPD during 1 year's treatment with tiotropium. Eur Respir J 2002; 19[2]:209–216).

dosed twice daily. Formoterol is available as a 12-μg/dose DPI preparation, which is also dosed twice daily. The regular use of LABAs by patients with COPD generally leads to improved lung function, a decrease in respiratory symptoms, and an enhanced quality of life. As for the effects on exacerbations, systematic review of eight trials evaluating LABAs on COPD found inconsistent results. Physicians prescribing LABAs should take note of recent changes in the labeling of these drugs, which highlight clinical studies linking regular use of salmeterol to an increased risk of serious asthma exacerbations and asthma-related deaths. Comparable studies are not available for COPD. The possibility that tachyphylaxis with regular use of long-acting β-agonists may underlie these adverse effects and is a topic of active research.

Combining β-Agonist and Anticholinergic Bronchodilators

The combination of β$_2$-agonists and anticholinergic agents has proven to provide superior bronchodilation and improvement in health status compared with the use of either of these agents individually. These benefits are seen both with the use of SABAs and LABAs (Figure 40-7). In patients who remain symptomatic with persistent dyspnea despite the use of a single class of bronchodilators, a combination of β-agonist and anticholinergic bronchodilators can be used simultaneously on an intermittent or regularly scheduled basis.

Theophylline

The methylxanthines, such as theophylline, are modest bronchodilators with additional properties that decrease respiratory symptoms in patients with COPD. Theophylline also has mild diuretic properties, stimulates the central respiratory drive, improves diaphragm function, reduces diaphragm fatigue, and also has antiinflammatory effects. A recent systematic review of the literature showed that theophylline significantly improves FEV$_1$, FVC, V$_{O_2max}$, Pa$_{O_2}$, and Pa$_{CO_2}$

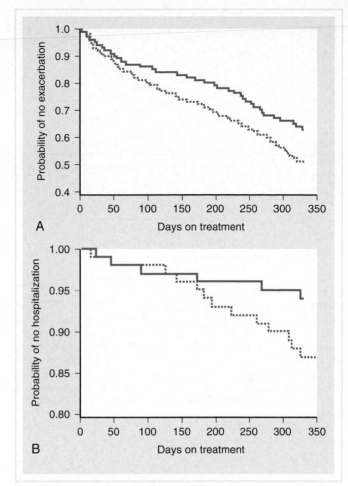

FIGURE 40-6 Effect of short-acting versus long-acting anticholinergic on risk for exacerbation and hospitalization. Tiotropium (*solid lines*) versus ipratropium (*dotted lines*). (From Vincken W, van Noord JA, Greefhorst AP, et al: Dutch/Belgian Tiotropium Study Group: Improved health outcomes in patients with COPD during 1 year's treatment with tiotropium. Eur Respir J 2002; 19[2]:209–216).

compared with placebo in patients with COPD. However, there is considerable potential for side effects, and the necessity for monitoring serum concentrations, together with theophylline being an inferior bronchodilator, has relegated it to second-line therapy. Although the mechanisms of action of theophylline are not known with certainty, studies in animals suggest that bronchodilatation is mediated by the inhibition of two isozymes of phosphodiesterase (PDE III and, to a lesser extent, PDE IV); nonbronchodilator prophylactic actions, however, are probably mediated through one or more different molecular mechanisms that do not involve inhibition of PDE III and might include antagonism of adenosine receptors. Theophylline is metabolized by the cytochrome P-450 mixed-function oxidases. The toxic-therapeutic ratio for this class of drugs is low. Maintaining levels less than 15 μg/mL will limit side effects, but physicians and patients should be alert to the fact that many other medications interfere with theophylline metabolism. Typical dosing for theophylline (targeting a serum concentration of 10 μg/mL) is 100–900 mg/day in a pill formulation. Higher blood levels produce only minimal additional bronchodilation. Side effects include nausea, vomiting, diarrhea, abdominal pain, gastroesophageal reflux (by inhibiting contraction of the lower esophageal sphincter), nervousness,

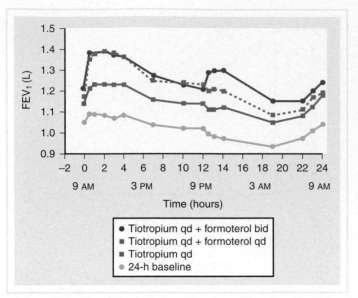

FIGURE 40-7 Effect of combined therapy with a long-acting anti-cholinergic and a long-acting β_2-agonist in COPD. Mean expired volume in 1 sec (FEV_1) before (24-h baseline) and at the end of 2-week treatment periods. (1) $P < .05$ tiotropium qd plus formoterol bid vs tiotropium qd at all time points. (2) $P < .05$ tiotropium qd plus formoterol qd vs tiotropium qd from 9 AM until 9 PM. (3) $P < .05$ tiotropium qd plus formoterol bid vs tiotropium qd plus formoterol qd from 9 PM until 9 AM. (From van Noord JA, Aumann JL, Janssens E, et al: Effects of tiotropium with and without formoterol on airflow obstruction and resting hyperinflation in patients with COPD. Chest 2006; 129[3]:509–517.)

headache, sleep disorders, muscle cramps, arrhythmias, including sinus and ventricular tachycardia and premature ventricular contractions, and seizures. Unfortunately, development of these side effects does not always correlate with elevated serum levels, and more serious problems (e.g., arrhythmia and seizures) may occur without being preceded by other symptoms. It is possible that the beneficial effects of theophylline, particularly the antiinflammatory effects, can be obtained by use of lower serum concentrations by altering histone deacetylase activity. Future studies that focus on lower serum concentrations in COPD may be associated with fewer adverse effects.

Theophylline should be considered for patients who remain symptomatic despite the use of inhaled bronchodilators, because the drug improves airflow when added to inhaled LABAs. Discontinuing the medication has decreased exercise capacity and increased symptoms in patients with severe COPD.

Second-generation inhibitors of phosphodiesterase-4 have shown some promise in preliminary studies. Newer formulations under study that maintain the bronchodilator and antiinflammatory properties with fewer GI side effects include cilomilast, piclamilast, and roflumilast.

CORTICOSTEROIDS

Corticosteroids are much less beneficial in treating chronic COPD than in treating asthma, and, accordingly, there is some controversy regarding their use in COPD. Oral steroids have a role in treating COPD exacerbations, because a 7–14-day course increases the rate of recovery and reduces the frequency of treatment failure. In stable COPD, however, only approximately 10% of patients have >30% increase in their FEV_1 after

a 2-week course of oral steroids; long-term use is not recommended because of their significant side effects.

A number of trials suggest that chronic use of *inhaled steroids* does not retard the rate of decline in FEV_1 over time, but they do reduce the frequency of acute exacerbations, particularly for patients with an FEV_1 of <50% predicted. In some studies, respiratory symptoms were reduced.

On the basis of these data, current international guidelines suggest that inhaled steroids should be considered for patients with an $FEV_1 <50\%$ predicted who have frequent exacerbations. Unfortunately, there are no good predictors of which patients will be steroid responsive. Oral steroid trials may not accurately predict the response to inhaled corticosteroids and, hence, are not recommended to assess the efficacy of inhaled corticosteroids as maintenance therapy. Other clinically important outcomes that may be improved with inhaled corticosteroids include bronchial responsiveness, patient symptoms, and health status. In the near future, the results of a large clinical trial that studied the effects of inhaled corticosteroids (and LABAs) on mortality in COPD will become available, and these results will further inform practice.

Inhaled corticosteroids come in a variety of formulations: fluticasone, budesonide, and mometasone are the most potent, and other formulations include beclomethasone, triamcinolone, and flunisolide. The most common side effects are a bitter taste in the mouth, oral thrush, and hoarseness. Concerns have also been raised about osteoporosis and cataracts as long-term adverse effects in older subjects. Inhaled steroids have not been approved by the Food and Drug Administration for use in COPD as monotherapy.

Inhaled corticosteroids may be used in combination with LABA. Studies have generally suggested improved lung function with administration of both agents compared with use of either agent alone. The FDA has approved fluticasone propionate, 250 µg, and salmeterol, 50 µg, inhalation powder for twice-daily maintenance treatment of airflow obstruction in patients with COPD associated with chronic bronchitis.

OTHER AGENTS

Mucolytics and Antioxidants

There does not seem to be a role for routine use of mucolytics (e.g., guaifenesin). DNAse was shown to reduce the frequency and duration of acute exacerbations of acute bronchitis in patients with cystic fibrosis but is ineffective in treating acute or chronic bronchitis in patients with COPD. A recent large randomized controlled trial of orally administered N-acetylcysteine, which was studied largely for its antioxidant effect, showed it to be ineffective in halting the deterioration of lung function and in preventing frequency of exacerbations in patients with COPD.

PULMONARY REHABILITATION

Despite a maximal medication program, many patients with COPD still have disabling symptoms, particularly dyspnea and poor exercise tolerance. This can limit their daily activities and impair their quality of life. In such situations, pulmonary rehabilitation is an effective therapeutic program that provides benefits over and above those that can be achieved with medications alone.

Pulmonary rehabilitation has been defined by a National Heart, Lung, and Blood Institute workshop as:

> A multidimensional continuum of services directed to persons with pulmonary disease and their families, usually by an interdisciplinary team of specialists, with a goal of achieving and maintaining the individual's maximum level of independence and functioning in the community. (Fishman AP: Pulmonary rehabilitation research: NIH workshop summary. Am J Respir Crit Care Med 1994; 149:825–833.)

Benefits of Pulmonary Rehabilitation

Substantial benefits can be achieved by comprehensive programs (Table 40-1). Pulmonary rehabilitation reduces dyspnea and improves exercise capacity. Present studies have also identified that pulmonary rehabilitation can reduce the length of hospital stay and decrease health care use. A small meta-analysis of 42 patients who attended pulmonary rehabilitation immediately in the setting of, or directly after a COPD exacerbation, showed nearly 39% fewer hospital admissions, 30% fewer hospital days, and 70% fewer emergency room visits 3 months after hospital discharge. Pulmonary rehabilitation has also been shown to decrease symptoms of depression and anxiety. These gains lead to an increased ability to perform daily activities with associated improvement in health-related quality of life (Figure 40-8).

A clear and concise description of the expected outcomes of rehabilitation should be used to convey the benefits to patients considering participating, physicians referring patients, and insurers providing payment for medical care. Pulmonary rehabilitation does not alter the underlying physiology of COPD, the spirometric indices of airflow limitation, or the degree of oxygenation. The education provided during a pulmonary rehabilitation program should improve compliance with prescribed medications and, accordingly, lead to an additional reduction in symptoms.

Principles of Pulmonary Rehabilitation

Two key principles guide the application of pulmonary rehabilitation:

1. The program should be tailored to meet the needs of each individual.
2. Multiple therapeutic components should be included.

Although comprehensive pulmonary rehabilitation programs usually have defined components that are carried out over a set time period for all participants, all forms of rehabilitation are tailored to the unique needs of each individual. This requires that the patient have input into designing the goals and directions of the program. An initial session conducted by the program coordinator should be devoted to assessing the individual's needs and desires. Establishing realistic and achievable goals enhances participation and optimal outcomes.

Universal components of pulmonary rehabilitation are listed in Box 40-2. Personnel with experience in each modality are most often integrated into a multidisciplinary team to provide a coordinated plan of therapy. Programs may include physical therapists, occupational therapists, social workers, psychologists, nurses, respiratory therapists, psychiatrists, and/or dietitians. The types of health care professionals used depend on the expertise available, the program's structure, and the needs of the individual patients. For example, because many patients with severe COPD and marked functional limitations experience some degree of anxiety and depressive symptoms, psychologic counseling is routinely included in most pulmonary programs. Counseling may be performed by nurses or other professionals, who are skilled and experienced in this area, or by psychologists or psychiatrists. For patients with signs of clinical depression, referral to a psychiatrist may be indicated for antidepressant medications and/or psychotherapy.

No studies have established the optimal duration for a pulmonary rehabilitation program. In general, most programs run sessions 2 or 3 days a week over a 6–12-week period, regardless

TABLE 40-1 Outcomes of Pulmonary Rehabilitation

Symptom/Therapy/Outcome	Outcome	Grade*	Recommendation
Dyspnea	Reduced dyspnea	A	Dyspnea outcomes should be routinely measured
Lower extremity exercise	Improved exercise tolerance	A	Exercise training of muscles of ambulation is recommended
Upper extremity exercise	Improved arm function with strength and endurance training	B	Arm exercise is recommended
Ventilatory muscle training	Improved respiratory muscle strength, but improved dyspnea and exercise muscle strength and dyspnea who remain symptomatic despite optimal therapy	B	Not an essential component of pulmonary rehabilitation; may be considered in selected patients with decreased respiratory tolerance only in some studies
Psychosocial and education	Decreased affective distress	C	Recommended based on expert opinion; cognitive and behavioral intervention enhance exercise adherence
Quality of life	Improved quality of life	A	
Health care utilization	Reduced hospitalizations in some uncontrolled studies	B	
Survival	Survival may be improved	C	

*Grade of evidence supporting recommendation: A, Evidence provided by controlled trials with statistically significant, consistent results. B, Evidence provided by observational studies or controlled trials with less consistent results. C, Expert opinion because of results or lack of controlled trials.

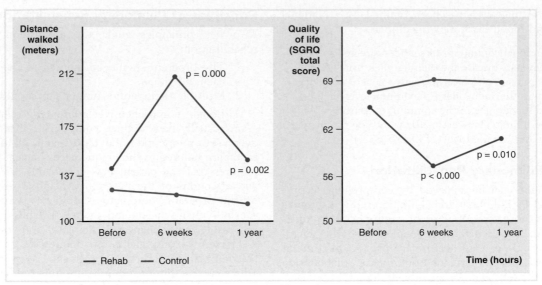

FIGURE 40-8 Outcomes of pulmonary rehabilitation. *Left,* Exercise (as measured by the shuttle walk distance) is increased immediately after rehabilitation (6 weeks) and at 1 year in patients with chronic obstructive pulmonary disease (COPD) randomly assigned to receive comprehensive pulmonary rehabilitation compared with patients receiving standard medical management. *Right,* Disease-specific quality of life (measured by the St. George's Respiratory Questionnaire [SGRQ] Total Score) is improved immediately after rehabilitation (6 weeks) and at 1 year in patients with COPD randomly assigned to receive comprehensive pulmonary rehabilitation compared with patients receiving standard medical management. Note that lower scores indicate improved health status. (Based on data from Griffiths TL, Burr ML, Campbell IA, et al: Results at 1 year of outpatient multidisciplinary pulmonary rehabilitation: A randomized controlled trial. Lancet 2000; 355:362–368.)

---

of disease severity. A recent meta-analysis of randomized control trials found, however, that patients with mild to moderate disease did better than controls in programs that were conducted over only 3–8 weeks. Patients with severe COPD showed substantial improvement compared with controls when the rehabilitation program lasted >6 months. In general, the benefits increase the longer one continues to follow an exercise program. In addition to their supervised training sessions, patients are encouraged to exercise on their own for a total of four to five sessions a week until optimal exercise level is achieved. After the formal program, patients should exercise three to four times each week to maintain the gains in performance.

Ideally, pulmonary rehabilitation should begin while patients are still hospitalized for an acute exacerbation as a recent meta-analysis of six trials including 230 patients enrolled 3–8 days after admission found a 38–96 m improvement in 6-min walk distance, and patients reported less fatigue on Borg Scores.

Patient Selection

Appropriate candidates have severe dyspnea, impaired exercise tolerance, and reduced quality of life despite being treated with a maximal medical program. In general, data support a benefit for those patients who are GOLD stage II or above. Other markers indicating the potential need for rehabilitation include frequent hospitalizations or emergency visits because of respiratory disease, frequent office visits, and suboptimal adherence to medical treatment or oxygen therapy. The degree of airflow limitation is an imprecise criterion for pulmonary rehabilitation, because the FEV_1 may not provide an accurate estimate of the patient's symptoms or quality of life. Nevertheless, the presence of severe airflow limitation (FEV_1 $\leq 35\%$ of predicted) should alert the physician to the potential need for pulmonary rehabilitation. Although controversial, many programs require that patients be nonsmokers before beginning therapy as evidence that they are committed to adhering with the recommended program. In fact, for those patients who remain active tobacco users, pulmonary rehabilitation can provide medical instruction and social support to facilitate smoking cessation. Significant comorbidities that may preclude exercise, such as coronary artery disease, should be excluded before referral, and comorbidities that may impair exercise training, such as arthritis, should be maximally treated. In addition, individuals with severe cognitive dysfunction and/or psychiatric illness who cannot participate in activities are not good candidates.

Although most commonly applied to patients with COPD, the principles of pulmonary rehabilitation can also be applied to patients with other respiratory disorders such as asthma, cystic fibrosis, interstitial lung disease, and pre/post lung transplantation.

Pulmonary Rehabilitation Components

Initial Assessment

The coordinator of the pulmonary rehabilitation program should enlist the cooperation of the patient in the development of specific patient-centered goals. Achievement of short-term goals is useful to enhance patient motivation and participation.

Exercise Training

Although even low-level exercise may be beneficial, more intensive training improves physiologic function and lessens dyspnea. The only form of exercise training that has been shown to have an established benefit is lower extremity aerobic training that often consists of walking or stationary cycling. Training programs should follow the principles of exercise duration, session frequency, and exercise intensity that have been shown to be useful in healthy individuals. A formal maximum exercise test is usually performed before training. This is useful to exclude the possibilities of coronary artery disease or exercise-induced arrhythmias that would preclude strenuous training and to determine whether the patient will need supplemental oxygen during the training program. Exercise that incorporates upper extremity strengthening is also useful.

Psychosocial Counseling

Depression and anxiety are frequently seen in patients with COPD. Psychologic assessment and counseling are designed to assist the patient and family in managing the psychologic stresses of the illness.

Control of Dyspnea

Breathing retraining can assist the patient in controlling and managing shortness of breath without overuse of medications. Pursed-lip breathing, diaphragmatic breathing, and controlled breathing also improve oxygenation, slow the respiratory rate, increase tidal volume, decrease air trapping, and reduce the work of breathing. Although used by some programs, inspiratory and expiratory muscle training is not generally considered a standard part of pulmonary rehabilitation, because there has been no consistent data to support benefit.

Instruction in daily activity performance is also useful. Coordinating breathing with specific activities, avoiding breathholding, and exhaling while doing tasks that require unusual effort all reduce dyspnea. Pacing breathing with activities such as stair climbing can also reduce dyspnea and improve performance of physical tasks.

Reducing energy requirements can enhance performance of activities in patients with limited respiratory reserve. Techniques such as the use of proper body mechanics, pacing of activities, and planning sufficient rest periods are useful.

Patients are also encouraged to maximize their bronchodilator therapy and oxygen supplementation while in training sessions, because these adjuncts have been shown to increase tolerated work rates and to sustain benefits of pulmonary rehabilitation.

Education

Education should be undertaken with the goal of improving patient adherence with the most effective health-enhancing behaviors. A behavioral approach requires education about specific details of the techniques and timing of medication use that can be successfully incorporated into the patient's daily schedule of activities to allow maintenance of a more normal lifestyle. Individual education for each patient about his or her medical program, combined with group instruction, is a key component of comprehensive rehabilitation programs.

Nutritional Counseling

Having a body weight less than 90% of ideal is a marker for increased mortality in COPD. Nutritional counseling in such patients may play a role in improving muscle mass necessary for normal daily activities. On the other hand, in overweight patients, weight loss may improve exercise. A diet adequate to meet caloric needs is required during exercise training. Accordingly, nutritional assessment and counseling are commonly provided during pulmonary rehabilitation.

Adherence rates for pulmonary rehabilitation are approximately 50%. Those who do not attend are more likely to have depression, live alone or in rented accommodations, are divorced or widowed, and remain active smokers. Some patients have further been influenced by the attitudes of their referring physician. When their doctor maintained a positive perspective on their participation, these patients were more inclined to attend and derived greater benefit from the sense of group support seen in their sessions. Lack of social support or negative views from their physician tended to interfere with attendance.

OXYGEN THERAPY (See Chapter 41)

The goals of oxygen therapy in patients with COPD are to:

1. Improve survival
2. Reduce dyspnea
3. Allow more exercise by eliminating exercise-induced hypoxemia

Studies reported in the 1980s conclusively demonstrated the survival benefit of long-term oxygen therapy in patients with hypoxia and COPD (Figure 40-9). The inclusion criteria from these studies have been adopted as indications for oxygen therapy by most health care insurers, including Medicare (Box 40-3): a PaO_2 $\leq$55 mmHg or a PaO_2 of 56–59 mmHg when there is also evidence of end-organ dysfunction secondary to chronic hypoxia (e.g., peripheral edema without another cause, pulmonary hypertension, or erythrocytosis [hematocrit $\geq$56%]). With the advent of pulse oximetry, the need for oxygen can also be suggested by oxygen saturation measurements (i.e., a saturation of $\leq$88% with the patient seated at rest or a saturation of 89% with other evidence of chronic hypoxemia). Although oximetry is less invasive and more easily performed than arterial blood gas analysis, oximetry readings are less accurate and reproducible, and can also be affected by factors such as poor vascular circulation, motion artifact, ambient light, and nail polish. In patients who meet these criteria, oxygen should be used continuously (during the day, with activity, and nocturnally), rather than when patients only experience symptoms of dyspnea.

The assessment for long-term oxygen therapy should be performed with patients seated, at rest, and breathing room air when they are in optimal medical condition rather than during an acute exacerbation. Patients should also be taking appropriate medications for COPD, including bronchodilators.

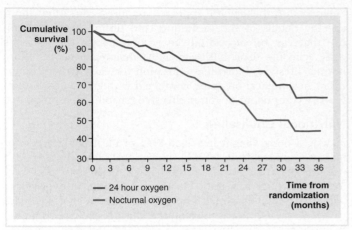

FIGURE 40-9 Survival in patients with chronic obstructive pulmonary disease and hypoxia randomly assigned to either continuous oxygen therapy or nocturnal oxygen therapy. Patients receiving continuous oxygen therapy during the day and night have better survival than those receiving oxygen only at night. (From Nocturnal Oxygen Therapy Trial Group: Continuous or nocturnal oxygen therapy in hypoxemic chronic obstructive lung disease: A clinical trial. Ann Intern Med 1980; 93:391–398.)

BOX 40-3 Indications for Ambulatory Continuous Oxygen Therapy in Patients with Chronic Obstructive Pulmonary Disease*

Stable chronic obstructive pulmonary disease on optimal medical therapy
and
$Pa_{O_2} \leq 55$ mmHg ($Sa_{O_2} \leq 88\%$) seated at rest
or
$Pa_{O_2} = 56$–59 mmHg
plus
Erythrocytosis: hematocrit $\geq 56\%$
Right heart dysfunction: P pulmonale, edema

These indications are based on the entry criteria for the Nocturnal Oxygen Therapy Trial (Nocturnal Oxygen Therapy Trial Group: Continuous or nocturnal oxygen therapy in hypoxemic chronic obstructive lung disease: A clinical trial. Ann Intern Med 1980; 93: 391–398) and are accepted by Medicare and most health care insurers.
Pa_{O_2}, Partial pressure of arterial oxygen; Sa_{O_2}, arterial oxygen saturation.
*Long-Term Oxygen Treatment in Chronic Obstructive Pulmonary Disease: Recommendations for Future Research: An NHLBI Workshop Report.

Continuous oxygen therapy also improves pulmonary hypertension dyspnea, depression, cognitive function, quality of life, exercise capability, and frequency of hospitalizations. The goal of chronic oxygen therapy is to increase the Pa_{O_2} to above 60 mmHg (an oxygen saturation of $\geq 90\%$). Pulse oximetry is useful while titrating the oxygen flow rate to achieve this result. Oxygen flows should be adjusted both at rest and during activity to achieve oxygen saturations of 90% or greater. Many patients with COPD require higher flows of oxygen with exercise to maintain the desired saturation. In the Nocturnal Oxygen Therapy Trial, which demonstrated a survival

benefit from long-term oxygen in COPD, the oxygen flow rate was increased at night by 1 L above that required at rest during the day. The prescription for oxygen should include flow rates at rest, during activity, and with sleep.

Oxygen prescriptions should include the number of hours of daily use, the amount required for ambulation, the type of oxygen system to use, and the method of delivery. In patients who meet the aforementioned criteria, oxygen should be prescribed for use 24 h each day. Many patients with COPD do not meet the criteria for oxygen at rest, however, but do have oxygen desaturation during exercise or during sleep, despite a negative evaluation for obstructive sleep apnea. Oxygen therapy provided during exercise in patients with desaturation to 88% or less decreases dyspnea and improves exercise capacity. Patients with nocturnal hypoxemia can have complications related to these episodes, such as daytime somnolence, cardiac arrhythmias, and pulmonary hypertension. Supplemental oxygen for patients with desaturation during sleep prevents oxyhemoglobin desaturation, and data from one observational study suggest that there may be a survival benefit. Thus, patients with exercise-induced hypoxemia and nocturnal hypoxemia may be prescribed oxygen during exercise or sleep, respectively. The use of short-burst oxygen therapy (defined as intermittent use for relief of breathlessness before activity or for recovery after exercise in the absence of hypoxemia or cor pulmonale) has not been found to be beneficial.

Oxygen sources include concentrators, compressed gaseous oxygen, and liquid oxygen. Electrically powered concentrators obtain oxygen by concentrating air and are the least expensive way of providing oxygen supplementation. Concentrators are typically stationary and for use at home; however, some newer models are adaptable for portable use. They may also generate considerable heat and noise. Compressed gas cylinders are available in various sizes, some of which may be used as portable oxygen sources. Liquid oxygen is the most costly supply system because it requires personnel visiting the patient's home, usually weekly, to refill the containers. For ambulation, lighter weight versions of the compressed gas oxygen systems and the liquid oxygen systems are the most convenient (Figure 40-10).

Oxygen has been most commonly delivered as a continuous flow of gas. However, oxygen reaches the lung only when the patient inhales; oxygen delivered during exhalation is wasted. Oxygen conservation devices have used this principle to reduce the amount of oxygen required and increase the duration of portable supply systems. Demand-delivery devices (also called pulse-dose systems) are available that administer a bolus of oxygen during the initial period of inhalation. Demand-delivery devices sense when patients begin to inhale and then trigger the delivery of oxygen. Flow ceases during exhalation, thereby reducing oxygen wastage. Demand-delivery devices have been incorporated into portable gaseous and liquid oxygen systems. Oxygenation that uses demand or pulse-dose oxygen delivery systems, however, is not always equivalent to continuous oxygen flow delivery. Accordingly, the appropriate oxygen flow rate for each patient should be determined with the specific delivery system the patient actually uses over the long term.

Patients frequently do not understand the role of supplemental oxygen. Some of the more common misunderstandings are that oxygen is required only for control of dyspnea, and that the use of higher doses will eliminate dyspnea. Thus,

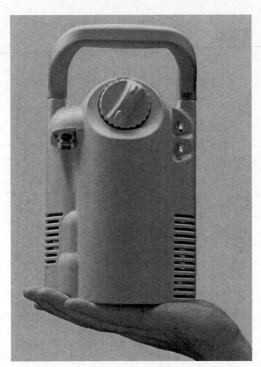

FIGURE 40-10 Example of a small, lightweight, portable liquid oxygen canister that incorporates demand delivery during inspiration only.

patient education is a prerequisite for proper use and adherence to therapy. Other barriers include patient vanity over appearance, denial of the illness, difficulty of use during ambulation, and fear that oxygen use will impair quality of life. These issues tend to reduce compliance with therapy. Education and pulmonary rehabilitation can address these concerns. In general, once a patient with COPD meets criteria for oxygen therapy, their life expectancy is poor, with a 5-year survival rate estimated at 40%. These figures are further influenced by additional comorbidities, older age, a body mass index <20, and evidence of cor pulmonale.

Lung Volume Reduction Surgery

Although it seems counterintuitive that removing part of the lung might be an effective therapy for patients with severe emphysema, the National Emphysema Treatment Trial (NETT) established this to be the case. The NETT, however, did identify a "high-risk" group (i.e., patients with an $FEV_1 \leq 20\%$ predicted and either homogenous distribution of emphysema or carbon monoxide diffusing capacity [DL_{CO}] $\leq 20\%$ predicted) who had significant operative mortality from lung volume reduction surgery (LVRS) that was not offset by the benefits and in whom LVRS is clearly not recommended. With this important caveat, recent follow-up data from the NETT indicate an overall survival advantage for LVRS versus medical therapy with a 5-year risk ratio for death of 0.86 ($P = .02$) improved maximal exercise through 3 years and health-related quality of life through 4 years. These results demonstrate that the benefits of LVRS are demonstrable and durable. Subgroup analyses indicated that patients without high-risk features can be further stratified into groups with clear benefit and groups with less certain benefit. Survival, exercise capacity, and quality of life are all clearly improved in the subset of patients with upper-lobe predominant disease and low exercise capacity; patients with upper-lobe predominant disease and high exercise capacity, however, have durable improvements in exercise capacity and quality of life but not in survival. Patients who have non-upper lobe predominant disease do not have sustained (>3 year) benefit in any of these outcomes, and the appropriateness of LVRS for these patients is questionable. Potential candidates for LVRS should be referred to centers that have experience with the procedure. Such centers usually are also experienced with lung transplantation and can, therefore, determine whether lung transplantation is a more appropriate option.

Lung Transplantation (See Chapter 78)

At present, COPD is the most common indication for lung transplantation. Depending on the recipients' age and severity of lung disease, single- or double-lung transplantation may be considered. Indications for transplantation include: (1) patients with advanced COPD who are symptomatic despite maximal medical therapy, (2) patients who are at high risk of death from their disease (within 2–3 years), (3) one or more of the following parameters: an FEV_1 <25–30% of predicted, pulmonary hypertension, right ventricular failure, and/or Pa_{CO_2} >55 mmHg, (4) severe functional limitation, and (5) an age <55 for heart/lung transplantation, age <60 for bilateral lung transplantation, or age <65 for single-lung transplantation. Contraindications include active malignancy within 2 years (except basal or squamous cell skin cancer), substance addiction within 6 months of surgery, dysfunction of extrathoracic organs, hepatitis B antigen positive, hepatitis C positive with proof of liver disease, and HIV infection (controversial).

Survival rates for patients with COPD undergoing lung transplantation seem to be somewhat better than those observed for other lung diseases. Although reports can differ, in general, the 1-year survival rate is approximately 90%. Two-year survival is 65–90%, and 5-year survival ranges from 41–53%. Significant improvements in pulmonary function, exercise capacity, and quality of life have been observed after transplantation. Primary complications are infection and/or related to rejection. Overall, the actual survival benefit remains unclear compared with those who wait for transplantation. Additional factors such as functional and quality of life benefit must be considered in the decision process. Recent changes to algorithms for organ allocation will likely lead to a decreasing number of lung transplants for COPD relative to other diseases in the coming years.

Summary

Smoking cessation has an important role in preventing progression of COPD and should be aggressively pursued in all smokers.

At present, bronchodilator therapy remains central to the management of symptomatic patients. The choice of bronchodilators allows physicians and patients to make decisions on the basis of many factors, such as effectiveness, cost, ease of use, and convenience. Ultimately, the best selections are those that optimize adherence. It is important to appreciate that the mechanisms of action of many of these drugs are complementary and that additional benefits may be obtained when they are used in combination.

For selected patients with severe disease, other therapies are effective. For those with a history of exacerbations, the addition of inhaled corticosteroids may prove beneficial. Long-term ambulatory oxygen therapy improves survival and reduces dyspnea in patients with documented hypoxia. LVRS is an option for carefully selected patients with CT evidence of upper lobe predominant emphysema. For patients with continued dyspnea and poor exercise tolerance, despite a maximal medication regimen, pulmonary rehabilitation is an effective therapeutic program that provides additional benefits.

SUGGESTED READINGS

American Thoracic Society: Pulmonary rehabilitation, 1999. Am J Respir Crit Care Med 1999; 159:1666–1682.

Croxton TL, Bailey WC: Long-term oxygen treatment in chronic obstructive pulmonary disease: Recommendations for future research: an NHLBI Workshop Report. Am J Respir Crit Care Med 2006; 174: 373–378.

Fiore MC, Bailey WC, Cohen SJ, et al: Clinical practice guideline: Treating tobacco use and dependence, Bethesda, MD: U.S. Department of Health and Human Services, Public Health Service; June, 2000.

Global strategy for the diagnosis, management, and prevention of chronic obstructive pulmonary disease: Available at www.goldcopd.com.

Naunheim KS, Wood DE, Mohsenifar Z, et al: Long term follow-up of patients receiving lung-volume reduction surgery versus medical therapy for severe emphysema by the National Emphysema Treatment Trial Research Group. Ann Thorac Surg 2006; 82:431–443.

Similowski T, Derenne J-P, Whitelaw WA, eds: Lung biology in health and disease. In Clinical Management of Chronic Obstructive Pulmonary Disease. New York: Marcel Dekker; 2002.

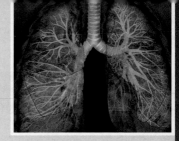

41 Oxygen Therapy

VICTOR KIM • GERARD J. CRINER

INTRODUCTION

Oxygen administration is a common supportive treatment for patients with acute respiratory failure and for those with chronic lung diseases and hypoxemia. The goal of this therapy is maintaining normal hemoglobin saturation so as to facilitate normal oxygen delivery to peripheral tissues. Oxygen therapy is generally safe and nontoxic; however, there are some concerns that long-term exposure to supranormal levels may lead to parenchymal lung injury and that it could cause hypercapnia in patients with chronic obstructive pulmonary disease (COPD). The goals of this chapter are to briefly describe indications for the acute and chronic administration of oxygen, oxygen delivery devices, physiologic effects of treatment, potential toxicities, and the effect on long-term morbidity and mortality.

EFFECTS OF HYPOXEMIA

Patients may have impaired judgment at low levels of hypoxemia, with progressive loss of cognitive and motor functions, and eventually loss of consciousness as severe hypoxemia ensues. Other nonspecific symptoms of hypoxemia include headache, breathlessness, palpitations, angina, restlessness, and tremor.

Minute ventilation increases when the PaO_2 falls below approximately 55 mmHg. Hypoxemia causes peripheral vascular beds to dilate, and this results in a compensatory tachycardia and a subsequent increase in cardiac output to improve oxygen delivery. Regional pulmonary vasoconstriction occurs in response to alveolar hypoxia in an effort to match ventilation and perfusion. Erythropoietin increases result in erythrocytosis, which increases oxygen-carrying capacity. These compensatory mechanisms can cause detrimental long-term effects, such as high blood viscosity, pulmonary hypertension, and right ventricular failure. On a cellular level, mitochondrial function declines, anaerobic glycolysis occurs, and the lactate/pyruvate ratio increases.

INDICATIONS FOR OXYGEN ADMINISTRATION

The overall goal of oxygen therapy is to avoid tissue hypoxia. Indications recommended by the American College of Chest Physicians and the National Heart, Lung, and Blood Institute are listed in Box 41-1. In the acute setting, the most common indication for oxygen administration is the presence of hypoxemia; however, oxygen administration is also justified for those in cardiac or respiratory arrest or those experiencing hypotension or respiratory distress. A reasonable therapeutic goal is to achieve an arterial oxygen tension of 60 mmHg or an SaO_2 of 90%, because the oxygen content of arterial blood rapidly falls at levels below these. The American Heart Association guidelines for Advanced Cardiac Life Support recommend that supplemental oxygen should be given to patients with an acute coronary syndrome regardless of the presence or absence of hypoxemia. Although hypoxemia is common in acute coronary syndromes, and oxygen administration is undoubtedly beneficial in this situation, the use of oxygen in normoxic patients with acute coronary syndromes is not supported by convincing data. Similarly, it is recommended that patients in sickle cell crisis be given supplemental oxygen to prevent or limit further sickling from tissue hypoxia, although, again, this comes without convincing supporting data.

Not all causes of hypoxemia are corrected with oxygen administration. The mechanisms of hypoxemia are summarized in Table 41-1. Ventilation-perfusion imbalance is the most common pathophysiologic cause of acute hypoxemia. The magnitude of response to supplemental oxygen depends on the degree of ventilation-to-perfusion mismatch in individual lung units. Hypoxemia from hypoventilation will also respond to oxygen administration. However, the mainstay of treatment is reversal of the underlying cause of hypoventilation that, depending on the degree of hypoventilation encountered, frequently involves initiating some form of mechanical ventilation. Decreased diffusing capacity and low FiO_2 also respond to supplemental oxygen. Right-to-left shunts, in which deoxygenated blood does not reach ventilated lung units where it can participate in gas exchange, shows no appreciable response to oxygen administration. When the shunt fraction is greater than 20–25%, hypoxemia may persist despite the use 100% oxygen. Determining the cause of hypoxemia predicts the response to oxygen therapy to other approaches to reverse the underlying disease process.

The indications for long-term oxygen therapy (LTOT) are summarized in Table 41-2. Approximately 800,000 patients are currently receiving LTOT in the United States at a cost of approximately $1.8 billion annually. In the United Kingdom, 865,000 people receive home oxygen at a cost of £19,310,000. The requirements for medical necessity for Medicare coverage have been based primarily on the entry criteria for the Nocturnal Oxygen Therapy Trial but have been refined on the basis of five consensus conferences on LTOT. These guidelines apply not only to hypoxemic COPD patients but also those with hypoxemia secondary to other pulmonary and cardiac diseases.

LTOT is indicated for patients who are hypoxemic at rest (i.e., have a PaO_2 <55 mmHg or a SaO_2 <88%) or for those with borderline hypoxemia (PaO_2 56–59 mmHg or SaO_2 89%) who also have evidence of cor pulmonale or polycythemia. Many patients with resting hypoxemia will have increased

TABLE 41-2 Indications for Long-Term Oxygen Therapy

Absolute	$PaO_2 \leq 55$ mmHg or $SaO_2 \leq 88\%$
In presence of cor pulmonale	PaO_2 55–59 mmHg or $SaO_2 \leq 89\%$, EKG evidence of "P" pulmonale, hematocrit $> 55\%$, congestive heart failure
Only in specific situations	$PaO_2 \geq 60$ mmHg or $SaO_2 \geq 90\%$ With lung disease and other clinical needs such as sleep with nocturnal desaturation not corrected by CPAP
If the patient is normoxemic at rest but desaturates during exercise or sleep	O_2 should be prescribed if PaO_2 falls below 55 mmHg during exercise or sleep Also consider nasal CPAP or bilevel positive airway pressure

Recreated from Criner GJ: Effects of long-term oxygen therapy on mortality and morbidity. Respir Care 2000; 45(1):105–118. With permission.

oxygen requirements during exertion and sleep, so it is prudent for the clinician caring for these patients to assess oxygen needs during these situations as well. In the United States, Medicare also allows oxygen to be prescribed during sleep if the PaO_2 is <55 mmHg, the SaO_2 is $<88\%$, or if there is a fall in $PaO_2 > 10$ mmHg or a fall in $SaO_2 > 5\%$ with signs or symptoms of hypoxemia. The latter indication is defined by the Center for Medicare and Medicaid Services as "impaired cognitive process, restlessness, or insomnia." Oxygen may also be prescribed during exercise if the PaO_2 falls to 55 mmHg or the SaO_2 falls to 88%.

SHORT-TERM EFFECTS OF OXYGEN ADMINISTRATION

Oxygen improves breathlessness during exercise in both normal subjects and in those with COPD. In COPD, the perceived decrease in breathlessness may be due to a decrease in exercise-induced increases in minute ventilation and resulting dynamic hyperinflation and/or to the alleviation of hypoxic pulmonary vasoconstriction resulting in improved hemodynamics. Oxygen flow may also stimulate upper airway and facial receptors of the trigeminal nerve and reflexively inhibit central nerve output, thereby decreasing the sensation of dyspnea. Finally, there also seems to be a direct effect of oxygen administration on the perception of dyspnea independent of any changes in minute ventilation.

Oxygen administration decreases minute ventilation and work of breathing during acute respiratory failure (ARF). A study in 20 patients with COPD found a fivefold increase in mouth occlusion pressure during ARF, which dropped by 40% after oxygen administration, demonstrating its effect on central respiratory drive. Oxygen also decreased minute ventilation by 14% in ARF, mostly by decreasing the respiratory rate without a compensatory increase in tidal volume. These effects may reduce the possibility of respiratory muscle fatigue developing during ARF.

METHODS OF OXYGEN DELIVERY

A summary of oxygen delivery devices is provided in Table 41-3. Low-flow oxygen systems (e.g., nasal cannulas, simple masks, and reservoir masks) deliver oxygen with variable amounts of FiO_2. High-flow oxygen systems are capable of delivering at least 40 L/min of conditioned gas, providing a precise and consistent FiO_2 regardless of the patient's breathing pattern. Both low-flow and high-flow systems can deliver a wide range of FiO_2; the terms "low" and "high" do not reflect

TABLE 41-1 Mechanisms of Hypoxemia

Cause	(A-a) Gradient	Response to Supplemental Oxygen	Examples
Low inspired O_2	Normal	Yes	High altitude, dense smoke inhalation
Alveolar hypoventilation	Normal	Yes	Narcotic overdose, neuromuscular weakness, obesity, hypoventilation
Ventilation-perfusion mismatch	Widened	Yes	COPD exacerbation, congestive heart failure (mild), pneumonia (mild)
Shunt, right-to-left	Widened	None substantial	Intracardiac right-to-left shunt, pulmonary arteriovenous fistula
Diffusion defect	Widened	Yes	Pulmonary vascular disease, interstitial lung disease

TABLE 41-3 Oxygen Delivery Devices

Device	Oxygen Flow Rate (L/min)	FiO_2
Nasal cannula	1	0.21–0.24
	2	0.23–0.28
	3	0.27–0.34
	4	0.31–0.38
	5–6	0.32–0.44
	6–8	Up to 50
Simple masks	5–6	0.30–0.45
	6–10	0.35–0.55
Venturi masks*	4	0.28
	6	0.28–0.31
	8	0.31–0.35
	12	0.40–0.50
Partial rebreathing masks	7	0.35–0.50
	≥8	≥0.60
Non-rebreathing masks	≥10	≥0.80

Recreated from Criner GJ, D'Alonzo GE: Critical care study guide. New York: Springer Verlag New York; 2002. With permission.
*The final FiO_2 varies according to the oxygen flow and to the total gas delivered, which is a function of the diluter jet and flow settings.

the delivered FiO_2 but describe the flow of gas delivered through the system.

The nasal cannula is the most common oxygen delivery system. It is well tolerated, but there is great variability in the final FiO_2 because of admixture with entrained ambient air. Use of flows greater than 6 L/min is discouraged, because it induces nasal mucosal dryness, crusting of secretions, and epistaxis despite humidification.

Similar to the nasal cannula, the simple mask (Figure 41-1) does not allow precise control of delivered oxygen concentration because of dilution with ambient air that is inspired through the exhalation ports. However, the mask can deliver higher FiO_2 (up to 55%), especially at higher flows (7–10 L/min), allows better humidification, and produces a good seal around the patient's nose and mouth. Low flows (<5 L/min) should be avoided because of the potential for rebreathing exhaled carbon dioxide when the mask dead space is not continuously flushed by a sufficient baseline flow of oxygen.

The Venturi mask (Figure 41-2) is characterized by its accurate delivery of oxygen concentration. It is designed to generate very high velocity flows of 100% oxygen through a narrow orifice that entrains a specific proportion of room air, thereby controlling the delivered oxygen concentration to within 2% of the set FiO_2. Patients with significant oxygen requirements who are at risk for worsening hypercapnia are the best candidates for this mask.

A partial rebreathing mask (Figure 41-3) is a simple oxygen mask with a large reservoir bag attached. High-flow oxygen directly feeds into this reservoir bag, and when the patient inhales, the gas is drawn from the bag as well as the from the exhalation ports. When the patient exhales, the first third of the exhaled tidal volume returns into the reservoir, and the rest dissipates through the exhalation ports. As long as the bag does not collapse by maintaining high flow rates, the partial rebreathing mask can deliver up to 60% inspired oxygen concentration.

A nonrebreathing mask (Figure 41-4) is distinguished from the partial rebreathing mask by the addition of two one-way

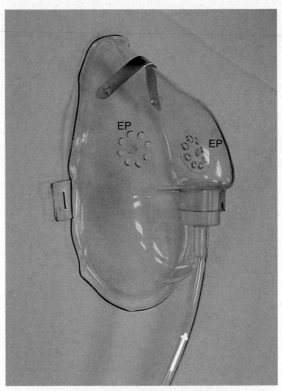

FIGURE 41-1 Simple mask. Oxygen is supplied through the tubing directly into the mask. The patient inhales the oxygen within the mask and exhales through the exhalation ports (EP).

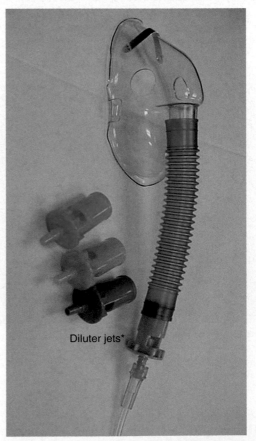

FIGURE 41-2 Venturi mask. Oxygen is supplied directly into the mask by means of an adjustable diluter jet that entrains ambient air, so that the FiO_2 inhaled is controlled.

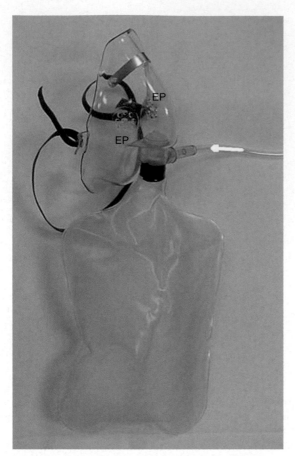

FIGURE 41-3 Partial rebreather mask. Oxygen is inhaled from the reservoir and the exhalation ports (EP) and exhaled through the EP and also partially into the reservoir.

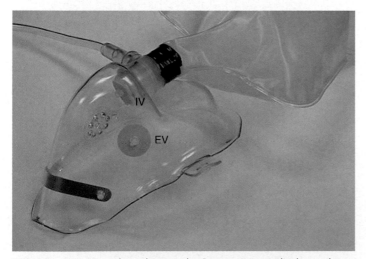

FIGURE 41-4 Nonrebreather mask. Oxygen is supplied to a large reservoir, the patient inhales high concentrations of oxygen through a one-way inhalation valve (IV), and then exhales through the one-way exhalation valve (EV).

valves, one on the inhalation and exhalation ports, respectively. These allow the patient to inhale oxygen from the reservoir but prevent backflow of the expired volume into the bag during exhalation, thereby avoiding entraining ambient air through the exhalation ports during inspiration. The

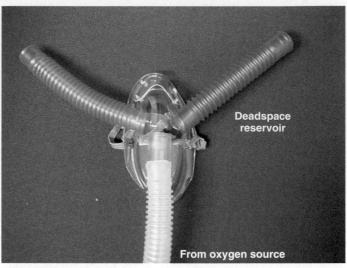

FIGURE 41-5 Tusk mask. Modification of a simple facemask with 6-inch tubing substituted for exhalation valves to prevent entrainment of room air during inspiration.

nonrebreathing mask can deliver close to 100% oxygen when adequate flow is maintained, and the mask has a good seal on the patient's face. Manufacturers of nonrebreathing masks avoid placing valves on both exhalation ports as a precautionary measure in the event of inspiratory valve malfunction, which would interrupt the flow of oxygen. To avert potential valve problems, some intensivists make up reservoir masks by adding additional dead space to simple masks to avoid entraining room air without the use of one-way valves (Figure 41-5). These "tusk masks" still require high flows of oxygen to flush all exhaled air from the mask dead space and minimize the entrainment of ambient air during inspiration.

EFFECT OF LONG-TERM OXYGEN THERAPY ON MORTALITY

Chronic hypoxemia leads to the development of cor pulmonale and portends a poor prognosis. Early noncontrolled studies showed a reduction in mortality in patients with COPD, cor pulmonale, and severe hypoxemia with the use of continuous oxygen therapy for 7–41 months. Two landmark studies performed in the late 1970s, the Nocturnal Oxygen Therapy Trial (NOTT) and the British Medical Research Council (MRC) Domiciliary Study, examined the effects of LTOT on survival and physiologic function in patients with severe chronic bronchitis and emphysema.

The British MRC Long-Term Domiciliary Oxygen Therapy Trial was conducted in the late 1970s and reported in March of 1981. It was carried out in three centers in the United Kingdom and enrolled 87 patients, all younger than the age of 70 years, who had chronic bronchitis or emphysema with irreversible airways obstruction (i.e., a forced expiratory volume in the first second [FEV_1] of 0.58–0.75 L), severe hypoxemia (i.e., arterial oxygen tension [PaO_2] of 49.4–51.8 mmHg), carbon dioxide retention (i.e., a $PaCO_2$ of 56–60 mm Hg), and a history of cor pulmonale (i.e., a mean pulmonary artery pressure of 32.3–35.0 mmHg). Patients randomly assigned to receive oxygen were given 2 L/min through nasal prongs for at least 15 h a day. In 5 years of follow-up, 19 of the 42 oxygen-treated patients died compared with 30 of the 45 control subjects. Mortality seemed to be highest in the subgroup of patients with the highest baseline Pa_{CO_2} and red cell mass. No significant differences were found in the rate of decrease of FEV_1, the increase in Pa_{CO_2}, the red cell mass, or the decreases in Pa_{O_2}, or increase in pulmonary artery pressures (but trends to improvements were seen in the latter two).

The NOTT study, sponsored by the National Heart, Lung, & Blood Institute, reported in 1980 the effects of continuous versus nocturnal oxygen therapy in hypoxemic COPD patients. This six-center study enrolled 203 patients with hypoxemic COPD, who were randomly allocated to receive either continuous oxygen therapy or 12 h of nocturnal oxygen therapy. All subjects were followed for at least 12 months. Overall mortality of the subjects assigned to continuous oxygen therapy and nocturnal oxygen therapy over 3 years of observation is shown in Figure 41-6. A total of 64 subjects died, 41 subjects in the nocturnal oxygen therapy group and 23 subjects in the continuous oxygen therapy group. At all six centers, mortality for the nocturnal oxygen therapy group exceeded that for the continuous oxygen therapy group. No differences were observed with respect to arterial blood gas values, lung volumes, FEV_1, maximum work attained, mean pulmonary artery pressures, or cardiac index, but the hematocrit was approximately 7% lower and pulmonary vascular resistance decreased 17.6% more in the group receiving continuous therapy.

Although both of the preceding studies showed improved survival, the patients were not comparable in the two studies (Table 41-4). Those in the MRC study tended to be more ill and had more hypercapnia and cor pulmonale and a substantial number continued to smoke while participating (27% in the control group and 44% in the placebo group). The NOTT trial made no comment on the incidence of continued smoking.

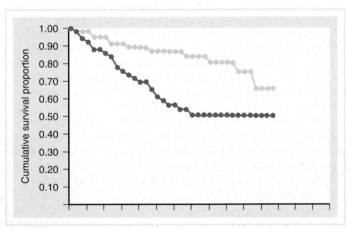

FIGURE 41-6 Overall mortality in the patients enrolled in the Nocturnal Oxygen Treatment Trial. Circles (*upper curve*) represent continuous oxygen therapy group. Squares (*lower curve*) represent nocturnal oxygen therapy group. Twelve-month mortality in the nocturnal oxygen group was 20.6% versus 11.9% in the continuous oxygen therapy group. Twenty-four-month mortality in the nocturnal oxygen group was 40.8% versus 22.4% in the continuous oxygen treatment group. (From Nocturnal Oxygen Therapy Trial Group: Continuous or nocturnal oxygen therapy in hypoxemic chronic obstructive lung disease: A clinical trial. Ann Int Med 1980; with permission.)

TABLE 41-4 Comparison of British Medical Research Council (MRC) and Nocturnal Oxygen Therapy Trial (NOTT) Long-Term Oxygen Treatment Trials

	MRC	NOTT
n	87	203
Study design	Prospective, controlled	Prospective, controlled
Protocol	No O_2 vs nocturnal use	Nocturnal vs continuous use
FEV_1	0.58–0.76 L	29% predicted
Percent female	24	20–23
Pa_{O_2} (mmHg)	49–51	51
Pa_{CO_2} (mmHg)	55–60	43
MPaP (mmHg)	32–35	30
Hours O_2 use/day	0 vs 15	12 ± 2.5 vs 17.7 ± 4.8
Smoking status	25–52%	?

Recreated from Criner GJ: Effects of long-term oxygen therapy on mortality and morbidity. Respir Care 2000; 45(1):105–118. With permission.

Despite these differences, these two prospective, controlled trials seem to establish that nocturnal oxygen therapy is better than no oxygen therapy at all and that continuous oxygen therapy is better than nocturnal oxygen therapy in severely hypoxemic patients with elevated hematocrit, pulmonary artery pressure, and respiratory acidosis.

In an attempt to determine whether the preceding findings extended to patients with less severe disease and only moderate hypoxemia, Gorecka and colleagues randomly assigned 135 patients with COPD with Pa_{O_2}s of 56–65 mmHg and a mean FEV_1 of 0.83 L to LTOT or no supplemental oxygen. The cumulative survival was 88%, 77%, and 66% at year 1, 2, and 3, respectively, and no differences were seen between the two groups.

OXYGEN THERAPY AND PULMONARY HEMODYNAMICS IN COPD

Substantial evidence suggests that the presence of secondary pulmonary hypertension in COPD increases the risk for hospitalization and is associated with worsened survival. Because of the known association of resting hypoxemia with the development of secondary pulmonary hypertension, investigators have focused on supplemental oxygen as treatment for pulmonary artery hypertension in patients with pulmonary hypertension and hypoxemic COPD. Although data from several studies show that oxygen in hypoxemic COPD patients is associated with favorable, but minimal, changes in the magnitude of pulmonary hypertension at rest and during exercise (particularly in those who receive oxygen continuously compared with those who receive it on an intermittent basis), it is difficult to attribute the improvements in survival of patients with COPD receiving continuous versus nocturnal oxygen therapy solely to changes in pulmonary hemodynamics. The response to acute administration of oxygen on pulmonary hemodynamics does not seem to predict the long-term effects of oxygen therapy on survival.

ACCENTUATION OF HYPERCAPNIA

Worsening hypercapnia and respiratory acidosis is of concern when oxygen is administered to patients with chronic carbon dioxide retention at baseline. The most commonly held theory explaining this phenomenon is blunting of the hypercarbic ventilatory drive leading hypoventilation when oxygen administration relieves any component of hypoxic drive. However, Aubier and colleges administered 100% oxygen to patients with COPD when they were in acute respiratory failure and found an acute 18% decrease in minute ventilation (V_E). However, within 15 min, V_E returned to 93% of its baseline value, but the $PaCO_2$ increased approximately 23 mmHg. Approximately 5 mmHg of the rise (22%) was attributed to the decrease in V_E, whereas 7 mmHg (30%) was attributed to the Haldane effect (i.e., a reduction of hemoglobin's affinity to bind and carry CO_2) and the largest component, 11 mmHg (48%) was attributed to increased dead space ventilation which, in turn, can be explained by oxygen improving alveolar O_2, thereby relaxing hypoxic vasoconstriction and increasing perfusion to alveoli with fixed alveolar ventilation. This is thought to occur much more commonly during acute exacerbations to the extent that the problem can generally be ignored when prescribing oxygen to relieve breathlessness and alleviate hypoxemia when patients are in their stable condition.

OXYGEN TOXICITY

In the 18th century, Lavoisier recognized that "when there is an excess of vital air [i.e., oxygen] animals undergo a severe illness." Hyperoxia promotes cellular injury through the increased production of reactive oxygen species, impairing the function of essential intracellular processes and provoking an inflammatory response that leads to tissue damage and cell death.

Hyperoxia has been associated with a multitude of pathophysiologic consequences, including depression of respiratory drive, pulmonary vasodilatation, ventilation perfusion imbalance, hypercapnia, absorption atelectasis, acute tracheobronchitis, diffuse alveolar damage, acute respiratory distress syndrome (ARDS), and bronchopulmonary dysplasia. The term *oxygen toxicity* is usually reserved to describe the airway and lung parenchymal injuries that occur as a result of hyperoxia.

High concentrations of oxygen rapidly damage airway epithelium, leading to tracheobronchitis and bronchopulmonary dysplasia. The syndrome of acute tracheobronchitis and mucociliary dysfunction was described initially in normal volunteers breathing 100% FiO_2 for more than 24 h with symptoms of retrosternal discomfort, cough, sore throat, nasal congestion, eye irritation, and fatigue, but large airway edema and erythema can be demonstrated bronchoscopically in most patients receiving an FiO_2 of 0.9 for 6 h, and the concentration of reactive oxygen species in exhaled breath condensate increases after only 1 h of breathing a FiO_2 of 28%. Bronchopulmonary dysplasia is characterized by fibrosis and destruction of acinar structures, resulting in scarring and emphysematous changes that develop in very low birth weight neonates and is attributed to hyperoxia, pulmonary edema, and/or mechanical ventilation–induced trauma.

Parenchymal lung injury attributed to hyperoxia is described pathologically as diffuse alveolar damage. Progressive airspace disease has been described in those with ARDS who have required prolonged periods of mechanical ventilation with a high FiO_2. It is difficult to discern whether the airspace disease is a result of the toxic effects of oxygen, the underlying disease process, or ventilator-induced lung injury. Absorption atelectasis occurs as a result of alveolar nitrogen washout from high concentrations of inspired oxygen. This tends to occur in alveolar units with a low ventilation/perfusion ratio. Oxygen may also interfere with the normal production of surfactant, thereby predisposing to atelectasis of affected areas.

It is still unclear what concentration of inspired oxygen causes toxicity, particularly in critically ill patients. The arbitrary threshold of 60% FiO_2 comes from studies conducted in normal volunteers in the 1950s. Other studies suggest that oxygen radical scavengers could be upregulated by the inflammatory response and/or by transient oxygen administration, and these could limit the toxicity of hyperoxia. It is extremely difficult to isolate the effects of oxygen amid multiple variables such as mechanical ventilation–induced alveolar overdistention, pneumonia, and sepsis. In general, attempts should be made to reduce FiO_2 to the least amount that maintains PaO_2 above 60 mmHg or SaO_2 above 90%. It is important to remember, however, that the immediate risk of hypoxemia is far more devastating than the potential for oxygen-induced lung injury.

CONTROVERSIES AND CONCERNS

The indications for LTOT were derived from entry criteria for the NOTT trial, as well as recommendations from several national consensus conferences. The data on which these indications are based are more than 25 years old, and no further studies have been performed to better refine the role of LTOT in COPD or other chronic hypoxemic states. There are several clinical scenarios in which long-term oxygen administration is of unproven benefit. For example, three studies have found no survival benefit in COPD and mild hypoxemia or in the absence of cor pulmonale or severe desaturation. The average use of oxygen in these studies was approximately 13.5 h/day, which may have been an inadequate duration of therapy. There may be other beneficial aspects of the use of oxygen therapy in this group, such as depression, neuropsychologic function, exercise capacity, and quality of life. Further studies are necessary to delineate which patients with mild hypoxemia would have a survival benefit and what other therapeutic benefits may be derived from oxygen therapy.

LTOT improves hemodynamics during exercise but only in those receiving it continuously (as opposed to just during the period of exercise). Although LTOT is approved for patients who are normoxemic while awake but who are hypoxemic during exercise, the long-term benefits of this approach have not been demonstrated.

A significant proportion of COPD patients with PaO_2 >60 mmHg during the day (up to 25%) can exhibit REM-related hypoventilation and subsequent hypoxemia, and LTOT is also approved for this use. Although LTOT may prevent hypoxemia during sleep, may prevent or delay the development of pulmonary hypertension, and improves sleep continuity and quality in those who desaturate, two recent studies found no improvement in survival with nocturnal oxygen (despite finding that oxygen reduced pulmonary artery pressures) and no delay in the time to prescription of continuous oxygen therapy. Given the lack of survival benefit, screening for nocturnal desaturation in normoxemic patients with

COPD should probably be reserved for those with evidence of pulmonary hypertension.

SUMMARY

Oxygen is an important supportive therapy for those with hypoxemia and acute and chronic respiratory failure. The clinical benefit of treating hypoxemia to prevent or reverse the ill effects of tissue hypoxia far outweighs the potential harm from oxygen toxicity or hypercapnia. As long as the FiO_2 is delivered in a controlled manner, hypoxemia can be treated without overwhelming concern for worsening hypercapnia in high-risk patients. It is also clear that the benefits of oxygen therapy extend beyond the reversal of hypoxemia. LTOT improves survival in hypoxemic COPD and may favorably affect neuropsychiatric function, exercise capacity, sleep continuity, pulmonary hemodynamics, and quality of life. Further studies are needed to better define the benefits of oxygen in hypoxemic lung diseases other than COPD and those with only mild hypoxemia.

SUGGESTED READINGS

Anonymous: Long term domiciliary oxygen therapy in chronic hypoxic cor pulmonale complicating chronic bronchitis and emphysema. Report of the Medical Research Council Working Party. Lancet 1981; 1(8222): 681–686.

Aubier M, Murciano D, Fournier M, et al: Central respiratory drive in acute respiratory failure of patients with chronic obstructive pulmonary disease. Am Rev Respir Dis 1980; 122:191–199.

Aubier M, Murciano D, Milic-Emili J, et al: Effects of the administration of O_2 on ventilation and blood gases in patients with chronic obstructive pulmonary disease during acute respiratory failure. Am Rev Respir Dis 1980; 122:747–754.

Chaouat A, Weitzenblum E, Kessler R, et al: A randomized trial of nocturnal oxygen therapy in chronic obstructive pulmonary disease patients. Eur Respir J 1999; 14:1002–1008.

Comroe JH, Dripps RD, Dumke PR, Deming M: The effect of inhalation of high concentrations of oxygen for 24 hours on normal men at sea level and at a simulated altitude of 18,000. JAMA 1945; 128:710.

Dean NC, Brown JK, Himelman RB, et al: Oxygen may improve dyspnea and endurance in patients with chronic obstructive pulmonary disease and only mild hypoxemia. Am Rev Respir Dis 1992; 146:941–945.

Fletcher EC, Luckett RA, Goodnight-White S, et al: A double-blind trial of nocturnal supplemental oxygen for sleep desaturation in patients with chronic obstructive pulmonary disease and a daytime PaO_2 above 60 torr. Am Rev Respir Dis 1992; 145:1070–1076.

Gorecka D, Gorzelak K, Sliwinski P, et al: Effect of long-term oxygen therapy on survival in patients with chronic obstructive pulmonary disease with moderate hypoxaemia. Thorax 1997; 52(8):674–679.

Nocturnal Oxygen Therapy Trial Group: Continuous or nocturnal oxygen therapy in hypoxemic chronic obstructive lung disease: A clinical trial Ann Int Med 1980; 93:391–398.

Sackner MA, Landa J, Hirsch J, Zapata A: Pulmonary effects of oxygen breathing: A 6-hour study in normal men. Ann Intern Med 1975; 82:40.

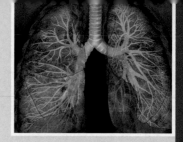

42 Pulmonary Rehabilitation

THIERRY TROOSTERS • RIK GOSSELINK •
DANIEL LANGER • MARC DECRAMER

INTRODUCTION

Generally, rehabilitation is defined as "restoration of human functions to the maximum degree possible in a person or persons suffering from disease or injury." Rehabilitation, therefore, is not confined to a specific organ or structure but rather to the functioning and interaction of a person in his or her environment. Pulmonary rehabilitation is a form of rehabilitation dealing with patients primarily with respiratory disorders and limited participation in daily life. The rehabilitation process, however, is not oriented at improving lung function but is aimed at improving the long-term systemic consequences patients with lung diseases may suffer. These so-called systemic consequences include, but are not limited to, muscle weakness, nutritional depletion, impaired mental state, exercise intolerance, and symptoms that are often out of proportion of the lung function abnormality.

The goals of pulmonary rehabilitation are patient and society centered in the sense that rehabilitation aims at improving symptoms, exercise tolerance, patient participation in daily life, and health-related quality of life, as well as at reducing the overall cost of care in these patients by reducing or postponing use of health care resources. To be efficient, rehabilitation programs should be an integral part of the overall care plan. Ideally, they facilitate communication between health care providers across lines of health care. In a recent document of the American Thoracic Society and the European Respiratory Society, pulmonary rehabilitation was explicitly put within the context of integrated care and was defined as "an evidence-based, multidisciplinary, and comprehensive intervention for patients with chronic respiratory diseases who are symptomatic and often have decreased daily life activities. Integrated into the individualized treatment of the patient, pulmonary rehabilitation is designed to reduce symptoms, optimize functional status, increase participation, and reduce health care costs through stabilizing or reversing systemic manifestations of the disease."

This definition acknowledges the significant evidence base for rehabilitation programs and recognizes that its primary aim is not enhancing lung function. The definition, however, is rather comprehensive, and it follows that a thorough discussion of all components of pulmonary rehabilitation is outside the scope of this chapter. Rather, after discussing the outcomes of pulmonary rehabilitation, this chapter focuses on one intervention, often referred to as the cornerstone of rehabilitation programs for patients with respiratory diseases: exercise training. In addition, most of the discussion pertains to patients with chronic obstructive pulmonary disease (COPD). Indeed, most research has been conducted in this large patient population. Finally, most of the discussed techniques can be transposed to patients with other lung diseases. In fact, many of the techniques are also used in other diseases, such as frailty, osteoporosis, and congestive heart failure.

OUTCOMES AFTER PULMONARY REHABILITATION

The success of achieving the goals of rehabilitation can be assessed through physiologic, psychosocial, and economic outcome measures. In a recent meta-analysis, the effects of pulmonary rehabilitation programs on exercise tolerance were systematically reviewed. In incremental tests, peak work rate improves on the average by approximately 20% compared with baseline, whereas peak oxygen uptake improves by 10% when the rehabilitation groups are compared with the respective controls. The effect of pulmonary rehabilitation on whole-body constant work rate exercise tolerance is much larger (80–100%). Exertional dyspnea is consistently reported to be reduced after pulmonary rehabilitation.

The clinical relevance of the benefit of pulmonary rehabilitation is illustrated by the improved functional capacity, as measured by the 6-min walk test. The pooled effect size of all randomized controlled studies of the results of pulmonary rehabilitation is approximately 50 m, with a 95% confidence interval of 26–72 m^2. The minimal clinically important difference (MCID) of the 6-min walking test has been estimated to be approximately 50 m. We calculated that the number needed to have one patient with a clinically significant benefit was 3 (95% CI, 1.7–6.4).

A review of the published literature shows that the improvement in health-related quality of life after pulmonary rehabilitation clearly exceeds the MCID. When disease-specific instruments were used, the lower limit of the 95% confidence interval exceeded the minimal clinically important difference. This means that almost all patients benefit to a clinically important extent from pulmonary rehabilitation in terms of health-related quality of life. To improve health-related quality of life, the effects of adding pulmonary rehabilitation to the treatment of a patient with COPD may be greater than adding another drug.

Interestingly enough, improved health-related quality of life is sometimes observed even in the absence of clinically significant improvements in exercise capacity. It is clear that the enhanced health-related quality of life is surely not only influenced by the physiologic benefits. Improved mental state, enhanced self-efficacy, enhanced symptom control, and ameliorated perception of symptoms are among the nonphysiologic pathways likely to contribute to an enhanced health-related quality of life. Long-term follow-up has shown that quality-of-life benefits are maintained above control levels if rehabilitation yields clinically significant effects on exercise tolerance.

Effects of rehabilitation on psychologic well-being (e.g., anxiety and depression) are less studied. Obviously, the effects of pulmonary rehabilitation on psychologic morbidity should be expected only in the 20–40% of patients referred for pulmonary rehabilitation with significant psychologic morbidity.

Few randomized controlled studies have examined the effectiveness of pulmonary rehabilitation programs on use of health care resources and assessed the cost-effectiveness of this intervention. To assess the cost-effectiveness of pulmonary rehabilitation, long-term follow-up is mandatory. In one well-conducted study, Griffiths and co-workers reported that patients with COPD spent fewer days in the hospital during a 1-year follow-up period. In fact, it was concluded from this study that it is very likely that pulmonary rehabilitation can be organized without an additional health care cost to society. Smaller recent studies of outpatient rehabilitation showed similar trends in reducing hospital days but lacked statistical power to confirm significance. Because several non-controlled studies also support the propensity of pulmonary rehabilitation to reduce hospital in-patient days, the main cost driver in COPD, we believe that the evidence is good enough to conclude that pulmonary rehabilitation is cost-effective. This benefit of rehabilitation programs may be attributed to the physiologic improvements or, alternately, to the improved knowledge of the disease and enhanced self-management. In a recent randomized controlled trial, hospital admissions were reduced by 40% in patients with a history of hospital admissions who followed a self-management program and in whom a "case manager" was assigned to follow-up the patients.

Interestingly, the effect of pulmonary rehabilitation programs on physical activity levels in daily life has been poorly investigated with objective measures. Clearly, objective assessment of physical activities is the "gold standard" for investigating the patients' engagement in everyday physical activities. Questionnaires have been shown to be inaccurate for objective analysis of the involvement of patients in activities. The results of studies that used activity monitors have, so far, been conflicting. All studies, so far, had unequivocally a number of patients that did not increase their physical activity levels, as is indicated by the variability in the outcome. Taken together the need for better insight on the effect of pulmonary rehabilitation on physical activity levels seems to be crucial, because enhanced activity levels may have a protective effect on morbidity and may be effective in maintaining the physiologic effects gained from an exercise training program. It may be that specific interventions are needed to enhance physical activity levels in patients with COPD. Giving patients feedback on their physical activity levels may enhance their engagement in daily physical activities. This is clearly an important avenue for future research.

THE EXERCISE TRAINING INTERVENTION

Rationale

From the definition of pulmonary rehabilitation it follows that "reversing the systemic consequences" of the lung disease renders the benefits of rehabilitation programs. As expected, exercise training does impact on cardiovascular function. Working at either a constant (steady state) work rate or at

progressive, high-intensity exercise training, the heart rate reduces for a given energy output with repetitive training. It has also been suggested that baroreflex sensitivity is altered favorably after exercise training. Whether exercise training also has favorable effects on vascular function, as in patients with heart failure or cardiac structure, has not been investigated. Exercise training aims at reversing the skeletal muscle abnormalities. Clinically, skeletal muscle strength has been reported to be reduced in severe COPD, in proportion to the skeletal muscle mass. Local endurance is even more impaired than skeletal muscle strength. The skeletal muscle of patients with COPD is also more rapidly fatigued during exercise, compared with healthy muscle, and deranged muscle bioenergetics have been reported. At the microscopic level, generalized skeletal muscle atrophy with a predominance of glycolytic fibers is seen. This pattern is slightly different from that observed with aging, where typically type II fiber atrophy is present. In addition, the number of capillary to fiber contacts is reduced. In the context of pulmonary rehabilitation two important findings at the molecular level deserve to be mentioned. First, the activity of two important enzymes, citrate synthase and HADH, is reduced in patients with COPD. These enzymes play an important role in the oxidative energy processes in skeletal muscle. As a result, the skeletal muscle has to rely on anaerobic glycolysis at abnormally low work rates. The produced lactate provides an additional drive to the compromised ventilatory system and leads to early ventilatory limitation (maximum exercise ventilation). Second, the skeletal muscle is more vulnerable to oxidative stress. In a subset of patients with a low body mass index (BMI), this may compromise the benefits of exercise training.

Most, if not all, skeletal muscle consequences of COPD are also seen after severe deconditioning. It seems likely that inactivity is the main driver of the skeletal muscle abnormalities seen in most patients. In subgroups of patients, however, other mechanisms may further impair skeletal muscle function. Such subgroups of patients include those with hypoxemia or hypercapnia, those rapidly losing body weight, or those treated with high doses of oral corticosteroids. Most of the deconditioning-induced abnormalities are at least partially reversible. After exercise training, skeletal muscle force is increased and the limb muscles are less prone to exercise-induced contractile fatigue. At the molecular and fiber level, oxidative enzyme capacity is enhanced and skeletal muscle fibers do hypertrophy and the number of capillary contacts per fiber increases.

Exercise Training, Practical Aspects

In general, exercise training in patients with COPD follows the principles of exercise training in the healthy elderly. Programs generally consist of a warmup, a core program in which at least 30 min of exercise is included, and a cooling down period. Close supervision and proper monitoring will ensure safety during the program. In fact, very few exercise-related events, and as far as the authors are aware, no fatal events have been reported after pulmonary rehabilitation in the published literature. Tables 42-1, A–C summarize a suggested training schedule in patients with COPD used in the authors' center.

Whole-Body Exercise

Exercise training has been included in virtually all studies investigating the benefits of pulmonary rehabilitation. To successfully increase skeletal muscle properties and render measurable physiologic benefits, it is important that patients do exercise at relative high work loads. To do so, the exercise training intervention can be adapted to the individual exercise potential of the patient. The conventionally used form to deliver exercise training to COPD patients is endurance training. In COPD patients with primarily moderate disease, exercise training conducted at approximately 75% of the peak work rate (60% of the difference between the lactate threshold and peak oxygen uptake) results in significant physiologic effects in patients across disease stages.

Interval exercise training has been shown to result in physiologic benefits comparable to those of endurance training. The advantage of interval training is that the ventilatory

requirements remain relatively limited. In our center, interval training is used in patients with severe ventilatory limitation or those not able to sustain long exercise bouts. It is important to adjust and increase the training load in every session. Trained personnel should be available to ensure close supervision on the training intensity. Training intensity can be monitored by use of Borg symptom scales. A score of approximately 4–6 is generally advised as an appropriate training intensity, provided the patients are familiar with the scale. Interestingly a given Borg symptom score is generally chosen by a patient at a fixed relative work rate relative to the peak work rate. Hence, as patients improve during training, the

TABLE 42-1A Training Scheme for the Treadmill Exercises Used in the Authors' Institute

(A) Endurance Training, Proposed Schedule on the Treadmill

WK	Duration	Training Load
1	10 min	75% 6 MWs
2	12 min	75% 6 MWs
3	12 min	80% 6 MWs
4	14 min	80% 6 MWs
5	14 min	85% 6 MWs
6	14 min	90% 6 MWs
7	16 min	90% 6 MWs
8	16 min	95% 6 MWs
9	16 min	100% 6 MWs
10	16 min	105% 6 MWs
11	16 min	110% 6 MWs
12	16 min	110% 6 MWs

6 MWs is the speed obtained during a 6-min walking test. Training week (WK) is displayed along with the duration of the block of exercise and the intensity relative to the maximal training load.

TABLE 42-1B Training Scheme for the Cycling Exercises Used in the Authors' Institute

(B) Interval Training Proposed Training Schedule on the Bicycle

WK	Duration	Number Blocks	Training Load
1	2 min	5×	60% Wmax
2	2 min	6×	60% Wmax
3	2 min	6×	65% Wmax
4	2 min	7×	65% Wmax
5	2 min	7×	70% Wmax
6	2 min	7×	70% Wmax
7	2 min	7×	75% Wmax
8	2 min	8×	75% Wmax
9	2 min	8×	80% Wmax
10	2 min	8×	80% Wmax
11	2 min	8×	85% Wmax
12	2 min	8×	85% Wmax

In between the different blocks patients are allowed to rest or they can continue cycling at reduced work rate.

Continued

TABLE 42-1C Training Scheme for the Resistance Training Exercises Used in the Authors' Institute

	(C) Schedule for the Resistance Training Program		
	WK	**Load**	**Reps**
	1	70% 1 R.M.	3×8
	2	70% 1 R.M	3×8
	3	76% 1 R.M	3×8
	4	82% 1 R.M	3×8
	5	88% 1 R.M	3×8
	6	94% 1 R.M	3×8
	7	100% 1 R.M	3×8
	8	106% 1 R.M	3×8
	9	112% 1 R.M	3×8
	10	115% 1 R.M	3×8
	11	118% 1 R.M	3×8
	12	121% 1 R.M	3×8

1 RM is the maximal weight a patient can lift once over the whole range of motion without compensatory movements. The number of repetitions (Reps) remains three series of eight repetitions throughout the training program.

same Borg rating will be achieved at higher absolute work rates. Because most patients are not limited by the cardiovascular system, use of the heart rate to guide exercise training is not advised.

Interventions to minimize the ventilatory burden during exercise training include the use of supplemental oxygen, the use of noninvasive ventilation, and the use of light-density gas mixtures (helium-oxygen). Oxygen reduces the ventilation for a given exercise intensity, hence application of supplementary oxygen may allow training at higher intensity at acceptable levels of pulmonary ventilation. Noninvasive mechanical ventilation reduces the work of breathing and has been used successfully in severe COPD as an adjunct to exercise training. In less severe COPD, however, the impact of the use of noninvasive mechanical ventilation is not significant. The use of noninvasive mechanical ventilation may increase the complexity of the training regimen disproportionately to the anticipated benefits, and this intervention should be restricted to very carefully selected patients. Last, the required ventilation can be reduced simply by reducing the amount of muscles put to work. If exercise is confined to one leg, ventilation is considerably reduced, allowing a significant increase in training load to those muscles. During cycling, for example, fewer muscles are recruited than with walking exercises, and it is not surprising that for a given oxygen consumption, cycling is more fatiguing to the skeletal muscles involved. It would be interesting to conduct a head-to-head comparison study on the physiologic effects of cycling versus walking exercises when applied in a rehabilitation program to check whether, on the basis of the larger potential to elicit muscle fatigue, cycling would be

a form of exercise training that results in larger physiologic effects than walking.

Obviously, optimal bronchodilator therapy also allows for better pulmonary ventilation during exercise. In one study, a potent long-acting anticholinergic drug, tiotropium, enhanced exercise training effects compared with the use of short-acting bronchodilators only.

Resistance Training

Another form of conventional training is resistance training. This form of exercise generally consists of weightlifting or—in less controlled forms—may consist of exercises against gravity (squat exercises or rising from a chair) or exercises with elastic bands. They can be used as the only form of training or in combination with whole-body exercises. Skeletal muscle strength was consistently increased more when resistance training was added to the exercise regimen. Increased muscle strength is an important treatment objective in patients with COPD who have muscle weakness. Indeed, many activities of daily life do require strength on top of muscle endurance. As mentioned previously, muscle weakness is an important factor related to morbidity and even mortality in COPD. It follows that patients with muscle weakness may be particularly good candidates to a resistance training program.

Resistance training is easy to apply in clinical practice. Patients are instructed to lift weights (generally on a multigym device). The weight imposed and the number of repetitions ensure overload of the skeletal muscle. In patients with COPD and several other chronic diseases, resistance training is started at approximately 70% of the weight a patient can lift once (i.e., the one repetition maximum). Proper warmup exercises are advised to prevent damage to joints and tendons in frail patients. The effects of resistance training programs may be enhanced in male hypogonadal patients by testosterone replacement therapy. Weekly intramuscular injections with testosterone, aiming at restoring testosterone levels to normal values, did enhance skeletal muscle force more than either of the interventions alone. Further studies, however, are required to investigate the long-term safety of this intervention. However, because skeletal muscle dysfunction is in itself a negative prognostic factor, short-term use of testosterone may be beneficial to result in a rapid restoration of this potentially harmful situation.

Another intervention used to specifically stimulate the peripheral muscles is neuromuscular electrical stimulation (NMES). Skeletal muscle force seems to increase more in patients treated with NMES, as monotherapy or in combination with general exercise training. It is important that the increased muscle function is engaged in functional exercises respecting the contraction time and intensity of daily life. Hence, we would advise the use of NMES only in combination with regular exercise training. NMES, however, may be a first approach to enhance skeletal muscle function in the most frail patients, who are too weak to take part in regular rehabilitation.

In summary, exercise training programs can be adjusted to the individual exercise limitations of patients with COPD. In individual patients, endurance training, interval training, or resistance training can be offered to keep the training stimulus attractive and with acceptable symptoms. Several interventions can be considered to further alleviate the ventilatory burden or specifically stimulate the peripheral muscles. An empirical flowchart that may guide the clinician to design the exercise intervention is given in Figure 42-1. It should be recognized that this flowchart is not directly validated but rather compiles the available knowledge and clinical expertise.

SPECIFIC RESPIRATORY MUSCLE TRAINING

The respiratory muscles have been specifically targeted for training in COPD. Inspiratory muscle training programs can be conducted at home by use of resistive breathing with target inspiratory pressures or target inspiratory flows or with threshold loading devices. Normocapnic hyperpnea has also been applied, albeit less frequently, in COPD. When the training load is appropriate (controlled and more than 30–40% of PI_{max}), inspiratory muscle training leads consistently to reductions in dyspnea and improved measures of inspiratory muscle performance. Programs are relatively inexpensive but require regular supervision. Whether inspiratory muscle training translates to increased exercise tolerance and quality of life is much less clear. Therefore, there has been some debate as to whether inspiratory muscle training should be part of rehabilitation programs in COPD, with most evidence-based guidelines concluding that it should not be a routine component.

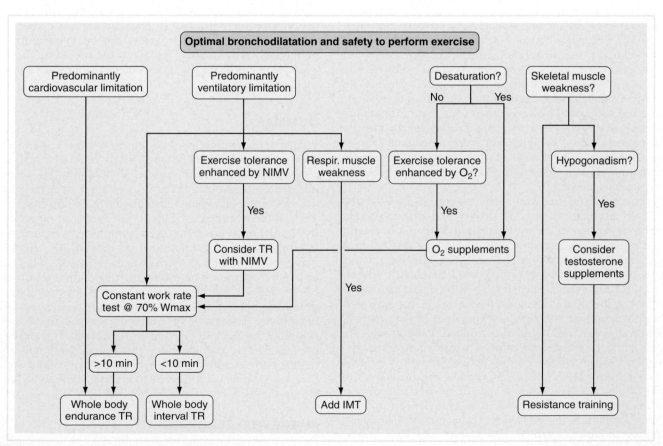

FIGURE 42-1 Empirical algorithm that could help the clinician to prescribe exercise therapy in individual patients on the basis of the exercise limitation of the patient (investigated in an incremental exercise test). With further clinical findings different training strategies or combinations can be prescribed. Typical cutoffs are: respiratory muscle weakness, PI_{max} <60% predicted; hypogonadism: total serum testosterone, <400 ng/dL^{-1}; desaturation, saturation on exercise <85%. Constant work rate test at 70% W_{max} is an exercise performed at 70% of the peak work rate from the incremental test. **IMT,** Inspiratory muscle training; **NIMV,** noninvasive mechanical ventilation; **TR,** training.

In patients with inspiratory muscle weakness, one can speculate that increasing respiratory muscle function may transform into functional benefits. Therefore, in patients with inspiratory muscle weakness, the prescription of strictly standardized inspiratory muscle training may be justified as an adjunct to exercise training, with the aim of improving exercise-induced symptoms of dyspnea. It should be noted, however, that whole-body exercise training, by itself, has improved inspiratory muscle force in some studies. Inspiratory muscle training as a stand-alone treatment is clearly inferior to general exercise training in COPD if the goal is to improve function or health-related quality of life.

OTHER INTERVENTIONS THAT ARE OFTEN PART OF PULMONARY REHABILITATION PROGRAMS

Given the prevalence of abnormalities in body composition (both overweight and underweight), psychologic morbidity, social isolation, poor self-management skills, and inappropriate management of daily life activities, other health care providers are crucial as members of a multidisciplinary rehabilitation team. Clearly, it is beyond the scope of this chapter to provide detail on the precise content of the interventions offered by these health care providers. Their actions are—as those offered by the exercise training specialists—structured and fit with the overall aims of the individualized rehabilitation program.

Nutritional specialists will focus on problems of underweight or overweight and will give advice as to balanced nutritional intake, taking into account the caloric and protein load of meals. Eventually, nutritional supplements can be considered in carefully selected patients. Meta-analysis clearly showed that providing nutritional supplements to unselected patients did not result in clinically meaningful improvements. If these interventions are successful, however, they contribute importantly to the enhanced survival. It remains challenging to identify which patients would benefit most from nutritional supplements. Although it is thought that patients with systemic inflammation are less responsive to nutritional interventions, more research is needed.

Psychologic counseling can focus on several issues. First, psychiatric morbidities, such as anxiety and depression, are potential targets for therapy. Compared with patients with chronic heart failure, patients with severe lung disease were shown to be more likely to have psychologic risk factors such as a psychiatric history, comorbid psychiatric illness, and stressful life events. Second, the psychologist may assist in achieving the desired behavioral changes in patients with COPD. In those who still smoke at the onset of the program, smoking behavior should clearly be tackled. Patients who are inactive could be assisted to achieve a more active lifestyle. Behavioral change toward a more active lifestyle is difficult and may require the use of several models and techniques to achieve this goal. Reliance on one specific theoretical construct is not likely to be successful in all patients. Changing physical activities depends on the physiologic capacities of the patient, psychological aspects such as mood state and self-efficacy, logistic, and cultural aspects.

Occupational therapists focus on the daily life situation of the patient. Home visits may reveal potentially nonergonomic physical activities. Improving the ergonomy does result in an enhanced efficiency with daily life tasks, which may result in fewer symptoms on performing activities. An occupational therapy intervention carried out at the home of severely disabled patients may improve the ability of patients to carry out daily tasks. This is obviously the core of any rehabilitation process, as mentioned previously. Specific training of physical activities of daily life has also been suggested to alleviate dyspnea more than just with exercise training alone. The occupational therapist could also investigate the pace at which patients perform their daily life activities. This pace should be adjusted to the physiologic possibilities (i.e., exercise tolerance, lung function, and hyperinflation) of the patient. Last, the occupational therapist may discuss tools to aid the patient in his or her daily life, for example, wheeled walking aids. These enhance the walking distance, reduce symptoms of dyspnea, and improve oxygen saturation, particularly in patients with poor walking efficiency and those walking at a slow pace. During exacerbations, wheeled walking aids may be used to assist in early mobilization of the patients.

Finally, patients often lack self-management skills to deal with their chronic condition. This is particularly true for patients after a recent hospital admission. Programs aimed at enhancing self-management have been shown to be successful in reducing hospital readmissions. These programs, in combination with a case manager, are cost-effective if a case manager could manage 50–70 patients. In these programs, patients get personalized advice on how to deal with issues related to their disease. The programs provide customer-tailored "action plans" specifying the steps to follow in particular situations, such as an exacerbation. In mild and stable patients, the benefits of acquiring self-management skills are less certain. Obviously, self-management programs can be integral part of a pulmonary rehabilitation program. A nurse specialist, for example, would have the ideal professional profile to integrate such a program.

SUMMARY

Pulmonary rehabilitation programs have been shown to be an "evidence-based" intervention. This is reflected in the most recent guideline on pulmonary rehabilitation and in a regularly updated meta-analysis. It has become clear over the past few decades that pulmonary rehabilitation is an essential cornerstone in the treatment of patients with reduced physical activity levels or with unresolved symptoms despite medical treatment. The program should be individually tailored and may vary in complexity from patient to patient. This chapter elaborated on the exercise training intervention, but it should be emphasized that rehabilitation involves, by definition, multiple disciplines of health care providers. Adequate and multidisciplinary assessment of patients is crucial to set out the rehabilitation track in individual patients. This review focused on the exercise training intervention, which should also be designed for each individual patient. To do so, knowledge of the exercise tolerance, exercise limitation, and muscle function seems crucial.

SUGGESTED READINGS

Bourbeau J, Julien M, Maltais F, et al: Reduction of hospital utilization in patients with chronic obstructive pulmonary disease: a disease-specific self-management intervention. Arch Intern Med 2003; 163:585–591.
Ferreira IM, Brooks D, Lacasse Y, Goldstein RS: Nutritional supplementation in stable chronic obstructive pulmonary disease (Cochrane review). Cochrane Database Syst Rev 2000; CD000998.

Griffiths TL, Burr ML, Campbell IA, *et al*: Results at 1 year of outpatient multidisciplinary pulmonary rehabilitation: a randomised controlled trial. Lancet 2000; 355:362–368.

Lacasse Y, Goldstein R, Lasserson TJ, Martin S: Pulmonary rehabilitation for chronic obstructive pulmonary disease. Cochrane Database Syst Rev 2006; CD003793.

Nici L, Donner C, Wouters E, *et al*: American Thoracic Society/European Respiratory Society statement on pulmonary rehabilitation. Am J Respir Crit Care Med 2006; 173:1390–1413.

O'Donnell DE, McGuire M, Samis L, Webb KA: General exercise training improves ventilatory and peripheral muscle strength and endurance in chronic airflow limitation. Am J Respir Crit Care Med 1998; 157:1489–1497.

Skeletal muscle dysfunction in chronic obstructive pulmonary disease: A statement of the American Thoracic Society and European Respiratory Society. Am J Respir Crit Care Med 1999; 159:S1–40.

Troosters T, Casaburi R, Gosselink R, Decramer M: Pulmonary rehabilitation in chronic obstructive pulmonary disease. Am J Respir Crit Care Med 2005; 172:19–38.

Troosters T, Gosselink R, Decramer M: Short- and long-term effects of outpatient rehabilitation in patients with chronic obstructive pulmonary disease: a randomized trial. Am J Med 2000; 109:207–212.

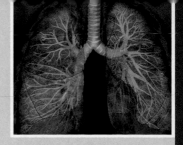

SECTION IX
AIRWAY DISEASES

43 Asthma: Epidemiology and Risk Factors

RICHARD HUBBARD

Asthma is one of the most common chronic illnesses in the developed world, and there is good evidence that it has become substantially more prevalent during the second half of the twentieth century. Despite a large number of research studies, the reasons some people have asthma develop and others do not and why asthma has emerged as a public health problem in some populations earlier than in others are not well understand. The aims of this chapter are to review the descriptive epidemiology of asthma, to understand how common the disease is and the extent of the health burden associated with asthma, and to consider epidemiologic studies of asthma etiology. Because defining asthma for epidemiologic studies has proved difficult, this chapter will start with a discussion section on asthma diagnoses.

THE PROBLEM OF DIAGNOSING ASTHMA FOR EPIDEMIOLOGIC STUDIES

> Asthma refers to the condition of subjects with widespread narrowing of the bronchial airways, which changes in severity over short periods of time either spontaneously or due to treatment and is not due to cardiovascular disease.
> CIBA Guest Symposium 1958

The central clinical feature of asthma is variation in airway caliber over time, and this is captured nicely in the definition of asthma that was developed during the CIBA Guest Symposium of 1958. The main advantage of this definition is that it is readily recognized and understood by both people with asthma and health care workers, and so it is useful clinically for diagnosing asthma and assessing response to treatment. It is perhaps not surprising, therefore, that most current definitions of asthma have evolved from this definition. The main drawback of this definition and others like it for research purposes is that it is not quantitative. It is not clear to what extent the degree of airflow obstruction needs to vary or over what time period.

The need to derive a practical definition of asthma for use in large-scale questionnaire-based epidemiologic research has led to a focus on asthma symptoms. In questionnaire surveys, the presence of asthma is often defined on the basis of responses to questions about symptoms of wheeze in the past 12 months, wheeze ever, and doctor-diagnosed asthma. This approach has been shown to have good short-term repeatability but may lack specificity, particularly in children, because other causes of wheezing illness, such as viral infection, may be misdiagnosed as asthma. Furthermore, there may be problems when questionnaires are translated into other languages, because direct translations of the word "wheeze" are not always available.

To validate questionnaire definitions of asthma, some researchers have used measures of bronchial hyperresponsiveness as a "gold standard" marker of asthma. The main drawback of this approach, however, is that rather than being a "gold standard" marker, bronchial hyperresponsiveness is just a marker of one physiologic characteristic of asthma. In addition, the presence of bronchial hyperresponsiveness is not specific to asthma, and in the general population only approximately half of the people who have bronchial hyperresponsiveness have respiratory symptoms consistent with asthma, whereas the other half are asymptomatic. Furthermore, only approximately half of the people defined as being asthmatic on the basis of a respiratory questionnaire or a physician diagnosis have bronchial hyperresponsiveness on the day of testing.

In summary, there is no perfect measure of asthma for use in epidemiologic studies, and when reading and interpreting data from epidemiologic studies, it is important to be clear what definition of asthma has been used to fully understand the data.

DESCRIPTIVE EPIDEMIOLOGY OF ASTHMA

Incidence of Asthma

The incidence of a condition describes the number of new instances of a condition occurring in a population over time, whereas the prevalence refers to the proportion of the population with the condition at one specific point in time. To generate incidence figures, a population needs to be under regular surveillance to determine exactly when the asthma starts. In reality, few studies have been able to achieve this for asthma. In some studies, such as analyses of the British Birth Cohorts, repeated cross-sectional surveys have been conducted in the same populations to give a measure of change in prevalence over time. Such studies do not give data on true disease incidence, however. One compromise has been to use the incidence of first time diagnoses of asthma recorded in primary care data sets. In these studies, date of first recorded diagnosis of asthma acts as a proxy for date of onset of asthma. By use of these methods, estimates from UK general practice data suggest that during the first 3 years of life the incidence of asthma is remarkably high at 73 per 1000 person-years. The incidence of asthma then declines progressively through childhood and into young adult life, and by the age of 25, the incidence has fallen to 2 per 1000 person-years. Incident asthma does occur throughout adult life, however, and a study in Minnesota revealed that the incidence of asthma in people older than the age of 65 years was 1 per 1000 person-years.

Prevalence

The prevalence of a condition provides a good measure of disease burden and is a useful statistic for planning health care provision. Because the prevalence of a condition will reflect both the incidence of new cases and the rates of resolution of existing cases, prevalence is not as useful a measure as incidence for etiologic studies. However, for the reasons detailed previously, most epidemiologic studies of asthma relate to prevalence rather than incidence.

Historically, there has been a wide range of prevalence figures reported for asthma varying between 1 and 30% of the population. This variation partly depends on the definitions of asthma that the studies have used but also reflects variations in the prevalence of asthma in different populations, the age group studied, and changes in asthma prevalence over time.

In 1991, in an effort to overcome these methodologic problems and to address similar issues for other allergic diseases, researchers from around the world started the International Study of Asthma and Allergies in Childhood (ISAAC). In 1998, the group published data on the prevalence of asthma for 463,801 children aged between 13 and 14 years living in 56 countries. Data were collected by use of a standardized questionnaire that asked about symptoms of wheeze in the last year, and in a subsample of countries this was validated against a video showing a child having an asthma attack. The results provided evidence of a marked variation in the prevalence around the world, with countries such as United Kingdom, Australia, New Zealand, and the Republic of Ireland having a prevalence of more than 25%, whereas the prevalence in Georgia, Romania, Albania, and Indonesia were less than 5%. The reasons for this wide variation have not been explained (Figure 43-1).

Prevalence of Asthma by Age and Gender

Asthma is present in all age groups, but the prevalence is generally highest in children and lowest in the middle-aged and the very elderly. For example, approximately 11% of 10-year-olds receive a prescription for a treatment for asthma each year in the United Kingdom, but only 5% of 40-year-olds do. The prevalence of the use of asthma medications increases from the age of 60, which is in keeping with evidence that new cases of asthma still occur in this age group, although these findings may also reflect some misdiagnosis of COPD as asthma (Figure 43-2).

Data from a number of sources including the 1958 British Birth Cohort, the Nottinghamshire School's survey, and the UK General Practice Research Database all demonstrate that in younger children asthma is more common in boys than girls, but around the age of puberty, this reverses, and throughout adult life asthma is more common in women than men. The reasons for this are not known (Figure 43-3).

Changes in Prevalence of Asthma Over Time and Asthma Epidemics

During the second half of the 20th century, it became apparent that studies of asthma in Europe and Australasia were reporting progressively higher and higher estimates of disease prevalence. Furthermore, a number of studies reported the emergence of asthma as a new public health problem in a

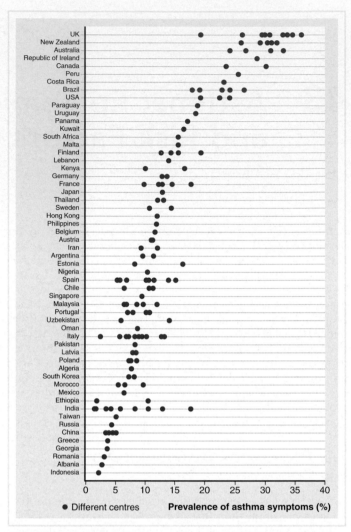

FIGURE 43-1 Twelve-month prevalences of self-reported asthma with a written questionnaire, for children ages 13 to 14 years. (Adapted with permission from the International Study of Asthma and Allergies in Childhood [ISAAC] Steering Committee: Lancet 351:1225–1232, 1998.)

number of African countries for the first time. It was not clear initially whether these reports reflected a true increase in asthma prevalence or were the result of shifts in diagnostic labeling or differences in method. As a result, a number of studies were repeated in the same population by use of the same methods, and these provided good evidence that a true increase in asthma prevalence was occurring in a number of countries around the world. In one example, a survey was conducted in 1973 of 12-year-old children living in South Wales by use of both a questionnaire and an exercise provocation test. The survey was then repeated by use of the same methods in 1988. The prevalence of current asthma on the basis of questionnaire responses increased from 4–9% between the two surveys, and this change was also reflected in an increased incidence of positive exercise tests. Another study used medical history and examination data collected from recruits to the Finnish Defence Force and showed a large increase in the prevalence of asthma from 1960 onward. A similar trend in the number of conscripts being discharged from the army because of asthma was found.

In 2006, the ISAAC phase 3 was published. This study is a follow-up study to ISAAC 1 completed at least 5 years after

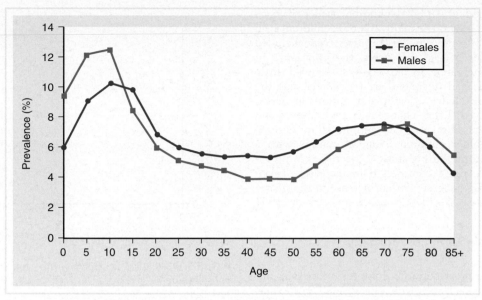

FIGURE 43-2 Prevalence of treated asthma in 1996, England and Wales.

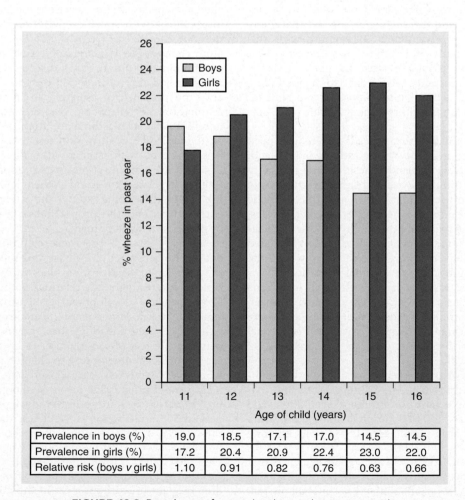

	11	12	13	14	15	16
Prevalence in boys (%)	19.0	18.5	17.1	17.0	14.5	14.5
Prevalence in girls (%)	17.2	20.4	20.9	22.4	23.0	22.0
Relative risk (boys v girls)	1.10	0.91	0.82	0.76	0.63	0.66

FIGURE 43-3 Prevalence of treated asthma in boys versus girls.

the first study. A total of 193,404 children aged 6–7 years from 66 centers in 37 countries and 304,679 children aged 13–14 years from 106 centers in 56 countries were included in the study. In children aged 6–7 years, the prevalence of asthma symptoms increased in 25 centers, showed little change in 27 centers, and decreased in 14 centers. For the older children, the prevalence of asthma symptoms increased in 42 centers, showed little change in 24 centers, and decreased in 40 centers. Similar trends were noted for eczema and hay fever. For older children living in centers with a high prevalence of asthma during study 1, decreases in prevalence over time were more common than increases. Taken together, these findings suggest that an increase in the prevalence of allergic disease worldwide occurred between 1991 and 2002.

Burden of Disease in Terms of Mortality and Morbidity

Asthma is one of the most common long-term illnesses, but only a few people die each year from this disease. For example, in the United Kingdom in 2004, 1381 deaths were registered as caused by asthma, which represents 0.2% of all deaths and 1% of deaths under the age of 35 years. Worldwide it has been estimated that asthma is responsible for 250,000 deaths each year. Data from the United Kingdom demonstrate that death from asthma is associated with socioeconomic disadvantage, and this highlights the fact that many asthma deaths may be preventable. In keeping with this finding, the Global Initiative for Asthma has suggested that approximately 50% of asthma deaths may be avoidable. There is evidence that mortality rates from asthma are falling in some countries, such as the United Kingdom and Finland, and it seems likely that these improvements result from better asthma management.

On two occasions in the past three decades, there have been substantial increases in mortality from asthma in England, Wales, Australia, and New Zealand. These asthma mortality epidemics have been attributed by some researchers to adverse effects arising from the use of high-dose sympathicomimetic bronchodilator use, but despite a number of research studies, there is still some doubt regarding the validity of this explanation. There is accumulating evidence that the use of inhaled corticosteroids may help to prevent deaths from asthma. In New Zealand, the introduction of inhaled corticosteroids during the early 1980s was associated with a fall in asthma mortality. Similar findings have also been reported from an analysis of the Saskatchewan, Canada, health databases, where the death rate from asthma fell by 21% with each additional canister of inhaled corticosteroid used in the previous 12 months (Figure 43-4).

Acute exacerbations of asthma represent an important public health problem. Each year in the United States, approximately 11 million people have an asthma exacerbation, and this leads to more than 400,000 hospital admissions. Data from Canada suggest that in people aged 15–34 years, the rate of hospital admissions per 100,000 person years is 150 for women and 70 for men. Again, there is good evidence that the use of inhaled corticosteroids is associated with a reduced risk of having an asthma exacerbation and hospital admission. Data coordinated by the WHO suggests that on a worldwide basis the number of DALYs lost each year because of asthma is 15 million. The current estimated asthma-related health care budget in the United States is $11.5 billion.

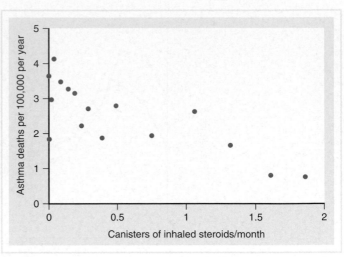

FIGURE 43-4 Asthma death rate by inhaled corticosteroid consumption.

Risk Factors for Developing Asthma

Atopy

People who are atopic have an increased tendency to have allergic hypersensitivity reactions develop when then come into contact with specific environmental allergens to which they are sensitized. There is not one unifying definition of atopy, but people who are atopic tend to have elevated levels of immunoglobulin E (IgE) directed against environmental allergens and also positive skin tests to these allergens. In general, the presence of atopy is an important risk factor for asthma, but not all people who are atopic have asthma, and not all people with asthma are atopic. When atopy is defined on the basis of a positive skin test to a common aeroallergen, it is associated with asthma with odds ratios in the region of 2–4, and it has been estimated that approximately 30–60% of asthma is related to atopy. When levels of antigen-specific IgE are used to define atopy, the strength of the association with asthma and the proportion of asthma cases explained by atopy is marginally higher.

In many studies, the most common allergens to which people are sensitized are house dustmite, grass, and cat, but the pattern of sensitization does vary between geographic regions. Interestingly, the relationship between early exposure to allergen and development of sensitization does not seem straightforward. For example, data from a birth cohort on Ashford, United Kingdom, has shown that the relationship between the risk of sensitization to both house dustmite and cat and the level of exposure to allergen is bell shaped. In other words, at low levels of exposure the risk of sensitization increases with increasing levels of allergen exposure, but very high levels of exposure seem to reduce the risk of sensitization, perhaps by inducing tolerance. These data are consistent with the findings of several other cohort studies that show that in populations where cat ownership is common, the risk of being sensitized to cats is lower in those children whose families own cats during the first few years of their life compared with children brought up without a cat in the house.

A number of studies have investigated whether reducing the level of exposure to allergens, in particular house dustmite, may improve the clinical outcome in people with asthma. In one trial, 1122 adults with asthma, of whom 65% had a positive skin test to house dustmite, were randomly allocated to receive a protective bed mattress cover or not. The cover was successful in reducing the level of allergen exposure in the intervention group, but even after 6 months of use, there was no improvement in peak expiratory flow rate or reduction in the use of inhaled corticosteroids in the active group. Similar negative findings have been reported in other studies in adults. The PIAMA study in The Netherlands randomly assigned 1282 babies at high risk of developing atopy by virtue of having an atopic mother to receive a protective bed cover, a placebo cover, or no intervention. Again, the bed cover resulted in lower levels of allergen exposure but this did not impact of the development of sensitization to house dustmite. In general then, studies of allergen avoidance have been disappointing in either improving asthma management for people with asthma or preventing the development of sensitization. Further research is required to understand the other factors that lead to the development of sensitization.

Family Structure and Genetics

One of the most consistent findings of epidemiologic studies over the past 25 years is that the presence of older brothers and sisters seems to reduce the risk of developing atopy, hay fever, and eczema. To explain these findings, David Strachan proposed the hygiene hypothesis in which he suggested that the protective influence of older siblings on the risk of allergic disease is mediated by infection. Support for this hypothesis came from immunologic studies that suggested that when babies are born their immune system is slanted toward TH2 responses, which favor the development of allergy, whereas early infection drives the immune system toward TH1 responses potentially reducing allergic sensitization.

The findings of research studies of birth order and asthma have been less consistent than those for hay fever and atopy, and this may reflect the more complex etiology of asthma. One potential reason for this is that the causes of early childhood asthma may be different from those later in childhood. For example, in a birth cohort analysis of primary care records for approximately 30,000 children, McKeever et al were able to show that the presence of older siblings increased the risk of diagnoses of asthma below the age of 2 years, but decreased the risk of developing asthma above this age in a dose-dependent manner. The authors concluded that the likely explanation for these findings was that diagnoses of asthma over the age of 2 years is related to atopy and thus shows the expected protective influence of increasing birth order, but those under the age of 2 years are related to viral illnesses, the frequency of which increases with increasing numbers of older children.

A number of studies have now investigated the hygiene hypothesis and attempted to demonstrate that early infection reduces the risk of developing allergic disease and explains the strong birth order effects. To date, the results are mixed, and in general, the evidence in support of the hygiene hypothesis is unconvincing. Furthermore, research that uses cord blood monocytes has shown that the risk of being sensitized to allergens at birth is related to the number of older siblings. This suggests that this protective effect of having older siblings on the risk of developing allergic disease is already present at the time of birth. Taken together these findings have led some researchers to start to look for other potential explanations for the strong birth order effects. A number of other diseases also show similar birth order effects. Perhaps the best example of this is acute lymphoblastic leukemia diagnosed in children

under the age of 5 years. It is possible, therefore, that the findings observed for allergic disease reflect a general influence of birth order on early immune development that we do not yet understand.

One interesting by-product of studies investigating the hygiene hypothesis has been the recognition from a number of studies in Europe that farmer's children seem to have a reduced risk of developing atopy and asthma. Detailed studies in Austria, Germany, Switzerland, and the United Kingdom have suggested that the protective influence of farming may be related to exposure to stables, livestock, and unpasteurized milk. These studies do not explain the influence of birth order on the risk of developing allergic disease, but they do highlight the fact that early life exposure to environmental allergens does have a lasting effect on the risk of allergic disease developing.

It is well recognized by both doctors and people with asthma that asthma tends to run in families. A number of studies have shown that if one parent has asthma, then the increased risk of the child having asthma is in the region of 50–100%. In most studies, this increase in risk is higher if the mother has asthma than if the father has asthma. Insights into the relative contribution of genetic and nongenetic contributions to the etiology of asthma can be gained by comparing the concordance rates for asthma and other allergic diseases in both monozygotic and dizygotic twins. In one of the largest twin studies to date, Strachan et al examined the risk of having asthma and other allergic diseases in 340 monozygotic and 533 dizygotic twins. Concordance rates for all allergic disease outcomes were higher in monozygotic twins than dizygotic twins, but although these differences were significant at the 5% level for hay fever, eczema, and the presence of specific IgE, they were not for self-reported diagnoses of asthma or symptoms of wheeze. The authors concluded that genetic factors influence the risk of developing sensitization to aeroallergens and clinical allergic disease but note that genetically identical twins were often discordant in their expression of atopy, suggesting an important modifying role for environmental factors.

There have now been more than 500 published studies that have tried to identify which genetic factors are important in the etiology of asthma. Although genetic studies are prone to false-positive results because of small sample sizes and multiple hypothesis testing, there are some consistencies in the findings, and 25 potential candidate genes have been identified in at least six studies and a further 79 genes have been identified in two or more studies. Potential candidate genes include CCR5δ32, CD14 C-159T, IL-12β, β-2 adrenoreceptor, IL-4, IL-13, IL-15, CD14, CD16, and TNF G-308A. One large family linkage study of families living in the United Kingdom and United States identified a region of chromosome 20 as being strongly linked to asthma. Further positional cloning studies identified a disintegrin and metalloprotease 33 (ADAM33) as the candidate gene responsible for the linkage signal. Subsequently, a number of studies have looked for a link between single nucleotide polymorphisms in the ADAM33 gene and the risk of asthma, and some, but not all, studies have reported a link. There is clearly more research needed to identify the relative importance of a number of different genes to the etiology and natural history of asthma and how these genes interact with environmental exposures.

Smoking

In children, exposure to environmental tobacco smoke has consistently been shown to increase the risk of asthma and wheezing illness developing. The detrimental impact of environmental tobacco smoke seems to be greatest in the first few years of life. It may also increase the severity of asthma in children who already have the condition. There is evidence that exposure to environmental tobacco smoke early in life, particularly *in utero*, leads to a small deficit in FEV_1 in school-aged children.

Cigarette smoking during adolescence slows lung growth such that peak FEV_1 values in early adult life tend to be lower in smokers than nonsmokers. In nonsmokers, FEV_1 values plateau during early adult life, before starting a slow decline. In contrast, smokers have no plateau in their lung function values and hence start to lose lung function at an earlier stage than nonsmokers. Furthermore, the rate of decline of FEV_1 in adult life in smokers is approximately twice that in nonsmokers. Cigarette smoking also increases bronchial hyperresponsiveness and the frequency and severity of asthma exacerbations.

Respiratory Infections

A number of viral infections, such respiratory syncytial virus (RSV) and influenza B, may cause wheezing illness in children. The Tucson Children's Respiratory Study, a birth cohort study of more that 1000 children, found that children who were infected with RSV before the age of 3 years were still at increased risk of wheezing illness at the age of 6, although no increase was present at the age of 11 years. These findings, and others like it, suggest that RSV infection may cause a prolonged wheezing illness in children that leads to a diagnosis of asthma but that eventually resolves.

A number of epidemiologic studies have demonstrated that respiratory infections early in life are a predictor of asthma later on. For example, McKeever *et al* showed that 54% of children are diagnosed as having a respiratory tract infection during the first year of life by their general practitioner and that these children have a 26% increased incidence of subsequent asthma diagnoses. What is not clear from these results, and similar findings from other groups, is whether the infection actually causes the asthma or is just a marker of as yet undiagnosed asthma.

Infection with measles virus has a specific impact on the immune system and may cause prolonged changes in cell-mediated immunity. Anecdotally, measles infection may lead to remission of nephritis and atopic diseases. In a study of young adults in Guinea-Bissau, Shaheen *et al* were able to demonstrate that among those individuals who had measles infection and survived, there was a reduced prevalence of atopy defined on the basis of a positive skin test.

During the 1990s, several studies in the United Kingdom and New Zealand suggested that routine childhood vaccination, particularly against *Bordetella pertussis*, might be associated with an increased risk of asthma. Further support for this hypothesis came from experimental data showing that *Bordetella pertussis* is a powerful adjuvant and can greatly enhance levels of antibody production against a specific allergen, and that in rodents the vaccine may act as a promoter of IgE production. However, two more recent detailed and large-scale studies have failed to demonstrate a link between childhood vaccination and allergic disease, and it seems unlikely that vaccination has an etiologic role in asthma.

Obesity

Obesity is an increasingly common problem in a number of countries around the world. For example, data from the 1999–2002 National Health and Nutritional Examination Survey in the United States found that approximately 65% of American adults were either obese or overweight. A number of cross-section studies have suggested a positive association between the presence of obesity and asthma. One major drawback to these studies, however, is the potential for reverse causation. It seems likely that people with asthma will have a reduced capacity for exercise and more exposure to corticosteroids than the general population, and it is possible that it is these factors that lead people to put on weight. To address this question, Camargo *et al* analyzed prospective cohort data from the Nurses Health Study and found evidence of a dose-response relationship between increasing body mass index (BMI) and the incidence of asthma such that the relative risk for asthma developing in women in the highest category of BMI was 2.7. Similar findings have subsequently been reported from a number of different cohorts in both children and adults. For reasons that are not clear, the impact of obesity is usually more marked in women than in men. Some studies have also shown an increased risk of having atopy with increasing BMI, and again this association tends to be stronger in women than men.

It is clear that if obesity is an important risk factor for asthma, then the rising prevalence of obesity will contribute to increasing the prevalence of asthma. Some intervention studies have looked at the potential for weight reduction programs to benefit people with asthma. In a randomized trial of 38 people with a BMI of more than 30 in Finland, a low-energy diet was associated with a marked loss of weight that was sustained at 1 year. This loss in weight led to a significantly higher lung function in the intervention group, and this benefit was sustained at 1 year. Similar improvements in respiratory symptom scores were found. A recent Cochrane review concludes that at present there is only a small amount of evidence to support the use of calorie-controlled diets in asthma. Given the large impact of both asthma and obesity on public health, it is clear that this is an area in need of more research.

Diet

The observation that higher levels of dietary salt are associated with hypertension, which may in part be mediated by an increase in vascular tone, led Burney to hypothesize that higher levels of salt may also be a risk factor for asthma. In an initial ecologic analysis, Burney found that regional mortality rates for asthma in men and children, but not women, were associated with regional table salt sales. In a follow-up clinical study of 138 men, Burney was also able to demonstrate an association between 24-h urinary excretion of sodium and bronchial reactivity. Subsequent epidemiologic studies of asthma and sodium have produced inconsistent results, however. A number of small clinical trials have assessed the short-term impact of either increasing or decreasing the salt in the diet of people with asthma, and some trials have shown benefits.

The work of Burney *et al* on salt was important, because it also opened up a new avenue of research in asthma epidemiology and led to a number of studies of other aspects of diet. Most of the evidence to date comes from large cross-sectional studies, and there have been relatively few longitudinal studies. Evidence is also available from some intervention studies, but most have included only small numbers of people and short-term interventions. When interpreting the results of the observational studies of diet, it is important to remember that diet is particularly difficult to measure accurately, and so these studies will be prone to random error.

Many studies have focused on the role of vitamin C in the diet, and, in general, the results suggest that higher dietary levels of vitamin C are associated better lung function. Similar results have been found for fresh fruit consumption. The results for vitamin E are less consistent, but data from the Nurses Health Study does suggest that higher levels of vitamin E intake are associated with a lower incidence of asthma. In a cross-sectional survey in the United Kingdom, the risk of having bronchial reactivity was inversely associated with levels of magnesium consumption, and there are clinical data that suggest that when given intravenously, magnesium is a bronchodilator. Evidence from an Australian cross-sectional survey showed that children who ate more oily fish had a lower risk of having asthma. Support for these findings comes from an analysis of the first National Health and Nutritional Examination Survey, which found that higher consumption levels of n-3 fatty acids was associated with higher spirometry readings. A small follow-up intervention study failed to find a benefit of the use of fish oils for children with asthma, but a trial is currently ongoing to assess the use of fish oils during pregnancy in atopic women.

As part of a case-controlled study of dietary antioxidants in asthma, Shaheen et al found that the use of paracetamol was associated with the risk of having asthma in a dose-dependent way, such that in people who use paracetamol every day the risk of having asthma was more than doubled. The same research group has demonstrated an association between maternal consumption of paracetamol during pregnancy and the risk of atopy and asthma in children contributing data to the UK ALSPAC cohort study, and, in an ecologic analysis of the ISAAC 1 data set, that the prevalence of asthma in a country is related to that country's national per capita sales of paracetamol. In an analysis of the Nurses Health Cohort in the United States, an association was present between the level of use of paracetamol and the incidence of asthma. Other groups have also reported similar findings including studies in Ethiopia.

Pollution

There is good evidence that both indoor and outdoor pollution can have an adverse effect on health. On days of high levels of outdoor pollution, there are increases in all-cause mortality and also mortality from respiratory and cardiovascular disease. Indoor pollution in the form of smoke from cooking stoves has been shown to be an important cause of pneumonia in children. There is an increasing amount of evidence that outdoor pollution can have an adverse effect on people with asthma. In one study from Hong Kong, ambient levels of PM10, PM2.5, nitrogen dioxide, and ozone were all associated with hospital admission rates for asthma. A number of studies have shown that the closer people live to main roads the more likely they are to report respiratory symptoms such as wheeze.

Although the preceding evidence suggests that pollution may have an adverse effect on asthma control, what is not clear is whether pollution is an important cause of asthma and/or allergic disease? Certainly, the ambient levels of most common air pollutants in the United Kingdom have decreased over the time period during which the prevalence of asthma has increased. Furthermore, a study from Germany has shown that the prevalence of asthma is similar in children living in Leipzig

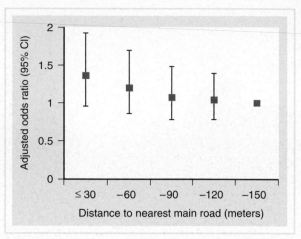

FIGURE 43-5 Living near a main road and the risk of wheezing in children. (From Am J Respir Crit Care Med 164[12]:2177–2180, 2001.)

and Munich even though there is a large difference in the levels of pollution between the two cities (Figure 43-5).

Birth Weight and Growth

Babies who are born prematurely have an increased risk of wheezy illness developing early in life. For example, in a birth cohort in the United Kingdom by use of data from general practice, children who were born prematurely had a 90% increase in the incidence of wheezing illness during the first 3 years of life. There is also good evidence from an analysis of the 1970 British Birth Cohort of an inverse relationship between birth weight and the risk of asthma developing. For example, symptoms of asthma were twice as common at the age of 26 years in people born with a weight of less than 2 kg than those born with a weight of between 3 and 3.5 kg. In the same study, no association was present between birth weight and either hay fever or eczema. The authors conclude that early lung growth, reflected in birth weight, has a lasting influence on the risk of developing asthma but not other allergic disease. Similar findings have been reported by others.

Occupation

A number of occupations are known to cause asthma. Car bodywork paint sprayers and bakers are good examples in the United Kingdom. As working patterns and processes change, a number of new occupations are identified as causes of occupational asthma. Despite this, there is relatively little information available of the number of new cases of asthma resulting from occupational exposures each year. One study from Japan suggests the figure is approximately 15%. However, accurate figures for Western countries are not known.

Role of Urbanization in Africa

Studies of asthma prevalence in Africa during the 1970s found that asthma was rare, particularly in more rural communities. For example, a study of Xhosa children from Cape Town in 1979 found that the prevalence of exercise-induced fall in peak expiratory flow rate was 3.2% in urban children but only 0.1% in rural children. More recent studies have reported higher

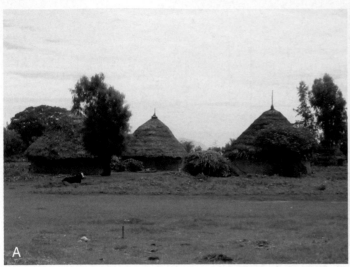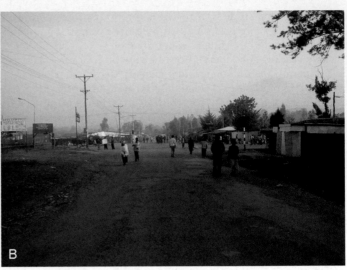

FIGURE 43-6 A, Rural and, **B,** urban Ethiopia.

levels of asthma, particularly in the urban centers, and the emergence of asthma as a public health problem. Taken together, the data from Africa suggest that an asthma epidemic has started in the continent and that a major factor driving the emergence of asthma is a move toward more urbanization. An increased prevalence of asthma in urban populations compared with rural populations is one of the most consistent epidemiologic findings, and it is clear that the increase occurs at a very early stage of urbanization. The reasons for this are not fully understood, but there is evidence to suggest that as people become more urbanized, the prevalence and severity of parasitic disease may drop and that some parasites, such as hookworm, may have a protective role in reducing the prevalence of asthma (Figure 43-6).

SUMMARY

- Asthma is an important cause of morbidity and avoidable mortality throughout the world.
- The prevalence of asthma is increasing around the world, and new epidemics of asthma seem to be evolving in a number of developing countries.
- The environmental exposures that are responsible for these changes have not yet been identified, highlighting the need for further research in this area.

SUGGESTED READINGS

Asher MI, Montefort S, Bjorksten B, *et al*, ISAAC Phase Three Study Group: Worldwide time trends in the prevalence of symptoms of asthma, allergic rhinoconjunctivitis, and eczema in childhood: ISAAC Phases One and Three repeat multicountry cross–sectional surveys. Lancet 2006; 368(9537):733–743.

Beuther DA, Weiss ST, Sutherland ER: Obesity and asthma. Am J Resp Crit Care Med 2006; 174:112–119.

Britton J: Symptoms and objective measures to define the asthma phenotype. Clin Exp Allergy 1998; 28(Suppl):2–7.

Fogarty A, Britton J: The role of diet in the aetiology of asthma. Clin Exp Allergy 2000; 30:615–627.

McKeever TM, Hubbard R, Lewis, S, Britton J: Birth order and asthma. In Busse W, Lemanske R, eds: Asthma prevention: Risk factor in the development of asthma. Lung Biology in Health and Disease series. Marcel Dekker; in press.

Message SD, Johnston SL: Viruses in asthma. Brit Med Bull 2002; 61:29–43.

Pearce N, Beasley R, Burgess C, Crane J: Asthma epidemiology—Principles and methods. Oxford: Oxford University Press; 1998.

Strachan DP, Cook DG: Parental smoking and childhood asthma: Longitudinal and case-control studies. Thorax 1998; 53:204–212.

Taussig LM, Wright AL, Holber CJ, *et al*: Tucson Children's Respiratory Study: 1980 to present. J Allergy Clin Immunol 2003; 111:661–675.

The International Study of Asthma and Allergies in Childhood (ISAAC) Steering Committee.: Worldwide variation in the prevalence of symptoms of asthma, allergic rhinoconjunctivitis and atopic eczema: ISAAC. Lancet 1998; 351:1225–1232.

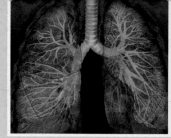

SECTION IX
AIRWAY DISEASES

44 Asthma: Cell Biology

RYAN H. DOUGHERTY • STEPHEN C. LAZARUS

Although asthma has long been thought of as a disease of airway smooth muscle, even early observers recognized that other cells in addition to muscle were involved. Clinicians had identified eosinophils, Creola bodies (clusters of airway epithelial cells), and Curschmann's spirals (spiral-shaped mucus plugs) in the sputum of patients with asthma exacerbations. Pathologists had described eosinophilic inflammation, mucus plugging of small airways, and "epithelial basement membrane thickening" in patients who died of asthma. However, it was not until the 1990s that histopathologic studies showed convincingly that all asthma has an inflammatory basis. Thus, patients with mild asthma, even if biopsied when they were not symptomatic and when their lung function was near normal, had too many eosinophils, mast cells, and lymphocytes in their airway tissues. Since that time, attention has focused on the cells involved in the pathogenesis of asthma and on the cell–cell interactions involved in the clinical manifestations. Various inflammatory cells and mediators have been implicated in the bronchoconstriction, bronchial hyperresponsiveness, and mucus hypersecretion that are the hallmarks of asthma, and new therapeutic interventions are aimed at interrupting some of these pathways.

CLINICOPATHOLOGIC CORRELATIONS

Although dyspnea and wheezing are the major symptoms associated with asthma, it is clear that these are not due solely to smooth muscle contraction. In many cases the submucosal region of the airway is edematous, there may be excessive mucus in the airway lumen, and small peripheral airways may be plugged with inspissated mucus, giving rise to ventilation-perfusion mismatch. In addition, the asthmatic airway has a tendency to contract too easily and too forcefully. This phenomenon is called bronchial hyperreactivity or bronchial hyperresponsiveness. In most cases, mucus hypersecretion and bronchial hyperresponsiveness correlate well with the degree of airway inflammation. In addition to the excessive number of eosinophils, lymphocytes, and mast cells that were identified previously, more recent studies have implicated neutrophils, macrophages, dendritic cells, and myofibroblasts in the pathophysiology of asthma.

CELLS INVOLVED IN THE DEVELOPMENT OF ASTHMA

Asthma is a complex disease, which almost certainly involves a heritable component and an environmental component. Various strategies have been used to identify asthma candidate genes, with controversial results. Similarly, studies of single nucleotide polymorphisms and of haplotypes have produced inconsistent outcomes. However, candidate loci linked to asthma, bronchial hyperresponsiveness, atopy, and IgE production have been identified and offer promise for future studies of this kind. It seems that, in the right genetic context, certain stimuli initiate the steps that lead to the development of atopy and asthma. These probably must occur relatively early in life, and there may be a relatively narrow window during which these events may be prevented.

Most data now suggest that a specific population of CD4-positive (CD4$^+$) T-helper lymphocytes play a critical role in the development of asthma (Figure 44-1). Under some circumstances, undifferentiated or naive T-helper (Th0) lymphocytes are directed toward this proatopic, proasthmatic T-lymphocyte phenotype (Th2). Exposure to certain microbes by infection (e.g., measles, TB) or from the environment (e.g., living near cattle) during early childhood may drive T lymphocytes toward a nonatopic, nonasthmatic phenotype (Th1). This has been termed the "hygiene hypothesis" and has led to attempts to prevent the development of asthma by feeding of probiotics to susceptible infants. Support for this theory comes from comparisons of asthma prevalence in East versus West Germany and in rural versus urban environments, suggesting that vaccinations, the use of antibiotics, and emphasis on cleanliness all lead to preferential expansion of Th2 rather than Th1 cell populations.

Th1 and Th2 lymphocytes are defined, on the basis of murine models, by the cytokines they produce. Among the major products of Th2 cells are interleukin-3 (IL-3), IL-4, IL-5, IL-13, and granulocyte macrophage colony-stimulating factor (GM-CSF). IL-5 and GM-CSF are important for the growth and differentiation and migration of eosinophils; IL-4 and IL-13 drive B-cell switching from IgG to IgE production; IL-4 and IL-5 also promote mast cell growth and differentiation. IL-4 and IL-13 are structurally similar (and share the same receptor); IL-13 signals through the alpha subunit of the IL-4 receptor. Thus, infants with a genetic predisposition to asthma or atopy who have little exposure to infections or environmental microbial organisms in the neonatal period may have the consequences of this Th2-type inflammation develop: eosinophilia, increased mast cell numbers, production of IgE, leading to the clinical asthma phenotype and a predisposition to exacerbations triggered by subsequent exposure to allergen, virus, or environmental triggers.

STEPS LEADING TO THE CLINICAL MANIFESTATIONS OF ASTHMA

Immune Mechanisms

In a sensitized individual, the process of allergen-induced airway inflammation begins with the uptake and processing of aeroallergens. Many cells, including airway epithelial cells,

559

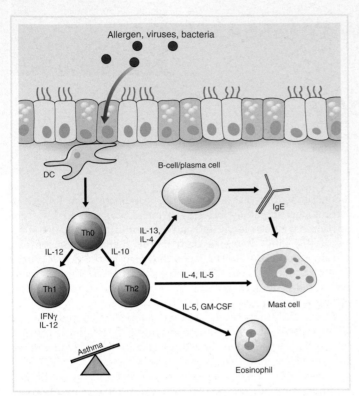

FIGURE 44-1 Early inflammatory events in asthma. On antigen encounter, dendritic cells (DC) are activated and induce the differentiation of T-helper 0 (Th0) cells into either Th1 or Th2 cells. In asthmatic subjects, this process leads to a preferential differentiation into a Th2 phenotype. These Th2 cells may mediate a wide range of events that contribute to the (allergic) inflammatory response, such as immunoglobulin E *(IgE)* production, mast cell development, and maturation and activation of eosinophils. *GM-CSF,* Granulocyte macrophage colony-stimulating factor; *IFN,* interferon; *IL,* interleukin.

macrophages, and dendritic cells, are capable of antigen presentation, but the dendritic cell is believed to be the most effective at this process. Dendritic cells are found within the epithelium and in the subepithelial tissue throughout the respiratory tract from the upper airways to the alveoli. When airway dendritic cells ingest allergen, they migrate to lymphoid tissue where antigen is presented to naive Th0 cells. Type I or myeloid dendritic cells release IL-12, which favors the differentiation of Th0 cells into Th1 cells. Type II or plasmacytoid dendritic cells secrete IL-10, which drives the differentiation of Th0 cells to Th2 cells. The number of dendritic cells in the blood and in airway tissue, both the epithelium and the subepithelial lamina propria, is increased in asthma and can increase very rapidly when allergen enters the airway of a sensitized individual. Most of these are type II or plasmacytoid dendritic cells. Recruitment of dendritic cells to the airway is thought to be achieved by elevated levels of chemokines and mediators such as RANTES (regulated on activation, normal T-cell expressed and secreted), monocyte chemoattractant proteins (MCP) 1–4, eotaxin, and platelet-activating factor (PAF).

T Cells

When a sensitized individual is exposed to allergen, Th2 cells accumulate in the airway, drawn by Th2-specific chemokines such as thymus and activation-regulated chemokine (TARC or CCL17). Activated Th2 cells and Th2-derived cytokines

such as IL-4, IL-5, and IL-13 are found in bronchoalveolar lavage fluid and airway biopsy samples from both atopic and nonatopic subjects with asthma. The presence of these Th2 cells and products correlates with asthma severity, eosinophilia, and bronchial hyperresponsiveness.

Temporal Sequence of Allergic Asthmatic Response

There is a well-described, stereotypic sequence that occurs when previously sensitized individuals are exposed to specific antigen (Figure 44-2). Cross-linking by antigen of adjacent IgE molecules bound to mast cells by high-affinity IgE receptors results in activation of mast cells with the release of both preformed and newly generated mediators, including histamine, tryptase, chymase, the cysteinyl leukotrienes LTC_4, LTD_4, and LTE_4, PGD_2, and PAF. These mediators are responsible for the immediate bronchoconstrictor response, referred to as the "early-phase response" (EPR), or the "early asthmatic response" (EAR), that occurs rapidly after allergen exposure and that usually resolves spontaneously within 1–2 h. In approximately 50–60% of patients, there is a second bronchoconstrictor response that occurs 4–12 h after allergen exposure (without additional exposure). This "late-phase response" (LPR), or "late asthmatic response" (LAR), is believed to be due to the migration into the airway of additional inflammatory cells and the release of mediators from those cells. Airway eosinophilia is common during the LPR, and this inflammatory response is associated with increased bronchial hyperresponsiveness, increased vascular permeability, submucosal edema, and mucus hypersecretion.

AIRWAY INFLAMMATION AND INFLAMMATORY CELLS

Eosinophils

In subjects with asthma, there are increased numbers of eosinophils in the sputum (Figure 44-3), blood, bronchoalveolar lavage fluid, and airway tissues. In general, the number of eosinophils in the airways correlates with the severity of asthma and with the magnitude of bronchial hyperresponsiveness. As described previously, the number of eosinophils in the airways increases during the asthmatic LPR after allergen challenge, and this increase is temporally related to the increase in bronchial hyperresponsiveness. Products of eosinophils are also increased in the airway tissues and secretions of subjects with asthma, and these increase further after allergen exposure and during exacerbations. Charcot–Leyden crystals, found commonly in the sputum of asthmatic patients, are a crystalline condensation product of eosinophil granule proteins. The major granule products of eosinophils are eosinophil cationic protein (ECP), major basic protein (MBP), eosinophil peroxidase, and eosinophil-derived neurotoxin. Epithelial damage in asthma has been attributed to these toxic proteins, although recent data suggest that they may have beneficial effects as well. In addition to these granule-associated proteins, eosinophils secrete a number of proteolytic enzymes, lipid mediators (especially cysteinyl leukotrienes LTC_4, LTD_4, LTE_4), oxygen metabolites, and cytokines, all of which contribute to the acute and chronic changes in the airway.

Various cytokines produced by Th2 cells can affect the growth and maturation of eosinophils and their recruitment to the airway, and elevated levels of IL-2, IL-3, IL-4, and

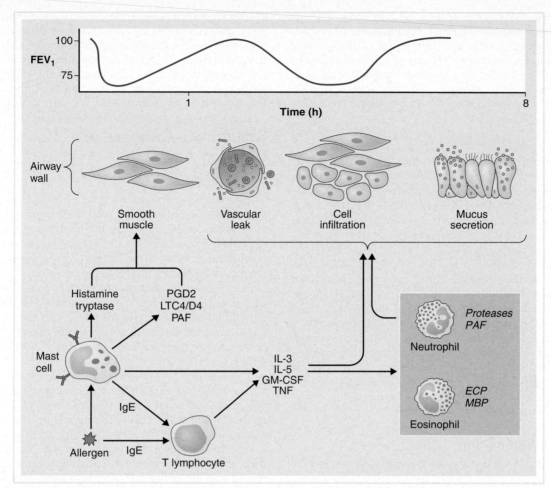

FIGURE 44-2 Mechanisms of the early-phase and late-phase responses to allergens. Allergic asthmatic subjects who inhale an aeroallergen to which they are sensitive have immediate bronchoconstriction develop, which usually resolves spontaneously within 1–2 h; in approximately 50% of the subjects, this immediate response is followed 3–12 h later by further bronchoconstriction and the development of airway inflammation and increased bronchial hyperresponsiveness. The mechanism of the early-phase and late-phase responses is thought to involve allergen-induced activation of mast cells (mediated by cross-linking of immunoglobulin [IgE] molecules bound via the high-affinity IgE receptors) and T cells (perhaps mediated by a mechanism involving CD23 and IgE receptors) that results in smooth muscle contraction, vascular leak, accumulation of activated eosinophils and mast cells, and degranulation of goblet cells. *ECP*, Eosinophil cationic protein; *LTC4/D4*, leukotriene C4/D4; *MBP*, major basic protein; *PAF*, platelet-activating factor; *PGD2*, prostaglandin D$_2$. (Adapted from Mason RJ, Broaddus VC, Murray JF, et al: Murray and Nadel's Textbook of Respiratory Medicine. 4th ed. Philadelphia: Saunders; 2005.)

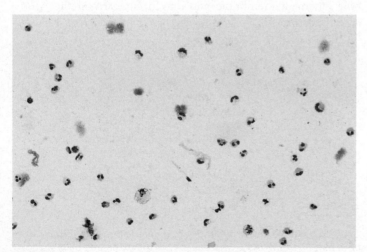

FIGURE 44-3 Sputum of asthmatic subjects obtained after sputum induction by hypertonic saline (a noninvasive method to study airway inflammation) contains high numbers of eosinophils.

IL-5 are found in airway secretions and tissues. Eotaxins 1, 2, and 3 and RANTES have also been linked to eosinophil recruitment. Of these, IL-5 seems to be the most important.

The exact role of the eosinophil in the development of asthma and bronchial hyperresponsiveness is controversial. The associations described previously have been observed in both animal models and in humans, but studies of monoclonal antibodies directed against IL-5 have demonstrated no clinical benefit and no change in bronchial hyperresponsiveness despite significant reduction in peripheral blood eosinophils and sputum eosinophils. This suggests a mechanism that is independent of eosinophils and that eosinophils may be a marker, rather than an effector, of these physiologic responses.

Neutrophils

Although asthma is generally thought of as an eosinophilic disease, up to 20% of patients with asthma have increased numbers of neutrophils in sputum and in the airway submucosa. Neutrophil predominance has been reported in fatal asthma, during acute exacerbations of asthma, and in some patients with chronic severe asthma. The increased number of neutrophils is often associated with increased levels of IL-8, a very potent neutrophil chemoattractant. Neutrophils probably contribute to airway epithelial damage and remodeling through the actions of neutrophil elastase, reactive oxygen species, and proinflammatory mediators and cytokines, including LTB_4, TNF-α, IL-1β, and IL-6.

Mast Cells

Mast cells (*Mastzellen* in German) were given their name by Ehrlich because they appeared to be stuffed full of metachromatic granules. These granules contain the proteoglycans heparin or chondroitin sulfate, the preformed mediator histamine, and the serine proteases tryptase or chymase. In addition, mast cells are capable of generating a number of newly formed mediators including LTC_4, LTD_4, PGD_2, PAF, and the cytokines IL-3, IL-4, IL-5, IL-6, and TNF-α. Mast cells express on their surface the high-affinity receptor (FcϵRI) for IgE. When allergen binds to and cross-links adjacent IgE molecules, the mast cell is activated, resulting in the very rapid release of preformed granule-associated mediators; secretion of newly generated mediators follows almost immediately. These various products contribute to the immediate manifestations of asthma and to airway remodeling. Mast cells are present in all normal tissues. In patients with asthma, they localize particularly to the airway smooth muscle, the airway epithelium, and airway submucosal glands.

Neurogenic Inflammation

Adrenergic receptors are distributed throughout the airways, and adrenergic agonists are widely used as bronchodilators. Cholinergic pathways contribute to airway smooth muscle tone, and anticholinergics can also be effective bronchodilators. However, neither of these neural pathways is thought to play a major role in airway inflammation or in the development of bronchial hyperresponsiveness. In contrast, the nonadrenergic noncholinergic (NANC) system is responsible for what is known as neurogenic inflammation. NANC nerves release bronchoactive tachykinins such as substance P and neurokinin (NK) A. Two classes of NK receptors have been described. Airway smooth muscle contraction is mediated by NK2 receptors; NK1 receptors are important in the regulation of submucosal gland secretion, vascular tone and permeability, and leukocyte adhesion. Elevated levels of neuropeptides have been described in the asthmatic airway, and asthmatic subjects have bronchoconstriction develop when exposed to aerosols of these peptides. Further evidence for the importance of this pathway is the presence in the airway epithelium of neutral endopeptidase, an enzyme that degrades tachykinins.

STRUCTURAL CHANGES IN CHRONIC ASTHMA

Remodeling

The earliest descriptions of airway histopathology came from autopsy studies of patients who died from asthma. Common findings included airway inflammation, inspissated mucus, epithelial desquamation, and thickening of the subepithelial basal lamina. In addition, there is hyperplasia and/or hypertrophy of epithelial goblet cells and airway smooth muscle. Collectively these changes are referred to as "airway remodeling" (Figure 44-4). They are thought to be consequences of chronic inflammation (Figure 44-5), but they are not present to the same degree in all patients with severe chronic asthma, and many of these changes have been described in patients with relatively mild asthma as well.

Desquamation of epithelial cells, leaving a denuded surface with diminished barrier function, is common, and clumps of columnar epithelial cells (Creola bodies) in expectorated sputum suggest that this is an ongoing process *in vivo*. Recent studies suggest that the airway epithelium in asthmatic patients is unusually fragile, leading to damage by mediators from inflammatory cells, by environmental irritants such as cigarette smoke and air pollutants, and by biopsy and fixation procedures. Goblet cell numbers are increased in the airway biopsy specimens of patients with mild, moderate, and severe asthma, and airway epithelial mucin stores are increased threefold over the levels found in control subjects.

Subepithelial Membrane

Early studies described what was interpreted as basement membrane thickening in the airways of patients with fatal asthma. This is now recognized as thickening of the subepithelial reticular layer (*lamina reticularis*) immediately beneath the basement membrane and may occur early in the course

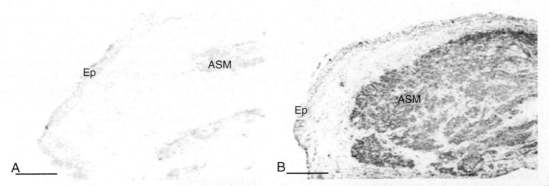

FIGURE 44-4 Airway remodeling in bronchial biopsy specimens of a control subject **(A)** and a patient with severe asthma **(B)**. Biopsy from the control subject shows normal epithelial *(Ep)* integrity and airway smooth muscle *(ASM)* area, whereas that of the asthmatic patient shows enlargement of the subepithelial basement membrane and increased ASM content. Scale bar = 200 μm. (Adapted with permission from Benayoun L, Druilhe A, Dombret M, *et al*: Airway structural alterations selectively associated with severe asthma. Am J Respir Crit Care Med 2003; 167:1360–1368.)

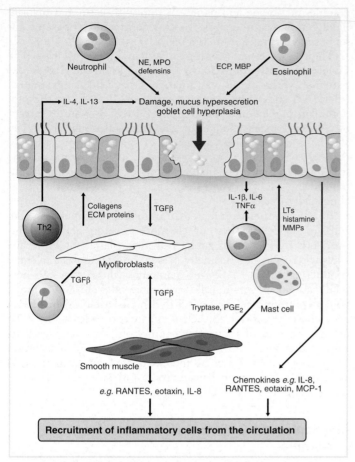

FIGURE 44-5 Inflammatory response and airway remodeling in asthma. Schematic representation showing the complex interaction between inflammatory cells and resident cells, resulting in enhanced airway inflammation and airway remodeling. The latter process is characterized by processes such as extracellular matrix (ECM) production, epithelial damage, and mucus differentiation. *ECP,* Eosinophilic cationic protein; *IL,* interleukin; *LT,* leukotriene; *MBP,* major basic protein; *MCP,* monocyte chemoattractant protein; *MMP,* matrix metalloproteinase; *MPO,* myeloperoxidase; *NE,* neutrophil elastase; *PGE₂,* prostaglandin E₂; *RANTES,* regulated on activation, normal T-cell expressed and secreted; *TGF,* transforming growth factor; *TNF,* tumor necrosis factor.

of asthma. This subepithelial fibrosis consists of abnormal amounts of type I and III collagen, fibronectin, and tenascin, probably secreted by myofibroblasts whose numbers are increased in the subepithelial region. Once thought to be a marker of severe asthma, thickening of the reticular layer has now been described in children with new asthma and in patients with nonasthmatic rhinitis and eosinophilia. Thus, the significance of this finding as a marker of either asthma severity or asthma chronicity is unclear.

Vascular Changes

Another feature of the asthmatic airway is an increase in both the number and size of blood vessels in the submucosal tissue. When these bronchial vessels dilate, as in response to mediators of allergic inflammation, they increase the density of the submucosal tissue and compress the adjacent airways.

At the same time, mediator-induced vascular permeability may lead to submucosal edema and further narrowing of the airway lumen.

Airway Smooth Muscle

Airway smooth muscle is increased in the asthmatic airway, especially in chronic severe asthma. Both hypertrophy and hyperplasia have been described. Hyperplasia seems to be more important, and studies have described a threefold increase in the number of airway smooth muscle cells in the asthmatic airway compared with controls. These cells demonstrate an exaggerated contractile response to inflammatory mediators such as histamine and cysteinyl leukotrienes, as well as to methacholine, leading to the use of methacholine bronchoprovocation as a diagnostic and quantitative measure of bronchial hyperreactivity. Airway smooth muscle cells seem to be primed to proliferate when exposed to mitogenic stimuli such as epidermal growth factor (EGF), fibroblast growth factor (FGF), mast cell proteases (tryptase), histamine, LTD₄, IL-1, and IL-11. Airway smooth muscle cells also have the capacity to synthesize a variety of substances that contribute to the inflammatory milieu of the asthmatic airway. These include eotaxin, IL-8, IL-11, RANTES, GM-CSF, and prostaglandins.

Remodeling is not just a marker of asthma progression. Thickening of the airway wall by increases in mucosal edema, blood vessel volume, subepithelial collagen, and airway smooth muscle mass changes the geometry such that a given amount of muscle shortening in a remodeled airway will increase airway resistance more than in a normal airway. Increased epithelial mucin stores lead to mucin hypersecretion during asthma exacerbations.

The Epithelial–Mesenchymal Trophic Unit

Evidence suggests that an abnormal epithelial repair process leads to remodeling. Transcription factors such as STAT1, AP-1, and NF-κB and various proinflammatory cytokines, chemokines, and growth factors (e.g., EGF, FGF, TGF-β) are upregulated in the airway epithelium and communicate to mesenchymal cells in the submucosa. As a result of this signaling, some of these mesenchymal cells are converted into myofibroblasts, with enhanced capacity to synthesize new extracellular matrix and smooth muscle mitogens. These interactions between epithelium and mesenchyme recapitulate interactions that occur during embryonic development, and, therefore, the term epithelial–mesenchymal trophic unit (EMTU) has been used to describe these phenomena. It is not known whether remodeling in asthma is due to persistence of this EMTU, or if the EMTU develops *de novo* as part of the pathophysiology of asthma.

Mucus Hypersecretion and Goblet Cell Hyperplasia

In the normal airway, ciliated cells predominate in the bronchial epithelium. Goblet cells are nonciliated, fewer in number, and line the upper and lower respiratory tract. Goblet cells are the primary source of mucus in noncartilaginous airways, whereas submucosal glands secrete mucus in the remaining cartilaginous, upper airways. Normally, mucus provides an important barrier of protection for the airway epithelium against inhaled toxins, infectious agents, and irritant particles. Mucus is a complex, dilute liquid composed of

1–2% aqueous solution of electrolytes, proteins, lipids, and carbohydrates. There is an upper gel layer and a lower aqueous sol layer in direct contact with beating cilia on the surface of epithelial cells. Inhaled particles are trapped in the gel and removed from the airway by the tips of beating cilia, a process referred to as "mucociliary clearance." Once trapped in mucus, foreign particles can also be removed forcefully by coughing. Increased production of mucus and altered viscoelastic properties of mucins, as often occurs in asthma, can contribute to mucus plugging (Figure 44-6), reduced airflow, and excessive cough.

Mucus solution contains approximately 2% high-molecular-weight mucin glycoproteins (MW 2–20×10^5 Da). Mucins are long, threadlike, highly glycosylated molecules connected end-to-end by disulfide bridges. The stiffness of these molecules confers viscoelastic properties to mucus, making it a "gel." Exocytosis of mucin from goblet cells is a multistep regulated cellular process that is an important target in understanding and controlling mucus hypersecretion in asthma. Mucins are densely packed, because the strong negative charge on mucins is shielded by Ca^{2+} ions within the granule. Exocytosis obeys first-order kinetics and is extremely rapid, taking merely tens of milliseconds once initiated. The cytoplasmic granule membrane fuses with the goblet cell apical membrane. Outflow of Ca^{2+} ions occurs by cooperative Ca^{2+}/K^+ ion exchangers on the membrane. At the same time, water uptake causes hydration of the mucin polymer network and the long, negatively charged mucins spring out of the goblet cell like a "Jack-in-the-box." The regulatory mechanisms for this process are not well understood, but it is clear that the myristoylated alanine-rich C kinase substrate (MARCKS) protein plays an integral role. Mucin secretagogues activate cell-surface receptors activating protein kinase C (PKC) and cyclic GMP–dependent protein kinase G (PKG). Activated PKC phosphorylates MARCKS, causing its translocation from the cell membrane into the cytoplasm. Simultaneously, PKG activates cytoplasmic protein phosphatase-2A (PP2A) that dephosphorylates cytoplasmic MARCKS, resulting in its attachment to the granule membrane and its interaction with actin and myosin, linking the mucin granule to the contractile apparatus for its journey to the cell membrane.

There are 18 known human mucin genes (MUCs). The molecular identity of MUCs within inspissated secretions from patients with status asthmaticus has been examined. MUC5AC and a low-charge isoform of MUC5B are the predominant mucins in asthmatic plugs. MUC2, a quite "insoluble" form typically found in the gastrointestinal tract, can also be detected at low quantities in sputum from asthmatic patients, whereas it is rarely expressed in the normal airway. It is possible that even small amounts of the relatively insoluble mucins, MUC5B and MUC2, can render asthmatic mucus abnormally thick.

In asthma, there are increased numbers of goblet cells, the cells are longer, and they contain more secretory granules. This process is referred to as goblet cell hyperplasia (GCH) in airways where they are normally present and metaplasia in small conducting airways (<2 mm diameter) where they are normally absent. Even in mild and moderate chronic asthma, goblet cell numbers can be 2.5-fold higher than normal, with an increase in stored epithelial mucin threefold higher than normal. Studies of induced sputum from asthmatic patients suggest that severe asthma involves increased mucin secretion from goblet cells, whereas increased stored mucin in mild asthma provides a mechanism for rapid airway obstruction during acute exacerbations.

Mechanism of Goblet Cell Hyperplasia in Asthma

Most of the evidence for mechanisms of goblet cell hyperplasia comes from animal models. In sensitized animals, airway allergen challenge causes marked goblet cell hyperplasia. Cytokines produced by Th2 CD4$^+$ T cells, including IL-4, IL-5, IL-9, and IL-13, seem to be responsible for this response. Increases in airway goblet cell numbers result from transdifferentiation of either the basal cells of the epithelium or a nonciliated cell type known as the Clara cell. Induction of MUC5AC in these cell types may be an early step in goblet cell differentiation.

An important regulator of this process seems to be the epidermal growth factor (EGF) cascade. The EGF receptor (EGFR) is activated by a variety of ligands, including transforming growth factor-alpha (TGF-α), heparin-binding EGF, amphiregulin, betacellulin, and epiregulin. These proteins are synthesized as transmembrane precursors and then cleaved proteolytically by metalloproteases to release mature growth factor that then binds and activates the EGFR. Of these, TGF-α seems most important. IL-13 induces expression and autocrine secretion of TGF-α by human bronchial epithelial cells. TGF-α binds directly to the EGFR, activating its cytoplasmic tyrosine kinase activity, resulting in changes in gene expression, including induction of MUC5AC and goblet cell differentiation. Not only does EGFR become activated in response to allergens and Th2 cytokines, but also to cigarette smoke, neutrophils, oxidative stress, mechanical irritation, and bacterial products. These cascades increase MUC5AC expression and drive differentiation of epithelial cells into goblet cells.

The calcium-activated chloride channel (hCLCA1) also plays a role in goblet cell hyperplasia. Induced by Th2 cytokine stimulation, overexpression of this channel in epithelial cells induces mucus cell metaplasia. Another important ion

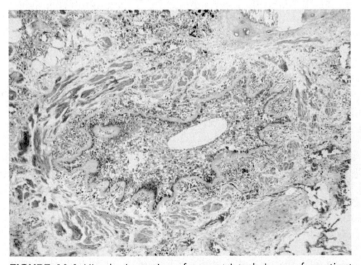

FIGURE 44-6 Histologic section of a constricted airway of a patient who died from asthma showing sloughing of the epithelium, prominent thickening of the subepithelial basement membrane, infiltration of the mucosa by inflammatory cells, and enlargement of the bronchial smooth muscle area. The airway lumen is filled with cell detritus and mucus plugs obstructing the airways.

channel is the sodium potassium chloride cotransporter (NKCC1). These different molecular pathways provide important therapeutic targets for reducing mucus hypersecretion in asthma.

Conclusions

Studies over the past 15–20 years have demonstrated convincingly that the pathophysiology of asthma involves far more than abnormal regulation of airway smooth muscle. We now know that a multitude of inflammatory cells are involved, not only in the clinical manifestations of the disease but also in its pathogenesis. Cell–cell interactions are an extremely important part of the regulatory process. The effects of some interactions are immediate (e.g., bronchoconstriction), others may set in place a path that evolves over time (e.g., Th2 cell bias); some effects are reversible, others are not. Despite these advances, gaps in our knowledge about the cell biology of asthma remain. Does the hygiene hypothesis explain pathogenesis, and if so, what is the critical time window for intervention? Is remodeling a marker of severe or poorly controlled asthma, or a phenomenon observed in a unique subset of patients, sometimes early in the disease? Are different asthma phenotypes the result of different inciting factors, or of different responses to the same stimulus? Finally, do asthma severity and asthma control relate to differences in the magnitude of the cellular responses or are the cell–cell interactions different? Understanding the cell biology of asthma is critical if we hope to develop novel therapy that is truly disease modifying.

SUGGESTED READINGS

Bradding P, Walls AF, Holgate ST: The role of the mast cell in the pathophysiology of asthma. J Allergy Clin Immunol 2006; 117:1277–1284.

Effros RM, Nagaraj H: Asthma: new developments concerning immune mechanisms, diagnosis, and therapy. Curr Opin Pulm Med 2007; 13:37–43.

Holgate ST, Holloway J, Wilson S, et al: Understanding the pathophysiology of severe asthma to generate new therapeutic opportunities. J Allergy Clin Immunol 2006; 117:496–506.

Jeffery PK, Haahtela T: Allergic rhinitis and asthma: inflammation in a one-airway condition. BMC Pulm Med 2006; 6(Suppl 1):S1–S5.

Kay A: The role of T lymphocytes in asthma. In Crameri R, ed: Allergy and asthma in modern society: A scientific approach. Basel: Karger; 2006.

Lambrecht BN, Hammad H: The other cells in asthma: Dendritic cell and epithelial cell crosstalk. Curr Opin Pulm Med 2003; 9:34–41.

Leckie MJ, ten Brinke A, Khan J, et al: Effects of an interleukin-5 blocking monoclonal antibody on eosinophils, airway hyperresponsiveness, and the late asthmatic response. Lancet 2000; 356:2144–2148.

Nadel JA: Innate immune mucin production via epithelial cell surface signaling: relationship to airway disease. Curr Opin Allergy Clin Immunol 2007; 7:57–62.

Schaub B, Lauener R, von Mutius E: The many faces of the hygiene hypothesis. J Allergy Clin Immunol 2006; 117:969–977.

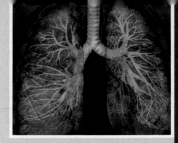
45 Asthma: Clinical Features, Diagnosis, and Treatment

MARTYN R. PARTRIDGE

Three hundred million people are estimated to have asthma worldwide. One hundred million more will develop the disease in the next two decades. The main clinical features of asthma are those of breathlessness, chest tightness, coughing, and wheezing, but these symptoms are not exclusive to asthma. Confirmatory objective diagnostic testing is not always possible and is usually not practical in the very young. Both overdiagnosis and underdiagnosis are likely to be common. Effective treatments for the condition exist, but even if correctly prescribed, they are often not taken. For most with asthma, the condition is a long-term condition, and somebody being diagnosed for the first time with asthma may live with it for 60, 70, or more years. Our approach needs to be cognizant of this fact, and the aim is to tackle asthma in partnership with the patient, recognizing that for most, self-management is the ideal.

As with most diseases, the condition results from an interaction between the host and the environment. Host factors are likely to be, in part, inherited, and we know that a family history of asthma or atopy represents an important risk factor for the development of asthma. There is, however, no simple inheritance pattern; some genes predispose to atopy and some predispose to airway hyperresponsiveness. The population's genetic constitution cannot, however, have changed over the past 20–30 years or so; whereas identification of the genes associated with asthma may be helpful in targeting future therapies, the rising prevalence must reflect environmental factors activating the inherited predisposition to asthma and other atopic diseases in more people now than previously. The rising prevalence of asthma (see Chapter 43) seems to be associated in some way with civilization, Westernization, or modern living. Studies in Zimbabwe and Ghana show increased frequencies of asthma in richer urban areas than rural areas, and in the Far East much higher rates of asthma are found in children who live in Hong Kong than among those of similar genetic constitution who live in the neighboring provinces of Southern China. Although prevalence seems to vary widely from country to country, in no country is the importance of asthma insignificant. In Pakistan, for example, 9% of school-aged children have asthma, and health services, therefore, have to tackle a rising prevalence of this and other "developed country" diseases, while still facing the burden of traditional infectious diseases.

The reasons asthma prevalence is increasing remain unclear. Maternal smoking is associated with an increased risk of the offspring developing a wheezing illness, but there are many other hypothetical causes. Higher rates of asthma occur in populations that take less magnesium and less oily fish in the diet, among those exposed to fewer infections in early life (e.g., the first born in a family), and in those who exhibit less tuberculin skin-test reactivity. Dietary factors, less breast-feeding, and a lack of early life exposure to infections may thus render a genetically susceptible individual more prone to asthma; this enhanced tendency may then be activated by other recent changes in our environment. These might include changes in our homes—in many countries more "closed," less well-ventilated housing allows increased concentrations of allergens or the exhaust gases associated with cooking. Other environmental changes may be those associated with poverty (increased exposure to cockroach allergen in poor housing), chlorine breakdown products in swimming pools, or increased traffic pollution. Recent studies have also highlighted an association between an increased risk of asthma and obesity. Whether such an association is truly causal remains uncertain. The mechanism for such an association is similarly unclear.

The major challenge is that of primary prevention of the condition—that is, to identify what activates asthma in increasing numbers of those born with a genetic susceptibility. Once identified, the hope is that suitable environmental avoidance procedures or vaccines can be used to reduce the prevalence. There is increasing evidence that there might be windows of opportunity for such primary prevention interventions; for example, exposure to domestic pets may be protective against asthma at one stage of fetal or neonatal life and have an adverse effect at a later age. Because primary prevention is not yet possible, the current aim remains restricted to that of secondary prevention—to ensure that those who have asthma benefit from current knowledge and from the treatments available. This involves well-educated health professionals working in a well-organized, adequately funded system, and offering treatment in a manner that makes that treatment likely to be taken. An overview of the scope for both primary and secondary prevention and of the basis of the clinical features of asthma is shown in Figure 45-1.

CLINICAL FEATURES

Asthma is defined in physiologic terms as "a generalized narrowing of the airways, which varies over short periods of time either spontaneously or as a result of treatment." As an airway disorder, asthma's clinical features are common to other airway disorders and may include cough, wheezing, tightness in the chest, and breathlessness, but the key feature is the variability of these symptoms and the tendency for them to be worse at night or in the early morning and to be worse after exercise (Table 45-1). The wheeze arises from vibration of

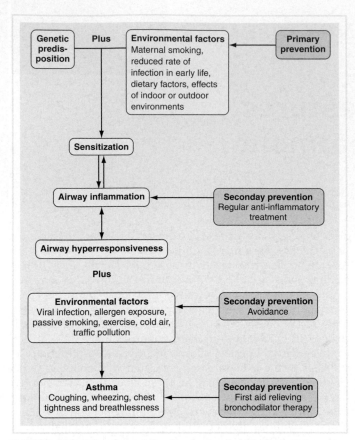

FIGURE 45-1 Overview of the factors involved in initiating asthma in those who have inherited a genetic susceptibility. The scope is shown for potential primary and secondary interventions.

the airway walls, the chest tightness and breathlessness reflect reduced airway caliber, and all of these and the cough reflect underlying airway inflammation and airway hyperresponsiveness (AHR). The factors that underlie the development of inflammation and AHR are shown in Figure 45-1. Characteristic pathologic features include the presence in the airway of inflammatory cells, plasma exudation, edema, smooth muscle hypertrophy, mucus plugging, and shedding of epithelium. Such features may be present even in those who have mild asthma, and the characteristic pathologic changes are frequently present even when no symptoms are found. Not only does the presence of these basic changes mean that clinical symptoms can develop at any time, but increasing indirect evidence also shows that the persistence of such untreated inflammatory change may lead to the airway narrowing becoming "fixed" with time. It is possible that such irreversible change may occur relatively early in the course of the disease.

Exacerbating Factors (Triggers)

The important risk factors for predisposition to asthma are detailed in Chapter 43. Several of these, and others, can also exacerbate or trigger asthma at some stage; a list is given in Table 45-2.

Infections

In children, viral infections (especially rhinoviruses, respiratory syncytial virus, and influenza virus) are some of the most common triggers of asthma, and the same most likely applies to adults. The adverse effects of such viruses are likely to be through the release from lung cells of similar chemical mediators as those that occur in asthma and through enhancement of the allergic response. Even in normal subjects, it is possible to demonstrate enhanced airway irritability for several weeks after viral infections, and it is not difficult to imagine how the addition of postviral AHR to the intrinsic AHR of asthma leads to enhanced symptoms.

Allergic Triggers

After an individual is sensitized to an allergen, subsequent reexposure is likely to worsen that individual's asthma. Common allergens are grass or tree pollen, pets, house dust, and

TABLE 45-1 Clinical Features Suggestive of Asthma*

Investigation	Outcome
Medical history	Episodic wheezing, chest tightness, shortness of breath, cough Symptoms worsen in presence of aeroallergens, irritants, or exercise Symptoms occur or worsen at night, awakening the patient Patient has allergic rhinitis or atopic dermatitis Close relations have asthma, allergy, sinusitis, or rhinitis
Physical examination	Hyperexpansion of the thorax Sounds of wheezing during normal breathing or a prolonged phase of forced exhalation Increased nasal secretions, mucosal swelling, sinusitis, rhinitis, or nasal polyps Atopic dermatitis/eczema or other signs of allergic skin problem

*Adapted from National Heart, Lung, and Blood Institute.

TABLE 45-2 Factors That May Exacerbate Asthma (Trigger Factors)

Factor	Comment
Smoking	Active and passive
Infections	Especially rhinoviruses, respiratory syncytial virus, influenza virus
Exercise	Especially on cold, dry days
Changes in the weather	Thunderstorms
Pollution	Ozone and sulfur dioxide
Allergens	Pet allergens, house dust and house dust mite, cockroach allergens, pollens
Drugs	Aspirin, nonsteroidal antiinflammatory agents, β-blockers (oral and ophthalmic)
Occupational factors	Dusty work places, "cold rooms"

mites. Exposure to only small quantities is sufficient to exacerbate the clinical condition. Although avoidance of allergens is a logical approach attractive to patient and health professional alike, it is, in reality, difficult to achieve. Cat allergen, for example, travels widely on other peoples' clothing and is found in circumstances in which cats are not found (e.g., on public transport, in hospital outpatient departments, or in a cinema). Other pet allergens include dogs and small mammals, which may be found not only in the home but also at school and in the workplace.

Indoor allergens include house dust mites and cockroaches. The former are globally distributed, but it is possible that changes in home design have enhanced exposure in some countries. House dust contains multiple organic and inorganic materials, but the most common domestic mite is the *Dermatophagoides* spp., which feed on human scales. The mites live in soft furnishings and especially thrive in warm, moist surroundings. In other environments, sensitization to cockroach allergen is more common, and lifestyle changes (e.g., increased use of central heating) have increased the number of environments in which cockroaches survive and thus enhanced the population's potential exposure to them. Molds may develop in damp housing, and this will cause asthma to deteriorate.

Air Pollution

Most people spend more than 95% of their lives indoors; therefore, the adverse effects of pollutants on the clinical features of asthma involve both indoor and outdoor pollution. Indoor pollutants include nitric oxide, nitrogen oxides, carbon monoxide, sulfur dioxide, carbon dioxide, and volatile organic compounds, which may arise from cooking, heating, or the use of insulation materials and paints. Outdoor pollutants may include visible smog or invisible agents that can damage respiratory epithelium, such as nitrogen oxides, ozone, sulfur dioxide, or particulate matter. The magnitude of the role of these agents in triggering attacks of asthma is unclear. Although they can certainly make asthma worse, the likelihood is that these triggers have significant effects only in those affected by more severe disease. However, it is possible that pollutants have an adverse synergistic effect, such that exposure to atmospheric pollution may enhance the risk of sensitization to allergens to which an individual is simultaneously exposed.

Exercise

Exercise is likely to exacerbate or provoke asthma at all ages and in all patients. How prominently exercise is quoted as a trigger depends on the intensity of the exercise and on whether the person with asthma has adjusted his or her lifestyle to avoid this trigger. Exercise-induced asthma is more likely to occur in cold, dry environments (e.g., cross-country running on frosty days) than in a heated indoor swimming pool, and this reflects its likely mechanism—water loss from the airway wall that results in increased osmolarity of surface liquid, which induces mediator release. Knowledge that exercise easily induces asthma has led to its frequent use as a diagnostic test.

Occupations

Occupational sensitizing agents may be responsible for the initiation of asthma, but certain occupational environments may also worsen the condition in those who already have it, as discussed in Chapter 66. It is essential that the possibility of occupational asthma is considered in all adults presenting for the first time with the disease and in those with unexplained worsening of their condition. Important questions to ask include whether their condition is better when away from work, on weekends, or on holidays.

Drugs

Some drugs may trigger attacks of asthma. The most severe reactions can be those with β-blocker tablets—topical β-blockers are also used in the treatment of glaucoma, and enough may be absorbed from this site to have severe or even fatal effects on airway function. Some studies have shown that just one drop of timolol to each eye may halve spirometry.

Up to 3% of those who have asthma may be aspirin sensitive, and aspirin (as well as other nonsteroidal antiinflammatory agents and possibly biphosphonates) may cause severe attacks. The patient may have previously taken aspirin with impunity, but within minutes to hours of a subsequent ingestion, fatal asthma may occur. Such adverse reactions may be more common in women than men and in those who have nasal polyps, but it can affect anyone who has asthma. However, the use of aspirin as a preventive agent in cardiac and cerebrovascular disease is increasingly recognized to be of value. Those with asthma should not, in general, be denied its use, but any suggestion of worsening of asthma after aspirin use should be taken seriously and further use avoided. Occasionally, desensitization to aspirin can be undertaken. It is important to note that aspirin sensitivity is often a marker of more severe asthma, in the same way as is fungal hypersensitivity. Typically, patients have rhinosinusitis and nasal polyps with loss of sense of smell and taste, and the severity of their asthma often necessitates long-term oral steroid therapy. In one study of more than 145 patients who had required mechanical ventilation for severe asthma, a quarter of them were subsequently shown to be aspirin sensitive. An additional problem may be cross-reactivity between aspirin sensitivity and use of parenteral hydrocortisone; aspirin-sensitive patients with asthma may have increased airway narrowing develop if given intravenous hydrocortisone for the treatment of an exacerbation of asthma. Because there is no evidence that parenteral steroids confer any advantage over steroid tablets, the use of intravenous steroids should be restricted to those who are unconscious or who may be vomiting or unable to swallow.

Premenstrual Asthma and Asthma in Pregnancy

Worsening of symptoms of asthma may occur in women in the premenstrual and menstrual phases. The peak of worsening symptoms occurs 2–3 days before menstruation begins and correlates with the late luteal phase of ovarian activity, when circulating progesterone and estrogen levels are at their lowest. Such an association may be overlooked by the patient or doctor, unless specifically questioned, and in severe cases, hospitalization has been shown to have always occurred around this time in an individual's cycle. For most patients, treatment remains of the standard type, if necessary increased in quantity, but progesterone supplementation (orally and by pessary) is necessary in a minority of patients.

Asthma may worsen, stay the same, or improve during pregnancy. The pattern may be repetitive in subsequent pregnancies. For those who experience a worsening of asthma, this is likeliest in the second and third trimester—but problems during labor are extremely unusual. Treatment for asthma should be the same during pregnancy as in the nonpregnant state, except that leukotriene antagonists should not be initiated during pregnancy. In the absence of appropriate advice, those with asthma may stop their medication on discovering they are pregnant, and it is important that pregnant women are reassured as to the safety of usual asthma therapies—both routine and those used for treatment of exacerbations. After delivery, breastfeeding should be encouraged; none of the commonly used asthma medications are secreted in breast milk to the degree that any alteration in treatment is necessary.

Associated Clinical Conditions

Several important conditions may exacerbate asthma or cause chronic deterioration to occur in association with it.

Rhinosinusitis. Asthma frequently coexists with rhinosinusitis; the latter may make asthma worse but also impair the patient's and health professional's assessment of the severity of the asthma. Allergic rhinitis often coexists not only with asthma but also with sinusitis, otitis media, and allergic conjunctivitis. The main features are of rhinorrhea, nasal obstruction, nasal itching, and sneezing. Correct diagnosis and management are essential and can lead to improvements in accompanying asthma (see Chapter 32). Nasal corticosteroids represent the most effective treatment for patients with persistent or moderate to severe rhinitis, but in those with milder or intermittent disease, antihistamines or chromones may have a role.

Churg–Strauss Syndrome. Originally described in 1951, this syndrome was characterized initially on the basis of histologic appearances that included vasculitis and extravascular granulomas occurring in patients with asthma and allergic rhinitis. Such a dependence on histologic characterization has the potential to delay diagnosis, and more recent understanding of the syndrome emphasizes the necessity for prompt diagnosis largely on the basis of clinical suspicion.

The criteria for diagnosis of Churg–Strauss syndrome (CSS) has been described as:

1. Presence of asthma
2. Peripheral blood eosinophilia (>1500 cells/mL)
3. Systemic vasculitis involving two or more extrapulmonary organs

Others have also included in their definition the presence of pulmonary infiltrates, sinus abnormalities, and demonstration of histopathologic changes. Those suggesting biopsy confirmation have done so because of a realization that rarely does CSS predate asthma or occur without marked eosinophilia. Although a biopsy of easily accessible affected tissue can be helpful, it should not delay institution of treatment (Figure 45-2). Antineutrophilic cytoplasmic antibodies are present in two thirds of cases but are not specific for CSS. The key to prompt diagnosis of CSS is to think of the condition especially when faced with an adult who is seen with allergic rhinitis, sinusitis, and worsening asthma followed by odd systemic features such as fever, rash (especially lower limb purpura), weight loss, or arthralgia. Other features include pulmonary infiltrates, peripheral neuropathy, cranial and other isolated nerve palsies, cerebrovascular incidents, abdominal pain, bloody diarrhea, and, occasionally, intestinal perforation. Renal disease occurs in a minority of patients and can be associated with hematuria, proteinuria, and hypertension. Cardiac involvement is one of the most feared and serious manifestations of CSS, with granulomatous eosinophilic infiltration of

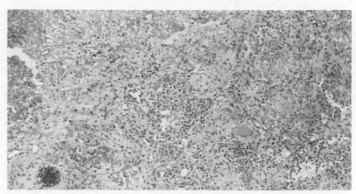

FIGURE 45-2 Histopathology of Churg–Strauss syndrome (CSS). This photomicrograph shows a combination of parenchymal necrosis and focally marked tissue eosinophilia in CSS. The inflammatory infiltrate includes a combination of eosinophils and variable numbers of epithelioid histocytes in a vaguely granulomatous appearance.

the myocardium and coronary vasculitis leading to heart failure and a risk of sudden death. These manifestations of disease may develop over a short period. In other cases, adult onset of upper airway problems is followed some time later by the onset of asthma, which later becomes severe, and, after a further variable time, systemic symptoms develop and other organs become involved. The differential diagnosis clearly depends on the manifestation of CSS occurring in that individual, but pulmonary manifestations may need differentiating from allergic bronchopulmonary aspergillosis (ABPA), other pulmonary eosinophilias, or pulmonary sarcoidosis. If and when vasculitis develops, differentiation is necessary from Wegener's granulomatosis, microscopic polyangiitis, and polyarteritis nodosa.

In the early stages of disease and with limited manifestations, the response to steroids alone may be very good. In others with more aggressive disease, additional treatment with cyclophosphamide is necessary. Prognosis reflects the degree of severity of the disease and its manifestations, with the worst outcomes being in cases in which cardiac decompensation or cerebrovascular manifestations develop.

The association of CSS with treatment of asthma by use of leukotriene antagonists has recently attracted attention. Although theoretically it is possible that any drug could induce a hypersensitivity vasculitis, the likeliest reason some have developed CSS after starting a leukotriene antagonist is that improved control of their asthma has led to a reduction in oral steroid dose and the unmasking of a previously inapparent systemic condition. In anyone with a history of difficult asthma in whom steroids are being reduced or tailed off, one should be alert to a risk of unmasking CSS, and inflammatory markers and eosinophil counts should be monitored.

Bronchopulmonary Aspergillosis. The fungus *Aspergillus* is globally distributed and found in soil and decaying leaf mold and vegetable matter. Fungal spores are dispersed by the wind, and peak levels are found during the winter. The size of the spores enhances inhalation and deposition within the lung, where body temperature is optimal for growth. The fungus can easily be found in sputum samples from those patients with a variety of lung conditions. Some patients with asthma develop hypersensitivity to *Aspergillus* on repeated exposure. These patients are likely to have other demonstrable sensitivities to common inhaled allergens such as house dust mite and pollen, but *Aspergillus* hypersensitivity may be associated with longer duration of disease and more severe disease. Other patients develop the condition known as allergic pulmonary aspergillosis, where, in addition to having asthma and *Aspergillus* hypersensitivity, they have pulmonary eosinophilia and infiltration with an intense allergic reaction in the proximal airways. This can result in bronchial occlusion, which may give rise to segmental or lobar collapse visible on the chest radiograph, predominantly in the upper lobes. Such episodes are manifest clinically as fever, worsening asthma, or chest pain. If untreated, such episodes can result in significant bronchial wall damage and the development of bronchiectasis of the proximal airways (Figure 45-3). Investigation of suspected ABPA includes the following:

1. Measurement of peripheral blood and sputum eosinophilia.
2. Demonstration of a positive immediate skin prick test to *Aspergillus fumigatus*.
3. Positive precipitins to *Aspergillus fumigatus*.
4. A raised total immunoglobulin E level.
5. Radiographic investigation; a chest radiograph may show lobar collapse and infiltrates, and CT scanning of the thorax can demonstrate bronchiectasis, which is classically worst in the proximal airways in this condition (Figure 45-4).

Although the acute syndrome associated with pulmonary infiltration is undoubtedly helped by oral corticosteroid therapy, the exact indication for long-term steroids is less clear. In most cases, it is preferable to treat episodes with courses of oral steroids and maintenance inhaled steroids between attacks. If the episodes of infiltration are frequent and severe, long-term maintenance corticosteroid therapy may be necessary. In such cases, a 4-month trial of the oral triazole antifungal agent itraconazole may decrease oral steroid requirements and improve asthma control.

Cryptogenic Eosinophilic Pneumonia. Eosinophilic pneumonia may occur as a complication of bronchopulmonary aspergillosis, as a result of the use of certain drugs (e.g.,

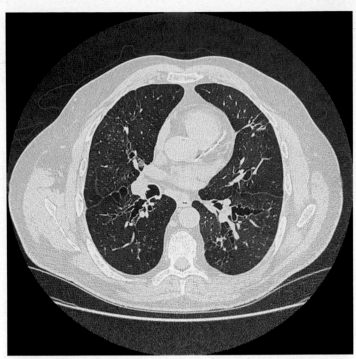

FIGURE 45-4 Computed tomography scan performed on a patient who has bronchopulmonary aspergillosis. Significant proximal airway bronchiectasis is shown.

nitrofurantoin, sulfasalazine), as a complication of parasitic infections, or represent a cryptogenic eosinophilic pneumonia (see Chapter 52). Although termed *cryptogenic*, this last condition is one that has a characteristic and consistent clinical presentation and has been recognized as a distinctive syndrome for more than 30 years. At least 50% of patients who have cryptogenic eosinophilic pneumonia already have asthma, and many develop it subsequent to the pneumonia. The characteristic presentation is of fever, breathlessness, weight loss, and profound and drenching night sweats; the chest radiograph shows a classic photographic negative of that seen in pulmonary edema, with the shadowing being mainly peripheral and most marked in the upper zones (Figure 45-5). The condition is sometimes mistaken for pulmonary tuberculosis; the important diagnostic differentiation is to measure the peripheral blood eosinophil count, especially when someone with asthma presents in this way.

Gastroesophageal Reflux. In some studies, one third of the normal population has been demonstrated to have gastroesophageal reflux at some stage. It may be more common in asthma and may make asthma worse, and some asthma therapies such as theophyllines may enhance reflux of acid into the esophagus. There is no evidence, however, that treatment of gastroesophageal reflux influences control of asthma.

DIAGNOSIS, DIFFERENTIAL DIAGNOSIS, AND ASSESSMENT OF SEVERITY

Asthma is a common disease with a high profile and awareness among both the general public and health professionals. This can lead to the potential for overdiagnosis. It is but one of many common respiratory conditions, but symptoms of

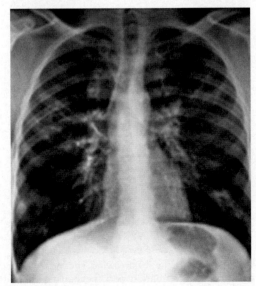

FIGURE 45-3 Allergic bronchopulmonary aspergillosis. Chest radiograph of a 21-year-old woman with asthma showing interstitial markings suggestive of bronchiectasis and patchy opacities (mucoid plugging) bilaterally.

respiratory diseases may be shared with disorders of other systems—breathlessness can be caused not only by lung disease, but also by heart disease, pulmonary vascular disease, diaphragm weakness, and systemic disorders such as anemia, obesity, or hyperthyroidism. A cough may similarly reflect an airway disorder but may also be due to diffuse parenchymal lung disease or treatment with an angiotensin-converting enzyme inhibitor. Even if one is relatively confident that a patient's symptoms reflect an airway disorder, remember that they are many in number (Table 45-3) and that airway obstruction may be localized (Figure 45-6) or generalized. Clinically, clues to the presence of a localized airway obstruction may be that the wheezing is asymmetric, monophonic rather than polyphonic, or there may be stridor emanating from the upper airways. Even when the wheezing and airway narrowing seems to be generalized, the list of differential diagnosis must be considered (see Table 45-3). Obliterative bronchiolitis is a rare cause of unexplained, generalized airway narrowing that can occur especially in women who have rheumatoid arthritis; it also occurs as a complication of rejection

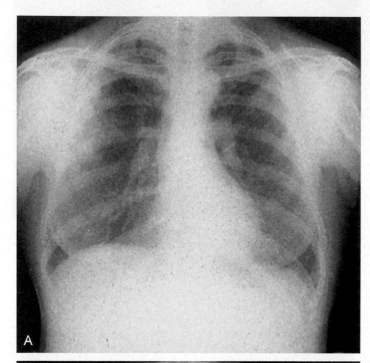

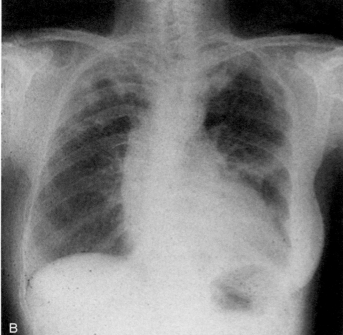

FIGURE 45-5 Chest radiographs of cryptogenic eosinophilic pneumonia. **A,** Predominantly peripheral upper zone shadowing. **B,** In this example, it is easier to see how cryptogenic eosinophilic pneumonia may be mistaken for tuberculosis unless the appropriate tests are performed.

TABLE 45-3 Differential Diagnosis of Airway Diseases in the Consideration of Asthma

Airway Diseases	
Localized	**Generalized**
Vocal cord paresis	Asthma
Laryngeal carcinoma	Chronic obstructive pulmonary
Thyroid enlargement	disease
Relapsing polychondritis	Bronchiectasis
Tracheal carcinoma	Cystic fibrosis
Bronchial carcinoma	Obliterative bronchiolitis
Bronchial carcinoid	
Post-tracheostomy stenosis	
Foreign bodies	
Bronchopulmonary dysplasia	
Obstructive sleep apnea	

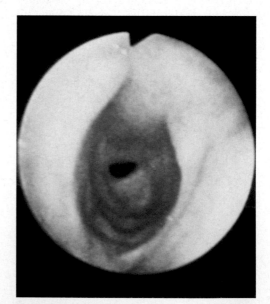

FIGURE 45-6 Severe tracheal narrowing secondary to prolonged previous endotracheal intubation and mechanical ventilation. The localized nature of this man's airway obstruction was overlooked for some time, and he was mistakenly treated for asthma by use of bronchodilators and inhaled corticosteroids.

after lung transplantation. In patients who produce large quantities of sputum, the alternate diagnosis of bronchiectasis is considered, and patients who have cystic fibrosis occasionally have late presentations and may be misdiagnosed as having asthma. After all of these diagnoses have been considered, in adults the final differentiation in many cases is that from chronic obstructive pulmonary disease (COPD), particularly because some with asthma are persistent smokers.

Differentiation of Asthma from Chronic Obstructive Pulmonary Disease

Some may argue that these conditions are a spectrum in which reversible airway obstruction occurs at one end and fixed narrowing at the other. Furthermore, many patients who have COPD exhibit some reversibility, and many who have asthma have a fixed component to the airway narrowing develop. Some of the treatments are also common to the two disorders. However, a more satisfactory approach seems to be to separate the two conditions.

The reasons for differentiation are that the cause of the two conditions is dissimilar (COPD being essentially the result of smoking), the pathologic processes can be quite different (emphysema does not occur in asthma), the natural history is different (progressive decline in airway caliber is likely in those patients who have COPD who continue to smoke), and the response to treatments is dissimilar in terms of both magnitude and type (for example, anticholinergic agents have no role in asthma other than during severe exacerbations). Taking a "prescription-oriented approach" to COPD can often cause harm (e.g., from side effects of corticosteroid therapies that have only a limited beneficial effect in COPD compared with asthma) and by deflection away from other issues that can help those who suffer COPD (e.g., correct selection of the right type of supplementary oxygen, attention to depression and social factors, and smoking cessation support). A summary of the key points of differentiation is shown in Table 45-4.

Vocal Cord Dysfunction

Vocal cord or glottic dysfunction is an important condition that can cause serious diagnostic difficulty in both adolescents and adults and, if not recognized, unnecessary overtreatment. Glottic wheezing or vocal cord dysfunction can occur within a spectrum of severity—at one extreme complicating genuinely troublesome asthma and at the other representing a conversion symptom or Münchhausen syndrome. A diagnosis of vocal cord dysfunction is made with considerable care, and in acute cases of wheezing, the diagnosis and treatment must always be regarded as that of pure asthma until that diagnosis is disproved.

Wheezing that arises from the glottis is heard throughout the lung fields when auscultation is performed with a stethoscope, but in cases of vocal cord dysfunction, the glottic origin can often be determined by removing the stethoscope from the ears and standing behind the patient and listening at neck level. The glottic origin of the noise (which often sounds more forced than usual wheezing) then becomes apparent. Direct visualization of the glottis by laryngoscopy may reveal the characteristic inspiratory apposition of the cords.

Sometimes those who have asthma make this noise because they subconsciously feel the need to impress on the doctor the severity of their condition. In other patients, the noise occurs for purely psychologic reasons, and no evidence of asthma is found. Patients may be of either gender, but are often women in the age range of 16–50 years who may have a paramedical background. Their "asthma" seems "resistant" to standard treatments and often they have been admitted to a hospital on many occasions and been treated with large doses of corticosteroids and other treatments.

TABLE 45-4 Differentiation of Asthma from Chronic Obstructive Pulmonary Disease

	COPD	Asthma
Age	Develops in 4th, 5th, and 6th decades	Often a history of childhood asthma (or wheezing in childhood, childhood bronchitis, or inability to take part in sports)
Symptoms	Shortness of breath is usually confined to exertion	Shortness of breath can occur at rest, or on exertion, and frequently awakens the patient in the early hours of the morning
Natural history	Progressive decline in exercise capacity especially if continues smoking	If treatment is adequate and instituted early in the course of the disease, normal lung function should be maintained in between attacks
Smoking history	History of current or previous smoking	May or may not be or have been a smoker
Atopic diseases	May or may not have a personal or family history of asthma, hay fever, or eczema	Likely to have a personal history of other atopic diseases, or a family history of asthma, hay fever, or eczema
Markers of inflammation		Likely to have increased exhaled NO levels, more eosinophils in blood, sputum, or airway samples than in those with COPD
Lung function	Likely to have higher residual volume and lower diffusing capacity than those with asthma, and flow volume curves may show pressure-dependent airway collapse	
Response to treatment	Limited reversibility with inhaled bronchodilators and steroids	Good reversibility with inhaled bronchodilators and steroids

Home peak-flow readings and attempts at spirometry may be variable but show little correlation with attacks or treatment. Flow-volume curves may show a characteristic "fluttering" of the inspiratory curve. Measurement of total airway resistance in a body plethysmograph may be diagnostic, because the panting maneuver necessary for such measurement abolishes the vocal cord adduction, and airway resistance can be shown to be normal. Occasionally patients end up being mechanically ventilated because of "severe" asthma, but once paralyzed, it can be seen that airway resistance is normal and there is no necessity for high inflation pressures.

Vocal cord dysfunction is probably much more common than appreciated and if underdiagnosed or mistaken for asthma, overtreatment is likely. Correct diagnosis is essential, and if vocal cord dysfunction is the sole or major part of the wheezing disorder, speech therapy can be helpful. As with other "conversion" symptoms, confrontation or challenge is best avoided, and attempts should be made to help the patient deflect stress away from the throat.

Difficult Asthma

Difficult asthma is often defined as patients with a diagnosis of asthma who remain symptomatic despite being on the top step of the asthma treatment guidelines. When assessing such patients, it is extremely important to remember that this condition is not synonymous with "treatment-resistant" asthma. Unless a protocolized approach is taken to these patients, misdiagnoses are common, and some studies have suggested that only 50% of these cases, after investigation, truly have severe asthma. A protocolized approach should involve careful reevaluation of the diagnosis, objective measurement of compliance, psychiatric or psychological assessment, and very careful review. In some series, 10% of those referred to a tertiary center turn out not to have asthma; in a higher proportion significant comorbidity is present, and it is this that accounts for the severity, and up to 30% of cases may be noncompliant to a significant degree with therapy. Misdiagnoses include everything from chronic obstructive pulmonary disease to vocal cord dysfunction, along with psychiatric comorbidity, cardiac disease, and localized airway tumors.

Investigations Used in the Diagnosis and Assessment of Asthma

The diagnosis of asthma is often far from easy, and there is no single diagnostic test, such as an elevated blood glucose estimation in diabetes. A suggestive clinical history (see Table 45-1) should lead to an attempt to make an objective corroboration of the diagnosis. Where this attempt involves prescription of a medication, it should be appreciated that such therapy represents a diagnostic trial, and the effect of the prescription should be monitored objectively. Because asthma is defined in physiologic terms, it is logical that physiologic tests are required to make the diagnosis, but other investigations may be helpful in some cases. The prime aim is to determine whether the patient fulfills the definition of "generalized airway narrowing that varies over short periods of time, either spontaneously or as a result of treatment." This definition may be fulfilled in a variety of ways, and these are summarized in Figure 45-7.

Peak Expiratory Flow Rate

In most cases, the diagnostic definition of asthma may be fulfilled by measurement of peak expiratory flow rate (PEFR) on more than one occasion in the clinic or surgery by use of a meter for recording two to three times daily at home, or, in cases of occupational asthma, at work (see Figure 45-7). Variability may be quantified and asthma diagnosed when there is greater than 20% diurnal variation on 3 or more days in a week for 2 weeks on a peak flow diary. Amplitude of peak flow variability is calculated as: highest PEFR − lowest PEFR/ highest PEFR × 100%. For example, $(500 - 400/500 \times 100 = 20\%$ PEF variability).

Spirometry

Although less generally available, spirometry is used as the standard measurement of dynamic airflow to detect the presence of airway obstruction and to test for reversibility of flow. Airflow obstruction is established if the forced expiratory volume in 1 second (FEV_1) is less than 80% predicted, or the ratio of FEV_1 to forced vital capacity is less than 75% or below the lower limit of normal. If evidence of airway narrowing is detected, response to a bronchodilator must be established, and if positive (greater than 15% response), a diagnosis of asthma is made. In other cases, little spontaneous variation of peak flow may occur over the period of observation, and the response to inhaled bronchodilators may be slight; in these cases, differentiation from COPD, for example, is difficult unless a trial of corticosteroid tablets (see Figure 45-7) is given. In some cases, a prolonged course of high-dose, inhaled corticosteroids (ICSs) can be used as an alternative test of corticosteroid responsiveness.

If peak expiratory flow rate and/or spirometry are normal at a time when patients are having symptoms, this suggests the need to consider an alternative diagnosis (Table 45-5). In other cases, when the patient is well when seen and has normal peak flow and spirometry, serial measurements are indicated, either by home peak flow monitoring or by spirometry performed on several occasions. An alternative is to establish whether the airway narrowing can be induced. In some suspected cases of occupational asthma, disease may be induced by careful exposure to small quantities of the probable incriminating agent (i.e., challenge testing). This should only be undertaken by those with appropriate specialist expertise, but more commonly an attempt can be made to induce airway narrowing by exercise. This is applicable to both adults and children old enough to perform forced expiratory maneuvers. It is best carried out by asking the patient suspected of having asthma to make some baseline peak flow readings and then to undertake 6 min of free running (see Figure 45-7).

Any postexercise fall in peak flow is abnormal, but a fall of greater than 15% is regarded as diagnostic of asthma. Peak flow readings are made at 2-min intervals for up to 20 min after exercise, and, if significant asthma is induced, bronchodilators are given. False-positive tests do not occur, but a false-negative result can happen; therefore, a negative exercise test does not exclude the possibility of asthma at other times.

Other Lung Function Tests

Detailed lung function may help in the differentiation of other conditions from asthma. The expiratory flow-volume curve is

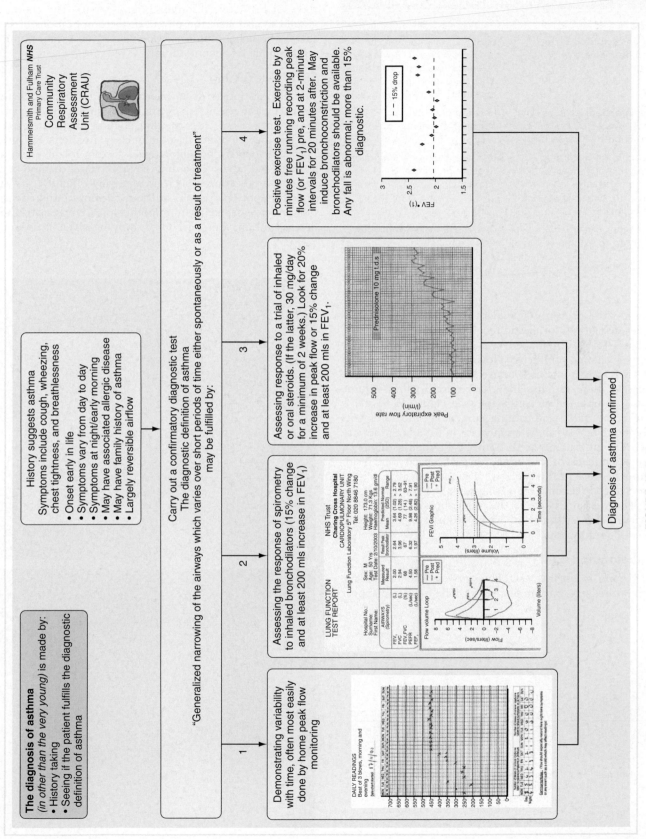

FIGURE 45-7 The diagnosis of asthma.

TABLE 45-5 Additional Tests for Suspected Asthma if the Diagnosis Is Uncertain

Reason	Test
Patient has symptoms, but spirometry is normal or near normal	Assess diurnal variation of peak flow over 1–2 weeks Consider bronchoprovocation with methacholine, histamine, or exercise
Suspect infection, large airway lesions, heart disease, or obstruction by foreign body	Chest radiograph and consider bronchoscopy
Suspect coexisting chronic obstructive pulmonary disease, restrictive defect, or central airway obstruction	Additional pulmonary function tests (e.g., diffusing capacity)
Suspect other factors that contribute to asthma	Allergy tests—skin or in vitro Nasal examination Gastroesophageal reflux assessment

useful to identify pressure-dependent reduction in expiratory flows—because of loss of elastic recoil forces seen in emphysema (Figure 45-8). The maneuver is also excellent for identifying upper airway problems. However, if the differential diagnosis is from chronic obstructive bronchitis (i.e., pure airway disease, with no emphysema), the expiratory flow-volume curve has a volume-dependent shape (see Figure 45-8) and is similar in both COPD and asthma. In general, measurements of lung volume tend to show an increase in total lung capacity with COPD, but patients with both COPD and asthma can show increased levels of functional residual capacity and residual volume because of the excessive gas trapping after expiration, the values in asthma increasing with the severity of the disease. The measurement of the single-breath gas transfer factor is normal in asthma but can be reduced in COPD and is reduced in emphysema.

Chest Radiograph

The radiograph in asthma can show airway wall thickening, best seen in the larger proximal airways. The lungs can appear

larger than normal because of gas trapping, with flattened diaphragms and horizontal ribs—they appear quite distinct from those of restrictive disorders (Figure 45-9). The chest radiograph can also alert the physician to complications of asthma such as bronchopulmonary aspergillosis, infection, pulmonary eosinophilia, or pneumothorax.

Skin Prick Testing

The demonstration of an allergic state by skin prick testing (or by measurement of specific immunoglobulin E) can help in the diagnosis by characterizing an individual as being atopic, and this may be useful in some unclear situations. Such testing may also identify possible trigger factors for an individual's asthma, and advice regarding environmental manipulation or avoidance procedures, such as removing a family cat, should probably not be given without demonstrating sensitization. Allergen-specific immunotherapy (hyposensitization or desensitization) can, of course, only be given if appropriate

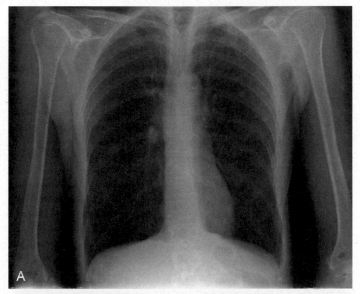

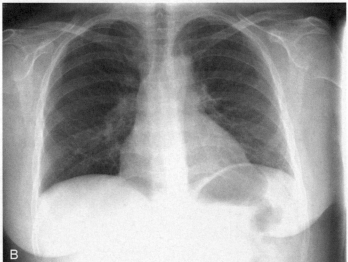

FIGURE 45-9 Comparative lung sizes on chest radiograph. **A,** Radiograph of a man who has hyperinflation secondary to severe airway narrowing. **B,** The small lungs (restrictive disorder) often seen in the very obese.

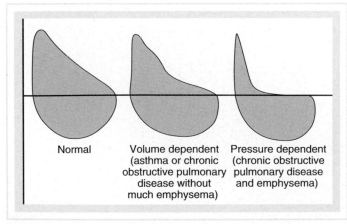

Normal

Volume dependent (asthma or chronic obstructive pulmonary disease without much emphysema)

Pressure dependent (chronic obstructive pulmonary disease and emphysema)

FIGURE 45-8 Flow-volume curves in some common diseases and their (limited) use in differentiating asthma from some other conditions.

allergens—mites, pollen, animal dander, or molds—have been identified.

Measurement of Airway Hyperresponsiveness

Measurement of airway hyperresponsiveness is a state in which there is an abnormal increase in airflow obstruction after exposure to a stimulus. Stimuli may be directly acting agents such as histamine, cholinergic agonists, leukotrienes, or prostaglandins, or act indirectly such as exercise, fog, metabisulfate, or cold air hyperventilation. Airway hyperresponsiveness is a cardinal feature of asthma, but it is not specific to it. It may also occur in a general population or in those with COPD, but failure to demonstrate airway hyperresponsiveness in someone with untreated suspected asthma should lead to reconsideration of the diagnosis. It is usually measured by use of histamine or methacholine. FEV_1 is initially measured and then remeasured after administration of saline to obtain a baseline value. Increasing doses of a constricting agent such as histamine or methacholine are then administered and FEV_1 measured after each increase in dose, and the test is stopped once a 20% fall in FEV_1 has been achieved. The result is expressed as the provocative dose or concentration that produces a 20% fall in FEV_1. In those with asthma, measurement reflects the degree of sensitivity of the airways and can reflect severity.

Sputum Examination and Measurement of Exhaled Nitric Oxide and Noninvasive Markers of Inflammation

The understanding that asthma is a chronic inflammatory disorder has developed over the past two decades, largely as a result of bronchial mucosal biopsy samples being taken from small numbers of individuals both when well and when troubled by asthma. Subsequently, other methods of assessing the degree of inflammation in the airways have been developed or refined and are now beginning to find a place in both the diagnosis and in the assessment of severity and, more recently, as a tool against which treatment may be titrated. These newer tools include assessment of airway inflammation by measurement of exhaled nitric oxide and by estimation of inflammatory cells in induced sputum samples. Correlation of these markers with measured airway hyperresponsiveness may occur in the untreated state but not necessarily in the treated state. Their exact role in the diagnosis and management of asthma remains unclear.

Nitric oxide is the most extensively studied exhaled marker of inflammation. Nitric oxide is made within bronchial epithelial cells by the action of nitric oxide synthase or L-arginine. An inducible isoform can be expressed in the presence of inflammation, leading to production of larger quantities of exhaled nitric oxide.

Exhaled nitric oxide may be elevated in a variety of lung diseases, but especially in asthma. An elevated level, therefore, is not specific for asthma, but it may be useful, for example, in determining the cause of a cough when an elevated level might suggest asthma as the cause, and it might be useful to monitor the course of disease and response to therapy. Nitric oxide may not necessarily correlate with other external markers of inflammation, and each marker may reflect the site of inflammation as well as type of inflammation present within the airway. Changes in sputum eosinophil counts may be a good marker of airway inflammation, and rises may predict imminent loss of asthma control. Treatment is currently adjusted according to symptoms or measurements that reflect airway caliber, and the relationship of these to the basic degree of inflammation present in the airways is tenuous. Recent work by use of sputum eosinophil counts to direct the dosing of inhaled steroid therapy has shown promise in terms of reduced asthma exacerbations and better asthma control without any overall greater use of therapy.

Grading of Severity of Asthma

The diagnosis of asthma is made by hearing a cough, wheeze, or breathlessness that is worse at night or in the early morning, and by demonstrating evidence of a reduced peak flow or obstructive spirometry that varies with time or after treatment. The same parameters may be used to assess severity, poor control, and the need for more treatment. These symptoms may be paralleled by peak-flow recordings that show severe morning "dips" (see Figure 45-7). The normal (or predicted normal) peak-flow rate depends on an individual's age, gender, and height; it is, therefore, important to relate assessment of severity to the predicted value (or to relate it to that individual's previous best reading when known). Advice for management in accident and emergency departments, for example, can then be made on the basis of relating an individual peak-flow rate to predicted values, so that a peak flow, for instance, greater than 75% of predicted is regarded as reflecting mild asthma, 50–75% as moderate, 33–50% severe, and less than 33% as life threatening. In anyone who has asthma, the presence of fatigue, exhaustion, or cyanosis represents critical severity. Measurements of oxygen saturation and blood gas partial pressures, although of no value in the routine management of asthma, are of greater importance in the management of acute severe asthma (see the following section). Several other classifications of asthma severity are available, most of which are based on PEFR or FEV_1 values plus symptoms. The Global Initiative for Asthma Classification of Asthma Severity by Clinical Features before treatment is shown in Box 45-1. How well the features of asthma are controlled can similarly be defined as uncontrolled, partly controlled, or fully controlled. These levels of asthma control are summarized in Table 45-6. One problem in assessing the control of an individual's asthma is that the doctor/patient interaction occurs only at one point in time. All too often a patient's recall of his or her condition expressed as "I am fine" does not reflect the true situation over the preceding days or weeks. This may lead to an underestimation of the severity of an individual's asthma and persisting unnecessary morbidity that, if detected, could have led to a change in therapy and better asthma control. This is why the British Guidelines on Asthma Management have adopted the recommendation of the Royal College of Physicians of London and suggested that at every consultation with a person with asthma, the following questions should be asked and the answers recorded in the notes.

Three questions to be asked at every consultation: In the last week or month,

1. Have you had any difficulty sleeping because of your asthma symptoms (including cough)?
2. Have you had your usual asthma symptoms during the day (cough, wheeze, chest tightness, or breathlessness)?
3. Has your asthma interfered with your usual activities (e.g., housework, work/school)?

Intermittent

Symptoms less than once a week
Brief exacerbations
Nocturnal symptoms not more than twice a month
- FEV_1 or PEV $\geq$80% predicted
- PEF or FEV_1 variability <20%

Mild Persistent

Symptoms more than once a week but less than once a day
Exacerbations may affect activity and sleep
Nocturnal symptoms more than twice a month
- FEV_1 or PEV $\geq$80% predicted
- PEF or FEV_1 variability <20–30%

Moderate Persistent

Symptoms daily
Exacerbations may affect activity and sleep
Nocturnal symptoms more than once a week
Daily use of inhaled short-acting β_2-agonist
- FEV_1 or PEV 60–80% predicted
- PEF or FEV_1 variability >30%

Severe Persistent

Symptoms daily
Frequent exacerbations
Frequent nocturnal asthma symptoms
Limitation of physical activities
- FEV_1 or PEV $\geq$60% predicted
- PEF or FEV_1 variability >30%

*Adapted from the Global Initiative for Asthma Guidelines (2006).

MANAGEMENT AND TREATMENT

In this section, drug treatments for asthma, environmental manipulations, immunotherapy, and complementary therapies are considered, with a brief description of the common inhalational devices available for use.

Other aspects of management, which include education and self-management, are considered in the section on prevention and organization of care.

The medicines available for the routine management of asthma are best divided into:

- Those taken to relieve symptoms when they occur
- Those that need to be taken regularly

In the future, this classification may require simplification. One type of combination inhaler, which contains an inhaled corticosteroid and a long-acting inhaled β-agonist, is taken regularly, but because the long-acting inhaled β-agonist that it contains also has a rapid onset, it has been approved in many countries for use both as regular maintenance therapy and a reliever.

The pharmacology of these interventions has been extensively reviewed in Chapters 36 and 37, and only clinical aspects are discussed here.

Inhaler devices may include:

- Pressurized metered-dose inhalers (pMDI)
- pMDIs plus a spacer device
- Breath-activated MDIs
- Breath-activated dry powder devices
- Nebulizers

Aerosols

Some knowledge of the properties of aerosols will aid in the understanding of their use. The size of aerosol particles and their distribution are expressed as if the aerosol were composed of a suspension of spheres with different diameters. The mass median diameter of the aerosol is the diameter about which 50% of the total particle mass resides. The mass median aerodynamic diameter (MMAD) is the product of the mass median diameter and the square root of the particle density. The MMAD of an aerosol has a profound effect on where most particles entering the lung will land and thereby act. Particle deposition is influenced by inspiratory flow—the higher the entry flow, the more central will be the deposition—because of inertial impaction, particularly of large particles (>6 mm). Smaller particles (<5 mm) will reach smaller airways and those of 2- to 3-mm size reach the alveoli. Small particles may not settle and will be expired. The relationship of site of deposition and particle size is shown in Figure 45-10. Deposition is also greatly affected by turbulent flow, and the deposition at airway bifurcations can be up to 100 times more than elsewhere. In general, inertial impaction of aerosols occurs with large particles in large airways where flow is high (i.e., nose, pharynx, larynx, trachea, and carina). Deposition is enhanced by turbulent flow that predominates in these central passages. Gravitational sedimentation is time dependent and affects the small particles. These settle in small

TABLE 45-6 Levels of Asthma Control*

Characteristic	Controlled (All of the following)	Partly Controlled (Any measure present in any week)	Uncontrolled
Daytime symptoms	None (twice or less/week)	More than twice/week	Three or more features of partly controlled asthma present in any week
Limitations of activities	None	Any	
Nocturnal symptoms/awakening	None	Any	
Need for reliever/rescue treatment	None (twice or less/week)	More than twice/week	
Lung function (PEF or FEV_1)[†]	Normal	<80% predicted or personal best (if known)	
Exacerbations	None	One or more/year[‡]	One in any week[§]

*Adapted from the Global Initiative for Asthma Guidelines (2006).
[†]Lung function is not a reliable test for children 5 years and younger.
[‡]Any exacerbation should prompt review of maintenance treatment to ensure that it is adequate.
[§]By definition, an exacerbation in any week makes that an uncontrolled asthma week.

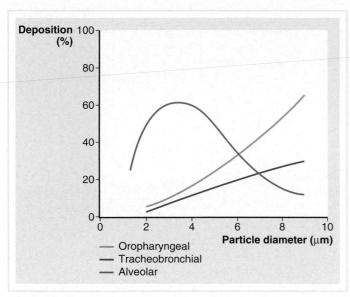

FIGURE 45-10 Relationship between percentage deposition in the respiratory tract and the diameter of the aerosol particles.

airways, provided time is sufficient (i.e., slow breathing or breath-holding). The combination of small particles, low flow, and short distances favors sedimentation. Thus, the mode of inhalation and type of breathing influences deposition. Fast inhalation enhances central inertial impaction and slow inhalation with breath-holding favors peripheral sedimentation.

Aerosol Production, Delivery, and Efficacy

Pressurized Metered-Dose Inhalers. The pMDI has been widely used in clinical practice since the early 1960s. It is composed of a canister and a plastic actuator. The drug is contained in the small canister either dissolved or suspended as crystals in a liquid propellant mixture. To prevent aggregation of the small particles, a low concentration of a surfactant is included to act as a lubricant. The aerosol released from the pMDI consists of large droplets of propellant enclosing the drug particles. The propellants boil off as soon as they leave the canister, and this breaks the liquid stream up into droplets that continue to evaporate as they move away at an initial velocity of 30 m/sec. Because of the high velocity of the drug particles, the effects of the evaporating propellants and the hygroscopicity of the drug itself, together with the curved anatomy of the upper respiratory tract, means that most of the drug impacts in the oropharynx and less than 25% of the released dose reaches the lungs. However, it is important to note that, because different drugs have different characteristics of hygroscopicity and electrostatic charge, although a pMDI will reproducibly emit a constant dose of a drug, it cannot be assumed that the same quantity of every drug administered by this system will reach the lungs. The same is true for the dry powder system. Under the international agreement known as the Montreal Protocol, ozone-depleting substances such as chlorofluorocarbons are to be banned, reformulation of most CFC-containing pMDIs is now well advanced with non-CFC propellants (hydrofluoroalkane; HFA). Some HFA formulations use ethanol to make the drug soluble rather than a

suspension stabilized by surfactants. Furthermore, the mean particle size (i.e., MMAD) of some of the newer non-CFC-containing pMDIs is approximately 2 mm compared with 3–4 mm for the CFC aerosols, making it likely that more drug may be delivered peripherally, with not as much to the bronchial tree. (Clinical aspects of the transition to non-CFC pMDIs are discussed on page 593.)

Use and Compliance. The most efficient way to use a pMDI is:

1. Shake the canister thoroughly and remove the cap.
2. Place mouthpiece of the actuator between the lips.
3. Breathe out steadily, taking care not to actuate the canister during exhalation.
4. Release the dose while taking a slow deep breath in.
5. Hold in the breath and count to 10.
6. Wait 1 min before repeating.

These instructions, although simple, are followed incorrectly in some way or another by most prescribed this device. There are pros and cons for the use of pMDIs (Table 45-7).

Large Volume Spacers. Increasing the distance from the actuator to the mouth allows the particles to evaporate and slow down before inhalation. The spacer device allows large particles of drug to impact on the surfaces of the chamber, minimizing oropharyngeal deposition and increasing the respirable fraction, nearly doubling drug deposition below the larynx. The large volume spacers also decrease the incidence of oropharyngeal candidiasis that occurs with pMDIs containing corticosteroids. The spacer causes little inconvenience when used twice daily with ICSs and long-acting bronchodilator devices. It would be less convenient for bronchodilator therapy taken on an as-required basis. The spacers are particularly useful in treating young children and are an alternative to nebulizers in chronic and severe acute asthma.

Tube spacers—tubelike attachments to the pMDI—with a much smaller internal volume than the large-volume spacers are also available to permit slowing down of the aerosol before reaching the mouth.

TABLE 45-7 The Pros and Cons of Using a Pressurized Metered Dose-Inhaler

Pros	Cons
Small doses	Difficult (young, elderly, arthritic)
Topically very active	Education needed
Stores up to 200 doses	Poor compliance
Easy to use	Hard-to-monitor compliance
Minimal side effects	Dose and deposition uncertain
Portable	Less effective with increased airway obstruction
Unobtrusive	Requires high inspiratory flow or deep breath
	Wide variation in particle size
	Oropharyngeal impaction
	Cough in up to 30% of users
	Can be difficult to know when cannister is empty

Attempts have been made to facilitate the use of the pMDI by making it breath actuated, because the most common problem is coordination of inspiration with the dose actuation. When primed, the valve is actuated by an inspiratory flow of above 30 L/min and is easier to use than the conventional pMDI. A further problem is the canister is enclosed within the device, making "shaking" useless for guessing the amount of drug remaining—a potential hazard when the patient needs "rescue" medication.

Drug Powder Inhalers

The drug powder inhaler (DPI) systems depend entirely on the patient's inspiratory effort and are generally easier to use than the pMDIs. They inherently require faster inspiratory flows to disimpact the powder and allow the inhaled fraction to be less than 5 μm. They now come as reservoir inhalers containing multiple doses, usually designed for use through 1 month.

Reservoir Drug Powder Inhalers

These devices are breath-actuated by breathing in as fast and as deeply as possible. Patients are sometimes disconcerted that, because only micronized drug is released, the dose is so tiny that they feel nothing. The two common devices are the Turbuhaler, which is a 50- to 200-dose DPI, and the Accuhaler or Diskus, which contains a ribbon of blisters containing micronized drug and lactose. It contains up to 120 doses, with a counter visible; the drug is released by pressing a "trigger" to puncture the blister and then inspiring deeply from the mouthpiece.

Nebulizers

There are two types of nebulizers: jet and ultrasonic. The latter produces quite large particles (3–10 mm) from high-frequency (1–2 MHz) sound waves induced by the vibration of a piezo-electric crystal, which, when focused on the surface of a liquid, creates a fountain of droplets. The mean particle size is inversely proportional to the frequency of the ultrasonic vibrations of the crystal. It has less clinical use than the jet nebulizer.

The jet nebulizer achieves its particulate mist from a stream of compressed air or oxygen that draws up the liquid drug through a capillary by the Venturi effect and then atomizes it into tiny fragments. More than 99% of these initial droplets are large particles that impinge on suitable baffles and drop back into the reservoir for further nebulization, leaving just small particles in the aerosol leaving the nebulizer. Approximately 1 mL of the original drug solution (usually 2 mL) is left on the baffles after completion of nebulization and constitutes dead volume that cannot be used. This inefficient characteristic can be improved by increasing the fill to 4–6 mL, but the period of nebulization is then considerably prolonged.

DEPOSITION AND EFFICACY

All three systems (pMDI, DPI, and jet nebulizer) are relatively inefficient, with only approximately 8–15% of the drug reaching the lung (Figure 45-11). The nebulizer system is also extremely wasteful, because the stream of aerosol mist is continuous, causing wastage during expiration, which in airway obstruction is often two thirds of the respiratory cycle. In general, therefore, nebulizers are, dose for dose, no more efficient

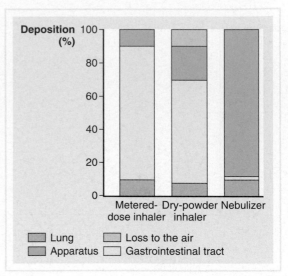

FIGURE 45-11 Deposition of aerosol delivered by pressurized metered-dose inhaler, dry-powder inhaler, and a nebulizer to different sites. (Adapted from Zainuddin *et al*, with permission of BMJ Publishing Group.)

than the pMDI or DPI systems. Studies comparing the clinical effect of bronchodilators administered by a nebulizer compared with multiple actuations from a pMDI through a spacer device show that nebulizer use may in children induce more tachycardia and prolong the duration of stay in an emergency department, and similarly in adults the nebulized route has been shown to have no advantage in those with moderate to severe episodes of worsening asthma. Comparable studies have not yet been performed in a randomized manner in those with life-threatening disease.

Medicines Taken to Relieve Symptoms ("Relievers" or "Rescue Medications")

Medicines taken to relieve symptoms are of two main types: β_2-agonists and anticholinergic agents. The former are the most important and most widely used.

β_2-Agonists

β_2-Agonists are advances on epinephrine (adrenaline) and iso-proterenol (isoprenaline), and the two most commonly used are albuterol (salbutamol) and terbutaline. Classified as having β_2-selectivity, all members of these classes have the potential to be beneficial bronchodilators but may also cause cardiac effects (tachycardia, increased cardiac output, peripheral vaso-dilatation, and arrhythmia) and systemic effects (hypokalemia, hyperglycemia, tremor, uterine relaxation). Such effects are dose-related and related to the method of administration—inhaled, ingested, or parenteral (subcutaneous, intramuscular, or intravenous). For routine use, these drugs are always recommended to be administered by the inhaled route wherever possible, so that high concentrations reach the airways where needed, and systemic side effects are minimized or avoided. The onset of action is also quicker by the inhaled route than that of tablet administration. Short-acting β-agonist relief inhalers are used only to relieve symptoms; the need for such medication on a regular basis reflects poorly controlled asthma and the need for more regular preventive therapy of different types. Increased use of these medicines thus indicates to the physician that a change in routine medication is needed, but is also a guide to the patient that change is needed; this advice is best given within the context of a written personal asthma action plan.

In acute attacks of severe asthma, the dose of albuterol (salbutamol) or terbutaline may be increased and administered either from the routine inhaler, from the routine inhaler plus a large volume-spacer device, or by nebulization. There is no evidence that nebulization has any advantage over the standard inhaler plus spacer device. Persistent use of nebulizers within secondary care probably reflects a perception that it is quicker for a nurse or therapist to start a patient on a nebulizer than to supervise multiple actuations from an inhaler through a spacer. However, availability of nebulization in hospitals may encourage patients to bypass primary care or to wrongly assume that self-treatment at home according to a written personal asthma action plan may lead to them omitting a useful medication.

With all inhaled medications, it is important that the cheapest, most effective device (or combination of devices) with which the patient is comfortable is used and that instructions as to correct use of the inhaler are reinforced frequently.

Anticholinergic Agents

The most common of these agents (whether called anticholinergic or antimuscarinic agents) is the short-acting ipratropium bromide, but there is now available tiotropium that needs only to be taken once daily. Anticholinergic agents are less effective in asthma than β-agonists, having a slower onset of action. The addition of ipratropium in high doses to β-agonists is, however, synergistic in the initial management of acute severe asthma.

Regular (Preventive) Therapies

Regular preventive therapy for asthma involves the use of either specific antiinflammatory agents (ICSs, cromones, and leukotriene modifiers) or regular bronchodilators (oral and inhaled long-acting β-agonists, and theophyllines).

Inhaled Corticosteroids. The exact mechanism of action of ICSs remains unclear (see Chapter 37), but they are potent antiinflammatory agents that interfere with arachidonic acid metabolism and synthesis of leukotrienes and prostaglandins and inhibit cytokine production and secretion. This results in less inflammatory cell infiltration, reduced vascular leakage and permeability, and increased responsiveness of airway smooth muscle β-receptors. Their use increases lung function; reduces AHR, symptoms, frequency of attacks of asthma, and the need for courses of corticosteroid tablets; and improves quality of life. Serial bronchial mucosal biopsy samples show that they also reduce markers of airway inflammation. Commonly used ICSs include beclomethasone, budesonide, flunisolide, triamcinolone, fluticasone, mometasone, and ciclesonide and all are available in the inhaled form from a similar range of inhaler devices as for the inhaled β-agonists. Flunisolide and triamcinolone are little used outside the United States.

Differences between the various formulations of ICSs in terms of efficacy, absorption, metabolism, and side effect profile are frequently claimed. Although such differences may be demonstrated according to the particular parameter or outcome studied, it seems unlikely that, for most patients who have asthma, there is much difference between the drugs. The exceptions are that inhaled fluticasone is as effective as beclomethasone and budesonide at half the dose when given

by equipotent delivery systems, and there is a suggestion that ciclesonide has a preferable risk/benefit profile. Fluticasone should be given at half the dose recommended for beclomethasone and budesonide. Also, budesonide given by a Turbuhaler device delivers approximately twice as much ICS to the lung, and doses should probably be halved when this device is used. One manufacturer's reformulation of beclomethasone with a non-CFC propellant is also claimed to enhance pulmonary deposition of the inhaled steroid, necessitating a similar halving of dosage.

Intervention with inhaled steroids early in the course of the disease probably improves the chances of maintaining good lung function. In one seminal study, in adults who had mild asthma and who had been treated for 2 years with either ICSs or an inhaled β-agonist, significant reduction in the need for rescue bronchodilation occurred. The β-agonist–treated group was then given ICSs and the former either a lower dose of ICSs or placebo. Placebo was ineffective, but low-dose ICSs were moderately effective at maintaining bronchial responsiveness at the level achieved with the previous higher-dose ICS. In the group that had previously received bronchodilators alone, a significant improvement occurred in spirometry and peak flow, but to a lesser degree than in those who had been treated with ICSs from the beginning of the study.

Cromoglycate and Nedocromil. These two medicines represent alternative antiinflammatory agents. Both are taken by the inhaled route—the former needs a four times daily medication regimen, the latter twice daily. The mechanism of action is unclear, but the medications inhibit activation of, and mediator release from, several types of inflammatory cells and may inhibit neuronal pathways. Both preparations reduce symptoms and improve lung function in those who have asthma, but their effectiveness is usually much less than that of ICSs and their role in adults is extremely limited. In children who have mild asthma, although less effective than ICSs, these medications remain an alternate antiinflammatory treatment.

Leukotriene Modifying Agents. Leukotrienes are inflammatory mediators that play a significant role in the causation of asthma. They are formed from arachidonic acid in the cell membrane by the action of an enzyme called 5-lipoxygenase. Leukotrienes that contain a cysteinyl molecule (cysteinyl leukotrienes) cause constriction of smooth muscle in the airway wall; swelling, edema, and leakage from blood vessels in the airway walls; mucus gland stimulation; and secretion of mucus. They also attract eosinophils into the airways.

Leukotriene modifiers work either by inhibiting 5-lipoxygenase (e.g., zileuton) or by acting as a leukotriene receptor antagonist (e.g., zafirlukast, montelukast). Leukotriene modifiers represent a medication worth trying in people whose asthma remains troublesome despite the use of ICSs and long-acting inhaled bronchodilators and also as an alternative to low doses of inhaled steroids for a minority of people.

Regular Bronchodilators

Regular bronchodilators include oral and inhaled longer-acting β-agonists and theophyllines.

Theophyllines. Theophyllines have been available for many years and have bronchodilator effects and may have mild antiinflammatory effects also. They can improve lung function and reduce symptoms, and when given in addition to antiinflammatory agents in slow-release form, they may help cases of persistent nocturnal asthma. However, at bronchodilator levels, side effects such as nausea and vomiting (and less likely seizure and tachycardia) are frequent occurrences in up to 50% of users. Recent studies suggest that levels of theophylline, traditionally thought to be below those needed to achieve bronchodilation, may increase asthma control when added to low-dose ICSs. This suggests that at these low doses theophylline may have some other nonbronchodilator antiinflammatory effect. Two such studies show that for patients who are poorly controlled on low-dose ICSs, the addition of low doses of theophyllines may prove as effective as the alternative strategy of the use of high doses of ICSs.

Long-Acting β-Agonists. Long-acting β-agonists include oral products such as slow-release albuterol or bambuterol or inhaled long-acting β-agonists such as salmeterol or formoterol. They have no antiinflammatory action and must not be used alone to treat asthma. Two high-dose ICSs versus low-dose ICSs plus salmeterol studies in adults showed that not only do both options work, but also that the salmeterol-containing option was slightly better in terms of both lung function and reduction in symptoms.

Formoterol, another long-acting, inhaled β-agonist with a similar duration of action to salmeterol, but a quicker onset of action, has also been shown to reduce symptoms and improve lung function when added to modest doses of ICSs. Whether in children or adults, inhaled, long-acting β-agonists are useful when taken with low-dose inhaled steroids as an alternative to high-dose inhaled steroids but also as an adjunct to high-dose ICSs when treatment with these alone is not sufficient.

Corticosteroid Tablets. Corticosteroid tablets may be lifesaving in the treatment of acute attacks of asthma. For a very tiny proportion of patients, corticosteroid tablets are needed in the long term to control the condition. In short courses, the side effects are usually negligible (indigestion, weight gain), but in the longer term they may typically cause osteoporosis, hypertension, skin thinning, muscle weakness, obesity, cataracts, and hypothalamic-pituitary-adrenal axis suppression. Maximal use of ICSs and other therapies should reduce the need for corticosteroid tablets, but, when essential, the dose must always be kept as low as possible and must be taken first thing in the morning to minimize adrenocortical suppression and sleep disturbance. In those patients being started on regular oral steroids and in those taking frequent courses of steroid tablets, consideration of bone protection is important. Use of systemic steroids is associated with a significantly increased risk of hip and vertebral fracture. The higher the dose, the higher the risk, but the risk is significant even at daily doses of 7.5 mg of prednisolone. Loss of bone mineral density occurs maximally soon after starting steroid tablets, and steroid-induced osteoporosis is more prone to be associated with bone fracture than age-related, postmenopausal osteoporosis. Measurement of bone mineral density should, therefore, be undertaken when starting most patients with asthma on regular oral steroid therapy, and good nutrition, adequate dietary calcium intake, and physical activity should be encouraged. Tobacco use and excess alcohol should be avoided. In the elderly and in those with a history of previous fractures, bone protective therapy should be started at the time of institution of oral steroid therapy. In others, a decision regarding the need for bone protective agents will need to be made according to the results of bone densitometry estimations.

Trends in the Use of Medications

Inhaled steroids were introduced for the management of asthma more than 30 years ago. Seminal work, much of it in Finland in the 1980s, emphasized the presence of persistent inflammation within the airways of those with asthma, even at times when they had little in the way of symptoms. Early guidelines on the management of asthma were, therefore, able to adopt a rather simplistic approach to the routine management of asthma that suggested that if bronchodilators were needed more than occasionally, one should take regular low-dose inhaled steroids. If, despite their use, asthma was not well controlled, high-dose inhaled steroids should be used. If these did not affect adequate asthma control, any other available medication should be added to the high-dose inhaled steroids; if the patient was still symptomatic, he or she should be treated with regular steroid tablets. Between 10 and 15 years ago, new studies emerged that suggested that the guidelines might be promoting a suboptimal strategy, and a plethora of trials showed that the use of long-acting β-agonists (whether salmeterol or formoterol) in addition to low-dose inhaled steroids could achieve results equal to or better than that obtained with high-dose inhaled steroids. This was true both for improvement in lung function and in terms of more days free of symptoms. Similar results were obtained for salmeterol and formoterol added to beclomethasone, budesonide, or fluticasone but also to a lesser extent with the addition of theophylline or bambuterol to low-dose inhaled steroids. Some studies suggested that the higher dose of inhaled steroids was still necessary for those with frequent exacerbations, and there is likely to be a subgroup of those with asthma who do not benefit from the addition of a long-acting inhaled β-agonist, and these should only be continued if better control of asthma has been achieved with their use. These studies have led to a trend toward guidelines, suggesting that for those not well controlled on low-dose inhaled steroids, a long-acting bronchodilator (usually an inhaled β-agonist) should be added before increasing the dose of inhaled steroids. An additional factor in this change in emphasis has been the recognition that the dose-response curve with inhaled steroids is rather flat and, although additional doses achieve only small increments in terms of benefit, they may increase the risk of side effects. Although the latter are negligible compared with those with steroid tablets or compared with the risk of poorly controlled asthma, high-dose inhaled steroids can be associated with skin purpura and possibly an excess of cataracts and glaucoma. Their long-term safety with regard to an effect on bone mineral density requires ongoing study, because the only evidence to date suggests a nonsignificant increase in hip fractures in women compared with matched controls.

On the contrary, in children, excessive doses outside the licensed range can undoubtedly affect the hypothalamic-pituitary-adrenal axis. Rare cases of adrenocortical insufficiency and collapse have been reported. The correct action, therefore, is to carefully minimize the doses of inhaled steroids used, where necessary, by the addition of alternative agents. More recently, in addition to long-acting inhaled β-agonists, leukotriene-modifying agents have become more widely used, usually as an adjunct to inhaled steroids, but in some countries as an alternative to low-dose inhaled steroids, although all guidelines suggest low-dose inhaled steroids as the preferred optimal treatment. Higher doses of inhaled steroids are often needed by those with asthma who continue to smoke. Not only does continued smoking leave the patient at risk of concomitant smoking-induced airway narrowing, but the habit seems to block the effect of inhaled steroids on glucocorticoid receptors.

All guidelines have always recommended the stepping down of treatment when asthma control is maintained and achieved. Unfortunately, human nature being what it is, a patient telling a doctor that he or she is "fine" leaves a health professional with a subconscious tendency not to risk altering a satisfactory situation with the result that many may remain on higher doses of inhaled steroids than are necessary. Recent studies have emphasized that an active stepdown approach can lead to significant reduction in dosages of inhaled steroids used without any increase in exacerbation rates. Other recent studies have shown similarly that teaching patients to vary their dose themselves can achieve significant reductions in doses of steroids used compared with those on fixed-dosage regimens. Such advice can and should be incorporated into written personal asthma action plans (see page 591). A recent extension of this variable dosing is the use of the same inhaler for maintenance and reliever therapy. This is, at present, only possible with a budesonide/formoterol combination inhaler, where several trials have shown that regular once- or twice-daily use with extra doses of the combination inhaler for relief of symptoms leads to better controlled asthma, with lower overall medication use and less need for unscheduled health care, compared with those on a fixed dosing regimen. As a result of these studies, this new way to use an existing medication has been approved in several, but not all, countries.

Novel Agents

Omalizumab is a humanized monoclonal antibody that can be used as an add-on therapy for those with persisting troublesome asthma, despite maximal traditional therapies. It may be indicated in those with clear evidence of allergic asthma, with persisting reduction in lung function, and persisting frequent symptoms or severe exacerbations. Not all patients with these criteria are suitable for this preparation, and the dosage is determined by baseline IgE level; the treatment is administered by two- to four-weekly subcutaneous injection.

Environmental Manipulation

Wherever possible, those people who have asthma must avoid identifiable triggers. The difficulty is that many are not identifiable or not avoidable (e.g., the common cold). Avoidance of animal allergens is practical; if a child is shown to have developed symptoms after acquiring a cat and shown to have positive skin-prick test reactions to cat allergens, removal of the cat is obviously preferable to drug therapy. Reducing exposure to cockroach allergens can be achieved by clearing infested homes and careful use of pesticides. Reducing the quantity of house dust mite exposure by having as few soft furnishings as possible, use of good ventilation, intermittent deep freezing of soft toys, and barrier bedding may improve the control of asthma in some individuals sensitive to house dust mites. Avoidance of drugs or occupational agents known to affect the individual adversely is essential. Avoidance of passive smoking is helpful to all. However, despite the logic behind environmental manipulation and the patients desire to undertake it, it is often of only limited benefit and an adjunct to drug therapy; only rarely is it a substitute for drugs.

Immunotherapy

Widely used some years ago, and still used in some countries, the role of specific immunotherapy in asthma remains unclear and is a subject that merits further study. Aimed at treatment of the underlying allergy, even when well performed, it can be associated with unexpected side effects, and most guidelines no longer recommend its routine use in asthma. However, refinements in technique and patient selection are redefining a limited role for immunotherapy in allergic rhinitis, and for asthma it may appear as an adjunctive therapy for a few specific instances when given by a specialist. The opinion of the NIH expert panel is that immunotherapy be considered when:

- Clear evidence is found of a relationship between symptoms and exposure to an unavoidable allergen to which the patient is sensitive.
- Symptoms occur all year or during a major portion of the year.
- Difficulty occurs with the control of symptoms by use of pharmacologic management because multiple medications are required or medications are ineffective or not accepted by the patient.

The course of allergen immunotherapy is typically 3–5 years.

Complementary Therapies

Six percent of patients with asthma reported current use of complementary therapies in one recent study. Such therapies may include homeopathy, acupuncture, breathing techniques, herbal therapies, and ionizers. Not all are free of side effects; pneumothoraces and hepatitis have been reported after acupuncture, and use of ionizers may increase nocturnal cough. The taking of Royal Jelly (propolis) has been claimed as being beneficial for those with asthma, but deaths from severe reactions have been reported after its use. Many studies of Chinese medicines and acupuncture have been reported, but design of appropriate trials is difficult, and no definite evidence of benefit can be concluded. Similarly, homeopathy has been assessed in several trials with conflicting results, and no recommendations for use can be made on the available information. Breathing exercises including yoga and the Buteyko technique have attracted much interest. Pranayama breathing can be associated with reduced airway hyperresponsiveness and the Buteyko technique associated with a reduced need for bronchodilators.

Perhaps of greater importance than the efficacy or lack of efficacy of complementary therapies is the reason why they remain popular among those with asthma. Studies have suggested that this often reflects dissatisfaction with the relationship of the patient with those offering traditional medicine. Complaints include those reflecting the quality of the doctor–patient relationship and a lack of time. Other reasons include dissatisfaction with treatment, "distrust" of drugs, dislike of regular medication, and a desire for a cure.

Management Strategies for the Use of Medicines in the Day-to-Day Management of Asthma

The short-term aims of asthma management can be defined as:

- Rapid resolution of symptoms
- Restoration of quality of life
- Reduction in risk of attacks

The long-term aims of asthma management can be defined as:

- Best possible lung function
- Minimal side effects from treatment

To achieve these two sets of aims, most guidelines support a stepwise approach to therapy, which is summarized in Figure 45-12 and Table 45-8. Two sets of guidelines apply to the management of chronic asthma in adults—one from the British Thoracic Society/Scottish Intercollegiate Guidelines Network (UK; see Figure 45-12) and the other from the NIH (US; see Table 45-8)—and both are very similar to the recommendations of the Global Initiative for Asthma. They follow very similar principles of therapy. Both sets aim at a gradual increase in ICS and emphasize the importance of stepping down the intensity of therapy once control has been achieved.

It is important to stress that these are guidelines as to how to manage asthma over the weeks and months—a more acute self-management plan may be administered in a zone fashion as a self-treatment plan (see the following section). When the stepwise approach is used, doctors must start at the step most appropriate to the severity of the individual's asthma at

FIGURE 45-12 Stepwise approach to treatment of adults who have asthma—British Asthma Guidelines. (Adapted with permission from British Thoracic Society/Scottish Intercollegiate Guidelines Network.)

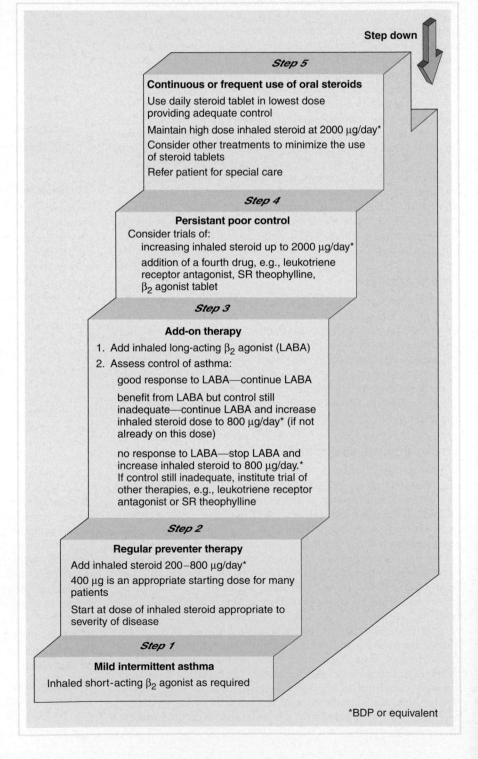

Step down

Step 5

Continuous or frequent use of oral steroids

Use daily steroid tablet in lowest dose providing adequate control

Maintain high dose inhaled steroid at 2000 µg/day*

Consider other treatments to minimize the use of steroid tablets

Refer patient for special care

Step 4

Persistant poor control

Consider trials of:

increasing inhaled steroid up to 2000 µg/day*

addition of a fourth drug, e.g., leukotriene receptor antagonist, SR theophylline, β_2 agonist tablet

Step 3

Add-on therapy

1. Add inhaled long-acting β_2 agonist (LABA)
2. Assess control of asthma:

   good response to LABA—continue LABA

   benefit from LABA but control still inadequate—continue LABA and increase inhaled steroid dose to 800 µg/day* (if not already on this dose)

   no response to LABA—stop LABA and increase inhaled steroid to 800 µg/day.* If control still inadequate, institute trial of other therapies, e.g., leukotriene receptor antagonist or SR theophylline

Step 2

Regular preventer therapy

Add inhaled steroid 200–800 µg/day*

400 µg is an appropriate starting dose for many patients

Start at dose of inhaled steroid appropriate to severity of disease

Step 1

Mild intermittent asthma

Inhaled short-acting β_2 agonist as required

*BDP or equivalent

TABLE 45-8	Stepwise Approach for the Management of Asthma in Adults and Children—National Institutes of Health*
Step 4 (Severe Persistent)	Daily medication: **Preferred treatment:** High-dose inhaled corticosteroids and long-acting inhaled β_2-agonists AND, if necessary Corticosteroid tablets or syrup (2 mg/kg/day, generally do not exceed 60 mg/day). (Make repeat attempts to reduce systemic corticosteroids and maintain control with high-dose inhaled corticosteroids.)
Step 3 (Moderate Persistent and Recurring Severe Exacerbations)	Daily medication: **Preferred treatment:** Low-to-medium dose inhaled corticosteroids and long-acting inhaled β_2-agonists **Alternative treatment:** Increased inhaled corticosteroids within medium-dose range or low-to-medium dose inhaled corticosteroids and either leukotriene modifier or theophylline
Step 2 (Mild Persistent)	Daily medication: **Preferred treatment:** Low-dose inhaled corticosteroids **Alternative treatment:** Cromolyn, leukotriene modifier, nedocromil, or sustained release theophylline to serum concentration of 5–15 μg/mL.
Step 1 (Mild Intermittent)	Daily medication: No daily medication needed Severe exacerbations may occur, separated by long periods of normal lung function and no symptoms. A course of systemic corticosteroids is recommended.
Quick Relief (all Patients)	Short-acting bronchodilator: 2–4 puffs short-acting inhaled β_2-agonists as needed for symptoms. Intensity of treatment will depend on severity of exacerbation; up to three treatments at 20-minute intervals or a single nebulizer treatment as needed. Course of systemic corticosteroids may be needed. Use of short-acting β_2-agonists > two times a week in intermittent asthma (daily, or increasing use in persistent asthma) may indicate the need to initiate (increase) long-term control therapy.

Preferred treatments are given in bold.
*Adapted from the National Heart, Lung, and Blood Institute.

the time of consultation and subsequently step up or step down to control the condition. At any time it may be necessary for the patient to take a short course of corticosteroid tablets to regain control. After control is achieved, the emphasis of management remains on stepping treatment down to the minimum level needed to maintain control.

MANAGEMENT OF ACUTE ASTHMA

Most acute asthma is not actually acute. Although it may be severe, the asthma "attack" suffered by many children and adults has often been developing for some time. In one study, 53% of adult patients admitted to the hospital with severe asthma had been waking because of asthma for at least 5 nights before admission. Half of these patients had sought advice from their primary care physician in the week before admission because of deteriorating asthma, but too often they received antibiotics or more bronchodilators rather than the corticosteroid tablets they probably needed. In another national survey of all patients who attended emergency departments because of asthma, one fifth had been waking because of "acute" asthma for 3 nights before attendance, and in a further Canadian study a fifth of those being admitted to the hospital with asthma were shown to have had symptoms of deteriorating asthma for at least 3 weeks before admission. An illustration of the size of this window of opportunity for better self-treatment in found in Figure 45-13. Data such as this suggests that many patients had adequate time to alter their treatment to prevent deterioration to crisis levels. Thus, undertreatment or inappropriate therapy is a major contributor to asthma morbidity and mortality. As a consequence,

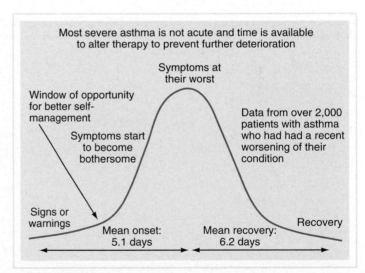

FIGURE 45-13 For most patients, the evolution of a severe attack of asthma occurs over several days, and a similar time period is needed for recovery. (Adapted from Partridge MR et al: BMC pulmonary medicine; 2006; 6:13.)

asthma is the third leading cause of preventable admissions to the hospital, and more than 5000 deaths per year in the United States and 1500 deaths per year in the United Kingdom are from asthma.

People who have asthma die because they, their loved ones, or their doctors underestimate the severity, because of delays in seeking medical treatment, and because of underuse of oxygen and corticosteroid tablets. The severity of an exacerbation, therefore, must be carefully assessed, and the outcome determines the treatment given and where it is given. Of children and adults seen in the accident and emergency departments who had asthma, fewer than half in one study received antiinflammatory therapy, and only few adults admitted had written plans to manage their asthma and control an exacerbation (Figure 45-14). Table 45-9 shows features associated with exacerbations of asthma of mild, moderate, severe, or critical nature. All but the mildest attacks require treatment with bronchodilators, corticosteroids, and oxygen, and careful follow-up and assessment of responses to each intervention (see Figure 45-14).

The criteria for admission to an intensive care unit include exhaustion; the most common reason those who have severe asthma require mechanical ventilation is that of exhaustion. The first warning of this may be a normal or raised arterial partial pressure of carbon dioxide ($PaCO_2$) on blood gas sampling—the normal picture in acute asthma being one of a low PaO_2 and a high $PaCO_2$.

The recognition and assessment of severe acute asthma begins at home, where it is often underestimated, sometimes by the patient, the caregiver, or the attending physician (Box 45-2; see also Figure 45-14 and Table 45-9). Symptoms and peak expiratory flow rate (PEFR) must be assessed immediately and the severity graded. Treatment is with bronchodilators that are repeated frequently if required, and the response to their use is monitored regularly by measurement of peak expiratory flow. In life-threatening asthma, bronchodilators (albuterol [salbutamol] 5–10 mg) and ipratropium bromide are administered by a nebulizer. Lesser degrees of severity (i.e., non-life-threatening asthma—moderate or severe asthma) is treated with four to six puffs of albuterol (salbutamol) from a pMDI by a large volume spacer plus ipratropium, four puffs from a pMDI and large volume spacer, both repeated as necessary, every 10–15 min. A good response (e.g., PEFR greater than 80% predicted or best) with symptom relief is followed by continuing regular β-agonists every 4 h for 24–48 h, increase the dose of ICS for 7 days, and review the patient within days.

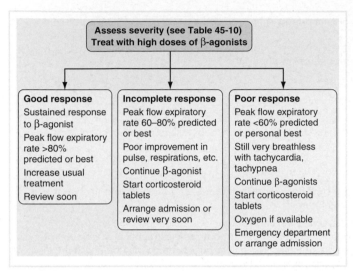

FIGURE 45-14 Home management of an acute exacerbation of asthma.

TABLE 45-9 Guide to the Severity of Asthma Exacerbations*

Symptoms	Mild	Moderate	Severe	Respiratory Arrest Imminent
Breathless	Walking Can lie down	Talking Prefers sitting	At rest Hunched forward	
Talks in	Sentences	Phrases	Words	
Alertness	May be agitated	Usually agitated	Usually agitated	Drowsy or confused
Respiratory rate	Increased	Increased	Often >30 breaths per minute	
Accessory muscles and suprasternal retractions	Usually not	Usually	Usually	Paradoxic thoracoabdominal movement
Wheeze	Moderate, often only end expiratory	Loud	Usually loud	Absence of wheeze
Pulse per minute	<100	100–120	>120	Bradycardia
Peak expiratory flow rate after initial bronchodilator (% predicted or % personal best)	Over 80	ca. 60–80	<60 (<100 L/min adults) or response lasts <2 h	
Arterial pressure of oxygen (PaO_2; on air)	Normal Test not usually necessary	>8.5 kPa (>60 mmHg)	<8.0 kPa (<60 mmHg) Possible cyanosis	
$PaCO_2$	<6 kPa (<45 mmHg)	<6 kPa (<45 mmHg)	>6 kPa (>45 mmHg) Possible respiratory failure (see text)	
Arterial oxygen saturation (%; on air)	>95	91–95	<90	

Hypercapnia (hypoventilation) develops more readily in young children than in adults and adolescents.
*Adapted from National Heart, Lung, and Blood Institute/World Health Organization Workshop.

BOX 45-2 The Recognition and Assessment in Hospital of Acute Severe Asthma

Features of Acute Severe Asthma

Peak expiratory flow rate (PEFR) ≤50% of predicted or best
Cannot complete sentences in one breath
Respirations ≥25 breaths per minute
Pulse > 110 beats per minute

Life-Threatening Features

PEFR <33% of predicted or best
Silent chest, cyanosis, or feeble respiratory effort
Bradycardia or hypotension
Exhaustion, confusion, or coma
If arterial saturation of oxygen <92% or a patient has any life-threatening features, measure arterial blood gases

Blood Gas Markers of a Very Severe, Life-Threatening Attack

Normal (5–6 kPa [36–45 mmHg]) or high arterial partial pressure of carbon dioxide ($Paco_2$)
Severe hypoxia, Pao_2 <8.0 kPa (60 mmHg) irrespective of treatment with oxygen
A low pH (or high H^1)

No Other Investigations are Needed for Immediate Management

Caution: patients who have severe or life-threatening attacks may not be distressed and may not have all these abnormalities — the presence of any should alert the doctor.

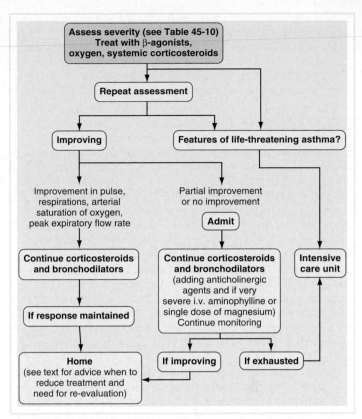

FIGURE 45-15 Management chart for the hospital treatment of acute severe asthma.

An incomplete response (PEFR 50–80% predicted or best) with persistent symptoms requires continuation of β-agonists every 2–4 h and prompt addition of oral corticosteroids. Either admission is arranged or the patient is seen again urgently (same day or next morning).

With a poor response (PEFR less than 60% predicted or best) with signs of distress, the patient is instructed to continue β-agonists, start oral corticosteroids, use oxygen if available, and proceed to the emergency department or call emergency services.

Acute Asthma in the Emergency Room

Proper recognition and assessment are vital (see Box 45-2)—an algorithm for further management is given in Figure 45-15—and severity must be assessed (see Table 45-9 and Box 45-2). Treatment is begun with β-agonists, high-flow oxygen, and systemic corticosteroids (e.g., prednisolone 30–60 mg orally daily) (see Figure 45-15). The aim is to achieve an arterial oxygen saturation (Sao_2) of greater than 92%. Ipratropium bromide can be added to albuterol (salbutamol). No sedatives of any kind can be given. A chest radiograph is indicated if a pneumothorax or consolidation is suspected, in life-threatening cases, if there is a failure to respond to initial treatment, or if there is a requirement for mechanical ventilatory support. If the Sao_2 does not reach 92% on high-flow oxygen or the PEFR is less than 100 L/min, arterial blood gas pressures are measured. If life-threatening features are present (see Box 45-2), the patient is transferred to the intensive care unit accompanied by a doctor prepared to intubate if any of the following occur:

- Deteriorating PEFR
- Worsening or persistent hypoxia or hypercapnia

- Exhaustion, feeble respirations, confusion, or drowsiness
- Coma or respiratory arrest

Intravenous aminophylline, 250 mg over 20 min, can be given if the patient is not taking regular oral theophyllines, followed by or starting with—if on oral theophylline—aminophylline 0.5 mg/kg/h as an infusion. A single dose of magnesium sulfate (1.2–2 g intravenous infusion over 20 min) has also been shown to be safe and effective in acute severe asthma.

Subsequent Management

Thereafter, the management includes:

- Repeated estimation of response to therapy by clinical assessment of peak flow measurement and oximetry every 15–30 min
- If improving, continue oxygen, oral corticosteroids four hourly, inhaled β-agonist
- If not improving after 15–30 min, continue corticosteroids and oxygen, give nebulized β-agonist every 30 min, add ipratropium, 500 µg nebulized, every 6 h
- If still not improving, commence aminophylline infusion if not already started
- Repeat arterial blood gas tensions if initial Pao_2 less than 8 kPa (60 mmHg) unless subsequent Sao_2 is greater than 92%, $Paco_2$ is normal, or the patient deteriorates.

On recovery, the patient should at discharge have:

- Been on discharge medication for 24 h
- Inhaler technique checked
- PEFR greater than 75% of predicted or better and PEFR diurnal variability less than 25% unless discharge agreed with respiratory physician

- Treatment with oral and inhaled corticosteroids in addition to bronchodilators
- Own PEF meter and a written personal asthma action plan
- Local follow-up arranged for within a week
- Follow-up appointment in chest clinic within 4 weeks

The reason(s) for the exacerbation and admission must be determined (Box 45-3) and details sent to the local physician, together with a discharge plan and potential best PEF.

The advice at discharge is most important. Patients need to be given clear advice as to how long to continue corticosteroid tablets, which should be continued in full dose until the patient is better and then either stopped suddenly (if the patient was not previously on corticosteroids and has taken them for less than 2 weeks) or tapered off. The length of course needed often reflects the length of deterioration of asthma before initiation of treatment; a short period of worsening asthma tends to respond more quickly than does an attack that followed a long period of poor control. For those patients treated with high doses of bronchodilators (whether from a nebulizer or a spacer device), it is important that they are not discharged from observation until the dose is reduced, for fear that the bronchodilator may mask signs of suboptimal control.

Every attack of severe asthma and every hospital admission or emergency room attendance must be regarded as a sign of failure of that patient's previous asthma management. After successful medical management of the attack comes the more important part—a review of the circumstances that led up to the attack. It is important to assess the patient's inhaler technique and self-monitoring skills. Was this a potentially life-threatening attack (Box 45-4)? What was the prodromal use and dose of antiinflammatory therapy? If a patient has been taking a regular preventive therapy, an attack of asthma generally indicates the need for at least a temporary increase in dose. Was there an avoidable cause for the attack (e.g., running out of inhalers), an occupational cause, premenstrual worsening, or a potentially life-threatening inadvertent use of a β-blocker? Finally, did the patient react appropriately to the deteriorating control of his or her asthma, and, if a self-management plan was available, had it been used? These issues are summarized in Box 45-3.

BOX 45-3 The Emergency Management of Asthma

Checklist for Use After an Emergency Attendance or Admission Because of Asthma

- Was this potentially fatal asthma? (see Table 45-13)
- Was the patient's inhaler technique satisfactory?
- Prior to the attack were they on, and were they taking, sufficient preventative therapy?
- Was there an avoidable precipitating cause (e.g., aspirin use, premenstrual worsening, alcohol, allergen exposure, or occupational cause)?
- Was this a genuine sudden severe (brittle) attack, and do they need to be taught the special first-aid measures needed by this group?
- Is the patient a poor perceiver of severity?
- Did the patient react appropriately to the impending attack, and did they have a written personal asthma action plan?

Note that every episode of severe asthma represents a potential failure of our previous management.

BOX 45-4 Features of Potentially Fatal Asthma

Any of the Following:
1. An episode of respiratory failure requiring intubation
2. Respiratory acidosis associated with an attack of asthma not requiring intubation
3. Two or more hospital admissions for asthma despite chronic use of oral steroids
4. Two episodes of pneumothorax (or pneumomediastinum) associated with an asthma attack

TABLE 45-10 Factors Associated with Noncompliance in Asthma

Type of Factor	Factor
Pharmacologic	Difficult multiple-drug, multiple-dose regimens Real or perceived side effects Inadequate instruction in use of inhaler devices
Nonpharmacologic	Misunderstanding Lack of information Dislike of regular medications Unexpressed fears or concerns Denial of diagnosis Denial of severity/risk Poor communication between patient and health professional

Prevention and Organization of Care

Not only must therapeutic methods of prevention be considered but so must the nonpharmacologic aspects of the management of what is, for most patients who have asthma, a long-term condition. This involves consideration of the important subjects of communication, patient education, and self-management.

Writing the correct prescription is only one small part of the treatment of asthma, but in a high proportion of cases the treatment is not taken in the way suggested by the doctor. The reasons for noncompliance (nonadherence) are given in Table 45-10; it is important to understand that often the reason is a simple failure of understanding or lack of information. Of patients who have asthma, 50% complain of lack of information, and in only a minority of cases do doctors write down for the patient or parent simple instructions as to which medication to use when. Such written advice is capable of dramatically increasing the proportion of patients, both children and adults, who can correctly describe their drug regimen—and writing down instructions for patients takes only a few seconds, especially if partially preprinted forms are used. However, up to 15% of adults attending hospital clinics and emergency rooms are functionally illiterate, and this has been shown to be associated with increased use of health service resources and with diminished ability to cope with inhaler techniques. Pictorial representation of the medication regimen may be helpful for these patients.

Reinforcement of spoken messages and acquisition of skills and techniques in inhaler use and in peak-flow monitoring can also be undertaken by use of written materials, loan of videotapes and audiotapes, and subsequent consultation with respiratory trained nurses. The messages offered to the patient by the entire health professional team need to be consistent and uniform, for nothing confuses a patient more than to be given apparently different messages from different people. The use of guidelines on asthma management provides a common text from which to teach patients. Even with a common text, however, it must be recognized that every person who has asthma is an individual and that the starting point for subsequent good communication and patient education is to recognize that each patient has a different set of needs and a different set of fears and concerns regarding the condition, as well as different expectations. A basic education regarding asthma should be offered to all, and the ground to be covered is shown in Box 45-5.

The importance of the effect of good communication on subsequent compliance cannot be underestimated. Many patients exhibit denial of either the diagnosis or its implications, and many have concerns regarding perceived or real side effects of treatment that need adequate airing if they are to feel happy taking treatment. Many express concerns at the unpredictable nature of asthma and express irritation at this uncertainty and the effect on quality of life.

Self-management education and the receipt of a written personal asthma action plan is one way of reducing patients' feelings of uncertainty and feelings of dependency. The patient or parent receives written advice from the health professionals as to how to adjust treatment in a variety of circumstances and when and from whom more urgent medical advice should be sought. These plans may be based on symptoms, or in adults on symptoms and objective monitoring of peak flow; a typical plan is given in Figure 45-16.

Most published studies on successful self-management education have involved patients monitoring their condition and detecting worsening by use of a combination of symptoms and peak-flow levels. However, results of other studies have

BOX 45-5 Suggested Content for an Asthma Educational Discussion

- Nature of the disease
- Nature of the treatment—differences between relievers and preventers
- Identify areas where patient wants treatment to have its effect
- How to use the treatment
- Acquisition of skills necessary to recognize worsening asthma
- Self monitoring
- Negotiation of goals and discussion regarding the future
- Appropriate allergen avoidance and environmental manipulation
- Receipt of a written personal asthma action plan written personal asthma action plan

ZONE 1*	ZONE 2	ZONE 3	ZONE 4
Your asthma is under control if	**Your asthma is getting worse if**	**Your asthma is severe if**	**It is a medical emergency if**
It does not disturb your sleep	You are having to use your ____ (reliever inhaler) more than usual	You are getting increasingly breathless	Your symptoms continue to get worse **and** Your peak flow readings have fallen to below ____
It does not restrict your usual activities **and** Your peak flow readings are above ____	You are waking at night with asthma symptoms **and** Your peak flow readings have fallen to between ____ and ____	You are having to use your ____ (reliever inhaler) every ____ hours or more often **and** Your peak flow readings have fallen to between ____ and ____	**Do not be afraid of causing a fuss. Your doctor will want to see you urgently.**
ACTION	**ACTION**	**ACTION**	**ACTION**
Continue your normal medicines	**Increase your usual medicines**	**Start a course of corticosteroid tablets**	**Get help immediately**
Your preventer is ____ You should normally take ____ puffs/doses ____ times every day (using a spacer), even when you are feeling well	Increase your ____ (preventer inhaler) to ____	Take ____ prednisolone (corticosteroid) tablets strength ____ (mg each) and then ____	Telephone your doctor straightaway on ____ or call an ambulance
Your reliever is ____ You should normally only take it when you are short of breath, coughing or wheezing, or before exercise	Continue to take your ____ (reliever inhaler) to relieve your asthma symptoms	Discuss with your doctor how and when to stop taking the tablets	Take ____ prednisolone (corticosteroid) tablets strength ____ (mg each) immediately
Your other medicines are ____		Continue to take your ____ (reliever and preventer inhalers) as prescribed	Continue to take your ____ (reliever inhaler) as needed, or every 5–10 minutes until the ambulance arrives

* If you are persistently in this zone, your doctor may reduce your usual medication.

FIGURE 45-16 Typical partially preprinted self-treatment plan.

suggested that subjective monitoring achieves similar results to objective monitoring. Yet another study showed that in 60% of patients, there is no significant correlation between how they feel and measurements of airflow, and those with the most severe asthma may be less able to perceive deterioration in airway caliber. Further studies may, therefore, be needed to better define the role of home peak-flow monitoring, but currently the decision should be to discuss objective monitoring with patients and to recommend it, as a minimum, for those with moderate to severe disease.

Self-management may mean any of the following:

- The use a relieving bronchodilator as required and seeking medical attention if its use becomes more frequent or exceeds, for example, every 4–6 h
- Requesting an early consultation if nighttime symptoms develop
- Increasing preventive therapy at the first sign of cold
- Increasing preventive therapy when bronchodilator use increases or nighttime symptoms occur
- Starting a course of corticosteroid tablets in response to deteriorating symptoms or falling peak flow

Most published plans suggest that suitable thresholds for therapeutic change on the basis of peak-flow readings would be:

- Peak flow greater than 85% of usual best: Continue normal therapy
- Peak flow 70–85% of usual best: Increase inhaled steroid to maximal dose
- Peak flow 50–70% of usual best: Start a course of steroid tablets
- Peak flow less than 50% of usual best: Seek urgent medical attention

Many recent studies and systematic reviews support the use of self-management. Two controlled studies recruited outpatients who had moderately severe asthma and followed them for 6 or 12 months after being given self-management advice. In each case, the intervention group had less need for emergency medical care, less time off work, and a better quality of life than did the control group. In one of the studies, the self-management group not only had better-controlled asthma but achieved it by use of lower overall doses of corticosteroid tablets over a 12-month period compared with the control group. This implies either that increasing ICSs at the first sign of deterioration is an important therapeutic step or that giving patients control of their condition enhances compliance so that they take their ICSs and are less likely to deteriorate to a point where they need corticosteroid tablets. Compliance with the self-management plans was remarkably high—on 77% of the occasions when circumstances suggested that patients needed to start corticosteroid tablets, they did so. Another study has shown that the collecting of prescriptions for inhaled steroids was significantly greater in a group of patients who had received self-management education and a written personal asthma action plan than in a group of control patients with asthma.

There is some controversy regarding whether doubling inhaled steroids at the first sign of deterioration is beneficial. Although two studies in which that was the only variable did not show a reduction in those subsequently needing steroid tablets or hospitalization, all of the self-management studies that have shown beneficial outcomes have included that action. It may be that including that action within a four-zone plan prompts some to restart the inhaled steroids they may not have been taking as prescribed. Other studies suggest that perhaps a simple doubling of inhaled steroids may be insufficient, and one study showed benefit of quadrupling the dose. Clearly, this depends on the initial starting dose, and advice needs to be tailored to the individual. If the basic principle of always using the lowest dose of medication that controls the disease is adopted, it is possible that patients may routinely be on very low doses of maintenance inhaled steroids (where necessary by the addition of long-acting inhaled β-agonists) but triple or quadruple the dose at the first sign of deterioration. Controversy regarding exact details of the intervention described on a personal asthma action plan should not be an excuse for not implementing the principle, especially in the face of more than 36 randomized control trials showing benefits from self-management education and regular follow-up.

Asthma is an increasingly common condition. The challenge for the future is to prevent more people from developing it, but in the meantime excellent therapies are available to control it. However, these have to be offered to the patient in a manner that makes it likely they will be used to maximal benefit.

PITFALLS AND CONTROVERSIES

Accurate Diagnosis

Until a patient carries the correct diagnosis, he or she is unlikely to receive the correct treatment—repeated chest infections usually are not such and should raise the suspicion of asthma. Persistent coughs in adults and children may also be the most prominent features of undiagnosed asthma, so persistent cough merits investigation and a trial of asthma therapy. An occupational cause should always be considered in an adult presenting for the first time with asthma. Over diagnosis must also be avoided; unfortunately, publicity regarding asthma has led to a situation in which every respiratory symptom (and some cardiac ones) is treated for asthma until proved otherwise. Constant reminders that asthma is only one of numerous respiratory diseases are necessary.

Self-Management Education

Doctors are good at writing prescriptions. They are often not as good at implementing nonpharmacologic interventions that may be of equal or greater benefit. Good communication, self-management education, and the offering of a written personal asthma action plan to all with asthma should become normal practice.

Use of Inhaled Steroids

There is little doubt that the single chemical entity that has most improved the situation for 300 million people with asthma worldwide over the last 30 years has been the introduction of inhaled steroids. However, for many with asthma in the less prosperous countries of the world, these basic medicines are either not available, not prescribed, cannot be afforded, or not used because of cultural misconceptions or barriers. In other countries where inhaled steroids are easily available, they may be used suboptimally because of steroid phobia and less efficient medications used in their place. In other cases, inhaled steroids may be misused, with excessive doses being used and "step down" not being practiced.

Transition to Chlorofluorocarbon-Free Metered Dose Inhalers

Withdrawal of CFC propellants from MDIs under the Montreal Protocol means that most patients are now in the process of being changed to CFC-free MDIs. Patients need to be forewarned that reformulation of their inhaled medicines with new HFA propellants may lead to the inhaler feeling or weighing differently from their predecessors, and the impact of the aerosolized medicines on the oropharynx is likely to be less. A difference in taste may also occur. For some products, reformulation involves a change in dose of the medicine administered. Patients need to be reassured that:

- Treatment is as safe as it was previously
- Treatment is as effective as it was previously
- Previous propellants were environmentally, and not individually, damaging
- New inhalers are very similar
- The active ingredient is the same

More trials have been undertaken with the new products than were ever undertaken with the original inhalers.

Successful Management

To offer treatment in a manner that makes it likely it will be taken involves:

- Eliciting the patients' understanding of the condition
- Eliciting their fears, concerns, and information needs
- Discussing common goals and clarifying the risks versus benefits of treatment or no treatment
- Giving control of the condition to the patient by means of a written personal asthma action plan
- Reinforcing the spoken word with personalized written information
- Offering regular follow-up during which reinforcement of these messages is given, as is further opportunity for discussion and reduction of therapy to the minimum necessary to control the condition.

SUGGESTED READINGS

British Thoracic Society/Scottish Intercollegiate Guideline Network: British guideline on the management of asthma. Thorax 2003; 58:1–94.

National Asthma Education and Prevention Program: NAEPP Expert Panel Report: Guidelines for the diagnosis and management of asthma—Update on selected topics (NIH Publication No. 02-5075), Bethesda, MD: National Institutes of Health; 2002.

National Institutes of Health. National Heart, Lung and Blood Institute: Global strategy for asthma management and prevention (update from NIH Publication No. 02-3659), Bethesda, MD: Global Initiative for Asthma (GINA); 2002.

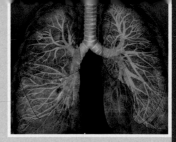

46   Cystic Fibrosis

FELIX RATJEN • ELIZABETH TULLIS

INTRODUCTION

Cystic fibrosis (CF) is a common, fatal, autosomal-recessive disorder. Its frequency varies between different populations with approximately 1 in 3300 live births in Caucasians, 1 in 15,000 in African Americans, and 1 in 32,000 in Asians. Although reports of CF exist from medieval ages, it was first described and recognized as a genetic disease by Anderson in 1938. Although the increase in sweat chloride and sodium concentrations was observed by Saint Agnese in the 1950s, it was not until 1983 that Paul Quinton described the defective chloride transport in sweat glands and respiratory epithelium as the underlying abnormality. The discovery of the causative, mutated gene encoding a defective chloride channel in epithelial cells in 1989 has improved our understanding of the pathophysiology and opened up new avenues of treatments. Despite these major advances, it is still not entirely clear how mutations in the cystic fibrosis transmembrane regulator (CFTR) gene cause the multiple facets of CF disease manifestations.

GENETICS

CF is caused by mutations in a gene on chromosome 7 encoding a protein that was subsequently named cystic fibrosis transmembrane regulator (CFTR). More than 1400 mutations have been described to date and reported to the Cystic Fibrosis Genetic Analysis Consortium. Most of these mutations are rare, and only four mutations occur in a frequency of more than 1%. CFTR mutations can be grouped into five classes: CFTR is not synthesized (I), is inadequately processed (II), is not regulated (III), shows abnormal conductance (IV), or has partially defective production or processing (V). Class I–III mutations are more common and associated with pancreatic insufficiency, whereas patients with the less common class IV–V mutations often are pancreatic sufficient (Figure 46-1).

The most common mutation worldwide found in approximately 66% of patients with CF is a class II mutation caused by a deletion of phenylalanine in position 508 (F508) of CFTR. F508$\triangle$ CFTR is misfolded and trapped in the endoplasmic reticulum and subsequently proteolytically degraded. However, small amounts of DF508$\triangle$ CFTR reach the plasma membrane of epithelial cells where it has been shown to have functional activity. These findings suggest that F508$\triangle$ CFTR rescue from ER degradation may be a potential therapeutic intervention.

CFTR belongs to a family of transmembrane proteins called ATP-binding cassette (ABC) transporters and functions as a chloride channel in apical membranes. However, CFTR possesses other functions in addition to being a chloride channel.

CFTR has been described as a regulator of other membrane channels such as the epithelial sodium channel (eNaC) and the outwardly rectifying chloride channel (ORCC). CFTR also transports or regulates HCO^{3-} transport through epithelial cell membranes and may act as a transporter for other proteins, such as glutathione.

There is a relationship between CFTR genotype and clinical phenotype in CF. Patients who carry 2 "severe" mutations that cause loss of function in CFTR (Class I, II, and III) have "classic" CF, which is characterized by pancreatic insufficiency, early age of diagnosis, and elevated sweat chloride. In contrast, patients who have at least 1 "mild" mutation with partial function in CFTR are typically diagnosed at an older age, have sweat chloride values that are closer to normal values, and are pancreatic sufficient.

Whereas class IV and V CFTR mutations are linked with pancreatic sufficiency, attempts to link specific mutations to the severity of lung disease have shown large phenotypic variability. This is best documented for patients homozygous for the F508$\triangle$ mutation who exhibit a wide spectrum in lung disease severity. This wide phenotypic variation suggests that environmental factors and/or genes other than CFTR influence the development, progression, and disease severity of CF (Figure 46-2).

PATHOPHYSIOLOGY

Although there is ongoing debate on how CFTR mutations cause disease, some of the fundamental questions have been clarified in recent years. CFTR is expressed in higher quantities in tissues that are clinically affected by CF such as sinuses, lungs, pancreas, liver, and reproductive tract, although low levels also occur elsewhere. Because lung disease is the most pertinent clinical feature of CF, we will focus on the pathophysiology of CF in the respiratory tract.

Airway epithelial cells secrete chloride and absorb sodium chloride, the balance of which is regulated through apical channels including CFTR (Figure 46-3). Ion secretion and absorption affect water transport, and a balance between secretion and absorption is thought to be important to maintain an adequate layer of airway surface liquid (ASL). The ASL supports the thin mucous layer on top of epithelial cells, which is constantly transported out of the lungs through ciliary movement. Lack or dysfunction of CFTR leads to reduced chloride secretion and sodium chloride hyperabsorption with depletion of ASL. In the absence of adequate ASL, respiratory cilia collapse, leading to breakdown of mucociliary transport. Mucus accumulates in the lower airways, and inhaled bacteria are trapped in this viscous mucous layer on top of respiratory epithelial cells.

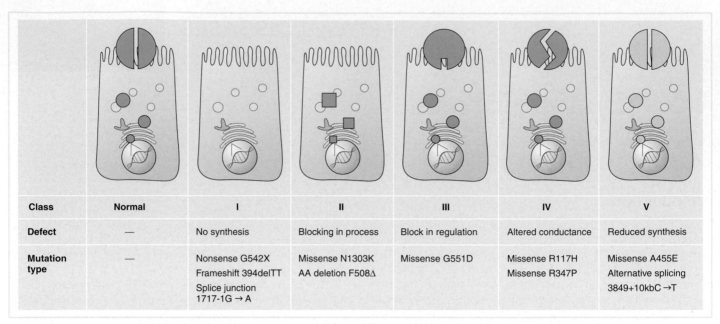

Class	Normal	I	II	III	IV	V
Defect	—	No synthesis	Blocking in process	Block in regulation	Altered conductance	Reduced synthesis
Mutation type	—	Nonsense G542X Frameshift 394delTT Splice junction 1717-1G → A	Missense N1303K AA deletion F508Δ	Missense G551D	Missense R117H Missense R347P	Missense A455E Alternative splicing 3849+10kbC →T

FIGURE 46-1 Major classes and molecular consequences of cystic fibrosis transmembrane conductance regulator (CFTR) mutations.

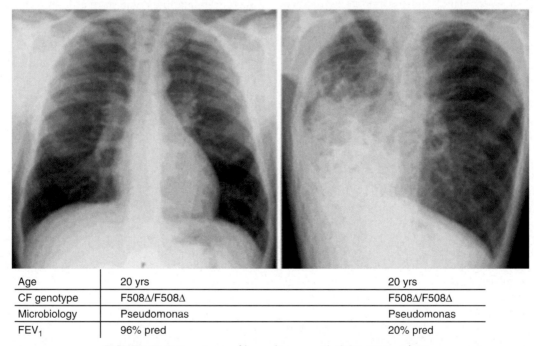

Age	20 yrs	20 yrs
CF genotype	F508Δ/F508Δ	F508Δ/F508Δ
Microbiology	Pseudomonas	Pseudomonas
FEV_1	96% pred	20% pred

FIGURE 46-2 Spectrum of lung disease with CXR, FEV, and age.

The spectrum of bacteria that are relevant for CF disease is relatively limited. Overall, *Pseudomonas aeruginosa* is the most common isolate, followed by *Staphylococcus aureus*, and *Haemophilus influenzae*. Later in the course of disease, multiresistant organisms such as *Stenotrophomonas maltophilia*, *Achromobacter (Alcaligenes) xylosoxidans*, and *Burkholderia cepacia* complex may be isolated. As in other chronic pulmonary diseases, nontuberculous mycobacteria (usually *M. avium-intracellulare* or *M. abscessus*) may be isolated. It is challenging to prove whether these organisms are causing ongoing disease and treatment is required or if they are just colonizing the damaged lung. For a more detailed discussion of nontuberculous mycobacteria (NTM) infections, see Chapter 31.

Stenotrophomonas maltophilia, *Alcaligenes xylosoxidans*, and *Burkholderia cepacia* complex are isolated in less than 10% of patients with CF. *B. cepacia* complex is an unusual organism that is found in the environment (soil and water) and causes chronic infection in only CF and chronic granulomatous disease. It is inherently multiresistant and difficult to treat and, in CF, is associated with a significantly worse prognosis. There is evidence for person-to-person spread in patients with CF. Approximately 10–15% of patients with CF who are infected with *B. cepacia* complex will have rapidly progressive deterioration, so-called cepacia syndrome, with necrotizing pneumonia, markedly elevated white blood cells (WBCs), bacteremia, and almost 100% mortality.

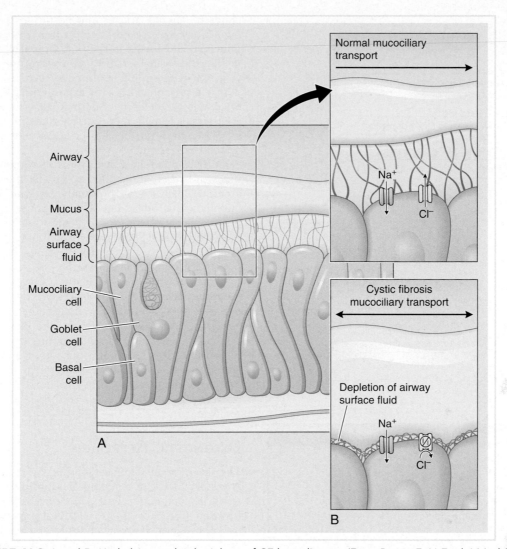

Airway

Mucus

Airway
surface
fluid

Mucociliary
cell

Goblet
cell

Basal
cell

A

Normal mucociliary
transport

Na^+

Cl^-

Cystic fibrosis
mucociliary transport

Depletion of airway
surface fluid

Na^+

Cl^-

B

FIGURE 46-3 **A** and **B,** Underlying pathophysiology of CF lung disease. (From Ratjen F: N Engl J Med 2006.)

The mucus in CF lacks oxygen, leading to anaerobic growth conditions for bacteria. These growth conditions trigger a switch of *S. aureus* and *P. aeruginosa* from nonmucoid to mucoid cell types, the predominant phenotype in CF lungs. These mucoid strains form biofilms in CF airways, which are resistant to killing by the host defense system, resulting in chronic infection. Inflammatory products, such as elastase, released by neutrophils, stimulate mucus secretion, perpetuating the cycle of mucus retention, infection, and inflammation.

There is evidence that inflammation is dysregulated in CF airways. Neutrophilic airway inflammation has been detected in infants with CF in the first months of life, as well as in CF fetal lung tissue. Whether or not inflammation is directly related to the CFTR defect is still disputed. However, an exaggerated, sustained, and prolonged inflammatory response to bacterial and viral pathogens is an accepted feature of CF lung disease. There is sufficient evidence that the persistent endobronchial inflammation is deleterious for the course of lung disease (Figure 46-4).

Exocrine pancreatic insufficiency is present in approximately 85–90% of patients with CF and linked to specific CFTR mutations. The exocrine pancreas has great functional reserve, and 98–99% of its function must be lost before

malabsorption will occur. Patients who are pancreatic sufficient do not have normal pancreatic exocrine function but have sufficient function to prevent fat malabsorption. Pancreatic disease begins *in utero* and is thought to result from decreased volume of pancreatic secretions with decreased concentrations of HCO^{3-}. Without sufficient fluid and HCO^{3-}, digestive proenzymes are retained within small pancreatic ducts and are prematurely activated, ultimately leading to tissue destruction, fibrosis, and fatty replacement. The resulting malabsorption contributes to the failure to meet the increased energy demands because of the hypermetabolic state associated with endobronchial infection. Lung infections may lead to anorexia and vomiting, promoting malnutrition. These factors may exacerbate lung infection leading to a vicious circle of malnutrition and infection.

CLINICAL FEATURES

Typical signs and symptoms for CF are listed in Box 46-1. Symptoms of CF may vary, with monosymptomatic cases often diagnosed late. It is, therefore, important to be aware of the spectrum of symptoms that may arise and initiate adequate diagnostic steps.

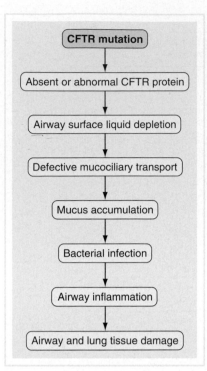

FIGURE 46-4 Sequence of CF pathophysiology.

BOX 46-1 Symptoms of Cystic Fibrosis

Chronic Airway Disease

Chronic productive cough
Airway colonization with CF pathogens (*Staph. aureus*, mucoid *P. aeruginosa*)
Persistent chest radiograph abnormalities
Airway obstruction
Clubbing
Pansinusitis
Nasal polyps

Gastrointestinal Disease

Meconium ileus, distal intestinal obstruction syndrome (DIOS), rectal prolapse
Pancreatic insufficiency, pancreatitis
Biliary cirrhosis
Failure to thrive, edema with hypoproteinemia, deficiency of fat-soluble vitamins

Salt Wasting with Metabolic Alkalosis

Infertility Caused by Obstructive Azoospermia

Although the classical presentation of CF is the combination of chronic productive cough, steatorrhea, and failure to thrive, approximately 10–15% of the patients do not have pancreatic insufficiency clinically. Because the lungs of patients with CF are normal at birth, pulmonary symptoms may not be obvious. Between 10% and 15% of newborn infants with CF may fail to pass meconium, leading to meconium ileus. Meconium ileus is linked to pancreatic insufficiency but per se not associated with more severe clinical disease.

Less common presentations of CF, such as prolonged jaundice in the newborn and rectal prolapse in infants and young children, should trigger diagnostic tests. Occasionally, an infant may have severe malnutrition with anemia, hypoalbuminemia, and edema in the first 4 months of life.

Infertility can be a presenting symptom in adult patients with CF with limited pulmonary symptoms; 98% of males with CF are infertile, with azoospermia secondary to atretic or absent vas deferens. Spermatogenesis and sexual potency are normal. Female reproductive function is normal, although a lower rate of fertility has been postulated because of dehydrated cervical mucus.

Initially pulmonary symptoms of cough will occur only at times of exacerbations, but eventually there is progression to a chronic daily cough productive of sputum. The sputum is initially white, but as infection continues, the mucus becomes thicker and purulent. Minor hemoptysis often occurs at times of exacerbations. Some patients will have an "asthmatic" component to their disease with wheezing, chest tightness, paroxysmal dry cough, and a degree of reversibility in airflow obstruction with bronchodilators. Over time, as pulmonary function declines, there is increasing dyspnea. Hypoxemia is not usually seen until FEV_1 is less than 35% predicted, and hypercarbia usually occurs when the FEV_1 is less than 25 or 30% predicted. Cor pulmonale occurs late in the illness.

Pansinusitis is found on sinus radiographs in most patients, although not all will have symptoms of recurrent sinusitis, headache, and postnasal drip. Nasal polyps are seen in approximately 20% of patients and tend to recur even after surgical removal.

DIAGNOSTIC APPROACH

The diagnosis of CF is established by clinical manifestations. A history of CF in a sibling or a positive newborn screening result in conjunction with laboratory evidence of CFTR dysfunction (see Box 46-1). CFTR dysfunction is documented by either elevated sweat chloride or characteristic abnormalities in nasal potential difference or by CF-causing mutations in the CFTR gene.

A diagnostic algorithm is presented in Figure 46-5. Abnormal ion transport is reflected in high sweat sodium chloride levels, and measurement of chloride concentration in sweat after iontophoresis of pilocarpine is used for diagnosis. Sweat testing must be done using standardized methods, by qualified staff, in an experienced laboratory. A sweat chloride concentration >60 mmol/L on repeated analysis is diagnostic for CF. A sweat chloride concentration of between 30 and 60 mmol/L is considered a borderline result but may be seen in patients with CF.

Diagnosis can be confirmed by genotyping of the most common CFTR mutations, which vary by ethnic origin of the population tested. More than 1500 mutations in CFTR have been reported to the CFTR database. Most commercial screening panels test for less than 50 mutations and will identify 85–90% of CF alleles.

The diagnosis of CF requires the presence of 2 CF-causing mutations. For a mutation to be considered CF causing, it must meet at least one of these criteria: (1) mutation must cause a change in the amino acid sequence that severely affects CFTR synthesis or function, (2) mutation must introduce a premature termination signal (insertion, deletion, or nonsense mutations), (3) mutation must alter the "invariant" nucleotides of intron splice sites (the first or last two nucleotides), or (4) mutation must cause a novel amino acid sequence that

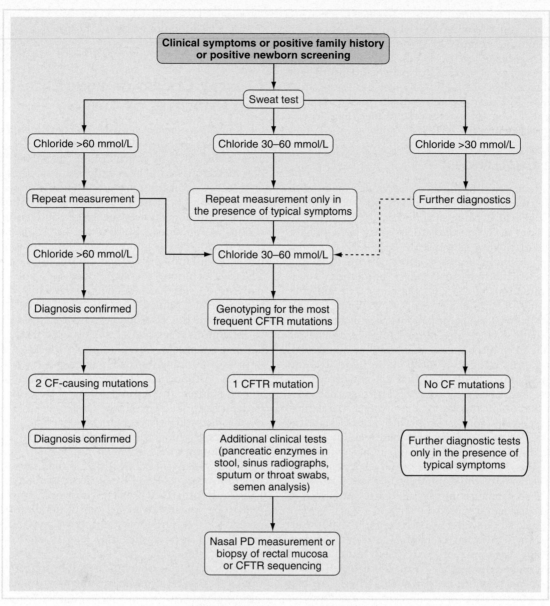

FIGURE 46-5 Diagnostic algorithm.

does not occur in the normal CFTR genes from at least 100 carriers of CF mutations from the patient's ethnic group. Of the more than 1500 CFTR mutations that have been reported, only approximately 30 are considered disease causing to date.

If CFTR genotyping or sweat test is not diagnostic, a second test of CFTR function such as nasal potential difference (NPD) measurement can be performed. The transport of sodium and chloride ions across the nasal mucosa creates a transepithelial electrical potential difference (PD). Changes in PD in response to stimulation or inhibition of ion channels by nasal perfusion can be measured, and there exists a typical normal or CF response. This test is technically difficult and requires a skilled and highly trained operator and thus may not be available in all CF centers. Other techniques to examine CFTR function include analysis of rectal mucosal biopsies in an Ussing chamber.

Clinical tests not directly assessing the CFTR defect can also aid in the diagnostic process. Most patients with CF are pancreatic insufficient, and a decreased concentration of chymotrypsin or pancreas-specific elastase in feces or 72-h stool collection and fecal fat analysis can confirm this. Most patients with CF have total opacification of their paranasal sinuses, and sinus radiography may be helpful. Bacterial pathogens typical for CF (e.g., mucoid *Pseudomonas*, *Staphylococcus aureus*) can be detected in sputum or throat swabs and suggest a CF diagnosis. Obstructive azoospermia is found in 98% of men with CF and is a result of congenital bilateral absence of the vas deferens (CBAVD). The finding of azoospermia or lack of vas deferens on careful urologic examination or transrectal ultrasound is very suggestive of CF.

Fifty percent of all patients with CF in North America are diagnosed by the age of 6 months, and ~90% by the age of 8 years. Neonatal screening has been proposed as early diagnosis and, therefore, earlier initiation of treatment may improve outcome. A randomized screening program in Wisconsin has shown that weight gain and early growth was better in patients diagnosed by neonatal screening. Because good nutrition is linked to a better prognosis, these data would favor the introduction of population-wide neonatal screening. Neonatal screening programs have now been introduced in many countries and are most commonly based on a two-step approach with immune reactive trypsinogen (IRT) in dried blood spots and confirmation by DNA analysis in positive cases. Blood trypsinogen is elevated in pancreatic-insufficient patients in the first weeks of life, but the rate of false-positive results of a single IRT test is high, which can be reduced substantially by inclusions of a second step, including genetic testing for the most common CFTR mutations.

DIAGNOSTIC CHALLENGES

In 5–10% of patients, the diagnosis of CF is not made until adulthood. An increased awareness has led, and will lead, to greater numbers of adults being diagnosed with CF. Most of these people will not have typical features of CF but will have subtle symptoms or single organ disease (CBAVD, recurrent acute pancreatitis, or bronchiectasis). Most patients diagnosed as adults are pancreatic sufficient, have "borderline" sweat tests, and have mutations in the CFTR gene that are not considered CF-causing. Commercial genetic screening panels may have diagnostic limitations for patients seen in adulthood, because they usually include the more common CF-causing mutations usually seen in patients diagnosed in childhood. Those individuals presenting in adulthood are more likely to have less common, "mild" mutations that are not part of the panel. Complete sequencing of the CFTR gene has now become feasible and offers an additional possibility to ascertain the diagnosis, especially for patients with equivocal sweat test results. Nasal PD measurement may be especially helpful in establishing a diagnosis of CF in these patients. Interpretation of these results should be done by an experienced CF physician, who is aware of the limitations of these tests.

Obstructive azoospermia is highly related to mutations in CFTR, and the finding of CBAVD should trigger genetic testing for CF, especially because assisted reproductive techniques allow these men to father children. Up to 80% of men with CBAVD may have one or two CFTR mutations but not other phenotypic features of CF. A diagnosis of CF should not be made in these cases unless diagnostic criteria are met (i.e., sweat test >60 mmol/L or 2 CF-causing mutations or NPD typical for CF). The long-term prognosis for these men is still not certain, including whether typical CF lung disease may develop over time, and thus it is recommended that these men receive appropriate clinical follow-up. The relationship between CFTR mutations and recurrent acute pancreatitis, bronchiectasis, or other sinopulmonary disease is not as strong as that seen with CBAVD. However, a higher than expected prevalence of CFTR mutations is found in these populations.

Despite all these tests, a small number of patients remain in whom a definite diagnosis cannot be made. Typical CF bronchiectasis may be seen in patients who have CFTR mutations that are not considered disease causing and who have a normal or borderline sweat test. Thus, it seems that CF lung disease may occur even with lesser degrees of dysfunction of CFTR. The important message is that presence of CFTR mutations may put patients at risk for significant CF disease developing later in life, and close follow-up is advised.

Discussion of this dilemma is made more confusing by lack of a common and standardized terminology for patients who have evidence of CFTR dysfunction without a definite diagnosis of CF. These patients are being referred to as "atypical CF," "mild CF," "nonclassic CF," or "CFTRopathy" or, if CFTR mutations exist in the absence of lung or gastrointestinal disease, "preCF."

CLINICAL COURSE OF LUNG DISEASE AND PRINCIPLES OF THERAPY

CF lungs are normal at birth. Pathologic studies have shown that the first abnormalities are usually detected in the small airways reflected by mucus plugs and dilatation distal to the obstructed airways. These early abnormalities are often focal and do not necessarily produce clinically apparent symptoms. The disconnect between pathologic abnormalities and pulmonary symptoms is now recognized and has important implications for treatment. Studies that use bronchoalveolar lavage have shown that ongoing airway inflammation is present in patients with mild disease and can be observed early in infancy. The lack of impressive symptoms does not mean that these patients do not have ongoing progressive disease requiring continuous treatment.

Although the traditional approach was to wait for symptoms, a more aggressive strategy is used today. This aggressive approach translates into continuous lifelong treatment, which is time consuming and labor intensive for patients and their families. Although the burden for individuals is considerable, it has changed the natural history of disease progression in patients with CF. The classic course of CF was characterized by chronic productive cough and a gradual, but steady, decline in pulmonary function. Most patients today have rather limited symptoms, and many do not regularly expectorate sputum. Now most patients with CF maintain their pulmonary function over years, reflected in an annual rate of decline in FEV_1 of less than 2% predicted per year. However, it is important to be vigilant about periods of deterioration that present as episodes of pulmonary exacerbations and, unless treated rapidly and aggressively, may lead to an irreversible loss in pulmonary function.

Pulmonary exacerbations are often triggered by viral infections but require prompt treatment with antibiotics directed against pathogens present in respiratory cultures. It is important to recognize the signs of a pulmonary exacerbation early on to avoid permanent damage to the lung. Symptoms of pulmonary exacerbation are outlined in Box 46-2. In general, any increase in symptoms lasting more than a few days, associated with a decline in FEV_1, requires antibiotic therapy. Because most patients are chronically infected with bacteria, suppression rather than eradication of organisms is the primary goal of therapy. Duration of therapy is not guided by changes in sputum bacteriology but rather by improvement in symptoms and pulmonary function.

Because many patients have normal lung function and the annual rate of decline in pulmonary function is rather limited, it has become difficult to assess lung disease by lung function alone. Despite this, FEV_1 remains the best predictor of outcome in patients with CF and is, therefore, used to follow the course of lung disease and to guide treatment. Chest radiographs are performed annually in most centers but have limited sensitivity to detect early abnormalities. High-resolution CT scans can detect abnormalities not detected by conventional radiographs but are associated with a higher cumulative radiation dose and are, therefore, not considered part of routine care at present. There is considerable interest in

BOX 46-2 Symptoms and Signs of a Pulmonary Exacerbation

Symptoms

Increased frequency, duration, and intensity of cough
Increased or new onset of sputum production
Change in sputum appearance
New onset or increased hemoptysis
Increased shortness of breath and decreased exercise tolerance
Decrease in overall well-being—increased fatigue, weakness, fever, poor appetite

Physical Signs

Increased work of breathing—intercostal retractions and use of accessory muscles
Increased respiratory rate
New onset or increased crackles on chest examination
Increased air trapping
Fever
Weight loss

Laboratory Findings

Decrease in FEV_1 of 10% or greater compared with best value in previous 6 months
Increased air trapping and/or new infiltrate on chest radiograph
Leukocytosis
Decreased Sa_{O_2}

Adapted from Gibson and Ramsey, AJRCCM 2003.

developing more sensitive outcome parameters assessing function, structure, infection, and inflammation that will help to guide treatment, but currently these tests have a limited role outside of research studies.

Fighting bacterial infections and avoiding lung function decline are key aspects of CF treatment; regular assessments not only of the clinical status, but also of lung function and sputum microbiology, are, therefore, warranted. Quarterly clinic visits, at which these tests are performed, are considered to be standard in CF care, but some patients require more frequent follow-up.

THERAPY

Gene Replacement Therapy and Pharmacologic Treatment of the Underlying Defect

CF is caused by deficient or absent CFTR, and it is, therefore, logical to attempt gene replacement therapy as a form of curative treatment. Gene therapy trials so far have targeted the respiratory tract directly. A number of vector systems have been tested in human trials, but adenoviruses and cationic lipids are the two most commonly used vectors. Even though some transient effect on CFTR expression and function has been achieved, no study could demonstrate a long-lasting effect. Viral vectors seem to be more efficient than cationic lipids but have the disadvantage of being immunogenic. Although attempts are ongoing to overcome these shortcomings, gene therapy is currently not a therapeutic option for patients with CF.

Another approach to treat the underlying defect is CFTR pharmacotherapy aiming to improve trafficking, expression, or function of CFTR. For patients carrying class I stop mutations, which lead to decreased mRNA production, treatment with aminoglycosides or derivatives have been shown to increase CFTR expression, and clinical trials are currently under way to assess the clinical benefits of this therapy. Because most patients do not carry stop mutations, this approach addresses only a small fraction of the CF population. For the most common mutation, DF508$\triangle$, misfolded CFTR is degraded in the endoplasmic reticulum before reaching the cell membrane. Because this misfolded CFTR does have chloride-conducting function, compounds that affect intracellular trafficking, called chaperones, may provide clinical benefit. Some studies have provided proof of concept. Compounds detected through high-throughput screening programs will be tested in clinical trials in the near future.

An alternative to CFTR pharmacotherapy is to activate other chloride channels present in the apical surface of epithelial cells or to inhibit sodium hyperabsorption. This concept seems attractive, because CF mice lacking CFTR do not develop lung disease, and this may be due to better function of alternative chloride channels. Two activators of alternative chloride channels are currently being tested in clinical trials, but efficacy data are not available to date.

Symptomatic Treatment

In the absence of a proven curative treatment regimen, symptomatic therapy is still the mainstay of CF therapy. Most of the treatment approaches are directed to interrupting the cycle of mucus retention, infection, and inflammation. Early initiation of treatment is important to avoid permanent damage to the lung.

Airway Clearance

Chest physiotherapy remains the backbone of airway clearance and is recommended for all patients. Short-term benefits have been demonstrated for many techniques, but long-term efficacy data are limited. The most commonly used techniques are manual percussion, positive expiratory pressure (PEP) mask therapy, and autogenic drainage. In addition, techniques that provide vibration to the airways actively or passively are being used. There is ongoing debate as to which technique provides the best efficacy for patients with CF. Physical activity and exercise are considered important adjuncts to physiotherapy, because impairments in exercise tolerance have been linked to poorer prognosis.

Airway secretions in CF are highly viscous, and it, therefore, intuitively makes sense to use drugs that reduce the viscoelasticity of sputum. Classic mucolytics such as N-acetylcysteine have little effect on lung disease in CF, although they are being revisited because of their potential benefit as antioxidants. Their ineffectiveness as a mucolytic may be because CF mucus contains little mucin and is mainly composed of pus. Recombinant human DNase (rhDNase) administered by inhalation has been found to reduce sputum viscosity, improve pulmonary function, and reduce the number of pulmonary exacerbations both in patients with moderate and mild lung disease. There are also data suggesting that it reduces inflammation in the airways. Hypertonic saline has been assessed as another potential drug to improve airway clearance, and recent studies suggest that it may also increase airway surface liquid. The effect on lung function seems to be smaller than that of rhDNase, but these therapies have different mechanisms of action and can, therefore, not be viewed as being virtually exclusive.

Management of Airway Infection

Aggressive treatment of airway infection is one of the main reasons for the increased life expectancy of patients with CF that has been achieved over the last decades. Bacterial pathogens in patients with CF are usually limited to a relatively small spectrum of pathogens with *S. aureus* or *H. influenzae* being most prominent in younger patients. Most patients go through phases of clinical stability with intermittent pulmonary exacerbations. A set of criteria is used to diagnose pulmonary exacerbations (see Box 46-2), but the threshold for initiating targeted antibiotic therapy should be rather low. Antistaphylococcal antibiotics are usually administered for periods of 2–4 weeks. Patients with CF have differences in drug clearance and require dosages approximately 50% higher than individuals without CF. Many CF physicians try to eradicate bacteria from CF airways with courses of oral antibiotics even in the absence of symptoms. Prophylactic antistaphylococcal therapy with flucloxacillin initiated from the time of diagnosis is also used in some centers. Although one small study has reported a lower rate of cough and hospital admissions during the first 2 years of life, continuous antistaphylococcal therapy was associated with a higher rate of *P. aeruginosa* acquisition in two other studies, in which mainly cephalosporins were used. *P. aeruginosa* infection increases pulmonary inflammation and has a negative effect on lung function, when this pathogen persists. At present, there is insufficient evidence to support the use of prophylactic antistaphylococcal therapy in patients with CF.

Overall *P. aeruginosa* is the major pathogen in CF lung disease. Its prevalence increases with age, and most adult patients are chronically infected with this organism. After an initial transient colonization period with nonmucoid strains, untreated patients generally become chronically infected with mucoid strains of *P. aeruginosa*. Antibiotic therapy usually fails to eradicate mucoid *P. aeruginosa* from the airways. High bacterial counts, low metabolic rate of pathogens in biofilms, poor penetration of antibiotics into airway secretions, as well as anaerobic conditions in sputum, are considered to be responsible for this finding. Chronic infection with mucoid strains has a negative impact on the subsequent course of lung disease.

Although eradication is virtually impossible in chronic infection, treatment has been shown to be effective in the early phase of *P. aeruginosa* infection. A major improvement in the fight against *P. aeruginosa* infection in patients with CF is early antibiotic therapy. Both inhaled antibiotic therapy with tobramycin alone and the combination of inhaled antibiotics with oral ciprofloxacin have been used successfully. Although the optimal treatment regimen for early *P. aeruginosa* infection has yet to be determined, this treatment regimen successfully reduces the incidence of chronic airway infection with *P. aeruginosa* in patients with CF.

To avoid adverse effects and to obtain high drug concentrations in airways, inhaled antibiotic therapy is the treatment of choice for maintenance therapy in patients infected with *P. aeruginosa*. The best evidence is currently available for inhaled tobramycin, which has been shown to improve lung function and reduce pulmonary exacerbations in chronically infected patients. In addition, colistin is being used off label for inhalation. Although colistin has the advantage that the rate of resistant strains is rather low, its short-term efficacy has been found to be inferior to inhaled tobramycin. In addition to inhaled antibiotics, azithromycin has been shown to improve pulmonary function and reduce pulmonary exacerbations in patients with *P. aeruginosa*–positive disease. Although macrolides have no efficacy against *P. aeruginosa* when tested in routine cultures, there is some evidence that they may affect *P. aeruginosa* growing in biofilms. Whether this explains their efficacy or whether this is due to antiinflammatory properties of macrolides is still unclear. Common treatment options for antibiotic therapy are displayed in Table 46-1.

Pulmonary exacerbations are usually treated with intravenous antibiotic therapy. Combination therapy with a semisynthetic penicillin (such as Piperacillin), a third-generation cephalosporin (i.e., ceftazidime), or a carbapenem (imipenem or meropenem) with an aminoglycoside (most frequently tobramycin) is administered for a period of 2–3 weeks. Oral ciprofloxacin is used for less severe exacerbations. Some centers treat chronically infected patients with routine

TABLE 46-1 **Options for Oral and Inhaled Antibiotic Therapy**			
Pathogen	**Antibiotic**	**Pediatric Dose**	**Adult Dose**
Staphylococcus aureus	Choose one:		
	Dicloxacillin	6.25–12.5 mg/kg four times daily	250–500 mg four times daily
	Cephalexin	12.5–25 mg/kg four times daily	500 mg four times daily
	Amoxicillin/clavulanate	12.5–22.5 mg/kg of amoxicillin component twice a day	400–875 mg of amoxicillin component twice a day
Haemophilus influenzae	Choose one:		
	Amoxicillin	25–50 mg/kg twice a day	500–875 mg twice a day
	Amoxicillin/clavulanate	12.5–22.5 mg/kg of amoxicillin component twice a day	400–875 mg of amoxicillin component twice a day
	Cefuroxime axetil	15–20 mg/kg twice a day	250–500 mg twice a day
Pseudomonas aeruginosa	Choose one:		
	Ciprofloxacin	10–15 mg/kg twice a day	750 mg twice a day
	Tobramycin by inhalation	300 mg by nebulizer, twice a day	300 mg by nebulizer, twice a day
	Colistin via inhalation	150 mg by nebulizer, twice a day	150 mg by nebulizer, twice a day

Adapted from Gibson and Ramsey, AJRCCM, 2003.

intravenous antibiotic therapy every 3 months regardless of respiratory symptoms, but this approach has not yet been supported by sufficient evidence.

Treatment of the less common gram-negative organisms (*Burkholderia cepacia complex*, *Alcaligenes xylosoxidans*, and *Stenotrophomonas maltophilia*) can be challenging. These organisms are inherently multiresistant. Although some species of the *B. cepacia* complex, such as *B. cenocepacia*, are associated with a more rapid decline and can also cause cepacia syndrome, a rapidly fatal septic syndrome, the relevance of other gram-negative bacteria is less clear, and it is not established at present whether they are responsible for causing disease.

For patients chronically infected with *B. cepacia* complex, doxycycline or trimethoprim-sulfamethoxazole is effective for minor exacerbations. For more severe infections, the best antibiotic combination is meropenem, high-dose inhaled tobramycin in combination with either ceftazidime, chloramphenicol, or trimethoprim-sulfamethoxazole. Treatment of exacerbations with *B. cepacia* may require prolonged antibiotic therapy (weeks to months) before a clinical response is seen. Use of pulmonary function, WBC, and markers of inflammation (CRP or ESR) may be helpful to guide therapy. Genotyping has shown that the organisms present at times of exacerbation are the same as when the patient is clinically stable, but the bacterial density is higher during exacerbations. Thus, choice of antimicrobial therapy on the basis of the most recent sputum cultures is indicated.

S. maltophilia can be treated with trimethoprim-sulfamethoxazole or doxycycline. Because *S. maltophilia* isolates can develop resistance during treatment, trimethoprim-sulfamethoxazole is commonly combined with a second antibiotic, such as ticarcillin-clavulanate or levofloxacin. *A. xylosoxidans* can be challenging to treat, but options include imipenem and piperacillin. Inhaled colistin may also be effective, because *in vitro* studies have demonstrated that high concentrations of colistin inhibit most strains of *A. xylosoxidans*.

Because patient-to-patient transmission of bacterial pathogens occurs, separation regimens have been implemented to prevent cross-infection in patients with CF. This is particularly important with *B. cepacia*, because person-to-person transmission has been proven, and chronic infection with this organism is associated with a worse clinical outcome. Vaccines are being developed against *P. aeruginosa*, but their efficacy is currently not proven.

Inflammation

CF is characterized by an intense, neutrophil-dominated airway inflammation. Early trials of antiinflammatory treatment have been performed with corticosteroids. Oral prednisone (1–2 mg/kg body weight every other day) was found to reduce lung function decline in *P. aeruginosa*–positive patients, but serious side effects such as glucose intolerance, growth retardation, and cataracts were found in prednisone-treated patients. Inhaled steroids, although widely used in patients with CF, have not been shown to improve lung function and airway inflammation. Treatment is, therefore, not indicated unless patients have demonstrated airway hyperreactivity that is present in 25–40% of patients with CF. High-dose ibuprofen has been shown to slow lung function decline in patients with CF in a single center trial, but this has not been replicated. Even though other drugs targeting specific elements of CF

airway inflammation have been studied, none has been proven to be both efficacious and safe.

Lung Transplantation

Double lung or heart lung transplantation is a therapeutic option for patients with CF with end-stage lung disease. Determining the timing for transplant remains challenging, and there have been many attempts to develop prediction models to help with this assessment. A patient must be ill enough that there would be a survival benefit from transplant, but not so sick that they would die on the waiting list. FEV_1 less than 30% predicted in a patient receiving maximal medical treatment has been found to be the best indicator, because generally it predicts a median survival of 2 years. However, one must also take into consideration the length of the waiting list for the transplant center. Generally, survival is better for adults than for children, but a survival benefit through lung transplantation has also been reported in children. Survival is significantly worse for patients infected with *B. cepacia* complex, particularly *B. cenocepacia*, and most centers consider *B. cenocepacia* infection a contraindication for transplantation. However, the Toronto group has shown that, even in these high-risk patients, transplantation improves survival. Currently, worldwide transplant experience (ISHLT data) has shown a 1-year survival after transplantation of 80%, 5-year survival of 55%, and 10-year survival of 35%.

Pancreatic Insufficiency and Malnutrition

Patients with CF with poor nutritional status are more prone to chest infections, and poor nutritional status is linked to worse prognosis. An aggressive approach to maintain normal weight in patients with CF is, therefore, warranted. This is achieved by assuring a high-fat, high-caloric diet with adequate replacement of pancreatic enzymes. If this cannot be achieved through oral intake, enteral feeding by nasogastric tube or gastrostomy tube is used to maintain adequate nutritional status and normal growth. Malabsorption is frequently not completely corrected with pancreatic enzyme replacement caused by multiple factors, including incomplete dissolution of the pH-sensitive enteric coating in the proximal small bowel because of lack of neutralization of gastric acid by pancreatic bicarbonate. Use of medications to reduce gastric acidity may improve the effectiveness of enzymes in some patients.

Infertility and Pregnancy

Although 98% of men with CF are infertile, with azoospermia secondary to absent vas deferens, spermatogenesis and sexual potency are normal and men with CF can become fathers with assisted reproductive techniques such as microscopic epididymal sperm aspiration in conjunction with *in vitro* fertilization.

Female reproductive function is normal, although a lower rate of fertility has been postulated because of dehydrated cervical mucus. In general, pregnancy is well tolerated in women with CF, and many studies have shown that pregnancy does not have a negative impact on survival. If women have reasonable lung function (FEV_1 >50% predicted), a stable clinical condition, and adequate nutritional status (BMI >19), the fetal and maternal outcomes are good. It is important to closely monitor maternal weight gain during pregnancy and to check for gestational diabetes in each trimester. Genetic testing for CF mutations in the partner is recommended for both men and women with CF who wish to have children.

COMPLICATIONS

Pulmonary Complications

Pneumothorax

Pneumothorax occurs in patients with more severe lung disease and lower lung function, and thus is usually seen in older children and adults. Rupture of emphysematous lung may result in spontaneous pneumothorax. Treatment is challenging, because it may be difficult to expand the fibrotic and infected lung. Pneumothoraces are often recurrent. Chest tube drainage is usually required, and a small-gauge tube is preferred to minimize pain. Good analgesia is necessary to allow chest physiotherapy to continue and prevent worsening pulmonary infection. Chemical pleurodesis with doxycycline, talc, or thoracoscopic surgery may be required to treat recurrent pneumothoraces, although this may not be effective in all cases. If there is an ongoing air leak despite these interventions, surgical pleurodesis may be necessary. Pleurodesis was considered a contraindication to lung transplantation because of problems with removal of the lung at transplant and bleeding complications, but now most centers will transplant patients who have had medical or surgical manipulation of their pleural space.

Hemoptysis

Chronic pulmonary infection leads to enlargement of the bronchial artery circulation supplying the lung. Hemoptysis is not uncommon even in patients with mild lung disease and usually indicates infection. Vitamin K deficiency caused by pancreatic insufficiency can contribute to the problem. Massive hemoptysis (defined as >250 mL of blood in 24 h) is less common but occasionally can be life threatening. (See Chapter 24.) Hemoptysis is usually treated with antibiotic therapy. Vitamin K and tranexamic acid may also be used. Ongoing massive hemoptysis requires bronchial artery embolization. Angiography is used to locate the abnormal bronchial artery vessels. These vessels are aberrant, and arteries arising from one side may supply contralateral segments of the lung. Because location of the bleeding does not always correlate with origin of abnormal bronchial arteries, bronchoscopy to locate source of bleeding is not helpful. However, bronchoscopy may be necessary to manage the airway in life-threatening hemoptysis. Embolization should be performed by experienced interventional radiologists because of potential complications of bronchial artery embolization, including infarction of the esophagus, lung parenchyma, or chest wall (causing dysphagia or severe chest pain), and transverse myelitis caused by accidental embolization of the spinal arteries.

Allergic Bronchopulmonary Aspergillosis (ABPA)

Although aspergillus is frequently detected in sputum cultures, most of these patients do not have symptoms that can be attributed to the presence of the fungus. A fraction of patients with CF have symptoms caused by hypersensitivity. This entity is called allergic bronchopulmonary aspergillosis (ABPA) and should be suspected in patients who have respiratory deterioration but do not respond well to antibiotic therapy. In addition to symptoms of chronic productive cough, ABPA is usually accompanied by asthmatic features (wheezing), and patients may expectorate gritty brown sputum ("sandy" sputum). Some of the features of ABPA are difficult to assess in CF, because bronchiectasis, wheezing, productive

cough, and the presence of *Aspergillus* in the sputum are common features of CF lung disease. Diagnosis is supported by elevated IgE (usually >1000 IU/mL), a positive skin test, and serum precipitins against *Aspergillus* (see Chapter 53). Treatment of symptoms and decline in lung function requires corticosteroids; high doses (1–2 mg/kg body weight) may be required initially before the dose can be tapered. Adjunctive antifungal therapy with itraconazole has been found to be efficacious in patients without CF with ABPA, but its efficacy in patients with CF remains to be proven. Duration of ABPA therapy is tailored to clinical response, improvement of FEV_1, and normalization of serum IgE levels.

Gastrointestinal Complications

Pancreas

Pancreatic insufficiency is present in most patients from birth and occurs when >98% of the pancreas has been destroyed. Malabsorption of fat leads to malnutrition and deficiency of fat-soluble vitamins (A, D, E, and K). Approximately 10–15% of patients have sufficient pancreatic function so that pancreatic enzyme replacement is not needed (pancreatic sufficiency [PS]). Acute pancreatitis, which may be recurrent, will develop in ∼20% of these patients with PS, and some will have ongoing destruction of the pancreas and become pancreatic insufficient (PI).

Distal Intestinal Obstruction Syndrome (DIOS)

Undigested fat, mucus from the gastrointestinal tract, swallowed sputum, and reduced water in the small bowel result in thick, sticky bowel contents. Partial bowel obstruction, usually at the ileocecal junction, can cause recurrent right lower quadrant (RLQ) pain and occasionally altered bowel habit. This condition occurs in ∼15–20% of patients and is called distal intestinal obstruction syndrome (DIOS). The diagnosis is made clinically from the history and palpation of a tender mass in the RLQ along with evidence of fecal collection in the RLQ on abdominal imaging. DIOS rarely causes complete bowel obstruction, elevated WBC, or fever, so if these features are present, other causes of abdominal pain such as intussusception, appendicitis/appendiceal abscess, and C. *difficile* colitis should be considered. Treatment requires large volumes of intestinal lavage solution (Golytely, Peglyte) to clear the bowel. Occasionally, enemas with water-soluble, osmotic agents such as Gastrografin or Hypaque (diatrizoate sodium) are needed. Prevention of recurrent DIOS should focus on adequate use of pancreatic enzyme replacement and use of mineral oil or polyethylene glycol.

Intussusception can occur in 1–2% of children and young adults with CF and may mimic DIOS. The location of the intussusception is usually ileo-ileo but may be ileo-colic. Intussusception may be recurrent and asymptomatic but can cause small bowel obstruction and be associated with intermittent severe colicky abdominal pain, a palpable mass, and vomiting.

CF Liver Disease

Infants may have cholestasis from abnormally concentrated and sticky bile. Fatty infiltration of the liver may be seen, but its significance is uncertain. CFTR is expressed in cells of the biliary tract and plugging of the small intralobular ducts, periductal inflammation and fibrosis can occur. Focal biliary cirrhosis is the most common feature of CF liver disease but is very difficult to detect. Autopsy studies suggest that it is present in up to 70% of adults with CF. Approximately one third of patients have abnormal liver function tests, but the presence of abnormality does not correlate very well with the presence or extent of liver disease. Hepatocellular function is generally preserved. Focal biliary cirrhosis progresses to multinodular cirrhosis and portal hypertension in ~5% of patients. Liver disease is a life-limiting factor in only a few patients, and liver transplantation is rarely indicated, because hepatocellular failure is very rare. A small, poorly functioning "micro gallbladder" is commonly found, and cholesterol gallstones develop in up to 10% of patients with CF. Choledocholithiasis is less common. Ursodeoxycholic acid has been shown to normalize elevated liver enzyme levels, but its long-term effect on the evolution of liver disease remains largely unproven.

CF-Related Diabetes

Langerhans cell function is initially retained, and diabetes mellitus is rare in the first decade in patients with CF. The prevalence of glucose intolerance and diabetes mellitus rises continuously with increasing age, and ~15–25% of adults with CF and PI will have diabetes requiring insulin therapy. CF-related diabetes (CFRD) shares features of both type I and II diabetes with a combination of decreased and delayed insulin secretion, as well as insulin resistance. Glucose intolerance can persist for many years before frank diabetes occurs. Control of diabetes is important to prevent protein catabolism and weight loss. Poorly controlled diabetes may increase pulmonary infections. Most patients will require treatment with insulin. During pulmonary exacerbations, increased insulin resistance can temporarily raise insulin needs threefold to fourfold. Patients with CFRD with poor blood glucose control develop microvascular complications but rarely show macrovascular complications.

Malignancy

A review of CF clinics in North America and Europe found that there was an increased prevalence of gastrointestinal malignancies in people with CF. The proposed etiology is the chronic injury/inflammation of the gastrointestinal tract. The increased risk starts in the third decade, and the malignancies are found in all parts of the gastrointestinal tract (colon, esophagus, small bowel, pancreas, liver, and biliary tree). The odds ratio for the risk of digestive tract malignancies in patients with CF is 6.5 (95% confidence interval, 3.5–11.1). Screening is difficult because of the widespread nature of the cancers and overall low prevalence but may be indicated in patients referred for lung transplantation, those with a family history of gastrointestinal cancers, and those with GE reflux. New gastrointestinal symptoms should trigger appropriate diagnostic tests.

CF-Related Bone Disease

Adults with CF have evidence of decreased bone density, including osteopenia and osteoporosis, as measured by bone dual energy X-ray absorptiometry (DEXA). Prevalence of low bone density in adults with CF ranges from 40–70%, and up to 50% of adults with severe lung disease who are awaiting transplantation will have osteoporosis. The etiology of the decreased bone density is multifactorial, and both failure of normal bone formation and excessive bone loss occur. Malnutrition, vitamin D and K deficiency, hypogonadism, increased bone loss because of elevated inflammatory cytokines from chronic pulmonary infection, and use of corticosteroids all may play a role in the development of low bone density. It is not completely clear whether DEXA scans predict fracture risk in patients with CF. A consensus report suggests treatment with calcium and vitamin D supplementation, treatment of hypogonadism if present, promotion of exercise, treatment of pulmonary infection, and use of bisphosphonates in patients with osteoporosis, those receiving corticosteroids, or those on the transplant list.

Hypertrophic pulmonary osteoarthropathy (HPOA) is a chronic proliferative periostitis and is associated with digital clubbing. It can cause severe bony pain and swelling especially in knees, ankles, and wrists. It frequently flares at times of pulmonary exacerbations, improving with treatment of the lung infection. Radiography confirms the typical periosteal new bone formation at the distal ends of long bones.

Episodic arthropathy occurs in approximately 5–10% of people with CF and presents as transient episodes of acute swelling and joint pain involving single or multiple large or small joints. These episodes do not necessarily correlate with pulmonary exacerbations. This is a nonerosive arthropathy and responds to nonsteroidal antiinflammatory drugs or corticosteroids.

Approximately 1–2% of patients with CF will have a cutaneous vasculitis develop that on biopsy is a leukocytoclastic vasculitis. Systemic involvement is very rare. It is usually seen on the lower extremities, and the rash consists of purpura that is usually painless. This typically resolves spontaneously and specific treatment is not required.

Prognosis

When CF was first described, the median survival was less than 2 years of age. With improvements in therapy, institution of a high-caloric, high-fat diet to optimize growth and nutrition, and establishment of multidisciplinary CF care centers, the survival has steadily improved (median survival, 37 years). CF should no longer be thought of as a pediatric disease as, in Canada, 50% of patients with CF are now adults.

A number of factors have been shown to influence prognosis in patients with CF. For many decades, there has been a gender gap noted, with males having better survival. Although this gender-related difference in survival is decreasing, it still exists. The etiology is unclear and does not seem to be related to pulmonary function or nutritional status. Other factors influencing survival in CF include nutritional status, socioeconomic status, and presence of chronic infection with *P. aeruginosa* or *B. cepacia complex*.

CONCLUSIONS

Overall, CF treatment has been one of medicine's success stories, because the increase in life expectancy achieved over the last decades has been rather impressive. Although the understanding of the disease process has greatly advanced with the definition of the underlying abnormality, treatment is still largely targeted at the downstream consequences of the CFTR defect (mucus retention, infection, and inflammation). There is considerable promise that in the near future therapies that will lead to partial or complete correction of CFTR function, as well as more efficient symptomatic therapies, will become available. Even if these therapies fail in completely correcting the underlying defect, they may be sufficiently efficacious to prevent clinical deterioration. Thus, CF may still continue to be a chronic disease requiring long-term treatment but may cease to be life shortening.

SUGGESTED READINGS

Borowitz D, Baker RD, Stallings V: Consensus Report on Nutrition for Pediatric Patients with Cystic Fibrosis. J Pediatr Gastroenterol Nutr 2002; 35:246–259.

Boucher RC: An overview of the pathogenesis of cystic fibrosis lung disease. Adv Drug Del Rev 2002; 54:1359–1371.

Davis PB: CF since 1938. Am J Respir Crit Care Med 2006; 173:475–482.

Gibson RL, Burns JL, Ramsey BW: Pathophysiology and management of pulmonary infections in cystic fibrosis. Am J Respir Crit Care Med 2003; 168:918–951.

Knowles MR, Durie PR: What is cystic fibrosis? N Engl J Med 2002; 347 (6):439–442.

Ratjen F, Döring G: Cystic fibrosis. Lancet 2003; 361:681–689.

Rosenstein RJ, Cutting GR: The diagnosis of CF: A consensus statement. J Pediatr 1998; 132:589–595.

Rowe SM, Miller S, Sorscher EJ: Mechanisms of disease: Cystic fibrosis. N Engl J Med 2005; 352:1992–2001.

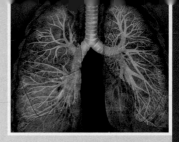

47 Lung Tumors

DAVID E. MIDTHUN • JAMES R. JETT

Lung cancer is now the most commonly diagnosed cancer worldwide according to the International Agency for Research. There are an estimated 1.35 million new cases per year, and at 1.18 million deaths annually, this is the leading cause of cancer death. This prevalence is alarming given that, at the turn of the twentieth century, lung cancer was a rare malignancy. The 5-year survival for lung cancer in the United States and Europe is currently approximately 16% and speaks to the devastation caused by this cancer (Figure 47-1). The frequent presence and lethal nature of lung cancer has established its position in the forefront of problems in pulmonary medicine.

The term *lung cancer* is used to describe cancer that arises in the airways or pulmonary parenchyma. Lung cancer is classified into primarily two subgroups: small-cell lung cancer (SCLC) and nonsmall-cell lung cancer (NSCLC). The distinction in subgroups is essential with regard to treatment and prognosis. Approximately 95% of all lung cancers fall into either SCLC or NSCLC categories (Table 47-1). Although lung cancer and bronchogenic carcinoma are terms often used synonymously, tumors of other rare cell types compose the other 5% of cancers that originate in the lung. Most of this chapter is devoted to a discussion of SCLC and NSCLC. Carcinoid tumor, lymphoma, mucoepidermoid carcinoma, adenoid cystic carcinoma, hamartoma, and lung metastasis are discussed at the end of the chapter.

EPIDEMIOLOGY, PATHOGENESIS, AND PATHOLOGY

Epidemiology

Cigarette smoke is by far the number one cause of lung cancer. The relationship between smoking and lung cancer was initially reported in the 1940s and was further established from epidemiologic research in the 1950s. The first U.S. Surgeon General's *Report on Smoking and Health* was published in 1964 and concluded that cigarette smoking was causally related to lung cancer.

In 1965, 52% of men and 34% of women in the United States older than age 18 years were cigarette smokers. The percentages of smokers have declined to current levels of approximately 25% for men and 19% for women. Smoking rates in many countries in Europe and Asia have been equivalent to or higher than in the United States. According to 2002 data from the World Health Organization, approximately one third of all men worldwide smoke, and approximately 15 billion cigarettes are sold daily. Smoking rates for men in China are 67% and for women 4%, and one in three cigarettes smoked daily worldwide is in China. Smoking rates in Europe vary by country with approximately 30–40% of men and 15–30% of women smoking. Worldwide each day 80,000–100,000 children start smoking, and approximately half of these are in Asia. Approximately 1 of every 5 deaths results from smoking, and long-term studies estimate that approximately half of all regular smokers are eventually killed by their habit.

According to most reported series, approximately 85–90% of lung cancer occurs in smokers or former smokers. Cigarette smoking is identified as the major cause of each of the histologic types of lung cancer: small cell, squamous cell, large cell, and adenocarcinoma. The risk of lung cancer developing increases with the number of cigarettes smoked, earlier age at which smoking started, and longer duration of smoking. Cigarette smoke contains more than 4000 chemical constituents, some of which have been identified as carcinogens. Smoking is also associated with the formation of cancers of the larynx, pharynx, mouth, esophagus, pancreas, and bladder. Current smokers of one pack a day for 20 years have a rate of lung cancer 10 to 15 times that of someone who has never smoked. The risk increases to 20 to 25 times if two or more packs per day of cigarettes are consumed for a similar duration (Figure 47-2). The British physician study showed the risk of lung cancer remains elevated long after smoking cessation and declines for 15 years to then remain approximately twice that of someone who has never smoked. Results of the Multiple Risk Factor Intervention Trial were similar. After 10.5 years of follow-up, 119 men who were smokers or former smokers at entry died of lung cancer compared with no lung cancer deaths among men who reported never smoking. The lag time for a significant reduction in lung cancer death from smoking cessation was many years. Even if cigarette consumption ceased today, the current epidemic of lung cancer would persist for decades.

Passive smoking is sidestream smoke that is unintentionally inhaled by someone in the presence of a smoker. A number of epidemiologic studies have evaluated passive smoking and the risk of lung cancer. Studies that involved women who never smoked but who lived with a smoking husband suggest a 1.2 to 2 times increase in lung cancer risk compared with nonsmoking women in smoke-free homes. There does not seem to be a threshold for tobacco carcinogenesis. Passive smoking is estimated to account for approximately 3000 new cases of lung cancer per year in the United States. Recognition of the deleterious effect of passive smoking has led many cities and a few states in the United States to pass bans on smoking in public places, including bars and restaurants.

Radon exposure is perhaps the greatest element of lung cancer risk for neversmokers who have not been exposed to asbestos. Radon is a decay product of naturally occurring radium, which, in turn, is a breakdown product of uranium.

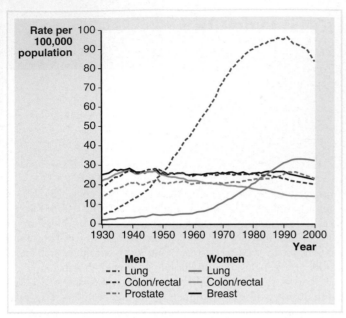

FIGURE 47-1 United States cancer death rates. (From Jemal A, Murray T, Samuels A, *et al*: Cancer statistics, 2003. CA, Cancer J Clin 2003; 53:5–26).

TABLE 47-1 Lung Cancer Classification

Category	Incidence (%)
Small-cell lung cancer	20
Non–small-cell lung cancer	75
Adenocarcinoma	35
Squamous cell carcinoma	30
Large-cell carcinoma	10
Others	5
Carcinoid tumors	—
Pulmonary lymphoma	—
Mucoepidermoid carcinoma	—
Adenoid cystic carcinoma	—
Sarcomas	—

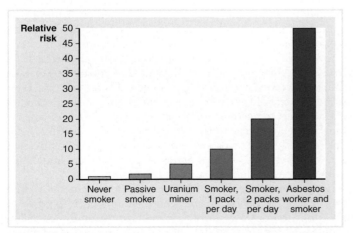

FIGURE 47-2 Approximate relative risk factors for lung cancer.

Radon is present in indoor and outdoor air, and the relative risk of lung cancer seems to increase linearly with exposure. The Committee on Biological Effects of Ionizing Radiation reported that radon in the general environment is responsible for 10% of all lung cancers in the United States, placing it as the second most frequent cause of lung cancer. The U.S. Environmental Protection Agency has established acceptable levels for annual exposure to radon and has advised that most houses be tested for radon.

Air pollution from motor vehicles, factory emissions, and wood and coal burning heaters has been shown to contain carcinogens. The degree of risk related to air pollution is difficult to quantify, but it is estimated to cause 1–2% of all lung cancer.

A clear association exists between asbestos exposure and lung cancer, although the increased risk is generally not observed until 20 or more years after the initial exposure. A naturally occurring, fibrous silicate ubiquitous in the soil, asbestos was commercially used in the construction industry and for its fire-retardant properties. There are different types of asbestos fibers, and some are more carcinogenic than others. A combination of asbestos exposure and cigarette smoking results in an approximate 50-fold increase in the risk of lung cancer compared with someone who has never smoked and has not been exposed to asbestos. Exposures to other materials that have been shown to cause lung cancer include chromium, nickel, and arsenic.

Dietary factors also seem to play a role in the eventual development of lung cancer. In retrospective case-controlled studies, fruit consumption was suggested to be protective, although results of prospective studies have been mixed. Vegetable consumption has been associated with decreased lung cancer risk. No protective role has been found for retinol, but studies support a protective role for beta-carotene and vitamin C. However, three randomized controlled trials failed to show a protective effect of supplementation with beta-carotene—an increased risk for lung cancer was found among heavy smokers in the alpha-Tocopherol beta-Carotene Cancer Prevention Study.

An inherited susceptibility for lung cancer has recently been established. A family history of lung cancer is recognized as predicting approximately a twofold increased risk after controlling for smoking, but a lung cancer gene per se has not yet been identified. Squamous cell carcinoma seems to be most associated with familial clustering of lung cancer. Women may be at greater risk than men who have an equivalent smoking history. An increasing number of genetic abnormalities are recognized in resected lung cancers. Genetic predisposition may result from a difference in carcinogen metabolism, genetic instability of DNA repair processes, or altered oncogene expression.

Studies have shown that chronic obstructive pulmonary disease is a risk factor for lung cancer over and above the risk from cigarette smoking. Presence of airflow obstruction on pulmonary function testing was associated with a four to six times greater risk of lung cancer when controlled for cigarette smoking. The association of airflow obstruction and lung cancer was further supported by the Lung Health Study, in which 5800 patients who had mild airway obstruction and a history of smoking were assessed for effectiveness of smoking cessation and anticholinergic therapy. Lung cancer was the leading cause of death during the 5 years of follow-up for this study. Whether airflow obstruction predisposes to lung cancer or whether both arise from a common factor is unclear.

PATHOGENESIS

The current understanding of the pathogenesis of lung cancer is that of a multistep process of carcinogen-induced genetic damage to cells that proceeds through the stages of initiation, promotion, and progression. The increased incidence of lung cancer with aging and the pathologic change of bronchial epithelium from dysplasia to carcinoma *in situ* in smokers are consistent with a multistep process. The mechanism by which smoking causes lung cancer is not completely understood. Components of cigarette smoke have been shown to initiate and promote the process of carcinogenesis. Genetic changes have also been demonstrated in respiratory epithelial cells of histologically normal appearance obtained from smokers.

Greater recognition of the genetic changes that occur in lung cancer will lead to a better understanding of its pathogenicity. Gene expression arrays have shown gene expression patterns in lung cancer are highly variable and upregulation or downregulation of genes is inconsistent. Early-stage cancers have shown a number of genetic and molecular alterations, including mutations in the p53 tumor suppressor gene and K-ras proto-oncogene, hypermethylation of the p16 tumor suppressor gene, and loss of chromosome heterozygosity. Both SCLC and NSCLC have been shown to contain certain chromosomal abnormalities. K-ras mutations are present in approximately 30% of adenocarcinomas and are uncommon in other cell types. Mutations of p-53 tumor suppressor gene are present in approximately 50% of NSCLC and 70% of SCLC. Overexpression of epidermal growth factor and its receptor is present in approximately 60% of NSCLC. Identification of critical, early molecular alterations may allow early detection of cancer through analysis of sputum, blood, or stool.

Although survival with lung cancer correlates best to the stage of disease, large survival discrepancies among patients within a single stage of disease are unexplained and may reflect specific tumor biology. Research in cancer biology has revealed a number of markers that may be significant in tumor behavior. Predictions of a good or bad outcome have been attempted on the basis of oncogene amplification; level of tumor-associated antigens, specific enzymes, and growth factors; rate of cell proliferation; and other biologic factors. Recognition of the genetic profile of a patient's lung cancer is now being used in research protocols to determine the biologic activity of the cancer in predicting survival. Tailoring patient-specific treatment on the basis of the genetic mutations is in its early stages; a good example is the response from gefitinib for those cancers showing epidermal growth factor receptor (EGFR) mutations.

Pathology

Histopathologic designation of lung cancer is based on the World Health Organization Classification System. Differing cell types are distinguished by their appearance under light microscopy. A correct histologic distinction between small-cell and non-small-cell is imperative to determine treatment and prognosis. An agreement between pathologists in the separation of SCLC and NSCLC occurs in greater than 95% of cases. NSCLC is further subdivided into squamous cell, adenocarcinoma, and large-cell carcinoma. Considerable variation in histologic differentiation in individual cases leads to differences in interpretation. Interobserver variation among pathologists in the recognition of NSCLC subtypes ranges as high as 25–40% of cases. This difficulty may become clinically significant as the treatment of NSCLC becomes more subtype specific. The genetic profile of NSCLC will likely be of greater importance than the histologic subset in predicting its biology.

Adenocarcinoma is the most frequent histologic cell type of lung cancer, and it composes approximately 40% of most lung cancer series. Studies of CT screening report that approximately 70% of cancers identified are adenocarcinomas and reflects the greater ability of CT to find nodular cancers in the periphery of the lung compared with centrally located tumors. Adenocarcinoma is the most common cell type among smokers and accounts for nearly all of lung cancer identified in patients who have never smoked. The most frequent location of adenocarcinoma is in the peripheral aspects of the lung parenchyma as a solitary nodule or mass (Figure 47-3). The histologic identification of adenocarcinoma requires evidence of neoplastic gland formation or the presence of intracytoplasmic mucin. Bronchoalveolar cell carcinoma (BAC) is a subtype of adenocarcinoma and may present as a nodule or mass that may be solid, part solid, or of ground-glass attenuation. BAC may also present as multiple nodules or with a pneumonia-like infiltrate (Figure 47-4). Histologic features of bronchoalveolar cell carcinoma include origin distal to grossly recognizable bronchi, well-differentiated cytologic features, and growth along intact alveolar septa.

Squamous cell carcinoma is the second most common cell type and comprises approximately 25% of lung cancer in most series. Squamous cell type correlates highly with smoking history and originates most often in association with the central airways—trachea, main stems, lobar, and the segmental bronchi (Figure 47-5). Patients who have squamous cell carcinoma often have symptoms of airway involvement such as cough and hemoptysis. Radiographic presence of squamous cell carcinoma may be suggested by evidence of airway obstruction such as a lobar collapse or postobstructive pneumonia. Because of the central location, the tumor may be radiographically occult and even unapparent in the early stage on CT. Squamous cell may present as a peripheral mass, and cavitation may be seen as it may in other types of NSCLC (Figure 47-6). The

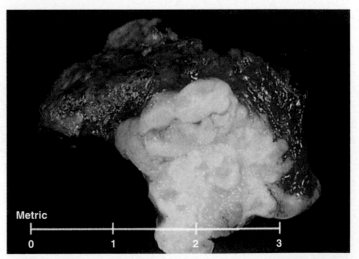

FIGURE 47-3 Peripheral adenocarcinoma. This wedge resection gross specimen of a peripheral nodule showed grade 2 adenocarcinoma. The patient underwent a lobectomy with formal lymph node dissection.

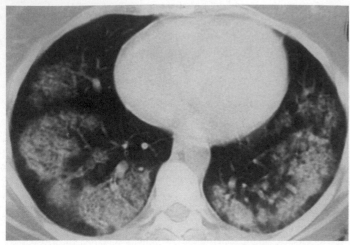

FIGURE 47-4 Bronchoalveolar cell carcinoma. Computed tomography scan of the chest in a patient who has unresolving pneumonia, showing bilateral alveolar infiltrates. Transbronchoscopic biopsy revealed bronchoalveolar cell carcinoma.

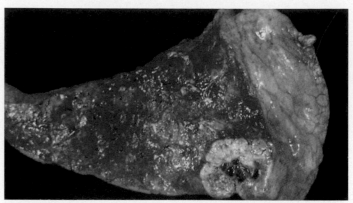

FIGURE 47-6 Cavitating squamous cell carcinoma. Gross specimen of the right lower lung showing a peripheral, thick-walled cavity with central necrosis. Histologic examination revealed squamous cell carcinoma.

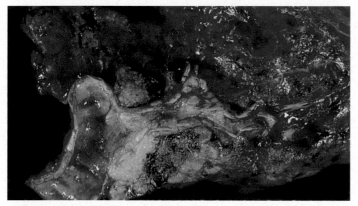
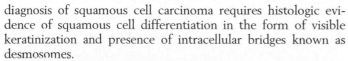

FIGURE 47-5 Squamous cell lung cancer. Gross specimen of the left lung showing obstruction of the left upper lobe bronchus by tumor and peribronchial extension. Histologic examination showed grade 2 squamous cell carcinoma.

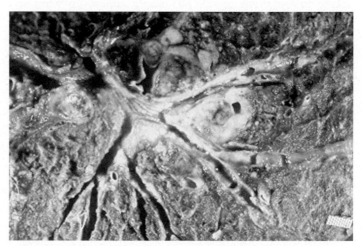

FIGURE 47-7 Small-cell lung cancer. Right lung gross specimen showing a lung mass with lymphadenopathy and extrinsic bronchial compression.

diagnosis of squamous cell carcinoma requires histologic evidence of squamous cell differentiation in the form of visible keratinization and presence of intracellular bridges known as desmosomes.

Large-cell, undifferentiated carcinoma is a cell type that is less well differentiated under light microscopy and lacks glandular or squamous differentiation. Large-cell tumors compose approximately 10% of most series, but considerable variability may occur between centers, depending on the nuances of the pathologist's interpretation of poorly differentiated carcinomas. Large-cell, undifferentiated carcinoma usually presents as a peripheral mass, and necrosis is often prominent.

Small-cell type accounts for approximately 20% of most series of lung cancer; SCLC is most highly associated with smoking and tends to occur in areas of the chest adjacent to the central airways and often with extensive adenopathy (Figure 47-7). Imaging not infrequently shows a large mediastinal mass that encompasses lymph nodes and the primary site of origin is unclear. SCLC is the most common lung cancer to

present with evidence of distant metastasis and, for the purposes of treatment, is considered a systemic disease even in limited stage—the sole exception being SCLC presenting as a peripheral nodule with no adenopathy. SCLC is the most frequent cell type to exhibit one of the distinct paraneoplastic syndromes. Histologic features include a pleomorphic population of small cells, which may be round, oval, or angulated and contain variable amounts of cytoplasm. The nuclei are typically hyperchromatic and have dispersed chromatin.

CLINICAL FEATURES

The clinical presentation of lung cancer is, unfortunately, a frequent occurrence. Prompt and thorough evaluation of a patient who has lung cancer may reveal an early-stage lesion and lead to curative treatment, or reveal evidence of advanced stage disease, and may avoid unnecessary surgery. Physicians need to maintain a high index of suspicion for this disease, particularly among smokers and former smokers.

Asymptomatic Presentation

In a nonscreened setting, approximately one fourth of patients who have lung cancer present with no symptoms. The desired situation is to detect a lesion early at a curable stage and before the onset of symptoms, although this discovery is often serendipitous. A nodule or mass may be identified on a chest radiograph carried out as part of a preoperative evaluation for unrelated surgery. Alternately, a nodule may be noted on imaging carried out in pursuit of other concerns, such as the spine or abdomen, in which part of the lungs are included (Figure 47-8). Screening sputum cytology, chest radiography, and CT have shown an ability to detect lung cancer at an early stage but have not proved a role in reducing mortality. As a result, the American Cancer Society, the American College of Radiology, and the National Cancer Institute have not recommended screening for lung cancer. CT screening has shown promise in that approximately three fourths of the cancers identified with CT screening are not visible on chest radiography done at the same time. CT screening is discussed as a subject of controversy toward the end of the chapter.

Symptomatic Presentation

Approximately three fourths of patients who have lung cancer in a nonscreened setting present with symptoms at the time of diagnosis. Symptoms from lung cancer may result from local extension, metastasis, or paraneoplastic effects. Most patients who present with symptoms show evidence of metastasis at the time of presentation and are unresectable.

Local Effects

Symptoms that stem from local effects of malignancy include cough, hemoptysis, chest pain, and dyspnea. Cough is present in 50–75% of patients who present with lung cancer and occurs most frequently with squamous cell and small-cell types because of central airway involvement. New onset of cough in a smoker or former smoker raises concern of bronchitis and obstructive airway disease as well as cancer. Lung cancer is uncommonly the cause of bronchiectasis because of rate of disease progression. Slow-growing neoplasms such as carcinoid tumor or hamartoma may present with bronchiectasis. Bronchorrhea or cough productive of large volumes of thin, mucoid secretions may be a feature of bronchoalveolar cell carcinoma and usually indicates advanced disease. Although bronchitis is the most common cause of hemoptysis, hemoptysis occurs in 25–50% of patients who are seen with lung cancer. Bronchoscopic series reveal bronchogenic carcinoma with incidences in the range of 2.5–9% in patients who had hemoptysis and an unsuspicious or normal chest radiograph. Any amount of hemoptysis can be alarming to the patient and, when in large volume, may be lethal. Death from hemoptysis results from asphyxiation from occlusion of the major airways rather than from exsanguination.

Chest pain is present in approximately one fourth of patients presenting with lung cancer and can be quite variable in character. Dull, aching, persistent pain may occur from mediastinal, pleural, or chest wall extension (Figure 47-9). Pleuritic pain may be the result of direct pleural involvement, obstructive pneumonitis, or a pulmonary embolus related to a hypercoagulable state. Pain is more often present on the side of the chest that contains the neoplasm and, importantly, the presence of pain may not preclude resectability. Patients with carcinomas that involve the chest wall in the absence of lymph node involvement have T3 lesions (see staging) and still a favorable survival after surgery.

Approximately 25% of patients have dyspnea when presenting with lung cancer. Dyspnea may be due to a variety of causes including, but not limited to, the following: extrinsic or endoluminal airway obstruction, obstructive pneumonitis or atelectasis, pleural effusion, lymphangitic metastasis, tumor emboli, pneumothorax, or pericardial effusion with tamponade (Figure 47-10). Partial obstruction of a bronchus may

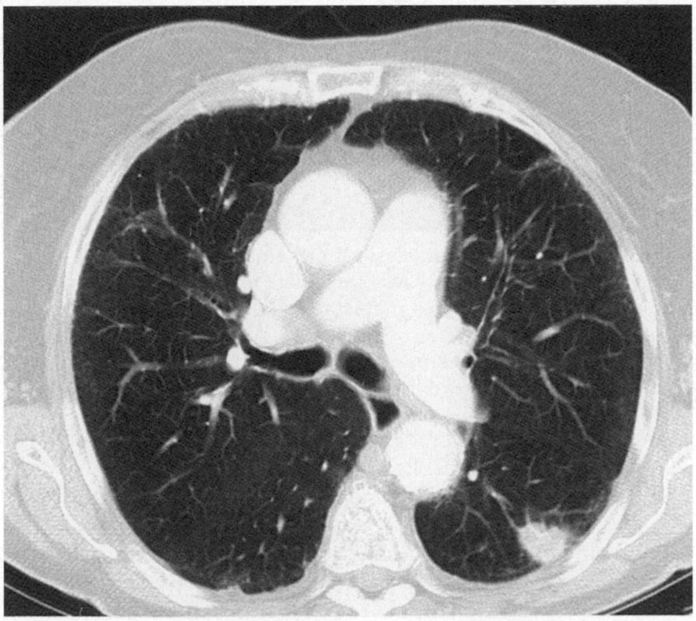

FIGURE 47-8 Solitary pulmonary nodule (SPN). The chest radiograph shows a 2-cm-long left, midlung SPN; resection revealed a stage IA adenocarcinoma.

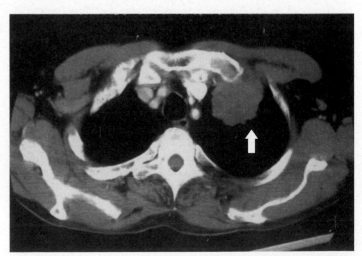

FIGURE 47-9 Stage IIB squamous cell carcinoma. Computed tomography scan showing a 4-cm diameter, left upper lobe mass (*arrow*) adjacent to the chest wall. Resection included aspects of the first and second rib, because histologic evidence of chest wall involvement was found. No lymph node involvement was found (T3N0M0, see text).

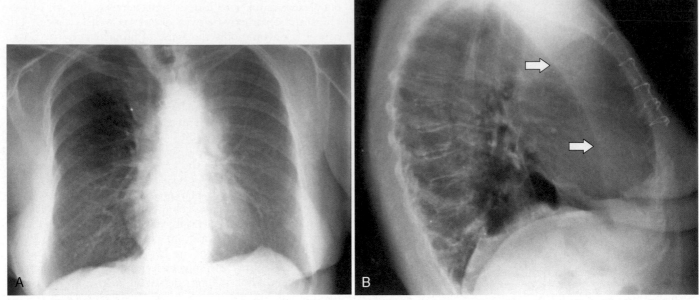

FIGURE 47-10 Squamous cell carcinoma causing lobar collapse. The posteroanterior **A,** and lateral chest **B,** radiographs show a left upper-lobe collapse (*arrows*) in a patient who presented with cough. Bronchoscopy revealed a squamous cell carcinoma that occluded the left upper-lobe bronchus.

cause a local wheeze, heard by the patient or by the physician on auscultation. Larger airway obstruction may cause stridor. Pulmonary function may be telling in a patient with dyspnea. Lung cancer may cause flattening of the inspiratory and/or expiratory flow-volume loop from presence of tumor in the trachea itself, from extrinsic compression, or from vocal cord paralysis.

Metastatic Effect

Hardly a body tissue is immune from the metastatic presence or effects of lung cancer. Lung cancer may spread by direct extension, through lymphatics, or hematogenously. The most frequent sites of distant metastasis are the liver, adrenals, bones, and brain.

Liver

Among patients diagnosed to have operable NSCLC in the chest, approximately 5% show CT evidence of liver metastasis. In the preoperative evaluation of patients thought to have resectable nonsmall-cell lung cancer, positron emission tomography (PET) identifies unsuspected metastases in the liver or adrenals in approximately 7% of patients preoperatively. The presence of hepatic metastasis late in the course of the disease is much higher. Autopsy studies have shown evidence of hepatic metastasis in greater than 60% of patients who have small-cell type and approximately 30% of those who have squamous cell carcinoma of the lung (Figure 47-11). Involvement of the liver is shown by CT in approximately 25% of patients who have SCLC at initial staging. Patients are often asymptomatic from the liver involvement, and evidence is usually found with CT, liver enzyme abnormalities, or with PET.

Adrenal

The usual scenario in the concern for adrenal metastasis is a unilateral adrenal mass found during staging CT for a known or suspected lung cancer. One series found that, of 330

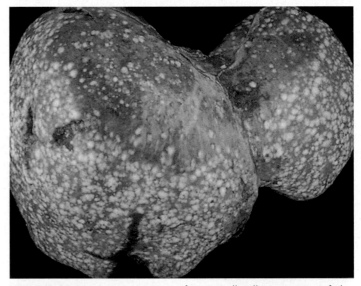

FIGURE 47-11 Liver metastases from small-cell carcinoma of the lung. The gross autopsy liver specimen from a 50-year-old male smoker shows innumerable metastatic foci of small-cell carcinoma.

patients who had operable NSCLC, 25 (7.5%) had isolated adrenal masses and 8 (2.4%) proved malignant. In other words, only approximately 25% of the adrenal abnormalities were actually due to a metastasis; benign causes of an adrenal mass include adenomas, nodular hyperplasia, or hemorrhagic cysts. The finding of a unilateral adrenal mass in a patient who has otherwise resectable disease requires a negative PET scan, an MR showing the characteristics of a benign adenoma, or a needle biopsy guided by CT to confirm the absence of metastasis. Metastasis to an adrenal gland is present at autopsy in 25–40% of patients who have lung cancer (Figure 47-12).

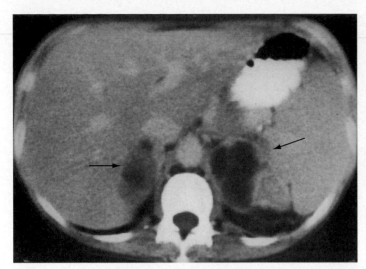

FIGURE 47-12 Adrenal metastases. Computed tomography scan of the abdomen showing large adrenal metastases (*arrows*) in a patient who has a lung mass and mediastinal adenopathy. Fine-needle aspirate of the adrenals showed adenocarcinoma.

Bone

Bone metastasis from lung cancer is most common from the small-cell type, but is not infrequent in the nonsmall-cell type. An osteolytic radiographic appearance is more frequent than an osteoblastic one, and vertebral bodies are the most common bones involved. In approximately 30–40% of patients initially staged for SCLC, evidence of bone metastasis will be identified by bone scan, PET, or bone marrow biopsy. Chest pain, skeletal pain, bone tenderness, and elevated levels of serum calcium or alkaline phosphatase are usually present in patients who have bony metastasis caused by NSCLC. Bone pain and elevated levels of serum calcium or alkaline phosphatase are often absent in patients who have SCLC and bone marrow involvement. PET scanning has improved the ability to identify metastases to many organs, including bone, with greater sensitivity than CT or bone scanning.

Nervous System

Neurologic manifestations of lung cancer include direct extension, metastatic effects, and paraneoplastic syndromes; the latter are discussed in the next section. The presence of central nervous system metastasis may be asymptomatic or cause headache, vomiting, visual field loss, cranial nerve deficit seizures, or hemiparesis. Squamous cell carcinoma has the least tendency to metastasize to the central nervous system and SCLC the greatest. Sequential resection may be feasible in selected cases that have operable NSCLC in the chest and a solitary brain metastasis. Various surgical series have shown 2-year survival rates of 25–45% in this setting. Autopsy series have shown brain metastasis in the range of 25–40% for patients who had lung cancer.

Isolated nerve dysfunction may be the result of regional extension of bronchogenic carcinoma. Neoplasm is the most common cause of unilateral vocal cord paralysis, and lung cancer is the most common malignancy. The onset of persistent hoarseness in a smoker raises concern for laryngeal cancer, of course, but also for lung cancer because of involvement of the recurrent laryngeal nerve as it courses under the arch of the aorta and back up to the larynx. Extension of lung cancer into the phrenic nerve may result in diaphragm paralysis; patients may report dyspnea or be asymptomatic.

Superior Vena Cava Syndrome

Bronchogenic carcinoma accounts for 65–80% of superior vena cava (SVC) syndrome in reported series. A sensation of fullness in the head and dyspnea are the most common presenting features of SVC syndrome. Cough, pain, and dysphagia are less frequent symptoms. Physical findings include dilated neck veins, a prominent venous pattern on the chest, facial edema, and a plethoric appearance (Figure 47-13). The chest radiograph typically shows widening of the mediastinum or a right hilar mass, but may be normal. For most patients who have SVC syndrome secondary to lung cancer, the symptoms resolve after radiation or chemotherapy. In a Cochrane meta-analysis of treatment of SVC obstruction caused by lung cancer, chemotherapy and/or radiotherapy relieved obstruction in 77% of small-cell and 60% of non-small-cell cancers. SVC stenting relieved obstruction in 95% of cases with immediate results and should be considered early in the treatment of SVC syndrome.

Pleura

Presence of carcinoma cells in the pleural fluid establishes the lung cancer as T4 (stage IIIB) disease and as unresectable. Of patients who have lung cancer, fewer than 10% have pleural involvement at presentation. Dyspnea and cough are common symptoms that occur with malignant pleural effusions; approximately one fourth of patients who have lung cancer and pleural metastases are asymptomatic (Figure 47-14). Malignant effusions are typically exudates and may be serous, serosanguineous, or grossly bloody. The simple presence of a pleural effusion in the setting of bronchogenic carcinoma does not establish unresectability. In the presence of a resectable lung cancer, a benign pleural effusion may result from lymphatic obstruction, postobstructive pneumonitis, or atelectasis. Presence of pleural metastasis needs to be confirmed or excluded so that a chance for curative resection is not missed (Figure 47-15). Documented cases of malignancy have shown the yield of pleural fluid cytology to be approximately 65%. Retrospective series have shown that yields from thoracentesis are similar for quantities of pleural fluid as small as 10 mL compared with as much as a liter. Pleural biopsy adds little to the yield of cytologic examination. In a patient suspected to have malignancy, repeat pleural fluid cytology with or without pleural biopsy is appropriate if the initial study is negative. Surgical (thoracoscopy) or medical pleuroscopy should follow two or three negative cytology examinations to further evaluate the pleural space.

Superior Sulcus Tumor

The superior sulcus is a groove created by the subclavian artery in the rounded vault of the pleura and apices of the upper lobes of the lungs. Presence of a superior sulcus neoplasm and the resulting syndrome of characteristic pain, Horner's syndrome, bony destruction, and atrophy of hand muscles were first described in the 1920s by Dr. Pancoast (Figures 47-16 and 47-17). Pancoast syndrome is most commonly caused by NSCLC (usually squamous cell) and only rarely by small-cell carcinoma. Pain resulting from superior sulcus tumors is most commonly located in the shoulder, followed by the forearm, scapula, and fingers. Patients often seek a chiropractor or

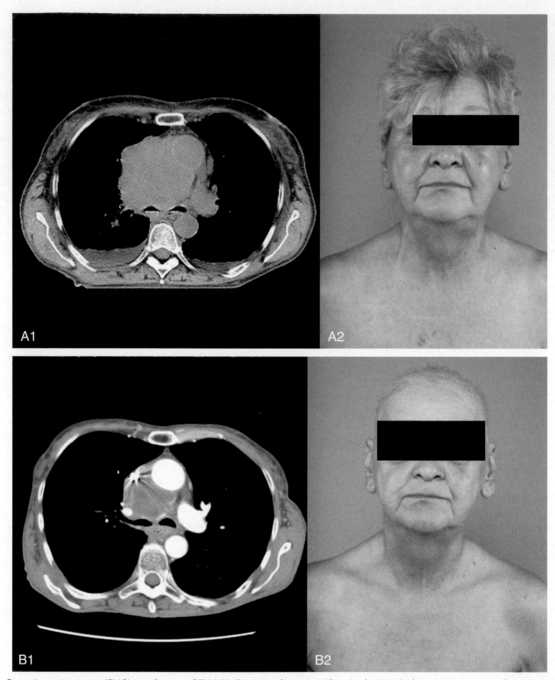

FIGURE 47-13 Superior vena cava (SVC) syndrome. CT **(A1)** shows as large mediastinal mass (adenocarcinoma on biopsy); the patient had a prominent venous pattern **(A2)** on chest from SVC obstruction. She received external beam radiation (6000 cGy) and concurrent chemotherapy with etoposide and cisplatin and her symptoms improved within 8 days. Follow-up at 2 months showed the mass on CT **(B1)** was smaller and her collateral venous pattern **(B2)** had resolved.

orthopedist before a diagnosis is made. Treatment is described later in this chapter.

Paraneoplastic Syndromes

Paraneoplastic effects of tumor are those remote effects that are not related to the direct invasion, obstruction, or metastasis. Paraneoplastic syndromes occur in approximately 10–20% of patients with a bronchogenic carcinoma (Table 47-2).

Musculoskeletal

Clubbing of the digits may be a paraneoplastic manifestation of lung cancer or be caused by other diseases. Clubbing may involve the fingers and toes and consists of selective enlargement of the connective tissue in the terminal phalanges (Figure 47-18). Physical findings include loss of the angle between the base of the nail bed and cuticle, rounded nails, and enlarged fingertips. Clubbing is an isolated finding and is usually asymptomatic. Nonmalignant causes of clubbing include pulmonary fibrosis, congenital heart disease, and bronchiectasis.

Hypertrophic pulmonary osteoarthropathy (HPO) is an uncommon process associated with lung cancer. HPO is characterized by painful arthropathy that usually involves the ankles, knees, wrists, and elbows and is most often symmetric. The pain and arthropathy are caused by proliferative periostitis that

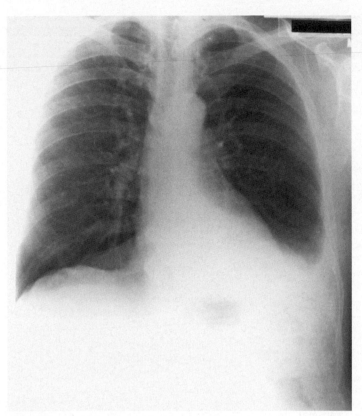

FIGURE 47-14 Malignant pleural effusion. Chest radiograph showing a left pleural effusion; thoracentesis revealed adenocarcinoma consistent with a lung primary tumor.

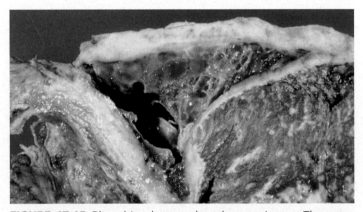

FIGURE 47-15 Pleural involvement by adenocarcinoma. The gross specimen shows malignant pleural involvement similar to the appearance of mesothelioma. Histologic examination revealed adenocarcinoma.

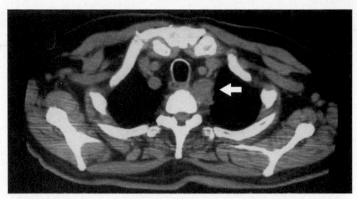

FIGURE 47-16 Superior sulcus tumor. Computed tomography scan from an 81-year-old man who was seen with left scapular pain shows a superior sulcus mass (*arrow*) in the left lung apex. Ptosis and myosis were also present. Transbronchoscopic biopsy revealed grade IV non-small-cell carcinoma.

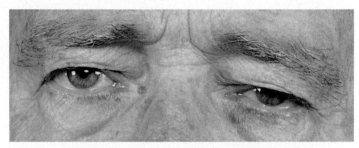

FIGURE 47-17 Ptosis as part of Pancoast syndrome. Drooping of this man's left eye is evident as part of Pancoast syndrome, and meiosis was also present. His computed tomography scan is shown in Figure 47-16.

involves the long bones, but may also involve metacarpal, metatarsal, and phalangeal bones. Patients with HPO may have clubbing of fingers and toes in addition to the painful arthralgia. The pathogenesis of HPO is uncertain, but it may arise from a humoral agent. For patients who smoke and have a new onset of arthralgias, HPO needs be considered. In a patient with HPO, a radiograph of the long bones (i.e., tibia and fibula) may show characteristic periosteal new bone formation. An isotope bone scan typically demonstrates diffuse uptake by the long bones (Figure 47-19). Large-cell and adenocarcinoma are the most common histologic types associated with HPO.

For unclear reasons, the symptoms of HPO may resolve after thoracotomy, whether the primary cancer is resected or not. For patients who are not operable, the usual treatment is with nonsteroidal antiinflammatory agents. Recently, there have been reports of selective benefit with use of a bisphosphonate, pamidronate.

Although still a topic of debate, population-based studies from Sweden and Australia suggest a frequency of malignancy of 15–25% in patients with dermatomyositis-polymyositis. The risk of malignancy is higher with dermatomyositis than polymyositis and is highest in the first 2 years after the diagnosis. A reasonable approach to cancer surveillance in these patients is a careful history and physical examination, chest radiograph, basic laboratory tests, and age-appropriate cancer screening examinations including mammography and colonoscopy. Other tests should be based on symptoms and abnormalities detected during the basic evaluation.

Hematologic

Anemia frequently occurs in patients who have lung cancer and may be caused by iron deficiency, chronic disease, or bone marrow infiltration. Anemia is also a frequent consequence of chemotherapy. Eosinophilia is more commonly associated with Hodgkin's disease but may occur in patients who have lung cancer. Production of various cytokines by neoplastic cells may result in eosinophilia, leukocytosis, or thrombocytosis, of which thrombocytosis is by far the most common.

TABLE 47-2 Paraneoplastic Syndromes

System	Paraneoplastic Syndrome	System	Paraneoplastic Syndrome
Musculoskeletal	Hypertrophic osteoarthropathy Polymyositis Osteomalacia Myopathy	Neurologic	Lambert–Eaton syndrome Peripheral neuropathy Encephalopathy Myelopathy Cerebellar degeneration Psychosis Dementia
Cutaneous	Clubbing Dermatomyositis Acanthosis nigricans Pruritus Erythema multiforme Hyperpigmentation Urticaria Scleroderma	Vascular/hematologic	Thrombophlebitis Arterial thrombosis Nonbacterial thrombotic endocarditis Thrombocytosis Polycythemia Hemolytic anemia Red cell aplasia Dysproteinemia Leukemoid reaction Eosinophilia Thrombocytopenic purpura Hypercoagulable state
Endocrinologic	Cushing's syndrome Syndrome of inappropriate antidiuretic hormone secretion Hypercalcemia Carcinoid syndrome Hyperglycemia/hypoglycemia Gynecomastia Galactorrhea Growth hormone excess Calcitonin secretion Thyroid-stimulating hormone	Miscellaneous	Cachexia Hyperuricemia Nephrotic syndrome

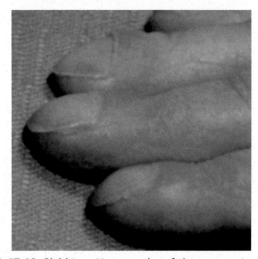

FIGURE 47-18 Clubbing. Hypertrophy of the connective tissue in the terminal phalanges of this patient who has lung cancer.

The association of deep venous thrombosis and malignancy was described by Trousseau more than a century ago, and lung cancer is the most common malignancy associated with Trousseau syndrome. The causes of the hypercoagulable state remain poorly understood. One large study documented clinically significant association of idiopathic thrombosis and the subsequent development of overt cancer; however, other investigators concluded that the literature does not enable firm recommendations about whether to screen for a malignant neoplasm in patients who have unexplained venous thromboembolism. A careful clinical evaluation that includes history, physical examination, routine laboratory tests, chest radiograph, and age-appropriate screening tests seems appropriate. Routine CT scans of the chest and abdomen are not generally accepted as being cost-effective. Thromboembolism in the patient who has malignancy is often refractory to warfarin

treatment. In patients with lung cancer (or any malignancy) and a reasonable quality of life, low molecular weight heparin has been shown to be superior to oral anticoagulation and is the treatment recommended by the Seventh American College of Chest Physicians Guidelines on Antithrombotic and Thrombolytic Therapy.

Hypercalcemia

Hypercalcemia in association with malignancy may arise from a bony metastasis or, less commonly, tumor secretion of a parathyroid hormone–related protein (PTHrP), calcitriol, or other cytokines, including osteoclastic activating factors. The most common cancers to cause hypercalcemia are those of the kidney, lung, breast, head and neck, and myeloma and lymphoma. In one study of 690 consecutive lung cancers, 2.5% had tumor-induced hypercalcemia. Squamous cell histology is the most common cell type associated with hypercalcemia, and generally patients have advanced disease (stage III or IV) and are seldom resectable. The median survival in patients who have hypercalcemia resulting from NSCLC is approximately 1 month. Symptoms of hypercalcemia include anorexia, nausea, vomiting, constipation, lethargy, polyuria, polydipsia, and dehydration. Confusion and coma are late manifestations, as are renal failure and nephrocalcinosis. Cardiovascular effects include shortened QT interval, broad T wave, heart block, ventricular arrhythmia, or asystole. Individual patients may manifest any combination of these signs and symptoms in various degrees.

Hypercalcemia of malignancy that is not caused by bony metastases results from accelerated bone resorption, decreased bone deposition, or increased renal tubular reabsorption of calcium. Accelerated bone resorption is caused by activation of osteoclasts by cytokines or PTHrP in most cases. PTHrP, calcitriol, or cytokines are secreted autonomously by the tumor. Serum parathyroid hormone levels are usually normal or low, but an elevated level of PTHrP can be detected in the

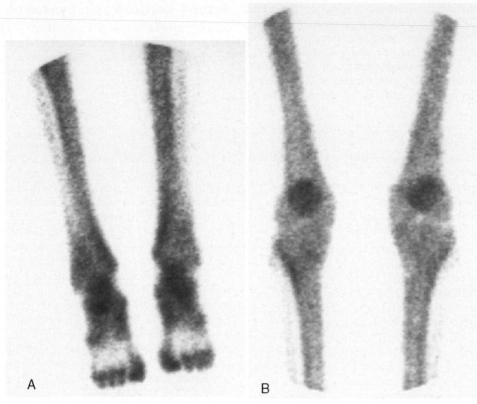

FIGURE 47-19 Hypertrophic pulmonary osteoarthropathy. The bone scan shows diffuse uptake of the ankles **(A)** and long bones **(B)** in this patient who had lung cancer.

serum in approximately one half of these patients. Cytokines or PTHrP are secreted autonomously by the tumor. Not only does PTHrP cause calcium readsorption, but it also interferes with renal mechanisms for readsorption of sodium and water with resultant polyuria. Polyuria and vomiting result in dehydration; decreases in glomerular filtration further aggravate the hypercalcemia.

Mild elevation of serum calcium may not require treatment, so the decision is based on the patient's symptoms. For patients who have widely metastatic and incurable malignancy, it may be most appropriate to give supportive care only and not treat the hypercalcemia. The average life expectancy in this situation is 30–45 days, even with aggressive treatment.

Most patients who have serum calcium of 12–13 mg/dL (3–3.25 mmol/L) or higher require treatment. The corrected serum calcium in such individuals who have low albumin is calculated by: measured serum calcium + 0.8 × [4 g/dL (or 40 g/L) – measured serum albumin] = corrected serum calcium.

The four basic goals of treatment are:

1. Correct dehydration
2. Increase renal excretion of calcium
3. Inhibit bone resorption
4. Treat the underlying malignancy

Because of the polyuria, patients with hypercalcemia are volume-contracted. Initial treatment is with intravenous normal saline, by use of 3–6 L/24 h as tolerated, with careful attention to volume status and urinary output. In the past, after hydration, loop diuretics were commonly used with only mild benefit. Loop diuretics have been displaced by more

effective treatment with calcitonin and bisphosphonates. The bisphosphonates have a high affinity for bone and inhibit osteoclast activity and are more potent than calcitonin. Zoledronate, a newer bisphosphonate, is the most effective; the usual dose is 4 mg given intravenously over 15 min. Normal calcium levels are achieved within 4–10 days in 85% of patients and are maintained a median of 30–40 days. Adverse effects are generally mild and transient and include fever, hypophosphatemia, and asymptomatic hypocalcemia. Occasional renal adverse events may occur with elevation of serum creatinine. Calcitonin inhibits bone resorption, increases renal calcium excretion, and has a rapid onset of action, but the duration of action is short-lived. Calcitonin is a relatively weak agent and, when used alone, generally lowers the serum calcium by a maximum of 1–2 mg/dL (0.3–0.5 mmol/L). Use of calcitonin is appropriate when the calcium needs to be lowered urgently (onset of action 4–6 h) while waiting for the more effective but slower-acting agents to take effect or when relief of bony pain is desired. The usual dose of calcitonin is 4 IU/kg given intramuscularly or subcutaneously every 12 h. The dose can be increased up to 6–8 IU/kg every 6–12 h. Intranasal calcitonin is not effective for hypercalcemia of malignancy. The efficacy of calcitonin may be limited to the first 48 h before tachyphylaxis occurs. The effects of calcitonin and bisphosphonates are additive and combined treatment is beneficial.

Syndrome of Inappropriate Antidiuretic Hormone Secretion

Causes of hyponatremia include tumors, pulmonary infections, central nervous system disorders, and drugs. Approximately 10% of patients who have SCLC exhibit the syndrome of inappropriate antidiuretic hormone secretion (SIADH); however, SCLC accounts for approximately 75% of cases of SIADH. Antidiuretic hormone (vasopressin) is secreted in the anterior hypothalamus and exerts its action on the renal collecting ducts by enhancing the flow of water from the lumen into the medullary interstitium, which results in the concentration of urine. The criteria for the diagnosis of SIADH include:

- Hyponatremia associated with a low plasma osmolality (<275 mOsm/kg)
- Inappropriately elevated urine osmolality (> 200 mOsm/kg) relative to serum osmolality
- Elevated urine sodium (usually >40 mEq/L)
- Clinical euvolemia without edema
- Normal renal (creatinine <1.5 times the upper limit of normal), adrenal, and thyroid function.

The serum uric acid is usually low, and the urine osmolality/serum osmolality ratio is frequently greater than 2.

The severity of symptoms is related to the degree of hyponatremia and the rapidity of the fall in serum sodium. In one large series of patients with SIADH, only 27% had signs or symptoms of hyponatremia despite a median sodium level of 117 mEq/L (range, 101–129 mEq/L). Symptoms of hyponatremia include anorexia, nausea, and vomiting. With rapid onset of hyponatremia, symptoms caused by cerebral edema may include irritability, restlessness, personality changes, confusion, coma, seizures, and respiratory arrest. In minimally symptomatic or asymptomatic patients, fluid restriction of 500–1000 mL/24 h is the initial treatment of choice. If further treatment is needed, oral demeclocycline 900–1200 mg/day is considered. Demeclocycline induces a nephrogenic diabetes insipidus and blocks the action of antidiuretic hormone on the renal tubule, thereby increasing water excretion. The onset of action varies from a few hours to a few weeks, so this drug is not recommended for acute emergency treatment. Renal function should be monitored, because nephrotoxicity can occur. In patients who have more severe or life-threatening symptoms (serum sodium of <115 mEq/L), treatment consists of intravenous fluids with 0.9% saline and supplemental potassium and diuresis with loop diuretics such as furosemide or ethacrynic acid. The efficacy of treatment with normal saline is variable and questioned by some experts. With severe CNS symptoms, it may be appropriate to treat with 300 mL of 3% saline given over 3–4 h in combination with a loop diuretic. Saline with no diuretic ultimately does not raise the sodium concentration. Rapid correction of the sodium may have life-threatening consequences, and caution is advised. The rate of correction of the sodium is best limited to 1 mEq/L/h or a maximum of 8 mEq/L/day in the first day and no more than 18 mEq/L in the first 48 h. Faster correction has been associated with the development of central pontine myelinolysis, which may result in quadriplegia, cranial nerve abnormalities that manifest as pseudobulbar palsy, alteration in mental status, and subsequent death. Accordingly, in the course of treating hyponatremia, serum sodium must be monitored frequently to ensure that correction is not too rapid. For patients with SIADH resulting from SCLC, treatment with chemotherapy should be initiated as soon as possible and is likely to result in improvement in the hyponatremia within a few weeks. After an initial response to chemotherapy, SIADH may recur when disease relapses.

Ectopic Corticotropin Syndrome

Ectopic production of corticotropin or corticotropin-releasing hormone with associated Cushing syndrome has been identified in patients who have SCLC; carcinoid tumors of the lung, thymus, or pancreas; and neurocrest tumors such as pheochromocytoma, neuroblastoma, and medullary carcinoma of the thyroid. In ectopic corticotropin secretion, SCLC accounts for 75% of cases. Cushing syndrome is seldom caused by NSCLC.

Classic features of Cushing syndrome include truncal obesity, striae, rounded (moon) face, dorsocervical fat pad (buffalo hump), myopathy and weakness, osteoporosis, diabetes mellitus, hypertension, and personality changes. However, the rapid growth of SCLC means that patients are more likely to present with edema, hypertension, and muscular weakness rather than with the classic symptoms. Hypokalemic alkalosis and hyperglycemia are usually present. Of patients who have SCLC, 2–5% have Cushing syndrome develop. Patients who have SCLC and Cushing syndrome seem to have a shortened survival period than patients who have SCLC without the syndrome, and this may be because of more frequent opportunistic infections. The best screen for Cushing syndrome is the 24-h urine free-cortisol measurement. Marked elevation of cortisol production (e.g., greater than 500 μg/24 h) and plasma corticotropin levels >200 pg/mL (40 pmol/L) are highly suggestive of ectopic corticotropin as the cause of Cushing syndrome. The plasma level of adrenocorticotropin hormone (ACTH) is elevated in many, but not all, patients.

Treatment of Cushing syndrome caused by ectopic corticotropin has included adrenal enzyme inhibitors such as metyrapone, aminoglutethimide, mitotane, or ketoconazole, given alone or in combination. Ketoconazole is the agent used most commonly in this setting. Ketoconazole given orally at a dosage of 400–1200 mg/day may control hypercortisolism within a few days to weeks, but the response is variable. The usual starting dose is 200 mg three times per day and increased rapidly up to 400 mg three times per day as a maximum dose. Dose adjustments are based on the serum and urinary cortisol levels. Liver function tests should be followed closely in patients treated with high-dose ketoconazole. If ketoconazole does not control the cortisol secretion, it should be maintained at 1200 mg/day and metyrapone added at 250 mg two or three times per day and the dose escalated as needed to a maximum dose of 4.5 g/day. Symptomatic hypoadrenalism may result from treatment, and some authorities recommend a replacement dose of dexamethasone 0.25–0.5 mg/day when there is evidence of cortisol secretion approaching normal. When Cushing syndrome arises from SCLC, it is advisable to proceed with appropriate chemotherapy and carefully watch for superimposed infections, as is necessary for any patient who takes high-dose corticosteroids. Cushing syndrome related to a bronchial carcinoid is best treated by surgical resection of the tumor.

Neurologic

The paraneoplastic neurologic syndromes associated with lung cancer, mostly small-cell type, are quite variable. They include Lambert-Eaton myasthenic syndrome (LEMS), subacute sensory neuropathy, encephalomyelopathy, cerebellar degeneration, autonomic neuropathy, retinal degeneration, and opsoclonus. The frequency of any of these neurologic syndromes in SCLC is approximately 5%, and neurologic symptoms may precede the diagnosis by months to years. Most patients who have SCLC and an associated paraneoplastic syndrome have limited stage disease that may or may not be obvious on initial evaluation. Careful radiographic evaluation of the lungs and mediastinum is indicated in a current or former smoker who has a suspected paraneoplastic neurologic syndrome. In this setting, even subtle abnormalities of the mediastinum require a biopsy. If a patient has a positive paraneoplastic blood test and the CT chest scan does not reveal an abnormality, it is recommended that a positron emission tomography (PET) scan be performed. A positive PET scan may help identify the lesion to facilitate biopsy confirmation of the diagnosis.

Paraneoplastic neurologic syndromes are thought to be immune mediated on the basis of the identification of a number of autoantibodies. The literature is confusing because of different names used by various investigators. The anti-Hu antibody is the same as the antineuronal nuclear-antibody type I (ANNA-1), and the anti-Ri antibody is identical to ANNA-2. Both of these antibodies, predominantly ANNA-1, have been associated with SCLC. Such antibodies should not be confused with the anti-Purkinje antibody (anti-yo), which is characteristically found in patients who have subacute cerebellar degeneration as a manifestation of gynecologic malignancy or breast cancer. The more recently described CRMP-5 antibody, also known as CV-2, has been associated with SCLC and thymomas. More than one of these paraneoplastic autoantibodies may be identified in some patients. These autoantibodies predict the patient's neoplasm but not a specific neurologic syndrome (Table 47-3).

In a review of 162 sequential patients who had ANNA-1, 142 (88%) were proven to have cancer, 132 of which were SCLC. In 97% of these cases, the diagnosis of SCLC followed the onset of the associated neurologic syndrome, usually by less than 6 months, but in 20% the period was more than 6 months. Of special note is that 90% of cases had disease limited to the lung or mediastinum (limited stage disease). In one large series, ANNA-1 antibodies were identified in 16% of SCLC cases. These antibodies were associated with limited stage disease, complete response to therapy, and longer survival than patients who had SCLC and no ANNA-1 antibody. These neurologic syndromes seldom improve with treatment, so the goal is to diagnose and treat the patient as soon as possible to prevent progression of the disease process.

Less common manifestations of neurologic paraneoplastic syndromes are orthostatic hypotension and intestinal dysmotility.

The ANNA-1 binds to the nucleus of all neurons in the central and peripheral nervous system, including the sensory and autonomic ganglia, myenteric plexus, and cells of the adrenal medulla. The gastrointestinal symptoms may present as nausea, vomiting, abdominal discomfort, or altered bowel habits suggestive of intestinal pseudo-obstruction. Many of these patients are seen with gastrointestinal symptoms and significant weight loss before the diagnosis of SCLC.

Proximal muscle weakness, hyporeflexia, and autonomic dysfunction characterize LEMS. Cranial nerve involvement may be present and does not differentiate LEMS from myasthenia gravis. LEMS has been strongly associated with antibodies directed against P/Q-type presynaptic voltage-gaited calcium channels of peripheral cholinergic nerve terminals. These antibodies have been identified in more than 90% of patients who have LEMS and block the normal release of acetylcholine at the neuromuscular junction. In contrast, myasthenia gravis is associated with antiacetylcholine receptor antibodies, which are present in approximately 90% of patients. Malignancy is present in approximately one half of patients who have LEMS, and SCLC is by far the most common histologic type. Of all patients who have SCLC, only 2–4% have LEMS. Calcium channel autoantibodies have also been identified in 25% of patients with SCLC who are not affected by neurologic problems. The diagnosis of LEMS is based on characteristic electromyographic findings that show a small amplitude of the resting compound muscle-action potential and facilitation with rapid, repetitive, supramaximal nerve stimulation or after brief exercise of the muscle. A single-fiber electromyograph is optimal for making the diagnosis.

Treatment of SCLC that induces remission of the cancer may result in attenuation or remission of the LEMS in some patients. LEMS is the predominant paraneoplastic neurologic syndrome that may improve with successful treatment of the associated lung cancer. The use of acetylcholinesterase inhibitors is of limited benefit in LEMS. Diaminopyridine enhances the release of acetylcholine and has been used with mixed results for treatment of both motor and autonomic deficits.

DIAGNOSIS AND STAGING

Diagnosis

The diagnosis of bronchogenic carcinoma requires histologic or cytologic examination. The asymptomatic patient found to

TABLE 47-3   Likelihood of Malignancy in Patients Presenting with Neurologic Symptoms and Paraneoplastic Neuronal or Cytoplasmic Autoantibodies

IgG	Total Patients	Patients with Proven Cancer	Lung Cancers Among Patients with Cancer		
			Overall	SCLC	NSCLC
ANNA-1	217	114 (80)	99 (87)	93	6
CRMP-5	208	84 (74)	60 (71)	53	7
PCA-1	101	62 (91)	0		
PCA-2	43	17 (89)	15 (88)	10	5
Amphiphysin	26	18 (86)	10 (56)	10	0
ANNA-2	17	8 (57)	5 (63)	3	2
ANNA-3	10	5 (62)	4 (80)	2	2

Adapted from Pittock SJ, Kryzer TJ, Lennon VA. Paraneoplastic antibodies coexist and predict cancer, not neurological syndrome. Ann Neurol 2004; 56:715-9.
ANNA-1, Antineuronal nuclear autoantibody type 1 (anti-Hu); *PCA-1,* Purkinje cell cytoplasmic autoantibody-type 1 (anti-Yo); *PCA-2,* Purkinje cell cytoplasmic autoantibody-type 2; *ANNA-2,* antineuronal nuclear autoantibody type 2 (anti-Ri); *ANNA-3,* antineuronal nuclear autoantibody type 3 (anti-Hu).

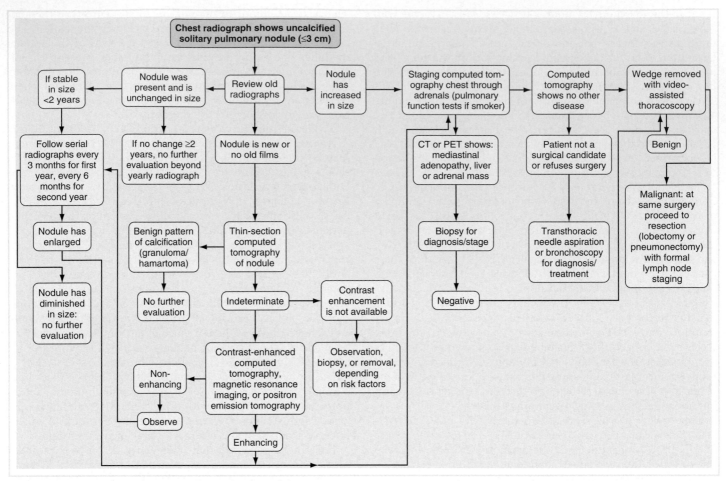

FIGURE 47-20 Evaluation algorithm for the solitary pulmonary nodule. Thin-section computed tomography (CT), contrast-enhanced CT, and staging CT may be carried out as a single study.

have a solitary pulmonary nodule (SPN) provides diagnostic challenges (Figure 47-20). By definition, an SPN is a solitary lesion surrounded by normal lung and not involved with atelectasis or hilar enlargement. The overall goal in evaluating an SPN is to promptly resect curable cancers and avoid removal of benign nodules. The likelihood that a nodule is malignant is greatly determined by the nodule size and also increases with advancing patient age, history of smoking, and prior history of malignancy. Every effort should be made to review prior chest imaging (chest radiographs, chest CTs, and sometimes abdominal CTs), because it may be helpful to identify whether the nodule is new, stable, or enlarging. Nodules shown to diminish in size are benign, and nodules shown to be stable in size over a 2-year period are considered benign by radiology criteria. Evidence of nodule enlargement is a reliable indicator of malignancy; although growth may occasionally be seen in a granuloma, the growth rate is usually much faster or slower than for malignancy.

Evaluation of focal pulmonary opacities has greatly improved with CT scans. Thin-section CT is more sensitive than plain film or plain tomography in the detection of calcium, and multiple nodules may be identified. The presence of calcification within a nodule is a reliable indicator that the nodule is benign, unless the calcification is eccentric, and then the nodule should still be considered indeterminate. A decision for close observation is appropriate for the newly detected nodule that is less than 8 mm. Follow-up usually requires CT, and the interval and duration of follow-up is determined by the size

of the nodule and the risk group of the patient. The recommendations from the Fleischner Society for low-risk patients (never smokers with no prior history of malignancy) is no follow-up for nodules <4 mm, 12 months for nodules 5–6 mm, and 6 months for nodules 7–8 mm. For high-risk patients (current or former smokers or history of malignancy), follow-up is recommended at 12 months for nodules <4 mm, 6 months for nodules 5–6 mm, and 3 months for nodules 7–8 mm. For nodules >8 mm further evaluation with contrast-enhanced CT, PET, or needle biopsy is generally recommended. Contrast enhanced CT is a weight-dependent dose of contrast injected at a specified rate with nodule enhancement measured at time 0, 1, 2, 3, and 4 min. Lack of enhancement (<15 Hounsfield Units) is an excellent indicator that a nodule is likely benign and only follow-up to assure lack of growth is all that is needed. Enhancing nodules are slightly more likely to be malignant than benign, and for this reason enhancement is less helpful in decision making. In a large meta-analysis evaluating solitary pulmonary nodules, PET had a sensitivity of 94% and a specificity of 86% for malignancy. Observation seems appropriate for a PET-negative nodule unless it has shown evidence of growth at a rate consistent with malignancy. Nodules that remain indeterminate after radiographic assessment require a decision between observation, biopsy, or removal.

Bronchoscopy and transthoracic needle aspiration are the two methods available for biopsy. Bronchoscopy is not appropriate for the evaluation of most SPNs. For nodules 2 cm or less in diameter, the yield from bronchoscopy is in the range of 10–20%. Bronchoscopy in the setting of an SPN rarely alters stage or identifies a synchronous tumor and is not needed for routine preoperative assessment. Presence of an air-bronchogram or bronchus leading into the nodule greatly increases the likelihood of diagnosis with bronchoscopy. Early results that used an electromagnetic navigation system to guide the bronchoscopist have improved diagnostic yield for pulmonary nodules but not to the level achieved with transthoracic needle aspiration (TTNA). TTNA has a yield of 80–90% for nodules 2 cm or smaller. Both procedures are limited by the frequent inability to make a specific benign diagnosis. A new spiculated nodule in a smoker may be best managed by proceeding to staging evaluation or to surgical resection without biopsy. The best management of an indeterminate SPN may be unclear, and it is important to inform and involve patients in the decision-making process.

Establishing cell type may be accomplished through bronchoscopy, needle aspiration, sputum cytologic examination, or surgery. Sputum cytologic examination is inexpensive and carries a high diagnostic specificity. Sputum cytologic examination in patients who have larger tumors, or tumors that are centrally located, has a higher likelihood of being positive. Sensitivity of a single sputum specimen for the detection of lung cancer is approximately 50% and increases with repeated specimens. Sputum cytologic examination is not often positive in patients who have small peripheral tumors. Radiographically occult squamous cell carcinomas may be detected at an early stage by sputum cytologic examination; however, positive sputum cytologic examination in the setting of adenocarcinoma is usually a poor prognostic sign.

Staging

When lung cancer is suspected on the basis of patient presentation, two main questions need to be answered: what is the cell type and what is the stage of the disease? The clinical evaluation for suspected lung cancer requires a careful history and physical examination, as well as complete blood count and serum chemistry panel that includes liver function tests and calcium. Localized pain, lymphadenopathy, or specific laboratory abnormalities direct the physician in further testing. Guidelines for staging are published by the American College of Physicians, the American Thoracic Society, and European Respiratory Society. These recommend that all patients who have lung cancer have a careful history and physical examination, basic blood parameters, and a CT scan of the chest that extends through the liver and adrenal glands. Pursuing tumor markers in the serum is not recommended. Pulmonary function testing should be obtained in patients who are considered for surgical resection. Quantitative ventilation-perfusion lung scan or cardiopulmonary exercise testing may assist in the selection of surgical candidates among patients who have marginal pulmonary function.

The role of PET in the evaluation of patients with known or suspected lung cancer is being defined, but several series have now shown that it will find unsuspected mediastinal or distant spread and avoid unnecessary thoracotomy in approximately one in five patients preoperatively. PET is based on the principle that cancer cells have a high rate of glycolysis and an increased cellular uptake of glucose because of an increased number of transport proteins compared with nonneoplastic cells. The PET tracer 18-fluoro-deoxyglucose (18-FDG) is taken up into cells, metabolically trapped, and accumulates. PET has been used to evaluate SPNs and has a sensitivity of approximately 90% and a specificity of 85% for determining

malignancy. These data are based on nodules 1 cm or larger. The resolution limit of nodules for PET evaluation is approximately 7–8 mm. False-positive PET scans have been reported with tuberculosis, fungal diseases, other infections, and sarcoidosis. Inflammatory disorders such as a rheumatoid nodule or cryptogenic organizing pneumonia may also cause false-positive PET scans. False-negative PET scans may occur with low-grade tumors such as bronchoalveolar cell carcinoma, carcinoid tumor, and tumors less than 1 cm in size. Hyperglycemia interferes with 18-FDG uptake and may result in a false-negative scan.

For evaluation of mediastinal lymph node metastasis, PET has a sensitivity and specificity of approximately 90% and 85%, respectively, on the basis of a meta-analysis of the literature. This compares favorably with the use of CT scan staging of the mediastinum where there is an approximately 30–40% rate of both false-positive and false-negative results. PET has also been shown to detect distant metastases in 10–15% of patients who are thought to be operable. Because of the 10–15% rate of false-positive PET scans, it is absolutely necessary to obtain a biopsy or other imaging proof of distant metastasis before deciding that the patient is inoperable. CT-PET integrates the CT and PET images and has been shown to have higher sensitivity and specificity for assessing lung cancer stage than CT and PET done separately. (For a more detailed discussion of PET see Chapter 2).

An important aspect of the clinical evaluation is to establish both resectability and operability. The history, physical examination, laboratory tests, and chest CT through the adrenals are used to try to establish whether resectable disease is present. Resectability is determined by stage: whether the tumor may be removed surgically and result in a survival benefit. The specifics of resectability are discussed in the following section on staging and in the section on treatment. Operability is determined by whether the patient can withstand the operation. In other words, stage I peripheral nodule may be resectable, but if the patient's pulmonary function is too poor, he or she may not be operable. Multiple factors are involved in operability, including functional status, pulmonary function, cardiac and other medical problems, and willingness to undergo surgery. Some of these are more quantifiable than others, and some may be modifiable. Regarding pulmonary function, the ability to tolerate resection is estimated by the predicted postoperative lung function (preoperative function minus resected function). Patients who have normal pulmonary function can be anticipated to tolerate pneumonectomy or a lesser resection. A quantitative lung scan may assist the prediction of postoperative lung function. If the postoperative predicted forced expiratory volume in 1 sec and diffusing capacity are greater than 40%, surgery is generally well tolerated. Additional exercise assessment, specifically aerobic capacity, may help predict the appropriateness of surgery in patients who have less than 40% predicted function. Some patients refuse to undergo surgery even when a good outcome is predicted.

In early stage disease, whether a diagnosis is needed before surgical removal or not depends on the clinical circumstance. A 2-cm growing lesion in a former smoker with a CT-PET showing uptake only in the lesion may not need to be biopsied before resection—the likelihood of identifying a specific benign diagnosis is low and a result that is nonspecific would lead to resection because of the high likelihood of malignancy. In advanced-stage disease, diagnosis and staging is best accomplished with a single invasive test. Rather than biopsy a mass in the lung for diagnosis and perform a subsequent liver biopsy to prove metastasis, the liver or other site establishing

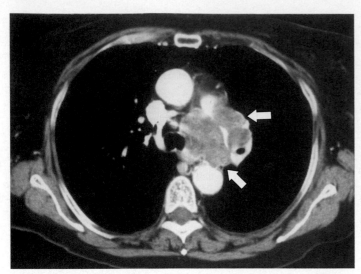

FIGURE 47-21 Small-cell lung cancer with mediastinal adenopathy. Computed tomography scan of the chest shows a large, left upper-lobe mass with extensive left hilar and mediastinal adenopathy (*arrows*) and extrinsic compression of the left main stem bronchus. Transbronchial needle aspiration revealed small-cell carcinoma.

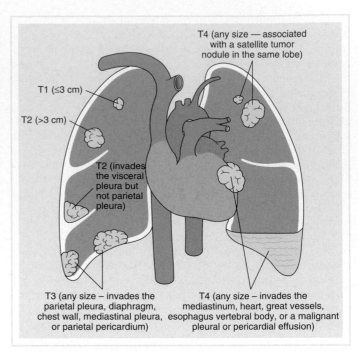

FIGURE 47-22 Primary tumor (T) staging classification in the lung.

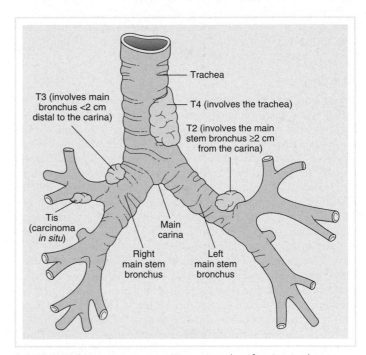

FIGURE 47-23 Primary tumor (T) staging classification in the airway.

the most advanced stage is best pursued initially. The appropriate staging test is determined by the location of apparent neoplastic involvement and the test most likely to achieve the information with the least risk. A cancer presenting as a large mass or central lesion is often easily diagnosed by bronchoscopy. Diagnostic yield approaches 100% with bronchial biopsy when the malignant lesion is present endobronchially. The visual extent of the tumor can guide surgical resection, or biopsy of involvement may establish lack of resectability. Transbronchial needle aspiration through the flexible bronchoscope may be used to sample lymph nodes in the paratracheal (stations 2 and 4, right and left), subcarinal (station 7), and hilar positions (Figure 47-21). In this way bronchoscopic needle aspiration may allow simultaneous diagnosis and staging of advanced-stage lung cancer. When abnormal nodes are identified by CT or PET, needle aspiration at the time of bronchoscopy is an underused technique. Several recent series have shown improvement in yields with endobronchial ultrasound (EBUS) compared with blind bronchoscopic needle aspiration. EBUS is real-time imaging of mediastinal nodes and allows the ability to see the needle in the node at the time of sampling. Yields of 90% for the paratracheal and subcarinal nodes have been reported. The addition of EBUS reduces the need for mediastinoscopy to stage N2 (ipsilateral mediastinal) and N3 (contralateral mediastinal) nodes. Sampling of mediastinal nodes by means of esophagoscopy with ultrasound-guided fine needle aspiration (EUS-FNA) is an alternative method for diagnosis and stage and is appropriate for subcarinal (station 7), left paratracheal stations 2 and 4, and paraesophageal (station 8) and pulmonary ligament (station 9) nodes. Diagnosis and stage may also be accomplished by cytologic examination of a pleural effusion and may establish T4 (stage IIB) disease.

Staging: Non-Small-Cell Lung Cancer

Staging of lung cancer is the most accurate means to estimate prognosis and guide treatment decisions. As previously mentioned, the diagnosis is best pursed by the test most likely to provide the answer to both diagnosis and stage. The characteristics of the primary tumor (T) (Figures 47-22 and 47-23),

regional lymph nodes (N) (Figure 47-24), and metastatic involvement (M) (Figure 47-25) are used to stage NSCLC according to the TNM system. Descriptors of the staging classifications are provided (Table 47-4), and the stage groupings are outlined (Table 47-5). The importance of this staging system is to improve uniformity and allow appropriate comparison of prognosis and treatment studies between institutions and between countries. A new revised TNM international staging system is due to be published in early 2009.

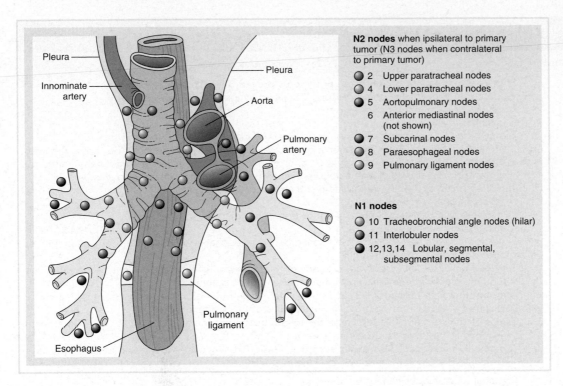

FIGURE 47-24 Lymph node stations (N) for lung cancer staging. (From Mountain CF, Dresler CM: Regional lymph node classification for lung cancer staging. Chest 1997; 111:1718–1723.)

N2 nodes when ipsilateral to primary tumor (N3 nodes when contralateral to primary tumor)

- 2   Upper paratracheal nodes
- 4   Lower paratracheal nodes
- 5   Aortopulmonary nodes
- 6   Anterior mediastinal nodes (not shown)
- 7   Subcarinal nodes
- 8   Paraesophageal nodes
- 9   Pulmonary ligament nodes

N1 nodes

- 10 Tracheobronchial angle nodes (hilar)
- 11 Interlobuler nodes
- 12,13,14   Lobular, segmental, subsegmental nodes

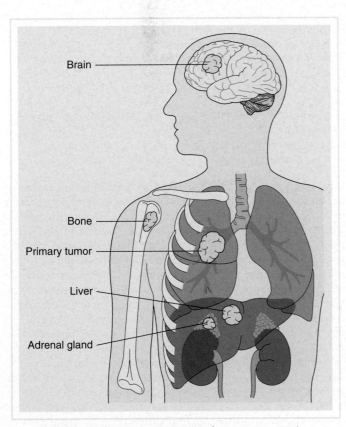

FIGURE 47-25 Metastases (M) in lung cancer staging.

Staging: Small-Cell Lung Cancer

The TNM staging system discussed previously is primarily used to stage NSCLC, and it can be applied to SCLC; however, the limitation is that less differentiation in survival is evident for the various stages. Accordingly, most physicians use the old Veterans Administration staging system of "limited" and "extensive"' disease categories (Figure 47-26). Limited disease is defined as disease confined to one hemithorax and the ipsilateral supraclavicular nodes. This stage of disease can be safely encompassed within the radiation field. Extensive stage disease is defined as disease that has spread beyond these confines and cannot be encompassed in a safe radiation field. Contralateral hilar lymph nodes, cervical lymph nodes, or distant organ metastasis is considered extensive stage disease. A pleural effusion that is cytologically positive for malignant cells or a bloody effusion in the setting of known SCLC is usually classified as extensive stage disease.

TREATMENT AND PROGNOSIS

Non-Small-Cell Lung Cancer

Stages 0, IA/B, and IIA/B

At initial presentation in a nonscreened population, only 15–25% of patients had resectable disease. Patients who have asymptomatic lung cancer at the time of diagnosis have a significantly better prognosis. The treatment of choice for stage 0 (carcinoma in situ), IA/B, or IIA/B NSCLC is surgical resection, provided the patient is medically fit. The 30-day operative mortality with lobectomy is 1–2% and 5–7% for pneumonectomy. The primary causes of operative mortality include pneumonia, respiratory failure, bronchopleural fistula, empyema, myocardial infarction, and pulmonary embolus. In recent years, the frequency of performing pneumonectomies at major cancer centers has decreased dramatically to 5% or less of all operations for lung cancer. Survival rates have been shown to be superior in centers that perform greater numbers of resections.

In the 1990s, video-assisted thoracoscopic (VATS) surgery developed rapidly and is now commonly used at most thoracic surgical centers. This method is useful for lung biopsies and

TABLE 47-4 The TNM (Primary Tumor, Regional Lymph Nodes, and Distant Metastasis) Lung Cancer Staging Descriptions

Aspect	Descriptor	Description
Primary tumor (T)	TX	Primary tumor cannot be assessed, or tumor is proved by the presence of malignant cells in sputum or bronchial washings but not visualized by imaging or bronchoscopy
	T0	No evidence of primary tumor
	Tis	Carcinoma *in situ*
	T1	Tumor ≤3 cm in greatest dimension, surrounded by lung or visceral pleura, without bronchoscopic evidence of invasion more proximal than the lobar bronchus (i.e., not in the main bronchus); the uncommon superficial tumor of any size with its invasive component limited to the bronchial wall, which may extend proximal to the main bronchus, is also classified T1
	T2	Tumor with any of the following features of size or extent: >3 cm in greatest dimension Involves main bronchus, ≥2 cm distal to the carina Invades the visceral pleura Associated with atelectasis or obstructive pneumonitis that extends to the hilar region, but does not involve the entire lung
	T3	Tumor of any size that directly invades any of the following: chest wall (including superior sulcus tumors), diaphragm, mediastinal pleura, parietal pericardium Tumor in the main bronchus <2 cm distal to the carina, but with no involvement of the carina Associated atelectasis or obstructive pneumonitis of the entire lung
	T4	Tumor of any size that invades any of the following: mediastinum, heart, great vessels, trachea, esophagus, vertebral body, carina Tumor with a malignant pleural or pericardial effusion, or with satellite tumor nodule(s) within the ipsilateral primary tumor lobe of the lung
Regional lymph nodes (N)	NX	Regional lymph nodes cannot be assessed
	N0	No regional lymph node metastasis
	N1	Metastasis to ipsilateral peribronchial and/or ipsilateral hilar lymph nodes, and intrapulmonary nodes involved by direct extension of the primary tumor
	N2	Metastasis to ipsilateral mediastinal and/or subcarinal lymph node(s)
	N3	Metastasis to contralateral mediastinal, contralateral hilar, ipsilateral or contralateral scalene, or supraclavicular lymph node(s)
Distant metastasis (M)	MX	Presence of distant metastasis cannot be assessed
	M0	No distant metastasis
	M1	Distant metastasis present (separate metastatic tumor nodule(s) in the ipsilateral nonprimary tumor lobe(s) of the lung also are classified M1)

(From Mountain CF: Revisions in the International System for Staging Lung Cancer. Chest 111:1710–1717, 1997)

TABLE 47-5 The TNM (Primary Tumor, Regional Lymph Nodes, and Distant Metastasis) Lung Cancer Stage Groupings

Stage	TNM Subset
0	Carcinoma *in situ*
IA	T1N0M0
IB	T2N0M0
IIA	T1N1M0
IIB	T2N1M0 T3N0M0
IIIA	T3N1M0 T1N2M0 T2N2M0 T3N2M0
IIIB	T4N0M0; T4N1M0 T4N2M0 T1N3M0; T2N3M0 T3N3M0; T4N3M0
IV	Any T; Any N; M1

(From Mountain CF, Dresler CM: Regional Lymph Node Clasification for Lung Cancer Staging. Chest 111:1718–1723, 1997.)

removal of nodules. VATS lobectomy has not been considered as standard treatment for lung cancer but is gradually gaining in acceptance with proper node dissection. Before the general availability of VATS, a prospective trial by the Lung Cancer Study Group in North America randomly assigned patients with lesions 3 cm in diameter or smaller to resection by lobectomy or a more limited resection (segmentectomy or wedge)—all patients underwent thoracotomy. Patients who had limited resection had three times as many local recurrences than those who underwent lobectomy. The survival difference was of borderline significance ($P = 0.08$, one-sided) in favor of lobectomy. On the basis of this trial and other reports in the literature, lobectomy is considered the surgical procedure of choice for lung cancer if it yields an adequate resection and the patient has sufficient pulmonary function to tolerate it. Ideally, lung cancer surgery is accompanied by sampling of lymph nodes from three or four different mediastinal stations or mediastinal lymph node dissection (see Figure 47-24). Failure to biopsy mediastinal lymph nodes results in suboptimal staging, which impedes adequate staging and decision making as to the need for additional therapy. In the twenty-first century, no patient should have lung cancer surgery without mediastinal lymph node sampling. Many surgeons advocate radical lymph node dissection rather than just nodal sampling. The survival results of a randomized trial comparing lymph

absolute survival advantage in patients with totally resected stage IIA/B and IIIA disease who received four cycles of adjuvant cisplatin-based chemotherapy versus those who received no adjuvant chemotherapy. Current trials are evaluating adjuvant chemotherapy in Stage IB and some Stage IA patients with poor prognosis genetic profiles in the resected cancer. Induction or preoperative chemotherapy (neoadjuvant) followed by surgical resection is still an area of investigation but must be considered unproven and experimental for Stage I and II disease at this time.

Stages IIIA and IIIB

The presence of metastasis to an ipsilateral mediastinal lymph node (N2) establishes stage IIIA disease and was generally considered to be inoperable disease; however, N2 lymph node involvement is no longer an absolute contraindication to surgery. In two recent randomized, prospective trials of carefully selected stage IIIA patients, patients were treated with preoperative chemotherapy followed by surgical resection or surgery alone. Both of these small, randomized trials showed highly statistically and clinically significant differences in survival in favor of the preoperative chemotherapy followed by surgical resection. Numerous other phase II trials used neoadjuvant therapy (preoperative treatment) with two or three cycles of systemic chemotherapy with or without thoracic radiotherapy before surgical resection. Most of these trials enrolled stage IIIA patients, but some included carefully selected stage IIIB patients. The 3-year survival in these trials was 25–35%. The potential negative aspects of the neoadjuvant approach in advanced stage disease are a higher rate of pneumonectomy and a 10–15% treatment-related mortality rate in some series. Recently, investigators from the Southwestern Oncology Group in North America completed a randomized phase III trial that compared the neoadjuvant treatment followed by surgery versus definitive treatment with chemotherapy and thoracic radiation alone. The preliminary results did not show a statistically significant survival advantage in those who received surgery after induction therapy. However, in subset analysis, those patients who underwent a pneumonectomy after induction therapy had a significantly worse survival than those treated with chemoradiotherapy alone. In contrast,

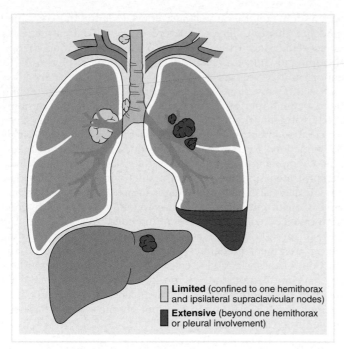

FIGURE 47-26 Staging classification for small-cell lung cancer.

node sampling versus mediastinal lymph node dissection are anticipated in the near future.

The 5-year survival for stage IA lung cancer is 70–80%; for stage IB, it is 50–60% in different series (Figure 47-27). For patients who have stage IIA disease, the 5-year survival is 40–55% and survival for stage IIB is approximately 40%. Stage IIB includes the patient who has a T3N0M0 lesion caused by chest wall involvement and is best treated by surgical resection. From 40–60% of patients who have stage IB, IIA, or IIB NSCLC have recurrences within the first 5 years of surgical resection. Postoperative thoracic radiotherapy has not improved survival in these patients and may actually be detrimental to survival. In the past 5 years, large randomized trials from Europe and North America have demonstrated an

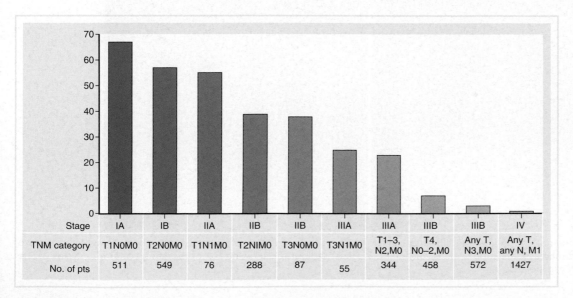

Stage	IA	IB	IIA	IIB	IIB	IIIA	IIIA	IIIB	IIIB	IV
TNM category	T1N0M0	T2N0M0	T1N1M0	T2NIM0	T3N0M0	T3N1M0	T1–3, N2,M0	T4, N0–2,M0	Any T, N3,M0	Any T, any N, M1
No. of pts	511	549	76	288	87	55	344	458	572	1427

FIGURE 47-27 Prognosis in non-small-cell lung cancer. (From Mountain CF: Revisions in the international system for staging lung cancer. Chest 1997; 111:1710–1717.)

those who underwent a lobectomy after induction therapy had a statistically significant better survival than those with chemoradiotherapy alone. The final publication of the results is pending.

Pancoast tumors or superior sulcus tumors are usually stage IIB, IIIA, or IIIB. Unresectable Pancoast tumors have been treated with thoracic radiotherapy alone, but, more recently, a combination of chemotherapy and concurrent thoracic radiation was shown to be superior to thoracic radiotherapy alone for lung cancer. When potentially resectable, Pancoast tumors have been treated by use of preoperative radiotherapy of 30–50 Gy (3000–5000 rad), followed by surgical resection. Higher doses of preoperative radiotherapy increase postoperative complications. The 5-year survival of Pancoast tumors treated by use of radiotherapy and surgical resection is 25–35%. A multicenter trial treated mediastinal lymph node (N2) negative patients with Pancoast tumors with two cycles of induction etoposide and cisplatin chemotherapy and concurrent thoracic radiotherapy of 45 Gy in 25 fractions followed by surgical resection 3–5 weeks later. The overall 5-year survival was 41%. A Japanese study has reported similar results, and accordingly this approach has been adopted as the standard of care.

For patients who have unresectable stage IIIA or IIIB NSCLC, thoracic radiotherapy alone had been the standard treatment in the 70s and 80s. The 5-year survival by use of radiotherapy alone is 3–5%; 70% of treatment failures occur within the field of radiation, and a 50–70% rate of distant metastasis occurs within the first 2 years. Investigators conducted randomized trials of thoracic radiotherapy alone versus combination chemotherapy and thoracic radiotherapy. By use of cisplatin-based chemotherapy, a number of multicenter trials demonstrated the superiority of combined modality therapy. Results are most favorable in patients who have better performance status and minimal weight loss. Meta-analyses of these trials show an approximate 10% absolute superiority in survival at 3–5 years by use of combination chemoradiotherapy. One of the North American Cooperative Groups reported a 7-year follow-up of their trial. The 5-year survival

was 6% for radiotherapy alone versus 17% for the combined modality therapy. The current recommended treatment for unresectable stage IIIA or IIIB NSCLC is combination chemotherapy and thoracic radiation if the patient is physically fit enough to tolerate this approach.

Radiotherapy alone may be indicated in the more debilitated patient (performance score ≥2). The most commonly used treatment schedule of radiotherapy when it is being given for curative intent is 60–65 Gy (6000–6500 rad) given in single daily fractions. Recent trials have evaluated the role of concurrent chemoradiotherapy versus sequential therapy and have demonstrated superior survival results with concurrent therapy but have also observed greater toxicity, especially esophagitis. Concurrent chemoradiotherapy in patients with good performance scores is the recommended treatment on the basis of the 2007 American College of Chest Physicians lung cancer treatment guidelines. Trials evaluating multiple daily fractions of thoracic radiotherapy with concurrent chemotherapy have not demonstrated superior survival to the once-daily fractions of radiotherapy with concurrent chemotherapy. The chemotherapy is platinum based, but no one regimen has been proven to be superior.

Stage IV

Approximately 50% of all patients who have NSCLC have distant metastasis (M1) at the time of initial diagnosis. No curative treatment is available for these individuals. The goal of therapy is to try to control their disease and palliate symptoms. Major response rates (more than 50% tumor shrinkage) of 20–30% have been reported with numerous combination chemotherapy regimens in patients who have this stage of disease. Almost all responses to treatment are partial; complete clinical remission is achieved in less than 5% of patients (Figure 47-28). Patients who respond to chemotherapy gain, on the average, an additional 6–9 months of life but eventually relapse and die of their disease. The median survival time for stage IV NSCLC with no treatment is 3–4 months, with a 1-year survival of approximately 15%.

As a result of the toxicity and lack of curative therapy, therapeutic nihilism has been prevalent among physicians

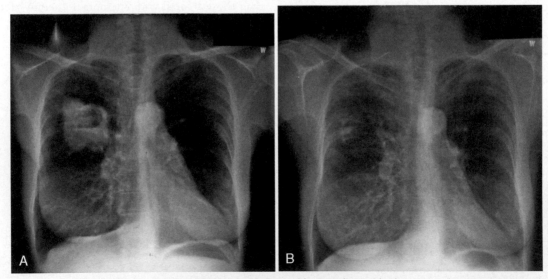

FIGURE 47-28 Response to chemotherapy in stage IIIB lung cancer. **A,** Chest radiograph showing a cavitary squamous cell carcinoma of the right lung. The patient had mediastinal lymph node involvement. **B,** Chest radiograph showing tumor regression after four cycles of chemotherapy with paclitaxel and carboplatin.

responsible for the care of these patients. A recent meta-analysis evaluated eight trials that enrolled more than 700 patients, and each of the trials randomly assigned patients to best supportive care versus chemotherapy by use of a cisplatin-based regimen. This analysis showed a benefit in survival to patients treated with chemotherapy. A reduction in the risk of death of 27% and an absolute improvement in survival of 10% at 1 year occurred in the chemotherapy-treated group. In the 1990s, a number of promising new chemotherapeutic agents were developed and used in patients who had stage IV NSCLC. These agents include paclitaxel, docetaxel, irinotecan, vinorelbine, and gemcitabine. Numerous phase III trials have been completed evaluating platinum-based combinations (cisplatin or carboplatin) with these newer chemotherapy agents. No one platinum doublet of chemotherapy has been shown to be superior. However, by use of platinum-based doublets, the median survival time is 8–9 months, and the 1-year survival is 30–35%. The results have been consistent in North America, Europe, and Japan.

Patients who are going to respond to systemic chemotherapy generally do so after the first two to three cycles of therapy. Randomized clinical trials have demonstrated that there is no advantage to treatment beyond four to six cycles with the same chemotherapy. Accordingly, it is reasonable to offer patients initial treatment with systemic chemotherapy and to treat for a maximum of four to six cycles, as long as no evidence of disease progression occurs. After the initial therapy, it is reasonable to observe until the patients have progressive disease develop. When progressive disease is evident, the risks and benefits of additional therapy with alternative agents need to be weighed. Pemetrexed, docetaxel, and erlotinib have all been shown to prolong survival when used as single agents in second-line treatment trials.

In the past 5 years, there has been great emphasis placed on the development of targeted agents for lung cancer. The first class of these novel agents that has been shown to be of benefit is the epidermal growth factor receptor (EGFR) tyrosine kinase inhibitor. The first drugs in this class were gefitinib and erlotinib. In 2004, it was discovered that a mutation in the EGFR tyrosine kinase domain predicted response to treatment with these agents. A Phase III trial with single agent erlotinib, in previously treated patients, demonstrated a survival advantage versus supportive care only. That trial was the basis for approval of erlotinib in second- or third-line treatment of advanced NSCLC. The EGFT-TKIs have not been shown to be of benefit when added to standard chemotherapy. The second class of novel agents approved for treatment of NSCLC (nonsquamous histology) is the antiangiogenesis drug, bevacizumab. This agent is an antivascular endothelial growth factor (VEGF) monoclonal antibody. A recent multicenter trial with paclitaxel, carboplatin with bevacizumab resulted in significantly better survival than the same chemotherapy alone. However, bevacizumab treatment was associated with a greater chance of fatal bleeding (4% vs 1%).

Quality of life (QOL) is difficult to evaluate and quantify. A number of questionnaires have been developed as QOL tools for cancer, including the Functional Living Index-Cancer Instrument, Functional Assessment of Cancer Therapy, and the Quality of Life Index. A positive correlation occurs between the baseline QOL score and survival in lung cancer patients. Trials have shown that patients who maintain or improve their QOL scores, on the basis of serial measurements, have superior survival to those whose QOL scores decrease. To date, no trials have shown serial QOL measurements in randomized trials of treatment versus supportive care only in patients who have advanced-stage lung cancer. In general, QOL decreases as the disease progresses, even without any associated toxicity from chemotherapy. Numerous trials that used chemotherapy have documented improvement of disease-related symptoms in those patients who achieve a disease regression, as well as in some patients who show no evidence of an objective tumor response. Improvement in symptoms such as cough, dyspnea, or pain undoubtedly results in improvement in the patient's QOL.

Bronchoscopic Treatment

In addition to its role in the diagnosis and staging of lung cancer, bronchoscopy is used to treat lung cancer by the methods of photodynamic therapy (PDT), laser therapy, and brachytherapy. Bronchoscopy may also be used to treat large airway compromise from the cancer with implantation of airway stents.

PDT is appropriate for superficial NSCLC, and the other bronchoscopic interventions may be applied to either NSCLC or SCLC. PDT uses photosensitivity in the form of toxic oxygen radicals that result in cancer cell death. After peripheral injection of hematoporphyrin derivatives, photosensitization is achieved by exposure to an argon-pumped dye laser carried by an optical fiber through the working channel of the flexible bronchoscope. Light energy is absorbed by the photosensitizer and produces cytotoxic tissue effects that are apparent over the next 6–48 h. The patient may expectorate necrotic tissue. Only cancers within the reach of the flexible bronchoscope and those that do not penetrate more than 4–5 mm into the bronchial wall may be effectively treated by PDT. Superficial squamous cell carcinomas that are radiographically occult seem to be most appropriate for this form of therapy. Superficial squamous cell carcinomas may be managed successfully with bronchoscopic PDT alone if they are smaller than 3 cm in surface area, are *in situ*, or have only a few millimeters of microinvasion and are located within the reach of the flexible bronchoscope. Studies to date include patients who are not surgical candidates for reasons other than tumor stage, as well as some patients who have potentially resectable tumors. After one or two PDT applications, 70–80% of patients achieve complete response rates and have subsequent recurrence rates of 10–15%. Generally, surgical excision is still deemed most appropriate for those lesions that are surgically resectable in a patient who is operable.

Various lasers have been used for palliative resection of endobronchial tumors, through both rigid and flexible bronchoscopes. The greatest clinical experience for this purpose is with the neodymium:yttrium aluminum garnet (Nd:YAG) laser, although lasers of other wavelengths, including CO_2 lasers, may be applied. Tissue effects from laser application include both photocoagulation and thermal necrosis. Initial experience with the Nd:YAG laser was at a power of 90 W, which occasionally resulted in significant hemorrhage and death. Subsequent use has reduced complications by using power in the range of 30–40 W with pulses of 0.5–1.0 sec. Appropriate patients for consideration of laser endobronchial malignant resection include those who are unresponsive to other treatment modalities, have lesions that involve the bronchial wall but do not obviously extend through the cartilage, have an identifiable bronchial lumen, and show evidence of functioning lung tissue beyond the level of the endobronchial obstruction. The success of laser treatment is greatest in proximal lesions of the trachea and main stem bronchi, because these are most easily accessible and provide the opportunity to regain the largest quantities of distal lung function. Palliation of symptoms is often immediate, although temporary, and median survival after laser resection is approximately 6 months. Survival improvement has been shown only in patients who undergo emergency laser therapy compared with similar patients who receive only external beam radiation.

Brachytherapy provides a means of intraluminal application of radiation and is generally used in patients who have previously received maximal doses of external beam radiation. Brachytherapy is appropriate for both intrinsic and extrinsic malignant airway obstruction when functioning lung may be maintained or regained by achieving airway patency. Radiation applications of low-dose and high-dose rate have been used successfully. The radiation is applied through a nylon catheter placed through the lesion endoscopically. Response rates range from 30–80%, with success more likely in those patients who had favorable response to previous external beam radiation. Median survival after brachytherapy is in the range of 4 months. Hemorrhage or fistula formations are the most frequent complications and occur in approximately 15% of patients.

Bronchoscopic placement of prosthetic airway stents has become popular for palliation of both intrinsic and extrinsic malignant obstruction. The largest international experience has been with a silastic stent, although metal stents, and combinations of metal and silastic and other materials are being used for stent composition. Stent insertion may be accomplished by use of the rigid or flexible bronchoscope, depending on the composition and delivery method of the prosthesis. Symptomatic improvement from regaining airway patency may be immediate and impressive. An attractive feature of the silastic stent is that it can be removed. Complications with the silastic stents include migration, mucus obstruction, and granulation tissue formation. The metal stents become incorporated into the bronchial wall and may be irretrievable or removed with great difficulty, and the formation of granulation tissue is more prevalent. Malignant growth may occur through the wall of the uncovered metal stents, or proximal or distal to either type of stent.

Small-Cell Lung Cancer

Approximately 15–20% of all lung cancer is SCLC. This cell type has the strongest association with cigarette smoking, and SCLC is rarely observed in an individual who has never smoked. Accordingly, if this diagnosis is made in an individual who has never smoked or has a minimal smoking history, a careful pathologic review should be undertaken to consider alternative diagnosis such as bronchial carcinoid tumor or lymphoma. This histologic type of cancer contains neuroendocrine granules identified by electron microscopy and is the cell type most commonly associated with ectopic hormone production and also is associated with many of the paraneoplastic syndromes.

Limited-Stage SCLC

Approximately one third of patients who have SCLC have limited-stage disease at diagnosis. Limited stage is highly responsive to treatment, with 80–90% response rates to conventional therapy. A complete clinical remission is obtained in 50–60% of limited-stage patients. The median survival time varies from 18–20 months in recent trials, with 2-year survival rates of 30–40% and 5-year survival of 15–25%.

Role of Surgery

Before the discovery of chemotherapeutic agents active against SCLC, surgery was used against this malignancy. The 5-year survival after surgery only was 1–2%. A randomized trial by the British Medical Research Council evaluated surgery versus thoracic radiotherapy alone for limited-stage disease and noted a median survival time of 199 days with surgical treatment versus 300 days with radiotherapy. This report, along with the discovery of active chemotherapeutic agents, resulted in the abandonment of surgical treatment for SCLC in the 1960s.

In the past decade, the role of surgery for very limited SCLC has been reexamined. Reports of highly selected, nonrandomized trials noted 5-year survival rates of 25–35% after surgical resection of SCLC that presented as a solitary nodule. The Lung Cancer Study Group in the United States has evaluated the role of surgery in a randomized prospective trial of patients who had limited-stage SCLCs. All patients received five cycles of cyclophosphamide, doxorubicin, and vincristine (CAV). Patients who showed at least a partial response were randomly assigned to either thoracotomy and resection or no surgery. All patients received identical thoracic radiotherapy. Survival rates on the two arms were identical ($P = .91$), which proved no survival advantage in treating the usual patient with limited-stage SCLC surgically.

The substantial 5-year survival rates after surgery in patients who have SCLC that presented as a pulmonary nodule indicate that it is advisable to treat these patients with surgical resection after appropriate staging to rule out distant metastasis. Occasionally, nodules diagnosed as SCLC after transthoracic needle aspiration or bronchoscopic biopsy are reclassified as a carcinoid tumor after resection. Patients who have SCLC that is completely resected should be treated with four cycles of adjuvant standard chemotherapy and thoracic radiotherapy sequentially. Preoperative evaluation of a peripheral SCLC should include magnetic resonance imaging of the brain or CT scan of the head with contrast, CT scan of the chest and upper abdomen, and PET scan or isotope bone scan to rule out distant metastasis. Ideally, such patients should undergo mediastinoscopy, and the lymph nodes should be negative for metastasis before proceeding to resection. Of all SCLC patients, less than 5% present as a peripheral nodule and are candidates for surgical treatment.

Chemotherapy and Radiation

In the 1970s, the treatment of choice was CAV chemotherapy. Subsequent randomized trials have shown similar survival, but less toxicity, by use of cisplatin and etoposide. The most common treatment regimens now are etoposide and cisplatin or etoposide and carboplatin. These regimens yield similar response rates and survival. The etoposide and carboplatin regimen is generally well tolerated, has been associated with less toxicity, and can be used in elderly patients.

Randomized trials in patients who have limited-stage disease compared chemotherapy alone versus combination chemotherapy and thoracic radiotherapy. A meta-analysis of 13 randomized trials that included more than 2000 patients showed that combined modality therapy resulted in a 14% decrease in the risk of death. The benefit in terms of absolute survival at 3 years was 5.4%. Accordingly, combined modality therapy with chemotherapy and thoracic radiation is considered standard for limited-stage SCLC.

The timing of thoracic radiotherapy is unclear. In a randomized trial from Canada, patients who received thoracic radiotherapy with cycle two of chemotherapy had a significantly better survival rate than those who received the radiotherapy with cycle six. The authors concluded that early radiotherapy was superior to delayed radiotherapy. At this time, it is generally thought that radiotherapy should be given earlier in the treatment course rather than later. Trials with concurrent chemotherapy and thoracic radiation have resulted in superior survival versus sequential therapy and are now the standard of care in North America.

The best treatment approach for limited-stage SCLC is combined chemotherapy by use of etoposide and cisplatin or etoposide and carboplatin and concurrent radiotherapy, with radiotherapy being administered early in the treatment program. With this approach, 50–60% of patients achieve a complete remission with 2-year and 5-year survivals of 40% and 20–25%, respectively. Unfortunately, 70% of the complete remissions relapse within 2 years. Second-line therapies for relapse SCLC yield only modest results.

There have been only modest improvements in survival for SCLC patients in the past 10 years. First, the beneficial role of thoracic radiotherapy in addition to chemotherapy has been substantiated. Second, concurrent chemotherapy and thoracic radiotherapy for limited-stage disease has resulted in improved survival compared with sequential therapy. Third, the number of chemotherapy cycles has decreased to 4 to 6 cycles (from the previous treatment that used 12 or more cycles). Randomized trials demonstrated that additional chemotherapy beyond four to six cycles does not improve long-term survival but adds to toxicity of the treatment. The proliferation of new treatments with novel mechanisms of action is the hope of the future.

Extensive-Stage Small-Cell Lung Cancer

Two thirds of all patients with SCLC have extensive-stage disease at diagnosis. Their response to chemotherapy is 60–80%, with a median survival time of 9–10 months and a 2-year survival of less than 10%. Virtually no patients survive for 5 years.

Approximately 20% of patients experience a complete clinical remission with treatment. The chemotherapeutic agents used are identical to those used for limited-stage disease. Virtually identical response rates and survival rates have been observed with regimens of etoposide and cisplatin; etoposide and carboplatin; etoposide, ifosfamide, and cisplatin; or cyclophosphamide, doxorubicin, and etoposide. Despite the high initial response rates with standard chemotherapy, the dismal 2-year survival rates emphasize the need to develop new active agents against this disease. Some of the cooperative oncology groups treat patients who have extensive-stage SCLC on phase II trials by use of promising new agents. In these trials, the major end point is response rate. The design of the trials allows for a rapid crossover of nonresponding or progressive-disease patients to standard therapy by use of the agents mentioned previously. This approach has not resulted in a significant survival disadvantage compared with initial treatment with standard chemotherapeutic regimens. Two newer agents for SCLC are paclitaxel and topotecan. Both of these agents showed good single-agent activity in previously untreated patients who had SCLC. The combination of paclitaxel and topotecan has yielded response rates and survival similar, but not superior, to standard chemotherapy. To date, no newer chemotherapy agents have been shown to be superior to standard chemotherapy.

Relapse

The median survival of SCLC patients after relapse from prior therapy is 3–4 months. No cures have occurred by use of second-line therapy. The chance of responding to second-line therapy is worse if the patient has not responded to first-line therapy with a platinum-containing agent, or if the relapse interval is less than 90 days since the prior therapy. If the patient's first-line therapy did not include a platinum-based regimen, the patient should be treated with etoposide and cisplatin or etoposide and carboplatin, in which case the chance of response to second-line therapy is 50% or greater. If patients show a good response to first-line therapy and have been in remission for 6 months or longer, it is reasonable to retreat them with the same chemotherapeutic agents that they received initially; the chance of response again is 50% or greater.

If patients relapse within 6 months of therapy by use of a platinum-based regimen or if they fail to respond to initial therapy, second-line treatment decisions are more difficult. Single-agent topotecan is the most common second-line chemotherapy in current use in North America. The chance of responding to second-line therapy is increased significantly if the patients responded to initial therapy and if they have been off this prior therapy for 3 months or longer. Because no standard second-line therapy is established for SCLC, these patients should, whenever possible, be enrolled in prospective clinical trials to evaluate new therapies.

CLINICAL COURSE AND PREVENTION

Among nonscreened patients who have lung cancer, the overall 5-year survival is 16%. Taking this into account, the clinical course of many patients who have lung cancer is unpleasantly predictable. For the advanced stages, the best efforts of the physician, surgeon, and medical and radiation oncologist do not often result in cure, but may have a significant impact in maintaining quality of life and prolonging survival. The two most important prognostic factors are tumor stage and performance scores. Resected stage IA NSCLC has a 5-year survival of approximately 70%; this compares with 10% for stage I tumors in patients who are not surgical candidates because of medical problems or refusal to undergo surgery. Long-term survival in patients at various stages of lung cancer detected in the absence of symptoms is 35% versus 10% among those detected in the presence of symptoms. To identify patients in the preclinical phase of lung cancer is desirable, but mortality reduction with a screening tool is yet to be established. Younger patients and those who have squamous cell type carry a better prognosis among those patients who have operable disease. The prognosis is less favorable for patients who have NSCLC beyond surgical resectability and in those who have SCLC.

After resection and possible cure for any stage of disease, the risk of a second primary lung cancer developing is 2–3% per year. Accordingly, patients are followed at intervals of 3–6 months for the first 2 years after treatment, and after this, patients are followed every 12 months for at least 5 years for the possible development of late recurrence or a new primary lung cancer. No specific follow-up protocol has been shown to be effective in improving survival.

Functional status has been shown to be an important predictor of survival. The Karnofsky Performance Status assesses activity and ability for self-care on a scale from 100–0. A performance status of 70 or less (one who is unable to work or pursue normal activities, but who lives at home and carries out self-care) is recognized as an independent predictor of shortened survival. Other performance status scales are in use and have similarly been shown to predict survival. These measures help to both refine the estimation of prognosis and determine when treatment is appropriate in advanced-stage disease. Weight loss of more than 10% of body weight and male gender are also independent predictors of shortened survival among patients who have unresectable disease. Poor prognosis is also associated with the presence of distant metastasis as is an elevated lactate dehydrogenase level. Within a single stage of lung cancer, considerable disparities arise in survival between patients, suggesting that other biologic factors are important in prognosis. Research into cancer biology has identified a number of markers that may play a role in tumor behavior but, at this point, the role is preliminary. A recent study showed that the presence of five genes (DUSP6, MMD, STAT1, ERBB3, and LCK) was an independent predictor of relapse-free survival and overall survival in a cohort of resected non-small-cell lung cancers.

Recurrence or progression of disease occurs in most patients who have lung cancer and often results in death. Patients who have squamous cell carcinoma have a higher rate of local failure and a lower rate of distant metastasis compared with those who have adenocarcinoma or large-cell carcinoma. Patients with small-cell carcinoma have a high rate of distant spread. Palliative care measures are frequently used in terminally ill patients with lung cancer. In one series hyperalimentation was administered in 90% of the patients, oxygen therapy in 78%, and morphine in 40%. The most frequent cause of death was respiratory failure caused by progression of cancer followed by infection and effusions of the pleura or pericardium. Hospice care effectively ensures the patient receives adequate pain control and other palliative measures, while it allows the patient to reside at home.

Lung cancer remains a highly preventable disease; approximately 85% of lung cancers occur in smokers or former smokers, and so primary prevention remains the avoidance of cigarettes. Efforts at early detection and treatment should not diminish the energy devoted to assist patients with smoking cessation. Smoking rates have fallen slowly in the United States and many other developed countries in the world. Unfortunately, cigarette smoking is highly addictive, and smoking cessation often proves difficult. Physicians may be important motivators to help patients quit smoking. A 3-min interview session with a physician can lead to a 5% success rate in smoking cessation when combined with antismoking reading materials and a follow-up visit. Use of supplemental nicotine, group therapy, behavioral training, hypnosis, or acupuncture achieves 1-year abstinence rates of approximately 20% in controlled trials. Recently, varenicline, a partial nicotine agonist, has shown superiority in randomized trials over sustained-release bupropion in smoking cessation with cessation rates at 12 weeks of 44.0%, 29.5%, and 17.7% for varenicline, bupropion SR, and placebo, respectively. Clearly, primary prevention by avoidance of smoking or through smoking cessation is the best way to prevent the devastating grip of this disease. Home radon testing may also play a role in reducing an individual's risk for lung cancer.

OTHER LUNG NEOPLASMS AND LUNG METASTASES

Carcinoid Tumor

Bronchial carcinoid tumors are low-grade malignant neoplasms composed of neuroendocrine cells and account for 1–2% of all tumors of the lung. Patients may be initially seen with hemoptysis, have evidence of bronchial obstruction, or be asymptomatic (Figure 47-29). The association of carcinoid syndrome (flushing and diarrhea) with bronchial carcinoid tumor is rare, as is ectopic production of adrenocorticotropic hormone and Cushing syndrome. Because carcinoid tumors are often endobronchial, bronchoscopy is an effective means to establish a diagnosis, but this is a relatively vascular tumor so caution in sampling is appropriate. Surgical resection is often curative, and in the absence of nodal metastasis, 10-year survival is greater than 90% for typical carcinoids. Prognosis is lessened in tumors larger than 3 cm or in the presence of nodal metastasis. The term *atypical carcinoid* is used when there is histologic evidence of increased mitotic activity, nuclear pleomorphism, and/or necrosis is present. These lesions tend to have a higher rate of metastasis and be larger at the time of diagnosis than typical carcinoid tumors. The 5-year survival with atypical carcinoid tumors is approximately 60–70%, and surgical treatment is desired when feasible. Carcinoid tumors are generally more refractory to chemotherapy and radiotherapy than non-small-cell lung cancers.

Pulmonary Lymphoma

Primary pulmonary lymphomas account for less than 1% of all lung cancer and are uniformly non-Hodgkin's lymphomas. In one series of 33 patients, 22 patients had small-cell lymphoma,

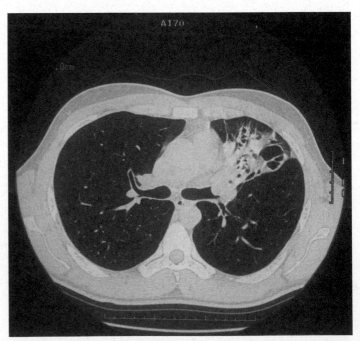

FIGURE 47-29 Carcinoid tumor. Computed tomography of the chest in a 34-year-old man with a 1-year history of recurrent left upper-lobe pneumonia and hemoptysis. Tumor obstructs the left upper-lobe bronchus with associated focal bronchiectasis. Bronchoscopy and subsequent resection revealed carcinoid tumor.

6 had large-cell lymphoma, and 5 had mixed-cell lymphoma. In these patients treated with surgery, surgery plus chemotherapy, or chemotherapy alone, 5-year survival was 77%. Surgical resection of a localized, primary non-Hodgkin's lymphoma may be curative, and chemotherapy seems effective in patients who have bilateral or disseminated disease.

Mucoepidermoid Carcinomas

Mucoepidermoid carcinoma is another rare airway neoplasm derived from minor salivary gland tissue in the proximal tracheobronchial tree. As a result of the central airway location, patients usually present with cough, hemoptysis, or obstructive pneumonia. Surgical resection remains the treatment of choice when feasible, and complete resection portends an excellent prognosis. Lesions of low-grade histology are uncommonly associated with nodal metastases.

Adenoid Cystic Carcinoma

Adenoid cystic carcinoma is the most common salivary gland-like tumor to occur in the lower respiratory tract and accounts for less than 1% of all primary lung cancers. Adenoid cystic carcinomas usually arise in the lower trachea, main stem, or lobar bronchi and are rarely peripheral. Presenting symptoms are usually cough, hemoptysis, or evidence of airway obstruction. Surgical resection is preferred; however, this cell type has a propensity to recur locally and metastasize, and resection is often incomplete. Delayed recurrence, as long as 15–20 years after initial resection, has been reported.

Hamartoma

Hamartoma is the most common benign neoplasm to occur in the lung. Histologically, the lesions consist of a combination of cartilage, connective tissue, smooth muscle, fat, and respiratory epithelium. Most hamartomas are detected as a smoothly bordered nodule by chest radiograph or CT when patients are asymptomatic. The highest incidence of hamartoma is in the sixth and seventh decade. A series of 215 patients reported that only 4 patients had symptoms related to the hamartoma. The classic CT appearance of popcorn-ball calcification occurs in only approximately 25% of hamartomas. Approximately 15% show evidence of fat on thin-section CT scanning (Figure 47-30). Radiographic recognition allows for simple observation in most instances; radiographically indeterminate lesions may be resected for confirmation. Multiple pulmonary hamartomas have been reported rarely.

Lung Metastases

The lung is a frequent site of metastasis from a variety of extrathoracic malignancies. Carcinomas recognized as frequent sources for pulmonary metastases include those of the head and neck, colon, kidney, breast, and thyroid, and melanoma. Approximately 10–30% of all malignant nodules resected from the lung are metastases. In addition to solitary or multiple nodules, metastatic patterns of carcinoma to the lung include lymphangitic, endobronchial, pleural, and embolic. The finding of multiple or innumerable nodules is the most common clinical situation (Figure 47-31). Depending on the size and location of the nodules, a diagnosis may be obtained by transthoracic needle aspiration or bronchoscopy. Surgical resection may be appropriate in the setting of a solitary pulmonary metastasis when evidence of other sites of metastatic disease have been excluded. Although randomized studies have not been performed, evidence suggests improved survival

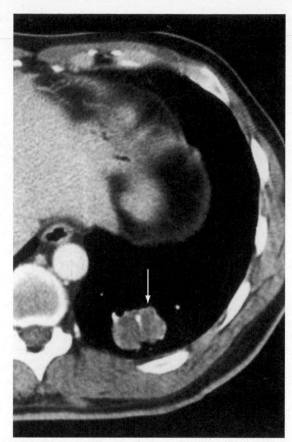

FIGURE 47-30 Hamartoma. Thin-section computed tomography through this solitary pulmonary nodule reveals evidence of calcification and fat consistent (*arrow*) with a hamartoma.

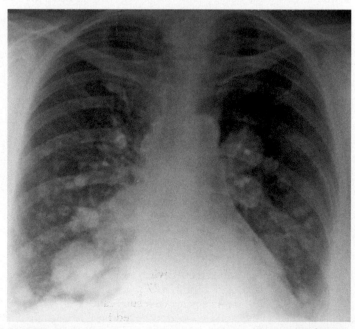

FIGURE 47-31 Pulmonary metastases. Chest radiograph of a 64-year-old woman showing innumerable nodules from metastatic adenocarcinoma of the thyroid.

in some patients who have solitary pulmonary metastasis from sarcomas, renal cell carcinoma, breast cancer, and colon cancer.

PITFALLS AND CONTROVERSIES

Screening for Lung Cancer

Screening for lung cancer with chest radiography or sputum cytologic examination has not been proven to reduce mortality. In the 1970s, the National Cancer Institute sponsored three large, randomized trials. Participants were men age 45 years or older who had smoked one pack of cigarettes per day or more within the year before enrollment. The Mayo Lung Project randomly assigned patients to a chest radiograph and 3-day pooled sputum cytologic examination every 4 months in the screened group, and the control group was advised to have an annual chest radiograph and sputum cytologic examination but had no scheduled follow-up. Johns Hopkins and Memorial Sloan-Kettering were the other two participating centers, and both randomly assigned patients to a dual screen with an annual chest radiograph and 3-day pooled sputum cytologic examination every 4 months versus an annual chest radiograph. None of these trials demonstrated a decrease in lung cancer mortality in the group screened at higher frequency, but none of the three centers had an untested control group. In each, the 5-year survival from lung cancer in the screened group was approximately 35%, which was more than double the historical precedent. A subsequent meta-analysis of studies evaluating chest x-ray screening showed that despite finding more cancers and more early-stage cancers, mortality was actually increased in those who received more frequent screening—more harm than good was done.

Computed Tomography Screening

The most sensitive image modality currently available for detecting pulmonary nodules is CT. Conventional chest CT requires radiation dosage and image-acquisition time that is impractical for screening purposes. The development of low-dose, fast-spiral CT greatly reduced the radiation dose and the scan time, making screening feasible. Conventional CT images are obtained at 140–300 milliamperes (mA) and are performed over many minutes by use of multiple breath holds. In contrast, low-dose, fast-spiral CT images may be obtained at 20–50 mA and the entire scan completed in 15 sec during a single breath hold.

Initial studies from Japan created excitement in suggesting the viability of low-dose spiral CT as a tool for early lung cancer detection. The first study screened a high-risk population for lung cancer with both low-dose spiral CT scanning and chest radiography. CT detected 15 cases of peripheral lung cancer; 11 of these were missed on chest radiography. An amazing 93% of the non-small-cell carcinomas identified were stage IA. In the United States, CT screening efforts were led by the Early Lung Cancer Action Project. The initial study enrollment included 1000 current or former smokers age 60 years or greater and screened with low-dose spiral CT and chest x-ray CT detected a total of 27 prevalence lung cancers; 23 of the 27 (85%) malignancies were surgical stage IA. A total of 559 noncalcified nodules were detected in 233 participants (23%). In the Mayo CT Screening study, 1520 participants age 50 years or older who were current or former smokers of more than 20 pack-years were enrolled and screened within

1 year. Baseline scanning revealed one or more noncalcified nodules in 51% of the participants; studies that used 10-mm collimation (CT slice thickness) found noncalcified nodules in approximately 25% of participants, and this number increases to 40–50% if 5-mm collimation is used. The high rate of nodule detection (false-positive scans) in these studies raises concern. The Mayo study reported that baseline and annual follow-up for 5 years revealed 66% of NSCLC cases detected were stage 1A. The largest single arm (no control group), observational report of CT screening combined the ELCAP and International Early Lung Cancer Action Program (IELCAP). Over 31,000 participants received a baseline scan and 27,000 repeat scans were performed. A total of 484 cancers were found and 85 percent of these were clinical stage I non-small cell carcinomas. Actuarial 10-year lung cancer survival was 80%, and the actuarial survival for those with stage 1 was 88%; median follow-up was 40 months.

Although these CT screening studies have shown a high percent of cancers are early stage and survival form diagnosis is long compared with nonscreened studies, these do not prove the effectiveness of screening. Screening introduces inherent biases of lead time length time and overdiagnosis; it is not clear whether the calculated survival is true improvement or just apparent improvement because of bias. By use of a validated prediction model, a recent study evaluation of screening studies from Mayo, Milan, and Moffet Cancer Center showed that CT found three times as many cancer as predicted, and most of these were early stage, but neither was there a reduction in the expected number of advanced stage cancers nor a reduction in lung cancer deaths. Randomized controlled trials of CT screening are currently under way in the United States and Europe and will hopefully definitively show mortality reduction with CT screening.

Evaluation of the Solitary Nodule

The optimal evaluation of an SPN is unclear (see Figure 47-20). Nodules that are indeterminate after radiographic investigations call for a decision between observation, biopsy, or removal. Newer radiologic techniques will, hopefully, ease the decision making and reduce the incision making. Contrast-enhanced CT, PET, and magnetic resonance imaging are useful in helping identify likelihood of malignancy in the setting of an SPN. A multicenter study has reported that CT enhancement has a sensitivity of 98% and a specificity of 73% in the identification of malignant neoplasms. The test involves the administration of conventional, iodinated contrast material at a specific rate with thin-section CT assessments through the nodule at 1-min intervals (Figure 47-32). Malignant neoplasms enhance significantly more (more than 15 Hounsfield units) than do granulomas and benign neoplasms. The overall negative predictive value of 96% establishes CT contrast enhancement as a valuable tool in the evaluation of indeterminate SPNs. This is perhaps best used as the initial test of evaluation after a nodule is identified on chest radiograph and, if negative (nonenhancing), is a strong predictor that the nodule is benign. PET scanning with ^{18}F-fluorodeoxyglucose has a sensitivity of approximately 95% and a specificity of 85% for identifying a nodule as malignant. PET and integrated CT-PET are becoming more widely available and also provide additional staging information in the setting of malignancy. The recently published guidelines from the Fleischner Society may be helpful in deciding the appropriate follow-up for small

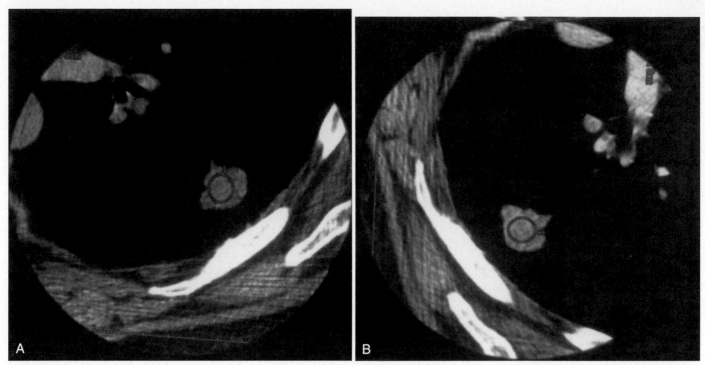

FIGURE 47-32 Evaluation of a solitary pulmonary nodule with computed tomography (CT) contrast enhancement. **A,** Before contrast injection. **B,** After injection of contrast according to protocol, CT scanning is carried out at 1-min intervals and shows an increase in nodule density of 63 Hounsfield units (HU). Enhancement by 15 HU indicates a higher likelihood of malignancy. Resection revealed stage IA (T1N0M0) NSCLC.

nodules identified on CT. These guidelines are described in more detail under the previous section on diagnosis.

Treatment: Stage IIIA

One important area that is unclear is the most appropriate treatment for stage IIIA NSCLC. The literature strongly suggests that surgery alone or radiotherapy alone is not an optimal treatment. If the patient has a negative mediastinoscopy or CT scan of the chest for adenopathy and is found to have stage IIIA disease at the time of thoracotomy, complete resection followed by adjuvant chemotherapy is recommended. The role of adjuvant thoracic radiotherapy for resected IIIA disease is less clear. In patients who are not operative candidates, the combination of concurrent chemotherapy and radiotherapy has been shown to be superior in those with good performance status and minimal weight loss.

Prophylactic Cranial Irradiation: Small-Cell Lung Cancer

Randomized trials have clearly documented that prophylactic cranial irradiation (PCI) reduces the rate of brain metastasis in patients who have SCLC. A large meta-analysis of PCI versus no PCI has shown a significant survival advantage with PCI. Ataxia, difficulty with concentration, memory problems, and dementia are occasionally observed in patients treated with cranial irradiation. Recent trials have used lower dose and fraction regimens, and preliminary reports have not noted any significant detrimental neurologic sequelae. Most medical and radiation oncologists now recommend PCI for patients in complete remission.

SUGGESTED READINGS

Alberg AJ, Samet JM: Epidemiology of lung cancer. Chest 2003; 123:21S–49S.

Bach PB, Jett JR, Pastorino U, et al: Computed tomography screening and lung cancer outcomes. JAMA 2007; 297:953–961.

Chen HY, Yu SL, Chen CH, et al: A five-gene signature and clinical outcome in non-small-cell lung cancer. N Engl J Med 2007; 356:11–20.

Devesa SS, Bray F, Vizcaino AP, Parkin DM: International lung cancer trends by histologic type: male:female differences diminishing and adenocarcinoma rates rising. Int J Cancer 2005; 117:294–299.

Jemal A, Siegel R, Ward E, et al: Cancer statistics, 2007. CA Cancer J Clin 2007; 57:43–66.

MacMahon H, Austin JH, Gamsu G, et al: Fleischner Society: Guidelines for management of small pulmonary nodules detected on CT scans: a statement from the Fleischner Society. Radiology 2005; 237:395–400.

Mountain CF: Revisions in the international system for staging lung cancer. Chest 1997; 111:1710–1717.

Parkin DM, Bray F, Ferlay J, Pisani P: Global cancer statistics, 2002. CA Cancer J Clin 2005; 55:74–108.

Pittock SJ, Kryzer TJ, Lennon VA: Paraneoplastic antibodies coexist and predict cancer, not neurological syndrome. Ann Neurol 2004; 56: 715–719.

Spiro SG, Silvestri GA: One hundred years of lung cancer. Am J Respir Crit Care Med 2005; 172:523–529.

van Tinteren H, Hoekstra OS, Smit EF, et al: Effectiveness of positron emission tomography in the preoperative assessment of patients with suspected non-small-cell lung cancer: the PLUS multicentre randomised trial. Lancet 2002; 359:1388–1393.

Winton T, Livingston R, Johnson D, et al: National Cancer Institute of Canada Clinical Trials Group; National Cancer Institute of the United States Intergroup JBR.10 Trial Investigators: Vinorelbine plus cisplatin vs. observation in resected non-small-cell lung cancer. N Engl J Med 2005; 352:2589–2597.

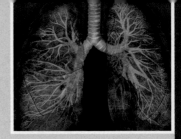

48 Disorders of the Mediastinum

DIANE C. STROLLO • MELISSA L. ROSADO-DE-CHRISTENSON

ANATOMY OF THE MEDIASTINUM AND GENERAL CONSIDERATIONS

The mediastinum is a central space within the thoracic cavity that is bounded by the sternum anteriorly, the pleura and lungs laterally, the vertebral column posteriorly, the thoracic inlet superiorly, and the diaphragm inferiorly. Although the mediastinum is often arbitrarily divided into compartments, true anatomic planes do not exist, and a mediastinal lesion can occupy more than one compartment. Anatomists and surgeons traditionally divide the mediastinum into four compartments: superior, anterior, middle, and posterior. The best-known imaging division of the mediastinum is based on the location of a mediastinal mass on the lateral chest radiograph. Because the initial imaging evaluation of mediastinal lesions is typically performed with radiography, localization of a mass in a radiographic mediastinal compartment allows the formulation of a focused differential diagnosis. This chapter divides the mediastinum into anterior, middle-posterior, and paravertebral compartments (Figure 48-1). The anterior mediastinum is defined by an imaginary line drawn along the anterior trachea and posterior cardiac border on a lateral chest radiograph. The paravertebral compartment is located posterior to an imaginary line drawn to connect the anterior aspects of the thoracic vertebrae. The middle-posterior mediastinum is the compartment located between the anterior and paravertebral compartments. Note that the paravertebral regions do not form part of the mediastinum proper. Mediastinal masses are generally described as being predominantly within one of the aforementioned compartments. Cross-sectional imaging allows more accurate localization of mediastinal abnormalities, characterization of the lesions, and visualization of their relationship with and effects on adjacent normal structures.

In adults, approximately 65% of primary mediastinal lesions are located in the anterior mediastinum, 10% in the middle-posterior, and 25% in the paravertebral compartment. In contrast, approximately 38% of childhood mediastinal lesions are located in the anterior, 10% in the middle-posterior, and 52% in the paravertebral compartment (Table 48-1). The most common mediastinal masses are neurogenic neoplasms, thymic lesions, cysts, lymphomas, and germ-cell neoplasms. Thymic and neurogenic neoplasms and foregut cysts are the most frequent lesions in adults, and neurogenic neoplasms, foregut cysts, and lymphoma are the predominant lesions in children. Less frequent mediastinal lesions include goiter, lymphangioma, intrathoracic hernia, pancreatic pseudocyst, extramedullary hematopoiesis, and meningocele. In addition, lung cancer may manifest as a mediastinal mass or as extensive mediastinal lymphadenopathy.

The nature of mediastinal diseases varies significantly with the patient's age and the clinical presentation. Overall, approximately one third of mediastinal neoplasms are malignant. The mediastinal neoplasms that affect children (40–50%) are more likely to be malignant than those affecting adults (25%). Most masses (80–90%) in asymptomatic individuals are benign, whereas approximately 50% of the lesions that produce symptoms are malignant. Conversely, approximately 75% of patients who have malignant neoplasms also have symptoms compared with less than 50% of patients with benign lesions. Patients with mediastinal masses may experience constitutional symptoms, paraneoplastic syndromes, and symptoms related to compression or invasion of adjacent mediastinal structures. The latter may herald a large, locally invasive or malignant lesion.

The initial evaluation of patients with mediastinal abnormalities includes a detailed history and physical examination targeted to discover specific symptoms and signs of various mediastinal disorders and associated diseases (Table 48-2). Posteroanterior (PA) and lateral chest radiography, computed tomography (CT), and occasionally magnetic resonance imaging (MRI) are used for lesion detection and characterization, usually followed by an invasive procedure for tissue diagnosis. However, some mediastinal lesions have a characteristic radiologic appearance, and biopsy may be unwarranted or contraindicated, as in congenital cysts and vascular lesions, respectively. In addition, laboratory evaluation to include a complete blood count, electrolytes, renal and liver function tests, and serologic tests for various autoantibodies and tumor markers may be useful in the initial evaluation and in posttherapy follow-up.

DISEASES OF THE ANTERIOR MEDIASTINUM

Mediastinal Neoplasms

Thymoma

Thymoma is the most common primary mediastinal neoplasm in adults and the most frequent tumor of the anterior mediastinum. It usually affects adults older than 40 years, with no gender predilection. Approximately 30% of patients with thymoma have thoracic symptoms of cough, dyspnea, and/or chest pain; 40–70% have symptoms related to one or more of the parathymic syndromes, typically myasthenia gravis (MG), but hypogammaglobulinemia, pure red-cell aplasia, and nonthymic malignancies may also occur. Some affected patients are asymptomatic and are discovered incidentally because of abnormal chest radiographs. Although the association of thymoma and MG is well recognized, approximately 85% of patients with MG have thymic lymphoid hyperplasia, and only 15% are found to have thymoma. In contrast, up to

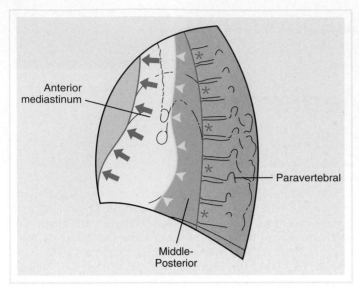

FIGURE 48-1 Mediastinal compartments on lateral chest radiography. The radiographic anterior mediastinum is situated anterior to an imaginary line drawn along the anterior trachea and continued inferiorly along the posterior heart border. The paravertebral compartment is situated posterior to an imaginary line that joins the anterior thoracic vertebral surfaces. The middle-posterior mediastinum is located between the anterior and the paravertebral compartments.

30–50% of patients with thymoma have MG develop. Hypogammaglobulinemia and pure red-cell aplasia occur in 10% and 5% of patients who have thymoma, respectively. Nonthymic malignancies occur in 12–20% of patients with thymoma and include thyroid carcinoma, bronchogenic carcinoma, and lymphoma.

Thymomas manifest on radiography as rounded, well-circumscribed, unilateral, anterior mediastinal masses (Figure 48-2). They are typically located anterior to the aortic root but may be found anywhere from the thoracic inlet to the diaphragm and rarely in the neck. On cross-sectional imaging, thymomas are often homogeneous, soft tissue masses (Figure 48-3) but may exhibit heterogeneity because of cystic change, hemorrhage, or necrosis, especially in large neoplasms. "Drop metastases" to the ipsilateral pleura, pericardium, or upper abdomen through a diaphragmatic hiatus are well documented and represent invasive disease. Pleural drop metastases may encase the lung and mimic diffuse malignant mesothelioma, although associated pleural effusion is infrequent. Lymph node and hematogenous metastases are rare. Mediastinal invasion may be detected with CT and may manifest as an irregular tumoral surface, contralateral extension of thymoma across the midline, and obvious invasion of mediastinal fat and structures. Imaging evidence of local invasion must be correlated with microscopic evidence of capsular transgression and tissue invasion, because encapsulated thymomas may produce fibrous adhesions to adjacent structures. MRI is more sensitive than CT in the detection of vascular invasion. CT-guided needle biopsy, mediastinotomy, mediastinoscopy, and/or video-assisted thoracoscopy may establish the diagnosis. However, histologic diagnosis before excisional surgery may not be required in classic cases of thymoma.

Thymomas represent neoplastic proliferation of thymic epithelial cells, intermixed with mature lymphocytes. The Revised 1999 World Health Organization (WHO) classification divides thymic epithelial neoplasms into three types (A, B, and C) on the basis of epithelial cell morphology, the ratio of lymphocytes to epithelial cells, and prognosis. Types A and B correlate with the traditional major histologic cell types of thymoma—epithelial, lymphocytic, mixed lymphoepithelial, and spindle cell. Type C refers to thymic carcinoma. Anatomic staging is based on the presence or absence of capsular invasion determined macroscopically during surgery and confirmed microscopically. Most thymomas are completely encapsulated; however, approximately 30% are invasive and grow through the capsule into surrounding adipose tissue, pleura, pericardium, great vessels, and/or heart. Encapsulated and invasive thymomas are microscopically identical and lack histologic features of malignancy, and thus the term "invasive" rather than "malignant" thymoma is used to denote capsular invasion.

The treatment of choice for encapsulated and invasive thymomas confined to the mediastinum is surgical resection. Postoperative radiation therapy is included in the treatment of invasive thymoma, but the role of preoperative irradiation is controversial. Chemotherapy with cisplatin-based regimens is generally recommended for metastatic or unresectable recurrent disease, with an overall response rate of 50–70% in small studies.

The prognosis of patients with thymoma varies with the stage and extent of surgical resection. Patients with completely resected, encapsulated lesions have the best prognosis. The overall 5- and 10-year survival rates in patients who have encapsulated thymomas are 75% and 63%, respectively, whereas patients with invasive thymoma have survival rates of 50% and 30%, respectively. Delayed recurrence of thymomas may occur, even in patients with completely resected encapsulated lesions, which emphasizes the importance of long-term follow-up.

The role of thymectomy in the treatment of parathymic syndromes is controversial. Thymectomy is more effective in patients with MG in the absence of a thymoma, with a clinical remission rate of approximately 35% and improvement in another 50%. Neurologic improvement is less likely when MG is associated with thymoma. Thymectomy in patients with pure red-cell aplasia results in a 40–50% remission rate, in contrast to those with hypogammaglobulinemia, who do not benefit from thymic resection.

Thymic Carcinoma

Thymic carcinomas are a heterogeneous group of aggressive, epithelial malignancies with a tendency for early local invasion and distant metastases. Men are more commonly affected (mean age, 46 years). The Revised 1999 WHO classification of thymic epithelial neoplasms describes thymic carcinomas as "nonorganotypic" malignancies (type C) that resemble carcinomas of extrathymic origin, such as lung carcinomas. By traditional histopathologic classification, the two most common cell types are squamous cell and lymphoepithelial-like carcinoma. Unlike thymoma, thymic carcinoma has malignant histologic features and typically manifests as a large, poorly defined, infiltrative, anterior mediastinal mass, frequently with regional lymph node and pulmonary metastases, and pleural and/or pericardial effusions (Figure 48-4).

The histologic grade and neoplastic staging determine the therapy and prognosis. Surgical resection, when feasible, is the preferred treatment. Adjuvant cisplatin-based chemotherapy and concurrent radiotherapy may be used. Response rates are generally poor, with 5-year survival rates of approximately 30%.

TABLE 48-1 Compartmental Classification of Mediastinal Disorders

Location	Source of Abnormality	Disorder Abnormality
Anterior Mediastinum	Disorders of thymus gland	Thymoma Thymic carcinoma Thymic carcinoid Thymolipoma Thymic cyst Thymic hyperplasia
	Lymphoma	Hodgkin disease Non-Hodgkin lymphoma

	Germ cell neoplasms	Benign—mature teratoma
		Malignant
		  Seminoma
		  Nonseminomatous germ cell neoplasms

	Thyroid	Intrathoracic goiter
	Parathyroid	Parathyroid adenoma
	Pericardial cysts	
	Miscellaneous	Mesenchymal neoplasms (lipoma, liposarcoma, angiosarcoma, leiomyoma) Cystic hygroma (mediastinal lymphangioma)

Middle — Posterior Mediastinum	Lymph node enlargement	Lymphoma
		Benign mediastinal lymphadenopathy
		  Granulomatous disease, infectious (tuberculosis, fungal infections)
		  Noninfectious (sarcoidosis, silicosis)
		Miscellaneous causes
		  Castleman disease
		  Amyloidosis
		Metastatic mediastinal lymphadenopathy
		  Lung, renal cell, gastrointestinal carcinoma, breast

	Cysts	Foregut cysts Bronchogenic and enteric cysts
	Esophageal disorders	Achalasia Benign tumors Esophageal carcinoma Esophageal diverticulum
	Vascular lesions	Aneurysms, hemangioma
	Miscellaneous	Herniations Pancreatic pseudocyst

Paravertebral Lesions	Neurogenic neoplasms	Peripheral nerve neoplasms:
		  Schwannoma, neurofibroma, malignant peripheral nerve sheath neoplasm
		Sympathetic ganglia neoplasms
		  Ganglioneuroma, ganglioneuroblastoma, neuroblastoma
		Paraganglionic neoplasms
		  Pheochromocytoma, paraganglioma

	Spinal	Lateral thoracic meningocele Paraspinal abscess (Pott's disease)
	Miscellaneous	Extramedullary hematopoiesis Thoracic duct cysts

Thymic Carcinoid

Thymic carcinoid is a rare, aggressive neuroendocrine neoplasm that typically affects men in the fourth and fifth decades. These are large, symptomatic, locally invasive neoplasms with frequent distant metastases. Approximately 35% of affected patients have endocrine abnormalities caused by ectopic hormone production develop, most commonly Cushing syndrome. Multiple endocrine neoplasia syndrome type I may also occur. However, the syndrome of inappropriate antidiuretic hormone secretion and the carcinoid syndrome are rare. Radiologically, thymic carcinoid is a large, lobular, heterogeneous, and usually invasive anterior mediastinal mass indistinguishable from thymic carcinoma or thymoma. There may be associated intrathoracic metastatic lymphadenopathy. Surgical resection, when feasible, is the treatment of choice, and response to chemotherapy and radiotherapy is poor.

Mediastinal Lymphoma

Lymphoma represents 10–20% of all mediastinal neoplasms in adults. Approximately two thirds of all lymphomas are

TABLE 48-2 Constitutional and Paraneoplastic Findings of Mediastinal Disorders

Diseases	Clinical Findings
Lymphoma	Fever, weight loss, night sweats, pruritus, hypercalcemia
Thymoma	Myasthenia gravis, hypogammaglobulinemia, pure red-cell aplasia
Thymic carcinoid	Cushing's syndrome, syndrome of inappropriate antidiuretic hormone secretion
Germ cell neoplasms	Gynecomastia, Klinefelter syndrome, hematologic neoplasms
Intrathoracic goiter	Hyper/hypothyroidism
Pheochromocytoma	Hypertension, hypercalcemia, polycythemia, Cushing syndrome
Autonomic ganglia neoplasms	Opsomyoclonus, hypertension, watery diarrhea, Horner syndrome
Sarcoidosis	Hypercalcemia

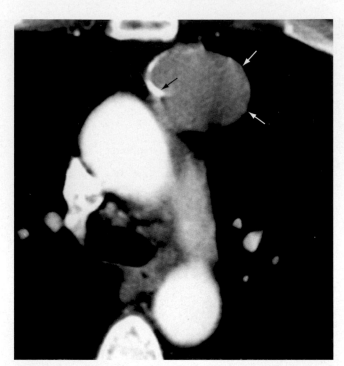

FIGURE 48-3 Contrast-enhanced chest computed tomogram (CT) (mediastinal window) of a patient with thymoma. A sharply marginated thymoma (*white arrows*) arises from the left thymic lobe and exhibits capsular calcification (*black arrow*).

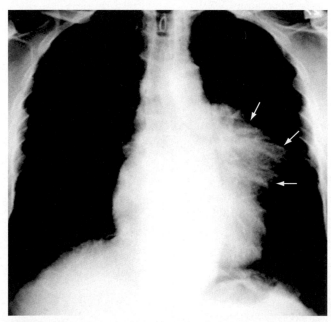

FIGURE 48-2 Posteroanterior (PA) chest radiograph of a patient with thymoma. A large, lobular, left anterior mediastinal thymoma (*arrows*) extends into the inferior mediastinum. Thymomas occur anywhere between the thoracic inlet and the diaphragm.

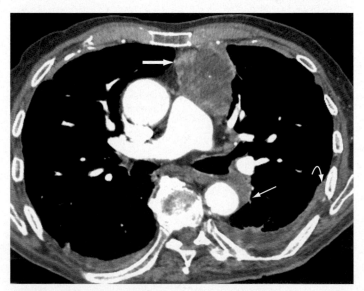

FIGURE 48-4 Contrast-enhanced CT (mediastinal window) of a patient with thymic carcinoma. A heterogeneous mass in the region of the thymic bed (*block arrow*) exhibits cystic change, peripheral nodular enhancement, and ipsilateral hilar (*thin arrow*) and pleural (*curved arrow*) metastases, bilateral pleural thickening, and small effusions.

non-Hodgkin's lymphoma (NHL). Mediastinal involvement typically denotes systemic lymphoma but may also represent primary disease. Although both Hodgkin's disease (HD) and NHL may affect the mediastinum, mediastinal involvement from systemic lymphoma is much more common in HD than in NHL. Nodular sclerosis is the most common subtype of HD to affect the mediastinum. Diffuse, large B-cell and lymphoblastic lymphomas represent the most common primary mediastinal subtypes of NHL. Patients affected by NHL have a higher incidence of systemic symptoms and concomitant involvement of extrathoracic and extranodal lymphoid tissue.

Hodgkin Disease

HD is most commonly seen in adults aged 20–30 years and in those older than 50 years. Even though the nodular sclerosis subtype is more common in women, HD in general does not exhibit a gender predilection in young patients. Patients who have mediastinal lymphoma tend to be younger. The usual presenting finding is cervical and supraclavicular lymphadenopathy. In less than 25% of patients, HD is limited to the thorax. Approximately one third of patients have systemic symptoms. Patients with mediastinal involvement are generally asymptomatic, although bulky lymphadenopathy may induce symptoms related to mediastinal compression.

Radiologically, most patients with HD have bilateral, asymmetric, mediastinal lymphadenopathy, which frequently involves the prevascular and paratracheal lymph nodes and rarely the posterior mediastinal or juxtacardiac lymph nodes. Nodular sclerosis HD can manifest as large, lobular, coalescent lymphadenopathy in the anterior mediastinum or as a discrete mass (Figure 48-5). Invasion, compression, and displacement of mediastinal structures, lung, pleura, and/or chest wall may occur. Affected lymph nodes usually exhibit homogeneous attenuation but may be heterogeneous because of hemorrhage, necrosis, or cystic change. *De novo* lymph node calcification rarely occurs but may develop 1–5 years after radiation therapy. Direct invasion of the lung occurs in 8–14% of untreated patients and is usually associated with hilar lymphadenopathy. The diagnosis is established with either core biopsy or surgical excision of affected palpable lymph nodes or masses found on imaging.

HD spreads by means of contiguous nodal chains and is staged anatomically according to the modified Ann Arbor Classification, combined with histologic staging (nodular sclerosis, mixed cellularity, lymphocyte predominant, lymphocyte depletion, and unclassified). Stages IA and IIA HD (asymptomatic disease on the same side of the diaphragm, without bulky lymphadenopathy) have historically been treated with radiation therapy alone. At this time, limited chemotherapy and limited radiotherapy are being evaluated for early stage disease. More advanced stages are treated with systemic chemotherapy. Bulky mediastinal lymphoma or HD is treated with chemotherapy followed by radiation therapy. Prognosis depends on the stage of the disease, with cure rates of more than 90% achieved in stage IA and IIA disease; even with diffuse or disseminated involvement of one or more extranodal tissues (stage IV), 50–60% of patients can be cured with combination chemotherapy. Recurrences may be cured with salvage chemotherapy.

Non-Hodgkin's Lymphoma

NHL typically affects older patients (compared with those affected by HD) and exhibits a slight male predilection. Diffuse, large B-cell and lymphoblastic lymphomas, the most commonly diagnosed subtype in the mediastinum, occur in younger patients. Diffuse large B-cell lymphoma is more common in females, and lymphoblastic lymphoma is more common in males and is frequently associated with acute lymphoblastic leukemia (Figure 48-6). Both may produce symptoms related to rapid growth and mediastinal invasion, including the superior vena cava syndrome. In addition, diffuse large B-cell lymphoma and lymphoblastic lymphoma may manifest as a primary mediastinal mass without extrathoracic lymphadenopathy. Most patients with NHL are initially seen with advanced disease and systemic symptoms, and approximately half have intrathoracic lymph node enlargement. Thoracic lymphadenopathy is typically isolated or noncontiguous and tends to occur in unusual sites, such as the posterior mediastinal, juxtacardiac, and retrocrural lymph node groups. Anterior mediastinal involvement is less common than in HD, but imaging features are similar to those of HD.

NHL is usually systemic on presentation and spreads unpredictably; thus, histologic classification has a better prognostic value than anatomic staging. According to the Revised European-American Classification of Lymphoid Neoplasms, NHL can be classified as indolent, aggressive, or highly aggressive.

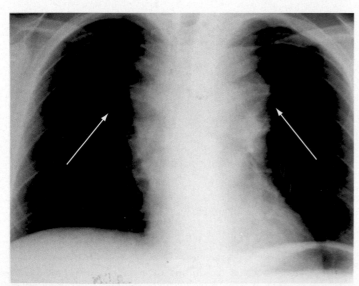

FIGURE 48-5 PA chest radiograph of a patient with Hodgkin's disease. A large predominantly anterior mediastinal mass *(arrows)* extends to both sides of midline.

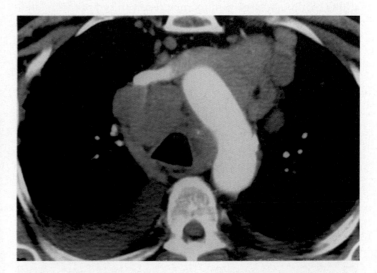

FIGURE 48-6 Contrast-enhanced chest CT (mediastinal window) of a patient with large B-cell non-Hodgkin's lymphoma. There is bulky, conglomerate anterior and middle-posterior mediastinal lymphadenopathy as well as bilateral pleural effusions.

Indolent NHLs are associated with a more favorable histology and a higher likelihood of nodal disease, but a more advanced clinical stage than the aggressive variety, with a propensity to transform into higher grade lymphomas. Aggressive NHLs have a less favorable histology, with a tendency for extranodal involvement. Although their prognosis is poor if untreated, they are potentially more curable than indolent lymphomas. The treatment of indolent NHLs is palliative, and use of radiotherapy and/or chemotherapy depends on disease stage.

Mediastinal Germ-Cell Neoplasms

The most common primary extragonadal site of germ-cell neoplasms is the anterior mediastinum. These lesions account for 10–15% of anterior mediastinal neoplasms in adults. Mediastinal germ-cell neoplasms are a diverse group of benign and malignant neoplasms, which may originate from ectopic primitive germ cells "misplaced" in the mediastinum during embryogenesis. Most neoplasms that occur in adulthood are benign, but childhood neoplasms are more commonly malignant. Adults in the third decade of life are most commonly affected. Benign, mature teratomas affect males and females equally, but most malignant mediastinal germ-cell neoplasms affect males. Although malignant germ-cell neoplasms that manifest as mediastinal masses are typically primary lesions, secondary neoplasia from a primary gonadal germ-cell neoplasm should be excluded. Elevation of serum levels of tumor markers, such as α-fetoprotein (AFP) and β-subunit of human chorionic gonadotropin (β-HCG), in a male with an anterior mediastinal mass strongly suggests the diagnosis of a malignant, nonseminomatous germ-cell neoplasm.

Mediastinal Teratomas

Teratomas represent the most common mediastinal germ-cell neoplasms, accounting for 60–70% of cases, and consist of tissues that may be derived from more than one of the embryonic germ-cell layers (Figure 48-7). Most teratomas are well differentiated and benign, hence the term *mature teratoma*. Uncommon categories include immature teratoma and malignant teratoma or teratocarcinoma.

Mature teratoma typically affects children and young adults. Although large tumors may result in symptoms related to local compression, patients with mature teratoma are frequently asymptomatic. Characteristic, but uncommon, symptoms include expectoration of hair (trichoptysis), sebum, or fluid as a result of communication between the tumor and the airways.

Radiologically, teratomas are spherical, lobular, well-circumscribed, anterior mediastinal masses that may exhibit calcification on radiography (Figure 48-8). CT typically demonstrates a multilocular cystic mass, and 75% of lesions contain fat attenuation. The treatment of choice is surgical excision, and the prognosis is excellent.

Seminomas

Mediastinal seminomas typically affect men in the third and fourth decades of life and represent 40–50% of mediastinal malignant germ-cell neoplasms of a pure histology. Most patients are symptomatic. β-HCG levels are elevated in 10% of the patients, but AFP level is normal in pure seminomas. The tumor manifests as a large, lobular, well-defined, anterior mediastinal mass. Invasion of mediastinal structures is uncommon, but lymph node, lung, and skeletal metastases may occur.

Cisplatin-based chemotherapy for four cycles has largely replaced previously used radiotherapy alone and results in cure rates of approximately 80%. Radiotherapy is still used in combination with chemotherapy to treat bulky disease and residual neoplasm after chemotherapy.

Nonseminomatous, Malignant Germ-Cell Neoplasms

Nonseminomatous, malignant germ-cell neoplasms affect young, symptomatic men and include choriocarcinoma, embryonal carcinoma, endodermal sinus (yolk sac) tumor, and mixed germ-cell neoplasms. Tumor markers (AFP and HCG) are elevated in most patients. A significantly elevated AFP level is usually found in endodermal sinus tumor and embryonal carcinoma, whereas HCG is typically elevated in choriocarcinoma. Nonseminomatous, malignant germ-cell neoplasms may be associated with various hematologic neoplasms, such as acute leukemia or myelodysplastic syndrome, and up to 20% of

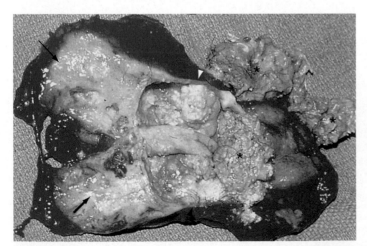

FIGURE 48-7 Gross specimen of mature cystic teratoma. The cut section demonstrates an encapsulated cystic mass with fat *(arrow)*, calcification *(arrowhead)*, and debris *(asterisk)*.

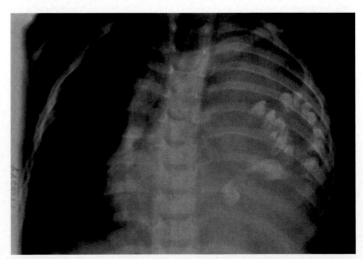

FIGURE 48-8 PA chest radiograph of a patient with mediastinal mature teratoma. A large mass occupies the entire left hemithorax with mass effect on the mediastinum. Well-formed teeth within the mass, although highly specific for the diagnosis, are an extremely unusual finding.

affected patients have Klinefelter syndrome. These tumors manifest radiologically as large heterogeneous masses with internal low attenuation areas corresponding to central necrosis surrounded by enhancing nodular irregular soft tissue. Invasion of adjacent structures, pleural and pericardial effusions, and lymph node and distant metastases are common.

Standard treatment involves systemic chemotherapy with cisplatin-containing regimens, followed by surgical resection of residual neoplasm if a positive response is achieved. Patients who respond to therapy are followed with serum tumor markers, which are expected to normalize after treatment. Compared with seminoma, the prognosis is less favorable; however, complete remission rates of 50–70% and 5-year survival rates of approximately 50% can be achieved.

Thymolipoma

Thymolipoma is a rare, benign thymic neoplasm composed of mature adipose and thymic tissues. It usually affects young adults and has no gender predilection. Thymolipomas grow slowly, frequently reaching a large size before diagnosis, and nearly half of the patients are asymptomatic. Thymolipomas manifest as large, anterior, inferior mediastinal masses that conform to adjacent thoracic structures and may mimic diaphragmatic elevation and cardiac enlargement on radiography. These lesions may also exhibit positional changes in shape. CT and MRI demonstrate soft tissue and adipose tissue components and establish an anatomic connection between the lesion and the thymus (Figure 48-9). The treatment of choice is surgical resection. The prognosis is excellent.

Cysts

Thymic Cyst. Thymic cysts are rare, anterior mediastinal masses that may be congenital or acquired. Congenital thymic cysts are usually found in the first two decades of life, whereas acquired thymic cysts are seen in association with the acquired immunodeficiency syndrome or thymic inflammation or malignancy, such as thymic carcinoma or HD. Radiologically,

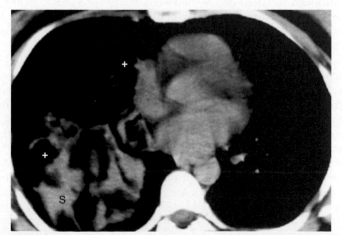

FIGURE 48-9 Unenhanced chest CT (mediastinal window) of a patient with thymolipoma. A large anterior mediastinal mass preferentially occupies the right inferior hemithorax. Note the anatomic connection with the thymus and an admixture of fat (+) and soft tissue (S) elements within the lesion.

thymic cysts are well-defined anterior mediastinal masses with cystic unilocular or multilocular appearances on cross-sectional imaging. Surgical excision is the recommended treatment. The diagnosis of cystic neoplasm should always be considered and excluded, and inflammatory cysts must be carefully examined to exclude associated malignancy.

Pericardial Cyst. Pericardial cysts, also termed *spring water cysts* or *clear water cysts* because of their clear fluid contents, are uncommon developmental lesions that occur in the radiographic anterior mediastinum. Most are discovered incidentally in asymptomatic middle-aged adults. These cysts are well circumscribed and usually abut the heart, the diaphragm, and the anterior chest wall, typically in the right cardiophrenic angle. CT typically demonstrates a nonenhancing cystic mass of water attenuation and an imperceptible wall (Figure 48-10). Unless significant symptoms or atypical imaging features are found, pericardial cysts are followed clinically and radiologically.

Glandular Disorders

Thymic Hyperplasia

Thymic hyperplasia most commonly occurs as a rebound phenomenon in patients who have received chemotherapy for treatment of lymphoma or germ-cell neoplasms. Diffuse hyperplasia occurs within 2 weeks to 12 months after chemotherapy and may manifest with mediastinal enlargement on radiography or may mimic thymic neoplasia on cross-sectional imaging. Differentiation from recurrent neoplasia is difficult, and close follow-up or biopsy is required.

Intrathoracic Goiter

Most intrathoracic goiters result from extension of cervical thyroid goiters into the mediastinum and typically affect women. Although patients are usually asymptomatic, compression of the trachea or esophagus rarely causes symptoms such as dyspnea or dysphagia. The risk of malignant degeneration is small. Most intrathoracic goiters are located in the anterosuperior mediastinum, usually on the right side, but other compartments may be affected. Ectopic intrathoracic goiter without a cervical component rarely occurs. Chest radiography often reveals a cervicothoracic mass that produces mass effect on the trachea. CT demonstrates a lobular, well-defined mass with heterogeneous attenuation resulting from hemorrhage, cystic change, and calcification (Figure 48-11). Intense and sustained contrast enhancement is common. In functioning goiters, uptake of radioactive iodine (iodine 123 [^{123}I] or iodine 131 [^{131}I]) and technetium 99m (^{99m}Tc) pertechnetate is diagnostic. Symptomatic or large goiters may be surgically excised.

Parathyroid Adenoma

Ectopic parathyroid glands in the mediastinum are usually located within or near the thymus gland. Most are encapsulated, functioning, benign adenomas, most commonly seen in older women who have persistent hyperparathyroidism after surgical parathyroidectomy. Because of their small size, they are rarely detected on chest radiography and frequently mimic lymph nodes on CT. Localization may be achieved by ^{99m}Tc sestamibi scintigraphy or dual isotope digital subtraction imaging with ^{99m}Tc pertechnetate and thallium-201 chloride. Scintigraphic (functional) localization is correlated with CT or MRI (anatomic) visualization of a mediastinal soft tissue nodule or mass. Selective venous

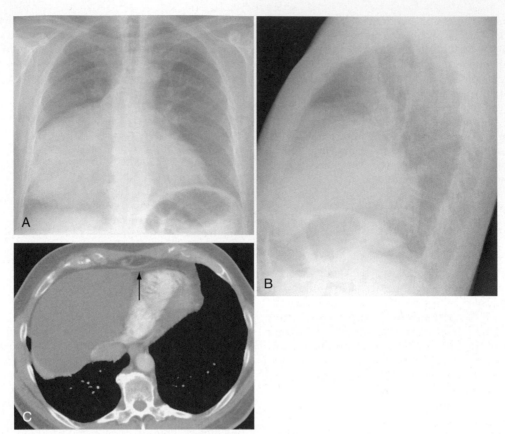

FIGURE 48-10 PA and lateral chest radiographs (**A** and **B**) and unenhanced chest CT (mediastinal window) (**C**) of an asymptomatic woman with a pericardial cyst. A sharply marginated mass in the right cardiophrenic angle exhibits water attenuation contents and an imperceptible wall and abuts the anterior chest wall, pericardium (*arrow*), and diaphragm.

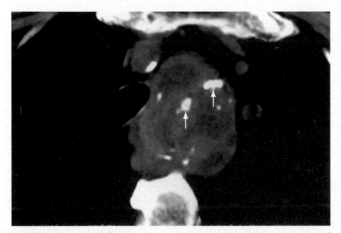

FIGURE 48-11 Unenhanced chest CT (mediastinal window) of a patient with intrathoracic goiter. A heterogeneous soft tissue mass has large flocculent calcification (*arrows*) and produces mass effect on the trachea.

sampling for parathyroid hormone levels may be necessary. Surgical excision is the treatment of choice.

DISEASES OF THE MIDDLE-POSTERIOR MEDIASTINUM

Benign Mediastinal Lymphadenopathy

Infectious and noninfectious granulomatous diseases may involve the mediastinal lymph nodes. Infectious granulomatous diseases include tuberculosis and fungal infections, such as histoplasmosis and coccidioidomycosis. The most important noninfectious granulomatous diseases include sarcoidosis and silicosis. Lymphadenopathy associated with granulomatous infection is usually unilateral and asymmetric, in contrast to bilateral and symmetric lymph node enlargement with sarcoidosis and silicosis. Many of these disorders cause lymph node calcification, which may exhibit an "eggshell" configuration, characteristic of silicosis and, less commonly, sarcoidosis. Although calcified lymph nodes generally represent a benign process, definitive exclusion of malignant lymphadenopathy may be impossible by CT alone, and histologic examination may be required.

Other benign causes of lymph node enlargement include reactive hyperplasia from bacterial or viral lung infections, amyloidosis, drugs such as phenytoin, and Castleman disease (angiofollicular lymphoid hyperplasia or giant lymph node hyperplasia). Castleman disease usually manifests in young, asymptomatic adults as incidental, large, well-circumscribed, middle mediastinal lymph nodes. Nodal hypervascularity results in intense, homogeneous enhancement after intravenous contrast administration on cross-sectional imaging. The hyaline vascular histologic type accounts for 80–90% of cases, whereas the plasma cell and multicentric types represent only 10%. Patients with the hyaline vascular type are typically asymptomatic, although symptoms of compression may occur. The plasma cell variety may be associated with constitutional symptoms and signs of fever, weight loss, fatigue, anemia, and hypergammaglobulinemia, which may improve after surgical excision. The multicentric type is rare and is associated with severe systemic symptoms in older patients, generalized lymphadenopathy, and hepatosplenomegaly, with eventual development of NHL.

Metastatic Mediastinal and Hilar Lymphadenopathy

Primary lung, breast, renal cell, gastrointestinal, and prostate carcinomas and malignant melanoma may metastasize to mediastinal and/or hilar lymph nodes and may manifest as a solitary mass, a dominant mass with lymphadenopathy, or multifocal enlarged lymph nodes. Ipsilateral mediastinal metastases from lung carcinoma represent N2 disease and may be operable. The diagnosis of metastases is established by a history of a known primary malignancy and confirmed by biopsy. The treatment depends on the underlying neoplasm and its stage.

Cysts

Foregut Cysts

Congenital foregut cysts represent 20% of mediastinal masses, and 50–60% of these are bronchogenic cysts. Enteric cysts, which include esophageal duplication and neurenteric cysts, account for approximately 10–15%. Up to 20% of foregut cysts cannot be histologically classified and, hence, are termed *nonspecific* or *indeterminate* cysts.

Bronchogenic Cysts

Bronchogenic cysts are thought to originate from abnormal ventral budding of the primitive foregut. Most are located in the mediastinum, most commonly in subcarinal or paratracheal locations. Up to 15% are reported to arise in the lung; other locations (pleura, diaphragm, pericardium) are rare. These cysts are usually lined by a pseudostratified, columnar, ciliated (respiratory) epithelium; exhibit cartilage and smooth muscle in their walls; and may contain serous fluid, mucus, milk of calcium, blood, or purulent material (Figure 48-12).

Bronchogenic cysts typically occur in adult males and females but may affect all age groups. Patients are commonly asymptomatic, but infection or bleeding eventually produces symptoms in up to two thirds of cases. Radiography usually reveals a well-circumscribed, spherical, middle mediastinal mass. On CT, these cysts are unilocular homogeneous, nonenhancing masses of variable attenuation, depending on the composition of the fluid (Figure 48-13). The cyst wall may contain calcification or enhance following the intravenous administration of contrast. A gas–fluid level within the cyst is exceptionally rare in mediastinal cysts but commonly occurs in pulmonary cysts and indicates communication with the airways or infection. Large cysts in children may compress the airways, with resultant atelectasis, bronchopneumonia, or air trapping. The treatment of choice is surgical resection (even in the absence of symptoms), although incidental cysts in asymptomatic adults have been followed clinically and radiologically. Bronchoscopic or thoracoscopic needle drainage of cyst fluid typically reveals mucus and bronchial epithelial cells and is reserved for patients with a high risk of surgical complications.

Enteric Cysts

Enteric (esophageal duplication and neurenteric) cysts originate from the dorsal foregut, are usually located in the middle or posterior mediastinum, and typically manifest in childhood. Enteric cysts are lined by squamous or enteric epithelium and

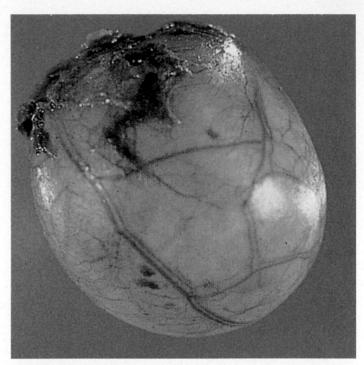

FIGURE 48-12 Gross specimen of bronchogenic cyst. The cyst has a spherical morphology and a thin wall that contains numerous vascular structures.

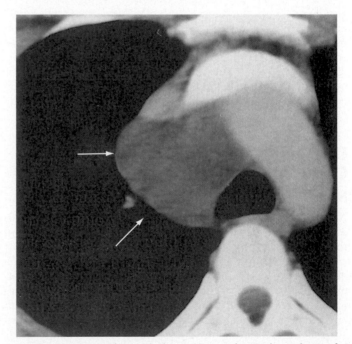

FIGURE 48-13 Unenhanced chest CT (mediastinal window) of a patient with bronchogenic cyst. A spherical mass (*arrows*) of water attenuation is closely related to the tracheal carina.

may contain gastric mucosa and/or pancreatic and neural tissue. The cyst walls have two well-defined, smooth muscle layers with a myenteric plexus. Esophageal duplication cysts almost always adhere to the esophagus or are located within its wall and can be associated with gastrointestinal malformations. Similarly, neurenteric cysts may be associated with gastrointestinal and/or cervical or upper thoracic vertebral anomalies, occasionally with a fibrous attachment to the spine or intraspinal extension.

Most enteric cysts are diagnosed during childhood. Hemorrhage or rupture may occur, especially when gastric epithelium or pancreatic tissue is present. The radiologic features of enteric cysts are similar to those of bronchogenic cysts. Esophageal duplication cysts are usually located close to the distal esophagus on the right side. Most neurenteric cysts are located in the posterior mediastinum, above the level of the carina on the right side, and approximately one half are associated with scoliosis, anterior spina bifida, vertebral fusion, hemivertebrae, and other vertebral anomalies. MRI is indicated to exclude intraspinal extension. Surgical excision is the treatment of choice. Prognosis after complete resection is excellent.

Vascular Lesions

Vascular lesions constitute approximately 10% of all mediastinal masses and may originate from the arterial or venous portions of the systemic or pulmonary circulation. They may mimic neoplasms on chest radiographs and should be considered in the differential diagnosis before biopsy is performed. The diagnosis is usually established with contrast-enhanced CT, MRI, and/or angiography.

Herniation

Hiatal hernias are common and result when an abdominal structure, usually the stomach, extends through the esophageal hiatus into the thorax and manifests as a retrocardiac mass. Morgagni hernias are congenital defects in the diaphragm that allow herniation of omentum or other abdominal contents into the thorax and typically manifest as right cardiophrenic angle masses. Diagnosis is typically established by visualization of abdominal contents in the hernia sac on cross-sectional imaging studies. Treatment of symptomatic cases is surgical.

DISEASES OF THE PARAVERTEBRAL COMPARTMENT

Neurogenic Neoplasms

Neurogenic neoplasms constitute 15–20% of adult and 40% of pediatric mediastinal tumors. Approximately 90% occur in the paravertebral region. Neurogenic neoplasms are the most common cause of a paravertebral mass and account for 75% of primary paravertebral "mediastinal" neoplasms. Approximately 50% of neurogenic neoplasms in children are malignant, whereas in adults most are benign. Approximately half of affected patients are asymptomatic. Neurogenic neoplasms are generally grouped into three categories according to their structure of origin: peripheral nerve, sympathetic ganglia, and paraganglionic neoplasms.

Peripheral Nerve Neoplasms

Schwannoma and Neurofibroma. Schwannoma (also termed *neurilemmoma*) and neurofibroma are the most common mediastinal neurogenic neoplasms. More than 90% are benign, and 10% are multiple. They are slow-growing neoplasms and usually arise from a posterior spinal nerve root but can involve any nerve in the thorax. Schwannoma and solitary neurofibroma affect men and women equally in the third and fourth

decades. Although these neoplasms may attain large sizes, most patients are asymptomatic. Approximately 30–45% of neurofibromas occur in individuals who have neurofibromatosis (von Recklinghausen disease). The presence of multiple neurofibromas or a single plexiform neurofibroma is pathognomonic of this disorder. Malignant transformation of a solitary schwannoma is extremely rare. Patients with neurofibromatosis and neurogenic neoplasms are at increased risk for malignant transformation of one or more lesions. Patients with neurofibromatosis may also have ganglion cell neoplasms develop.

Radiologically, schwannomas and neurofibromas are sharply marginated, spherical, and occasionally lobular paravertebral masses, which usually span one to two rib interspaces but can attain large sizes. Up to one half of the cases cause splaying and benign pressure erosion of the ribs, vertebral bodies, and neural foramina. Approximately 10% of schwannomas and neurofibromas grow through and widen adjacent neural foramina and expand on either end with a "dumbbell" or "hourglass" configuration (Figure 48-14). Typically, CT reveals a heterogeneous mass, which may contain punctate calcification or areas of low attenuation. MRI should always be performed to exclude intraspinal growth of the neoplasm (Figure 48-15). The treatment of choice is surgery. Recurrences are uncommon, even when excision is incomplete.

Malignant Peripheral Nerve Sheath Neoplasms

Malignant peripheral nerve sheath neoplasms are a rare group of spindle cell sarcomas thought to represent the malignant counterparts of schwannomas and neurofibromas. They occur equally in men and women in the third to fifth decades, and approximately half occur in individuals who have neurofibromatosis. The incidence of malignant degeneration of neurogenic

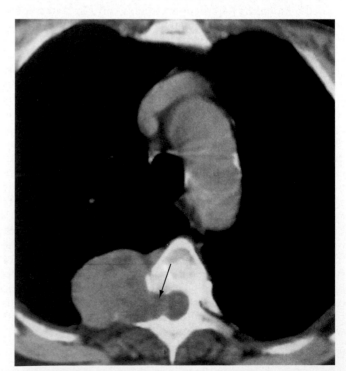

FIGURE 48-14 Unenhanced chest CT (mediastinal window) of a patient with neurofibroma. A spherical mass of heterogeneous attenuation exhibits intraspinal extension *(arrow)* with enlargement and pressure erosion of the adjacent neural foramen.

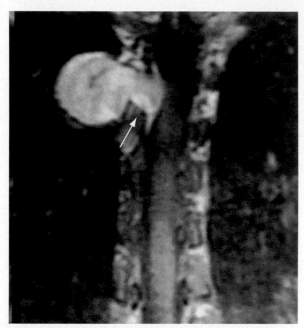

FIGURE 48-15 Gadolinium-enhanced coronal T1-weighted MRI of a patient with neurofibroma. A spherical heterogeneously enhancing paravertebral mass exhibits intraspinal extension (arrow) and mass effect on the spinal cord.

neoplasms in patients with neurofibromatosis is approximately 5%. Malignant peripheral nerve sheath neoplasms may also occur sporadically or be induced by radiation. Pain and an enlarging mass are common at presentation. Radiologically, mediastinal malignant peripheral nerve sheath neoplasms manifest as sharply marginated, spherical, heterogeneous masses on cross-sectional imaging and may exhibit explosive growth.

Sympathetic Ganglia Neoplasms

Neoplasms of sympathetic ganglia affect both children and young adults, but malignant lesions are most common in children. Ganglioneuroma and ganglioneuroblastoma usually arise in the sympathetic ganglia of the paravertebral region. Approximately one half of neuroblastomas arise from the adrenal glands, and one third are located in the mediastinum, the most common extraabdominal location.

Ganglioneuromas

Ganglioneuromas are benign neoplasms that affect males and females equally. Affected patients are older children (typically older than 5 years of age) and young adults. One half of the patients are symptomatic from local effects of the tumor or intraspinal growth. Radiologically, they are well-circumscribed, oblong, paravertebral masses that usually span three to five vertebrae and may exhibit skeletal displacement or pressure erosion. MRI is indicated to exclude intraspinal extension. Surgical excision is the treatment of choice and may necessitate a combined thoracic and neurosurgical approach.

Ganglioneuroblastomas

Ganglioneuroblastomas are malignant neoplasms that usually affect children younger than 10 years of age, with no gender predilection. They demonstrate composite histologic, biologic, and radiologic features of ganglioneuromas and neuroblastomas

and are not usually distinguishable on imaging. Symptoms, when present, are caused by local mass effect, invasion of adjacent structures, or metastases. Staging and treatment are the same as for neuroblastomas. The prognosis of these lesions is generally more favorable than that of neuroblastomas.

Neuroblastomas

Neuroblastomas are highly malignant neoplasms that affect children younger than 5 years of age, typically boys. Neuroblastomas in children older than 5 years have no gender predilection. Two thirds of patients have constitutional symptoms, pain, cough, dyspnea, paraplegia, opsoclonus, and Horner syndrome. Systemic effects, such as hypertension, tachycardia, perspiration, flushing, and severe watery diarrhea, may result from elevation of catecholamine and vasoactive intestinal peptide levels. Radiologically, the masses are paravertebral, occasionally with local invasion, contralateral extension, and/or skeletal erosion. Approximately 10% exhibit extensive calcification on radiography. On CT, the tumors are heterogeneous because of hemorrhage and necrosis, and calcification may be detected in 80% of cases. MRI should always be used to exclude intraspinal extension and vascular or skeletal involvement. Metaiodobenzylguanidine scintigraphy (^{123}I or ^{131}I) may demonstrate uptake in both primary and metastatic sites.

Neuroblastomas and ganglioneuroblastomas are treated with surgical resection. Adjuvant chemotherapy and irradiation may be used for residual disease or as a primary treatment modality in advanced cases. Radiotherapy in children can lead to delayed complications such as myelitis and scoliosis. The prognosis is generally poor and depends on the age at diagnosis, the size, the degree of histologic differentiation, and the neoplastic stage. Patients with congenital and thoracic lesions have the best prognosis.

Paraganglionic Neoplasms

Pheochromocytoma. Pheochromocytomas are functioning paragangliomas that most commonly arise from the adrenal glands and occur more frequently in men in the third to fourth decades of life. Approximately 10% of pheochromocytomas are extraadrenal, and less than 2% are intrathoracic; the latter tend to be more aggressive and multicentric. Symptoms relate to excessive systemic catecholamines or local mass effect. Pheochromocytomas may be part of a multisystem endocrine syndrome, such as type 2a or 2b multiple endocrine neoplasia syndrome. Diagnosis can be established by measurement of urine catecholamines and their metabolites (vanillyl mandelic acid, homovanillic acid, metanephrine, and normetanephrine). Typically, CT and MRI reveal a well-delineated, enhancing, posterior mediastinal mass. The neoplasm is typically ^{123}I and ^{123}I metaiodobenzylguanidine avid. Treatment includes sympathetic α- and β-blockade for 1–2 weeks, followed by surgical excision. Chemotherapy and/or radiotherapy can be used to treat metastatic disease.

Paraganglioma. Paragangliomas are rare neoplasms of paraganglionic tissue. Most are benign, asymptomatic, and nonfunctioning. Radiologically, they typically manifest as sharply marginated, middle or posterior mediastinal nodules or masses, usually located adjacent to the aorta, pulmonary arteries, heart, or costovertebral sulci or within the left atrial wall. They are hypervascular lesions and demonstrate marked contrast enhancement. The treatment is surgical excision.

Lateral Thoracic Meningocele

Lateral thoracic meningoceles are rare and consist of redundant meninges that protrude through the neural foramen and contain cerebrospinal fluid. They do not exhibit a gender predilection and typically occur in association with neurofibromatosis. Patients are usually asymptomatic adults in the fourth to fifth decades of life. Radiologic studies demonstrate a well-circumscribed, paravertebral, cystic lesion, frequently associated with vertebral erosion, kyphoscoliosis, and/or widening of adjacent neural foramina. Cross-sectional imaging may demonstrate continuity with the thecal sac. CT demonstrates a homogeneous nonenhancing mass of water attenuation, and MRI shows signal intensity equal to that of adjacent cerebrospinal fluid. Symptomatic lesions are treated with surgical excision.

MISCELLANEOUS DISORDERS OF THE MEDIASTINUM

Mediastinitis

The term *mediastinitis* is used to refer to a variety of infectious and inflammatory conditions. Acute mediastinitis is more common than the chronic form and may be caused by esophageal or tracheobronchial perforation, penetrating chest trauma, postoperative sternal wound infection, extension of an oropharyngeal infection or a paravertebral or vertebral abscess, radiation therapy, malignancy, and, rarely, anthrax.

Patients with acute mediastinitis usually have had sudden onset of high fever, chills, chest pain, dyspnea, and dysphagia. Physical examination may reveal systemic toxicity, respiratory distress, Hamman sign, subcutaneous emphysema, chest-wall tenderness, and edema. Chest radiography and CT show mediastinal widening, pneumomediastinum, mediastinal air–fluid levels or fluid collections, and pleural effusions. An esophagram may reveal perforation. Acute mediastinitis is a generally diffuse process but may be localized when secondary to sternal wound infection. The treatment includes surgical drainage, débridement, repair of the traumatic injury, and broad-spectrum antibiotics. The mortality rate is high, especially when the diagnosis is delayed.

Chronic mediastinitis, also termed *fibrosing mediastinitis* or *granulomatous mediastinitis*, is caused by various infectious and inflammatory processes. Histoplasmosis and tuberculosis account for most cases. Noninfectious causes include mediastinal hematoma, radiation therapy, and drugs such as methysergide and hydralazine. Chronic mediastinitis can be associated with various idiopathic and autoimmune diseases, such as retroperitoneal fibrosis, Riedel's thyroiditis, pseudotumor of the orbit, sclerosing cholangitis, systemic lupus erythematosus, and rheumatoid arthritis. Dense fibrous tissue, most commonly located in the paratracheal, carinal, and hilar regions, compresses and obstructs mediastinal structures such as the superior vena cava, pulmonary vessels, airways, and esophagus. Superior vena cava syndrome is the most common clinical manifestation. Chest radiographs, CT, MRI, and perfusion scintigraphy, in addition to endoscopy, help to suggest the diagnosis. The typical CT finding is an infiltrative mediastinal soft tissue mass with calcification and coexistent pulmonary or hepatosplenic calcified granulomas. Noncalcified lesions present a diagnostic dilemma and require exclusion of malignancy. Histologic examination of mediastinal tissue may be necessary to exclude a malignant neoplasm or active infection.

Treatment is ineffective and mostly palliative; the benefit of corticosteroids is controversial. In the presence of viable fungal organisms or rising serum antibody titers, antifungal agents can be administered. With superior vena cava syndrome, long-term anticoagulation and vascular stents may be very effective.

Pneumomediastinum

Pneumomediastinum is typically caused by overdistention and rupture of alveoli because of increased intrathoracic volume or pressure that results from mechanical ventilation, blunt trauma, asthma, or spontaneous rupture. Air dissects along the pulmonary interstitium into the peribronchovascular tissues and mediastinum and frequently decompresses into the soft tissues of the neck. Less commonly, pneumomediastinum can be secondary to tracheobronchial or esophageal perforation, a gas-forming infection, traumatic direct entry of air, cervical soft tissue air, or pneumoperitoneum that tracks into the mediastinum.

Mediastinal Hemorrhage

Mediastinal hemorrhage can be spontaneous from rupture of a thoracic or other vascular aneurysm or dissection or can result from blunt or penetrating trauma or invasive medical procedures. Chest radiography typically reveals mediastinal widening. Unenhanced chest CT may show hyperdense areas within the mediastinum or aortic wall, and contrast-enhanced chest CT may reveal an intimal flap or dissection, a contained pseudoaneurysm, or frank extravasation of blood into the mediastinum, pericardium, and/or pleural space. The treatment depends on the cause and location of the source of bleeding and typically involves surgical repair, especially when the ascending thoracic aorta is involved.

Differential Diagnosis

Many mediastinal masses are benign and are found incidentally in asymptomatic patients. Large lesions may manifest with symptoms related to compression of adjacent structures. Aggressive or malignant neoplasms may produce constitutional symptoms, paraneoplastic syndromes, invasion of adjacent structures, or metastases. The radiologic evaluation of affected patients begins with chest radiography and is followed by cross-sectional imaging with CT and occasionally MRI. CT is useful in excluding vascular lesions and some benign causes of mediastinal widening such as lipomatosis. In addition, confident diagnosis of some lesions such as mature teratoma, mediastinal goiter, pericardial cyst, foregut duplication cyst, herniations, and lateral thoracic meningocele can be established. Adjacent structures may also be evaluated for mass effect or invasion. Patients with primary mediastinal masses and cysts usually undergo surgical resection. The presence of lymphadenopathy (in cases of lymphoma and metastatic disease) or certain positive tumor markers may prompt limited biopsy sampling of the lesion followed by oncologic consultation and chemotherapy and/or radiation therapy when appropriate. Resection of residual neoplasm will follow in some cases.

The most common primary anterior mediastinal masses are thymoma, teratoma, substernal goiter, and lymphoma. All other lesions are extremely rare. In the correct clinical setting, patients with an anterior mediastinal mass should have serologic evaluation for detection of antibodies to acetylcholine receptors or elevation of AFP and β-HCG to exclude MG and nonseminomatous malignant germ-cell neoplasm, respectively. Most primary thymic neoplasms arise in one lobe of the thymus and exhibit unilateral growth; thus, an anterior mediastinal mass that extends across the midline is likely an aggressive neoplasm or diffuse malignant lymphadenopathy. Whereas thymoma typically manifests as a homogeneous unilateral thymic mass, invasive thymoma may exhibit irregular margins, invasion of mediastinal tissue planes and structures, and/or drop metastases. Mature teratoma typically manifests as a large unilateral multilocular cystic mass that often exhibits intrinsic fat and/or calcification. Intrathoracic goiter almost always results from contiguous extension of a cervical goiter. Lymphoma may affect any mediastinal compartment and classically manifests as lymph node enlargement. The diagnosis is frequently made by biopsy of a palpable peripheral lymph node, and mediastinal involvement is determined by cross-sectional imaging studies. Diagnostic problems may arise when lymphoma manifests with primary mediastinal lymphadenopathy or focal mass. Pericardial cysts are often followed clinically and on imaging.

Middle-posterior mediastinal masses include lesions from many causes. Mediastinal lymphadenopathy is common and may be of benign or malignant etiology to include lymphoma and advanced lung cancer. Mediastinal cysts are typically congenital, classically affect predominantly the middle mediastinal compartment, and are often surgically excised because of the high incidence of symptoms and complications. Radiologic characteristics can establish the diagnosis of congenital cysts in most cases.

Neurogenic neoplasms are common paravertebral masses. On the basis of morphology, patient age, and presence or absence of symptoms or associated conditions, a prospective diagnosis can usually be established. Lesions of peripheral nerve origin typically affect asymptomatic adults, have a spherical morphology, and are cured by excision. Multiple lesions suggest the diagnosis of neurofibromatosis. Neoplasms of sympathetic ganglial origin usually affect children and young adults, have an elongate morphology, and have a variable prognosis because of higher frequency of malignant histologic types. Preoperative assessment usually includes MRI to exclude intraspinal extension and exclusion of elevated levels of serum and urine catecholamines in some cases to exclude malignancy or clinically active neoplasms. Lateral thoracic meningoceles may mimic neurogenic neoplasms on radiography but are readily diagnosed on cross-sectional imaging.

SUGGESTED READINGS

Aquino SL, Duncan G, Taber KH, et al: Reconciliation of the anatomic, surgical, and radiographic classifications of the mediastinum. J Comput Assist Tomogr 2001; 25:489–492.

Chalabreysse L, Roy P, Cordier JF, et al: Correlation of the WHO schema for the classification of thymic epithelial neoplasms with prognosis: A retrospective study of 90 tumors. Am J Surg Pathol 2002; 26: 1605–1611.

Jeung M-Y, Gasser B, Gangi A, et al: Imaging of cystic masses of the mediastinum. RadioGraphics 2002; 22:S79–S93.

Jung K-J, Lee KS, Han J, et al: Malignant thymic epithelial tumors: CT-pathologic correlation. AJR 2001; 176:433–439.

Lonergan GJ, Schwab CM, Suarez ES, Carlson CL: Neuroblastoma, ganglioneuroblastoma, and ganglioneuroma: Radiologic-pathologic correlation. RadioGraphics 2002; 22:911–934.

Moeller KH, Rosado-de-Christenson ML, Templeton PA: Mediastinal mature teratoma: Imaging features. AJR Am J Roentgenol 1997; 169:985–990.

Strollo DC, Rosado-de-Christenson ML: Tumors of the thymus. J Thorac Imaging 1999; 14:152–171.

Strollo DC, Rosado-de-Christenson ML: Primary mediastinal malignant germ cell neoplasms: Imaging features. Chest Surg Clin North Am 2002; 12:645–658.

Strollo DC, Rosado-de-Christenson ML, Jett JR: Primary mediastinal tumors. Part I. Tumors of the anterior mediastinum. Chest 1997; 112:511–522.

Strollo DC, Rosado-de-Christenson ML, Jett JR: Primary mediastinal tumors. Part II. Tumors of the middle and posterior mediastinum. Chest 1997; 112:1344–1357.

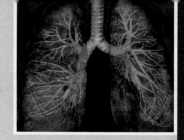

49 Approach to Diagnosis of Diffuse Lung Disease

ATHOL WELLS

The term *diffuse lung disease (DLD)* covers infiltrative lung processes that involve the alveolar spaces or lung interstitium. This definition is fundamentally unsatisfactory because it groups together a wide variety of diverse disorders, some of which (such as cryptogenic organizing pneumonia) are not diffuse, strictly speaking, but patchy and sometimes limited in extent. Furthermore, many secondary infiltrative abnormalities, including bacterial infection and malignancy, are excluded, whereas others, such as pulmonary involvement in connective tissue disease, are retained in most DLD classifications. The DLDs are grouped for historical reasons; in early series, they presented most frequently with widespread clinical and chest radiographic abnormalities. However, with increasing clinician awareness of the possibility of DLD, the diagnosis is often made when chest radiographic findings are limited or disease is apparent only on high-resolution computed tomography (HRCT).

The diagnostic difficulties resulting from the multiplicity of disorders contained within the DLDs are exacerbated by semantic confusion. Synonymous terms abound for some of the more frequently encountered DLDs, such as:

- Cryptogenic organizing pneumonia (bronchiolitis obliterans organizing pneumonia, proliferative bronchiolitis)
- Idiopathic pulmonary fibrosis (IPF, cryptogenic fibrosing alveolitis)
- Hypersensitivity pneumonitis (extrinsic allergic alveolitis)

This problem has been partially addressed by the reclassification of the idiopathic interstitial pneumonias by a joint American Thoracic Society/European Respiratory Society (ATS/ERS) international consensus committee, discussed in detail in Chapter 50. However, the term *cryptogenic fibrosing alveolitis (CFA)* continues to cause difficulties. As defined in the ATS/ERS reclassification, CFA is strictly synonymous with idiopathic pulmonary fibrosis (IPF). The diagnosis of IPF/CFA now requires the presence of usual interstitial pneumonia at surgical biopsy or typical appearances on HRCT, in association with a compatible clinical picture. This represents a radical change: in historical series, a wide variety of disorders presenting with a clinical picture of IPF was grouped together as IPF/CFA. The entity of "clinical CFA syndrome" is still necessary for epidemiologic studies but should not be viewed as a final diagnosis in clinical practice.

In routine practice, a simplified pragmatic approach to diagnosis is essential; consideration of a checklist of the more commonly encountered diseases is often useful. The classification of DLDs by their disease burden was addressed most definitively in a study from Bernalillo County, New Mexico, in which the incidence and prevalence of individual DLDs was quantified by use of a variety of methods (Table 49-1). New cases were estimated to occur in 32/100,000 years in males and 26/100,000 years in females; thus, although less common than lung infection, malignant disease or obstructive airway disease, the DLDs are responsible for a considerable disease burden. Moreover, the work load for the pulmonary physician is disproportionate, because the diagnosis of individual DLDs is often uncertain despite more intensive investigation than is generally required in obstructive airways disease, malignancy, or chronic lung suppuration.

A consideration of the differential diagnosis of DLD, on the basis of prevalence alone, is merely a starting point, for two reasons. First, clinical information at initial evaluation profoundly alters diagnostic probabilities; therefore, a lengthier checklist of the DLDs, on the basis of the possible underlying cause, is indispensable. Second, the length to which a specific diagnosis is pursued, with particular reference to surgical biopsy, is critically dependent on the importance of discriminating between likely differential diagnoses in individual cases. This crucial point is discussed in detail in the concluding section of the chapter.

INITIAL CLINICAL EVALUATION

Even before chest radiography and HRCT findings are considered, a wealth of diagnostic information can be obtained from initial evaluation. A possible underlying cause is often apparent, although environmental and drug exposures occurring many years earlier and apparently limited exposures are difficult to interpret in isolation in many cases. A great deal of information can often be obtained on the longitudinal behavior of disease from the evolution of symptoms, serial chest radiographic data, and, less frequently, serial spirometric volumes. The presence of associated systemic disease and/or prominent airway-centered symptoms may provide useful diagnostic clues. Less frequently, physical examination may serve to broaden the differential diagnosis. In addition to chest radiography and HRCT (considered in separate sections), certain noninvasive ancillary tests should be performed in selected cases, including autoimmune serology, measurement of precipitins, and echocardiography.

Clinical History

The identification of an underlying cause is the single most important contribution made by clinical evaluation. A checklist of the more important causes of DLD is provided in

TABLE 49-1 Prevalence and Incidence of Interstitial Lung Diseases in Bernalillo County, New Mexico

Cause	Interstitial Lung Disease	Prevalent Cases, n (%)	Incident Cases, n (%)
Occupational and environmental	Pneumoconiosis	8 (3.1)	—
	Anthracosis	3 (1.1)	—
	Asbestosis	17 (6.6)	15 (7.4)
	Silicosis	8 (3.1)	6 (3.0)
	Hypersensitivity pneumonitis	—	3 (1.5)
Drug/radiation	Drug-induced interstitial lung disease	5 (1.9)	7 (3.5)
	Radiation fibrosis	1 (0.4)	3 (1.5)
Pulmonary hemorrhage syndromes	Goodpasture's syndrome	—	1 (0.5)
	Vasculitis	—	1 (0.5)
	Hemosiderosis	2 (0.8)	—
	Wegener's granulomatosis	2 (1.2)	6 (3.0)
Connective tissue disease	Mixed connective tissue disease	2 (0.8)	2 (1.0)
	Systemic lupus erythematosus	6 (2.3)	1 (0.5)
	Rheumatoid arthritis	14 (5.4)	10 (5.0)
	Scleroderma	9 (3.5)	3 (1.5)
	Sjögren's syndrome	—	1 (0.5)
	Dermatomyositis/polymyositis	2 (0.8)	1 (0.5)
	Ankylosing spondylitis	—	—
Pulmonary fibrosis	Pulmonary (chronic) Fibrosis/postinflammatory	43 (16.7)	28 (13.9)
	Idiopathic/interstitial fibrosis	58 (22.5)	63 (31.2)
	Interstitial pneumonitis	8 (3.1)	12 (5.9)
Sarcoidosis		30 (11.6)	16 (7.8)
Other	Alveolar proteinosis	1 (0.4)	—
	Amyloidosis	—	—
	Bronchiolitis obliterans	—	1 (0.5)
	Chronic eosinophilic pneumonia	3 (1.2)	1 (0.5)
	Eosinophilic (granuloma) infiltration	2 (0.8)	—
	Infectious/postinfectious interstitial lung disease	3 (1.2)	1 (0.5)
	Lymphocytic infiltrative lung disease	1 (0.4)	—
	Interstitial lung disease, not otherwise specified	29 (11.1)	20 (9.8)
Total		**258**	**202**

Table 49-2. A careful occupational history is essential and should include details of all previous occupations, including short-term employment. Asbestos exposure is often extensive in railway rolling-stock construction, shipyard workers, power station construction and maintenance workers, naval boiler-men, garage workers (involved in brake lining), and other occupations in which asbestos exposure is overt; generally, workers in these occupations are well aware of their asbestos exposure. However, other workers, including joiners, electricians, carpenters, and manual workers in the building trade, who handle asbestos in the form of roofing and insulation material are often unaware of significant exposure. Other occupations associated with DLD include coal mining (coal workers pneumoconiosis), metal-polishing (hard-metal disease), and sandblasting (silicosis).

A careful history will also disclose exposure to organic antigens known to cause hypersensitivity pneumonitis. The two most prevalent forms of hypersensitivity pneumonitis are farmer's lung (in which the offending antigen, thermophilic actinomycetes, is contained within moldy hay) and bird fancier's lung, in which avian proteins are inhaled by those breeding birds, or, more commonly, those who keep birds as domestic pets. However, a wide range of other exposures also cause hypersensitivity pneumonitis, and particular attention should be paid to molds (often arising in sites of water damage); bathroom molds (as in "basement shower syndrome" and "hot-tub lung" are easily overlooked. Hobbies should also be considered (e.g. "cheese-maker's lung," "wine-maker's lung"). There are now more than 100 known causes of hypersensitivity pneumonitis, and because it is unrealistic to hope to memorize these, an up-to-date list of the 50 more frequent causes of hypersensitivity pneumonitis, such as that provided by Bertorelli, is highly useful.

A detailed drug history is also essential. The drugs most frequently causing DLD are probably amiodarone, methotrexate (at doses used in connective tissue disease), and antineoplastic agents, especially bleomycin. However, a wide variety of other agents (more than 200 at present) cause DLD, although often in only a small number of cases, and the list increases year by year. Fortunately, there is now an international web site devoted to drug-induced lung disease (www.pneumotox.com), through which all medications should be routinely checked in patients with DLD. Other therapeutic modalities causing DLD include radiotherapy and exposure to high concentrations of oxygen (especially in those previously receiving bleomycin). Paraquat ingestion (causing acute or delayed proliferative bronchiolitis), inhalation of crack cocaine or heroin (causing eosinophilic pneumonia, diffuse alveolar hemorrhage, organizing pneumonia, or pulmonary edema), and intravenous drug abuse (causing venoocclusive disease) are also relevant.

TABLE 49-2 Frequently Encountered Diffuse Lung Diseases with Identifiable Underlying Cause

Cause	Differential Diagnosis	
Occupational or other inhalant-related, inorganic	Coal worker's pneumoconiosis Asbestosis Silicosis Talc pneumoconiosis Aluminum oxide fibrosis	Metal polisher's lung/hard metal fibrosis Berylliosis Baritosis (barium) Siderosis (iron oxide) Stannosis
Occupational or other inhalant-related, organic	Bird fancier's lung Farmer's lung Bagassosis (sugar cane) Coffee worker's lung Tobacco grower's lung Fishmeal worker's lung	Mushroom worker's lung Maple bark stripper's lung Malt worker's lung Tea grower's lung Pituitary snuff-taker's lung
Collagen vascular disease related	Systemic lupus erythematosus Rheumatoid arthritis Scleroderma Polymyositis Dermatomyositis	Ankylosing spondylitis Mixed connective tissue disease Primary Sjögren's syndrome Behçet's syndrome Goodpasture's syndrome
Drug related	Amiodarone Propranolol Tocainide Nitrofurantoin Sulfasalazine Cephalosporins Gold Penicillamine Phenytoin Mitomycin Bromocryptine	Bleomycin Busulfan Cyclophosphamide Chlorambucil Melphalan Methotrexate Azathioprine Cytosine arabinoside Carmustine Lomustine
Physical agents/toxins	Radiation/radiotherapy High concentration oxygen Paraquat toxicity	Cocaine inhalation Intravenous drug abuse
Neoplastic disease	Lymphangitis carcinomatosis Bronchoalveolar cell carcinoma	
Vasculitis related	Wegener's granulomatosis Giant cell arteritis Churg–Strauss syndrome	
Disorders of circulation	Pulmonary edema Pulmonary veno-occlusive disease	
Chronic infection	Tuberculosis Aspergillosis Histoplasmosis	Viruses Parasites
Smoking induced	Emphysema Langerhans cell histiocytosis Alveolar cell carcinoma Respiratory bronchiolitis with associated interstitial lung disease	Desquamative interstitial pneumonia Respiratory bronchiolitis Non-specific interstitial pneumonia

Smoking-related DLD is increasingly diagnosed; diseases other than COPD that are caused by smoking include Langerhans cell histiocytosis, respiratory bronchiolitis associated with interstitial lung disease (RBILD), desquamative interstitial pneumonia, and nonspecific interstitial pneumonia. Recently, HRCT evaluation has made it clear that all these processes may co-exist in the same patients. Furthermore, both sarcoidosis and hypersensitivity pneumonitis are very rare in current smokers. Because RBILD and hypersensitivity pneumonitis often have overlapping clinical and HRCT features, the smoking history is an important discriminator between these two disorders.

A great deal of information on likely longitudinal behavior is often available. The distinction between acute and chronic disease is important, because acute infection, heart failure, and disseminated malignancy may all simulate DLD clinically and radiologically. The duration of dyspnea and cough, pattern of symptomatic progression, and previous responsiveness (or nonresponsiveness) to corticosteroid therapy may provide valuable diagnostic clues. Variable dyspnea and cough over a number of years, responding to steroid therapy, is compatible with hypersensitivity pneumonitis or sarcoidosis, whereas inexorably progressive dyspnea for 2–3 years, not responding to steroid therapy, is typical of IPF. A perusal of previous chest radiographs may be highly useful, with unchanging appearances over many years a frequent finding in sarcoidosis, but not in IPF. Previous full pulmonary function tests are seldom available, but serial spirometry is sometimes performed in general practice (because asthma is often suspected when the first symptoms of DLD occur); thus, it is sometimes possible to draw useful conclusions from the rapidity of decline (or, conversely, the duration of stability) of spirometric volumes.

Relevant systemic diseases associated with DLD include malignancy (lymphangitis carcinomatosis or multiple metastases) and connective tissue diseases complicated by DLD, especially rheumatoid arthritis, systemic sclerosis, systemic lupus erythematosus, polymyositis/dermatomyositis, and Sjögren's syndrome. Lung disease may precede systemic manifestations in all the connective tissue diseases (most frequently in polymyositis/dermatomyositis) or may develop concurrently with systemic manifestations. Thus, a full history should include details of arthritis/arthralgia, myositis, skin disorders, Raynaud's phenomenon, and dryness of the eyes or mouth. A subgroup of patients with autoimmune disease fail to meet formal criteria for an individual disorder, are considered to have "undifferentiated connective tissue disease," but may, nonetheless, develop DLD.

Airway-centered symptoms may help to refine the differential diagnosis. Cough occurs frequently in IPF, but prominent wheeze is more suggestive of hypersensitivity pneumonitis or, less frequently, sarcoidosis. Wheeze is also an important feature of some of the pulmonary vasculitides, especially Churg–Strauss syndrome and, occasionally, Wegener's granulomatosis. Hemoptysis is the most frequent pulmonary symptom at presentation in Goodpasture's syndrome; however, the volume of hemoptysis is not a good guide to disease severity, because hemoptysis may be trivial or even absent, despite considerable alveolar hemorrhage.

Clinical Examination

Physical examination tends to beless fruitful than the history and HRCT findings in refining the differential diagnosis of DLD. Bilateral predominantly basal crackles on auscultation are a defining feature of IPF and are very frequent in other forms of idiopathic interstitial pneumonia and asbestosis but are seldom present in sarcoidosis. Clubbing is a useful sign, because it points strongly to IPF or asbestosis; clubbing is rare in sarcoidosis, hypersensitivity pneumonitis, and pulmonary fibrosis associated with connective tissue (with the possible exception of rheumatoid arthritis). However, no diagnostic conclusions can be drawn from the absence of clubbing. Mid to late inspiratory squawks, an underrecognized sign, are strongly indicative of an underlying bronchiolitic disorder, including hypersensitivity pneumonitis (in which the bronchiolitic component may be prominent). Central cyanosis, tachypnea, and pulmonary hypertension are nonspecific findings in end-stage DLD; when pulmonary hypertension is associated with limited DLD, underlying connective tissue disease (especially systemic sclerosis and systemic lupus erythematosus) should be suspected.

Blood Tests

In most cases, specific diagnostic tests for DLD are confined to autoimmune serology and precipitins against organic antigens. Serologic evidence of rheumatoid arthritis and the other major connective tissue diseases should be sought in any patient with apparently idiopathic DLD, in whom the diagnosis is uncertain. This is particularly important when the diagnosis seems to be cryptogenic organizing pneumonia, because underlying connective disease is frequent and, when present, the prognosis is not always good and prolonged treatment may be required. In the antisynthetase syndrome, characterized by

Jo1 antibody positivity, polymyositis/dermatomyositis and progressive pulmonary fibrosis, lung disease often precedes systemic manifestations. However, although antibodies to extractable nuclear antigens tend to be disease specific, antinuclear antibodies and rheumatoid factor levels are often moderately increased in idiopathic pulmonary fibrosis and are less useful diagnostically unless titers are markedly elevated. The presence of precipitins to organic antigens increases the likelihood of hypersensitivity pneumonitis but should never be considered diagnostic in isolation. Positive precipitins denote exposure to an antigen, with immune recognition, but are not, in themselves, indicative of clinically significant DLD; bird breeders often have avian precipitin positivity without overt lung disease. Moreover, in many patients with convincing exposure histories and a histologic diagnosis of hypersensitivity pneumonitis, the appropriate precipitins are not present; avian antigens, for example, vary between bird species and even between individual birds.

Pulmonary Function Tests

Most DLDs are characterized by a restrictive ventilatory defect, a reduction in gas transfer, and variable hypoxia at rest or on exercise. A pure obstructive defect is often present in Langerhans cell histiocytosis and lymphangioleiomyomatosis and is sometimes a feature of fibrotic pulmonary sarcoidosis. A mixed ventilatory defect, which usually denotes an airway-centered component, is often present in hypersensitivity pneumonitis, sarcoidosis, and connective tissue disease (in which bronchiolitis or bronchiectasis may co-exist with pulmonary fibrosis). Paradoxically, normal lung volumes in association with severe reduction in gas transfer levels are the hallmark of the combination of emphysema and pulmonary fibrosis. The often-cited phenomenon of a marked increase in gas transfer (measured by use of single breath techniques) because of diffuse alveolar hemorrhage is rarely clinically useful, because this abnormality persists for only 36 h after hemorrhage. The most diagnostically useful pulmonary function pattern is preservation of gas transfer in association with irreversible airflow obstruction, a combination that points strongly toward intrinsic airways disease (i.e., bronchiolitis) rather than emphysema. However, the pattern of pulmonary function impairment seldom makes a major diagnostic contribution.

Chest Radiography

With recent attention focused on the diagnostic value of HRCT, it is often forgotten that the plain chest radiograph provides invaluable information in diffuse lung disease. Sometimes the chest radiograph points strongly toward a specific diagnosis. Sarcoidosis, the most prevalent DLD encountered in clinical practice, can be diagnosed with confidence, in many cases from the clinical and chest radiographic features at presentation; HRCT seldom adds useful diagnostic information in this context.

Several chest radiographic features have useful positive predictive values. The presence of hilar lymphadenopathy on chest radiography is particularly strongly predictive of sarcoidosis in the correct clinical context, although the radiographic differential diagnosis includes tuberculosis and malignancy, especially when hilar lymphadenopathy is asymmetric. Pleural effusions are an occasional feature of connective tissue disease, lymphangioleiomyomatosis, and asbestos-related disease (as well as disease processes that sometimes mimic DLD, including heart failure, infection, and malignancy). The distribution of disease on chest radiography is also diagnostically useful; granulomatous diseases (tuberculosis, sarcoidosis, hypersensitivity pneumonitis) tend to be more prominent in the mid to upper zones, whereas fibrotic diseases (IPF, fibrotic nonspecific interstitial pneumonia, asbestosis) have a predominantly lower zone distribution.

However, apart from a large subgroup of patients with sarcoidosis, diagnoses based on chest radiography are seldom confident. Chest radiography is sometimes insensitive; in the often-quoted series of Epler and colleagues, 10% of patients with biopsy-proven DLD had normal chest radiographic appearances. The superior diagnostic accuracy of HRCT, compared with chest radiography, has been documented in numerous series, and the increased confidence associated with an HRCT diagnosis is a considerable aid to management. The classification of chest radiographic abnormalities as nodular, reticulonodular, or reticular provides relatively little diagnostic information. Predominantly basal honeycombing on chest radiography (which is invariably associated with honeycombing on HRCT) may be diagnostically useful in increasing the likelihood of IPF but is radiographically overt in surprisingly few patients with that disease. It is now generally accepted that, except in patients with obvious sarcoidosis, routine HRCT is almost always warranted in DLD, although occasional exceptions exist (e.g., elderly patients with obvious lower zone honeycombing on chest radiography, indicative of IPF; patients with long-standing pulmonary fibrosis on serial chest radiography; and an obvious underlying cause, such as coal mining).

Two chest radiographic appearances pose particular diagnostic difficulties. *Persistent unexplained multifocal consolidation* has usually been treated unsuccessfully for community-acquired pneumonia and has a wide differential diagnosis. Serial chest radiography tends to be more useful than HRCT in refining investigation, since the crucial diagnostic distinction lies between fixed infiltrates (nonbacterial infection including tuberculosis, alveolar cell carcinoma, and other malignant processes) and changing infiltrates in which these diagnoses are effectively excluded. However, immunologically mediated diseases (including eosinophilic pneumonia, cryptogenic organizing pneumonia and vasculitic disorders) may give rise to either fixed or evanescent radiographic abnormalities and a histologic diagnosis is often warranted. *Diffuse alveolar filling processes* giving rise to widespread airspace consolidation are generally indicative of life-threatening disease. Although this picture may represent DLD (e.g., acute interstitial pneumonitis, acute eosinophilic syndromes, drug-induced pulmonary infiltration), it is essential to broaden the differential diagnosis beyond DLD to include diffuse pulmonary infection, toxic inhalation, severe aspiration, opportunistic infection (especially pneumocystis pneumonia), diffuse alveolar hemorrhage syndromes, mitral stenosis and, above all, heart failure. In both of these radiographic presentations, successful management often depends on consideration of a wide differential diagnosis from the outset.

HIGH-RESOLUTION COMPUTED TOMOGRAPHY

HRCT has been the most important diagnostic advance in diffuse lung disease in the past two decades. Numerous studies have confirmed the overall diagnostic accuracy of HRCT against findings at surgical biopsy, with a striking increase in

sensitivity and specificity for individual diseases compared with chest radiography. However, academic series understate the impact of HRCT, because the most important benefit has been to increase clinician confidence in noninvasive diagnosis, with a corresponding reduction in the numbers of patients needing to undergo surgical biopsy. Before HRCT, diagnoses based on clinical data and chest radiographic findings were seldom confident, and management was necessarily tentative in many cases. The combination of clinical and HRCT information now provides a confident first choice diagnosis in most patients, and in many other cases, the realistic differential diagnosis is shortened to two or three disorders. This allows surgical biopsy to be reserved for cases in which the distinction between a small group of possible disorders has important management implications and for occasional cases in which HRCT appearances are not suggestive of any single disorder. Thus, routine surgical biopsy, as a diagnostic "gold standard," can no longer be justified in the HRCT era.

Histospecific diagnosis aside, HRCT sometimes plays an important role in detecting diffuse lung disease. The superior sensitivity of HRCT, compared with chest radiography, has been an invariable finding in studies of a wide range of disorders. This feature of HRCT is particularly useful when symptoms or lung function impairment are associated with normal chest radiographic appearances. In connective tissue disease, pulmonary involvement is now the leading cause of death, and early treatment of progressive lung disease is desirable; by identifying limited pulmonary fibrosis, HRCT allows clinicians to select patients in whom more intensive monitoring is required, even when immediate treatment is not warranted. In workers previously exposed to asbestos, HRCT often discloses pulmonary fibrosis that is obscured on chest radiography by concurrent pleural disease. However, it should be stressed that the sensitivity of HRCT occasionally creates its own difficulties. When interstitial abnormalities are limited, their clinical significance is sometimes difficult to rationalize; disease that is evident only on HRCT should not be extrapolated, in terms of natural history and management, to the more extensive disease described in historical clinical series. It is essential that HRCT findings are integrated with other clinical and investigative features and not interpreted in isolation.

The distinction between predominantly inflammatory and predominantly fibrotic disease can generally be made with reasonable confidence from HRCT. Anatomic distortion and reticular abnormalities are strongly indicative of irreversible fibrotic disease, and this is invariably true of honeycomb change (Figure 49-1). Consolidation is usually reversible, although it may occasionally represent dense fibrosis, especially in sarcoidosis. Ground-glass attenuation is often more difficult to interpret. In early work, this HRCT sign was shown to identify a substantial increase in the likelihood of significant inflammation, especially in the absence of concurrent reticular abnormalities. However, it is now clear that ground-glass attenuation denotes fine fibrosis in many cases, and this is especially the case in nonspecific interstitial pneumonia, in which ground-glass attenuation is the cardinal HRCT feature (Figure 49-2), and in sarcoidosis. Traction bronchiectasis is a key HRCT discriminator, because it is invariably indicative of underlying fibrosis. Thus, reversible inflammatory disease is likely only when ground-glass attenuation is not associated with traction bronchiectasis or admixed with reticular abnormalities.

A wide range of HRCT profiles, encompassing the distribution and pattern of disease, are strongly suggestive of individual diffuse lung diseases. The cardinal findings in the more

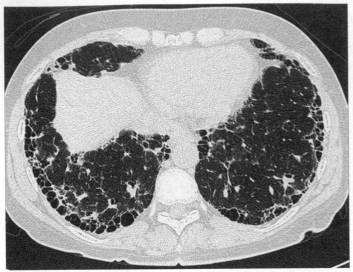

FIGURE 49-1 High-resolution computed tomography appearances in a patient with idiopathic pulmonary fibrosis (IPF). There is prominent subpleural honeycombing with no ground-glass attenuation. In the correct clinical context, this picture is virtually pathognomonic of IPF.

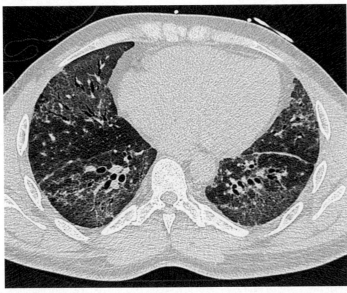

FIGURE 49-2 In a patient with nonspecific interstitial pneumonia, the predominant abnormalities on high-resolution computed tomography are ground-glass attenuation, with variable admixed fine reticular abnormalities and traction bronchiectasis. Notably, there is no honeycomb change.

BOX 49-1 High-Resolution Computed Tomography Features Recognized as Typical of Selected Diffuse Lung Diseases

Idiopathic pulmonary fibrosis: Lower zone, subpleural predominance, maximal posterobasally, predominantly reticular pattern with associated honeycombing.

Nonspecific interstitial pneumonia: Two frequent appearances. The variant that overlaps with idiopathic pulmonary fibrosis in disease distribution: ground-glass attenuation predominates, with a variable fine reticular component and traction bronchiectasis, but no honeycombing. The variant that overlaps with cryptogenic organizing pneumonia: consolidation with surrounding ground-glass attenuation and a variable fine reticular pattern.

Desquamative interstitial pneumonia: Ground-glass attenuation, sometimes diffuse, sometimes basal and peripheral centered, frequent associated fibrotic cysts with anatomic distortion and traction bronchiectasis.

Acute interstitial pneumonia: Widespread ground-glass attenuation admixed with features of fibrosis, usually with airspace consolidation, and occasional emphysema.

Respiratory bronchiolitis–interstitial lung disease: Patchy ground-glass attenuation, poorly defined centrilobular nodules, occasional mosaic attenuation, prominent bronchial wall thickening.

Sarcoidosis: Highly variable. Nodules distributed along bronchovascular bundles, interlobular septa, and subpleurally including the fissure; ground-glass attenuation that may represent either inflammation or fine fibrosis; reticular abnormalities, representing fibrosis; distortion most commonly occurring in upper zones with posterior displacement of the upper lobe bronchus; air trapping; associated hilar and mediastinal lymphadenopathy.

Subacute hypersensitivity pneumonitis: Widespread ground-glass attenuation, often containing poorly defined centrilobular nodules, admixed with areas of black lung (mosaic attenuation), representing air trapping and enhanced on expiratory high-resolution computed tomography.

Cryptogenic organizing pneumonia: Bilateral patchy consolidation, subpleural and predominantly basal in the majority, occasional peribronchial distribution, associated often sparse nodules up to 1 cm in diameter.

Constrictive bronchiolitis: Patchy areas of hyperlucency enhanced on expiration, which might not change in cross-sectional diameter on full expiration; associated bronchiectasis and bronchial wall thickening.

Langerhans cell histiocytosis: Bizarre cyst shapes and associated nodules throughout the lung fields but sparing the costophrenic angles and tips of the lingula and middle lobes. Associated emphysema is common.

Pulmonary lymphangioleiomyomatosis: Homogeneously distributed, thin-walled parenchymal cysts, varying from a few millimeters to several centimeters in diameter; associated with retrocrural adenopathy, pleural effusion, thoracic duct dilatation, pericardial effusion, and pneumothorax.

---

commonly encountered diffuse lung diseases are summarized in Box 49-1. As with all other applications of HRCT, it is essential that HRCT findings are integrated with the pretest diagnostic probability, distilled from the history, clinical signs, previous natural history or treated course, and investigative findings (especially chest radiography, pulmonary function tests, and serology for autoimmune disease and environmental antigens). The role of HRCT in diagnosis is critically dependent on the presence or absence of a likely cause. In patients with appropriate environmental antigen or drug exposures (hypersensitivity pneumonitis, pneumoconioses, drug-induced lung disease), malignant disease (lymphangitis carcinomatosis), clinical or serologic evidence of connective tissue disease, or a heavy smoking history (Langerhans cell histiocytosis, RBILD), the diagnostic weighting required from HRCT can be reduced. In these contexts, HRCT appearances that are merely compatible (and not classical) often allow a sufficiently confident diagnosis to obviate diagnostic surgical biopsy.

By contrast, the diagnostic role of HRCT is much greater in idiopathic disease, but unless the pretest diagnostic probability is high, confident diagnosis requires the presence of typical HRCT appearances. The optimal diagnostic use of HRCT in apparently idiopathic DLD can be distilled in a simple pragmatic algorithm:

1. The first step is to determine whether HRCT abnormalities are predominantly fibrotic on the basis of the presence of honeycombing, reticular abnormalities, anatomic distortion, or, in patients with prominent ground glass, the presence of traction bronchiectasis.
2. If disease is fibrotic, as in most cases, the next important question is whether HRCT findings are typical of IPF. As stated in the recent American Thoracic Society/ European Respiratory Society (ATS/ERS) recommendations, IPF can be diagnosed confidently on HRCT when there is honeycombing with little ground-glass attenuation in a predominantly basal and subpleural distribution. It is logical to focus on IPF, because it is the most prevalent idiopathic fibrotic disease among cases in which the diagnosis is not obvious from clinical and chest radiographic findings (most cases of sarcoidosis are diagnosed without recourse to HRCT [Figure 49-3]). Furthermore, IPF has a much worse prognosis than other fibrosing processes and is, therefore, the most important diagnosis to confirm or exclude from the outset. It is now known that HRCT appearances considered typical of IPF by experienced thoracic radiologists have a positive predictive value of more than 95%.

3. If appearances are not typical of IPF, the five most important differential diagnoses (on the basis of their prevalence in routine practice) are IPF with atypical HRCT appearances, sarcoidosis, nonspecific interstitial pneumonia, hypersensitivity pneumonitis (with the antigen unknown), and the fibrotic sequelae of cryptogenic organizing pneumonia. Among these, IPF with atypical HRCT appearances is the most prevalent disorder in most populations; up to 30% of IPF cases have atypical HRCT features. Atypical IPF is especially likely when HRCT appearances are not typical of any of the other four disorders.

The weighting given to HRCT in the diagnosis of diffuse lung disease varies from case to case but can usually be considered in three categories. In some patients, HRCT appearances are virtually pathognomonic; this includes many cases of IPF, Langerhans cell histiocytosis, sarcoidosis, and lymphangitis carcinomatosis. Often, HRCT findings are diagnostic when combined with clinical information. A good example is the combination of widespread ground-glass attenuation (often with poorly defined centrilobular nodules) in combination with mosaic attenuation, which may be strongly indicative of hypersensitivity pneumonitis in nonsmokers with a compatible exposure history but may also represent RBILD in smokers (Figure 49-4). Finally, even when not conclusive in its own

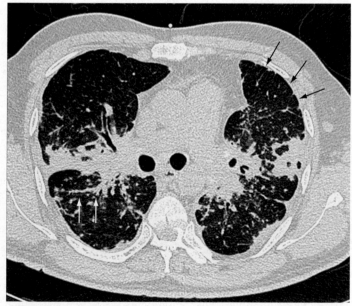

FIGURE 49-3 In this high-resolution CT scan from a patient with sarcoidosis, abnormalities suggesting the diagnosis include multiple, well-defined nodules, surrounding bronchovascular beading (*white arrows*), micronodules (especially in the left anterior lung, indicated by black arrows), septal thickening (by granulomatous infiltration), and areas of dense consolidation that may be reversible (coalescence of granulomata) or irreversible (fibrosis). This combination of abnormalities is virtually pathognomonic of sarcoidosis.

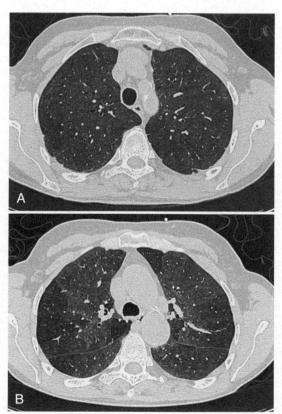

FIGURE 49-4 A, In hypersensitivity pneumonitis, abnormalities on inspiratory high-resolution computed tomography (HRCT), consisting of widespread ground-glass attenuation, often with poorly formed centrilobular nodules, are often extremely subtle, and HRCT appearances may be virtually normal. B, However, on expiratory HRCT, striking regional variation in lung attenuation is often apparent, with areas of darker lung representing gas trapping (because of the bronchiolitic component of the disease).

right, HRCT may also be invaluable when considered in conjunction with diagnostic surgical biopsy. The histologic entity of nonspecific interstitial pneumonia (NSIP) is found in a variety of clinicoradiologic contexts, including entities overlapping clinically with IPF, fibrosing organizing pneumonia, and hypersensitivity pneumonitis; HRCT evaluation is central to the distinction between these variants.

BRONCHOSCOPIC PROCEDURES

Although endobronchial and transbronchial biopsies are straightforward and relatively noninvasive procedures, the volume of tissue taken is small, and only bronchial and peribronchial tissue is sampled. Thus, both procedures have a high yield in diseases that have a peribronchial distribution, especially sarcoidosis and lymphangitis carcinomatosis. Occasionally, transbronchial biopsy findings can help to cement a diagnosis of hypersensitivity pneumonitis, although bronchoalveolar lavage (BAL) tends to be more rewarding in this regard. Bronchoscopic biopsy procedures have little or no diagnostic value in the idiopathic interstitial pneumonias. Hemorrhage and pneumothorax (with transbronchial biopsy) are the important risks associated with bronchoscopic procedures. Major hemorrhage is rare, but pneumothoraces complicate transbronchial biopsies in 1–2% of procedures, although intercostal tube drainage is not always required.

In the 1980s, BAL was regarded by many as an important part of the diagnostic algorithm in diffuse lung disease. The distinction between a BAL neutrophilia (suggestive of IPF) and a BAL lymphocytosis (as in sarcoidosis or hypersensitivity pneumonitis) was held to be particularly useful. However, as experience accumulated, it became apparent that diagnoses distinctions on the basis of BAL in large groups of patients were insufficiently reliable in individual cases. The advent of HRCT, with the wealth of additional diagnostic information that it provided, also limited the role of BAL, which had been more influential in the pre-HRCT era, when most noninvasive diagnoses were tentative. There are currently no published evaluations of the diagnostic value added by BAL, once HRCT findings are taken into account. However, in the past 5 years, BAL has enjoyed a renaissance in some centers. In recent ATS/ERS recommendations, compatible BAL findings (i.e., no lymphocytosis) are a requirement for the noninvasive diagnosis of IPF; this criterion reflects the diagnostic value of BAL findings when HRCT appearances are suggestive of IPF but are not definitive. However, a BAL lymphocytosis has an even greater diagnostic impact in some patients with sarcoidosis or hypersensitivity pneumonitis; when significant fibrosis supervenes in these disorders, HRCT appearances often become atypical, and IPF is frequently the preferred diagnosis before the performance of BAL. A BAL lymphocytosis in the setting of fibrotic diffuse lung disease is sometimes an important justification for diagnostic surgical biopsy. Thus, BAL continues to play a useful diagnostic role in a significant subset of patients when clinical and HRCT features are inconclusive, although it adds little to diagnosis in most DLD cases.

SURGICAL BIOPSY

Surgical biopsy, formerly performed as an open procedure but now widely obtained by use of video-assisted thoracoscopic surgery (VATS), was once regarded as the diagnostic reference standard and, until recently, was advocated as a routine diagnostic procedure by some authorities. However, routine surgical biopsy is impracticable outside referral centers, and in the 1980s, even before HRCT had a significant diagnostic impact, it was performed in less than 15% of patients with IPF in the United Kingdom. Even in referral centers, the performance of diagnostic surgical biopsies has been radically reduced with the application of HRCT. In one UK referral center (the Royal Brompton Hospital), biopsy was performed in more than 50% of IPF cases in the 1980s but in less than 25% of IPF cases in the mid 1990s. Moreover, it is increasingly clear that open or VATS biopsy is not a true diagnostic "gold standard." Variation between 10 thoracic pathologists in assigning a histologic diagnosis in DLD was recently found to be considerable, with agreement only moderate (kappa coefficient of agreement of 0.38). In more than 20% of biopsies, the first choice diagnosis was assigned with low confidence.

Thus, although biopsy procedures add invaluable information in selected cases, and a pattern of usual interstitial pneumonia is usually diagnostically definitive, a histologic diagnosis in isolation should no longer be viewed as a diagnostic "gold standard."

Sometimes, the histologic diagnosis is at odds with clinical and HRCT information and must be integrated with other information. In some patients with fibrotic hypersensitivity pneumonitis, a histologic pattern of usual interstitial pneumonia (which is normally indicative of IPF) is disclosed at biopsy, despite clinical, HRCT, BAL features of hypersensitivity pneumonitis and an indolent course during follow-up. Similarly, in a cohort of more than 100 patients with IPF or fibrotic NSIP reported by Flaherty et al., a combination of histologic and HRCT findings provided more accurate prognostic information than either modality in isolation. Thus, surgical biopsy is now best viewed, like HRCT, as a diagnostic "silver standard" and can often be avoided when HRCT and clinical features are typical of an individual DLD.

The morbidity and mortality associated with surgical biopsy in DLD are low in patients with an adequate pulmonary reserve but increase significantly in severe disease. In the series of Utz et al., patients with advanced IPF (with a mean gas transfer level of less than 35% of predicted) had a mortality ascribable to biopsy of 15%. Although this figure is generally regarded as an overstatement of the risk of the procedure, on the basis of other series and widespread anecdotal experience, a surgical biopsy should not be performed unless central to management if the gas transfer is less than 30% of predicted. Moreover, in advanced idiopathic fibrotic disease, the prognostic value of a histospecific diagnosis diminishes. In the series of Latsi et al., mortality was identical in IPF and fibrotic NSIP when the gas transfer was less than 35%, despite major differences in survival in less severe disease.

Thus, in younger patients (younger than the age of 60) presenting with a typical clinical picture of severe IPF and HRCT features suggestive of fibrotic NSIP, immediate referral for consideration of lung transplantation is warranted without a histologic diagnosis. The exception is the patient presenting with overwhelmingly severe acute DLD, in which the diagnosis is unclear, and realistic differential diagnoses include acute interstitial pneumonia, severe infection (including opportunistic infection), and malignancy. BAL may be required to exclude infection, and occasionally a histologic diagnosis is required to rationalize management. Both procedures can be performed in ventilated patients, and if disease is slightly less severe, elective mechanical ventilation may be warranted to investigate appropriately.

INTEGRATED DIAGNOSIS IN DIFFUSE LUNG DISEASE

The central diagnostic challenge for the clinician is to integrate the information just discussed into a final diagnosis, without overemphasizing any single clinical or investigative feature in isolation. Indeed, only the clinician is able to play this role, because both histologic and HRCT diagnoses made without reference to other information are seriously flawed in a significant proportion of cases. The most difficult dilemma, when noninvasive evaluation discloses two or more realistic diagnoses, is whether to accept diagnostic uncertainty without investigating further or to resort to invasive (surgical biopsy) or semiinvasive (BAL, transbronchial biopsy) procedures.

This decision should be made pragmatically and not by protocol. The value of a specific diagnosis in DLD is that the clinician is informed of the probable natural history and the likelihood that treatment will play a useful role; from these considerations, the optimal approach to monitoring disease during follow-up will usually be apparent. Thus, the essential purpose of pursuing a diagnosis is to identify probable disease behavior with and without treatment. Broadly, with occasional exceptions, longitudinal disease behavior in DLD can be subdivided into the five patterns listed in Table 49-3. When an individual patient can be subclassified confidently into one of these groups, invasive investigation will often add little to short- and long-term management. Three strands of information are of particular value in making these distinctions: the underlying cause (if any), a morphologic assessment by use of HRCT (and histologic evaluation in selected cases), and observed longitudinal disease behavior.

The identification of an underlying cause is vital, because it may, when considered in conjunction with HRCT appearances, allow disease to be classified confidently as self-limited inflammation (e.g., acute drug-induced lung disease, hypersensitivity pneumonitis, respiratory bronchiolitis with associated interstitial lung disease in smokers), with a good outcome, provided that the offending agent is removed. In long-standing disease, knowledge of a cause often allows the clinician to classify fibrotic abnormalities on HRCT as stable fibrotic disease (e.g., the fibrotic sequelae of nitrofurantoin lung, silicosis, and other pneumoconioses); the confidence of this conclusion is increased by the documentation of stable longitudinal disease behavior on the basis of previous chest radiographs, symptoms, and, occasionally, pulmonary function tests. In both self-limited inflammation and stable fibrotic disease, invasive diagnostic investigations are seldom warranted, and potentially toxic treatments can usually be minimized.

A histologic diagnosis is required more frequently in apparently idiopathic disease to draw two essential distinctions: between inherently stable and potentially progressive fibrotic disease and between major inflammation (with a high risk of evolution to fibrosis with undertreatment) and inexorably progressive fibrotic disease. In both scenarios, therapeutic intervention may be the key to a substantially better outcome. Knowledge of likely intrinsic disease behavior is invaluable, because it allows decisive management and increases patient confidence considerably. A confident diagnosis of hypersensitivity pneumonitis, nonspecific interstitial pneumonia, or

TABLE 49-3 The Most Frequent Patterns of Longitudinal Disease Behavior in Diffuse Lung Disease with Selected Examples of Underlying Diagnoses That May Appear in Several Categories*

Self-limited inflammation	Drug-induced lung disease (acute onset) Hypersensitivity pneumonitis (usually short-term exposure) Sarcoidosis (distinct subset with, usually, acute onset)
Stable fibrotic disease	Drug-induced lung disease (residual fibrosis after cessation) Hypersensitivity pneumonitis (after prolonged exposure) Sarcoidosis (residuum of burnt-out disease) Nonprogressive pneumoconioses after exposure (e.g., silicosis)
Major inflammation, risk of fibrotic progression	Drug-induced lung disease (unusually florid reactions) Hypersensitivity pneumonitis (usually continuing exposure) Sarcoidosis (prolonged severe inflammation)
Inexorably progressive fibrosis	Drug-induced lung disease (continuing exposure) Hypersensitivity pneumonitis (antigen usually unknown) Sarcoidosis (small subset of patients) Progressive pneumoconioses after exposure (e.g., asbestosis)
Explosive acute diffuse lung disease	Drug-induced lung disease

*Excluding the idiopathic interstitial pneumonias, covered in Table 49-4.

cryptogenic organizing pneumonia associated with significant fibrosis justifies aggressive intervention with a higher risk of drug toxicity, because the treated outcome is often good. By contrast, in IPF, in which the benefits of treatment may be marginal, a more cautious therapeutic approach is often warranted, and in younger patients, the timing of consideration of transplantation can be rationalized. As a general principle, BAL and/or surgical biopsy should always be pursued in patients fit for these procedures (as judged by age, disease severity, and comorbidity) if a confident management strategy, based on disease behavior, cannot be constructed from noninvasive evaluation.

These principles apply especially to the most common presentation of nongranulomatous idiopathic DLD: the CFA clinical syndrome. In previous decades, underlying histologic appearances have tended to be lumped together, but the recent ATS/ERS reclassification of the idiopathic interstitial pneumonias (Table 49-4) has provided a framework for the separation of a number of disease entities with strikingly diverse natural histories and treated outcomes. In an evaluation by Nicholson *et al.* of biopsy diagnoses of "cryptogenic fibrosing alveolitis" made in the 1980s, in patients presenting with the CFA clinical syndrome, an alternative histologic diagnosis was evident on review (associated with a much better observed outcome) in more than 50% of cases. The ATS/ERS classification system is logical and pragmatic, because, as

TABLE 49-4 ATS/ERS Consensus Classification of the Idiopathic Interstitial Pneumonias and the Most Frequent Patterns of Longitudinal Behavior Associated with Individual Diagnoses

Clinicopathologic Diagnosis	Likely Longitudinal Behavior Idiopathic Pulmonary Fibrosis/ Inexorably Progressive Fibrosis Cryptogenic Fibrosing Alveolitis
NSIP	Cellular NSIP: self-limited or major inflammation Fibrotic NSIP: stable or progressive fibrosis
Cryptogenic organizing pneumonia	Self-limited or major inflammation
Acute interstitial pneumonia	Explosive acute disease
Desquamative interstitial pneumonia	Self-limited or major inflammation
Respiratory bronchiolitis–associated	Self-limited inflammation interstitial lung disease
Lymphocytic interstitial pneumonia	Self-limited or major inflammation

NSIP, nonspecific interstitial pneumonia.

shown in Table 49-4, each individual entity tends to fall into a particular category of longitudinal disease behavior (although a certain amount of overlap is inevitable). Thus, when a confident noninvasive diagnosis is unattainable in patients with idiopathic interstitial pneumonia, surgical biopsy should always be considered.

In the recent influential study of Flaherty *et al.,* in which the final diagnosis was multidisciplinary, two conclusions highly relevant to routine diagnosis were apparent. When a confident pre-biopsy diagnosis of IPF was made by clinicians or radiologists, the diagnosis virtually never changed with the addition of histologic data. By contrast, in the remaining cases, diagnoses made by clinicians and radiologists changed in approximately 50% of cases when biopsy data were considered. However, it should also be stressed that the final diagnosis differed from the histologic diagnosis in 25% of cases. It is now widely accepted that a multidisciplinary diagnosis, negotiated between clinicians, radiologists, and (in biopsied cases) pathologists, is the diagnostic reference standard in DLD.

SUGGESTED READINGS

American Thoracic Society: Idiopathic pulmonary fibrosis: Diagnosis and treatment. International consensus statement. Am J Respir Crit Care Med 2000; 161:646–664.

American Thoracic Society/European Respiratory Society: American Thoracic Society/European Respiratory Society international multidisciplinary consensus classification of the idiopathic interstitial pneumonias. Am J Respir Crit Care Med 2002; 165:277–304.

Bertorelli G, Bocchino V, Olivieri D: Hypersensitivity pneumonitis. Eur Respir Monogr 2000; 14:120–136.

Coultas DB, Zumwalt RE, Black WC, Sobonya RE: The epidemiology of interstitial lung diseases. Am J Respir Crit Care Med 1994; 150:967–972.

Epler GR, McLoud TC, Gaensler EA, et al: Normal chest radiographs in chronic diffuse infiltrative lung disease. N Engl J Med 1978; 298:934–939.

Flaherty KR, Thwaite EL, Kazerooni EA, et al: Radiological versus histological diagnosis in UIP and NSIP: Survival implications. Thorax 2003; 58:143–148.

Flaherty KR, King TE Jr., Raghu G, et al: Idiopathic interstitial pneumonia: what is the effect of a multidisciplinary approach to diagnosis? Am J Respir Crit Care Med 2004; 170:904–910.

Hunninghake GW, Zimmerman MB, Schwartz DA, et al: Utility of a lung biopsy for the diagnosis of idiopathic pulmonary fibrosis. Am J Respir Crit Care Med 2001; 164:193–196.

Latsi PI, Du Bois RM, Nicholson AG, et al: Fibrotic idiopathic interstitial pneumonia: The prognostic value of longitudinal functional trends. Am J Respir Crit Care Med 2003; 168:531–537.

Nicholson AG, Colby TV, du Bois RM, et al: The prognostic significance of the histologic pattern of interstitial pneumonia in patients presenting with the clinical entity of cryptogenic fibrosing alveolitis. Am J Respir Crit Care Med 2000; 162:2213–2217.

Utz JP, Ryu JH, Douglas WW, et al: High short-term mortality following lung biopsy for usual interstitial pneumonia. Eur Respir J 2001; 17:175–179.

Wells AU: High resolution computed tomography in the diagnosis of diffuse lung disease: A clinical perspective. Semin Respir Crit Care Med 2003; 24:347–356.

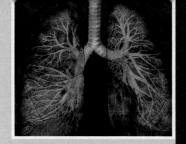

50 Idiopathic Pulmonary Fibrosis and Other Idiopathic Interstitial Pneumonias

ULRICH COSTABEL

INTRODUCTION

In the past, the term idiopathic pulmonary fibrosis (IPF) has been used as an umbrella label to describe all patients with pulmonary fibrosis of unknown cause, regardless of differences in histologic patterns. Today, IPF refers to a distinct form of the idiopathic interstitial pneumonias associated with the histologic pattern of usual interstitial pneumonia (UIP), as presented in the International Consensus Statement on IPF of 2000 and the American Thoracic Society/European Respiratory Society (IRS/ERS) Consensus Classification of 2002 (Table 50-1). IPF is the most common form of the idiopathic interstitial pneumonias accounting for 50–60% of cases, followed by nonspecific interstitial pneumonia (NSIP) that represents 20–40%; the remaining conditions are much more rare. IPF has the worst prognosis after acute interstitial pneumonia (AIP), with a median survival of only 2.8 years. Cryptogenic organizing pneumonia (COP) and lymphoid interstitial pneumonia (LIP), which is rarely idiopathic, are covered in Chapter 53.

Historically, Hamman and Rich were the first to describe pulmonary fibrosis of unknown cause. In 1944, they reported on four patients with acute diffuse interstitial fibrosis who died within 1–6 months. It is now clear that these patients had AIP, and not IPF as defined today.

Definition of IPF

The definition, as written in the ATS/ERS Statement of 2000, reads as follows:

- IPF is a specific form of chronic fibrosing interstitial pneumonia of unknown etiology, limited to the lung and with the histopathological appearance of UIP on surgical lung biopsy with:
  - The exclusion of known causes of interstitial lung disease such as drug toxicities, environmental exposures, and connective tissue diseases
  - Abnormal pulmonary function tests with evidence of restriction and/or impaired gas exchange
  - Characteristic abnormalities on chest radiography or high-resolution computed tomography (HRCT) scans.

In the absence of a surgical lung biopsy, the diagnosis of IPF is less secure. However, in the immunocompetent adult, the presence of all of the following major diagnostic criteria, as well as at least three of the four minor criteria, increases the likelihood of a correct clinical diagnosis.

Major Criteria

- Exclusion of known causes (see preceding section)
- Abnormal pulmonary function tests with evidence of restriction and impaired gas exchange
- Bibasilar reticular abnormalities with minimal or no ground-glass opacities on HRCT scans
- Transbronchial biopsy or bronchoalveolar lavage showing no features to support an alternative diagnosis

Minor Criteria

- Age older than 50 years
- Insidious onset of otherwise unexplained dyspnea on exertion
- Duration of illness more than 3 months
- Bibasilar inspiratory crackles on chest auscultation

In clinical practice, surgical lung biopsy is performed in only 15–30% of patients with IPF. HRCT can confidently secure the diagnosis in most patients.

EPIDEMIOLOGY

Patients with IPF are usually between 50 and 70 years of age, with a mean age at diagnosis of 67 years, and approximately two thirds of patients older than the age of 60 years. Patients with the other idiopathic interstitial pneumonias, such as desquamative interstitial pneumonia (DIP), NSIP, or AIP, usually are younger at presentation (Table 50-2). Men are affected slightly more frequently than women.

Data on the incidence and prevalence of IPF are scant and variable. Most are based on older studies that did not distinguish between IPF and the other forms of the idiopathic interstitial pneumonia. There is evidence that the incidence is increasing on the basis of the mortality statistics from England and Wales. The incidence has been estimated at 10.7/100,000 per year for males and 7.4/100,000 for females, and the prevalence at 20.2/100,000 for males and at 13.2/100,000 for females in the early 1990s in New Mexico. The nationwide prevalence of IPF in Finland as defined by the new ATS/ERS criteria was recently estimated to be 16–18/100,000. The incidence and prevalence of IPF increases markedly with age (e.g., prevalence 2.7/100,000 for age 35–44 years; prevalence 250/100,000 for age older than 75 years).

Routine mortality statistics for IPF did not become available until 1979, when the introduction of the ninth revision of the

International Classification of Diseases provided a specific code for this disease for the first time, but the code does not distinguish between IPF and the other forms of idiopathic interstitial pneumonias. Registered mortality from IPF has since risen substantially in many countries (Figure 50-1) to a degree that seems unlikely to be purely an artifact of increased recognition or a change in diagnostic labeling.

RISK FACTORS

Several risk factors for IPF have been identified, in particular, occupational exposure to metal or wood dust. Organic solvents, mycotoxins, hydrogen peroxide, and various other occupational exposures have also been implicated. Epstein–Barr virus, influenza, cytomegalovirus, and hepatitis C virus infections have also been suggested to have a role in etiology,

although the evidence is not yet conclusive. IPF is more common among cigarette smokers and ex-smokers than nonsmokers, and it has recently been suggested that IPF may be related to use of some of the antidepressant drugs. The prevalence of chronic aspiration secondary to gastroesophageal reflux is increased in patients with IPF.

PATHOGENESIS

The traditional concept in regard to the pathogenesis of IPF was that the initial event is an inflammatory process (alveolitis characterized by infiltration of inflammatory cells such as macrophages, lymphocytes, and neutrophils). Inflammation was believed to lead to recruitment of fibroblasts and

TABLE 50-1 American Thoracic Society and European Respiratory Society Classification of Idiopathic Interstitial Pneumonias	
Histologic Pattern	Clinical-Radiologic-Pathologic Diagnosis
Usual interstitial pneumonia	Idiopathic pulmonary fibrosis or cryptogenic fibrosing alveolitis
Nonspecific interstitial pneumonia	Nonspecific interstitial pneumonia (provisional)
Organizing pneumonia	Cryptogenic organizing pneumonia (synonymous with idiopathic bronchiolitis obliterans organizing pneumonia)
Diffuse alveolar damage	Acute interstitial pneumonia
Respiratory bronchiolitis	Respiratory bronchiolitis interstitial lung disease
Desquamative interstitial pneumonia	Desquamative interstitial pneumonia
Lymphocytic interstitial pneumonia	Lymphocytic interstitial pneumonia

Unclassifiable interstitial pneumonias: Some cases of interstitial pneumonia are unclassifiable for a variety of reasons. Such cases constitute a heterogeneous group with poorly characterized clinical and radiologic features.

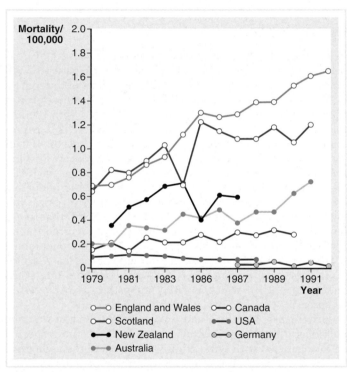

FIGURE 50-1 Crude mortality rates for idiopathic pulmonary fibrosis (IPF) in seven countries. (Adapted with permission from Coultas DB, Zumwalt RE, Black WC, Sobonya RE: The epidemiology of interstitial lung diseases. Am J Respir Crit Care Med 1994; 150:967–972.)

TABLE 50-2 Contrasting Clinical Features of Idiopathic Interstitial Pneumonias							
	IPF	NSIP*	DIP	RB-ILD	AIP	COP	LIP
Age (y)	65	55	40	35	50	55	50
Occurrence in children	No	Occasional	Rare	No	Rare	No	Rare
Onset	Chronic	Subacute/chronic	Chronic	Chronic	Acute	Acute/subacute	Chronic
Clubbing	Frequent	Occasional	Frequent	No	No	No	Rare
Fever	Rare	10–30%	No	No	50%	70%	Occasional
Mortality (%)	70–90	11–60	0–27	0	80	13	?
Mean survival	2.8	4–13 y	12 y	Not reduced	1.5 months	>10 years	?
Response to corticosteroids	Poor	Good	Good	Good	Poor	Good	Good

AIP, Acute interstitial pneumonia; COP, chronic organizing pneumonia; DIP, desquamative interstitial pneumonia; IPF, idiopathic pulmonary fibrosis; NSIP, nonspecific interstitial pneumonia; RB-ILD, respiratory bronchiolitis–interstitial lung disease; LIP, lymphocytic interstitial pneumonia.
*NSIP has a variable prognosis: favorable for cellular type, intermediate for fibrotic type.

myofibroblasts and finally to collagen formation and irreversible fibrosis. The new theory implies that IPF is a primary epithelial and fibroblastic disease, and inflammation is, in fact, an epiphenomenon of the fibrotic pathway.

The current hypothesis suggests that after an initial injury to the alveolar epithelial cells, these cells themselves can release a number of fibrogenic cytokines such as transforming growth factor-β–1, platelet-derived growth factor, basic fibroblast growth factor, and tumor necrosis factor-alpha. Under the influence of theses cytokines, fibroblasts are attracted to the site of injury; they start to proliferate and to transform into myofibroblasts. Also, a phenotypic change of the epithelial cell is believed to induce "epithelial/mesenchymal transition" and is considered as one mechanism by which fibroblasts appear. The fibroblasts in IPF seem to be more resistant to apoptosis than normal fibroblasts, whereas the alveolar epithelial cells seem to undergo apoptosis at an increased rate.

A further mechanism that may potentiate the fibrotic process is increased production of oxidants and diminished levels of antioxidants such as glutathione in the lung of patients with IPF, providing the basis for an antioxidant approach in the treatment of IPF.

GENETICS

Some evidence suggests that genetic factors may contribute to the risk of IPF developing. Reported associations with the HLA-antigen phenotype have not proved consistent, but the increased prevalence of autoantibodies in individuals with IPF is well recognized. The significance of this association, either in etiologic or pathogenetic terms, is not yet established. So far, no genetic factors have been conclusively associated with sporadic IPF or other forms of idiopathic interstitial pneumonias.

Familial pulmonary fibrosis that is rare and accounts for only 0.5–3.5% of all IPF cases has provided the best evidence for a genetic predisposition of the disease. Surfactant protein C-gene mutations have been observed as a cause of UIP in 14 individuals in a family spanning six generations. The largest study on familial pulmonary fibrosis, reporting the results of a nationwide collaborative approach in the United States, recruited 111 families having 309 affected and 360 unaffected individuals. This study showed that familial pulmonary fibrosis is inherited as an autosomal-dominant trait with a variable penetrance. Older age, male sex, and having ever smoked cigarettes was associated with the development of familial pulmonary fibrosis, very similar as is known for sporadic IPF. Forty-five percent of affected individuals were phenotypically heterogeneous, the dominant HRCT/histopathologic subtype being UIP with 80%. Overall, the clinical features and survival rates of familial IPF are similar to those of sporadic IPF.

CLINICAL FEATURES

Idiopathic Pulmonary Fibrosis

Typically, IPF is seen in older patients and usually has an insidious onset and slow disease progression. The most common presenting symptoms are exertional dyspnea and dry cough of gradual onset. Hemoptysis is uncommon and, if present, should raise the suspicion of an underlying lung cancer, the relative risk of which increases 7- to 14-fold in IPF. On physical examination, the most frequent signs are bilateral fine crackles

on auscultation (in 96% of patients in one series). They are typically end-inspiratory and most prevalent in the lung bases but tend to extend to the upper lung zones with progression of the disease. Finger clubbing is present in approximately 50%, and arthralgia or arthritis, in the absence of more overt clinical evidence of connective tissue disease, in approximately 20%. Constitutional symptoms, including malaise and weight loss, are recognized but uncommon. Fever is rare, and its presence suggests an alternative diagnosis. In more advanced disease, cyanosis and cor pulmonale may also be present.

The chest radiograph is abnormal at presentation in virtually all patients with IPF. Typical chest radiograph appearances are of bilateral, linear (reticular), or reticulonodular shadowing, predominantly at the periphery and at the lung bases and usually associated with reduced lung volume (Figure 50-2). In most cases, the shadowing leads to a loss of definition of the cardiac and diaphragmatic outline. In more advanced disease, the reticular shadowing combines with multiple cystic translucencies to produce the appearance of honeycomb lung.

High-resolution computed tomography (HRCT) now has a central role in the diagnostic approach to diffuse lung diseases. It can reveal disease before the chest radiograph becomes abnormal, helps to narrow the differential diagnosis on the basis of the CT pattern, and allows the identification of associated emphysema. The primary role of HRCT in suspected idiopathic interstitial pneumonia is to separate patients with the typical findings of IPF from those with the less specific findings associated with other idiopathic interstitial pneumonias. The typical HRCT changes of IPF consist of a reticular pattern, in a subpleural and peripheral distribution, usually heterogeneous (patchy) and bilateral with a predilection for the basilar regions (Figure 50-3). A variable amount of

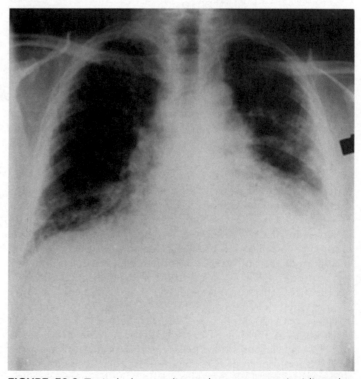

FIGURE 50-2 Typical chest radiograph appearance in idiopathic pulmonary fibrosis (IPF), with reticular and some nodular shadowing at both bases and some reduction of lung volume. (Radiograph courtesy of Dr. Andrew Evans, Nottingham City Hospital, UK.)

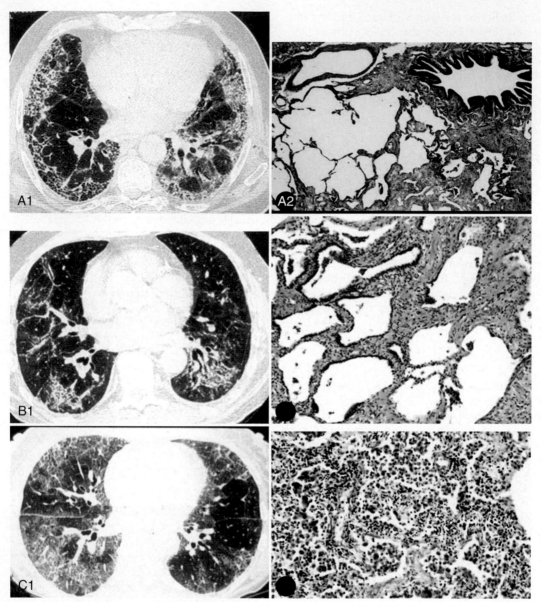

FIGURE 50-3 Typical HRCT scans and histopathologic patterns. **A,** IPF and UIP. **B,** NSIP. **C,** DIP. The patterns are described in detail in Table 50-3. (Histology courtesy of Dr. Dirk Theegasten, Department of Pathology, Ruhr University, Bochum, Germany.)

ground-glass opacity may be present, but this is usually minor and limited in extent to the areas of involvement by the reticular pattern. The distribution is most predominant posteriorly at the bases but becoming more anterior with progression of disease. As the disease becomes more severe, it spreads centrally and to the upper zones. In areas of more severe involvement, traction bronchiectasis and subpleural cysts (honeycombing) are often seen. Consolidation and nodules are absent. When all of these radiologic features are present (characteristic IPF/UIP pattern), the changes are virtually pathognomonic, and the diagnosis of IPF is correct in more than 90% of cases (specificity ranging between 90 and 97% in various studies). Extensive ground-glass opacities on CT should prompt consideration of a diagnosis other than IPF, particularly DIP, but also RBILD, NSIP, extrinsic allergic alveolitis, or alveolar proteinosis (Table 50-3). The role of HRCT in prognosis and response to treatment is discussed later in this chapter.

The characteristic lung function abnormalities in IPF are restrictive, with reduction of total lung capacity, vital capacity, forced expiratory volume in 1 second (FEV_1), and residual volume. Often at presentation, the impairment of FEV_1 and forced vital capacity (FVC) is relatively minor, but measures of gas transfer show a more marked reduction. With coexisting emphysema, lung volumes may be normal, and measures of gas exchange, such as DL_{CO} and oxygenation, are disproportionally reduced compared with the rather well-preserved lung volumes. Arterial blood gas tensions may be normal in patients with early disease but more commonly demonstrate hypoxemia. Exercise tests show arterial desaturation even when arterial blood gas measurements are normal at rest. A 6-min walk test may be helpful to assess the extent of impairment, the need for supplemental oxygen, and to determine evolution of the disease over time. Six-month follow-up investigation is important to assess the rate of deterioration. Patients with rapid declines in lung function have a worse prognosis. It has

TABLE 50-3 Contrasting Histopathologic and HRCT Characteristics of Idiopathic Interstitial Pneumonias

Histologic Pattern	Histopathologic Findings	Usual CT Findings
Usual interstitial pneumonia	Architectural destruction, fibrosis with honeycombing, fibroblastic foci. Nonuniformity of these changes within biopsy specimen (temporal heterogeneity)	Peripheral, subpleural, and basal distribution. Irregular reticular changes with honeycombing, traction bronchiectasis and architectural distortion. Focal, but minimal, ground-glass change.
Nonspecific interstitial pneumonia	Variable interstitial inflammation and fibrosis. Uniformity of changes within biopsy specimen. Fibroblastic foci inconspicuous/absent	Peripleural, peribronchial, basal; subpleural sparing possible. More ground-glass attenuation. Reticular changes and traction bronchiectasis seen, but honeycombing is not prominent. Little consolidation may be present.
Lymphocytic interstitial pneumonia	Extensive lymphocytic infiltration in the interstitium often associated with peribronchiolar lymphoid follicles (follicular bronchiolitis)	Centrilobular nodules, ground-glass attenuation, septal and bronchovascular thickening, thin walled cysts.
Diffuse alveolar damage	Diffuse. Alveolar septal thickening, airspace organization, hyaline membranes	Gravity-dependent consolidation, ground-glass opacification—often with lobular sparing. Traction bronchiectasis occurs later
Organizing pneumonia	Lung architecture preserved. Patchy distribution of intraluminal organizing fibrosis in distal air spaces	Patchy consolidation and/or nodules. May have a ground-glass component.
Desquamative interstitial pneumonia	Uniform involvement of parenchyma. Alveolar macrophages filling the alveoli with little interstitial disease	Peripheral, subpleural, basal distribution. Ground-glass attenuation, minor reticular changes, "geographic pattern."
Respiratory-bronchiolitis associated interstitial lung disease	Bronchocentric alveolar macrophage accumulation, minor inflammation and fibrosis	Patchy ground glass. Bronchial wall thickening with centrilobular nodules.

recently been shown that decreases in vital capacity of 10% or more and in DLco of 15% or more from baseline over a period of 6–12 months are associated with an increased risk of death.

Bronchoalveolar lavage differential cell counts in a patient with typical IPF usually shows elevated neutrophils and eosinophils. This pattern may be helpful in narrowing the differential diagnosis but is not diagnostic of IPF, because it is also observed in other fibrosing lung conditions. A neutrophilia is noted in 70–90% of patients, an associated increase in eosinophils in 40–60%, and a mild additional lymphocytosis in 10–20%. Higher percentages of lymphocytes (<30%) are uncommon in IPF, and, when present, other disorders should be excluded (e.g., granulomatous infectious disease, sarcoidosis, hypersensitivity pneumonitis, COP, NSIP, or LIP).

Transbronchial biopsy is not useful to diagnose the pattern of UIP but may suggest an alternative specific diagnosis (e.g., malignancy, infections, sarcoidosis, hypersensitivity pneumonitis, COP, eosinophilic pneumonia, or Langerhans cell histiocytosis).

Up to a third of patients have antinuclear antibodies or rheumatoid factor in their serum at presentation, despite the conventional exclusion of patients who show overt clinical evidence of connective tissue disease from the diagnosis of IPF.

Other Idiopathic Interstitial Pneumonias

Idiopathic NSIP shows similar clinical characteristics to IPF, with some exceptions. The patients are on average 10 years younger than patients with IPF, show clubbing less frequently (between 10% and 50% in various series), and may have a fever in up to one third of cases. The predominant HRCT pattern of NSIP is ground-glass opacification, often associated with

reticular changes and traction bronchiectasis, sometime with subpleural sparing and/or lower lobe shrinkage. Honeycombing is not prominent and turns out to be very predictive of UIP when a predominance of ground-glass opacity is absent. Bronchoalveolar lavage may show an increase in lymphocytes in addition to increased proportions of neutrophils or eosinophils, whereas a predominance of lymphocytes is absent in IPF.

RBILD and DIP are strongly associated with a history of cigarette smoking. RBILD is exclusively a disease of cigarette smokers, whereas DIP can be also seen in nonsmokers (80% active or former cigarette smokers, 20% nonsmokers). Both diseases affect patients in their fourth decades of life and are more common in men than in women, by a ratio of 2:1. Finger clubbing is absent in RBILD, but it is seen in half of the patients with DIP. Pulmonary function tests in RBILD may demonstrate obstructive and restrictive physiology, whereas pure restriction is the usual finding in DIP. RBILD usually shows minor changes on HRCT, the most common changes being bronchial wall thickening, centrilobular nodules, and patchy ground-glass opacities, without clear anatomic predilection. Associated centrilobular emphysema is common but not severe. Caused by the bronchiolar component of the disease, areas of decreased attenuation because of air trapping may be seen. The HRCT changes of DIP are more extensive than in RBILD, with widespread ground-glass opacification in a subpleural and basal distribution, often showing a geographic pattern. Bronchoalveolar lavage findings may show an increase in neutrophils, and particularly in eosinophils, in patients with DIP, whereas the predominance of pigmented smoker's alveolar macrophages is a characteristic finding of both RBILD and DIP. The contrasting clinical features of idiopathic interstitial pneumonias are summarized in Table 50-2.

DIAGNOSIS

The diagnostic process in a patient suspected of having an idiopathic interstitial pneumonia is dynamic (Figure 50-4). The first question is whether the disease is idiopathic or associated with known causes of interstitial fibrosis, or whether it represents another form of interstitial lung disease of unknown cause such as Langerhans cell histiocytosis, eosinophilic pneumonia, and others. The next question is whether the disease is IPF or one of the other interstitial pneumonias.

The clinical diagnosis of IPF depends primarily on the identification of symptoms and signs of breathlessness, basal crackles, finger clubbing often seen on examination; the characteristic radiographic appearances; and the demonstration of restrictive lung function. The clinical history must, however, also explore and exclude other possible causes of interstitial fibrosis, such as the occupational exposure or exposure to drugs, allergens, and other substances outlined in Chapter 49. It is, therefore, especially important to establish details of occupations in which the patient has worked, as well as to illicit a history of recreational activities, to establish whether the patient has been exposed to birds, moldy hay, or other known causes of extrinsic allergic alveolitis. It is also important to obtain a drug history to identify potentially relevant current or previous drug exposures. The examiner should also seek evidence of skin rashes, arthritis, or arthralgia as markers of connective tissue disease, and general markers of other contributors to breathlessness such as chronic obstructive pulmonary disease, respiratory infections, cardiac disease, primary or metastatic lung cancer, pulmonary embolus or hemorrhage, sarcoid, and so on. A full smoking history is also important, because smoking is a risk factor for IPF and because lung function test data in these patients may show a mixed obstructive and restrictive defect.

HRCT has a central role in the evaluation of a patient with idiopathic interstitial pneumonia (see Figure 50-4). If on the basis of the history, physical examination, chest radiograph, and lung function tests, a patient possibly has idiopathic interstitial pneumonia, the next and obligatory step is to perform HRCT. This may also provide clues to the presence of non-idiopathic interstitial pneumonias such as sarcoidosis, extrinsic allergic alveolitis, lymphangioleiomyomatosis, Langerhans cell histiocytosis, and alveolar proteinosis. In a patient with a confident CT diagnosis of IPF with consistent clinical features (see the major and minor ATS/ERS criteria), a surgical lung biopsy is not necessary. A transbronchial biopsy and/or BAL may be helpful in identifying alternate diagnoses, but the limited size of a transbronchial biopsy does not usually yield a sufficiently substantial sample to make a confident diagnosis of UIP or any other idiopathic interstitial pneumonia.

In summary, the diagnosis of IPF requires combined clinical, radiologic, and pathologic effort. A surgical biopsy can no longer be considered the "gold standard" in making the diagnosis of IPF. The histopathologic pattern of UIP (Table 50-4) is not specific for IPF and may also be associated with collagen vascular disease, drug toxicity, chronic hypersensitivity pneumonitis, and asbestosis. Along the same lines, the NSIP pattern can be associated with no detectable cause (idiopathic NSIP) or may be seen in collagen vascular disease, hypersensitivity pneumonitis, drug-induced pneumonitis, infections, and immunodeficiency, including HIV infection. The same is true for the organizing pneumonia pattern (see Chapter 53) and the diffuse alveolar damage pattern in acute interstitial pneumonia, which is also associated with infection, collagen vascular disease, drug toxicity, and inhalation of toxic substances. Given the importance of a confident diagnosis in determining possible treatment and defining the prognosis, a clear diagnosis should be obtained early in the course of illness or before commencement of therapy.

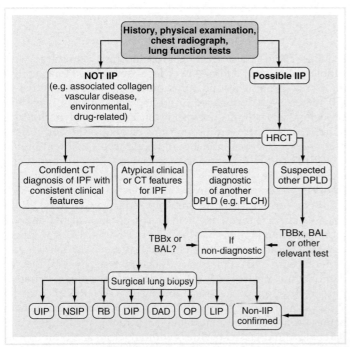

FIGURE 50-4 Suggested diagnostic algorithm for the evaluation of patients with diffuse parenchymal lung disease (DPLD). The importance of the HRCT is highlighted. *BAL*, Bronchoalveolar lavage; *DAD*, diffuse alveolar damage; *DIP*, desquamative interstitial pneumonia; *IIP*, idiopathic interstitial pneumonia; *LIP*, lymphocytic interstitial pneumonia; *NSIP*, nonspecific interstitial pneumonia; *OP*, organizing pneumonia; *PLCH*, pulmonary Langerhans cell histiocytosis; *RB*, respiratory bronchiolitis; *TBBx*, transbronchial biopsy; *UIP*, usual interstitial pneumonia. (Adapted with permission from Travis WD, King TE, Bateman ED, et al: ATS/ERS international multidisciplinary consensus classification of idiopathic interstitial pneumonias. General principles and recommendations. *Am J Respir Crit Care Med* 2002; 165:277–304.)

TREATMENT

There is no established optimal treatment for IPF. The usual treatment strategy is antiinflammatory, and this is unsuccessful in preventing the progression of IPF in most patients. Better therapy is urgently needed, and new strategies are targeted at developing truly antifibrotic drugs.

Despite the widespread use of corticosteroids to treat IPF, no definitive evidence shows that these drugs improve either survival or quality of life. The available evidence on corticosteroid effects is based entirely on observational or retrospective comparative studies, none of which has involved a randomized, placebo-controlled, double-blind design. In addition, many of these included patients with other idiopathic interstitial pneumonias. Corticosteroid therapy is associated with significant morbidity, with adverse effects reported in a quarter of those treated. Typical corticosteroid doses are 40–60 mg of prednisone per day, for at least a month, tapering down

TABLE 50-4   Key Differences among the Histopathologic Features of Usual Interstitial Pneumonia, Nonspecific Interstitial Pneumonia, and Desquamative Interstitial Pneumonia

Usual Interstitial Pneumonia	Nonspecific Interstitial Pneumonia	Desquamative Interstitial Pneumonia
Dense fibrosis and honeycombing	Preserved architecture, variable fibrosis, and cellularity	Intraalveolar macrophage accumulation
Fibroblastic foci prominent	Few fibroblastic foci	No fibroblastic foci
Patchy, heterogeneous pattern	Temporally homogenous	Uniform involvement
Subpleural, paraseptal distribution	Inconsistent distribution	Diffuse distribution

within 3 months to approximately 10 mg/day. Prophylaxis against corticosteroid-induced osteoporosis with calcium and vitamin D_3 should be started early.

The suggestion to use prednisone in combination with azathioprine or cyclophosphamide is based on small randomized controlled trials that likely included patients with other idiopathic interstitial pneumonias. Improved survival relative to prednisone therapy, albeit to borderline level of statistical significance, has been reported for treatment with a combination of azathioprine and modest doses of corticosteroids. A similar study in a small number of patients found no significant benefit from the addition of cyclophosphamide to prednisone. Evidence of benefit from colchicine, penicillamine, or cyclosporin is limited to small uncontrolled trials.

The ATS/ERS Consensus Statement recommends that treatment offered to a patient with IPF be combined therapy, including corticosteroids and either azathioprine or cyclophosphamide (Box 50-1). If therapy is offered to a patient, it should be started early, at the first identification of clinical or physiologic evidence of impairment or documentation of decline in lung function. Treatment should be limited to those patients who have been given adequate information regarding the advantages and risks of treatment. The combined therapy should be continued for at least 6 months, and close monitoring every 3–6 months is recommended. If the patient's condition is found to be improved or stable, which occurs transiently in 10–30% of patients, and this can be regarded as a beneficial effect of treatment, the combined therapy should be continued with the same doses of medication. In patients in whom the disease progresses, treatment can be modified by switching to a different cytotoxic agent, or an alternative therapy or lung transplantation may be considered.

As disease progresses, patients with IPF can derive some benefit from more general approaches to the management of dyspnea and respiratory failure, such as supplemental oxygen, help with mobility outside and inside the home, opiates for respiratory distress, and other general social and nursing support.

Lung transplantation is also an option for some patients and provides improved quality of life and survival for those who have advanced disease but is of limited availability and often contraindicated in patients of older age and significant associated comorbidities. Because patients with IPF have the highest mortality on the waiting list, early referral for lung transplantation is important. Patients without contraindications should be listed for lung transplantation when they have significant functional impairment defined as a DLco <39% predicted or rapid disease progression with decline in FVC of 10% during 6 months of follow-up.

N-acetylcysteine (NAC) at a high dose of 600 mg tid significantly decreased disease progression in terms of loss of lung

BOX 50-1   American Thoracic Society and European Respiratory Society Recommendations for Treatment of Idiopathic Pulmonary Fibrosis

Corticosteroid (prednisone or equivalent)
0.5 mg/kg of body weight per day orally for 4 weeks
0.25 mg/kg/day for 8 weeks
Taper to 0.125 mg/kg/day or 0.25 mg/kg/day on
   alternate days
plus
Azathioprine
2–3 mg/kg/day
Maximum dose 150 mg daily
Begin dosing at 25–50 mg/day; increase in 25-mg increments
   every 1–2 weeks until the maximum dose is achieved
or
Cyclophosphamide
2 mg/kg/day
Maximum dose 150 mg daily
Begin dosing at 25–50 mg/day; increase in 25-mg increments
   every 1–2 weeks until the maximum dose is achieved

function after 1 year compared with placebo in a large randomized controlled trial involving 155 patients, all receiving the standard therapy of prednisone and azathioprine. On the basis of the outcome of this trial, which is the first in IPF that showed positive effects on the predefined primary end points, this drug can be recommended for all patients who do not wish or do not qualify to participate in a clinical trial.

Potential opportunities for therapeutic intervention in the future include the use of antifibrotic agents such as pirfenidone and bosentan, antiproliferative drugs such as rapamycin, and antagonists to cytokines such as TNFα, and to growth factors thought to be involved in the pathogenesis of pulmonary fibrosis. Multicenter clinical trials with such agents are underway; their results are currently awaited. Interferon-gamma is no longer an option in the treatment of IPF, a large randomized controlled trial involving more than 800 patients failed to meet primary and secondary end points

There are no prospective trials on treatment of the other idiopathic interstitial pneumonias. Therapy of fibrotic NSIP is suggested to be the same as of IPF. The suggested treatment of the other chronic idiopathic entities is prednisone with the addition of other immunosuppressants later if necessary. Acute interstitial pneumonia and acute exacerbation of IPF requires intravenous high-dose corticosteroids and/or cyclophosphamide. Patients with DIP and RBILD should also stop cigarette smoking.

CLINICAL COURSE AND PREVENTION

The clinical course of IPF is variable but in most cases involves a progressive deterioration to death from respiratory failure. Life expectancy as estimated from follow-up of populations of patients with IPF who attended specialist clinics has usually been approximately 5 years, but these figures can be substantially biased by the inclusion of other idiopathic interstitial pneumonias and by the tendency for longer-term survivors to be overrepresented in such populations. Typical survival in newly presenting cases of IPF is now probably closer to 3 years, which compared with individuals of similar age and sex, represents a reduction in normal life expectancy of approximately 7 years. Most of the excess mortality in these patients is directly or indirectly attributable to IPF, but there may also be an increased risk of death from cardiovascular conditions, infections, and lung cancer.

The histologic diagnosis of UIP is the most important factor determining survival in patients with suspected idiopathic interstitial pneumonia. All other histologic entities except AIP have a significantly better prognosis (Figure 50-5). The presence of honeycombing on HRCT is a good surrogate for UIP and could be useful in diagnosing patients unable to undergo surgical lung biopsy or in those in whom the recent ATS/ERS criteria for making a confident clinical diagnosis are fulfilled. Patients with NSIP are more likely to respond or remain stable on therapy with prednisone. Patients whose condition remains stable after prednisone therapy have the best prognosis.

Markers of a poor prognosis of IPF include a relatively low FVC, diffusing factor for carbon monoxide, or arterial oxygen level at presentation, desaturation to less than 88% in the 6-min walk test, male sex, older age, lack of lymphocytosis in BAL, and high counts of fibroblastic foci on biopsy. During follow-up investigations, a rapid decline in FVC or in DL_{CO} over 6 months indicates poor prognosis. Evidence of improvement after a trial of corticosteroid therapy is associated with a favorable prognosis and may, in turn, be more likely in those with a relatively cellular histologic pattern on lung biopsy or a predominantly ground-glass pattern on HRCT of the lung. Extensive ground-glass shadowing is, however, atypical for IPF and likely indicative of another diagnosis. Current cigarette smoking at the time of diagnosis has been associated with improved survival—a finding that remains unexplained.

Acute exacerbation of IPF has now been recognized as a disease-specific catastrophic event that may occur for no obvious reason at any point of time during the course of disease. The condition is characterized by a sudden increase in dyspnea over a month, worsening hypoxia, new infiltrates on chest radiograph or HRCT, and rapid development of respiratory failure, after exclusion of other conditions causing respiratory decompensation such as cardiac, thromboembolic, aspiration, or infectious processes. The frequency is approximately 10% in a 2-year period of follow-up. Histopathology shows diffuse alveolar damage superimposed on UIP. Acute exacerbations are treated by use of high-dose corticosteroids, such as methylprednisolone, 500 mg daily for 3 days, this strategy being based on case studies only. The mortality of an acute exacerbation of IPF is high; patients who survive may stabilize at a significantly lower level of lung function for a limited period of time.

Because the cause of IPF is not understood, prevention is not feasible. A number of potentially avoidable risk factors, such as occupational exposure to metal or wood dust and the use of common drugs, have now been identified, but none has yet been established with sufficient confidence to justify attempts at primary prevention. Secondary prevention is also not currently a practical option for IPF, although the implication of viral infections in the pathogenesis of IPF presents potential opportunities for future investigations.

PITFALLS AND CONTROVERSIES

The major pitfall in the management of patients with idiopathic interstitial pneumonias is to misdiagnose the disease as idiopathic when there is an association with drugs or with exposure to organic antigens causing extrinsic allergic alveolitis. The insidious form of bird fancier's lung may mimic IPF, and even biopsy or HRCT may show a UIP pattern in these patients. BAL may be helpful in this regard. A significant increase in lymphocytes <30% may direct the examiner to take a better recreational history of the patient that may reveal the relevant exposure. Similarly, drug exposure may cause any of the histopathologic patterns of the idiopathic interstitial pneumonia, and if there is any doubt, the suspected drug should be withdrawn.

Some confusion has emerged from the new classification of the idiopathic interstitial pneumonias, because clinicians have used the name of the histologic pattern for the clinical diagnosis. This is not correct. For example, the term for the final diagnosis should be IPF, and not UIP, which is just the histologic pattern and by some authors also used to describe the HRCT pattern. Neither the pathologist nor the radiologist can make the diagnosis of IPF without knowing about the history and the clinical findings of the patients. It is important to recognize the necessity of a multidisciplinary clinical/radiologic/pathologic approach in making the final diagnosis of an idiopathic interstitial pneumonia.

In regard to the classification, it has been debated whether RBILD should be included among the idiopathic interstitial pneumonias, because this entity is associated with cigarette

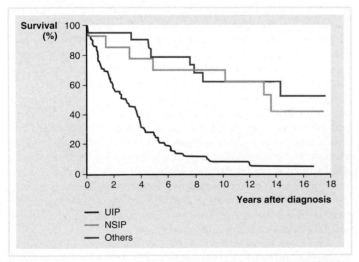

FIGURE 50-5 Survival in idiopathic interstitial pneumonias according to histopathologic subgroups. Patients with UIP had a significantly worse survival compared with the other subgroups. Median survival for UIP patients was 2.8 years. *NSIP*, Nonspecific interstitial pneumonia; *UIP*, usual interstitial pneumonia. (Adapted with permission from Bjoraker JA, Ryu JH, Edwin MK, et al: Prognostic significance of histopathologic subsets in idiopathic pulmonary fibrosis. Am J Respir Crit Care Med 1998; 157:199–203.)

smoking in 100% of cases, so that there is a known cause that contradicts the term idiopathic. This is in contrast to DIP, which is not exclusively seen in smokers. Further controversies existed regarding whether NSIP and DIP reflect early stages of IPF. Now most researchers believe that these three histologic patterns also reflect three different entities.

Another controversial issue is whether the histopathologic evaluation can still be considered as the "gold standard" for diagnosis. It seems increasingly difficult to justify a surgical biopsy when the clinical and HRCT features are typical of IPF. In this setting, biopsy would reveal the UIP pattern in almost 100% of cases. By contrast, the clinical/radiologic diagnosis of NSIP is less reliable; in most cases, the histology will still reveal the UIP pattern. Two problems are associated with surgical biopsy as the "gold standard." The first is the problem of sampling error: divergent histopathologic diagnoses in two or more biopsy sites. The second is the large interobserver variation between histopathologists, with a low to moderate kappa coefficient of agreement. At best, surgical biopsy can be considered as a "silver standard" today.

The final controversy is related to treatment: there are nihilists who do not believe in any effect of antiinflammatory therapy and do not treat their patients. Others, such as the author of this article, have seen individual patients who deteriorated after they needed to be withdrawn from their ongoing standard therapy with prednisone and azathioprine plus NAC before being randomly assigned into a clinical trial. After reinstitution of the antiinflammatory therapy, the patients improved again. These single-case observations strongly suggest that there is some effect of the antiinflammatory regimen in individual patients, at least transiently. There seem to exist transcontinental differences, the North American colleagues are more reluctant to use prednisone today, whereas the standard therapy plus NAC is more frequently applied in Europe.

SUGGESTED READINGS

Demedts M, Behr J, Buhl R, et al: High-dose acetylcysteine in idiopathic pulmonary fibrosis. N Engl J Med 2005; 353:2229–2242.

Flaherty KR, Andrei AC, Murray S, et al: Idiopathic pulmonary fibrosis. Prognostic value of changes in physiology and six-minute-walk test. Am J Respir Crit Care Med 2006; 174:803–809.

Flaherty KR, Toews GB, Travis WD, et al: Clinical significance of histological classification of idiopathic interstitial pneumonia. Eur Respir J 2002; 19:275–283.

Hunninghake GW, Zimmermann MB, Schwartz DA, et al: Utility of a lung biopsy for the diagnosis of idiopathic pulmonary fibrosis. Am J Respir Crit Care Med 2001; 164:193–196.

King TE, Costabel U, Cordier JF, et al: ATS/ERS International Consensus Statement. Idiopathic pulmonary fibrosis: diagnosis and treatment. Am J Respir Crit Care Med 2000; 161:646–664.

Latsi PI, du Bois RM, Nicholson AG, et al: Fibrotic idiopathic interstitial pneumonia. The prognostic value of longitudinal functional trends. Am J Respir Crit Care Med 2003; 168:531–537.

Nicholson AG, Fulford LG, Colby TV, et al: The relationship between individual histologic features and disease progression in idiopathic pulmonary fibrosis. Am J Respir Crit Care Med 2002; 166:173–177.

Raghu G, Weycker D, Edelsberg J, et al: Incidence and prevalence of idiopathic pulmonary fibrosis. Am J Respir Crit Care Med 2006; 174:810–816.

Selman M, King TE Jr, Pardo A: Idiopathic pulmonary fibrosis: prevailing and evolving hypotheses about its pathogenesis and implication for therapy. Ann Intern Med 2001; 134:136–151.

Travis WD, King TE, Bateman ED, et al: ATS/ERS international multidisciplinary consensus classification of idiopathic interstitial pneumonias. General principles and recommendations. Am J Respir Crit Care Med 2002; 165:277–304.

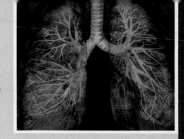

51 Sarcoidosis

LORI SHAH • ALVIN S. TEIRSTEIN • MICHAEL C. IANNUZZI

In the 130 years since Jonathan Hutchinson first described sarcoidosis as a skin disorder, involvement of every organ has been reported. The central abnormality in sarcoidosis is granuloma accumulation, leading to altered organ architecture and function. Although the inciting events in sarcoidosis remain unknown, in general, granulomas form to confine pathogens, restrict inflammation, and protect surrounding tissue. Clinical, epidemiologic, and family-based studies support the hypothesis that sarcoidosis is triggered by airborne exposure in a genetically susceptible individual. The diagnosis is established when compatible clinical and radiologic findings are supported by evidence of noncaseating epithelioid cell granulomas in one or more organs in the absence of organisms or particles. Clinically, sarcoidosis is characterized by frequent remissions and occasional exacerbations causing diverse pulmonary and extrapulmonary symptoms. Few randomized controlled treatment trials in sarcoidosis exist. Corticosteroids remain the therapeutic cornerstone for those with organ-threatening or chronic progressive disease.

EPIDEMIOLOGY

Sarcoidosis occurs worldwide and may affect any individual at any age, although more than 80% of patients are diagnosed between ages 20 and 50 years. In the United States, African Americans are three and a half times more commonly affected, with an age-adjusted incidence of 35.5/100,000 persons compared with 10.9/100,000 in whites. African American women are most commonly affected with a lifetime risk of approximately 2.7%. African Americans also more often have chronic disease and more organs involved. The incidence in most European nations has been reported at less than 1/100,000. In Scandinavian countries such as Sweden and Finland, incidence ranges from 11–64/100,000. In Japan, <10/100,000 new sarcoidosis cases occur annually. The Japanese, however, have a particular susceptibility to cardiac involvement.

ETIOLOGY AND RISK FACTORS

No single environmental sarcoidosis trigger has been identified. Recently, the multicenter A Case Control Etiologic Sarcoidosis Study (ACCESS) found modest (odds ratio ~ 1.5) increased risk with exposure to pesticides, moldy environments, working with building materials, hardware, or industrial organic dusts. Sarcoidosis was not associated with exposure to rural residence, wood dusts, or heavy metals.

Several microorganisms and viruses have been suggested as potential sarcoid antigens and include *Mycobacteria*, *Borrelia burgdorferi*, *Chlamydia pneumoniae*, *Rickettsia helvetica*, *Rhodococcus equi*, *Nocardia*, *Propionibacterium*, fungi, spirochetes, *Tropheryma whippelii*, *Corynebacterium*, and human herpesvirus-8. None have been consistently supported in well-controlled studies. A possible explanation for the difficulty in identifying an infectious cause for sarcoidosis is that an insoluble bacterial protein serves as antigen long after the infecting organism has been cleared.

Socioeconomic status does not affect risk, but low income and other financial barriers to care are associated with sarcoidosis severity at presentation.

GENETIC FACTORS

Racial differences in incidence rates and disease clustering in families support the hypothesis that heredity contributes to sarcoidosis etiology. Sibs of patients with sarcoidosis have approximately a fivefold increased risk than the general population. Several human leukocyte antigen (HLA) associations with sarcoidosis have been reported (Table 51-1), but HLA seems more likely to influence phenotype than susceptibility. The major histocompatibility complex (MHC) class I allele HLA-B8 is associated with acute sarcoidosis. HLA-DQB1*0201 and HLA-DRB1*0301 are strongly associated with acute disease and good prognosis.

Investigators have studied non-HLA candidate genes that influence antigen processing, antigen presentation, macrophage and T-cell activation, and cell recruitment. Table 51-2 lists non-HLA candidate genes studied to date. Although these candidates are logical on the basis of function, their associations with sarcoidosis have not been consistently reproduced.

To date, two genome scans for sarcoidosis have been reported: one in German Caucasians, with the strongest linkage signals at chromosomes 3p and 6p, and the other in African Americans with signals at chromosomes 5p and 5q. So far, one candidate gene from the linked regions, butyrophilin-like 2 (BTNL2) gene on chromosome 6p, has been confirmed to be associated with sarcoidosis. Butyrophilin was initially cloned from cattle mammary epithelial cells and is a B7 family member, which functions as a negative costimulatory molecule.

PATHOPHYSIOLOGY

Despite advances in understanding the immunologic and molecular mechanisms leading to granuloma formation, how environmental exposure, immune response, or genetics interact to cause sarcoidosis remains to be defined. The events leading to granuloma formation likely begin with antigen presented to T lymphocytes by way of MHC class II peptide (Figure 51-1). The T-cell CD4/CD8 ratio in bronchoalveolar fluid obtained from patients with sarcoid is as high as 10:1 compared with the 2:1 ratio found in healthy individuals, indicating a predominate

TABLE 51-1 **Summary of HLA Association Studies of Sarcoidosis**

HLA	Risk Alleles	Finding
HLA-A	A*1	Susceptibility
HLA-B	B*8	Susceptibility in several populations
HLA-DPB1	*0201	Not associated with sarcoidosis
HLA-DQB1	*0201	Protection, Löfgren's syndrome, mild disease in several populations
	*0602	Susceptibility/disease progression in several groups
HLA-DRB1	*0301	Acute onset/good prognosis in several groups
	*04	Protection in several populations
	*1101	Susceptibility in whites and African Americans
		Stage II/III chest X-ray
HLA-DRB3	*1501	Associated with Löfgren's syndrome
	*0101	Susceptibility/disease progression in whites

CD4 response. The T-cell repertoire in sarcoidosis (α/β and δ/γ receptors) is oligoclonal, suggesting that the triggering antigens favor progressive accumulation and activation of selective T-cell clones. Early on, macrophage activation occurs and CD4 lymphocyte release Th1-predominant cytokines such as interferon-γ, interleukin-2, interleukin-12, interleukin-15, and tumor necrosis factor-α (TNF-α). Macrophages, in the face of chronic cytokine stimulation, differentiate into epithelioid cells, gain secretory and bactericidal capability, lose some phagocytic capacity, and fuse to form multinucleated giant cells. In more mature granulomas, fibroblasts and collagen encase the ball-like cell cluster. As granulomas accumulate, alteration in organ architecture and function occurs. One clinical curiosity is that granulomas can still form in instances with marked T-cell suppression such as sarcoidosis patients receiving cyclosporine after transplantation and in patients with AIDS.

Granulomas can resolve with little consequence or progress to fibrosis. Acute granulomatous and chronic fibrotic sarcoidosis likely represent different immunopathogenic processes, which remain to be defined (Figure 51-2). A switch from Th1 to Th2 cytokine profile along with other mediators, such as interleukin-6, transforming growth factor-β, osteopontin,

TABLE 51-2 **Non-HLA Candidate Genes Evaluated in Sarcoidosis**

Candidate Gene	
Angiotensin converting enzyme (ACE)	Increased risk for ID and DD genotypes. Moderate association between II genotype and radiographic progression.
C-C Chemokine receptor 2	Associated with protection/Löfgren's syndrome
Chemokine receptor 5	CCR5Δ32 allele more common in patients treated with corticosteroid. Refuted with haplotype analysis and larger sample.
CD80, CD86	No association detected
Clara cell 10-KD protein	An allele associated with sarcoidosis and with progressive disease at 3 years follow-up.
Complement receptor 1	Association with the GG genotype for the Pro1827Arg (C[5507]G) polymorphism
Cystic fibrosis transmembrane regulator (CFTR)	R75Q increases risk
Cytotoxic T-lymphocyte antigen 4 (CTLA-4)	No association with sarcoidosis
Heat shock protein 70 like	HSP(+2437)CC associated with susceptibility/Löfgren's syndrome
Inhibitor κBα	Associated with -297T allele. Allele -827T in stage II.
IL1α	The IL-1 α-889 1.1 genotype increased risk.
IL-4 receptor	No association detected
IL-18	Genotype -607CA increased risk over AA
Interferon gamma	IFNA17 polymorphism (551T→G) and IFNA10 [60A]- IFNA17 [551G] haplotype increase risk
Macrophage migration inhibitory factor	No association with 5-CATT in Irish population
Natural resistance associated macrophage protein (NRAMP)	Protective effect of (CA)(n) repeat in the immediate 5' region of the NRAMP1 gene
Toll-like receptor 4	Asp299Gly and Thre399Ile mutations associated with chronic disease
Transforming growth factor (TGF)	TGF β2 59941 allele, TGFβ3 4875 A and 17369 C alleles were associated with fibrosis on chest X-ray
Tumor necrosis factor-α	Genotype -307A allele associated with erythema nodosum/Löfgren's syndrome and -857T allele with sarcoidosis. -307A not associated in African Americans
Vascular endothelial growth factor	+813 CT and TT genotypes associated with protection
Vitamin D receptor (VDR)	*Bsm*I allele associated with sarcoidosis

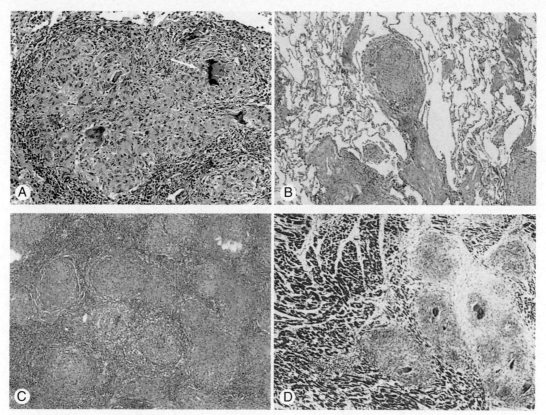

FIGURE 51-1 Noncaseating granulomatous inflammation in sarcoidosis. **A,** Closeup of epithelioid granuloma with giant cells and mononuclear cell infiltration. **B,** Open lung biopsy showing granulomas, giant cells, and lymphocytic infiltrates in lung parenchyma and within interlobular septal and subpleural regions. **C,** Lymph node biopsy showing extensive replacement with typical sarcoid-type epithelioid granulomas. Fibrinoid necrosis, but not overt caseation, may be seen in the center of granulomas. **D,** Myocardial biopsy showing patchy granulomatous inflammation with giant cells.

and insulin growth factors (IGF) is suggested to result in fibrosis. In summary, one could say that the affected organs in sarcoidosis are the staging ground for a "hereditary frustrated phagocytosis."

CLINICAL FEATURES

The clinical presentation of sarcoidosis varies. Up to two thirds of patients are asymptomatic and have sarcoidosis diagnosed incidentally on the basis of radiographic findings of hilar lymphadenopathy. In ACCESS, just more than half the patients were initially seen with pulmonary symptoms. Skin manifestations were present in 24%, and constitutional symptoms were present in 12% of patients. The presence of pulmonary symptoms actually resulted in a delay in diagnosis, possibly because of considering alternative diagnoses such as asthma or bronchitis that also present with cough and dyspnea.

Two well-recognized acute, febrile presentations of sarcoidosis are Löfgren's syndrome (arthritis, erythema nodosum, and bilateral hilar adenopathy) and Heerfordt's syndrome (uveitis, parotid gland enlargement, and facial nerve palsy). Both syndromes are uncommon in African Americans. These acute presentations portend a good prognosis with disease resolution within 1–2 years.

Pulmonary

More than 90% of patients with sarcoidosis have pulmonary involvement. Common complaints include dry cough, vague

chest discomfort, and dyspnea, particularly with exertion. Pleuritic chest pain is uncommon. Wheezing may occur with endobronchial involvement or hyperreactive airways. Sputum production and hemoptysis occur in advanced fibrocystic disease.

Chest auscultation may reveal fine, late, or mid-expiratory crackles, but comparatively less than what may be heard in pulmonary fibrosis. In view of the marked chest radiographic abnormalities, physical examination of the lungs is surprisingly unrevealing. Clubbing is rare, but when present, is usually associated with advanced bronchiectasis or liver disease.

Pulmonary Hypertension

The prevalence of pulmonary arterial hypertension and right ventricular dysfunction ranges from 4–28%. In most cases, sarcoidosis-related pulmonary arterial hypertension is mild to moderate or is manifest only with exercise. Severe pulmonary hypertension and right heart failure usually occur in association with severe fibrotic parenchymal disease. Right ventricular failure has been reported in up to 30% of sarcoidosis-related deaths. Interestingly, only approximately one fifth of patients with sarcoidosis with pulmonary arterial hypertension have signs and symptoms such as elevated jugular venous pressure, S3 or S4 right heart sound, hepatojugular reflux, lower extremity edema, and/or right ventricular heave. Approximately 60% of patients with pulmonary arterial hypertension demonstrate stage IV chest X-ray pattern, characterized by honeycombing, hilar retraction, bulla, cysts,

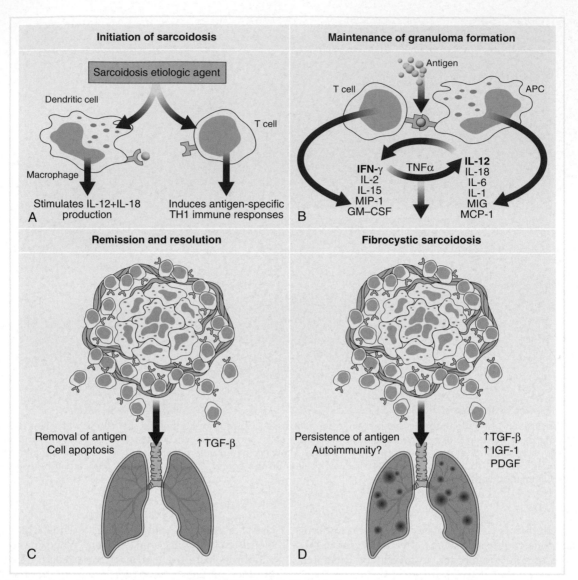

FIGURE 51-2 Model of the immunopathogenesis of sarcoidosis. **A,** Initiation of sarcoidosis involves stimulation of IL-1218 production from mononuclear phagocytes and dendritic cells and adaptive T-cell immunity to an inciting agent. **B,** Maintenance of granuloma formation by a TH1 immune response driven by IFN-γ and IL-1218. **C,** Resolution of sarcoidosis after removal of stimulating antigen, suppression of T-cell responses by TGF-β and other mediators, and granuloma resorption by cell apoptosis. **D,** Fibrotic outcome from persistent, possibly autoimmune, antigenic stimulation in the presence of TGF-β and other profibrotic mediators.

and/or emphysema. These findings highlight the need to suspect pulmonary arterial hypertension in patients with suggestive clinical, radiographic, and pulmonary function testing abnormalities.

Chest Radiology

Chest radiographs are classified into four patterns (Figure 51-3). Unfortunately, these radiographic patterns have been termed stages, leading to the erroneous assumption that they represent "disease stages" rather than "chest X-ray patterns." Patients with radiographic pattern I may have had disease for many years, and patients with radiographic pattern III may have acute disease. Only radiographic pattern IV (broad fibrotic bands, bulla, hilar retraction, bronchiectasis, and

diaphragmatic tenting) has temporal significance, indicating chronic disease.

Stage 0: Absence of radiographic abnormalities
Stage I: Bilateral hilar and/or mediastinal adenopathy without pulmonary parenchymal abnormalities
Stage II: Hilar and/or mediastinal lymphadenopathy with pulmonary parenchymal abnormalities (generally a diffuse interstitial pattern)
Stage III: Diffuse parenchymal disease without nodal enlargement
Stage IV: Pulmonary fibrosis with evidence of volume loss, cystic or honeycomb changes

Intrathoracic lymphadenopathy and parenchymal infiltrates (stage II chest X-ray) are the most commonly encountered

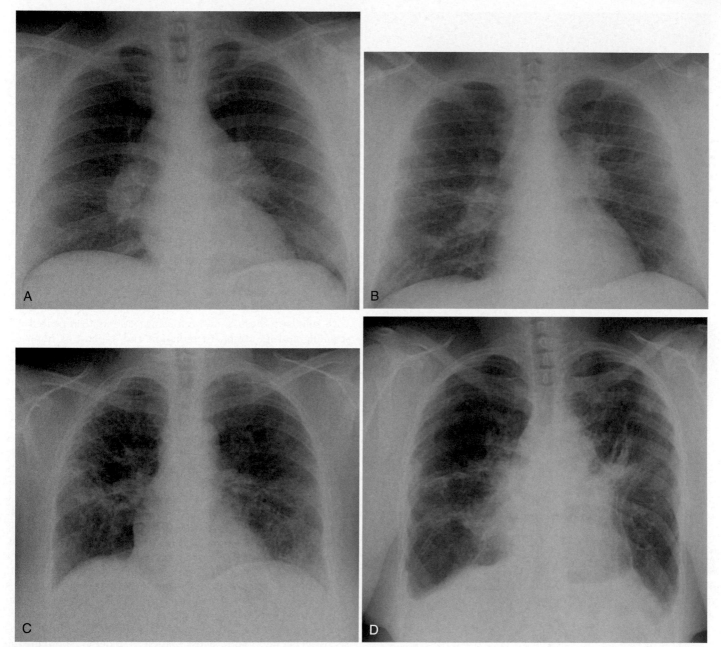

FIGURE 51-3 Chest radiography stages of sarcoidosis. **A,** Stage I sarcoidosis CXR with bilateral hilar lymphadenopathy. **B,** Stage II CXR with bilateral lymphadenopathy and reticulonodular infiltrates. **C,** Stage III CXR with bilateral infiltrates without adenopathy. **D,** Stage IV CXR with upward hilar retraction, large cystic and bullous changes, and fibrocystic disease.

radiographic finding, occurring in 85% of patients. The pulmonary parenchymal changes have a strong predilection toward the upper lung fields, unlike those noted in other diffuse parenchymal diseases such as pulmonary fibrosis, which are basilar predominant. In addition, lung inflation on chest radiograph tends to be preserved compared with other causes of pulmonary fibrosis, where small lung volumes are most often seen.

Chest computed tomography (CT) scans demonstrate enlarged lymph nodes and pulmonary infiltrates with more sensitivity than plain chest radiographs. Chest CT often reveals infiltrates in a patient with a "Stage I" chest-X-ray or lymph node enlargement in a patient with "Stage III" chest X-rays. High-resolution CT scan typically demonstrates symmetric

mediastinal or hilar lymphadenopathy, parenchymal changes with upper lobe predominance, or multiple small nodules in a perivascular distribution, along with thickened bronchovascular bundles and interlobular septa. More unusual patterns of lung infiltrates may occur in some patients. Larger, more well-defined nodular infiltrates may mimic malignancy (Figure 51-4). Chest CT may also reveal bronchiectasis (Figure 51-5). In patients with fibrocystic lung disease (Figure 51-6), mycetomas may occur. Remarkable discrepancy between radiographic findings, pulmonary function testing abnormalities, and severity of symptoms often exist.

Although chest CT scans yield a detailed anatomic map, CT scans do not often aid in diagnosis or therapy when compared

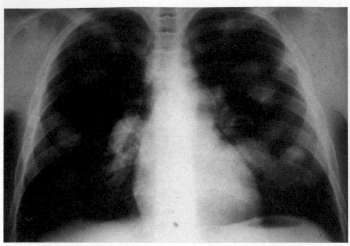
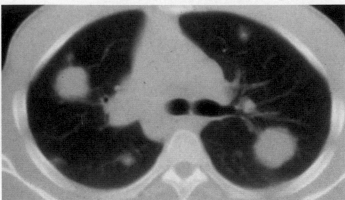

FIGURE 51-4 Nodular sarcoidosis with multiple bilateral pulmonary nodules.

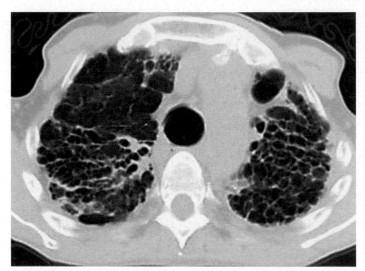

FIGURE 51-5 Fibrotic bronchiectasis: Upper lobes with multiple small cystic areas called honeycombing.

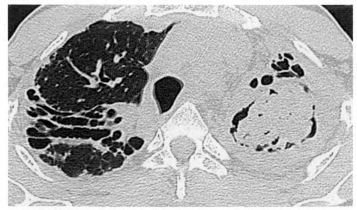

FIGURE 51-6 Fibrotic honeycombed upper lobes with left upper lobe aspergilloma filling a large bullae.

with standard chest X-ray. Exposing patients to repeated CT scanning and its attendant radiation and expense is unnecessary. CT scans are indicated in the following scenarios: (1) hemoptysis, (2) a radiographic pattern or new finding that does not suggest sarcoidosis, (3) evaluation for transplant candidacy, (4) search for a mycetoma.

Pulmonary Function Testing

Pulmonary function testing offers a more accurate evaluation of the impact of pulmonary sarcoidosis than chest radiographic patterns. The two most common abnormalities are reductions in lung volume and vital capacity representing a restrictive ventilatory defect, with a reduction in diffusing capacity (DL_{CO}). A decreased DL_{CO} is generally the first abnormal test detected and the last to return to normal in those individuals whose disease resolves. Obstructive ventilatory defects may also be seen in up to 30% of nonsmokers with sarcoidosis and are believed to represent endobronchial involvement. In addition, obstructive defects are increasingly seen with fibrosis and bullous transformation. Tests for bronchial hyperreactivity are positive in up to 30% of patients.

The prognosis in patients with isolated pulmonary sarcoidosis is generally good. Most patients undergo spontaneous remission or disease stabilization within 2–5 years after diagnosis. Patients with stage I chest radiographs have a >80% rate of radiographic resolution compared with patients with stage II (60%) or stage III (30%). A small number of patients may progress to end-stage lung disease. For those patients with progressive decline in pulmonary function, assessment for oxygen desaturation with exertion should be performed with consideration for oxygen therapy. It should be emphasized that it has been estimated that most patients lead asymptomatic lives without ever discovering they are affected by sarcoidosis.

Extrapulmonary Sarcoid

Sarcoidosis may affect any organ system. The most commonly involved organs include the skin (30%), eyes (25%), lymph nodes, liver, and spleen (20%). Abnormalities in calcium metabolism (hypercalciuria followed by hypercalcemia) are detected in approximately 15% of patients. Clinically apparent cardiac and nervous system involvement has been said to occur in approximately 5% of patients, but MRI and PET scans demonstrate these organs are more commonly involved. In general, patients who are initially seen with extrapulmonary disease have a worsened prognosis.

Skin

Cutaneous involvement, one of the most common manifestations of extrapulmonary sarcoidosis, is quite varied and includes erythema nodosum, plaques, nodules, papules, macules, vitiligo, ulcerations, psoriasis-like, and acneiform lesions. Lesions may be single or occur in crops, arise in scars and tattoos, and commonly involve the trunk, scalp, nape of the neck, and extremities (Figure 51-7). Skin lesions in African American patients frequently leave scars, pits, and pale depigmented areas.

Erythema nodosum occurs in approximately 10% of patients and usually manifests as tender, subcutaneous nodules, often on the anterior tibial surface (Figure 51-8). The onset of erythema nodosum is usually sudden and accompanied by constitutional symptoms such as fever, malaise, and polyarthralgias. Erythema nodosum usually lasts 3 weeks and can recur. Biopsy of erythema nodosum will show nonspecific septal panniculitis and does not histologically support the diagnosis of sarcoidosis. Biopsy of skin lesions other than erythema nodosum usually yields granulomas.

Lupus pernio (Figure 51-9) presents as a violaceous, indurated lesion affecting the mid-face, particularly the nose, nasal alae, malar and periorbital areas, and areas around the eyes. Lupus pernio can erode into underlying cartilage and bone and be extremely disfiguring. It is more common in women and is associated with chronic disease.

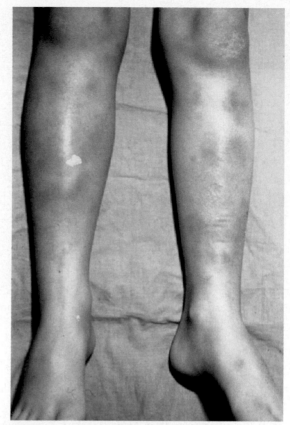

FIGURE 51-8 Erythema nodosum of the anterior tibia. Raised tender nodules on anterior tibial surface.

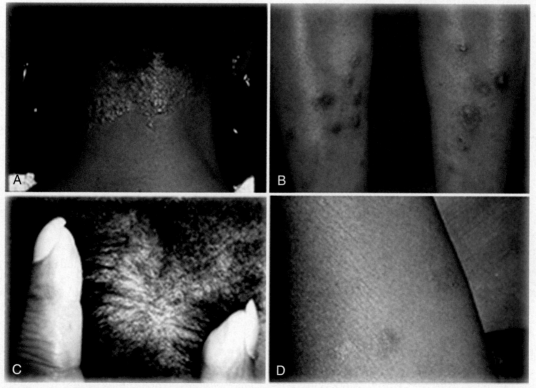

FIGURE 51-7 Skin lesions. **A,** Cluster of waxy papules on nape of the neck. **B,** Raised darkened granulomatous nodules. **C,** Dark, crusting scalp nodules. **D,** Red, nontender nodules.

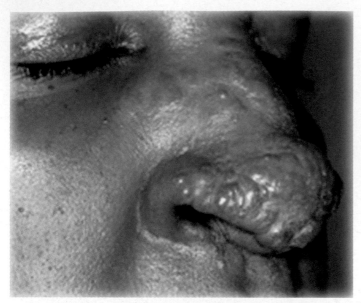

FIGURE 51-9 Lupus pernio. Raised, bulbous, nodular, crusting, disfiguring nasal granulomas.

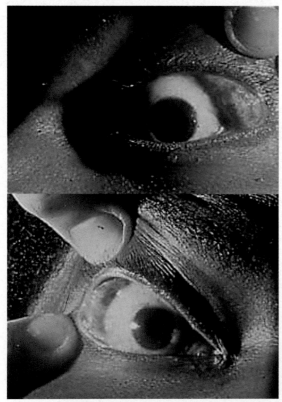

FIGURE 51-10 Enlarged, nodular lacrimal glands.

Lacrimal gland involvement is common and usually asymptomatic (Figure 51-10). All of the uveal tract (iris, ciliary body, choroid) may be involved. Anterior (iritis, iridocyclitis) is more common than posterior uveitis (choroiditis). Acute anterior uveitis presents with photophobia, eye pain, and blurry vision. Chronic anterior uveitis is much more insidious and

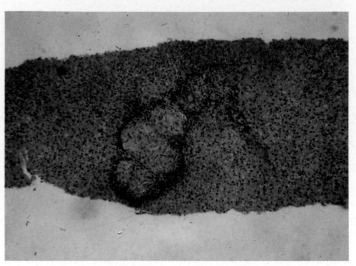

FIGURE 51-11 Liver granuloma.

may silently result in vision loss and glaucoma. Chronic anterior uveitis is more common than acute. Approximately 15% of patients with ocular involvement have both anterior and posterior uveitis. Routine dilated funduscopic examination and slit-lamp examination by an ophthalmologist is recommended.

Liver and Spleen

Between 51% and 80% of patients with sarcoidosis will have granulomas present on liver biopsy (Figure 51-11). Liver involvement in African Americans is at least twice as common as in Caucasians. The liver is palpable in 15% of patients. Sarcoid liver disease includes asymptomatic liver enzyme elevation, chronic cholestasis, portal hypertension with variceal bleeding, hepatopulmonary syndrome with refractory hypoxemia, and cirrhosis with liver failure. Granulomatous hepatitis in sarcoidosis often results in marked constitutional symptoms such as fever, night sweats, anorexia, and weight loss. If liver function testing is abnormal, a viral hepatitis screen and anti-mitochondrial antibodies to rule out viral hepatitis and primary biliary cirrhosis should be obtained. The serum alkaline phosphatase and γ-glutamyl transferase are elevated proportionally higher than aspartate aminotransferase, alanine aminotransferase, and bilirubin.

Palpable splenomegaly occurs in 6% of patients. Abdominal ultrasound and CT scan may reveal a characteristic hypodense nodular pattern.

Lymphatics

Although intrathoracic lymph node enlargement is the most common lymphatic manifestation, all lymph node–bearing sites may be involved. Peripheral lymph nodes may be small or grow to several centimeters and are usually mobile and nontender.

Heart

Cardiac sarcoidosis seems to be more common in Japan, with one autopsy series demonstrating cardiac sarcoidosis in almost 50% of cases. In the United States, clinically apparent cardiac involvement occurs in approximately 5–10% of sarcoidosis patients; however, newer imaging techniques such as MRI and PET scanning suggest that cardiac inflammation may be more common in North Americans than previously appreciated.

The left ventricular free wall is most commonly involved followed by the basal septum. Conduction abnormalities ranging from first-degree atrioventricular (AV) block to complete heart block are common cardiac abnormalities. Complete heart block occurs in 30% of affected patients, often heralded by syncope. The most feared extrapulmonary complication is sudden death because of ventricular fibrillation or tachycardia. Because this complication may occur in any patient with sarcoidosis, complaints of dizziness, palpitations, or abnormalities on ECG such as first-degree AV block should trigger additional studies. Other less common cardiac manifestations include mitral regurgitation, ventricular aneurysms, pericarditis, pericardial effusions, and tamponade.

Every patient should have a routine electrocardiogram on initial assessment. Further cardiac evaluation may include an echocardiogram, right and/or left cardiac catheterization, electrophysiologic study, and cardiac MRI or PET scan to identify myocardial irritability, left ventricular dysfunction, or pulmonary arterial hypertension. Oral corticosteroid therapy and the need for pacemaker/automatic implantable cardiac defibrillator placement should strongly be considered in patients with arrhythmias or markedly diminished left ventricular function.

Neuroophthalmologic

Neurosarcoidosis occurs in 5–15% of patients. The most common manifestation is cranial neuropathy, with unilateral or bilateral seventh nerve palsy seen in 50–70% of cases. Cranial neuropathies may resolve spontaneously or with corticosteroids and rarely recur. Optic neuritis, the second most common neuropathy, can result in blurred vision, field defects, and blindness. Central nervous system involvement also includes mass lesions, aseptic meningitis, obstructive hydrocephalus, and hypothalamic and/or pituitary dysfunction. Seizures, headache, change in mental status, confusion, and diabetes insipidus may be presenting symptoms.

Calcium Metabolism

Sarcoid granulomas result in increased conversion of 1-hydroxy-vitamin D_3 to the active, 1, 25- dihydroxyvitamin D_3. Hypercalcemia is present in 5% of patients, often presenting as kidney stones. Hypercalcuria is more common than hypercalcemia, and a 24-h urine collection for total calcium should be included in the initial evaluation. Occasionally, patients are initially seen with signs and symptoms of severe hypercalcemia. Typically, calcium abnormalities respond to relatively low doses of corticosteroids.

Other Organ Systems

Patients may complain of nasal and sinus congestion, hoarseness, and noisy breathing because of nasopharyngeal mucosa, sinus, and vocal cord granulomatous infiltration. Sarcoidosis of the upper respiratory tract is associated with chronic disease. Parotid and salivary gland enlargement occur in approximately 10% of patients. Bone and muscle involvement is often asymptomatic, but MRI with gadolinium often locates abnormalities in patients with persistent muscle, joint, or bone pain. Direct bone marrow involvement with cytopenia is not uncommon.

Quality of Life

Sarcoidosis may adversely affect the quality of life. One study revealed that 60% of patients reported symptoms of clinical depression. A patient's insurance status, income, and access to medical care were all highly correlative with depressive symptoms. Other studies indicate that quality of life worsens when patients are placed on corticosteroid therapy. Sarcoidosis impacts quality of life and is associated with stress, fatigue, pain, and sleep disturbances. This makes improved communication between physicians and patients with sarcoidosis essential.

DIAGNOSIS

Because sarcoidosis presents with nonspecific signs and symptoms, it may be difficult to diagnose. Differential diagnoses include infectious causes such as tuberculosis, fungal infections, and other specific infections like brucellosis, chlamydia, tularemia; and autoimmune disorders such as Wegener's granulomatosis, Churg–Strauss syndrome, and malignancies. Occupational and environmental-induced diseases such as chronic beryllium disease, hypersensitivity pneumonitis, and drug-induced lung disease should also be considered.

Chronic beryllium disease (CBD), an occupational hypersensitivity disorder, is elicited by beryllium exposure. Historically, workplace exposure has been seen in the defense, nuclear, aerospace, computer, and electronic industries. CBD is characterized by noncaseating granulomas within affected organs, predominantly lung and skin. Differentiating berylliosis from sarcoidosis can be extremely difficult and relies on a thorough occupational history and demonstrating beryllium sensitization with the beryllium lymphocyte proliferation test. Unsuspected CBD may be misdiagnosed as sarcoidosis, especially in patients with ongoing exposure and presumed corticosteroid resistance. CBD prognosis is worse than sarcoidosis, with an estimated 25% mortality. Progression to clinical disease seems to depend on length and exposure type. CBD resolution has been reported after termination of exposure. Thus, after establishing the diagnosis of CBD, beryllium avoidance is the first recommended therapeutic measure.

In suspected sarcoidosis, a diagnosis should be established with biopsy whenever possible. The key pathologic finding is the granuloma. Fiberoptic bronchoscopy (FOB) is an important tool for diagnosis. FOB can identify endobronchial lesions through direct airway visualization (Figure 51-12). The sensitivity of transbronchial lung biopsy, with 4–6 pieces collected, ranges from 40–90%, and is operator dependent. Additional endobronchial biopsies, transbronchial needle aspiration (TBNA), or endoscopic ultrasonography (EUS)–guided biopsy of lymph nodes can improve yield to up to 90%. In the appropriate clinical settings, TBNA and EUS-guided biopsy may supplant mediastinoscopy. One limitation is that needle aspiration/biopsy does not allow for evaluation of nodal architecture and may not deliver adequate material for thorough investigation to rule out infection. The CD4:CD8 ratio of bronchoalveolar lavage (BAL) in patients with sarcoid should be greater than 3.5 and can assist in making a diagnosis; however, BAL cell counts are neither diagnostic nor prognostic.

No specific diagnostic blood test for sarcoidosis exists. Mild anemia, lymphopenia, hypercalcemia, elevated total protein, and abnormal liver function testing may be seen.

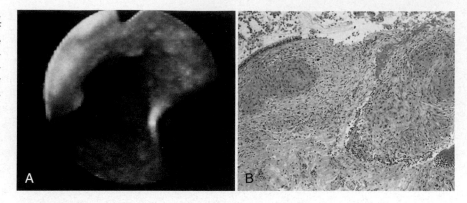

FIGURE 51-12 Endobronchial sarcoidosis. **A,** Bronchoscopic view shows extensive nodularity of bronchial mucosa, that is, "cobblestoning" of the airway. Rarely, Wegener's granulomatosis, tuberculosis, or fungal disease demonstrates similar airway abnormalities. **B,** Endobronchial biopsy demonstrating several granulomas and giant cells beneath bronchiolar epithelium.

Elevated serum angiotensin converting enzyme (SACE) levels are present in 50–75% of cases but have low sensitivity and specificity.

TREATMENT (Table 51-3)

Corticosteroids

Sarcoidosis is often a mild, self-limited disease and frequently does not require treatment. Clinical assessment, radiography, and sequential lung function testing with particular attention to any significant decline in gas transfer (DLCO) provide a sound basis on which to gauge treatment decisions. Some advantage is gained from laboratory tests, but little from measurement of BAL fluid cell populations. Taken overall, serial radiographic and sequential lung function tests are most likely to be helpful in the recognition of those patients likely to have chronic progressive pulmonary disease develop and, thereby, enable the provision of early treatment for them. Corticosteroid treatment is indicated when patients are dyspneic and the lung function tests commensurately poor and in those showing deterioration of health as judged clinically, radiologically, and particularly by progressive impairment of lung function tests. Corticosteroids suppress disease activity, and their use produces symptomatic, radiographic, and functional improvement. Uncertainty remains with regard to their effect on the overall natural history of the condition. When treatment is required, corticosteroids are the first line of therapy. Although corticosteroids have been shown to improve symptoms and may correct laboratory, radiographic, or pulmonary function abnormalities, long-term benefit remains unproven; no current evidence exists to demonstrate that corticosteroids significantly alter the natural history of disease or improve survival. Some extrapulmonary disease may respond better to nonsteroidal therapies.

Early experience of the use of steroids in patients with sarcoidosis showed that manifestation of activity both constitutional and organ related were favorably affected in the short term and that in those with persistent hypercalcemia serum levels became normal. Moreover, repeat biopsies during cortisone administration generally showed revisions of granulomas. However, cessation of short-term treatment was almost always followed by resurgence of the active manifestations.

Subsequent uncontrolled studies of patients treated with prednisolone for longer periods confirmed the early findings in that extrathoracic lesions were usually partially or completely suppressed and enlarged lymph nodes in the mediastinum diminished in size whereas in the lungs apparently nonfibrotic lesions showed diminution or clearing of radiographic shadows, although functional impairment usually showed only partial improvement that was more evident in ventilatory than in gas exchange tests. Longer standing fibrotic lung changes showed little objective change, although hypocalcemia and hypercalcuria were usually controlled by moderate doses of prednisolone. The improvement noted during limited periods of treatment is maintained after its cessation, but in many there is a resurgence of the sarcoidosis within a few months towards its former state or occasionally to a worse one. The sequence of events may be repeated after further periods of treatment, and occasionally new manifestations appear shortly after the end of a period of corticosteroid treatment. Thus, the effect of corticosteroids is usually one of simply suppression of the manifestations of sarcoidosis.

There have been a number of controlled situations in which the progress of patients with pulmonary sarcoidosis receiving specific regimens of corticosteroid treatment have been compared with that of similar groups not receiving corticosteroids. These comparative studies in patients who were treated for periods up to 18 months with corticosteroids confirmed that corticosteroids could suppress active granulomas and relieve symptoms, but in none was there evidence that the treatment improved long-term prognosis.

The British Thoracic Society (BTS) Sarcoidosis Study was conducted on a multicenter basis to try to determine the effects of long-term corticosteroid therapy in patients with pulmonary sarcoidosis. Fifty-eight patients were allocated to long-term treatment with the aim of producing as normal a chest radiograph as possible and were allocated to a treatment schedule of 30 mg prednisolone daily for 1 month, followed by 20 mg daily for 1 month, and thereafter 10 mg daily for 9 months. After 1 year of treatment, the use of prednisolone was tapered in a stepwise manner over 6 months. Thirty-one patients were allocated to selected treatment; in these, treatment was reserved for use only if warranted by the development of symptoms or deteriorating lung function. The initial dose of prednisolone was 30 mg daily for 1 month with gradual tapering and withdrawal of treatment over 6–9 months. The average follow-up for the two groups was close to 5 years. Prolonged treatment with the aim of optimizing radiographic appearance resulted in a significantly better long-term functional outcome, although the improvements in symptoms, lung function, and radiographic appearance among the patients in the two groups at final analysis was not large.

TABLE 51-3 Treatment of Sarcoidosis

Drug Group and Indications	Specific Drug	Dosage and Duration	Side Effects
Corticosteroids for pulmonary or systemic sarcoidosis	Prednisone	Initial regimen: 40 mg q24h for 2 weeks 30 mg q24h for 2 weeks 25 mg q24h for 2 weeks 20 mg q24h for 2 weeks 10–15 mg q24h for 6–8 months Taper to 2.5 mg every 2–4 weeks; if relapse, reinstitute lowest prior effective dose	Increased appetite, weight gain Cushingoid habitus Hyperglycemia Adrenal axis suppression Emotional lability, depression Psychosis, pseudotumor cerebri Hypertension Sodium, fluid retention Glaucoma, cataracts Osteoporosis, osteonecrosis Compression fractures Myopathy Pancreatitis Striae, easy bruisability, acne
Antimalarials for mucocutaneous sarcoidosis	Chloroquine phosphate	500 mg q24h for 2 weeks, then 500 mg q48h for 6 months, followed by 6-month drug-free period	Retinopathy Gastrointestinal upset Headache Discoloration of nailbeds Reversible dermatitis
	Hydroxychloroquine sulfate	200 mg q12h or q24h, may be given indefinitely	Retinopathy (rare) Gastrointestinal symptoms Dermatitis
Alternative therapies for: Mild disease or as corticosteroid-sparing agent Severe, refractory sarcoidosis and as corticosteroid-sparing agent	Pentoxifylline	400 mg q6h or q8h, may be given indefinitely	Gastrointestinal upset Headache
	Azathioprine	50 mg q24h for 2 weeks Increase by 50 mg every 2–4 weeks Maximum suggested: 150–200 mg q24h	Bone marrow suppression Hepatic toxicity Gastrointestinal toxicity Carcinogenicity Opportunistic infections
	Methotrexate	10–20 mg once a week plus folic acid 1 mg/day	Hepatic toxicity Gastrointestinal toxicity Pulmonary toxicity (hypersensitivity pneumonitis) Bone marrow suppression Opportunistic infections
Experimental	Doxycycline Minocycline Thalidomide	200 mg/day 200 mg/day 100–150 qhs	Photosensitivity Gastrointestinal upset Teratogenicity Peripheral neuropathy Sedation Skin reactions
	Infliximab	Infusion	Infusion reactions Opportunistic infections Tuberculosis fungal infections, serious infections, sepsis Hypersensitivity reactions
	Etanercept	Injection	Injection site reactions serious infections, sepsis, death Gastrointestinal upset CNS demyelination disorders

In summary, views with regards to the management of pulmonary sarcoidosis remain divided. Most physicians favor a long-term schedule of treatment, although some consider only short-term therapy with the additional aim of minimizing the side effects of corticosteroids to the patient.

Oral corticosteroid therapy should be strongly considered in the following situations:

1. Hypercalcemia or hypercalciuria
2. Central nervous system involvement
3. Anterior or posterior uveitis that is unresponsive to local therapy
4. Active cardiac involvement
5. Progressive involvement in any organ system (i.e., progressive respiratory symptoms, abnormal pulmonary function parameters such as reduced diffusion or vital capacity, or worsening radiographic abnormalities)

The optimal dose and duration of corticosteroid treatment has not been determined in randomized, prospective trials.

The treatment regimen is individualized on the basis of symptoms and response rate. For pulmonary sarcoidosis, the initial dose is generally 30–40 mg/day of prednisone, observing for either symptomatic or radiographic response, or improvement in pulmonary function parameters at 1–3 months. Patients who fail to respond to an initial 3-month course are unlikely to respond to a more prolonged therapeutic course. Among responders, the prednisone dose may be slowly tapered, but treatment should be continued for 9–12 months and tapered thereafter if appropriate. Symptoms or radiographic abnormalities occur frequently after discontinuing treatment. Some studies have found that more than one third of patients experience symptom recurrence within 2 years of discontinuing therapy.

Relapse Rates

In a nonrandomized prospective study over a 4-year period, corticosteroid-treated patients, who relapsed after clinical stability with symptoms severe enough to warrant treatment after a remission of more than a month, were compared with those of a group who had shown spontaneous remission without treatment. A 74% relapse rate was observed among 103 patients in the induced remission group compared with 8% among 118 patients who had achieved a spontaneous remission. Relapse rates were similar in Caucasians and African Americans, but Caucasian patients maintained a sustained remission with twice the frequency of African Americans. Another retrospective report evaluated the rate and pattern of relapses among 239 patients originally from a consecutive series of 702 patients with histologically confirmed sarcoidosis. A relapse severe enough to require further treatment was seen in 30; 25 of these relapsed within the first year, and in none of these 30 patients was prednisolone subsequently withdrawn successfully. Low-dose corticosteroid therapy is usually well tolerated, but because of an extensive adverse effect profile, patients should be counseled regarding known immediate effects, including weight gain, insomnia, glucose intolerance, and euphoria. Long-term use effects include early cataracts or glaucoma and reduced bone density resulting in osteoporosis or osteonecrosis. Judicious use of calcium or vitamin D therapy is important to prevent hypercalcemia and hypercalciuria. Bisphosphonate therapy is often used, especially when bone density scanning clarifies reduced bone density.

The role of bisphosphonates in the prevention of glucocorticoid-induced osteoporosis has been studied. Alendronate and intravenous pamidronate gave promising results in the preservation of bone density of the spine and hip relative to baseline measurements and placebo. Accordingly and where appropriate, it is usual to prescribe one or the other over the medium or longer term.

Although *Pneumocystis* pneumonia is rare, with doses exceeding 20 mg/day, prophylaxis is reasonable.

Although multiple randomized controlled trials have been conducted to assess the efficacy of inhaled corticosteroids in pulmonary sarcoidosis, there is a lack of consistent data to support their use, and if so, in which patient populations (i.e., in patients with obstructive vs restrictive pulmonary function testing patterns, patients with bronchial hyperresponsiveness, or patients with endobronchial granulomas). Most authorities recommend inhaled corticosteroids for persistent cough.

IMMUNOSUPPRESSIVE AND OTHER ALTERNATIVE THERAPIES

Various immunomodulatory and immunosuppressive therapies may be used if either corticosteroid therapy is poorly tolerated, as augmentation for corticosteroid-resistant cases, or as steroid-sparing agents.

Hydroxychloroquine

The antimalarial drug hydroxychloroquine may be an effective steroid-sparing agent and is particularly useful in neurosarcoidosis cases, skin involvement, and abnormalities in calcium metabolism. Beneficial effects have also been reported in the treatment of hypercalcemia, and it has a specific effect on the sarcoid granuloma and is not simply acting as a nonspecific antiinflammatory agent. It is contraindicated for use in patients with posterior uveitis, because retinitis is a potential toxic effect. For patients placed on hydroxychloroquine, ophthalmologic examinations should be conducted every 3–6 months during therapy to monitor for this potential rare ocular toxicity. As with the cytotoxic agents discussed later, women of childbearing age should be counseled to use birth control while taking hydroxychloroquine.

Azathioprine, Methotrexate, and Cyclophosphamide

Azathioprine, methotrexate, and cyclophosphamide have all been used in treatment of sarcoidosis. Although these agents benefit selected patients, no studies exist that clearly delineate when these drugs should be used for therapy. Systematic reviews could identify only four randomized trials comparing these agents, and the results were largely inconclusive. Methotrexate has been shown to be useful in uveitis. New agents that are currently being investigated include leflunomide, a methotrexate analog, which has been shown to be effective and may have less pulmonary toxicity.

Tetracyclines

Doxycycline and minocycline may benefit some with cutaneous sarcoidosis but have not been shown to be effective for other organ involvement.

Antitumor Necrosis Factor Therapy
Pentoxifylline

Although pentoxifylline inhibits TNF, clinical experience indicates that the drug has limited efficacy but may be helpful as a corticosteroid-sparing agent or to lessen systemic symptoms such as fatigue. Gastrointestinal side effects may limit dosing.

Thalidomide

Small clinical series have found that thalidomide may be beneficial in cutaneous sarcoidosis, particularly lupus pernio. Sedation, peripheral neurotoxicity, and teratogenicity limit its usefulness.

TNF Alpha-Blockers

Infliximab, a monoclonal antibody directed against soluble and membrane bound TNF-α has recently been shown to be effective in refractory sarcoidosis, specifically ocular disease.

Interestingly, etanercept, another TNF-α blocker was found ineffective. There is clearly a need for additional randomized controlled trials to investigate these agents' role in sarcoidosis.

Lung Transplantation

Lung transplantation is an appropriate option for patients with sarcoidosis with severe physiologic impairment refractory to medical therapy. Timing of transplantation for patients with sarcoidosis is challenging, because mortality rates are high (27–53%) among patients with sarcoidosis awaiting lung transplant. Furthermore, models predicting mortality have not been validated. The most recently published guidelines for lung transplant candidate selection do not delineate disease-specific guidelines for referral. Extrapolating from idiopathic pulmonary fibrosis, the following recommendations for lung transplantation have been suggested: (1) a forced vital capacity (FVC) less than 60% predicted, (2) diffusing capacity less than 50% of predicted, (3) rest or exercise-induced hypoxemia, or (4) failure to maintain lung function despite treatment with steroids or other immunosuppressive agents. These recommendations seem reasonable, because the mortality rate for patients with sarcoidosis on the lung transplant waiting list is similar to patients with pulmonary fibrosis.

Specific risk factors for mortality in sarcoidosis patients awaiting lung transplantation have been identified. One study showed an elevated right atrial pressure as the only variable independently associated with mortality in multivariate analysis. A right atrial pressure of >15 mmHg resulted in a 5.2-fold increase in risk of death. Interestingly, the mean pulmonary artery pressure (mPAP) at the time of lung transplant was significantly higher than at the time of listing. Almost all the patients studied had marked progression of pulmonary hypertension while awaiting transplantation, suggesting that more careful right ventricular hemodynamic monitoring can predict who is at increased risk for death. Although repeated right heart catheterizations may not be feasible, repeat echocardiograms and/or monitoring B-type natriuretic peptide (BNP) levels may be helpful to identify worsening pulmonary hypertension.

A recent review of 405 patients with sarcoidosis listed for lung transplantation in the United Network for Organ Sharing (UNOS) database indicated that there was no significant difference between pulmonary function testing parameters in survivors and nonsurvivors. However, underlying pulmonary hypertension, the amount of supplemental oxygen required, and African American race are significant mortality predictors. Although mPAP was elevated both in survivors and nonsurvivors, mPAP of patients who died on the waiting list was 33% higher. The marked pulmonary hypertension noted in nonsurvivors was not thought to reflect either cardiac sarcoidosis or chronic left ventricular dysfunction, because of the nearly normal cardiac indices and pulmonary capillary wedge pressures. These data suggest that referral guidelines should be modified to include these particular risk factors, at least until further prospective studies are performed.

Early referral allows for timely evaluation for possible listing. If the risks specific to transplantation in sarcoidosis are considered and carefully evaluated, outcomes match those of other diagnoses. Recurrent sarcoidosis in the lung allografts can occur but does not affect survival or risk for complications.

CLINICAL COURSE

Between 30 and 60% of patients with sarcoidosis are symptomatic. African Americans tend to have more severe disease at presentation. Up to two thirds of patients have spontaneous resolution or improvement in disease activity. Of those with remission, one third have symptom resolution within 1 year and 85% within 2 years. Some patients can have remission as long as 5 years after presentation. Only 1–5% of patients die of sarcoid-related disease, which is usually a result of severe pulmonary, cardiac, or neurologic dysfunction. Earlier studies have outlined multiple risk factors associated with worsened prognosis in sarcoidosis (Box 51-1). Multisystem involvement and the effect it has on the psychosocial well-being highlights the need for a multidisciplinary approach.

To assist in following patients and choosing therapy, patients should be phenotyped at each visit. One phenotyping scheme is present in Box 51-2. SACE generally decreases in response to modest corticosteroid doses even when the disease is active or patients remain symptomatic. In those patients with elevated levels, SACE decline may be used as a marker of corticosteroid compliance.

Hemoptysis and Mycetomas

Fibrocystic sarcoidosis may be complicated by bronchiectasis, extensive cavitation, and mycetoma development within cavities, particularly with *Aspergillus* species (Figure 51-13). As a result, hemoptysis may occur and become life threatening. Most episodes of hemoptysis resolve with cough suppression, antibiotics, moderate corticosteroid doses, and discontinuing aspirin or other nonsteroidal antiinflammatory drugs. Angiographic embolization may be required. Surgical resection is often not feasible, because these patients generally have limited lung function reserve.

BOX 51-1 Sarcoidosis Risk Factors

Risk Factors Associated with Worsened Outcomes in Sarcoidosis

African-American race
Lupus pernio
Chronic uveitis
Age of onset after 40
Chronic hypercalcemia
Nephrocalcinosis
Progressive or prolonged symptoms >6 mo
Absence of erythema nodosum
Splenomegaly
Nasal mucosal involvement
Cystic bone lesions
Neurosarcoidosis
Myocardial involvement
Involvement of >3 organ systems
Stage III/IV pulmonary disease

Risk Factors Associated with Mortality on Lung Transplant Waiting List

Elevated right atrial pressure
Underlying pulmonary hypertension
Amount of supplemental oxygen required
African-American race

BOX 51-2 Sample Phenotyping Model

Phenotyping
Date of symptom onset
Year diagnosed
Biopsy results
Organ involvement
Physiologic impairment
 Ophthalmologic exam
 Pulmonary function
 Cardiac function
Blood test results
 CBC
 Liver profile
 ACE
Calcium metabolism

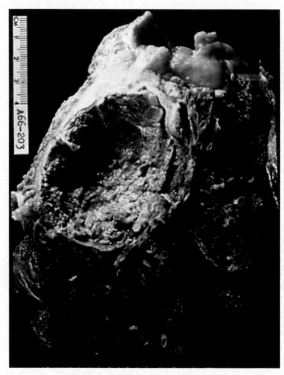

FIGURE 51-13 Fibrocystic cavity.

Pregnancy

Because sarcoidosis most commonly affects women in their childbearing age, physicians should be prepared to counsel patients on how sarcoidosis affects pregnancy. Patients should be told that sarcoidosis does not affect pregnancy and that pregnancy does not affect sarcoidosis. The more important issue relates to therapeutic options for those patients who are considering pregnancy or who are pregnant. Most therapy, such as immunosuppression and hydroxychloroquine, is contraindicated in pregnancy. Corticosteroids, as in asthma, are viewed as safe.

PITFALLS AND CONTROVERSIES

The diagnosis of sarcoidosis should be considered early during the evaluation of systemic and respiratory complaints, particularly with additional clues of uveitis, peripheral lymphadenopathy, skin rash, or cranial nerve involvement. The least invasive approach should be considered to histologically confirm the diagnosis. Biopsy of skin, lacrimal gland, peripheral lymph node, and lung through bronchoscopy has a high diagnostic yield. Bronchoscopy with endobronchial and transbronchial biopsies even in patients with a stage I chest X-ray has more than a 60% yield and should be considered before mediastinoscopy. Cardiac sarcoidosis should be considered in those individuals without risk for coronary artery disease, who have unexplained arrhythmias and cardiac dysfunction.

The lack of randomized, controlled treatment trials limits treatment options. Corticosteroids remain the most commonly used therapy. The role of corticosteroid-sparing medications continues to evolve. When corticosteroids are not tolerated in serious disease, hydroxychloroquine, methotrexate, azathioprine, and anti-TNF agents are used.

WEB RESOURCES FOR GUIDELINES AND PROTOCOLS

www.Sarcoidosis.org

SUGGESTED READINGS

Baughman RP: Lower, steroid-sparing alternative treatments for sarcoidosis. Clin Chest Med 1997; 18:853–864.

Hunninghake GW, Costabel U, Ando M, et al: ATS/ERS/WASOG statement on sarcoidosis. American Thoracic Society/European Respiratory Society/World Association of Sarcoidosis and other Granulomatous Disorders. Sarcoidosis Vasc Diffuse Lung Dis 1999; 16:149–173.

Judson MA: An approach to the treatment of pulmonary sarcoidosis with corticosteroids: The six phases of treatment. Chest 1999; 115:1158–1165.

Judson MA, Iannuzzi MC, Guest editors: Sarcoidosis: Evolving concepts and controversies. Semin Respir Crit Care Med 2007; 28 Vol 1.

Judson MA, Thompson BW, Rabin DL, et al: The diagnostic pathway to sarcoidosis. Chest 2003; 123:406–412.

Judson MA, Baughman RP, Thompson BW, et al: Two year prognosis of sarcoidosis: the ACCESS experience. Sarcoidosis Vasc Diffuse Lung Dis 2003; 20:204–211.

Koyama T, Ueda H, Togashi K, et al: Radiologic manifestations of sarcoidosis in various organs. Radiographics 2004; 24:87–104.

Padilla ML, Schilero GJ, Teirstein AS: Sarcoidosis and transplantation. Sarcoidosis Vasc Diffuse Lung Dis 1997; 14:16–22.

Rybicki BA, Iannuzzi MC, Frederick MM, et al: Familial aggregation of sarcoidosis: a case-control etiologic study of sarcoidosis (ACCESS). Am J Respir Crit Care Med 2001; 164:2085–2091.

Yeager H, Rossman RD, Baughman RP, et al: Pulmonary and psychosocial findings at enrollment in the ACCESS study. Sarcoidosis Vasc Diffuse Lung Dis 2005; 22:147–153.

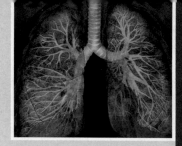

52 Eosinophilic Lung Disease

JEAN-FRANÇOIS CORDIER • VINCENT COTTIN

THE EOSINOPHILIC LEUKOCYTE AND EOSINOPHILIC PNEUMONIA

The eosinophilic lung diseases are characterized by prominent infiltration of the lung structures by eosinophils leading to several distinct clinical disorders, especially eosinophilic pneumonia (EP) (Box 52-1).

The Eosinophil Leukocyte

The eosinophil that is normally involved in nonspecific inflammatory responses and protection against infectious, especially parasitic, organisms may be the major culprit of tissue injury in eosinophilic disorders. It has many biologic properties directed by T-helper lymphocytes and interacts with mast cells and basophils, endothelial cells, macrophages, platelets, and fibroblasts. Mediators released by the eosinophil and/or surface enzymes, receptors for cytokines, chemokines, complement proteins, and other chemoattractants participate in various allergic and/or inflammatory processes.

Eosinophil precursors differentiate in the bone marrow under the action of several cytokines, including interleukin (IL)-5, IL-3, and granulocyte macrophage colony-stimulating factor (GM-CSF), and mature into eosinophils, which then circulate in the blood before being recruited into target tissues such as the lung. Recruitment of eosinophils involves cell adhesion and attraction, diapedesis, and chemotaxis by cytokines (mainly IL-5 and eotaxin). In tissues, the eosinophils may release active mediators on activation, including proinflammatory cytokines, arachidonic acid–derived mediators, enzymes, reactive oxygen species, and toxic substances. Activation and degranulation of the eosinophil releases specific proteins, including major basic protein (MBP), eosinophil cationic protein (ECP), eosinophil-derived neurotoxin (EDN), enzymatic protein eosinophil peroxidase (EPO), and the recently described MBP homolog.

Pathology of Eosinophilic Pneumonia

EP is characterized by the prominent infiltration of the lung structures by eosinophils. The lung interstitium is infiltrated by eosinophils, and essentially the alveolar spaces are filled with eosinophils and a fibrinous exudate, with conservation of the global architecture of the lung. In addition, eosinophilic microabscesses and a nonnecrotizing vasculitis are common in idiopathic chronic eosinophilic pneumonia (ICEP) and idiopathic acute eosinophilic pneumonia (IAEP). Macrophages and scattered multinucleated giant cells may be present within the infiltrate.

Diagnosis of Eosinophilic Pneumonia

The diagnosis of EP relies on both characteristic clinical-imaging features and the demonstration of alveolar eosinophilia with or without peripheral blood eosinophilia. Bronchoalveolar lavage (BAL) is a noninvasive surrogate of lung biopsy for the diagnosis of EP. The percentage of eosinophils at BAL is <2% in normal controls, and a differential cell count of eosinophils of 2–25% may be found in nonspecific conditions. Therefore, a cutoff of ≥25% eosinophils at BAL, and preferably ≥40%, is recommended for the diagnosis of EP. The presence of markedly elevated peripheral blood eosinophilia ($>1 \times 10^9$/L and preferably 1.5×10^9/L) together with typical clinical radiologic features obviates the need for lung biopsy in EP. Peripheral blood eosinophilia may be absent at presentation, especially in IAEP and in patients receiving corticosteroid treatment.

EP may be separated into EP of undetermined origin, which usually may be included within well-individualized syndromes, and EP with a definite cause (mainly infection and drug reaction) (see Box 52-1). Potential causes must be thoroughly investigated, because identification of a cause may lead to effective therapeutic measures.

EOSINOPHILIC LUNG DISEASES OF DETERMINED ORIGIN

Eosinophilic Pneumonia in Parasitic Diseases

Parasite infestation is the main cause of EP in the world. Clinical manifestations are nonspecific.

Tropical pulmonary eosinophilia is a disease of decreasing prevalence caused by the filarial parasites *Wuchereria bancrofti* and *Brugia malayi* deposited in the skin by mosquitoes. The clinical features of tropical EP largely result from an immune response of the host to the antigenic constituents of circulating microfilariae trapped in the lung vasculature (cough that may be associated with fever, weight loss, and anorexia). The chest X-ray shows bilateral infiltrative opacities. Blood eosinophilia is greater than 2×10^9 eosinophils/L at the early stage. The diagnosis of filariasis may be established by a strongly positive serologic evaluation in patients residing in an endemic area with persisting blood eosinophilia greater than 3×10^9/L and IgE levels exceeding 10,000 ng/mL, and it is further supported by clinical improvement in the weeks after treatment with diethylcarbamazine; the addition of corticosteroids may be beneficial in severe cases.

The nematode *Ascaris lumbricoides* is the most common helminth infecting humans. The disease is transmitted through food contaminated by human feces containing parasitic eggs. Löffler syndrome (transient mild EP) may develop during the migration of the larvae through the lung. Symptoms are often limited to cough, wheezing, and transient fever, which resolve in a few days, but blood eosinophilia may last for several weeks.

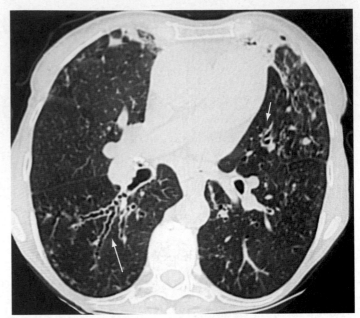

FIGURE 52-1 Bilateral bronchiectasis *(arrows)* in a patient with allergic bronchopulmonary aspergillosis (associated with some infiltrative opacities).

Allergic Bronchopulmonary Mycoses

Allergic bronchopulmonary aspergillosis (ABPA) (Figure 52-1) results from a complex allergic and immune reaction in the bronchi and the adjacent lung parenchyma in response to antigens from *Aspergillus* colonizing the airways of patients with asthma. A pattern of allergic bronchopulmonary mycosis similar to ABPA has rarely been reported with other fungi or yeasts. The immunologic response to the fungus combining both type-I and type-III hypersensitivity results in progressive damage to the bronchial and pulmonary tissue. Mucus plugs containing *Aspergillus* obstruct the airways with subsequent atelectasis, bronchial wall damage, and proximal bronchiectasis predominating in the upper lobes. The presence of bronchiectasis on CT in a patient with asthma is highly suggestive of ABPA.

ABPA occurs mainly in adults with preexisting asthma and in patients with cystic fibrosis.

The early ABPA is characterized by fever, expectoration of mucus plugs, peripheral blood eosinophilia greater than 1×10^9/L, and pulmonary infiltrates caused by EP, or segmental or lobar atelectasis caused by mucus plugging. Chronic ABPA is characterized by asthma, eosinophilia, and bronchopulmonary manifestations including bronchiectasis (see Figure 52-1 and Box 52-2). The expectoration of mucus plugs, the presence of *Aspergillus* in sputum, and late skin reactivity to *Aspergillus* antigen are also common at this stage.

The treatment of exacerbations of ABPA by corticosteroids may contribute to preventing the progression of the disease to the fibrotic end stage. Inhaled corticosteroids may reduce the need for long-term oral corticosteroids. Oral itraconazole is a useful adjunct to corticosteroids, allowing reduction of the corticosteroid oral dose and reducing the rate of exacerbations.

Eosinophilic Pneumonias Secondary to Drugs, Toxic Agents, and Radiation Therapy

Drugs taken in the weeks preceding the clinical syndrome of EP must be thoroughly investigated, including illicit drugs (cocaine or heroin). EP has been reported in association with

Visceral larva migrans syndrome caused by *Toxocara canis* occurs throughout the world. Humans and especially children become infected after ingestion of eggs released in feces of infected dogs (especially in the soil of public playgrounds in urban areas). Fever, seizures, fatigue, and pulmonary manifestations may occur (cough, dyspnea, wheezes or crackles at pulmonary auscultation, and pulmonary infiltrates at chest X-ray). Blood eosinophilia may be present initially or may develop only in the following days. Symptomatic treatment is recommended, whereas the use of antihelmintics is controversial.

Strongyloides stercoralis is an intestinal nematode, the larvae of which infect humans through the skin by contact with humid soil. Eosinophilia present in recently infected patients is often absent in disseminated disease. Strongyloidiasis may cause severe disease, affecting all organs (hyperinfection syndrome), especially in immunocompromised patients, sometimes years after the initial infection, with or without peripheral eosinophilia, and bilateral patchy infiltrates on chest X-ray. Treatment with thiabendazole is recommended.

BOX 52-2 Diagnostic Criteria of Allergic Broncho-Pulmonary Aspergillosis in Patients with Asthma

Criteria for ABPA-Central Bronchiectasis

1. Asthma — Yes
2. Central bronchiectasis (inner two thirds of chest CT field) — Yes
3. Immediate cutaneous reactivity to *Aspergillus* species or *A. fumigatus* — Yes
4. Total serum IgE concentration >417 kU/L (1000 ng/mL) — Yes
5. Elevated serum IgE–*A. fumigatus* and/or IgG–*A. fumigatus* — Yes
6. Chest roentgenographic infiltrates — No
7. Serum precipitating antibodies to *A. fumigatus* — No

Criteria for the Diagnosis of ABPA-Seropositive

1. Asthma — Yes
2. Immediate cutaneous reactivity to *Aspergillus* species or *A. fumigatus* — Yes
3. Total serum IgE concentration >417 kU/L (1000 ng/mL) — Yes
4. Elevated serum IgE–*A. fumigatus* and or IgG–*A. fumigatus* — Yes
5. Chest roentgenographic infiltrates — No

BOX 52-3 Drugs That Cause Eosinophilic Pneumonia*

Acetylsalicylic acid
Captopril
Carbamazepine
Diclofenac
Ethambutol
Fenbufen
Granulocyte monocyte-colony stimulating factor (GM-CSF)
Ibuprofen
L-Tryptophan
Minocycline
Naproxen
Para (4)-aminosalicylic acid
Penicillins
Phenylbutazone
Piroxicam
Pyrimethamine
Sulindac
Sulfamides, sulfonamides
Tolfenamic acid
Trimethoprim-sulfamethoxazole

*A more detailed list of drugs reported to cause eosinophilic pneumonia may be found at www.pneumotox.com.

many drugs, but causality has been confidently shown in fewer than 20 (Box 52-3).

Drug-induced EP may develop progressively and manifest as chronic EP, as transient pulmonary infiltrates with eosinophilia (Löffler syndrome), and occasionally as acute EP sometimes requiring mechanical ventilation.

Corticosteroids are often given concomitantly with drug withdrawal to accelerate clinical improvement. When present, associated cutaneous rash or pleural effusion increases the likelihood of the diagnosis.

Chronic EP similar to ICEP has been described after radiation therapy for breast cancer in women similar to the organizing pneumonia syndrome.

Other Lung Diseases with Associated Eosinophilia

Eosinophilia may be found in other bronchopulmonary disorders where EP is not prominent.

Eosinophilic inflammation of the airways is a pathologic feature defining a phenotype of asthma. Some mild increase of eosinophils in peripheral blood and BAL differential cell count (usually fewer than 5%) may be found in asthma. Monitoring of the sputum eosinophil count may help in adapting the treatment and reducing asthma exacerbations and hospital admissions. More important blood eosinophilia (i.e., $>1.5 \times 10^9$/L) may occasionally occur in the absence of any determined cause or context of systemic disease. The disease may evolve to ICEP or overt Churg–Strauss syndrome (CSS), or it may remain solitary, with frequent dependency on oral corticosteroids.

Eosinophilic bronchitis (without asthma) with a high percentage of eosinophils (up to 40%) in sputum is a well-individualized cause of chronic cough responsive to corticosteroid treatment. Patients usually have normal lung function.

Bronchocentric granulomatosis is a rare condition with nonspecific clinical and radiologic manifestations (fever, cough, and blood eosinophilia generally greater than 1×10^9 eosinophils/L), diagnosed by lung biopsy. Corticosteroids represent the mainstay of treatment.

Mildly increased levels of eosinophils may be found at BAL differential cell count in idiopathic interstitial pneumonias, a finding associated with a poor prognosis. Focal EP has been reported in cases of usual interstitial pneumonia. The typical clinical and imaging features of cryptogenic organizing pneumonia may closely mimic ICEP (some clinical or pathologic overlap may exist between these two diseases). Eosinophilia (usually mild) may be present in pulmonary Langerhans cell histiocytosis and in sarcoidosis.

EOSINOPHILIC LUNG DISEASE OF UNDETERMINED ORIGIN

Idiopathic Chronic Eosinophilic Pneumonia
(Figure 52-2)

ICEP is characterized by the progressive development of respiratory and systemic symptoms over several weeks. Cough, dyspnea, and chest pain are often accompanied by prominent fatigue, malaise, fever, and weight loss. Wheezes or crackles are found in one third of patients. Chronic rhinitis or sinusitis is present in approximately 20% of patients.

Most patients are nonsmokers. ICEP predominates in women (2:1 female/male ratio), with a mean age of 45 years at diagnosis, and a prior history of atopy in approximately half of the patients. Prior asthma is present in up to two thirds of the patients (it may get worse after the occurrence of ICEP), but it may also occur concomitantly with the diagnosis of ICEP or develop after it. Nonrespiratory minor manifestations are possible in ICEP, suggesting an overlap with CSS.

Imaging features of ICEP characteristically consist of alveolar opacities, with ill-defined margins and a density varying from ground-glass to consolidation. Migration of the infiltrates

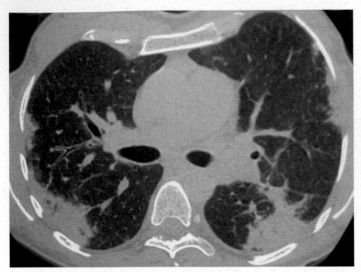

FIGURE 52-2 Bilateral peripheral patchy opacities in a patient with idiopathic chronic eosinophilic pneumonia.

highly suggestive of the diagnosis occurs in approximately a quarter of the cases. A peripheral predominance of the lesions (described as the classic pattern of "photographic negative of pulmonary edema") is seen in approximately one fourth of patients. On high-resolution computed tomography (HRCT), the opacities are almost always bilateral and predominate in the upper lobes, with co-existing peripheral ground glass and consolidation opacities (see Figure 52-2). In addition, septal line thickening, bandlike opacities parallel to the chest, or mediastinal lymph node enlargement may be seen.

High-level peripheral blood eosinophilia is the key to the diagnosis (mean blood eosinophilia approximately 5.5×10^9/L). Alveolar eosinophilia usually >40% at BAL differential cell count is a hallmark of ICEP. C-reactive protein is elevated. Total blood IgE level is increased in approximately half the cases.

Lung function tests in ICEP show an obstructive ventilatory defect in approximately half and a restrictive ventilatory defect in half the cases. Usually mild hypoxemia is present in most of the patients.

ICEP responds dramatically to corticosteroid treatment. We use an initial dose of 0.5 mg/kg/day for 2 weeks, followed by 0.25 mg/kg/day for 2 weeks, then corticosteroids are progressively reduced and stopped. Improvement of the symptoms occurs within 2 days, and chest X-ray opacities clear within 1 week and eventually disappear without sequelae in almost all patients. Relapses occur in most patients while decreasing or after stopping the corticosteroid treatment and respond very well to resumed corticosteroid treatment. Most patients need corticosteroids for more than 6 months, and often several years. Relapses of ICEP might be less frequent in patients who receive inhaled corticosteroids after stopping maintenance oral corticosteroids.

Idiopathic Acute Eosinophilic Pneumonia

IAEP differs from ICEP not only by its acute onset and severity, but also by the absence of relapse after recovery. This acute pneumonia develops in previously healthy individuals, with possible respiratory failure (see Figure 52-4). Blood eosinophilia often lacking at presentation contrasts with frank alveolar eosinophilia at BAL. Current diagnostic criteria are listed in Box 52-4.

IAEP occurs mainly in young adults, with a male predominance and no prior asthma history. In several cases, IAEP developed soon after the initiation of tobacco smoking. Potential respiratory exposures within the days before onset of disease have been reported (cave exploration, heavy dust inhalation, etc.). Inhalation of smoke or any nonspecific injurious agent likely contributes to the disease.

IAEP presents with the acute onset of cough, dyspnea, fever, and chest pain, sometimes with abdominal complaints or myalgias. Tachypnea, tachycardia, and crackles are present on examination. Chest X-ray shows bilateral infiltrates (Figure 52-3), with mixed alveolar interstitial and opacities, especially Kerley lines. Chest CT mainly shows ground-glass opacities and airspace consolidation, together with poorly defined nodules, interlobular septal thickening, and bilateral pleural effusions.

Whereas blood eosinophilia is usually lacking at presentation, the BAL eosinophilia is usually greater than 25%, obviating the need for a lung biopsy. The peripheral blood eosinophil count often rises during the course of disease, an evolution

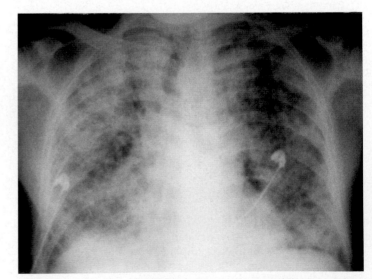

FIGURE 52-3 Diffuse infiltrative pulmonary opacities in a patient with idiopathic acute eosinophilic pneumonia with respiratory failure.

suggestive of the diagnosis. Eosinophilia may be also found in pleural effusion or sputum. High levels of IgE may be present. Lung function tests, when done in the less severe cases, may show a mild restrictive ventilatory defect, a reduced transfer factor, and increased alveolar-arterial oxygen gradient. Severe hypoxemia may be present, with most patients fulfilling diagnostic criteria for acute lung injury (including a $PaO_2/FIO_2 \leq$ 300 mmHg) or for acute respiratory distress syndrome ($PaO_2/FIO_2 \leq$ 200 mmHg), with mechanical ventilation necessary in most of them. In contrast with ARDS, extrapulmonary organ failure is exceptional.

Lung biopsy (when done) shows acute and organizing diffuse alveolar damage together with interstitial alveolar and bronchiolar infiltration by eosinophils, intraalveolar eosinophils, and interstitial edema. Although recovery without corticosteroid treatment may occur, a corticosteroid treatment is usually given for 2–4 weeks. Complete clinical and radiologic recovery occurs rapidly on corticosteroid treatment, with no relapse (in contrast with ICEP).

Churg–Strauss Syndrome (Figure 52-4)

CSS is included in the group of small vessel vasculitides and defined as an eosinophil-rich and granulomatous inflammation involving the respiratory tract and necrotizing vasculitis affecting small- to medium-sized vessels; it is associated with asthma and eosinophilia. All the pathologic lesions are seldom found on a single biopsy, and abnormalities are often limited to an eosinophilic perivascular infiltration of the tissues characteristic of the early (prevasculitic) phase of the disease.

CSS is a very rare disorder, occurring especially in the fourth and fifth decades, with no gender predominance. The natural history of CSS usually follows three phases: rhinosinusitis and asthma; blood and tissue eosinophilia; and emergence of vasculitis. Rhinitis of the allergic type is often accompanied by paranasal sinusitis and nasal polyps. Asthma progressively becomes corticodependent, usually preceding the onset of vasculitis by several years (however, these may be contemporary). The severity of asthma may attenuate with the onset of the vasculitis. The chest X-ray may remain normal throughout the course of the disease, but lung opacities mainly consisting of ill-defined pulmonary infiltrates, sometimes migratory and transient, are present in more than half of patients. Pleural effusion present in approximately one fourth of patients must be distinguished from that associated with cardiac failure resulting from cardiac eosinophilic involvement. HR-CT mainly shows areas of ground-glass attenuation or airspace

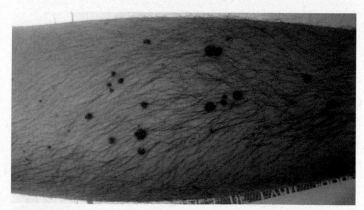

FIGURE 52-4 Vasculitic palpable purpura in a patient with Churg–Strauss syndrome.

consolidation, with peripheral predominance or random distribution. Centrilobular nodules, bronchial wall thickening or dilatation, interlobular septal thickening, and hilar or mediastinal lymphadenopathy are less common.

Blood eosinophilia greater than 1.5 and often $5 \times 10^9/L$ usually parallels disease activity. It disappears rapidly after the initiation of corticosteroid treatment. Eosinophilia, sometimes greater than 60%, is also present at BAL differential cell count. IgE levels are usually markedly increased. High levels of urinary EDN might represent an indicator of disease activity.

Extrapulmonary manifestations of CSS usually include asthenia, weight loss, fever, arthralgias, and/or myalgias. Nervous involvement typically consists of mononeuritis multiplex or asymmetric polyneuropathy. Cardiac involvement with eosinophilic myocarditis (or more rarely coronary arteritis) is often insidious and asymptomatic and may lead to dilated cardiomyopathy, although it may improve markedly with corticosteroid treatment. Pericardial effusion is common, but tamponade is rare. Digestive tract involvement usually manifests as isolated abdominal pain or diarrhea, but intestinal vasculitis (with ulcerations, perforations, or hemorrhage) and cholecystitis may occur. Cutaneous lesions present in approximately half of patients mainly consist of palpable purpura (see Figure 52-4) of the extremities, subcutaneous nodules, erythematous rashes, and urticaria. Renal involvement present in a quarter of cases is usually mild.

Currently used diagnostic criteria for CSS include (1) asthma, (2) eosinophilia exceeding $1.5 \times 10^9/L$, and (3) systemic vasculitis of two or more extrapulmonary organs (biopsy proven or not). Antineutrophil cytoplasmic antibodies (ANCA) may also be considered a major diagnostic criterion when present. A pathologic diagnosis of CSS may be obtained from skin, nerve, or muscle biopsies. Lung biopsy and transbronchial biopsies are not helpful.

ANCA are present in only approximately 40% of patients, mainly consisting of perinuclear ANCA (P-ANCA), with a specificity for myeloperoxidase on ELISA, whereas other ANCA (especially cytoplasmic ANCA with proteinase-3 specificity) are very rare in CSS. Interestingly, ANCA seem to distinguish two phenotypes of CSS: patients with ANCA have a vasculitic phenotype (with more frequent vasculitis on biopsy, renal involvement, peripheral neuropathy, and purpura), whereas patients without ANCA have more frequent cardiac and pulmonary involvement.

Corticosteroids are the mainstay of treatment of CSS, starting with 1 mg/kg/day of prednisone with progressive tapering over several months. Approximately half the patients without poor prognostic factors at onset achieve complete remission with corticosteroid treatment alone and do not have a relapse. Relapses of CSS must be distinguished from relapse or persistence of difficult asthma (with generally less than $0.5 \times 10^9/L$ blood eosinophils). Immunosuppressive treatment (such as oral azathioprine or intravenous pulses of cyclophosphamide) in addition to corticosteroids is reserved for a minority of patients with poor prognostic factors at onset (proteinuria greater than 1 g/day; renal insufficiency with serum creatinine greater than 15.8 mg/L; gastrointestinal tract involvement; cardiomyopathy; central nervous system involvement) and to those with relapses under more than 20 mg of prednisone daily. Subcutaneous interferon-α has been successfully used in patients with CSS with severe disease. The prognosis of CSS has improved considerably over the years, with presently 80% of patients alive at 5 years.

The possible role of triggering or adjuvant factors such as vaccines or desensitization in the development of CSS has been suspected. Drug-induced eosinophilic vasculitis with pulmonary involvement has been occasionally reported. The possible responsibility of leukotriene-receptor antagonists in the development of CSS is still debated, and these agents must be avoided in patients with asthma and eosinophilia and/or extrapulmonary manifestations.

Idiopathic Hypereosinophilic Syndromes

The historical definition of the idiopathic HES included a persistent eosinophilia greater than 1.5×10^9/L for longer than 6 months, a lack of evidence for a known cause of eosinophilia, and presumptive signs and symptoms of organ involvement. Recent studies have demonstrated that HES may result especially from clonal proliferation of lymphocytes or of the eosinophil cell lineage itself (Table 52-1).

HES, as described in older series, was much more common in men than in women (9:1), occurred between 20 and 50 years of age, and had an insidious onset of weakness, fatigue, cough, and dyspnea, with mean eosinophil count at presentation up to 20×10^9/L. Nonrespiratory manifestations of the HES mainly target the skin, heart, and nervous system.

Cardiac involvement present in 60% of patients is mainly characterized by endomyocardial fibrosis, often associated with intracavitary thrombi developing along the endocardium, and clinically associated with restrictive cardiomyopathy. Echocardiography shows the classic features of mural thrombus, ventricular apical obliteration, and involvement of the posterior mitral leaflet.

Lung involvement present in 40% of patients is nonspecific. Cough may be the predominant feature. Pleural effusion and pulmonary opacities on chest CT (interstitial infiltrates, ground-glass attenuation, small nodules) have been reported. The pulmonary manifestations of HES have not been reevaluated since the recent description of the two variants of HES. These must be distinguished from pleural effusion secondary to cardiac failure.

The "lymphocytic variant" of HES is a T-cell disorder resulting from the production of chemokines (especially IL-5) by clonal Th2 lymphocytes bearing an aberrant antigenic surface phenotype (such as $CD3^- CD4^+$). IgE level is elevated in most cases as a consequence of IL-4 and IL-13 production by Th2 lymphocytes. Most patients initially have cutaneous papules or urticarial plaques infiltrated by lymphocytes and eosinophils. The lymphocytic variant may account for approximately 30% of patients with HES. Lymphocyte phenotyping to detect a phenotypically aberrant T cell subset, and analysis of the rearrangement of the T-cell receptor genes in search of T-cell clonality, should be performed on the peripheral blood and bone marrow.

The "myeloproliferative variant" of HES is distinguished on the basis of clinical and biologic features common with chronic myeloproliferative syndromes, including hepatomegaly, splenomegaly, anemia, thrombocythemia, increased serum vitamin B_{12} and leukocyte alkaline phosphatase, and circulating leukocyte precursors. Mucosal ulcerations may be prominent. Severe cardiac manifestations are frequent and may resist corticosteroid treatment. The myeloproliferative variant of HES is attributed to a constitutively activated tyrosine kinase fusion protein (*Fip1L1-PDGFRα*) because of an interstitial chromosomal deletion in 4q12. Imatinib, a tyrosine kinase inhibitor used to treat chronic myelogenous leukemia, proved efficient in patients with the myeloproliferative variant of HES.

Only approximately half of the patients with HES respond to corticosteroid treatment. Other treatments include chemotherapeutic agents (hydroxyurea, vincristine, etoposide), cyclosporin, interferon-α (particularly in the myeloproliferative variant), and the anti-IL-5 antibody mepolizumab. Imatinib has become the major drug used in patients with the myeloproliferative variant of HES, especially when the FipL1-PDGFRα fusion protein is present. The prognosis of HES has improved markedly with approximately 70% survival at 1 year.

Pitfalls and Controversies

- The diagnosis of parasitic diseases in patients with eosinophilic pneumonia may be difficult and requires appropriate serologic tests and repeated search of parasites in the feces. It must be considered in any patient who lived in or visited an endemic area.

TABLE 52-1 Distinctive Characteristics of the Lymphocytic and the Myeloproliferative Variants of the Hypereosinophilic Syndromes

	Lymphocytic Variant	Myeloproliferative Variant
Distinctive clinical features	Skin manifestations: cutaneous papules or urticarial plaques	Male predominance Cardiac involvement Hepatomegaly, splenomegaly Mucosal ulcerations
Distinctive biologic features	Elevated serum IgE Hypergammaglobulinemia (polyclonal) Clonal peripheral lymphocytes with aberrant $CD3^- CD4^+$ surface phenotype Elevated serum IL-5	Anemia, thrombocythemia Increased serum vitamin B_{12} Increased leukocyte alkaline phosphatase Circulating leukocyte precursors Increased serum tryptase Identification of activated tyrosine kinase fusion protein
Pathogeny	T-cell clonal proliferation producing the Th2 cytokine IL-5	*FipL1 – PDGFRα* fusion protein resulting from interstitial deletion on chromosome 4q12
Main treatment considerations	Corticosteroids Interferon-α Anti-IL-5 (mepolizumab)	Imatinib Hydroxyurea Interferon-α Anti-IL-5 (mepolizumab)

- Eosinophilic pneumonia has been reported in association with a variety of drugs, but causality has been confidently established in fewer than 20.
- The dose and duration of treatment of ICEP with corticosteroids have not been established. Disease control must be balanced with treatment side effects.
- How respiratory exposure, including recent tobacco smoking, contributes to the pathogenesis of "idiopathic" acute eosinophilic pneumonia is unknown.
- There are currently no established diagnostic criteria for CSS. ANCA are present in fewer than 50% of patients, and true vasculitis is not present in all the patients.
- Asthma is a common denominator in most patients with ICEP and CSS.

SUGGESTED READINGS

Chitkara RK, Krishna G: Parasitic pulmonary eosinophilia. Semin Respir Crit Care Med 2006; 27:171–184.

Cordier JF: Eosinophilic pneumonias. In Schwarz MI King TE, Jr, eds: Interstitial Lung Disease, 4th ed. London: B.C. Decker Inc; 2003: 657–700.

Guillevin L, Cohen P, Gayraud M, et al: Churg-Strauss syndrome. Clinical study and long-term follow-up of 96 patients. Medicine (Baltimore) 1999; 78:26–37.

Keogh KA, Specks U: Churg-Strauss syndrome. Semin Respir Crit Care Med 2006; 27:148–157.

Marchand E, Etienne-Mastroïanni B, Chanez P, et al: the Groupe d'Etudes et de Recherche sur les Maladies "Orphelines" Pulmonaires: Idiopathic chronic eosinophilic pneumonia and asthma: How do they influence each other? Eur Respir J 2003; 22:8–13.

Marchand E, Reynaud-Gaubert M, Lauque D, et al: Idiopathic chronic eosinophilic pneumonia. A clinical and follow-up study of 62 cases. The Groupe d'Etudes et de Recherche sur les Maladies "Orphelines" Pulmonaires (GERM"O"P). Medicine (Baltimore) 1998; 77:299–312.

Pagnoux C, Guilpain P, Guillevin L: Churg-Strauss syndrome. Curr Opin Rheumatol 2007; 19:25–32.

Philit D, Etienne-Mastroïanni B, Parrot A, et al: Idiopathic acute eosinophilic pneumonia: A study of 22 patients. The Groupe d'Etudes et de Recherche sur les Maladies "Orphelines" Pulmonaires (GERM"O"P). Am J Respir Crit Care Med 2002; 166:1235–1239.

Rothenberg ME, Hogan SP: The eosinophil. Annu Rev Immunol 2006; 24:147–174.

Roufosse F, Goldman M, Cogan E: Hypereosinophilic syndrome: lymphoproliferative and myeloproliferative variants. Semin Respir Crit Care Med 2006; 27:158–170.

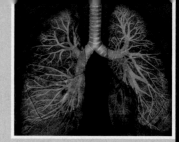

SECTION XII
DIFFUSE LUNG DISEASES

53 Organizing Pneumonia

JEAN-FRANÇOIS CORDIER • VINCENT COTTIN

DEFINITION

Organizing pneumonia (OP) is the name given to a pathologic pattern resulting from organization of an inflammatory exudate in the lumen of alveoli when resolution of pneumonia (e.g., pneumococcal pneumonia) does not occur. This characteristic pathologic pattern consists of intraalveolar buds of granulation tissue with fibroblasts and myofibroblasts intermixed with loose connective matrix (Figures 53-1 and 53-2). Similar lesions may be present within the lumen of the bronchioles, from which the previous term *bronchiolitis obliterans with organizing pneumonia (BOOP)* was derived. The latter nomenclature has been abandoned, because OP (and not bronchiolitis) is clearly the major lesion, and, furthermore, the term *bronchiolitis obliterans* in a source of confusion with bronchiolitis with airflow obstruction occurring, for example, after lung or hematopoietic stem cell transplantation.

OP is a nonspecific consequence of interstitial inflammation that may be present as an accessory finding in many disorders, including nonspecific interstitial pneumonia, usual interstitial pneumonia, organizing diffuse alveolar damage, aspiration pneumonia, vasculitides, or distal obstruction of the airways. Some histopathologic overlap may exist with chronic eosinophilic pneumonia or the OP-like variant of Wegener's granulomatosis. OP may be secondary to various defined agents or inflammatory disorders (e.g., connective tissue diseases) or may be cryptogenic (idiopathic). Additional findings suggestive of another diagnosis in secondary OP include necrosis or microabscesses (infectious process, necrotizing vasculitis).

However, OP is especially the major pathologic lesion underlying a characteristic clinical pathologic entity, namely cryptogenic organizing pneumonia (COP). COP has been included in the American Thoracic Society/European Respiratory Society international consensus classification of the idiopathic interstitial pneumonias (although it is not strictly interstitial).

PATHOGENESIS

The first event of the sequence leading to the formation of intraalveolar buds is alveolar epithelial injury with necrosis of pneumocytes (especially type I). The epithelial basal laminae are denuded and injured with the formation of gaps. Capillary endothelial injury is often associated. The consequence of alveolar injury is the flooding in the alveolar lumen by plasma proteins (permeability edema), including coagulation factors. The balance between coagulation and fibrinolysis is clearly in favor of coagulation (especially because of decreased fibrinolysis), thus leading to fibrin deposits that are soon populated by inflammatory cells and fibroblasts.

Fibroblasts differentiate into myofibroblasts and organize into fibroinflammatory buds. Inflammatory cells and fibrin are progressively replaced by aggregated fibroblasts/myofibroblasts intermixed with a loose connective matrix tissue rich in collagen (especially collagen III) and fibronectin. This process resembling that of cutaneous wound healing is similarly reversible without significant sequelae. It is likely that the relative preservation of the alveolar basal laminae is crucial in determining the reversibility of the lesions.

Animal models of intraluminal inflammation have been developed with a reovirus. Lesions similar to OP have been obtained by intranasal inoculation of moderate doses of virus in specific strains of mice (CBA/J) but not in other strains. Interestingly, diffuse alveolar damage with hyaline membranes was obtained with the same animal model when higher doses of virus are used. These experimental studies suggest that the intensity of the initial epithelial injury and yet undetermined factors inherent to the host may influence the evolution to either OP or diffuse alveolar damage. The mechanism by which corticosteroids facilitate the rapid resolution of OP is unclear.

CLINICAL FEATURES

Cryptogenic Organizing Pneumonia

The mean age of onset of COP is approximately 50–60 years. It is more common in nonsmokers or ex-smokers, with no gender predominance. The initial manifestations are fever, cough, malaise, anorexia, and progressive weight loss, with a subacute onset over a few weeks. Dyspnea is usually mild. Hemoptysis, chest pain, and severe dyspnea are rare. Crackles may be heard at pulmonary auscultation over involved areas. Finger clubbing is exceptional. The duration of symptoms before diagnosis is usually less than 2 months. In many patients the diagnosis is considered after they have received antibiotics without improvement.

The imaging pattern of typical COP consists of multiple patchy alveolar opacities (Figure 53-3). These are usually bilateral, located at the periphery of the lung, and sometimes migratory (with some opacities attenuating or clearing, whereas others appear in different areas), with a density ranging from ground glass to consolidation with air bronchogram. The size of the opacities may vary from 1–2 cm to lobar opacities. This imaging pattern of typical COP with multiple patchy alveolar opacities and especially being migratory are so characteristic that

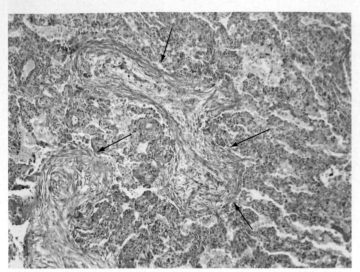

FIGURE 53-1 Buds of granulation tissue *(arrows)* in the lumen of alveoli. (Courtesy of F. Thivolet-Béjui, Lyon.)

they should immediately suggest the diagnosis. The main differential diagnosis at this stage is with idiopathic chronic eosinophilic pneumonia (in the latter, blood eosinophilia usually >1.5 G/L is present).

The other imaging patterns of COP are less characteristic and less frequently encountered. The infiltrative pattern associates interstitial opacities, with small superimposed alveolar opacities on HRCT (with possible perilobular pattern consisting of bowed or polygonal opacities with poorly defined margins bordering the interlobular septa) (Figure 53-4). Honeycombing is not present. Infiltrative COP may overlap both pathologically and on imaging with idiopathic nonspecific interstitial pneumonia (NSIP), where the pathologic lesions are alveolar interstitial uniform cellular inflammation (with more or less fibrosis), with the possible presence of foci of organizing pneumonia.

Another imaging pattern of COP is a solitary focal nodule or mass. It is often located in the upper lobes and is usually asymptomatic. An air bronchogram may be present. Diagnosis is often made by surgical resection of the lesion suspected to be a lung carcinoma, especially because OP may be associated with hypermetabolism on positron emission tomography. Solitary focal COP likely represents nonresolving infectious pneumonia in a number of cases.

Several less common imaging presentations of COP have been occasionally reported, including multiple nodules, cavitary opacities, nodules with reversed halo sign, and linear subpleural bands. Mediastinal lymphadenopathy is not rare in COP. Pleural effusion is uncommon.

Whereas mimics of COP with typical imaging features are few, mimics of COP presenting as nodules, masses, or infiltrative lung diseases are many (Box 53-1).

Lung function tests in COP show a mild restrictive ventilatory pattern and may occasionally be normal. The transfer coefficient for carbon monoxide is within normal limits, whereas the transfer factor is decreased in proportion with the restrictive defect. Hypoxemia is usually mild. When present, severe hypoxemia may be associated with diffuse infiltrative opacities or right-to-left shunting in perfused areas of lung consolidation.

Blood tests often show moderate leucocytosis and increased C-reactive protein but no significant peripheral blood eosinophilia.

Secondary Organizing Pneumonia

Secondary OP may result from a determined cause or occur in the context of systemic disorders (e.g., connective tissue disease) or other peculiar conditions. The clinical and imaging pattern of secondary OP parallel those of COP. A careful etiologic inquiry is thus necessary in any OP without evident cause. In most cases of secondary OP, corticosteroid treatment is effective.

Secondary OP of Determined Cause

A histopathology of OP prompts a search for a number of potential underlying causes, including a variety of infectious agents (bacteria, viruses, fungi, parasites). Diagnosis of the infection (which is no longer active at the time of OP) may be difficult and is based on the clinical history, the rise of antibody titers against the infectious agent, or occasionally on the direct identification of the infectious agent by use of specific stains and the pathologic analysis of the lung specimens.

Several drugs have been reported to cause OP (Box 53-2). All drugs taken in the weeks or months preceding the symptoms must be systematically recorded. Any drug suspected to be a cause of OP should be withdrawn if possible (rechallenge should be avoided). The diagnosis of drug-induced OP may be difficult, however, because it has no specific clinical radiologic presentation.

Radiation therapy to the breast after tumorectomy for cancer may precipitate the development of OP with an incidence of approximately 2.5% treated women and a mean delay of approximately 3–6 months after the completion of irradiation. In contrast with radiation pneumonitis, the alveolar opacities of OP (often migratory) may also appear in nonirradiated areas of the lungs. The opacities respond well to corticosteroid treatment, but relapses are common when corticosteroids are reduced or stopped. Interestingly, radiation therapy to the breast is followed by bilateral lymphocytic alveolitis at BAL, with only a minority of patients developing OP. This suggests that a "second trigger" and/or genetic susceptibility is necessary for OP to occur, in addition to radiation-primed lymphocytic alveolitis.

Secondary OP Occurring Within a Specific Context

OP occurs mainly in dermatomyositis-polymyositis and rheumatoid arthritis (it is less common in systemic lupus and Sjögren syndrome, and is exceptional in systemic sclerosis). OP may precede the development of the connective tissue disease or occur concomitantly, although it occurs more frequently during the course of the disease.

Multiple causes or clinical settings of secondary OP have been reported, a nonexhaustive list of which is reported in Box 53-3.

DIAGNOSIS OF ORGANIZING PNEUMONIA

When nonspecific clinical manifestations associated with typical imaging features suggest the diagnosis of COP, fiberoptic bronchoscopy (which excludes any bronchial obstruction) with BAL and transbronchial biopsies is necessary.

The BAL differential cell count in COP often shows a mixed pattern with increased levels of lymphocytes (20–40%), neutrophils (approximately 10%), and eosinophils (5%) (some mast cells and plasma cells may be present). The transbronchial lung biopsy specimens may show typical buds of granulation tissue within alveoli. The search for infectious agents on BAL differential cell count fluid and transbronchial biopsy specimens (by use of specific stains) must be systematically performed. The association of a typical clinical radiologic pattern and a mixed pattern at BAL differential cell count is considered highly suggestive of OP (and COP in the appropriate clinical context). A decreased ratio of CD4$^+$/CD8$^+$ lymphocytes in BAL has been reported in COP.

Because their small size does not allow exclusion of other pathologic patterns, informative transbronchial biopsies should be considered diagnostic of OP only in patients with a typical clinical and imaging profile. In addition, the diagnosis should be reconsidered whenever the outcome is unusual (especially in case of incomplete response to corticosteroids or relapse despite >20 mg/d of oral prednisone). The "gold standard" for the diagnosis of OP remains videothoracoscopic lung biopsy to obtain specimens of sufficient size to both definitely make the diagnosis of OP and exclude other processes. When performed, the biopsy should be done before corticosteroids are initiated. Microbiologic analysis may also be performed on the lung specimen.

TREATMENT OF COP

Corticosteroid treatment represents the current standard and results in rapid clinical and imaging improvement in typical COP. Pulmonary opacities on chest imaging usually completely resolve within a month. The doses and duration of treatment have not been established, and treatment should aim at the optimal balance between disease control and side effects. We start with prednisone, 0.75 mg/kg/d for 4 weeks, then progressively decrease for a total duration of treatment of 24 weeks, a treatment that limits intense and prolonged corticosteroid treatment with ensuing risk of iatrogenic complications. Relapses are common (up to 60% of cases) on decreasing or after stopping treatment, and these may be treated by doses of 20 mg/d of prednisone and progressively decreased. Relapses of the disease should prompt a search for a persisting cause of OP, especially drug intake. The overall prognosis of COP is excellent. Of note, spontaneous improvement or after treatment with macrolides has been reported in COP.

SEVERE ORGANIZING PNEUMONIA

Cases of severe COP have been reported, with potential severe respiratory failure requiring mechanical ventilation. Such cases only exceptionally correspond to pure OP pathologic lesions. They usually represent overlap of COP with one of the following: acute respiratory distress syndrome (ARDS) with pathologic features of diffuse alveolar damage undergoing organization; acute fibrinous and organizing pneumonia; or usual

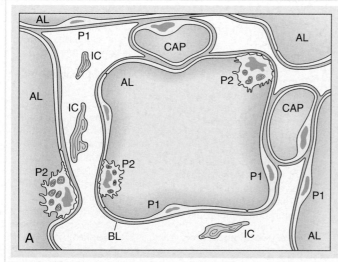

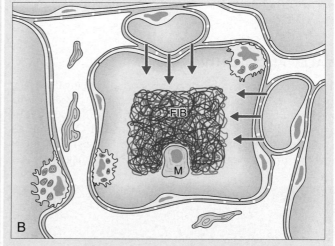

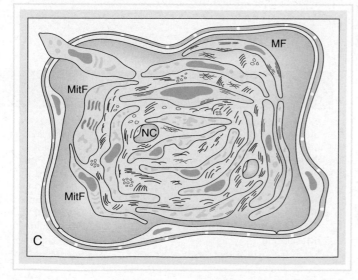

FIGURE 53-2 Formation of the intraalveolar buds of granulation tissue characterizing organizing pneumonia. **A,** Structure of the normal alveolar space (*CAP,* capillaries; *P1,* type 1 pneumocytes; *P2,* type 2 pneumocytes; *IC,* interstitial cells; *AL,* alveolar lumen; *BL,* basal laminae). **B,** Alveolar injury with alteration and necrosis of alveolar epithelial cells (especially type 1 pneumocytes), denudation of basal laminae with formation of gaps, and leaking of plasma proteins, especially coagulation factors (*arrows*) with formation of fibrin (FIB) within the alveolar lumen. Some inflammatory cells and macrophages are present. **C,** The intraluminal alveolar fibrin network has been colonized by fibroblasts *(F)* (*Mit. F,* mitotic fibroblast), with some of them acquiring a myofibroblast *(MF)* phenotype characterized by myofilaments beneath the cytoplasmic membrane. Fibroblast and myofibroblasts have a developed rough endoplasmic reticulum and produce a loose connective matrix (composed of collagens I and III, fibronectin, proteoglycans) interspersed between the cells. Neoformed capillaries *(NC)* are present within this intraalveolar bud of granulation tissue resembling wound healing.

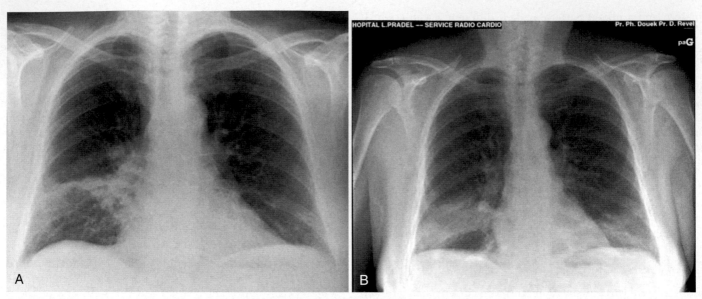

FIGURE 53-3 A, Patchy alveolar opacity. **B,** Six days later, the distribution of the right lower lobe opacity changed, a new contralateral basal opacity appeared.

interstitial pneumonia exacerbation. In such cases, the response to corticosteroids is not as favorable as in classical COP. Immunosuppressive agents (especially cyclophosphamide) are usually added to corticosteroids (often used at a higher dose, starting with 1–2 mg/kg/d of intravenous methylprednisolone) with variable outcome.

PITFALLS AND CONTROVERSIES

- OP is a nonspecific pathologic pattern found in many disorders, especially nonresolving infectious pneumonia. Assessing its clinical significance may be difficult. OP may be difficult to distinguish pathologically from occasional areas of OP present as an accessory finding in another disorder (e.g., nonspecific interstitial pneumonia, organizing diffuse alveolar damage).

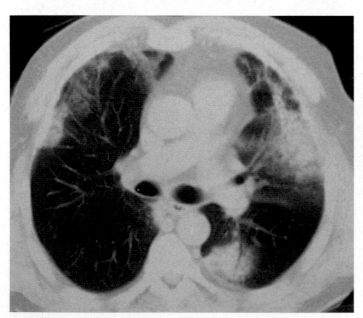

FIGURE 53-4 HRCT of typical COP. Bilateral peripheral patchy opacities (with an air bronchogram in the left opacities).

BOX 53-1 Mimics of COP on Chest Imaging

Multiple patchy alveolar opacities

Eosinophilic pneumonia (especially chronic idiopathic)
Bronchioloalveolar carcinoma
Primary pulmonary lymphoma (low-grade B-cell lymphoma of the mucosa associated lymphoid tissue, MALT)
Others: infectious pneumonia; Wegener's granulomatosis; diffuse alveolar hemorrhage; multiple infarction; aspiration pneumonia

Solitary focal nodule or mass

Bronchogenic carcinoma

Round pneumonia or abscess
Inflammatory pseudotumors
Others: all causes of coin lesions or masses

Diffuse infiltrative opacities

Idiopathic interstitial pneumonias, especially nonspecific interstitial pneumonia and idiopathic pulmonary fibrosis (especially in the exacerbation phase)
Others: all causes of infiltrative opacities especially of infectious or neoplastic origin

---

BOX 53-2 Main Drugs as Cause of Organizing Pneumonia

5-Aminosalicylic acid	Methotrexate
Acebutolol	Minocycline
Amiodarone	Nilutamide
Bleomycin	Nitrofurantoin
Busulfan	Rituximab
Carbamazepine	Sirolimus
Fluvastatin	Sulfasalazine
Interferon-α	Tacrolimus
Interferon-β	Thalidomide
Mesalazine	Trastuzumab

BOX 53-3 Miscellaneous Causes or Clinical Settings of Organizing Pneumonia

Aerosolized textile dye Acramin FWN; mustard gas
Paraquat (ingested)
Occult aspiration pneumonia
Connective tissue disease
Transplantation (lung, liver, bone marrow)
Primary biliary cirrhosis
Hematologic malignancies (leukemias, myeloblastic, lymphoblastic myelomonocytic, T-cell; Hodgkin disease)
Cancers and postthoracic radiotherapy
Inflammatory bowel diseases (ulcerative colitis; Crohn disease)
Others: common variable immune deficiency; Sweet syndrome; polymyalgia rheumatica; Behçet disease; thyroid diseases; sarcoidosis

---

- What differentiates the pathogenic fibrosing process of OP (which resolves with corticosteroids) from that of idiopathic pulmonary fibrosis (resistant to steroids) is poorly understood.
- The diagnostic value of BAL in COP has not been formally evaluated.
- The dose and duration of treatment with corticosteroids have not been established. Disease control must be balanced with treatment side effects.

SUGGESTED READINGS

American Thoracic Society/European Respiratory Society: Classification of the idiopathic interstitial pneumonias. International multidisciplinary consensus. American Thoracic Society/European Respiratory Society. Am J Respir Crit Care Med 2002; 165:277–304.

Beasley MB, Franks TJ, Galvin JR, et al: Acute fibrinous and organizing pneumonia: a histological pattern of lung injury and possible variant of diffuse alveolar damage. Arch Pathol Lab Med 2002; 126:1064–1070.

Colby TV: Pathologic aspects of bronchiolitis obliterans organizing pneumonia. Chest 1992; 102:38S–43S.

Cordier JF: Cryptogenic organising pneumonia. Eur Respir J 2006; 28: 422–446.

Cordier JF, Loire R, Brune J: Idiopathic bronchiolitis obliterans organizing pneumonia. Definition of characteristic clinical profiles in a series of 16 patients. Chest 1989; 96:999–1004.

Costabel U, Teschler H, Guzman J: Bronchiolitis obliterans organizing pneumonia (BOOP): The cytological and immunocytological profile of bronchoalveolar lavage. Eur Respir J 1992; 5:791–797.

Crestani B, Valeyre D, Roden S, et al, and the Groupe d'Etudes et de Recherche sur les Maladies Orphelines Pulmonaires (GERM"O"P): Bronchiolitis obliterans organizing pneumonia syndrome primed by radiation therapy to the breast. Am J Respir Crit Care Med 1998; 158:1929–1935.

Davison AG, Heard BE, McAllister WAC, Turner-Warwick ME: Cryptogenic organizing pneumonitis. Q J Med 1983; 52:382–394.

Epler GR, Colby TV, McLoud TC, et al: Bronchiolitis obliterans organizing pneumonia. N Engl J Med 1985; 312:152–158.

Lazor R, Vandevenne A, Pelletier A, et al, and the Groupe d'Etudes et de Recherche sur les Maladies "Orphelines" Pulmonaires (GERM"O"P): Cryptogenic organizing pneumonia. Characteristics of relapses in a series of 48 patients. Am J Respir Crit Care Med 2000; 162:571–577.

Lohr RH, Boland BJ, Douglas WW, et al: Organizing pneumonia. Features and prognosis of cryptogenic, secondary, and focal variants. Arch Intern Med 1997; 157:1323–1329.

Peyrol S, Cordier JF, Grimaud JA: Intra-alveolar fibrosis of idiopathic bronchiolitis obliterans-organizing pneumonia. Cell-matrix patterns. Am J Pathol 1990; 137:155–170.

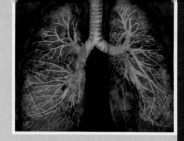

54 LAM and Other Diffuse Lung Diseases

ERIC J. OLSON • JEFFREY L. MYERS • JAY H. RYU

The term *diffuse lung diseases* encompasses a broad array of disorders, many of which are covered in other chapters. This chapter focuses primarily on four distinct and uncommon diffuse lung diseases: pulmonary lymphangiomyomatosis (LAM), pulmonary Langerhans cell histiocytosis (PLCH), lymphoid interstitial pneumonia (LIP), and pulmonary alveolar proteinosis (PAP). The unique epidemiologic, pathophysiologic, clinical, radiographic, management, and prognostic features will be described. In addition, this chapter briefly reviews several other rare forms of diffuse lung disease.

The terms *lymphangiomyomatosis*, *lymphangioleiomyomatosis*, and *pulmonary lymphangiomyomatosis* are used interchangeably. This process may involve pulmonary and/or extrapulmonary sites, including the mediastinal or retroperitoneal lymphatic system and abdominopelvic organs such as the uterus and kidneys. The discussion will concentrate on pulmonary LAM, which is the most common presentation. LAM is characterized by atypical smooth muscle proliferation in the lung that results in diffuse cystic changes and airway obstruction, recurrent pneumothoraces, and chylous pleural effusions. PLCH is the preferred term for the disease characterized by the proliferation and infiltration of the lung by Langerhans cells, with or without involvement of other organs, superseding other terms such as *primary pulmonary histiocytosis X*, *pulmonary eosinophilic granuloma*, *Langerhans cell granulomatosis*, *Letterer–Siwe disease*, and *Hand–Schüller–Christian disease*. Diffuse cystic changes in the lungs, airways obstruction, and recurrent pneumothoraces may also be seen with PLCH; in adults, this condition is strongly associated with smoking. LIP, initially described by Liebow and Carrington as a subtype of the idiopathic interstitial pneumonias, is marked by diffuse interstitial infiltration of the lung with lymphocytic and plasma cell components. It may be associated with a variety of underlying disorders; idiopathic LIP is considered rare. PAP, also called *alveolar proteinosis*, *alveolar phospholipidosis*, *alveolar lipoproteinosis*, and *pulmonary alveolar phospholipoproteinosis*, is a process characterized by accumulation of lipoproteinaceous material in the alveolar spaces (Figure 54-1).

EPIDEMIOLOGY, RISK FACTORS, AND PATHOPHYSIOLOGY

LAM is almost exclusively a disease of women of childbearing age, with the onset of symptoms typically occurring in the third and fourth decades of life. However, several cases have been reported in postmenopausal women, sometimes in association with postmenopausal hormone replacement, and biopsy-confirmed disease has also been documented in a man (with tuberous sclerosis complex). The cause of LAM is unknown, but its predilection for women, association with postmenopausal hormonal therapy, and occasional acceleration during pregnancy suggests a pathogenic role for estrogenic hormones. Most LAM cases occur sporadically but can also occur in subjects with tuberous sclerosis complex (TSC). TSC is an autosomal-dominant disorder characterized by hamartoma formation in multiple organ systems, including the central nervous system (cortical tubers; subependymal nodules; subependymal giant cell astrocytomas), skin (facial angiofibromas; periungual or ungual fibromas), eye (retinal nodular hamartomas), and abdominal viscera (renal angiomyolipomas [AMLs]). Up to 30–40% of women with TSC may have radiographic changes consistent with LAM. Alternately, patients with sporadic LAM may have some of the extrapulmonary manifestations seen in TSC, such as renal AMLs, thoracoabdominal lymphadenopathy, and abdominopelvic lymphangioleiomyomas, but they do not have evidence for hamartomatosis in other organ systems and thus do not fulfill the diagnostic criteria for TSC. The pathophysiologic basis of sporadic LAM (Figure 54-2) and TSC-LAM—namely, atypical smooth muscle cell proliferation—is believed to be similar and related to shared genetic factors (see "Genetics"). Prevalence of sporadic LAM has been estimated at approximately 2 cases per million women in the United States.

Dendritic cells are a diverse group of antigen-presenting cells that are classified according to their location, surface markers, and function. Langerhans cells are a specific population of dendritic cells that are present in normal lung, almost exclusively intercalated between epithelial cells of the airways. Their role is to engage inhaled antigens, then migrate to regional lymph nodes to stimulate a specific lymphocytic inflammatory response (see Chapter 11). Langerhans cells are distinguished by their characteristic pentilaminar, platelike cytoplasmic organelles (Birbeck granule or X-body) (Figure 54-3) seen on electron microscopy and their strong expression of the CD1a antigen on the cell surface. They also stain with S-100 and CD45 antibodies. PLCH is part of the spectrum of Langerhans' cell histiocytosis, diseases characterized by the unrestrained growth and infiltration of organs by Langerhans cells. The cause of the excessive proliferation of Langerhans cells in PLCH is not known, although the strong association with cigarette smoking suggests a causal link. Most studies have shown that more than 90% of PLCH patients are current or previous cigarette smokers. Furthermore, PLCH may regress with smoking cessation. It is postulated that cigarette smoking leads to recruitment and proliferation of Langerhans cells in the lung

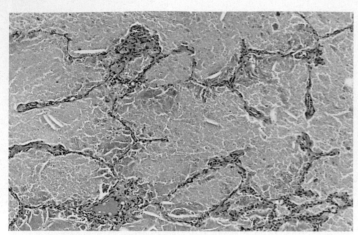

FIGURE 54-1 Histopathology of pulmonary alveolar proteinosis (PAP). Photomicrograph of PAP showing alveolar spaces filled with amorphous granular eosinophilic debris. The proteinaceous exudate includes scattered cell "ghosts." Alveolar septa are only minimally thickened in this predominantly airspace lesion.

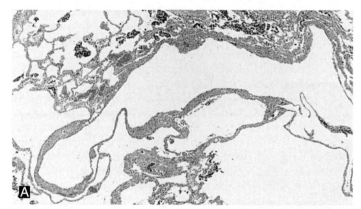

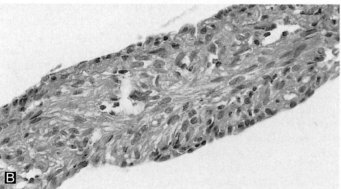

FIGURE 54-2 Histopathology of lymphangiomyomatosis (LAM). **A,** Low-magnification photomicrograph of LAM showing cystic spaces surrounded by a variably thick wall containing proliferating spindle cells. Hemosiderin pigment is present in adjacent air spaces, which attests to the presence of alveolar hemorrhage. **B,** Higher magnification photomicrograph showing smooth muscle cells within thickened peribronchiolar interstitium in LAM.

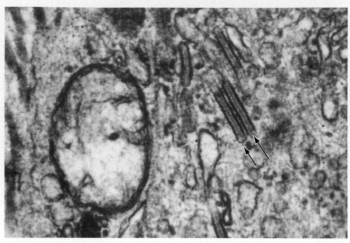

FIGURE 54-3 Langerhans cell histiocytosis. Electron micrograph showing Birbeck granules (*arrows*).

parenchyma. In extrapulmonary sites, Langerhans' cell proliferation may be monoclonal; however, most cases of PLCH seen in adults are believed to represent a reactive, not neoplastic, process. Morphologic studies show proliferating Langerhans cells involved in a bronchocentric process accompanied by mixed cellular infiltrates (Figure 54-4). Adjacent blood vessels and lung parenchyma are also involved. As this granulomatous-like reaction evolves, collagen fibrosis and scarring occur, with associated paracicatricial airspace enlargement that accounts for the concomitant cystic changes. The incidence and prevalence of PLCH are not well defined. Most cases occur in Caucasians between the ages of 20 and 40 years. Early studies suggested a male predominance, whereas more recent studies indicate higher involvement in women.

The classification of LIP has varied over time from an interstitial pneumonia to a lymphoproliferative disorder. Because its histologic pattern is that of an interstitial pneumonia and very few cases develop into lymphoma, the American Thoracic Society/European Respiratory Society consensus classification includes LIP in the list of idiopathic interstitial pneumonias. It seems, however, that LIP is rarely idiopathic and more commonly is associated with a variety of underlying conditions, including immunodeficiencies (human immunodeficiency virus [HIV] infection; severe combined immunodeficiency), collagen vascular disease (Sjögren's syndrome; rheumatoid arthritis; systemic lupus erythematosus), and other immunologic disorders (Hashimoto's thyroiditis; chronic active hepatitis; primary biliary cirrhosis; myasthenia gravis; pernicious anemia; and autoimmune hemolytic anemia). LIP is uncommon. From January 1985 to December 1999, just 15 patients with surgical lung biopsy-proven LIP (of 1167 surgical lung biopsies) were identified at the National Jewish Medical and Research Center (Denver, CO), and only 3 patients were classified as "idiopathic." The Epstein–Barr virus genome has been identified in some patients who have LIP. Most HIV-negative patients who have LIP are adults in their fourth to seventh decades. Women are more commonly affected than men. However, those who have LIP in association with HIV infection tend to be younger, with a male predominance.

PAP affects men about twice as often as women, and the disorder has been encountered in virtually all industrialized countries. The estimated incidence and prevalence are 0.36

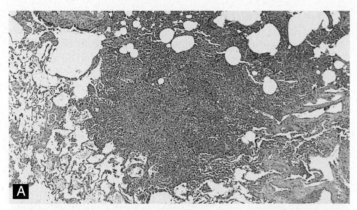

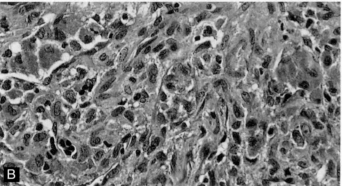

FIGURE 54-4 Histopathology of pulmonary Langerhans cell histiocytosis (PLCH). **A,** Low-magnification photomicrograph showing stellate, bronchocentric nodule in PLCH. **B,** High-magnification photomicrograph showing a polymorphic, interstitial infiltrate in PLCH. The cellular infiltrate includes a mixture of mononuclear cells and eosinophils. Langerhans cells predominate and are differentiated by highly convoluted nuclei with nuclear grooves, which result in nuclear configurations that resemble crumpled paper or coffee beans.

and 3.70 cases per million population, respectively. PAP is restricted to the lungs and is characterized by accumulation of periodic acid–Schiff (PAS)–positive, acellular, lipoproteinaceous surfactant component material in the alveolar spaces with negligible interstitial inflammation. PAP occurs most commonly as a primary acquired disorder but can also occur as a congenital disorder or as a secondary form in association with pulmonary infections, exposure to inhaled chemicals (insecticides) and minerals (silica; aluminum dust; titanium), immunodeficiency disorders (severe combined immunodeficiency disorder; immunoglobulin A deficiency; HIV), and hematologic disorders (lymphoma; leukemia). Pathogenesis primarily involves disrupted clearance of surfactant material by alveolar macrophages that, in some situations, seems related to impaired action of granulocyte-macrophage colony-stimulating factor (GM-CSF).

GENETICS

LAM and TSC are separate disorders, but they seem to share some genetic features as they do clinical traits. TSC results from mutations of either the hamartin *(TSC1)* gene on chromosome 9 or the tuberin *(TSC2)* gene on chromosome 16, both tumor suppressor genes. Hamartin and tuberin form a complex that is a negative regulator of the cell cycle. Inactivating mutations and loss of heterozygosity in the *TSC2* gene,

and, less commonly, mutations in *TSC1* gene have also been found in the cells of sporadic LAM patients, supporting a role for *TSC* genes in LAM pathogenesis. It remains unclear how *TSC1* or *TSC2* mutations correlate with the expression of LAM clinical features. Tracking of *TSC2* mutations has raised the possibility that LAM cells can metastasize. Renal AML cells and pulmonary LAM cells in sporadic LAM have been shown to contain the identical *TSC2* mutation not present in other, normal cells. LAM cells from recurrent disease in an engrafted lung have been shown to contain the same *TSC2* mutation present in native LAM cells before transplant, and the *TSC2* mutation was also found in four separate mediastinal lymph nodes. LAM cells, as defined by loss of heterozygosity of the *TSC2* gene, have also been detected in body fluids, such as blood and pleural/abdominal chyle.

PLCH is thought to be a reactive, polyclonal process usually provoked by cigarette smoking in susceptible individuals. Most cases occur sporadically. No predisposing genetic factors have been identified, yet there have been rare reports of familial clustering of cases.

The genetic aspects of LIP are not well defined.

The serendipitous observation that GM-CSF knockout mice develop lung disease similar to human PAP suddenly raised awareness of the important role of GM-CSF surfactant homeostasis. GM-CSF binding to specific receptors on alveolar macrophages is an important step in the degradation of surfactant. The primary acquired form of PAP seems to be due to GM-CSF neutralizing autoantibodies that functionally impair the GM-CSF–macrophage interaction and thereby diminish clearance of surfactant material by alveolar macrophages. Decreased GM-CSF stimulation probably also contributes to the other functional defects shown by alveolar macrophages in PAP, which results in an increased risk of pulmonary infections in this disorder. Congenital PAP is an autosomal-recessive, usually fatal, disorder of infants and children. Genetic alterations that have been described in these patients include mutations in the surfactant protein B gene, resulting in surfactant protein B deficiencies, mutations in the ATP-binding cassette transporter A3 sequence possibly resulting in abnormal surfactant phospholipids, and mutations in the GM-CSF receptor likely leading to a reduced effect of GM-CSF on alveolar macrophages. A rare genetic disorder, lysinuric protein intolerance, which results in impaired cellular amino acid transport, may lead to secondary PAP. Several mechanisms may explain PAP in the context of hematologic malignancies, including numerical deficiencies in normal macrophages because of impaired bone marrow production of peripheral blood monocytes (the precursors of alveolar macrophages) or displacement by functionally impaired alveolar macrophages derived from the leukemic clone.

CLINICAL FEATURES

To learn more about its clinical characteristics, a national LAM registry was established by the National Institutes of Health (NIH) (Bethesda, MD) in 1997. From 1998 to 2001, 243 patients with either new or established LAM were enrolled at six participating clinical centers. Thirteen patients had already undergone lung transplant and were excluded from the report of clinical features at time of enrollment. All subjects were women, with ages ranging from 18 to 76 years. The average age at symptom onset was 39 years and at diagnosis

41 years. The most common symptoms were breathlessness (73%), wheezing (47%), cough (31%), hemoptysis (34%), phlegm production (27%), and chyloptysis (7%). The sentinel event leading to LAM diagnosis was usually a pulmonary condition and included spontaneous pneumothorax (36%), other pulmonary symptoms (including dyspnea and wheezing) (28%), abnormal chest radiograph (20%), renal AML (4%), and pleural effusion (3%). Overall, 56% reported at least one spontaneous pneumothorax, 38% renal AMLs, and 21% pleural effusion. Sixty-seven percent had been pregnant and of those who could recall symptoms, 22% had experienced worsening of respiratory symptoms during pregnancy. TSC was present in 15%. Those with LAM-TSC were younger, were more likely to have renal AMLs, had less impaired pulmonary function, and were less likely to be treated with a progesterone derivative than those with sporadic LAM. There were no significant differences between the groups with respect to respiratory symptoms. Physical examination is usually unremarkable except for signs of pleural effusion or pneumothorax (if present) or occasional wheeze or basal crackles. Patients with TSC-LAM usually show pathognomonic findings of TSC, such as facial angiofibromas, and periungual or ungual fibromas.

The clinical presentation of PLCH most commonly includes dyspnea and nonproductive cough in a current or former smoker. A history of spontaneous pneumothorax is obtained in approximately 10–20% of patients, with a similar percentage of patients having no symptoms or only mild, nonspecific symptoms in the early stages of disease. Other symptoms may include wheezing, fever, fatigue, weight loss, and chest pain. Hemoptysis is uncommon (<5% of patients). Examination sometimes reveals crackles, wheeze, and digital clubbing. Approximately 15% of patients have extrapulmonary manifestations, including diabetes insipidus from hypothalamic involvement, pain from bone involvement, adenopathy from lymph node infiltration, rash from cutaneous involvement, and abdominal discomfort from hepatosplenic involvement.

Patients with LIP are usually symptomatic at presentation, most commonly reporting gradually progressive dyspnea and cough over a 3-year or greater period. Less common symptoms include weight loss, fever, chest pain, fatigue, and arthralgias. On examination, bibasilar crackles are heard in most patients, whereas digital clubbing and pneumothorax are unusual. Physical signs of associated conditions, such as connective tissue disorders, should be sought, because idiopathic LIP is considered a rare entity. Dysproteinemia, most commonly polyclonal hypergammaglobulinemia, monoclonal increase in IgG or IgM, or hypogammaglobulinemia, is found in more than 75% of patients. Rheumatoid factor and antinuclear antibody titers may be elevated in those who have Sjögren's syndrome in association with LIP.

Clinical presentation of PAP is nonspecific, with progressive dyspnea of insidious onset and a dry cough in most patients. Less common symptoms include chest pain, hemoptysis, weight loss, chills, fatigue, and arthralgias. Fever is also unusual and should raise suspicion for a superimposed process, such as infection. Crackles may occur over the involved areas of lung in approximately 20% of patients. Digital clubbing is uncommon and cyanosis is seen with severe disease. A review of the PAP cases reported to date indicated the median duration of symptoms before diagnosis was 7 months, the median age at diagnosis was 39 years, and most patients were smokers at symptom onset. Mildly elevated serum lactate dehydrogenase level is common, and increased levels of lung

surfactant A and D (SP-A and SP-D) and mucin-like glycoprotein (KL-6) in the serum have also been found in PAP; however, these findings are not specific. Patients affected by PAP may have PAS-positive material or elevated SP-A levels in their sputum, but these findings are also nonspecific. Serologic testing for GM-CSF autoantibodies is not routinely performed.

Chest radiographs of LAM patients are usually abnormal and show diffuse reticular and nodular densities, without sparing of the costophrenic angles (Figure 54-5). As the disease progresses, cystic changes may become apparent, together with signs of hyperinflation. Pneumothorax and/or pleural effusions may accompany infiltrates. However, early in the disease the chest radiograph may be entirely normal. High-resolution computed tomography (HRCT) of the chest reveals well-defined cystic spaces throughout both lungs, even in those patients with normal chest radiographs (Figure 54-6). Cystic changes are diffuse, with no sparing of the costophrenic angles. The cysts have uniformly thin walls and measure a few millimeters to several centimeters in diameter. Most are round, but they can coalesce into bizarre shapes as the disease progresses. Pleural effusions, pneumothoraces, and mediastinal adenopathy, which sometimes are not apparent on the chest radiograph, may also be seen. Most of the lung parenchyma between the cystic spaces appears normal. No difference is found in the appearance of the lungs of patients who have sporadic LAM versus those who have TSC-LAM. When CT of the chest is performed in a woman suspected of having LAM, it is useful to extend the scanning to the pelvis to look for renal AMLs, retroperitoneal lymphangiomyomas, or adenopathy.

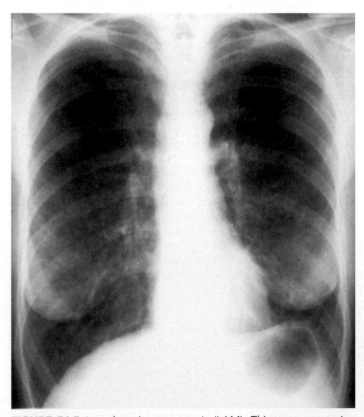

FIGURE 54-5 Lymphangiomyomatosis (LAM). This posteroanterior chest radiograph of a 37-year-old woman with LAM shows hyperinflation and diffuse reticular infiltrates.

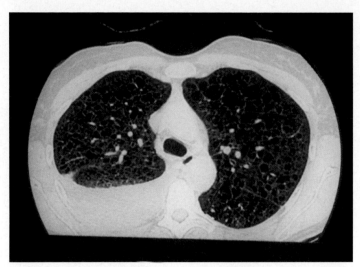

FIGURE 54-6 Lymphangiomyomatosis (LAM). High-resolution computed tomogram of a 42-year-old woman with tuberous sclerosis complex (TSC) with lung involvement (lymphangiomyomatosis) showing diffuse cystic changes and a right pleural effusion (chylothorax).

The typical chest radiographic finding in PLCH is reticulonodular infiltrates, most prominent in the middle and upper zones (Figure 54-7). The lung volume appears normal or increased, which helps distinguish PLCH from other diffuse lung diseases (except LAM) that usually produce reduced lung volumes. Sparing of the costophrenic angles helps distinguish PLCH from LAM. As the disease advances, cystic changes and bullae appear that may be difficult to distinguish from emphysema. Pleural disease (except for pneumothorax) and adenopathy are uncommon. Predilection for the middle and

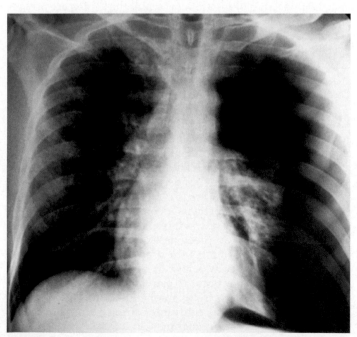

FIGURE 54-7 Pulmonary Langerhans cell histiocytosis. Posteroanterior chest radiograph of a 25-year-old male smoker with dyspnea. Massive left pneumothorax and interstitial infiltrates are seen in the right lung.

upper lung zones is confirmed by HRCT of the chest, which also shows thin-walled cysts and nodules (with or without cavitation), reticular densities, and some areas of ground-glass opacity (Figure 54-8). The cysts are irregularly shaped and more complex than those seen in LAM.

Chest radiography reveals basilar-predominant reticulonodular opacities in patients with LIP. Superimposed, patchy alveolar (Figure 54-9) or nodular infiltrates are present in approximately half of the patients. HRCT of the chest patterns include ground-glass opacities, interlobular septal thickening, centrilobular nodules, diffuse consolidation, cystic airspaces, and, in advanced cases, honeycombing. Mediastinal or hilar adenopathy and pleural effusions are infrequent in HIV-negative patients. However, intrathoracic adenopathy may be seen in up to one third of HIV-infected patients with LIP.

The intraalveolar buildup of surfactant-like material in patients with PAP results in bilateral, patchy airspace infiltrates on chest radiographs (Figure 54-10). Less commonly, an interstitial pattern may be seen. Infiltrates are often more prominent in the perihilar regions, and this "bat-wing" pattern may be mistaken for pulmonary edema. The radiographic differential diagnosis can include sarcoidosis, infections, bronchoalveolar cell carcinoma, pneumoconiosis, and other diffuse

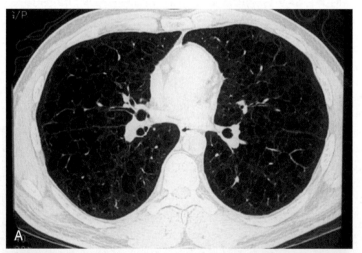
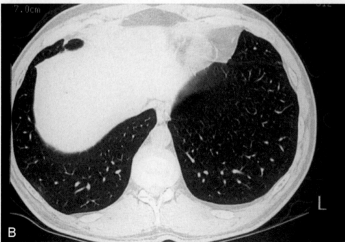

FIGURE 54-8 Pulmonary Langerhans cell histiocytosis. High-resolution computed tomograms of the same patient shown in Figure 54-7 taken 6 years after presentation. **A,** Diffuse cystic changes are seen with **(B)** relative sparing of bibasilar regions.

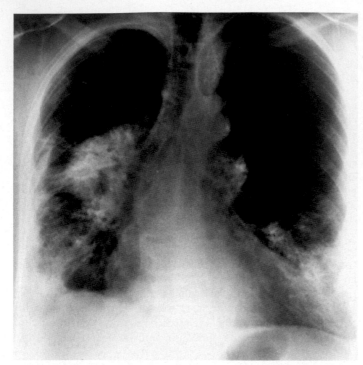

FIGURE 54-9 Lymphoid interstitial pneumonia (LIP). Posteroanterior chest radiograph of a 73-year-old woman with LIP showing consolidative infiltrates in the right midlung and lung base as well as the left lung base.

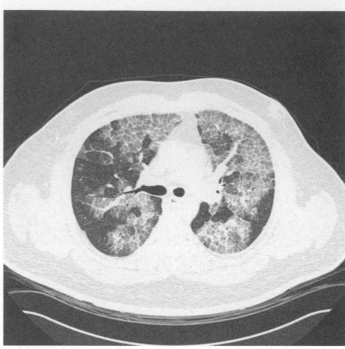

FIGURE 54-11 Pulmonary alveolar proteinosis (PAP). High resolution computed tomogram of a 39-year-old man with PAP shows the "crazy-paving" pattern of infiltration

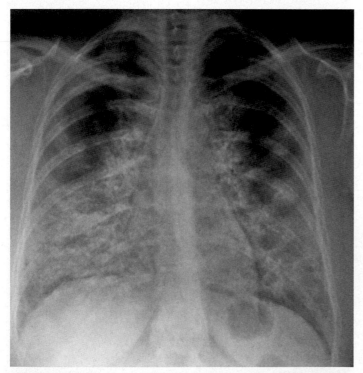

FIGURE 54-10 Pulmonary alveolar proteinosis (PAP). Posteroanterior chest radiograph of a 53-year-old woman with PAP shows diffuse alveolar infiltrates. She was initially seen with progressive exertional dyspnea of 1.5 years' duration.

diseases. Approximately one third of patients have asymmetric or unilateral infiltrates. HRCT of the chest demonstrates ground-glass and/or consolidative infiltrates in patchy or diffuse distributions. Distinct central or peripheral distribution is usually not seen, but sharp demarcation of the infiltrates from surrounding normal lung tissue is commonly observed. Reticular opacities or interlobular septal thickening are present within the airspace infiltrates, creating a "crazy-paving" pattern (Figure 54-11). This pattern is characteristic of, but not specific for, PAP and can be seen in diffuse alveolar damage superimposed on usual interstitial pneumonia, acute interstitial pneumonia, acute respiratory distress syndrome (ARDS), cardiogenic pulmonary edema, and drug-induced lung disease.

The results of pulmonary function testing in patients with LAM may vary. In the LAM Registry (of which 40% of subjects were either past or current smokers), the most common pulmonary function abnormality was obstruction that was present in 57% of subjects. The obstruction was mild (FEV_1 > 70% predicted) in 12%, moderate ($FEV_1 \geq 50$ and $\leq 70\%$ predicted) in 20%, and severe ($FEV_1 < 50\%$ predicted) in 25%. Seventeen percent of patients demonstrated bronchodilator responsiveness. Spirometry was normal in 34%, and thus normal spirometry should not preclude consideration of LAM in a young women presenting with spontaneous pneumothorax. The diffusing capacity was low in 57%. Obstructive and/or restrictive changes may occur in patients with PLCH. The relative contributions of cigarette smoking and the disease itself may be difficult to define. Diffusing capacity is usually abnormal and correlates with impairment in exercise performance. Restrictive changes with diffusion capacity reduction are found in patients with LIP and PAP. Hypoxemia is common in PAP patients, resulting from shunt physiology.

DIAGNOSIS

LAM, PLCH, LIP, and PAP may be strongly suspected on the basis of epidemiologic, clinical, radiographic, and physiologic features. For example, diffuse interstitial infiltrates in a non-smoking woman of childbearing age who has a history of recurrent pneumothoraces and/or chylous pleural effusions strongly suggests LAM. Similarly, the combination of cystic lesions and nodules in the middle and upper lung fields with sparing the costophrenic angles, and normal or increased lung volume in a young adult smoker strongly suggests the diagnosis of PLCH. A history of never having smoked makes the diagnosis of PLCH very unlikely. Predominantly bibasilar reticulonodular infiltrates with superimposed patchy alveolar opacities in a middle-aged individual with dysproteinemia suggest LIP. The diagnosis of PAP should be considered in a patient who has persistent perihilar alveolar infiltrates without evidence of congestive heart failure or infection.

The diagnosis of these four disorders generally requires histologic confirmation, but whether bronchoscopic or surgical lung biopsy is necessary depends on the extent to which the clinical and HRCT findings are classic. The finding of diffuse cystic lung changes without sparing of the costophrenic angles on HRCT in a young woman with a renal AML is pathognomonic for LAM, and no biopsy is necessary. The presence of lung cysts alone without other clinical features of LAM is not sufficient for diagnosis, and lung biopsy would be indicated to differentiate LAM from PLCH and metastatic sarcoma. Transbronchial lung biopsy may suffice, especially if the lung biopsy specimen stains positively for HMB-45, a highly sensitive and specific marker for LAM cells.

In the case of a smoker with HRCT findings of characteristic middle and upper lung zone–predominant cysts and nodules that spare the lung bases, a biopsy may not be necessary to establish the diagnosis of PLCH, especially if symptoms are mild and no immediate therapy beyond smoking cessation is anticipated. Bronchoalveolar lavage (BAL) may be considered in this context to confirm the diagnosis. Although Langerhans cells can be found in other disorders, which include idiopathic pulmonary fibrosis, the presence of at least 5%

CD1a-positive cells in the BAL fluid is highly specific for PLCH. When the clinical and radiographic features are not archetypical, BAL and transbronchial biopsy should be attempted, although the yield of transbronchoscopic lung biopsy is in the range of just 10–40% because of the patchy nature of the PLCH lesions and the small tissue yield. A high index of suspicion and an experienced pathologist are required for proper interpretation. If neither the BAL nor biopsy is positive, surgical lung biopsy or biopsy of bone lesions, if present, should ensue.

Although a transbronchial biopsy may occasionally suffice, the diagnosis of LIP usually requires a surgical lung biopsy (Figure 54-12). Infectious processes should be excluded. Immunohistochemical stains are valuable in distinguishing the dense interstitial lymphoid infiltrate of LIP from other lymphoproliferative disorders, such as lymphoma, diffuse lymphoid hyperplasia, nodular lymphoid hyperplasia, chronic lymphocytic leukemia, and multiple myeloma. BAL typically shows a nonspecific lymphocytosis.

In an appropriate clinical setting, the diagnosis of PAP may be made by BAL, which typically yields a milky effluent (Figure 54-13). Under light microscopy, this fluid shows large amounts of PAS-positive lipoproteinaceous material. Transbronchial biopsy also provides the diagnosis in most cases and demonstrates accumulation of granular, PAS-positive, lipoproteinaceous material within the alveolar spaces with alveolar architecture usually preserved, although thickening of the alveolar septa and interstitial fibrosis may occur in some cases. In the absence of a superimposed infection, very few inflammatory cells are seen in the lung tissue. Surgical biopsy is now less frequently required to confirm a PAP diagnosis.

TREATMENT

There are no proven therapies to reverse or prevent lung damage in LAM. The traditional treatment for LAM has been estrogen antagonism by intramuscular medroxyprogesterone, gonadotropin-releasing hormone analogs, such as leuprolide, tamoxifen, or oophorectomy. Overall, 54% of LAM Registry participants were being treated with a progesterone derivative

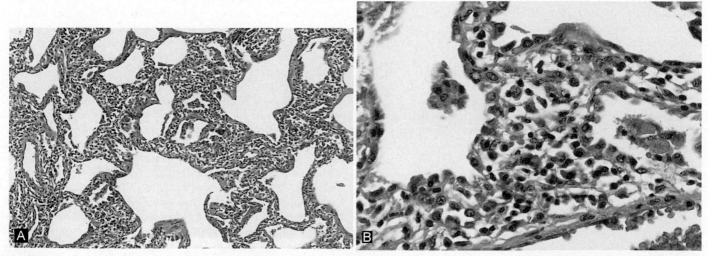

FIGURE 54-12 Histopathology of lymphoid interstitial pneumonia (LIP). **A,** Low-magnification photomicrograph demonstrating features of LIP. Alveolar septa are diffusely expanded by a cellular infiltrate characterized by a combination of lymphocytes and plasma cells. **B,** High-magnification photomicrograph showing LIP. The expanded alveolar septum contains an infiltrate of mononuclear cells that, in this example, includes mainly mature plasma cells.

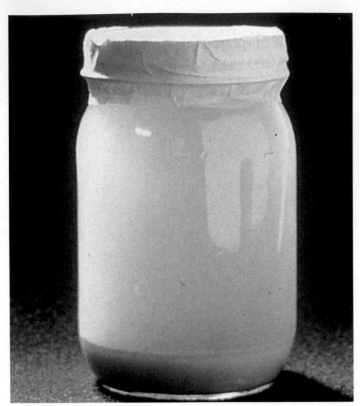

FIGURE 54-13 Lung lavage fluid in pulmonary alveolar proteinosis (PAP). A sample of lung lavage fluid in PAP showing the typical cloudy appearance and sediment that forms over 30 min.

at enrollment and 27% had undergone oophorectomy. The data regarding hormonal manipulation are weak and conflicting. Properly designed clinical trials of progesterone have not been performed. A retrospective review of lung function changes in 275 patients with LAM followed for approximately 4 years at the NIH suggested neither oral nor intramuscular progesterone slow the decline of lung function. Inhaled bronchodilators should be considered for those with wheezing, spirometric airflow limitation, and bronchodilator responsiveness. Neither inhaled nor systemic corticosteroids are helpful in LAM. Supplemental oxygen should be considered for those hypoxemic at rest, with exercise, and/or during sleep. Lung transplantation is an option for patients affected by advanced LAM.

Smoking cessation should be the initial intervention in all smokers with PLCH and may be all that is required. Corticosteroids are initiated for progressive or systemic disease despite smoking cessation, although data are insufficient to definitively support their role. Radiation therapy for bone lesions provides symptomatic relief. In those patients who have progressive disease despite smoking cessation and corticosteroids, options include cytotoxic drugs, which generally are of limited benefit, and lung transplantation. 2-Chlorodeoxyadenosine (2-CDA) has shown promise in several patients with progressive, multisystem disease. However, few of these patients had pulmonary involvement. Therefore, the role for 2-CDA in PLCH remains undefined.

Most patients affected by LIP are treated with corticosteroids. The response is variable, and optimal dosing of corticosteroids has not been defined. In the recently reported retrospective series of 15 LIP patients, 14 subjects were treated with corticosteroids and/or cytotoxic drugs, including cyclophosphamide, azathioprine, and cyclosporin A. In the nine subjects with follow-up data, four showed clinical improvement, four remained stable, and overall median survival was 11.5 years. Vigilance for and prompt treatment of superimposed pulmonary infections are important.

The treatment standard for PAP is whole lung lavage. This is performed with the patient under general anesthetic by means of a bronchoscope passed through a double-lumen endotracheal tube. The procedure typically lasts 1–2 h, during which repeated instillation and drainage of the lung with up to 20–30 L of isotonic saline is performed until the runoff is clear. Only one lung is usually lavaged at a session, with the other lung treated similarly 2–3 days later if necessary, although single-session, sequential, bilateral whole lung lavage has been performed. Chest percussion during the lavage may help. Approximately 85% of patients show improvement after lung lavage. The median duration of clinical benefit is approximately 15 months. Eventually, 60–70% of patients require repeat lavage, and the median total number of procedures is two. Lung lavage is associated with improved survival. Consistent with its proposed importance in surfactant clearance, preliminary experience with GM-CSF administration in PAP has shown potential with small studies to date, indicating favorable responses in 40–50% of patients, some enjoying a complete response. In these small studies, GM-CSF has either been administered subcutaneously (dose range, 5–20 µg/kg/day) or by aerosolization (dose range, 250–500 µg twice daily every other week). Corticosteroids have no beneficial effect.

CLINICAL COURSE AND PREVENTION

The clinical course varies greatly among these four diffuse lung diseases. Most patients with LAM experience slow progression of their disease. However, recent studies report survival rates of 38–78% at 8.5 years after the onset of symptoms, figures better than previously reported. Our experience suggests that the rate of progression varies among patients with LAM. In the cohort of patients with LAM followed by the NIH, the average yearly rates of decline in diffusing capacity and FEV_1 were $2.4 \pm 0.4\%$ predicted (0.69 ± 0.07 mL/min/mmHg) and $1.7 \pm 0.4\%$ predicted (75 ± 9 mL), respectively. In terms of predictors of decline, patients with higher initial diffusing capacity and FEV_1 tended to have a greater rate of decline in diffusing capacity. Conversely, patients with higher initial diffusing capacity and FEV_1, as well as older patients, experienced a lower rate of decline in FEV_1. Exogenous estrogens may exacerbate the disorder and should be avoided. Recurrent and contralateral pneumothoraces are very common. Chemical (sclerosing agent by a chest tube) or surgical pleurodesis are equally effective at reducing the recurrence rate of ipsilateral pneumothorax to approximately 30%, whereas the recurrence rate after conservative therapy (simple aspiration or chest tube without pleurodesis) is greater than 60%. Therefore, pleurodesis should be considered for the initial pneumothorax in LAM. A review of 34 patients with LAM who underwent lung transplantation revealed survival rates of 69% and 58% at 1 and 2 years after transplantation, respectively—values similar to transplant experience with other chronic pulmonary conditions. Approximately half the patients had substantial pleural adhesions that caused intraoperative difficulties, but prior pleurodesis does not prohibit successful lung transplantation. Recurrent pneumothorax in the remaining native lung and chylothorax were the main postoperative problems. Recurrent LAM was found in one patient in this series.

Substantial variation is also found in the natural history of PLCH. Some patients stabilize or spontaneously improve, whereas others have progressive lung disease, pulmonary hypertension, cor pulmonale, and respiratory failure develop. A retrospective review from Mayo Clinic (Rochester, MN) of 102 patients with histopathologically confirmed pulmonary LCH and with median follow-up of 4 years reported 33 deaths (15 caused by respiratory failure) and overall median survival of 12.5 years. Univariate analysis revealed poorer prognosis with older age and greater impairment of pulmonary function. Patients affected by only pulmonary involvement follow a more benign course. Cigarette smoking must be discouraged. PLCH has recurred in transplanted lungs, with or without smoking cessation.

The clinical course of LIP includes progression to diffuse pulmonary fibrosis in one third of cases. Some patients diagnosed with LIP probably have lymphoma from the outset, but cases in which LIP has transformed to lymphoma have occurred. Death may result from progressive lung involvement with cor pulmonale, malignant lymphoma, or complications of treatment. Those individuals with LIP in the setting of HIV usually die from complications of the HIV infection. Spontaneous improvement of LIP may occur.

Five- and 10-year survival rates in PAP are 75% and 68%, respectively. Death is most likely at the extremes of age but is overall uncommon and usually related to respiratory failure or uncontrolled infection. Superimposed infection, especially with opportunistic pathogens such as *Nocardia*, may occur and disseminate. There are no known disease-related or patient-related factors that are associated with risk for opportunistic infection. Spontaneous resolution of PAP has been reported in up to one third of patients with PAP with a median time from diagnosis to resolution being approximately 20 months. No features have been identified that reliably predict whose disease will spontaneously remit. Whether lung function and surfactant homeostasis truly return to normal or whether these patients have residual subclinical defects is unclear. Lung transplantation is an option in those individuals affected by progressive disease. Recurrent PAP after double lung transplantation has been reported.

PITFALLS AND CONTROVERSIES

The risks of pregnancy and air travel in LAM patients are not fully defined, and counseling must be handled on a patient-by-patient basis. The optimal timing for initiation of progesterone therapy remains unclear. Eight women in a cohort of 250 sporadic patients with LAM were found to have brain lesions compatible with meningiomas, a finding of concern because progesterone is a putative growth factor for meningiomas. Whether all patients with LAM require screening for meningiomas and how this information should influence treatment decisions remains unclear.

There may be an increased risk for neoplasms in PLCH. In the Mayo Clinic series, six hematologic cancers were diagnosed, so clinicians are advised to be mindful of malignancy in these patients, especially those with hemoptysis. The diagnosis of LIP should not be made without immunohistochemical staining to exclude lymphoma. It is likely that some cases diagnosed as the transformation of LIP to lymphoma represented lymphoma *de novo*.

OTHER RARE DIFFUSE LUNG DISEASES

The remaining disorders described in this section are a diverse group of diseases the pulmonary manifestations that stem from excessive accumulation of various types of material in the respiratory system.

Neurofibromatosis

Neurofibromatosis (NF) is a variably expressed autosomal-dominant disorder characterized by café-au-lait spots, subcutaneous neurofibromas, axillary freckling, and iris hamartomas (Lisch nodules). There are two distinct forms of NF: NF type 1, related to *NF 1* gene on chromosome 17, which codes for neurofibromin; and NF type 2, related to the *NF 2* gene on chromosome 22, which codes for merlin. *NF1* and *NF 2* are tumor-suppressor genes. Descriptions of chest involvement have included intrathoracic neurogenic neurofibromas, meningoceles, kyphoscoliosis, and parenchymal lung disease in the form of interstitial lung disease and/or cystic airspaces. The three largest series suggested parenchymal lung involvement by chest X-ray in 7–23% adult patients with NF. However, a recent review of 156 patients with NF seen at Mayo Clinic revealed bilateral interstitial infiltrates in only 3 (1.9%) patients and emphysematous changes in just 3.8%. All those with interstitial changes had other potential causes for the infiltrates, such as smoking-related interstitial lung disease, rheumatoid lung disease, recurrent pneumonias, and a history of ARDS. All those with bullae or cystic airspaces also had smoking-related emphysema. These findings cast doubt on the link between NF and parenchymal lung disease.

Pulmonary Alveolar Microlithiasis

Pulmonary alveolar microlithiasis results from the extensive intraalveolar deposition of concentrically lamellated calcium phosphate spheres, which produces a distinctive calcific, micronodular ("sandstorm") infiltrate on the chest radiograph (Figure 54-14). It is an autosomal-recessive disorder that is caused by mutations in the SLC34A2 gene on chromosome 4 that encodes a sodium phosphate cotransporter. The gene is highly expressed in type II alveolar cells, and mutations inactivate the normal gene function. A recent literature review of 576 cases revealed more than 50% of patients were asymptomatic; the remainder reported dyspnea, cough, and chest pain. One third of the cases were familial. The mean age of diagnosis was 35 years, and the age range of patients spanned from newborn to 80 years. Progression was slow, and patients usually died from cardiopulmonary failure. Microlith expectoration is uncommon. Supporting evidence can be obtained by transbronchial lung biopsy or by the demonstration of extensive pulmonary uptake during [99m]technetium diphosphonate scanning. No consistently effective therapy is known, although lung transplantation has been attempted, and regression of the calcific infiltrates has been reported in pediatric patients treated with a bisphosphonate.

Amyloid

Amyloid, a fibrillar, homogeneous, proteinaceous material usually derived from immunoglobulin light chains, can deposit in the tracheobronchial tree or pulmonary parenchyma in either localized or diffuse patterns. This accumulation can be part of a systemic process (primary systemic amyloidosis, secondary amyloidosis, familial amyloidosis) or can be isolated to the lung (localized pulmonary amyloidosis). The incidence

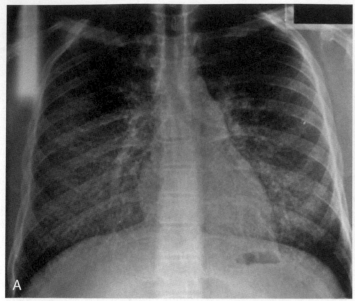

FIGURE 54-14 Pulmonary alveolar microlithiasis. **A,** Posteroanterior chest radiograph of an 18-year-old asymptomatic man who has pulmonary alveolar microlithiasis showing numerous tiny opacities present throughout both lungs. **B,** Magnified view of the right lower lung showing numerous opacities that measure less than 1 mm.

of pulmonary amyloid deposition with secondary and familial amyloidosis is low, whereas pulmonary involvement by primary systemic amyloidosis is common and usually takes the form of diffuse, alveolar, septal amyloid accumulation that manifests radiographically as reticular or reticulonodular infiltrates. Pleural effusions may also occur because of simultaneous pleural involvement or from heart failure caused by cardiac amyloid deposition. Prognosis is poor for patients with primary systemic amyloidosis who have pulmonary involvement.

A diffuse interstitial pattern is rare with localized pulmonary amyloidosis. Instead, pulmonary parenchymal involvement manifests as single or multiple nodules that are often detected incidentally on the chest radiograph. These nodules may grow slowly, cavitate, or calcify. Isolated amyloid masses or multifocal, submucosal plaques characterize the tracheobronchial forms of localized pulmonary amyloidosis. Diffuse endobronchial involvement is recognizable bronchoscopically as shiny, pale plaques with scattered focal stenoses. Symptoms depend on the extent of luminal compromise and include dyspnea, cough, hemoptysis, wheeze, atelectasis, and recurrent pneumonia. Severe localized stenosis can be treated with repeated bronchoscopic resection, perhaps incorporating laser ablation or surgery. Other pulmonary manifestations of amyloid deposition, whether caused by a systemic or localized process, are mediastinal and/or hilar adenopathy, mediastinal masses, and macroglossia that results in obstructive sleep apnea.

Tracheobronchial and diffuse parenchymal forms of pulmonary amyloidosis can be safely diagnosed at bronchoscopy, although the endoscopist must be prepared for potential bleeding. Lung nodules are diagnosed by needle aspiration or resection. Biopsy material reveals the characteristic apple-green birefringence with polarized microscopy after staining with Congo red.

Hermansky–Pudlak Syndrome

The Hermansky–Pudlak syndrome is a triad of oculocutaneous albinism, platelet aggregation dysfunction, and visceral ceroid deposition. It is an autosomal-recessive disorder with a high frequency among Puerto Ricans. At least four different genes may cause HPS. Mutations in the *HSP1* gene are associated with a progressive interstitial fibrosis that may develop during the second and fourth decades and for which there is no reliable treatment. The interstitial lung disease is thought to be related to the interaction of alveolar macrophages with ceroid, a material derived from incompletely processed lysosomal membranes. Such ceroid-laden macrophages have been demonstrated by Fontana–Masson staining of BAL fluid.

Lipoid Storage Disorders

Several autosomal-recessive, inborn errors of sphingolipid metabolism may have pulmonary manifestations that result from the intracellular accumulation of metabolic products induced by enzymatic defects. Gaucher's disease is caused by a deficiency of β-glucosidase, which leads to the formation of the characteristic Gaucher cell, a reticuloendothelial cell packed with glucose-1-ceramide. With Niemann–Pick disease, deficiencies in sphingomyelinase or cholesterol esterification lead to the development of foamy-appearing cells. Reticular or reticulonodular infiltrates can occur in Gaucher's and Niemann–Pick disease, as alveolar macrophages filled with material accumulate in the interstitium and alveolar spaces. Patients who have Fabry's disease, an X-linked sphingolipidosis caused by the absence of α-galactosidase A, may exhibit airflow obstruction and reduced diffusing capacities. In general, the pulmonary manifestations in these metabolic disorders are incompletely described, have a variable course, may occur in childhood, and are often overshadowed by the extrapulmonary manifestations.

Erdheim–Chester Disease

Erdheim–Chester disease (ECD) is a rare, nonfamilial disorder of unknown etiology characterized by the infiltration of non-Langerhans cell histiocytes. The disease is usually heralded by long bone pain caused by bilateral, symmetric osteosclerotic diaphyseal and metaphyseal lesions. Approximately 50–60% of patients with ECD will have extraosseous disease, with the pattern and extent variable. Sites of extraosseous involvement include the retroorbital and periorbital tissues, central nervous system, skin, kidney, liver, spleen, retroperitoneum, testis, and breast. Approximately 25% of the reported ECD cases in the literature have had pulmonary involvement, usually in the form of diffuse, bilateral, chronic interstitial infiltrates on chest radiography. ECD involvement of the lung is considered to be a distinct disease entity from PLCH. The most common pulmonary symptom is dyspnea, the gender distribution for pulmonary involvement by ECD appears equal, and most cases arise in middle age. Diagnosis rests on the demonstration of tissue infiltration by foamy histiocytes with non-Langerhans features (CD1a-negative and absence of Birbeck granules). There may be advanced fibrosis. In the lung, the histiocytic infiltration and associated fibrosis have a striking lymphatic distribution. Accordingly, chest CT reveals interlobular septal and visceral pleural thickening with patchy reticular and centrilobular opacities, as well as ground-glass attenuation. Other described intrathoracic manifestations of ECD include periaortic fibrosis ("coated aorta"), pericardial effusion resulting in cardiac tamponade in some cases, coronary artery infiltration leading to myocardial infarction, venal caval and pulmonary artery obstruction caused by extraluminal compression, right atrial tumor, cardiac valvular disease, and one case of subglottic stenosis. Prognosis is variable and depends on the degree of extraosseous disease. There are no reliable treatments. Given its role in promoting terminal differentiation of histiocytes, α-interferon has been tried with some success. External beam radiotherapy may provide short-term palliation.

SUGGESTED READINGS

American Thoracic Society/European Respiratory Society International Multidisciplinary Consensus Conference of the Idiopathic Interstitial Pneumonias. Am J Respir Crit Care Med 2002; 165:277–304.

Cha S-I, Fessler MB, Cool CD, et al: Lymphoid interstitial pneumonia: clinical features, associations and prognosis. Eur Respir J 2006; 28: 364–369.

Egan AJ, Boardman LA, Tazelaar HD, et al: Erdheim–Chester disease: Clinical, radiologic, and histopathologic findings in five patients with interstitial lung disease. Am J Surg Pathol 1999; 23:17–26.

Garay SM, Gardella JE, Fazzini EP, Goldring RM: Hermansky–Pudlak syndrome: Pulmonary manifestations of a ceroid storage disorder. Am J Med 1979; 66:737–747.

Long RG, Lake BD, Pettit JE, et al: Adult Niemann–Pick disease. Am J Med 1977; 62:627–635.

Mariotta S, Ricci A, Papale M, et al: Pulmonary alveolar microlithiasis: Review on 576 cases published in the literature. Sarcoidosis Vasc Diffuse Lung Dis 2004; 21:173–181.

Riccardi VM: Von Recklinghausen's neurofibromatosis. N Engl J Med 1981; 305:1616–1627.

Rosenberg DM, Ferrans VJ, Fulmer JD, et al: Chronic airflow obstruction in Fabry's disease. Am J Med 1980; 68:898–904.

Ryu JH, Moss J, Beck GJ, et al: The NHLNI lymphangioleiomyomatosis registry: characteristics of 230 patients at enrollment. Am J Respir Crit Care Med 2006; 173:105–111.

Seymour JF, Presneill JJ: Pulmonary alveolar proteinosis: progress in the first 44 years. Am J Respir Crit Care Med 2002; 166:215–235.

Utz JP, Swensen SJ, Gertz MA: Pulmonary amyloidosis: the Mayo Clinic experience from 1980 to 1993. Ann Intern Med 1996; 124:407–413.

Vassallo R, Ryu JH, Colby TV, et al: Pulmonary Langerhans'-cell histiocytosis. N Engl J Med 2000; 342:1969–1978.

Vassallo R, Ryu JH, Schroeder DR, et al: Clinical outcomes of pulmonary Langerhans'-cell histiocytosis in adults. N Engl J Med 2002; 346: 484–490.

Wolsen AH: Pulmonary findings in Gaucher's disease. AJR Am J Roentgenol 1975; 123:712–715.

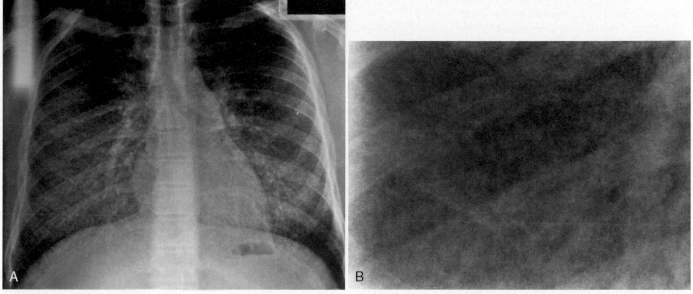

FIGURE 54-14 Pulmonary alveolar microlithiasis. **A,** Posteroanterior chest radiograph of an 18-year-old asymptomatic man who has pulmonary alveolar microlithiasis showing numerous tiny opacities present throughout both lungs. **B,** Magnified view of the right lower lung showing numerous opacities that measure less than 1 mm.

of pulmonary amyloid deposition with secondary and familial amyloidosis is low, whereas pulmonary involvement by primary systemic amyloidosis is common and usually takes the form of diffuse, alveolar, septal amyloid accumulation that manifests radiographically as reticular or reticulonodular infiltrates. Pleural effusions may also occur because of simultaneous pleural involvement or from heart failure caused by cardiac amyloid deposition. Prognosis is poor for patients with primary systemic amyloidosis who have pulmonary involvement.

A diffuse interstitial pattern is rare with localized pulmonary amyloidosis. Instead, pulmonary parenchymal involvement manifests as single or multiple nodules that are often detected incidentally on the chest radiograph. These nodules may grow slowly, cavitate, or calcify. Isolated amyloid masses or multifocal, submucosal plaques characterize the tracheobronchial forms of localized pulmonary amyloidosis. Diffuse endobronchial involvement is recognizable bronchoscopically as shiny, pale plaques with scattered focal stenoses. Symptoms depend on the extent of luminal compromise and include dyspnea, cough, hemoptysis, wheeze, atelectasis, and recurrent pneumonia. Severe localized stenosis can be treated with repeated bronchoscopic resection, perhaps incorporating laser ablation or surgery. Other pulmonary manifestations of amyloid deposition, whether caused by a systemic or localized process, are mediastinal and/or hilar adenopathy, mediastinal masses, and macroglossia that results in obstructive sleep apnea.

Tracheobronchial and diffuse parenchymal forms of pulmonary amyloidosis can be safely diagnosed at bronchoscopy, although the endoscopist must be prepared for potential bleeding. Lung nodules are diagnosed by needle aspiration or resection. Biopsy material reveals the characteristic apple-green birefringence with polarized microscopy after staining with Congo red.

Hermansky–Pudlak Syndrome

The Hermansky–Pudlak syndrome is a triad of oculocutaneous albinism, platelet aggregation dysfunction, and visceral ceroid

deposition. It is an autosomal-recessive disorder with a high frequency among Puerto Ricans. At least four different genes may cause HPS. Mutations in the *HSP1* gene are associated with a progressive interstitial fibrosis that may develop during the second and fourth decades and for which there is no reliable treatment. The interstitial lung disease is thought to be related to the interaction of alveolar macrophages with ceroid, a material derived from incompletely processed lysosomal membranes. Such ceroid-laden macrophages have been demonstrated by Fontana–Masson staining of BAL fluid.

Lipoid Storage Disorders

Several autosomal-recessive, inborn errors of sphingolipid metabolism may have pulmonary manifestations that result from the intracellular accumulation of metabolic products induced by enzymatic defects. Gaucher's disease is caused by a deficiency of β-glucosidase, which leads to the formation of the characteristic Gaucher cell, a reticuloendothelial cell packed with glucose-1-ceramide. With Niemann–Pick disease, deficiencies in sphingomyelinase or cholesterol esterification lead to the development of foamy-appearing cells. Reticular or reticulonodular infiltrates can occur in Gaucher's and Niemann–Pick disease, as alveolar macrophages filled with material accumulate in the interstitium and alveolar spaces. Patients who have Fabry's disease, an X-linked sphingolipidosis caused by the absence of α-galactosidase A, may exhibit airflow obstruction and reduced diffusing capacities. In general, the pulmonary manifestations in these metabolic disorders are incompletely described, have a variable course, may occur in childhood, and are often overshadowed by the extrapulmonary manifestations.

Erdheim–Chester Disease

Erdheim–Chester disease (ECD) is a rare, nonfamilial disorder of unknown etiology characterized by the infiltration of non-Langerhans cell histiocytes. The disease is usually heralded by long bone pain caused by bilateral, symmetric osteosclerotic diaphyseal and metaphyseal lesions. Approximately

chylothorax were the main postoperative problems. Recurrent LAM was found in one patient in this series.

Substantial variation is also found in the natural history of PLCH. Some patients stabilize or spontaneously improve, whereas others have progressive lung disease, pulmonary hypertension, cor pulmonale, and respiratory failure develop. A retrospective review from Mayo Clinic (Rochester, MN) of 102 patients with histopathologically confirmed pulmonary LCH and with median follow-up of 4 years reported 33 deaths (15 caused by respiratory failure) and overall median survival of 12.5 years. Univariate analysis revealed poorer prognosis with older age and greater impairment of pulmonary function. Patients affected by only pulmonary involvement follow a more benign course. Cigarette smoking must be discouraged. PLCH has recurred in transplanted lungs, with or without smoking cessation.

The clinical course of LIP includes progression to diffuse pulmonary fibrosis in one third of cases. Some patients diagnosed with LIP probably have lymphoma from the outset, but cases in which LIP has transformed to lymphoma have occurred. Death may result from progressive lung involvement with cor pulmonale, malignant lymphoma, or complications of treatment. Those individuals with LIP in the setting of HIV usually die from complications of the HIV infection. Spontaneous improvement of LIP may occur.

Five- and 10-year survival rates in PAP are 75% and 68%, respectively. Death is most likely at the extremes of age but is overall uncommon and usually related to respiratory failure or uncontrolled infection. Superimposed infection, especially with opportunistic pathogens such as *Nocardia*, may occur and disseminate. There are no known disease-related or patient-related factors that are associated with risk for opportunistic infection. Spontaneous resolution of PAP has been reported in up to one third of patients with PAP with a median time from diagnosis to resolution being approximately 20 months. No features have been identified that reliably predict whose disease will spontaneously remit. Whether lung function and surfactant homeostasis truly return to normal or whether these patients have residual subclinical defects is unclear. Lung transplantation is an option in those individuals affected by progressive disease. Recurrent PAP after double lung transplantation has been reported.

PITFALLS AND CONTROVERSIES

The risks of pregnancy and air travel in LAM patients are not fully defined, and counseling must be handled on a patient-by-patient basis. The optimal timing for initiation of progesterone therapy remains unclear. Eight women in a cohort of 250 sporadic patients with LAM were found to have brain lesions compatible with meningiomas, a finding of concern because progesterone is a putative growth factor for meningiomas. Whether all patients with LAM require screening for meningiomas and how this information should influence treatment decisions remains unclear.

There may be an increased risk for neoplasms in PLCH. In the Mayo Clinic series, six hematologic cancers were diagnosed, so clinicians are advised to be mindful of malignancy in these patients, especially those with hemoptysis. The diagnosis of LIP should not be made without immunohistochemical staining to exclude lymphoma. It is likely that some cases diagnosed as the transformation of LIP to lymphoma represented lymphoma *de novo*.

OTHER RARE DIFFUSE LUNG DISEASES

The remaining disorders described in this section are a diverse group of diseases the pulmonary manifestations that stem from excessive accumulation of various types of material in the respiratory system.

Neurofibromatosis

Neurofibromatosis (NF) is a variably expressed autosomal-dominant disorder characterized by café-au-lait spots, subcutaneous neurofibromas, axillary freckling, and iris hamartomas (Lisch nodules). There are two distinct forms of NF: NF type 1, related to *NF 1* gene on chromosome 17, which codes for neurofibromin; and NF type 2, related to the *NF 2* gene on chromosome 22, which codes for merlin. *NF1* and *NF 2* are tumor-suppressor genes. Descriptions of chest involvement have included intrathoracic neurogenic neurofibromas, meningoceles, kyphoscoliosis, and parenchymal lung disease in the form of interstitial lung disease and/or cystic airspaces. The three largest series suggested parenchymal lung involvement by chest X-ray in 7–23% adult patients with NF. However, a recent review of 156 patients with NF seen at Mayo Clinic revealed bilateral interstitial infiltrates in only 3 (1.9%) patients and emphysematous changes in just 3.8%. All those with interstitial changes had other potential causes for the infiltrates, such as smoking-related interstitial lung disease, rheumatoid lung disease, recurrent pneumonias, and a history of ARDS. All those with bullae or cystic airspaces also had smoking-related emphysema. These findings cast doubt on the link between NF and parenchymal lung disease.

Pulmonary Alveolar Microlithiasis

Pulmonary alveolar microlithiasis results from the extensive intraalveolar deposition of concentrically lamellated calcium phosphate spheres, which produces a distinctive calcific, micronodular ("sandstorm") infiltrate on the chest radiograph (Figure 54-14). It is an autosomal-recessive disorder that is caused by mutations in the SLC34A2 gene on chromosome 4 that encodes a sodium phosphate cotransporter. The gene is highly expressed in type II alveolar cells, and mutations inactivate the normal gene function. A recent literature review of 576 cases revealed more than 50% of patients were asymptomatic; the remainder reported dyspnea, cough, and chest pain. One third of the cases were familial. The mean age of diagnosis was 35 years, and the age range of patients spanned from newborn to 80 years. Progression was slow, and patients usually died from cardiopulmonary failure. Microlith expectoration is uncommon. Supporting evidence can be obtained by transbronchial lung biopsy or by the demonstration of extensive pulmonary uptake during [99m]technetium diphosphonate scanning. No consistently effective therapy is known, although lung transplantation has been attempted, and regression of the calcific infiltrates has been reported in pediatric patients treated with a bisphosphonate.

Amyloid

Amyloid, a fibrillar, homogeneous, proteinaceous material usually derived from immunoglobulin light chains, can deposit in the tracheobronchial tree or pulmonary parenchyma in either localized or diffuse patterns. This accumulation can be part of a systemic process (primary systemic amyloidosis, secondary amyloidosis, familial amyloidosis) or can be isolated to the lung (localized pulmonary amyloidosis). The incidence

50–60% of patients with ECD will have extraosseous disease, with the pattern and extent variable. Sites of extraosseous involvement include the retroorbital and periorbital tissues, central nervous system, skin, kidney, liver, spleen, retroperitoneum, testis, and breast. Approximately 25% of the reported ECD cases in the literature have had pulmonary involvement, usually in the form of diffuse, bilateral, chronic interstitial infiltrates on chest radiography. ECD involvement of the lung is considered to be a distinct disease entity from PLCH. The most common pulmonary symptom is dyspnea, the gender distribution for pulmonary involvement by ECD appears equal, and most cases arise in middle age. Diagnosis rests on the demonstration of tissue infiltration by foamy histiocytes with non-Langerhans features (CD1a-negative and absence of Birbeck granules). There may be advanced fibrosis. In the lung, the histiocytic infiltration and associated fibrosis have a striking lymphatic distribution. Accordingly, chest CT reveals interlobular septal and visceral pleural thickening with patchy reticular and centrilobular opacities, as well as ground-glass attenuation. Other described intrathoracic manifestations of ECD include periaortic fibrosis ("coated aorta"), pericardial effusion resulting in cardiac tamponade in some cases, coronary artery infiltration leading to myocardial infarction, venal caval and pulmonary artery obstruction caused by extraluminal compression, right atrial tumor, cardiac valvular disease, and one case of subglottic stenosis. Prognosis is variable and depends on the degree of extraosseous disease. There are no reliable treatments. Given its role in promoting terminal differentiation of histiocytes, α-interferon has been tried with some success. External beam radiotherapy may provide short-term palliation.

SUGGESTED READINGS

American Thoracic Society/European Respiratory Society International Multidisciplinary Consensus Conference of the Idiopathic Interstitial Pneumonias. Am J Respir Crit Care Med 2002; 165:277–304.

Cha S-I, Fessler MB, Cool CD, et al: Lymphoid interstitial pneumonia: clinical features, associations and prognosis. Eur Respir J 2006; 28: 364–369.

Egan AJ, Boardman LA, Tazelaar HD, et al: Erdheim–Chester disease: Clinical, radiologic, and histopathologic findings in five patients with interstitial lung disease. Am J Surg Pathol 1999; 23:17–26.

Garay SM, Gardella JE, Fazzini EP, Goldring RM: Hermansky–Pudlak syndrome: Pulmonary manifestations of a ceroid storage disorder. Am J Med 1979; 66:737–747.

Long RG, Lake BD, Pettit JE, et al: Adult Niemann–Pick disease. Am J Med 1977; 62:627–635.

Mariotta S, Ricci A, Papale M, et al: Pulmonary alveolar microlithiasis: Review on 576 cases published in the literature. Sarcoidosis Vasc Diffuse Lung Dis 2004; 21:173–181.

Riccardi VM: Von Recklinghausen's neurofibromatosis. N Engl J Med 1981; 305:1616–1627.

Rosenberg DM, Ferrans VJ, Fulmer JD, et al: Chronic airflow obstruction in Fabry's disease. Am J Med 1980; 68:898–904.

Ryu JH, Moss J, Beck GJ, et al: The NHLNI lymphangioleiomyomatosis registry: characteristics of 230 patients at enrollment. Am J Respir Crit Care Med 2006; 173:105–111.

Seymour JF, Presneill JJ: Pulmonary alveolar proteinosis: progress in the first 44 years. Am J Respir Crit Care Med 2002; 166:215–235.

Utz JP, Swensen SJ, Gertz MA: Pulmonary amyloidosis: the Mayo Clinic experience from 1980 to 1993. Ann Intern Med 1996; 124:407–413.

Vassallo R, Ryu JH, Colby TV, et al: Pulmonary Langerhans'-cell histiocytosis. N Engl J Med 2000; 342:1969–1978.

Vassallo R, Ryu JH, Schroeder DR, et al: Clinical outcomes of pulmonary Langerhans'-cell histiocytosis in adults. N Engl J Med 2002; 346: 484–490.

Wolsen AH: Pulmonary findings in Gaucher's disease. AJR Am J Roentgenol 1975; 123:712–715.

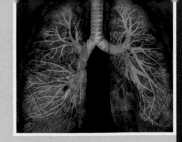

55 Extrinsic Allergic Alveolitis

STELLA E. HINES • CECILE S. ROSE

BACKGROUND

Extrinsic allergic alveolitis (EAA), also known as hypersensitivity pneumonitis (HP), refers to a constellation of granulomatous, interstitial, bronchiolar, and alveolar lung diseases that result from an immunologic reaction to a wide variety of inhaled organic dusts and chemical antigens. EAA is a complex syndrome of varying intensity, clinical presentation, and outcome.

Pathophysiology and Epidemiology

EAA is characterized by the presence of activated T lymphocytes in bronchoalveolar lavage (BAL) and an interstitial mononuclear cell infiltrate. The pathogenesis of EAA involves (1) repeated antigen exposure; (2) immunologic sensitization of the host to the antigen; and (3) immune-mediated damage to the lung. The immune inflammation resulting in lymphocytic alveolitis and granulomatous pneumonitis involves a combination of immune complex-mediated, humoral, and, most importantly, cell-mediated or delayed (type IV) immune reactions.

Although little is known about the true incidence and prevalence of EAA, rates seem to be low relative to more common lung diseases such as asthma, COPD, and sarcoidosis. Low disease rates are likely due in part to underrecognition and misdiagnosis. Most epidemiologic studies have focused on farmer's lung disease. Incidence and prevalence rates vary by geographic region and case definition, but typically range from 2–8% of farmers. Reported prevalences of bird fancier's lung range from 0.5–21%. Attack rates in some exposed populations are even higher, affecting 52% of office workers exposed to a contaminated humidification system in one report, and up to 65% in an outbreak of EAA among lifeguards at an indoor swimming pool.

Environmental, Host, and Genetic Factors

The wide range of specific antigens causing EAA (Table 55-1) can be grouped into three general categories: microbial agents, animal and plant proteins, and low-molecular weight chemicals. Although many people are exposed to environmental antigens associated with EAA, disease develops in only a small percentage. Exposure factors such as antigen concentration, complex mixtures (e.g., multiple microbial agents and their component parts), duration of exposure before symptom onset, frequency and intermittency of exposure, particle size, antigen solubility, use of respiratory protection, season and climate, and variability in work practices likely affect disease risk. For example, farmers lung is most common in regions with heavy rainfall, where feed is likely to become damp, and in harsh winter conditions, where damp hay is fed to animals in indoor barns with limited ventilation. Bird fanciers lung occurs

more frequently during the summer sporting season when exposures are at their highest. Summer-type hypersensitivity pneumonitis (HP), the most prevalent form of EAA in Japan, occurs mainly during the wet, summer months associated with microbial contamination of indoor furnishings.

Host susceptibility factors likely also influence risk for and prevalence of EAA. As with other granulomatous lung diseases, EAA occurs more frequently in nonsmokers. Viral infection may be a cofactor in triggering disease onset. Viral factors that may promote EAA include impaired mucociliary function, alterations of alveolar macrophage phagocytic function, and increased secretion of chemokines that enhance recruitment of lymphocytes to the lungs.

Genetic factors that modify susceptibility to EAA are not well characterized. Most research has been focused on the major histocompatibility complex (MHC). Several alleles and haplotypes of the MHC class II alleles seem to confer susceptibility or resistance to bird fanciers lung. For example, polymorphisms in the 5′ promoter region of the TNF-α gene may promote more rapid onset of disease after exposure and a more robust inflammatory response. In one study, promoter variants in tissue inhibitor of metalloproteinase-3 (TIMP-3) protected against susceptibility to bird fanciers lung compared with both normal controls and controls exposed to avian antigens without clinical disease.

Diagnosis and Clinical Features
Proposed Diagnostic Criteria

A number of diagnostic criteria have been proposed, but none have been validated. Recent diagnostic criteria proposed by the Hypersensitivity Pneumonitis Study Group include the following six clinical variables: (1) exposure to a known antigen; (2) positive precipitating antibodies; (3) recurrent episodes of symptoms; (4) inspiratory crackles; (5) symptoms 4–8 h after exposure; and (6) weight loss (Table 55-2). Presence of all six variables was associated with a diagnostic sensitivity of 86% and specificity of 86%. However, strict adherence to these criteria may result in underrecognition of mild disease, as well as failure to identify new antigens associated with EAA.

Signs and Symptoms

Symptoms of EAA may present with acute, subacute, or insidious onset. Acute symptoms occur within 4–12 h after exposure. Cough, dyspnea, chest tightness, fever, chills, malaise, and myalgias are common. Physical examination may reveal fever, tachypnea, tachycardia, and crackles. In the subacute and chronic presentations of EAA, symptom onset is more insidious, with progressive dyspnea on exertion, dry or minimally productive cough, fatigue, malaise, anorexia, and weight loss. The temporal relationship between exposure and symptom

TABLE 55-1 Three Major Categories of Antigens Causing EAA, with Exposure Source and Syndrome

Antigen	Exposure	Syndrome
Microbioal agents		
Bacteria		
Thermophilic bacteria		
Micropolyspora faeni	Moldy hay	Farmer's lung
Thermoactinomycetes vulgaris	Moldy sugarcane	Bagassosis
T. sacchari	Mushroom compost	Mushroom worker's lung
Streptomyces albus	Soil, peat	Farmer's lung
Non-thermophilic bacteria		
Bacillus subtilis, B. cereus	Water	Humidifier lung
Mycobacterium avium complex	Hot tubs	Hot tub lung
Mycobacterium sp.	Metal working fluids	
Endotoxin	Indoor pools	Lifeguard Lung
Fungi		
Aspergillus sp.	Moldy hay	Farmer's lung
	Water	Ventilation pneumonitis
	Animal bedding	Dog house disease
	Esparto grass	Espartosis
Aspergillus clavatus	Barley	Malt worker's lung
Penicillium casei, P. roqueforti	Cheese	Cheese washer's lung
Alternaria sp.	Wood pulp	Wood pulp worker's lung
Cryptostroma corticale	Wood bark	Maple bark stripper's lung
Graphium, Aureobasidium pullulans	Wood dust	Sequoiosis
Penicillium frequentans	Cork dust	Suberosis
Aureobasidium pullulans	Water	Humidifier lung
Cladosporium sp.	Hot tub mist	Hot tub HP
Trichosporon cutaneum	Damp wood and mats	Japanese summer-type HP
Cephalosporium sp	Sewage	Sewage worker's lung
Lycoperdon sp.	Puffballs	Lycoperdonosis
Mucor stolonifer	Paprika	Paprika splitter's lung
Botrytis cinera	Wine grapes	Spaetlese lung
Lentinus edodes (Shiitake), *Hypzigus marmoreus* (Bunashimeji)	Exotic mushrooms	Mushroom worker's lung
Animal and plant proteins		
Avian proteins	Bird droppings, feathers (bloom)	Bird fancier's lung
Urine, serum, pelts	Rats, gerbils	Animal handler's lung
Wheat weevil (*Siltophilus granarius*)	Infested flour	Wheat weevil lung
Fish	Meal	Fish-meal worker's lung
Pituitary extracts (bovine, porcine)	Pituitary snuff	Snuff taker's lung
Animal furs	Hair	Furrier's lung
Plants		
Coffee	Coffee bean dust	Coffee worker's lung
Trees (i.e. *Gonystylus bacanus*)	Wood dust	Woodworker's Lung
Cotton	Bract of cotton flower	Byssinosis
Low-Molecular Weight Chemicals		
Toluene diisocyanate (TDI)	Paints, resins, polyurethane foams	Isocyanate HP
Diphenylmethane diisocyanate (MDI)	Paints, resins, polyurethane foams	Isocyanate HP
Hexamethylene diisocyanate (HDI)	Paints, resins, polyurethane foams	Isocyanate HP
Trimellitic anhydride	Plastics, resins, paints	TMA HP
Copper sulfate	Bordeaux mixture	Vineyard sprayer's lung
Sodium diazobenzene sulfate	Chromatography reagent	Pauli's reagent alveolitis
Pyrethrins	Pesticide	Pyrethrum HP
Drugs	Amiodarone, gold, procarbazine	Drug-induced HP
Methyl methacrylate	Dental laboratories	

From Lacasse Y, Selman M, Costabel U, et al: Clinical diagnosis of hypersensitivity pneumonitis. Am J Respir Crit Care Med 2003; 168:952–958.

TABLE 55-2 Predictors of Hypersensitivity Pneumonitis Based on 2003 HP Study Group Findings

Variable	Odds Ratio (95% CI)
Exposure to known antigen	38.8 (11.6–129.6)
Positive precipitating antibodies	5.3 (2.7–10.4)
Recurrent episodes of symptoms	3.3 (1.5–7.5)
Inspiratory crackles	4.5 (1.8–11.7)
Symptoms 4–8 h after exposure	7.2 (1.8–28.6)
Weight loss	2.0 (1.0–3.9)

onset may be difficult to elicit. Physical examination findings may be scarce and can include basilar crackles. In patients with advanced fibrotic lung disease, signs of right heart failure and cyanosis may exist. Clubbing is a poor prognostic sign.

Laboratory Studies and Serum Precipitins

Most laboratory tests for EAA are nonspecific and may include mild elevations of the erythrocyte sedimentation rate, C-reactive protein, lactate dehydrogenase, and immunoglobulins. A mild neutrophilic leukocytosis with lymphopenia may occur. With recurrence of acute symptoms, ACE levels may be elevated.

The finding of precipitating antibodies in a patient with other clinical findings of HP is helpful to confirm the diagnosis and identify a relevant exposure, but serum precipitins are often neither sensitive nor specific. These antibodies are markers of exposure and have been reported in 30% of asymptomatic farmers and 50% of asymptomatic pigeon breeders. Moreover, precipitins may not be demonstrable in patients with known EAA. In the HP Study Group's evaluation of diagnostic criteria, 78% of patients with EAA had positive precipitins. In a study of patients with farmers lung, 40% had no detectable antigens. Reasons for such variability include poorly standardized antigens, improper quality controls, insensitive techniques, incorrect choice of antigen, or underconcentrated sera. A newer method of antigen detection called co-immunoelectrodiffusion had a sensitivity and specificity of 95.5% and 98.7%, respectively, among cases exposed to birds compared with controls with similar exposures. This approach may offer improved diagnostic sensitivity, but its general usefulness in the diagnosis of EAA awaits further study.

Pulmonary Physiology

Pulmonary function testing classically demonstrates a restrictive pattern, with decreased forced vital capacity, total lung capacity, and diffusion capacity. However, resting pulmonary function may be normal. Airflow limitation is not uncommon and was described in one study in 42% of patients with farmer's lung after 6 years of follow-up. Methacholine challenge is often positive. A mixed pattern of restriction and obstruction may be seen in subacute and chronic EAA. Hypoxemia may be present, and an exercise-induced decline in PaO_2 is an early sign of functional impairment. A 4- to 6-week period may be required for resolution of physiologic abnormalities after acute exposure.

Routine inhalation challenge is not recommended in most patients with suspected EAA. Inhalation challenge with the putative antigen usually induces a transient inflammatory response without long-term complications. In general, specific inhalation challenge is not performed because of lack of standardized antigens and limited access to an experienced center to conduct the study.

Imaging

Because of improvements in diagnostic imaging, plain chest radiographs now have a sensitivity of only approximately 10% in the diagnosis of EAA. The chest radiograph in acute or subacute illness may be normal or show diffuse ground-glass opacification and fine reticulonodular infiltrates (Figure 55-1). Consolidation is rare. In chronic EAA, fibrosis with upper lobe retraction, reticular opacity, volume loss, and honeycombing may be seen.

CT for EAA should always include thin sections spaced at 1–2-cm intervals, with high-resolution technique (HRCT). Expiratory HRCT images should be obtained and prone images performed whenever there is opacity in the dependent lungs on supine images. The sensitivity of HRCT for EAA is still only 45%, but specificity is 81%. The HRCT findings of EAA are multiple and are loosely correlated with histologic and pulmonary function abnormalities (Table 55-3).

Centrilobular Nodules. Nodules are the most frequent HRCT finding in EAA. They are often profuse (with a middle to lower lung zone predominance variably reported), round, poorly defined, and <5 mm in diameter. Centrilobular nodules probably reflect a cellular bronchiolitis and may not be associated with pulmonary function abnormality.

Ground-Glass. Hazy opacities that obscure underlying bronchovascular margins occur most commonly in acute EAA but may be present in subacute or chronic disease, especially if there is ongoing exposure. Opacities may be patchy or diffuse and are reversible. The imaging findings of ground-glass opacity probably represent histologic findings of active alveolitis or early fibrosis.

Consolidation. Although rare, consolidation may occur during acute EAA and often resolves with treatment.

Fibrosis. Interstitial fibrosis manifests in chronic EAA as irregular linear opacities, traction bronchiectasis, lobar volume loss, and irreversible honeycombing. A midlung predominance has been reported, but upper or lower lobes may be affected. Honeycombing is seen in up to 50% of chronic bird fancier's lung but is less commonly reported in other forms of EAA. The CT features of chronic EAA may resemble those of nonspecific interstitial pneumonitis (NSIP) or usual interstitial pneumonitis (UIP). Imaging features that favor EAA over IPF include upper or mid zone predominance, presence of ground-glass abnormality, and lower likelihood of honeycombing.

Cysts. Thin-walled cysts are present in up to 13% of patients with subacute EAA. These cysts resemble those seen in lymphocytic interstitial pneumonia, and their pathogenesis is uncertain.

Mosaic Attenuation/Expiratory Air Trapping. Mosaic pattern includes a patchwork of regions of differing attenuation associated with air-trapping. Air trapping reflects failure of

ACUTE/SUBACUTE HP: CT FEATURES

- Usually diffuse
- Profuse, poorly defined centrilobular nodules
- Tree-in-bud appearance
- Ground-glass attenuation
- Air trapping

CHRONIC HP: CT FEATURES

- Upper, mid, or lower lung predominance
- Centrilobular nodules
- Irregular lines
- Ground glass
- Air trapping
- Reticular opacity
- Honeycombing

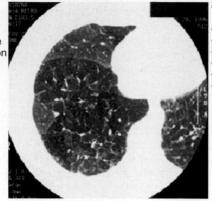

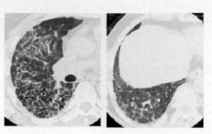

A

B

FIGURE 55-1 **A** and **B**, HRCT findings in acute and chronic extrinsic allergic alveolitis.

TABLE 55-3 Radiographic Abnormalities in EAA and their Associations with Pulmonary Function and Histologic Abnormalities

HRCT Abnormality	Physiologic Correlate	Histologic Correlate
Centrilobular nodules	None	Cellular bronchiolitis
Ground glass	Restriction, decreased diffusion capacity	Active alveolitis, fine fibrosis
Consolidation	Decreased diffusion capacity	Alveolar filling
Linear opacities, honeycombing, traction bronchiectasis	Restriction, decreased diffusion capacity	Fibrosis
Cysts	None	Unknown
Mosaic attenuation/air trapping	Obstruction	Bronchiolitis
Emphysema	Obstruction, decreased diffusion capacity	Emphysema, bronchiolar inflammation and obstruction

an area to increase in attenuation on expiratory imaging and probably represents bronchiolitis.

Emphysema. Emphysematous changes on HRCT have been reported more frequently since the 1990s. In multiple studies, emphysema has been more prevalent than fibrosis in chronic farmers lung, even when adjusted for smoking status. The pattern of emphysema seems to be similar to that of smoking-related emphysema. Although the mechanism for development of emphysema in EAA is unclear, it is probably associated with bronchiolar inflammation and obstruction.

Fiberoptic Bronchoscopy

BAL often shows a lymphocytic alveolitis in patients with EAA, typically without significant eosinophilia or neutrophilia. Although there are inconsistencies in lymphocyte subsets between different forms of EAA, a $CD8^+$ predominance occurs primarily in nonsmokers with acute or subacute HP, whereas a $CD4^+$ predominance tends to occur in smokers or in chronic EAA. The BAL lymphocytosis may persist for years despite clinical improvement and may occur in exposed patients without disease, thus limiting the specificity of BAL alone as a diagnostic tool. There seems to be little correlation between BAL findings and other clinical abnormalities such as radiographic changes, pulmonary function abnormalities, and the presence of serum precipitins.

Histopathology

Although lung biopsy is not necessary in cases of EAA when clinical findings are classic, the overlap of EAA with other inflammatory lung diseases often requires histologic confirmation. The classic pathologic triad of EAA includes: (1) cellular bronchiolitis, (2) an interstitial mononuclear cell infiltrate, and (3) scattered, small, poorly formed granulomas. However, all three findings may not be present in every case, and histologic findings are often nonspecific. In one case series of bird fancier's lung, granulomas were found in only 17%, although other reports describe granulomas in approximately two thirds of cases. Typical biopsy findings in subacute and chronic EAA include a patchy infiltrate of alveolar walls with mononuclear cells in a bronchocentric distribution, poorly formed granulomas or giant cells, and foamy macrophages. Intraalveolar foci of organizing pneumonia are often noted. Other histologic features of chronic EAA include UIP-like lesions (with the distribution of fibrosis more commonly in centriacinar and perihilar regions) or a fibrotic or cellular NSIP picture.

Treatment

The cornerstone for treatment of EAA is removal from exposure to the offending antigen. Antigen elimination is the most effective approach. For example, maple bark stripper's lung and bagassosis are now rare because of changes in handling of organic substrates that minimize growth of microorganisms. Sources of moisture leading to microbial contamination indoors, such as humidifiers, leaking pipes, or appliances and indoor hot tubs, should be eliminated. Removing pet birds from the home is the first step in exposure remediation for bird fanciers lung and should be followed by thorough cleaning of surfaces and ventilation systems. Removal of carpets and other fleecy furnishings may be helpful, because bird proteins may persist and are difficult to eliminate with cleaning or vacuuming alone. Efforts to ensure exposure abatement are often expensive and difficult to assess for adequacy. It is, therefore, important that patients with EAA receive regular clinical follow-up of symptoms, pulmonary function, and imaging to assess disease progression and to direct further efforts to minimize exposure.

In addition to antigen avoidance, pharmacologic treatment may be helpful. Oral corticosteroids are often used as first-line agents in severe or progressive disease. They are probably unnecessary in patients with mild pulmonary function abnormalities who are likely to recover with removal from exposure. Corticosteroid therapy may shorten duration of acute illness, but no documented improvement in long-term prognosis has been demonstrated. Typical treatment regimens begin with 40–60 mg of daily prednisone for 2–4 weeks, with monitoring for improvement in symptoms and pulmonary function. Pulmonary function tests should be obtained within 4–6 weeks of starting treatment. If there is improvement, steroids should be gradually tapered to minimal sustaining dose. If there has been no improvement, steroids should be tapered and discontinued. If airflow limitation is present, long-acting, inhaled β-agonists and steroids should be considered. Supplemental oxygen may be necessary in severe cases.

In refractory EAA, cytotoxic therapy has been used in regimens similar to those for idiopathic pulmonary fibrosis and connective tissue lung diseases. Although clinical trials have not been done, cyclophosphamide and azathioprine have had anecdotal success and should be continued if tolerated for at least 6 months. In patients unresponsive to medical therapy, lung transplantation may need to be considered.

Clinical Course and Prevention

The natural history of EAA is variable, but if the disease is recognized early, prognosis for recovery is excellent. Acute symptoms of fevers, chills, and cough resolve within days after exposure ceases, but malaise, fatigue, and dyspnea may persist for several weeks. Vital capacity and diffusion capacity improve within the first 2 weeks after an acute attack, but mild pulmonary function abnormalities may persist for months. Single episodes are normally self-limited, but continued symptoms and progressive lung impairment have been reported after recurrent acute attacks and even after a single severe attack. Persistent airways hyperreactivity or emphysema may complicate long-term recovery from EAA.

Long-term mortality rates for patients with chronic EAA range from 1–10%. Prognosis is poorer when disease is recognized late in it course. Prognostic factors include age, duration of exposure after onset of symptoms, and time of exposure before diagnosis. Continued antigen exposure is associated with an accelerated decline in lung function. Symptomatic pigeon breeders had a fourfold average rate of decline in lung function compared with expected rates. There are no current biomarkers that predict disease outcome or progression, but

downward trends in serum lactate dehydrogenase levels may parallel resolution.

Prevention largely begins with recognition of sentinel cases, because others exposed to the same environment are at risk for disease. Environmental control of microbial antigens involves controlling moisture through removal of sources of water intrusion and eliminating aerosol humidifiers and hot tubs. Indoor relative humidity should be maintained at less than 70%. High-efficiency filters should be used in ventilation systems, and the amount of outdoor air should be optimized. Efforts to decrease the incidence of farmer's lung have included the efficient drying of hay and cereals before storage, use of mechanical feeding systems, and better ventilation of farm buildings.

Pitfalls and Controversies

Because there is no single "gold standard" for the diagnosis of EAA, clinicians considering this diagnosis are often challenged by the wide range of diagnostic possibilities. Although understanding exposure is important in patient care, it is not uncommon that the antigen causing illness remains uncertain. Moreover, even when the relevant antigen is identified, eliminating exposure often remains challenging to both the patient and the provider. There are few guidelines regarding dose and duration of therapy, and decision-making is guided by individual patient responses.

Continued debate exists as to whether hot tub lung represents an infectious or hypersensitivity lung disease related to nontuberculous mycobacterial (NTM) aerosols and whether treatment with antimycobacterial drugs is necessary. The pathogenic potential of NTM in immunocompromised hosts is well known. Immunocompetent patients, however, tend to respond well to removal from exposure to hot tub aerosols and use of corticosteroids. Thus, for most immunocompetent patients with EAA caused by hot tub exposure, antimycobacterial therapy is probably not necessary.

SUGGESTED READINGS

Camarena A, Juarez A, Mejia M, *et al:* Major histocompatibility complex and tumor necrosis factor—A polymorphism in pigeon breeder's disease. Am J Respir Crit Care Med 2001; 163:1528–1533.

Cormier Y, Brown M, Worthy S, *et al:* High-resolution computed tomographic characteristics in acute farmer's lung and in its follow-up. Eur Respir J 2000; 16:56–60.

Fink JN, Ortega HG, Reynolds HY, *et al:* Needs and opportunities for research in hypersensitivity pneumonitis. Am J Respir Crit Care Med 2005; 171:792–798.

Glazer CS, Rose CS: Clinical and radiologic manifestations of hypersensitivity pneumonitis. J Thoracic Imaging 2002; 17:261–272.

Gupta A, Rosenman KD: Hypersensitivity pneumonitis due to metal working fluids: sporadic or under reported? Am J Indust Med 2006; 49:423–433.

Hanak V, Kalra S, Aksamit TR, *et al:* Hot tub lung: Presenting features and clinical course of 21 patients. Respir Med 2006; 100:610–615.

Lacasse Y, Selman M, Costabel U, *et al:* Clinical diagnosis of hypersensitivity pneumonitis. Am J Respir Crit Care Med 2003; 168:952–958.

Rose CS: Hypersensitivity pneumonitis. In Mason RJ, Broaddus VC, Murray JF, Nadel JA, Eds: Murray and Nadel's Textbook of Respiratory Medicine, 4th ed. Philadelphia: Elsevier Saunders; 2005.

Selman M: Hypersensitivity pneumonitis: A multifaceted deceiving disorder. Clin Chest Med 2004; 25:531–547.

Toubas D, Aubert D, Villena I, *et al:* Use of co-immunoelectrodiffusion to detect presumed disease-associated precipitating antibodies, and time-course value of specific isotypes in bird-breeder's disease. J Immunol Meth 2003; 272:135–145.

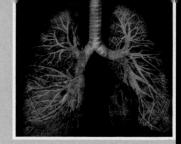

SECTION XIII

PULMONARY MANIFESTATIONS OF SYSTEMIC CONDITIONS

56 Connective Tissue Disorders

J.C. GRUTTERS • J.M.M. VAN DEN BOSCH

INTRODUCTION

Connective tissue disorders (CTDs) are generally referred to as a group of systemic diseases with abnormalities in the collagen and elastin holding tissues. Usually, they are characterized by the presence of overactivity of the immune system by unknown causes, which results in the production of autoantibodies. Specific entities include rheumatoid arthritis (RA), systemic sclerosis (SSc), dermatomyositis/polymyositis (DM/PM), mixed connective tissue disease (MCTD), systemic lupus erythematosus (SLE), Sjögren's syndrome (SS), relapsing polychondritis, and ankylosing spondylitis.

Pathologic changes are commonly seen in the lungs of these patients and may sometimes be the site of initial manifestation of the systemic disease. All compartments of the respiratory system can be involved, from pleura, airways, and the alveolar parenchyma through the pulmonary vasculature, and these anatomic regions can be affected either in isolation or in combination, producing a variety of clinical presentations. Furthermore, the pulmonary manifestations of CTDs need to be separated from the effects of therapy (i.e., drug reactions and opportunistic infections).

EPIDEMIOLOGY

RA is the most common CTD and occurs worldwide in approximately 1% of the adult population. The prevalence of SSc is ±10 in 100,000, with a female preponderance of between 4:1 and 9:1. PM/DM is relatively rare, affecting 2–10 per 1 million people and has a bimodal age distribution, with an early peak at 5–15 years and a later peak at 50–60 years of age. It occurs three to four times more commonly in women. SLE occurs in up to 1 in 2000 individuals, with a female/male ratio of 10:1. The prevalence of primary SS is approximately 0.5–1% in the general population and 10–30% in patients with other autoimmune disorders (secondary SS). SS affects predominantly middle-aged women. The prevalence of MCTD has not been precisely defined but probably approximates 1 in 10,000. The disease is more common in women than in men, and most patients present in the second or third decade of life.

Pulmonary Involvement

Estimates of the prevalence of pulmonary involvement in CTDs vary widely, depending on the investigated cohort and the methods used to detect lung abnormality. For parenchymal disease, the highest prevalence is seen in histologic or autopsy studies and HRCT evaluation that often demonstrates abnormalities not seen on the chest radiograph.

SSc shows the highest prevalence of interstitial pneumonias (IPs) (±80% being nonspecific IP [NSIP]) and of vascular disease among CTDs. Autopsy studies indicate that at least some degree of pulmonary fibrosis is present in up to 75% of patients, and vascular disease occurs in approximately 30%. RA and PM/DM also show relatively high prevalences of certain degrees of lung fibrosis, but clinically overt disease is less frequent and similar to that of SSc (approximately 5%). Compared with SSc, patients with RA and PM/DM complicated by lung fibrosis show higher frequencies of usual interstitial pneumonia (UIP) and organizing pneumonia (OP). Of all pulmonary manifestations in CTDs, pleural disease is probably the most common, especially in RA and SLE. Table 56-1 summarizes the relative frequencies of the major respiratory complications, including interstitial pneumonia (IP) subtypes, across the various CTDs.

GENETICS

There is increasing evidence of a genetic predisposition for CTDs. For example, RA is strongly associated with the class II major histocompatibility (MHC) gene product HLA-DR4; up to 70% of patients with definite RA express HLA-DR4 compared with 28% of control subjects. Evidence for genetic factors in SSc is supported by the observation of familial clustering, increased prevalence in twin studies, the high frequency of autoimmune disorders and autoantibodies in family members of patients with systemic sclerosis, and differences in prevalence and clinical manifestations among different ethnic groups. Strong genetic associations have been found between HLA-DRB1*11 and HLA-DPB1*1301 and diffuse systemic sclerosis, and there is some evidence to suggest that it is an amino-acid motif shared by the different class II susceptibility alleles that may be pivotal in predisposing to autoantibody formation.

Genetic Risk Factors for Pulmonary Complications

In SSc and RA in particular, a number of genetic factors have been shown to be specifically associated with pulmonary complications. In SSc, carriage of HLA-DRB1*11(04) and DPB1*1301 alleles is associated with lung fibrosis and DRB1*04 and DRB1*08 with pulmonary hypertension, which is linked to the presence of anticentromere autoantibodies (ACA). ACA positivity has also been shown to associate with carriage of a functional TNF promoter variant (i.e., TNF - 863A). This and other genetic findings have no clinical implication yet, but in the case of TNF-α, they suggest a different pathogenetic role of this cytokine across different SSc subsets. In RA, there is an association between obliterative bronchiolitis (OB) and the expression of histocompatibility antigens HLA-B40 and DR1, which implicates a genetic risk factor.

TABLE 56-1 Relative Frequencies of Pulmonary Manifestation in CTDs

Pulmonary Manifestation	RA	SSc	DM/PM	MCTD	SLE	SS
Interstitial pneumonias	++	+++	++	++	+	+
Usual interstitial pneumonia	++	+	+	+	+	+
Nonspecific interstitial pneumonia	+	+++	++	+	+	+
Organizing pneumonia	+	±	++	+	+	+
Diffuse alveolar damage	±		±	±	+	
Lymphocytic interstitial pneumonia	+				±	++
Follicular bronchiolitis	±					+
Constrictive bronchiolitis	+		±	±	±	
Bronchiectasis	++				±	±
Pleural involvement	+++			++	+++	±
Pulmonary hypertension		+++	+	++	++	±
Alveolar hemorrhage	±				+	
Respiratory muscle weakness		±	++		++	

+++, Common; ++, fairly frequent; +, occasional; ±, rare or very rare.

PATHOGENESIS

Interstitial Fibrosis

In CTDs, the current concept is that interstitial fibrosis occurs in response to a persistent inflammatory stimulus causing extended or repetitive tissue damage and that can be considered as an inappropriate response to injury or excessive wound healing. Activation and interaction of both the innate and adaptive immune system and interaction with extravascular tissue promote the production and secretion of inflammatory mediators, such as free radicals, cytokines, and chemokines, as well as growth factors and proteolytic enzymes that together modulate mesenchymal cell phenotypes and induce synthesis, deposition, and accumulation of extracellular matrix (ECM) components within the affected tissues. As part of the regulatory process, there is often an upregulation of connective tissue matrix protein breakdown enzymes, such as collagenase, and other metalloproteinases and serine proteases, such as elastase, which can cause damage to the original architecture. Over time these processes cause extensive tissue remodeling and a substitution of normal tissue architecture and structures with scar tissue.

Numerous lines of evidence suggest that autoimmune antibodies play a key role in the inflammatory process that precedes the development of fibrosis. Reactivity to the nuclear autoantigen topoisomerase I (Scl70) is rarely seen other than with SSc and strongly associated with the occurrence of lung fibrosis. Recently, it has been found that the serum of SSc patients contains stimulatory antibodies to the platelet-derived growth factor receptor, which can selectively induce intracellular transcription factors and reactive oxygen species, stimulate type I collagen-gene expression and myofibroblast phenotype conversion in human normal fibroblasts.

Vascular Disease

Pulmonary vessels may be involved by inflammation (vasculitis) or by concentric fibrosis formation. Vasculitis can affect all levels of the pulmonary circulation. Pulmonary capillaritis usually manifests as diffuse alveolar hemorrhage. The exact pathogenesis of vasculitis is not known, but in some syndromes such as SLE, it is thought to be due to immune complex deposition.

Concentric fibrosis of small arterioles will give rise to pulmonary arterial hypertension (PAH). The pathogenesis of PAH in CTDs is very complex, and at present no single unifying hypothesis explains all aspects of it. Potential etiologies are autoimmune antibodies (e.g., antifibrillarin, antiendothelial, or anticentromere antibodies) and enhanced vasoreactivity. Several reports have suggested that dysregulation of the pulmonary vascular tone may contribute to CTD-related pulmonary hypertension ("pulmonary Raynaud's hypothesis"). The observation of decreased nitric oxide (NO) production in the lungs of patients with SSc and pulmonary hypertension supports the concept that endothelial dysfunction contributes to altered regulation of pulmonary vascular tone and the development of PAH. Besides, other etiologies might be involved, including increased endothelin-1 (ET-1), platelet activation, and oxidant stress.

LUNG PATHOLOGY

Airway Pathology

CTDs may affect all parts of the airways. Usually, the pathology is characterized by diffuse inflammatory infiltrates in and around the walls of the larger and smaller airways and sometimes in their lumina. It is usually chronic in nature but may be a mixture of acute and chronic. Persistent inflammatory activity can cause damage to normal airway structures, which may induce wound-healing responses that lead to the accumulation of scar tissue in and around airways. In some conditions, there may be involvement of specific anatomic structures, such as in relapsing polychondritis.

Chronic Bronchitis/Bronchiolitis

This condition refers to a variable intense nonspecific chronic inflammatory cell infiltrate within the bronchial or bronchiolar walls. In Sjögren's syndrome, there is a predilection for the infiltrate to involve the seromucinous glands, leading to glandular atrophy and a "dry" trachea.

Follicular Bronchitis/Bronchiolitis

Follicular bronchitis/bronchiolitis (FB) is characterized by prominent peribronchial/bronchiolar lymphoid follicles with a minor interstitial inflammatory component. Compression of the airway lumina can lead to obstruction and a resultant intraluminal acute inflammatory cell infiltrate, plus pneumonia in some cases. FB is part of the spectrum of pulmonary lymphoid hyperplasia, with FB at one end being peribronchiolar in localization and lymphocytic interstitial pneumonia (LIP) showing interstitial predominance. Both FB and LIP are only rarely found in an idiopathic setting, and its recognition should always prompt for investigations for an underlying CTD.

Obliterative Bronchiolitis

Obliterative bronchiolitis (OB) is thought to begin with damage of the respiratory epithelium of terminal bronchioles, leading to the formation of chronic inflammatory granulation tissue, often laid down in a circumferential pattern causing narrowing of the airways. When the disease progresses, terminal bronchioles are obliterated by dense fibrous tissue, with sparing of the respiratory bronchioles and alveoli (Figure 56-1). Organizing pneumonia (OP) has been confused with OB and is one of the seven entities that comprise interstitial pneumonia. This confusion is caused by its older term of bronchiolitis obliterans organizing pneumonia (BOOP). In organizing pneumonia, however, there is patchy filling of alveoli with buds of granulation tissue that may extend into respiratory bronchioles but not terminal bronchioles.

Bronchiectasis

Bronchiectasis is defined as a permanent abnormal dilatation of the airways, usually associated with an inflammatory cell infiltrate. It has many causes, including most CTDs.

Parenchymal Pathology

Alveolar parenchymal disease in CTDs usually involves the IPs and sometimes other rare conditions such as alveolar hemorrhage and amyloidosis.

Interstitial Pneumonias

Interstitial pneumonias (IPs) is now used as a term to indicate the presence of diffuse inflammatory and/or fibrosing lung disease, either idiopathic or in the context of CTDs. In the past,

the term *fibrosing alveolitis* has often been used for this condition. During the past decade, there has been considerable refinement in the recognition of pathologic patterns of IPs. For idiopathic IPs, there are presently seven histologic patterns: usual interstitial pneumonia (UIP), nonspecific interstitial pneumonia (NSIP; with a cellular and fibrotic subgroup), organizing pneumonia (OP), diffuse alveolar damage (DAD), lymphocytic interstitial pneumonia (LIP), desquamative interstitial pneumonia (DIP), and respiratory bronchiolitis (RB). Use of this classification seems consistent and reliable and provides prognostic information for idiopathic disease. In cases with UIP on lung biopsy and high-resolution computed tomography (HRCT) characteristics compatible with UIP, and with no known cause or association, the diagnosis of idiopathic UIP (idiopathic pulmonary fibrosis [IPF]) is justified and carries a bad prognosis, especially when compared with idiopathic NSIP. However, this prognostic difference between idiopathic UIP and NSIP is not necessarily the case in patients with CTD. Those with a UIP pattern on biopsy have a better chance of response to treatment and better prognosis than their counterparts with idiopathic disease. Of note, DIP and RB are strongly associated with smoking and might not belong in the "idiopathic" IP classification system. Moreover, only small numbers of patients with histologic patterns of DIP and RB have been reported in series relating to CTDs, and many of these were smokers. Therefore, these two IP entities are unlikely to be causally related to CTD. A summary of the histopathologic characteristics of the IPs commonly seen in CTDs is given in Table 56-2.

Other Parenchymal Disorders

Other parenchymal disorders that can sometimes be found in CTDs include diffuse alveolar hemorrhage, amyloidosis, eosinophilic pneumonia, and alveolar proteinosis. In alveolar

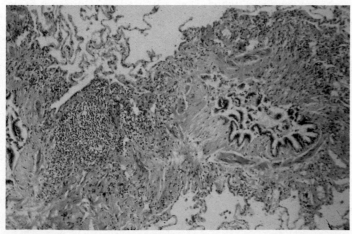

FIGURE 56-1 Lung biopsy of a patient with rheumatoid arthritis showing constrictive bronchiolitis.

TABLE 56-2 Interstitial Pneumonias in CTD Summary of the Major Histopathologic Characteristics

Type of Interstitial Pneumonia	Histopathologic Characteristics
Usual interstitial pneumonia	Fibrosis with honeycombing, fibroblast foci; anatomic destruction; little inflammatory cell infiltrate; normal/near-normal intervening lung parenchyma (temporal heterogeneity)
Nonspecific interstitial pneumonia	Variable interstitial inflammation and fibrosis; fibroblastic foci absent or very scarce; uniformity of changes within biopsy specimen
Organizing pneumonia	Patchy filing of alveoli by buds of granulation tissue that may extend into bronchioles (also termed Masson bodies); preservation of lung architecture
Lymphocytic interstitial pneumonia	Extensive lymphocytic infiltration in the interstitium often associated with peribronchiolar lymphoid follicles (follicular bronchiolitis)
Diffuse alveolar damage	Diffuse alveolar septal thickening by inflammatory cell infiltrate, hyperplastic pneumocytes, hyaline membranes, airspace organization

hemorrhage, biopsy shows a combination of intra-alveolar hemorrhage and hemosiderosis. The hemosiderin, which provides evidence of previous bleeding, is largely contained within alveolar macrophages but may also impregnate elastin in a blood vessel. Alveolar hemorrhage is usually caused by small vessel vasculitis of the lung, which is a rare pulmonary manifestation of CTDs, especially in SLE.

Amyloidosis is characterized by extracellular deposition of a proteinaceous substance that can be visualized under polarized light after staining with Congo red. This is most commonly seen in relation to SS, where it can be present in association with lymphoid hyperplasia to cause cystic changes.

Eosinophilic pneumonia is characterized by the expansion of alveoli by eosinophils, macrophages, and fibrinous debris, often with eosinophils involving the interstitium. There may also be focal intra-alveolar organization. This condition may often be related to drug exposure in patients with CTD, but it has also been attributed to RA itself.

Finally, alveolar proteinosis, which is marked by the accumulation of acellular finely granular lipoproteinaceous in alveolar spaces, has been described in dermatomyositis.

Pulmonary Hypertension

The histologic features in CTD-associated pulmonary arterial hypertension (PAH) vary in relation to the degree of raised pulmonary arterial pressure. In mild PAH, the histologic features are typically those of medial hypertrophy. With progression of the disease, marked intimal fibrous thickening and eventually plexiform lesions can be found. These histologic changes are essentially the same as those in primary pulmonary hypertension. Early changes need to be distinguished from secondary changes related to an associated interstitial pneumonia.

Pulmonary Malignancy

There is an increased risk for lung cancer in CTDs, especially in patients with lung fibrosis who also smoke. The most commonly seen neoplasm in SSc is adenocarcinoma, not infrequently with a bronchoalveolar pattern. Patients with Sjögren's syndrome have an increased risk of pulmonary lymphoma. This is usually a marginal zone non-Hodgkin's lymphoma of mucosa-associated lymphoid tissue (MALT). Preexisting follicular bronchiolitis/LIP is a risk factor (±5% may develop lymphoma).

CLINICAL FEATURES

Rheumatoid Arthritis

The clinical hallmark of rheumatoid arthritis (RA) is a small and large joint inflammatory erosive arthritis. Although rheumatoid factor (RF) has a reasonable sensitivity (60%), its specificity is often low (90%). Recently, anticyclic citrullinated peptide (CCP) antibodies have been identified that combine a high sensitivity (75%) with an excellent specificity (97%) for the diagnosis of RA. Extra-articular manifestations of RA are associated with RF, but interestingly not with anti-CCP antibodies. RA can involve any part of the respiratory tract, including the cricoarytenoid joint, the airways, the parenchyma, and the pleura. Usually, only one of these disorders is predominant in a single individual, although parenchymal changes are often associated with airway disease (on HRCT).

Pleural Disease

RA-associated pleural disease can be asymptomatic, although presenting symptoms and signs can include fever, pleuritic chest pain, and shortness of breath. Pleural effusions are generally small and unilateral, but rarely may occur in large volume or bilaterally. The fluid is exudative, with high protein and lactate dehydrogenase levels and low glucose concentration. Rheumatoid effusions usually have a low pH (<7.2) and are often paucicellular (<10,000/mL), with lymphocytic or polymorphonuclear predominance. Cytologic examination may reveal lipid droplets in the cytoplasm of neutrophils, similar to the phagocytes seen in the joint fluid of arthritic patients and known as RA cells, but these may occur in other conditions. Immunocytochemistry may reveal IgM (RF) and/or phagocytosed immune complexes in granulocytes and/or histiocytes. Thoracoscopy sometimes reveals a fine granular appearance to the pleural wall. Histopathologic examination of these micronodules may show a linear granulomatous reaction with the mesothelium replaced by palisading histiocytes. Histologic examination can also show fibrosis with often prominent chronic inflammation, including hyperplastic lymphoid follicles. In general, however, pleural biopsy will be especially helpful for exclusion of other causes of pleural disease.

Airways Disease

Bronchiectasis is a frequent finding on HRCT in patients with RA (up to 70%), but in most patients, it is asymptomatic.

Obliterative bronchiolitis is a serious complication of RA. It seems to be more common in women and usually occurs in patients who are RF positive and have well-established joint disease. In the past, penicillamine, which is rarely used now, has been associated with the development of OB in patients with RA. Also, a relationship with gold therapy has been suggested. Patients most often are initially seen with dyspnea and a nonproductive cough, which can worsen rapidly. The chest radiograph is usually normal but may show signs of hyperinflation (Figure 56-2) and in later stages fibrobullous degeneration (Figure 56-3). The diagnosis of OB should be considered in any patient with RA with progressive dyspnea and cough who has rapidly progressive air flow obstruction. Characteristic HRCT findings of OB consist of areas of decreased attenuation and vascularity with blood flow redistribution, resulting in areas of increased lung attenuation and vascularity ("mosaic perfusion" pattern), which is accentuated on expiratory scans (Figure 56-4). The prognosis is poor.

Interstitial Pneumonias

The prevalence of clinically significant IP in patients with RA is estimated at approximately 5%. It is seen more often in men than in women, especially in the context of a high RF titer and severe articular disease. The pathologic patterns are diverse, but in contrast to other CTDs, a UIP pattern is relatively common. Symptoms are nonspecific and include progressive dyspnea and nonproductive cough. Dyspnea may appear late because of physical inactivity secondary to polyarthritis. Most patients have fine bibasilar crackles, but clubbing is less common than in patients with idiopathic pulmonary fibrosis (IPF). Lung function tests usually reveal a restrictive defect with normal airflow and reduced DLco. HRCT is the most appropriate investigation for the detection

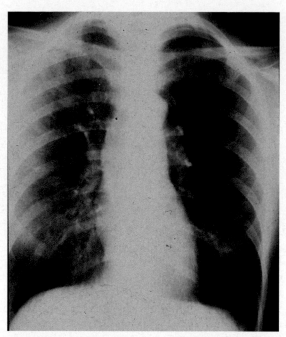

FIGURE 56-2 Chest radiograph of a patient with rheumatoid arthritis showing hyperinflation caused by constrictive bronchiolitis.

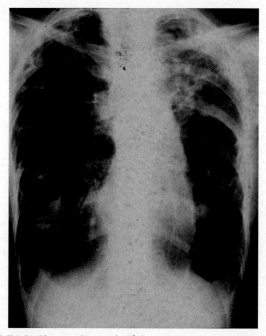

FIGURE 56-3 Chest radiograph of the same patient as in Figure 56-2 a few years later, showing evolution toward fibrosis and bullous degeneration.

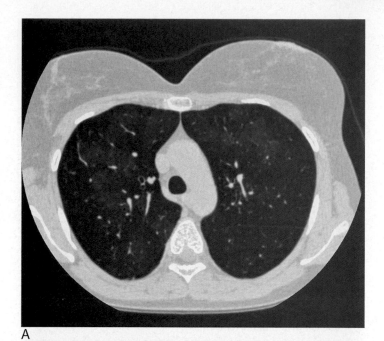

A

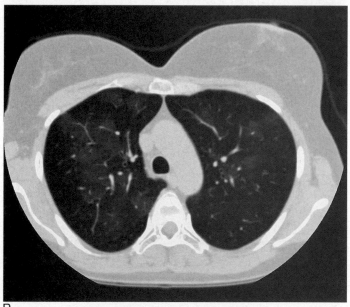

B

FIGURE 56-4 Characteristic findings on HRCT scan in a 36-year-old woman with rheumatoid arthritis and severe constrictive bronchiolitis (FEV$_1$ 35% predicted): inspiratory HRCT shows a geographic pattern, with areas of increased (normal) and decreased (air trapping) attenuation **(A)**, that is accentuated on the expiratory scan **(B)**.

of IP but is also useful in the follow-up. UIP patterns on HRCT appear similar in RA and IPF, but coexistence of pleural effusion and/or (necrobiotic) nodules may help in the differential diagnosis. In general, UIP associated with RA tends to follow a more benign course than the idiopathic form, but patients may develop end-stage respiratory failure.

Pulmonary Nodules

Pulmonary nodules are an uncommon manifestation in RA. Their occurrence is strongly associated with positivity for RF and with the presence of extrapulmonary (i.e., subcutaneous) rheumatoid nodules. Sometimes they may antedate clinical arthritis. Their radiologic appearance is not specific and may mimic malignancy, especially if the lesion is solitary. They may vary in size from millimeters to 7 cm. The nodules are most commonly found in the subpleural regions of the upper lung zones but may also be found in other parts of the lung (Figure 56-5). Histologically, they show a central zone of fibrinoid necrosis surrounded by a palisading rim of epithelioid histiocytes together with lymphocytes and plasma cells (necrobiotic nodule). Sometimes cavitation occurs, which

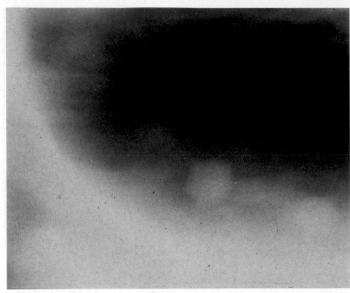

FIGURE 56-5 Chest X-ray showing multiple necrobiotic nodules in a patient with rheumatoid arthritis.

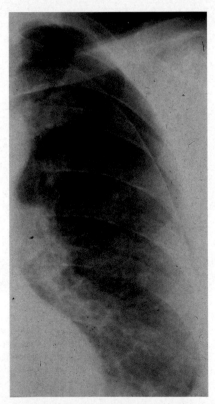

FIGURE 56-6 Pneumothorax in a patient with rheumatoid arthritis caused by perforation of a subpleural necrobiotic nodule.

can lead to complications like hemoptysis, secondary infections, or pneumothorax in the case of perforation to the pleura (Figure 56-6). During follow-up, uncomplicated pulmonary nodules may spontaneously resolve and recur, often in association with the size of extrapulmonary nodules and depending on disease activity status.

Caplan's syndrome is the coexistence of RA with pneumoconiosis, typically coal worker's pneumoconiosis or silicosis. They differ from rheumatoid nodules by their large size and

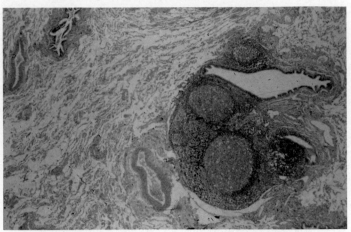

FIGURE 56-7 Lung biopsy showing hyperplasia of bronchus-associated lymphoid tissue (BALT) in a patient with rheumatoid arthritis.

by the presence of circumferential bands or arcs of dust within the necrotic centers of the lesions.

Lymphoid Hyperplasia

Hyperplasia of lymphatic tissue is commonly seen in RA. Especially lymph nodes, spleen, and bronchus associated lymphatic tissue (BALT) can be found to be hyperplastic (Figure 56-7).

Systemic Sclerosis

SSc can be classified according to criteria set up by the American Rheumatism Association. One major and two or more minor criteria are necessary to establish a diagnosis of SSc. Bibasilar pulmonary fibrosis is one of the minor criteria. A further subclassification can be made in limited (cutaneous) SSc (lSSc) and diffuse (cutaneous) SSc (dSSc). Limited SSc is characterized by skin involvement limited to hands, feet, face and/or forearms; the presence of anticentromere autoantibodies (ACA; 60–70%); the existence for years of Raynaud's phenomenon; and a significant incidence of pulmonary hypertension. The acronym CREST (*c*alcinosis, *R*aynaud's phenomenon, *e*sophageal dysmotility, *s*clerodactyly, and *t*elangiectasia) fits into this subclassification. Diffuse SSc is characterized by skin involvement on the upper arms and trunk, the presence of antitopoisomerase antibodies (Scl70; 40%), and a high incidence of interstitial lung disease. Furthermore, it is associated with hypertensive crises and renal failure, diffuse gastrointestinal disease, and myocardial involvement.

Interstitial Pneumonias

Most patients with SSc have pulmonary manifestations develop. Patients with diffuse scleroderma and antitopoisomerase I autoantibodies especially are at high risk for interstitial lung fibrosis. However, the clinical course of it may vary considerably. Although some patients have stable lung function parameters for years, others may have incapacitating or even fatal pulmonary fibrosis.

Lung fibrosis associated with SSc used to be expressed as fibrosing alveolitis (FA)SSc. It was believed that FASSc was indistinguishable from cryptogenic fibrosing alveolitis (CFA) or IPF. The histopathologic substrate of IPF is usually interstitial pneumonia (UIP). Various studies over the past decade have, however, clearly demonstrated that histologic and HRCT features of lung fibrosis in SSc are more similar to those found in idiopathic NSIP.

NSIP is the most common type of lung fibrosis in SSc, with incidence rates ranging from 55% to 77% of cases. In NSIP, fibrosis and inflammation are more diffuse in involved areas and of the same age throughout the affected lung. On HRCT, fibrotic changes are less coarse, and the proportion of ground-glass opacification is greater than in UIP. A UIP pattern, which is characterized by honeycomb changes and hardly any ground glass, can also be found in SSc. In contrast to the idiopathic equivalents, UIP and NSIP in SSc do not seem to behave differently in terms of response to immunosuppressive treatment or prognosis, but further studies are needed to investigate this observation more thoroughly.

The course of pulmonary fibrosis in SSc is variable and can range from indolent to rapidly progressive. Careful monitoring of longitudinal change of lung function is still regarded as one of the best means of evaluating disease behavior. BAL eosinophilia has also been linked to the progressiveness of lung fibrosis in SSc. The prognosis further depends on the severity of disease at presentation; patients with greater impairment in lung function and more extensive disease on HRCT have a higher mortality.

Pulmonary Hypertension

Pulmonary hypertension is typically seen in patients with the CREST syndrome. It is usually caused by a precapillary disease process leading to pulmonary arterial hypertension. In some patients, pulmonary hypertension is caused by veno-occlusive disease or related to severe interstitial fibrosis with hypoxemia. In addition, diastolic dysfunction of the left ventricle, possibly because of cardiac fibrosis, may lead to pulmonary hypertension. PAH is defined as a mean pulmonary artery pressure higher than 25 mmHg at rest or higher than 30 mmHg during exercise in the absence of left-sided heart disease, defined as a pulmonary wedge pressure >15 mmHg. Pulmonary hypertension, both isolated and in association with interstitial lung disease, occurs in approximately 30% of patients with diffuse scleroderma. In patients with limited scleroderma (CREST syndrome), it is found in up to 60% of patients. In both cases, the presence of PAH significantly worsens the prognosis. Reported survival in patients with SSc and pulmonary hypertension is similar to patients with primary pulmonary hypertension (i.e., 2-year survival of approximately 50%).

Other Thoracic Diseases in SSc

In addition to lung fibrosis and pulmonary vascular disease, SSc can be complicated by aspiration pneumonia because of regurgitation of pooled contents from a fibrotic, ectatic esophagus (Figure 56-8). Aspiration-related infection can be worsened by immunosuppressive treatment, architectural distortion, and traction bronchiectasis caused by fibrotic lung disease, which hinders normal protective clearance mechanisms and increases bacterial colonization of the airways.

Rarely, basal pleural thickening is found, but pleural effusions are very unusual.

Dermatomyositis/Polymyositis

Polymyositis and dermatomyositis (PM/DM) are rare inflammatory myopathies. Major criteria include symmetric muscle weakness; a muscle biopsy showing inflammatory cell infiltrates and necrosis; elevated muscle enzymes; and a characteristic electromyogram (EMG). The most common pulmonary

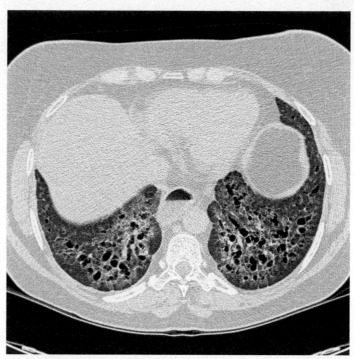

FIGURE 56-8 HRCT of the chest of a patient with systemic sclerosis showing extensive interstitial fibrosis with traction bronchiectasis and ectatic (dilated) esophagus.

complications derive indirectly from neuromuscular weakness and directly from diffuse inflammatory manifestations of PM/DM in the lung parenchyma. Furthermore, it may be complicated by pulmonary or extrapulmonary malignancies (PM relative risk, 1.7; DM relative risk, 3.8). Of note, PM/DM may also present as a paraneoplastic syndrome (up to 20% of cases), so it may be difficult to determine which condition arose first.

As in other CTDs, autoantibodies are frequently found in patients with PM/DM. Autoantibodies to a group of cellular enzymes, transfer RNA (tRNA) synthetases (anti-Jo1, anti-PL7, anti-PL12) are present in ±30% of patients with PM/DM and are rarely present in other CTDs. Presence of anti-tRNA synthetase antibodies is strongly associated with the occurrence of IPs.

Pulmonary Complications of Muscular Weakness

Muscular weakness can give rise to aspiration pneumonia (as a result of discoordinated swallowing) or respiratory insufficiency (reflecting respiratory muscle dysfunction). Airway protection is critical in patients with PM/DM and severe dysphagia; in severe cases, tracheotomy may be necessary while awaiting the impact of treatment for the underlying myopathy. Clinically significant respiratory muscle weakness has been cited in 7–22% of patients with PM/DM, sometimes leading to respiratory insufficiency requiring mechanical ventilatory support or death. Rarely, bilateral diaphragmatic paralysis has been reported. Respiratory muscle weakness may be the initial presentation of PM/DM, but this is rare. Serial measurements of forced vital capacity (FVC), maximal static inspiratory, and expiratory pressures (PI_{max} and PE_{max}) are useful to diagnose respiratory muscle weakness and monitor the course of the disease.

Interstitial Pneumonias

NSIP and OP are the most common forms of interstitial lung disease in PM/DM. Rarely, other types of IP are found. IP can occur at any point in the course of the disease. IP onset precedes PM/DM in approximately 20% of cases, but this may be higher, because treatment with immunosuppressive drugs may mask the myopathy, delaying the diagnosis for weeks or even years. Rarely, patients present more acutely, with fevers, dyspnea, and cough evolving over a few days or weeks. In this context, progression to acute respiratory failure may occur. This syndrome resembles idiopathic acute interstitial pneumonia (AIP) and is associated with a histopathologic pattern of DAD (Figure 56-9).

In PM/DM, the occurrence of IP is strongly associated with the presence of circulating antisynthetase antibodies (50–100% of cases). In contrast, antisynthetase antibodies are found in less than 5% of cases without diffuse lung disease. This clinical combination, which also includes arthritis, is known as the antisynthetase syndrome.

Mixed Connective Tissue Disease

MCTD is characterized by the presence of overlapping features of more than one CTD (e.g., Raynaud's phenomenon, synovitis, and/or myositis) and the presence of high titers (>1:1600) of circulating autoantibodies to a nuclear ribonucleoprotein antigen (anti-U1-RNP). Currently, there are different classification systems in use for the diagnosis of MCTD, causing difficulty in comparing populations and standardizing clinical evaluation. This is further complicated by the term *overlap syndrome*, which is often used for the presence of features of more than one CTD not in the context of high anti-U1-RNP titers, and by the fact that some patients have only a few features that defy categorization into one of the major CTDs but progress to exhibit typical findings of SSc, DM/PM, or SS over time.

Pulmonary complications and their pathologic features resemble those seen in other CTDs. The three most frequent are pleural effusion, interstitial pneumonia, and pulmonary hypertension. Pleural disease in MCTD occurs most frequently in patients with SLE-like clinical features; the pleura are seldom involved in SSc or PM/DM. Interstitial fibrosis most closely resembles interstitial lung involvement in SSc (i.e., showing a histologic pattern of NSIP). OP seems to be relatively infrequent in MCTD, despite a high prevalence in PM/DM. The most serious complication is progressive pulmonary arterial hypertension and cor pulmonale; rapid deterioration and death can occur despite intensive medical intervention. Other causes of pulmonary hypertension include pulmonary vasculitis and pulmonary thromboembolism, especially in MCTD with SLE-like features and circulating antiphospholipid antibodies.

Systemic Lupus Erythematosus

SLE is characterized by polyclonal B-cell activation and the production of autoantibodies directed against nuclear targets (i.e., double-stranded DNA and anti-Sm antibodies). In contrast, T-cell functions are impaired, resulting in a greater susceptibility to infectious complications.

Pleural disease with or without effusion is the most common pulmonary manifestation of SLE. Diaphragmatic dysfunction or shrinking lung syndrome is a rare disorder characterized by reduced lung volumes and normal parenchyma, probably caused by progressive pleural fibrosis and/or respiratory muscle weakness. Infection is the most common cause of parenchymal disease. Clinically significant interstitial pneumonia is a relatively rare complication in patients with SLE (±5%), and, usually, the course is slowly progressive with stabilization over time. Although difficult to demonstrate, immunohistochemistry may reveal characteristic granular patterns of IgG and complement at the alveolar capillary membrane (Figure 56-10). SLE-associated pulmonary hypertension should not be overlooked, especially in the presence of antiphospholipid antibodies. It has been reported in 4–14% of patients with SLE, with an overall mortality rate of 25–50% at 2 years from the time of diagnosis of pulmonary hypertension. In SLE, the pulmonary vasculature may be directly involved or pulmonary hypertension may be related to interstitial lung disease, diffuse alveolar hemorrhage, airways disease, or thromboembolic disease. Acute lupus pneumonitis/alveolar hemorrhage is a rare pulmonary manifestation in SLE.

Antiphospholipid Syndrome

The antiphospholipid syndrome (APS) is a systemic autoimmune disorder characterized by a combination of arterial and/or venous thrombosis, recurrent fetal loss (often accompanied by a mild-to-moderate thrombocytopenia), and elevated levels of antiphospholipid antibodies, namely the lupus anticoagulant and/or anticardiolipin antibodies, and/or antibodies to β_2-glycoprotein 1. The APS may be divided into two categories. Primary APS occurs in patients without and secondary APS occurs in patients with clinical evidence of a major autoimmune disorder (i.e., mainly SLE). Pulmonary manifestations that may be associated with APS include pulmonary embolism and infarction, primary thrombosis of large and small lung vessels, pulmonary capillaritis, pulmonary hypertension, and

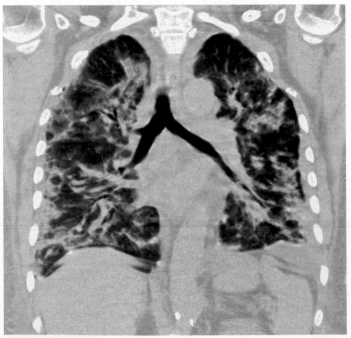

FIGURE 56-9 HRCT section (coronal plane) of a 73-year-old woman presenting with diffuse alveolar damage and organizing pneumonia (proven by VATS lung biopsy) as a first manifestation of antisynthetase syndrome (Jo1).

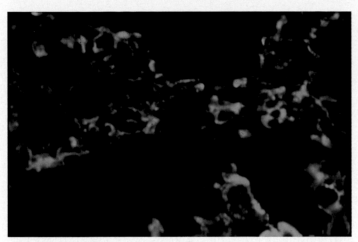

FIGURE 56-10 Immunohistochemical analysis of lung tissue of a patient with systemic lupus erythematosus complicated by interstitial pneumonia showing characteristic granular patterns of IgG and complement at the alveolar capillary membrane.

> **BOX 56-1 Pulmonary Manifestations in Sjögren's Syndrome**
>
> Upper airways disease
>   Nasal mucosa infiltration and dryness ("rhina sicca")
>   Oral cavity salivary gland involvement (xerostomia)
> Lymphocytic infiltration of the tracheobronchial submucosal glands (xerotrachea)
> Subepithelial bronchial and bronchiolar lymphocytic infiltration (lymphocytic bronchitis/bronchiolitis)
> Lymphoproliferative disorders
>   Diffuse lymphoid hyperplasia of the lungs (follicular bronchiolitis/lymphoid interstitial pneumonia, LIP)
>   Pseudolymphoma
>   Lymphomatoid granulomatosis
>   Malignant B-cell non-Hodgkin's lymphoma
> Other diffuse interstitial pneumonias
>   Usual interstitial pneumonia (UIP)
>   Nonspecific interstitial pneumonia (NSIP)
>   Organizing pneumonia (OP)
> Multiple lung cysts (often in association with LIP)
> Vasculitis and pulmonary hypertension
> Pulmonary amyloidosis
> Pleural disease (mainly in secondary Sjögren's syndrome)

> **BOX 56-2 Commonly Used Clinical Criteria for the Diagnosis of Relapsing Polychondritis***
>
> Bilateral auricular chondritis
> Nonerosive, seronegative inflammatory polyarthritis
> Nasal chondritis
> Ocular inflammation
> Respiratory tract involvement (upper and/or lower part)
> Cochlear with or without vestibular abnormality

*The presence of three or more criteria is required (according to McAdem and Zeuner)

adult respiratory distress syndrome (ARDS). Also, fibrosing alveolitis has been associated with APS. When multiple organs, systems, and/or tissues are involved and manifestations develop simultaneously or in less than 1 week, this is known as *catastrophic APS*, which has a mortality of >50% despite treatment with full anticoagulation, high-dose corticosteroids and immunosuppression, and intravenous immunoglobulins. There is some evidence that therapeutic plasma exchange might improve survival for patients with catastrophic APS.

Sjögren's Syndrome

Sjögren's syndrome (SS) is a slowly progressive autoimmune inflammatory disease affecting the exocrine glands and epithelia in multiple sites, leading to diminished or absent glandular secretions and to a more or less generalized mucosal dryness. SS presents with a wide spectrum from lacrimal and salivary exocrinopathy to systemic disease, including lung manifestations, and sometimes an associated B-cell lymphoma (±5%). The disease can occur alone (primary SS) or in association with almost all of the other CTDs (secondary SS). Pulmonary manifestations have been reported in both the primary and the secondary form of the syndrome. In the latter case, the coexisting CTD influences the pattern of pulmonary expression. A summary of the pulmonary manifestations of SS is given in Box 56-1.

Relapsing Polychondritis

Relapsing polychondritis is a very rare (<5 cases per million) multisystem disease in which recurrent progressive inflammation of cartilaginous structures results in widespread degenerative change. It is considered an autoimmune process, and autoantibodies directed against cartilage and type II collagen have been found. The condition may affect all parts of the body containing cartilage (e.g., the nose, ears, joint, and ribs). Involvement of the tracheobronchial tree may be found in up to 50% of cases. The diagnosis is generally clinical. The most widely applied diagnostic criteria are summarized in Box 56-2. CT may be a helpful radiologic procedure, because it commonly discloses smooth thickening of airway walls, as well as increased airway wall attenuation, with or without calcification. Airway collapse and lobar air trapping can be found in half of patients

examined with expiratory CT. Biopsy of affected cartilage is not generally required for a diagnosis but may be pivotal in atypical cases; auricular biopsy is the most frequent procedure, but rarely biopsy of the tracheal rings may be indicated. Finally, measurement of anti-type II collagen antibody may also be helpful, because it is fairly specific, although only positive in one third of patients.

Inflammation and destruction of the respiratory cartilage may lead to destruction and obstruction of the glottis, trachea, and/or bronchi, causing inspiratory and/or expiratory flow rate limitations, atelectasis, and secondary infections. Pulmonary parenchymal disease is rare with the exception of vasculitis, which may be present but is often subclinical. Treatment depends on disease severity. Mild cases may be controlled with nonsteroid anti-inflammatory agents, whereas relapses may require short-term, high-dose corticosteroids. In life-threatening disease, steroid-resistant disease, and the case of repeated relapses, corticosteroid therapy in combination with an immunosuppressive agent such as cyclophosphamide should be considered. Tracheostomy may be required for severe glottic or subglottic obstruction, and stenting is occasionally indicated for airway collapse or refractory airway stenosis.

Ankylosing Spondylitis

Ankylosing spondylitis (AS) is a chronic seronegative spondyl-arthritis strongly associated with the MHC antigen HLA-B27. HLA-B27 is present in 7% of whites and 95% of patients with AS. AS is a disease of white males with a prevalence of approximately 0.15%. AS is primarily a chronic inflammatory disease of the vertebral column, but involvement of other parts of the body is common. Nongranulomatous anterior uveitis occurs in up to 25% of patients, and asymptomatic inflammation of the thoracic aorta is present in 20–30%. In 10% of patients with AS, clinically important aortic incompetence or dilatation of the ascending aorta develops. Pulmonary complications take the form of extrapulmonary restriction or parenchymal disease. Apical fibrobullous disease, with or without cavitation and hilar distortion, is found in a few percent of patients, almost exclusively in males. However, AS should always be considered in patients seen with upper lobe fibrosis, being present in more than 20% of cases. Of note, a variety of other nonapical parenchymal diseases, like NSIP, can sometimes be found in patients with AS (Figure 56-11).

There is no effective treatment to retard the development of apical fibrosis; resistance to corticosteroids is usually seen. In most patients, careful observation without treatment is appropriate, with specific antimicrobial therapy when infectious complications occur. One of the greatest therapeutic dilemmas is the patient with major hemoptysis caused by aspergilloma development in a cavity. First treatment options should include the administration of antifungal agents and bronchial artery embolization. When not controllable, there may be no option but to proceed to surgical resection of the cavity (usually by means of lobectomy). However, this operation carries a high risk of postoperative bronchopleural fistula or empyema and may lead to a fatal outcome.

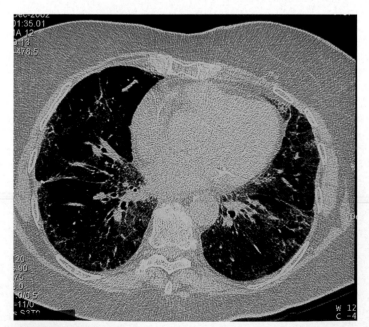

FIGURE 56-11 HRCT of the chest in a patient with ankylosing spondylitis complicated by diffuse parenchymal lung disease that histologically proved to be a nonspecific interstitial pneumonia (NSIP).

Marfan Syndrome

Marfan syndrome is an inheritable disorder of connective tissue. The condition affects all races and both sexes equally, and its prevalence is estimated at 1 in 5000 (0.02% of the population). The mode of inheritance is autosomal dominant with variable penetrance, and approximately 15–30% of all cases are due to *de novo* mutations. The disorder has been linked to a defect in the FBN1 gene on chromosome 15, which encodes the glycoprotein fibrillin-1. Fibrillin is essential for the formation of the elastic fibers found in connective tissue, because it provides the scaffolding for tropoelastin.

Affected individuals often have long limbs (arm span to height ratio >1.05) and involvement of the ocular system (e.g., ectopia lentis), cardiovascular (e.g., dilatation or dissection of the ascending aorta), and skeletal system involvement (e.g., pectus carinatum or excavatum, scoliosis, or spondylolisthesis). Pulmonary involvement occurs in approximately 10% of patients and involves apical emphysematous and cystic changes, and bullous degeneration that may lead to spontaneous pneumothorax. In some cases, upper lobe fibrosis has been described.

Behçet's Disease

Behçet's disease is an inflammatory disorder of unknown etiology affecting blood vessels of nearly all sizes and types, ranging from small arteries to large ones and involving veins and arteries. Disease prevalence varies from 1 in 10,000 to 1 in 300,000 worldwide, and it is most common in eastern Mediterranean countries and the Far East. It occurs mainly in young adults with the mean age of onset between 25 and 30 years and is associated with HLA-B51.

Because of the diversity of blood vessels that can be affected, manifestations of Behçet's disease may occur at many sites throughout the body. Mucocutaneous ulceration is the clinical hallmark, with aphthous oral and genital ulceration seen in almost all patients. Besides ocular lesions (anterior or posterior uveitis or retinal vasculitis) and skin lesions like erythema nodosum, pseudofolliculitis and papulopustular lesions often occur. Other features include marked arthralgias with synovitis, a predilection to thrombosis, and central nervous system involvement (headaches, meningoencephalitis, cranial nerve palsies, and seizures).

Pulmonary involvement is seen in <10% of patients. Symptoms include dyspnea, chest pain, and recurrent hemoptysis that can be life threatening. Pathology typically involves aneurysms of the pulmonary artery because of outpouchings of the blood vessel wall caused by inflammation (Figure 56-12). Also, arterial and venous thrombosis with pulmonary thromboembolism, pulmonary infarcts, and, sometimes, pleural effusions may occur. In case of hemoptysis, it is very important to distinguish between aneurysms of the pulmonary artery (with pulmonary–bronchial fistula formation) and pulmonary thromboembolism, because catastrophic pulmonary hemorrhage can occur if the wrong patients are anticoagulated. Glucocorticoids and other immunosuppressive agents such as cyclophosphamide and azathioprine are the mainstay of therapy to control the vasculitis. In life-threatening situations, lobectomy or pneumonectomy might be considered.

A form fruste of Behçet's disease is known as Hughes–Stovin syndrome (HSS), which has been defined as the presence of pulmonary artery aneurysm in the setting of systemic thrombosis without extrapulmonary features consistent with Behçet's disease.

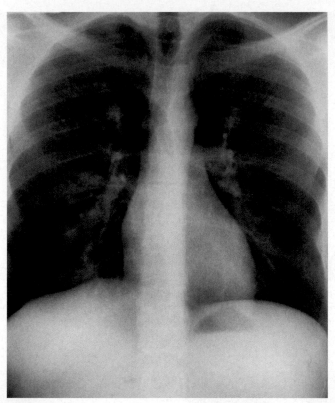

FIGURE 56-12 Chest radiograph of a 27-year-old Moroccan man with Behçet's disease initially seen with hemoptysis. There are multiple coin-sized consolidations present close to central vessels of the lung hili that proved to be aneurysms on angiography of the pulmonary artery.

DIAGNOSTIC TESTS AND FLOW CHARTS

Pulmonary Function Tests

Pulmonary function tests (PFTs) are very useful in the identification of clinically relevant parenchymal manifestations of CTDs. Pulmonary fibrosis leads to restrictive lung disease and interferes with gas exchange, resulting in decreased TLC, VC, and DL_{CO}, but often no decreased flow rates. Follow-up of lung function during the first 6 years of scleroderma symptoms seems helpful for the evaluation of disease progressiveness. It has been shown that the mean loss of percent vital capacity occurring over three 2-year time periods in patients whose initial pulmonary function tests were performed during the first 5 years of SSc were 32%, 12%, and 3% respectively. Thus, careful monitoring of lung function early in the disease, when the greatest loss of lung function occurs, may help identify patients likely to respond to new therapy.

PFT data also provide important prognostic information: SSc patients with FVC < 50% predicted have the worst prognosis, with a cumulative 10-year survival close to 50%. Furthermore, DL_{CO} < 70% predicted in combination with proteinuria and elevated ESR has been shown to accurately predict mortality over 5 years in patients newly presenting with scleroderma.

A reduction in DL_{CO} does not necessarily point to underlying interstitial lung disease but can also be a manifestation of pulmonary vascular disease or a combination of both. The ratio of VC5 predicted over DL_{CO}% predicted might be helpful; in pure fibrotic disease, the ratio is approximately 1, in isolated pulmonary arterial hypertension it is usually larger than 1.8, and when there is a mixture of both fibrosis and vasculopathy, the VC is moderately decreased but the DL_{CO} is even lower, also resulting in an elevated ratio.

Chest Radiography

Chest radiography should be performed in every patient with CTD, regardless of whether they have pulmonary complaints or findings. The pattern of abnormalities might help in the differential diagnosis of some of the CTDs. If any parenchymal abnormality is seen, HRCT should be performed.

High-Resolution CT Scans

Currently, HRCT is the imaging method of choice in evaluating patients with CTD with interstitial lung disease. It identifies more disease than the chest radiograph, is more specific, and has a greater ability to demonstrate co-existing pleural disease, small airway disease, bronchiectasis, and pulmonary nodules, but can also provide diagnostic clues like esophageal dilatation. In addition, HRCT can also be helpful in choosing the best site for open or thoracoscopic lung biopsy. HRCT has revolutionized the subcategorization of interstitial pneumonias in terms of histopathologic-radiologic patterns, especially in idiopathic disease. Similar patterns can be found in CTDs. Recently, 16-slice CT technologies have enabled postprocessing strategies (i.e., minimal intensity projection [minIP]) that may further improve the evaluation of parenchymal disease patterns. Table 56-3 summarizes the major characteristics of the different types of IPs, and Figures 56-13 to 56-16 illustrate HRCT patterns of UIP, NSIP, OP, and LIP.

TABLE 56-3 Interstitial Pneumonias in CTD Summary of the Major HRCT Characteristics

Type of Interstitial Pneumonia	HRCT Characteristics
Usual interstitial pneumonia	Peripheral, subpleural, and basal distribution; irregular reticular changes with honeycombing; traction bronchiectasis and architectural distortion; minimal ground-glass changes (focal)
Nonspecific interstitial pneumonia	Symmetric, peripheral distribution; basal predominance; more ground-glass attenuation; reticular changes and traction bronchiectasis; honeycombing is not dominant
Organizing pneumonia	Patchy consolidations and/or nodules and/or perilobular opacities; may have a ground-glass component
Lymphocytic interstitial pneumonia	Diffuse ground-glass attenuation; centrilobular nodules; septal and bronchovascular thickening; thin walled cysts
Diffuse alveolar damage	Gravity-dependent consolidation; ground-glass opacification—often with lobular sparing; traction bronchiectasis occurs later

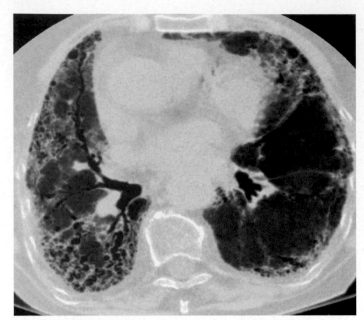

FIGURE 56-13 HRCT of usual interstitial pneumonia (UIP) in minimal intensity projection. (Courtesy of Dr. H. W. van Es, St. Antonius Hospital, Nieuwegein, The Netherlands.)

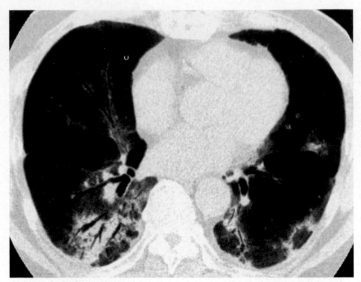

FIGURE 56-15 HRCT pattern of organizing pneumonia (OP) in minimal intensity projection. (Courtesy of Dr. H. W. van Es, St. Antonius Hospital, Nieuwegein, The Netherlands.)

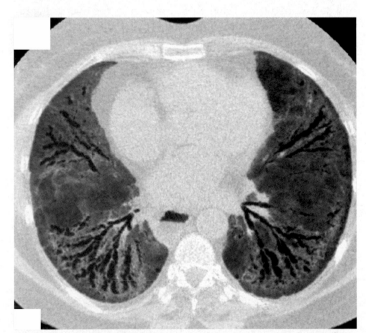

FIGURE 56-14 HRCT of nonspecific interstitial pneumonia (NSIP) in minimal intensity projection. (Courtesy of Dr. H. W. van Es, St. Antonius Hospital, Nieuwegein, The Netherlands.)

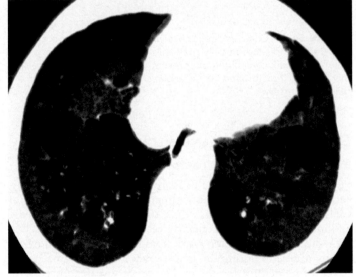

FIGURE 56-16 HRCT pattern of an lymphocytic interstitial pneumonia (LIP). (Courtesy of Dr. H. W. van Es, St. Antonius Hospital, Nieuwegein, The Netherlands.)

Bronchoalveolar Lavage (BAL)

BAL is a valuable diagnostic tool to rule out infection and confirm the presence of (fibrosing) alveolitis, and it can provide a specific diagnosis, as in cases of diffuse alveolar hemorrhage. Also, it can be particularly helpful in the differentiation of follicular bronchiolitis.

In SSc, differential cell count of BAL is also a valuable prognostic. In one study of 49 SSc patients with fibrosing alveolitis who were followed up for 2 years, only those with BAL granulocytosis (>3% neutrophils and/or >0.5% eosinophils) at baseline showed a significant disease progression with a marked reduction of DLco, whereas almost all patients with normal BAL findings or BAL lymphocytosis had stable lung function parameters during the study period.

HRCT also offers particular benefit in the assessment of the severity of diffuse lung and airway diseases. In addition, the pattern of abnormality may frequently be informative in terms of likelihood of response to treatment. A ground-glass pattern denotes predominantly inflammatory disease and is generally associated with improvement. A reticular pattern, particularly honeycombing, correlates well with the presence of established fibrosis.

Lung Biopsy

An important clinical question is when to biopsy for IPs in CTD. If patients are known to have a CTD and have respiratory symptoms, HRCT and lung function testing are most appropriate to detect or exclude with reasonable confidence diffuse interstitial lung disease. BAL might provide further clues for specific diagnosis and is especially helpful for exclusion of other diagnoses such as infections. In many cases, HRCT findings will also allow, with reasonable confidence, the diagnosis of one of the IP subsets. If this is not the case or HRCT findings are atypical beforehand, a surgical lung biopsy should be considered. However, there is relative lack of prognostic data in biopsy specimens taken from patients with CTD-associated interstitial pneumonia. Therefore, the decision to biopsy should be primarily reserved for cases with an atypical presentation and when a diagnosis other than IP is being considered (e.g., amyloidosis). Patients may also be taking immunosuppressive drugs, and histopathologic examination may be necessary to distinguish parenchymal manifestations of CTD from drug-induced lung disease and/or opportunistic infections. Finally, biopsies may be undertaken to investigate for associated malignancies, especially in LIP.

Diagnostic Flowchart

On the basis of the relatively high prevalence of parenchymal and vascular complications in patients with SSc, it is advisable to routinely screen for these complications at presentation of disease. In other CTDs, evaluation of pulmonary manifestations will usually take place in patients who are symptomatic. Figure 56-17 gives a diagnostic flowchart.

TREATMENT AND SCHEDULES

Treatment of pulmonary complications in CTDs is primarily based on the type of lung disease and not on the specific type of CTD. In most cases, there are no controlled data available for evidence-based decision making. Because CTDs are auto-immune-based inflammatory diseases and corticosteroids exert a broad range of immunosuppressive actions, they remain the mainstay of therapy despite their long list of potential side effects. Other well-known drugs are cyclophosphamide, azathioprine, and methotrexate (MTX). These drugs have immunocytotoxic properties but are also associated with more serious side effects. In particular, MTX has a small (±3%) risk of pulmonary toxicity. Furthermore, cyclosporine A and tacrolimus are of therapeutic value, because they can provide strong and specific T-cell suppression, but careful monitoring of blood levels is needed to minimize side effects.

Diffuse Lung Disease

Corticosteroids are widely used in the treatment of IPs associated with CTDs, although there is hardly any proof from randomized controlled trials that they prevent progression of interstitial pneumonias and/or reverse fibrosis. Despite this lack of evidence, they remain the mainstay of therapy, with usual doses of prednisone between 0.5–1.0 mg/kg in nonacute situations. It should be noted, however, that medium-dose corticosteroid therapy (i.e., 15 mg/day prednisone or equivalent) is associated with the development of scleroderma renal crisis, which may lead to irreversible renal failure.

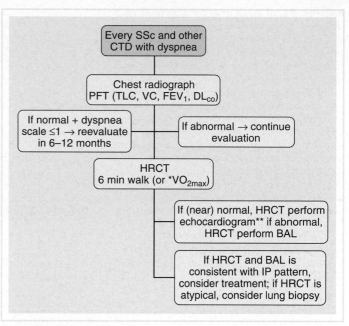

FIGURE 56-17 Diagnostic flowchart for the evaluation of pulmonary manifestations in CTDs. All patients with SSc and patients with other CTDs and respiratory symptoms can be evaluated for pulmonary complications according to this flowchart. Dyspnea scale is proposed by ATS/ERS: 0 = no breathlessness except with strenuous exercise; I = shortness of breath when hurrying or walking up a gradually sloping hill; II = walking slower than people of the same age because of breathlessness, or stopping for breath when walking at a normal pace on a level surface; III = stopping for breath after walking ±100 meters, or after a few minutes on a level surface; IV = being too breathless to leave the house or breathless when dressing or undressing. *VO_{2max} is recommended, because it provides more objective determination of functional capacity and impairment. It identifies factors limiting exercise capacity. **Routine echocardiography is recommended in SSC because of high risk of cardiac involvement and pulmonary hypertension.

Of the other immunosuppressive drugs, there are now randomized controlled data available in scleroderma diffuse lung disease only for cyclophosphamide. The North-American Scleroderma Lung Study investigated the effects of 12 months of 2 mg/kg oral cyclophosphamide versus placebo in patients with signs of interstitial lung fibrosis. Lung function was significantly preserved in the active treatment arm, although absolute changes were small. Interestingly, as well, there was an improvement in the skin score. There was a greater frequency of leukopenia and/or neutropenia in the cyclophosphamide group, but the difference between the two groups in the number of serious adverse events was not significant.

Vascular Disease

Treatment options for patients with CTD-associated pulmonary arterial hypertension are almost similar to those for primary pulmonary hypertension and are presented in Figure 56-18. Although patients with CTD may not respond as well to therapy as patients with primary pulmonary hypertension, aggressive therapy may improve functional status and quality of life.

Immunomodulatory therapy (i.e., corticosteroids with or without cyclophosphamide), long-term plasma exchange and autologous stem cell transplantation have also been reported to improve or stabilize pulmonary hypertension in patients

FIGURE 56-18 Algorithm for the treatment of pulmonary arterial hypertension in connective tissue disorders. The algorithm is focused on patients in World Health Organization functional class III or IV. Class III = patients with pulmonary hypertension (PH) resulting in marked limitation of physical activity; they are comfortable at rest; less than ordinary activity causes undue dyspnea or fatigue, chest pain, or near syncope. Class IV = patients with PH with inability to carry out any physical activity without symptoms; these patients manifest signs of right-heart failure; dyspnea and/or fatigue may even be present at rest; discomfort is increased by any physical activity. CCB = calcium channel blockers; levels of evidence: A = at least 2 RCTs that do not contradict, B = at least 1 RCT, C = efficacy evidence from observational studies, no RCTs available. RCT = randomized controlled trial.

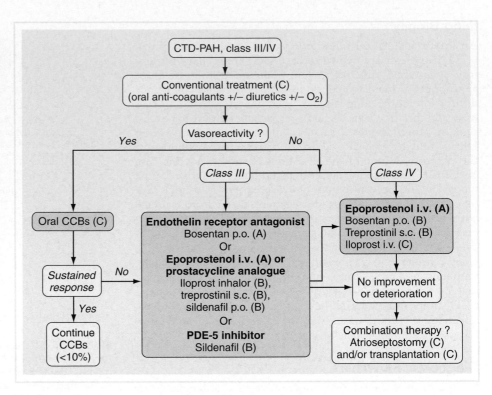

with CTDs. However, these reports represent case reports or retrospective case studies, and no prospective study of immunosuppressive therapy has been completed so far.

Lung Transplantation

Lung transplantation is now considered an accepted treatment in patients with end-stage pulmonary or cardiopulmonary disease, although chronic rejection still remains a key problem that precludes long-term survival. According to the recent International Society of Heart Lung Transplantation registry, pulmonary fibrosis caused by systemic diseases, such as scleroderma, sarcoidosis, histiocytosis X, and lymphangioleiomyomatosis (LAM), make up approximately 5% of all cases of lung transplantation. Provided that patients with systemic disease have no active disease in other organs and that other organ functions are preserved, the results after transplantation are similar to other disease conditions like IPF and emphysema.

Clinical Course and Prevention

Can early treatment of systemic disease prevent irreversible lung scarring or development of pulmonary hypertension? Through the widespread use of HRCT, there has been an increase in the detection of early lung disease in patients with CTDs. It is unclear what management strategy can be best applied in these cases, which are often asymptomatic and have normal or near-normal pulmonary function. In theory, these patients might benefit from early introduction of treatment to prevent further irreversible damage. However, most of these cases of subtle disease might never show progression. At present, these patients can only be considered "at risk" for intrinsically progressive disease and should be monitored carefully, especially in the first years after presentation.

Does the clinical course of IPs in the context of CTDs differ from their idiopathic counterparts? Currently, it is not clear that histologic distinctions between IP patterns are as important in CTD as in idiopathic IPs. In systemic sclerosis, in particular, it seems that outcome differs little between UIP and NSIP, once baseline disease severity is taken into account, not justifying routine biopsy in most patients.

Pitfalls and Controversies

Activity Versus Severity

The first question here is "What is disease activity?" Activity usually means "something is going on." In the context of CTDs and lung complications, this means "the underlying pathophysiologic process in the pulmonary tissue is still going on and has not (yet) come to a rest (i.e., complete remission)." Complete remission is, however, not synonymous with resolution of disease, because it may have caused severe damage to the tissue leaving scars (i.e., irreversible fibrosis).

Disease severity can best be defined in terms of symptoms and functional limitations of the patient. Sometimes pulmonary complications in CTDs are severe because of direct danger to life, such as diffuse alveolar hemorrhage.

In IPs, treatment decisions are primarily guided by severity of disease. In most of these processes, lung function impairment will be the upshot of the ongoing interstitial inflammatory process and irreversible fibrosis. However, in some cases, the inflammatory phase of the disease might have burnt out, leaving only extensive scar tissue. It is likely that it is the proportion of active disease that will determine success of immunosuppressive treatment. However, at present, there are no validated biomarkers or imaging technologies that can be used to dissect reversible inflammatory disease from irreversible fibrosis. Watchful follow-up of disease evolution is still considered the most important strategy to overcome these limitations.

WEB RESOURCES FOR GUIDELINES/PROTOCOLS

http://www.eustar.org/
This web site is an initiative of the EUSTAR group. EUSTAR stands for European League Against Rheumatism (EULAR) Scleroderma Trials and Research. The aim is to foster the study and the care of scleroderma and to achieve a consensus on evidence-based standards for the management of patients with scleroderma throughout Europe.

http://www.eular.org/
The European League Against Rheumatism (EULAR) is the organization that represents the patient, health professional, and scientific societies of rheumatology of all the European nations. EULAR endeavors to stimulate, promote, and support the research, prevention, treatment, and rehabilitation of rheumatic diseases.

http://www.rheumatology.org/
This is the web site of the American College of Rheumatology.

SUGGESTED READINGS

American Thoracic Society/European Respiratory Society: International multidisciplinary consensus classification of the idiopathic interstitial pneumonias. Am J Respir Crit Care Med 2002; 165:277–304.

Badesch DB, Abman SH, Ahearn GS, et al: Medical therapy for pulmonary arterial hypertension. ACCP evidence-based clinical practical guidelines. Chest 2004; 126:35S–62S.

Baroni SS, Santillo M, Bevilacqua F, et al: Stimulatory autoantibodies to the PDGF receptor in systemic sclerosis. N Engl J Med 2006; 354: 2667–2676.

Fagan KA, Badesch DB: Pulmonary hypertension associated with connective tissue disease. Pulmonary Circulation: Diseases and Their Treatment, 2nd ed., London: Arnold; 2004.

Jimenez SA, Derk CT: Following the molecular pathways toward an understanding of the pathogenesis of systemic sclerosis. Ann Intern Med 2004; 140:37–50.

Tashkin DP, Elashoff R, Clements PJ, et al: Cyclophosphamide versus placebo in scleroderma lung disease. N Engl J Med 2006; 354:2655–2666.

Verleden GM, Demedts MG, Westhovens R, Thomeer M: Pulmonary manifestations of systemic diseases. European Respiratory Monograph 34. Sheffield: ERS Journals Ltd; 2005.

Wells AU, Denton CP: Pulmonary Involvement in Systemic Autoimmune Diseases, 1st ed. Oxford: Elsevier Ltd; 2004.

Witt C, Borges AC, John M, et al: Pulmonary involvement in diffuse cutaneous systemic sclerosis: broncheoalveolar fluid granulocytosis predicts progression of fibrosing alveolitis. Ann Rheum Dis 1999; 58:635–640.

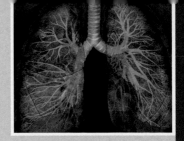

SECTION XIII
PULMONARY MANIFESTATIONS OF SYSTEMIC CONDITIONS

57 Pregnancy

STEPHEN E. LAPINSKY

The pregnant patient who has pulmonary disease is unique because of altered maternal physiology, the occurrence of diseases specific to pregnancy, and the need to consider two patients in all therapeutic decisions. In this chapter, the focus is on the changes in pulmonary physiology associated with pregnancy, certain pregnancy-specific disorders, and other pulmonary problems encountered in the pregnant patient.

PULMONARY PHYSIOLOGY

Physiologic Changes in Pregnancy

Hormonal changes in pregnancy affect the upper respiratory tract and cause airway hyperemia and edema resulting in symptoms of rhinitis. Estrogens are likely responsible for many of these effects because they produce capillary congestion and mucus gland hyperplasia. Changes to the thoracic cage result from both the enlarging uterus and from hormonal effects producing ligamentous laxity. The diaphragm is displaced cephalad by up to 4 cm, but the potential loss of lung capacity is partially offset by an increase in the anteroposterior and transverse diameters and by widening of the subcostal angle (Figure 57-1). Despite these anatomic changes, diaphragmatic function remains normal, diaphragmatic excursion is not reduced, and the maximum transdiaphragmatic inspiratory pressures that can be generated near term are similar to values generated by patients who are not pregnant. The changes in the chest wall return to normal within 6 months of delivery, although the costal angle may remain widened.

The aforementioned changes in the thorax produce a progressive decrease in functional residual capacity (FRC) by 10–25% by term (Figure 57-2). Residual volume decreases slightly, but the major change is in expiratory reserve volume. These alterations are measurable as early as 16–24 weeks of gestation and progress to term. The increased diameter of the thoracic cage and the preserved respiratory muscle function allow the vital capacity to remain unchanged, and total lung capacity decreases only minimally. Measurements of airflow and lung compliance are not affected, but chest wall and total respiratory compliance are reduced in the third trimester because of the chest wall changes and increased abdominal pressure. Inconsistencies in results reported in studies of diffusing capacity during pregnancy likely arise from the effects of anemia, variable changes in intravascular volume, and the increase in cardiac output. A small increase may be noted in early pregnancy with a subsequent decrease to normal values by term.

Minute ventilation increases markedly in pregnancy, beginning in the first trimester and reaching 20–40% above baseline at term (see Figure 57-2), produced mainly by an increase in tidal volume of approximately 30–35%. These changes are mediated by the increase in respiratory drive that results from elevated serum progesterone levels. A respiratory alkalosis with compensatory renal excretion of bicarbonate results, with $PaCO_2$ falling to 3.8–4.3 kPa (28–32 mmHg) and plasma bicarbonate falling to 18–21 mEq/L. Alveolar-to-arterial oxygen tension differences (PAO_2-PaO_2) are similar to nonpregnant values, and mean PaO_2 usually exceeds 13 kPa (100 mmHg) at sea level throughout pregnancy. Mild hypoxemia and an increased PAO_2-PaO_2 may develop in the supine position because of airway closure, because FRC diminishes near term. One study suggests that shunt is normally increased in the third trimester to approximately 15% and is not changed significantly by posture. Oxygen consumption increases, beginning in the first trimester, and reaches 20–33% above baseline by the third trimester because of fetal demands and maternal metabolic processes. The combination of a reduced FRC and increased oxygen consumption lowers oxygen reserve, which renders the pregnant patient susceptible to the rapid development of hypoxia in response to hypoventilation or apnea.

During labor, hyperventilation increases and tachypnea (caused by pain or anxiety) may result in marked respiratory alkalosis, augmented in some patients by volume depletion and/or vomiting. Alkalosis adversely affects fetal oxygenation by reducing uterine blood flow. In some patients, severe pain and anxiety may lead to rapid, shallow breathing with alveolar hypoventilation, atelectasis, and mild hypoxemia. Achieving adequate pain relief with narcotics or epidural analgesia blunts the ventilatory response and can correct the gas exchange abnormalities associated with active labor. The pregnancy-associated changes in lung function reverse significantly in the first 72 h postpartum and return to baseline within a few weeks.

Dyspnea in Pregnancy

Dyspnea is a common complaint in women who have otherwise normal pregnancies. Although a number of mechanisms have been proposed, the symptom most likely arises from a normal perception of the increased minute ventilation accompanying pregnancy. The diagnosis of this benign condition is based on the presence of isolated dyspnea not usually affecting daily activities, the absence of associated symptoms, and the exclusion of other pathologic conditions. Pregnancy also can be associated with increased exercise-induced dyspnea.

PREGNANCY-SPECIFIC DISORDERS

Amniotic Fluid Embolism
Epidemiology and Pathophysiology

Amniotic fluid embolism is a rare obstetric complication (between 1/8000 and 1/80,000 live births) that has a mortality

729

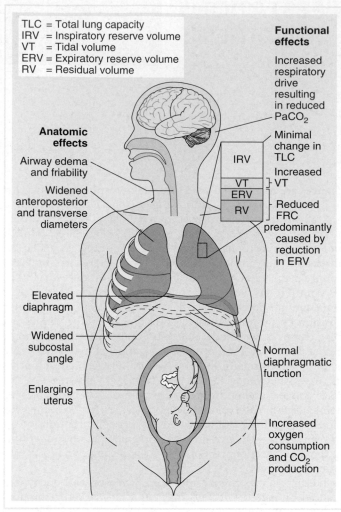

FIGURE 57-1 Pulmonary physiology in pregnancy: anatomic and functional effects of pregnancy that influence pulmonary physiology.

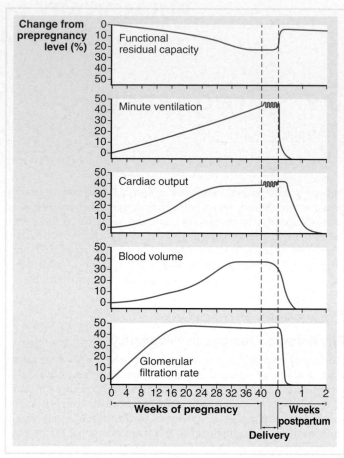

FIGURE 57-2 Physiologic changes in pregnancy. Shown are some of the physiologic changes that occur during pregnancy and the postpartum period. (Reproduced with permission from Lapinsky SE, Kruczynski K, Slutsky AS: Critical care in the pregnant patient. Am J Respir Crit Care Med 1995; 152:427–490.)

rate of 10–86% and may account for 10% of maternal deaths. Amniotic fluid embolism is usually associated with labor and delivery, but it may also occur with uterine manipulations or uterine trauma or in the early postpartum period. The mechanism seems to involve amniotic fluid that enters the vascular circulation through endocervical veins or uterine tears. Particulate cellular contents or humoral factors in the amniotic fluid produce acute pulmonary hypertension, both by obstructing the pulmonary vessels and by causing vascular spasm (Figure 57-3). Acute left ventricular dysfunction may also occur, either secondary to the initial pulmonary embolic event or in response to humoral events mediated by cytokines. The cardiovascular changes of amniotic fluid embolism resemble those of anaphylaxis, and sensitivity to amniotic fluid contents may be responsible.

Clinical Features and Diagnosis

The clinical presentation usually involves the sudden onset of severe dyspnea, hypoxemia, and cardiovascular collapse, often accompanied by seizures. Less common presentations include hemorrhage caused by disseminated intravascular coagulation and fetal distress. Up to one half of the patients

may die within the first hour, and cardiac arrest during this period is common.

The diagnosis of amniotic fluid embolism is usually made on the basis of observing the typical clinical picture. Fetal squames in a wedged pulmonary capillary aspirate have been used to confirm the diagnosis, but this does not seem to be a specific finding. Less invasive diagnostic tests such as maternal serum zinc coproporphyrin or sialyl-Tn levels have been investigated but are not currently in use.

The differential diagnosis includes septic shock, pulmonary thromboembolism, abruptio placentae, tension pneumothorax, or myocardial ischemia.

Treatment and Clinical Course

Treatment involves routine resuscitative and supportive measures, with prompt attention to adequate oxygenation, mechanical ventilation, and inotropic support. No specific therapy has been shown to be effective, but some suggest a role for corticosteroids. In view of the inconsistent hemodynamic findings, invasive monitoring may be of value. Survivors of the initial resuscitation are likely to experience the complications of disseminated intravascular coagulation or acute respiratory distress

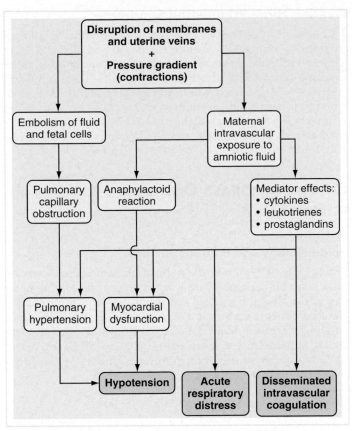

FIGURE 57-3 Pathophysiology of amniotic fluid embolism: proposed pathophysiologic mechanisms for the development of circulatory shock caused by amniotic fluid embolism.

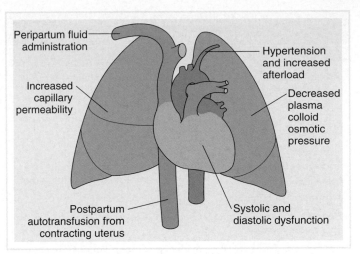

FIGURE 57-4 Pathophysiologic mechanisms responsible for the development of pulmonary edema in preeclampsia.

syndrome (ARDS). Neurologic damage caused by hypotension and hypoxemia is common.

Preeclampsia and Pulmonary Edema

Epidemiology and Pathophysiology

Pulmonary edema may rarely occur in association with preeclampsia (i.e., perhaps 3% of preeclamptic patients). The preeclamptic patient is usually volume depleted, and pulmonary edema most commonly occurs in the early postpartum period and is often associated with aggressive, intrapartum fluid replacement. Other factors that may contribute to the pathogenesis include reduced serum albumin, elevated left ventricular afterload, and systolic and diastolic myocardial dysfunction (Figure 57-4). Increased capillary permeability may also occur, aggravated by concomitant conditions such as sepsis, abruptio placentae, or massive hemorrhage.

Pulmonary edema has been described in chronically hypertensive, obese, pregnant patients in whom preeclampsia develops. Diastolic left ventricular dysfunction results from both the hypertension and the obesity, and pulmonary edema is precipitated by volume overload of pregnancy and hemodynamic stresses of preeclampsia.

Clinical Features and Diagnosis

Preeclampsia is characterized by hypertension, proteinuria, and peripheral edema, usually in the third trimester. The presentation of pulmonary edema is with acute respiratory distress in the preeclamptic patient, often in the early postpartum period.

Treatment and Clinical Course

The standard approach is to restrict fluid, administer diuretics cautiously, and provide ventilatory support if necessary. Invasive monitoring may be useful if inotropic or vasodilator therapy becomes necessary, particularly in the presence of renal dysfunction. Aggressive diuresis must be avoided, because filling pressures should not be reduced to the point of compromising cardiac output and reducing placental perfusion. Volume replacement may be necessary in preeclampsia, particularly if vasodilators are used, because these patients may be markedly volume depleted. Excessive fluid replacement may precipitate pulmonary or cerebral edema, however. The ultimate treatment of preeclampsia is delivery of the fetus.

Tocolytic Pulmonary Edema

Epidemiology and Pathophysiology

β-Adrenergic agonists, particularly ritodrine and terbutaline, may be used to inhibit uterine contractions in preterm labor. Use of these agents has become less common, however, because a number of studies have demonstrated that tocolysis does not improve neonatal outcome. A complication of β-agonists that is unique to pregnancy is the development of pulmonary edema. The frequency of tocolytic-induced pulmonary edema varies from 0.3% to 9%. Postulated mechanisms include prolonged exposure to catecholamines causing myocardial dysfunction, increased capillary permeability, large volumes of intravenous fluid administration (often in response to maternal tachycardia), reduced osmotic pressure, and/or hypotension induced by β-stimulation. Glucocorticoids are often administered in preterm labor to enhance fetal lung maturity and may compound fluid retention.

Clinical Features and Diagnosis

The clinical presentation is of acute respiratory distress with features of pulmonary edema. No specific features characterize this condition. The diagnosis is a clinical one, made in the presence of acute pulmonary edema occurring in the appropriate clinical situation. The differential diagnosis includes cardiogenic pulmonary edema, amniotic fluid embolism, and other conditions (Table 57-1). Failure of the pulmonary edema to resolve in 12–24 h requires a search for alternative causes.

TABLE 57-1 Acute Respiratory Distress Caused by Complications of Pregnancy and Labor

Disorder	Distinguishing Features
Amniotic fluid embolism	Cardiorespiratory collapse, seizures, disseminated intravascular coagulopathy
Pulmonary edema caused by preeclampsia	Hypertension, proteinuria
Tocolytic pulmonary edema	Tocolytic administration, rapid improvement with discontinuation
Aspiration pneumonitis	Vomiting, aspiration
Peripartum cardiomyopathy	Gradual onset, signs of heart failure
Venous thromboembolism	Evidence of deep venous thrombosis; radiologic investigations
Pneumomediastinum	Occurs during delivery, subcutaneous emphysema
Air embolism	Related to sexual intercourse or cesarean section, associated hypotension

Treatment and Clinical Course

The β-agonist must be discontinued, whereupon pulmonary edema should resolve rapidly; additional treatment is supportive and includes diuresis. Early recognition and management should reduce the need for invasive hemodynamic monitoring and mechanical ventilation.

Peripartum Cardiomyopathy

Cardiac failure may occur in the absence of preexisting heart disease as a result of the hypertension of pregnancy or from peripartum cardiomyopathy. This idiopathic dilated cardiomyopathy presents in the last month of pregnancy or in the postpartum period. The diagnosis is made by demonstrating impaired left ventricular function in the absence of other causes of cardiomyopathy. During labor and the early postpartum period, tachycardia and increased cardiac output may precipitate pulmonary edema. Pulmonary thromboembolic events are a common complication of this condition. Management is with diuretics and afterload reduction, bearing in mind that angiotensin-converting enzyme inhibitors should not be used during pregnancy because of the development of fetal renal dysfunction. Anticoagulation is recommended in all patients. Recovery occurs in approximately half of patients within 6 months, but persistent or progressive cardiac failure develops in a significant proportion. Because the latter group has a mortality rate in the range of 12–18%, cardiac transplantation may be considered.

Gestational Trophoblastic Disease

Pulmonary hypertension and pulmonary edema may complicate benign hydatidiform mole, caused by trophoblastic pulmonary embolism. This most commonly occurs during evacuation of the uterus, and the incidence of pulmonary complications is higher in later gestations. Molar pregnancy may be associated with choriocarcinoma, which can produce multiple, discrete pulmonary metastases, and occasionally pleural effusions.

Ovarian Hyperstimulation Syndrome

This syndrome, associated with the administration of gonadotrophins to stimulate ovulation for *in vitro* fertilization, may present with gastrointestinal or respiratory symptoms. Increased capillary permeability results in bilateral pleural effusions and ascites, associated with intravascular volume depletion. Complications include respiratory compromise because of the effusions, shock and renal failure caused by the volume depletion, as well as pulmonary emboli. Treatment is supportive, with fluid resuscitation and drainage of effusions.

OTHER PULMONARY DISORDERS IN PREGNANCY

Asthma

Epidemiology and Pathophysiology

Asthma affects 5–10% of the population and is, therefore, the most common pulmonary disorder in pregnancy. During pregnancy, the altered hormonal milieu may affect asthma control variably; patients may improve, worsen, or remain unchanged. Although pregnancy does not affect airflow in normal subjects, airway hyperreactivity in asthmatic subjects can be increased. Asthma severity usually returns to prepregnancy levels within 3 months postpartum.

Clinical Features and Diagnosis

The clinical features of asthma during pregnancy are the same as those in patients who are not pregnant. To differentiate from the dyspnea of pregnancy, objective assessment that uses pulmonary function tests to assess the degree of airflow limitation is essential. Gastroesophageal reflux is increased in both frequency and severity during pregnancy, and the symptoms of this condition should be sought as a contributing factor.

Treatment and Clinical Course

Management is similar to that in patients who are not pregnant (Table 57-2) and includes adequate monitoring, avoidance of precipitating factors, and patient education. Although physicians may be reluctant to prescribe medications during pregnancy, poorly controlled asthma is potentially more dangerous for the fetus. Inhaled corticosteroids remain the mainstay of therapy. The use of a spacer device is encouraged to reduce local side effects and systemic absorption. Although animal data suggest a small risk of cleft palate with systemic corticosteroid use, this has not been demonstrated in humans. Short courses of prednisone should be used to manage poorly controlled asthma when clinically indicated. Inhaled β-agonists seem safe and should be used as required for symptomatic relief. Gastroesophageal reflux, a potentially preventable cause of worsening asthma, is frequently overlooked. Antireflux measures may markedly reduce asthmatic symptoms. Acute attacks are treated by ensuring adequate oxygenation, closely monitoring the fetus, and administering appropriate medications. Concerns over fetal effects of drugs should not cause physicians and patients to avoid use of effective pharmacologic therapy. Updated management algorithms are available through the National Asthma Education and Prevention Program.

Poor asthma control has been reported to increase the incidence of preterm birth, low birth weight, and perinatal mortality. Acute exacerbations may be associated with hypoxemia, which may, in turn, compromise the fetus.

TABLE 57-2 Asthma Therapy in Pregnancy

Drug	Food and Drug Administration Classification
Inhaled bronchodilators	
Albuterol (Salbutamol)	C
Terbutaline	B
Ipratropium	B
Salmeterol	C
Formoterol	C
Tiotropium	C
Inhaled corticosteroids	
Beclomethasone	C
Budesonide	B
Fluticasone	C
Leukotriene antagonists	
Zafirlukast	B
Montelukast	B
Other	
Theophylline	C
Cromolyn	B
Systemic corticosteroids	C

Food and Drug Administration classification of drug safety in pregnancy. Category A, Human studies fail to demonstrate fetal harm; B, animal studies fail to demonstrate harm, but no human studies or animal studies demonstrate risk not shown in human studies; C, animal studies demonstrate risk or insufficient data available, drugs may be used if benefit outweighs risk; D, human studies demonstrate risk, drugs may be used if benefits justify the risks; X, contraindicated in pregnancy.

Pulmonary Thromboembolic Disease

Epidemiology and Pathophysiology

The incidence of venous thromboembolic disease related to pregnancy is 200/100,000 woman-years. The incidence is five times greater in the postpartum period than during pregnancy, and it remains an important cause of maternal mortality. It results from a hypercoagulable state associated with pregnancy, as well as from hormonally mediated venous stasis and local pressure effects of the uterus on the inferior vena cava. Pulmonary embolism occurs more frequently in the early postpartum period than during pregnancy, particularly after cesarean section.

Clinical Features and Diagnosis

The presentation is similar to that in the patient who is not pregnant. However, the clinical diagnosis of deep venous thrombosis and pulmonary embolism is notoriously inaccurate. An overwhelming predilection for left leg deep venous thrombosis in pregnancy occurs because of anatomic factors.

Investigation of suspected pulmonary embolism follows a similar approach to that in the patient who is not pregnant, and the diagnosis must be pursued aggressively. Duplex ultrasonography is useful for the diagnosis of deep venous thrombosis, although venous Doppler can give false-positive results because of venous obstruction by the gravid uterus. Ventilation-perfusion scanning can be performed with less than 0.5 mGy (<50 mrad) exposure to the fetus and, if necessary, a computed tomography pulmonary angiogram may be carried

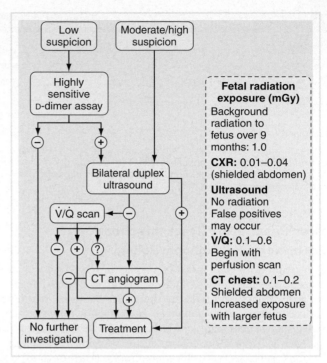

FIGURE 57-5 Diagnostic approach to thromboembolic disease in pregnancy and the radiation exposure of diagnostic tests. +, Positive test; −, negative test; ?, nondiagnostic test.

out with similarly low fetal exposure (Figure 57-5). Teratogenicity is generally thought to require exposure >50–100 mGy (5–10 rad), but an increased incidence of childhood leukemia has been documented with fetal radiation exposures of 20–50 mGy (2–5 rad).

The use of radiologic investigations during pregnancy remains a concern for the fetus. It is, nevertheless, important to establish a diagnosis of pulmonary embolism because of the major implications if such a diagnosis is missed and the potential effects of unnecessary therapy on the health of mother and fetus.

Treatment and Clinical Course

Warfarin therapy during the first trimester has been associated with an embryopathy, and central nervous system abnormalities have been described with second- and third-trimester exposure. Accordingly, warfarin is usually avoided (Table 57-3). The anticoagulant of choice is heparin, which does not cross the placenta, is not associated with adverse fetal outcome, and can be readily reversed. Low-molecular-weight heparins do not seem to cross the placenta and are both safe and effective in pregnancy.

When administered with adequate precautions, streptokinase, urokinase, and tissue plasminogen activator have been used successfully without major hemorrhagic complications or significant adverse effects on the fetus or placenta. Use of these agents should, nevertheless, be limited to life-threatening situations. When clinically indicated, transvenous placement of an inferior vena cava filter can be performed, although there is some risk of dislodgment because of the dilated venous system and pressure effects during labor.

Women who have a known hypercoagulable state and those who have had a previous thromboembolism are at increased risk and should receive prophylaxis with anticoagulation throughout pregnancy.

TABLE 57-3 Management of Thromboembolic Disease in Pregnancy

Therapy	FDA Classification	Comments
Heparin	C	Bone demineralization after prolonged use
Low molecular weight heparin	B/C	Good evidence of safety
Warfarin	D/X	Teratogenic, central nervous system abnormalities and bleeding occur, although the risk appears low. Sometimes used in the mid-trimester
Alteplase (r-tPA)	C	Consider in acute, life-threatening situations

FDA classification of drug safety in pregnancy. Category A, Human studies fail to demonstrate fetal harm; B, animal studies fail to demonstrate harm, but no human studies or animal studies demonstrate risk not shown in human studies; C, animal studies demonstrate risk or insufficient data available, drugs may be used if benefit outweighs risk; D, human studies demonstrate risk, drugs may be used if benefits justify the risks; X, contraindicated in pregnancy.

Lower Respiratory Tract Infections

Epidemiology and Pathophysiology

Lower respiratory tract infections are an infrequent occurrence but an important cause of indirect obstetric death. The pregnant patient is susceptible to the usual bacterial pathogens such as *Streptococcus pneumoniae*, *Haemophilus influenzae*, and *Mycoplasma pneumoniae* and is at increased risk of complications such as respiratory failure and empyema. Less common infections such as varicella pneumonia (Figure 57-6) and coccidioidomycosis may be associated with more severe disease than in nonpregnant patients. *Pneumocystis jirovecii* (previously *Pneumocystis carinii*) pneumonia may be seen in human immunodeficiency virus–positive patients. Pregnancy does not seem to affect the course or incidence of reactivation of tuberculosis.

Clinical Features and Diagnosis

The clinical features are similar to those in patients who are not pregnant. Although dyspnea and increased minute ventilation are common in pregnancy, the respiratory rate is not significantly elevated by the pregnant state.

A chest radiograph is essential for the diagnosis of lower respiratory tract infections and must be considered in any pregnant woman who has a clinical presentation suggestive of pneumonia. Delay in obtaining radiographic imaging may be in part responsible for the increased morbidity in the pregnant population. Further diagnostic investigations include the usual microbiologic cultures, sputum microscopy, and serologic tests as indicated.

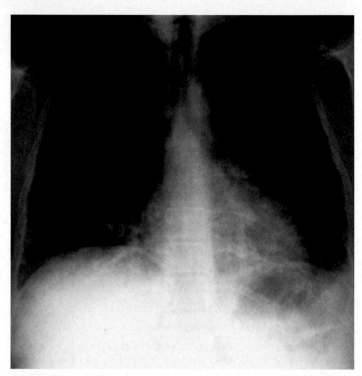

FIGURE 57-6 Chest radiograph of a woman with varicella pneumonitis that developed at 29 weeks' gestation. Note the diffuse, bilateral, fluffy nodular infiltrate. (Courtesy of Dr. M. Steinhardt, Mount Sinai Hospital, Toronto.)

Treatment and Clinical Course

Usual antibiotic guidelines may be followed, although tetracyclines should be avoided in pregnancy. Quinolones are usually avoided in pregnancy because of an association with arthropathy, but the risk seems to be low. Treatment of varicella pneumonitis is with acyclovir, which decreases mortality and has not been associated with fetal anomalies. Coccidioidomycosis is associated with an extremely high mortality rate, and disseminated disease should be treated with antifungal agents. *P. jirovecii* pneumonia requires treatment with trimethoprim-sulfamethoxazole with folate supplementation, as well as with corticosteroids, if indicated, clinically. Although folic acid antagonists and sulfa drugs carry risks for the fetus, pentamidine is associated with higher risks for mother and fetus. Tuberculosis treatment is with isoniazid and rifampin (rifampicin), which have a low risk of adverse fetal effects, as well as ethambutol initially, until sensitivities are available. Pyrazinamide has been used in pregnancy and is recommended by some authorities.

Although pneumonia is associated with an increased risk of mortality, this is probably attributable to underlying diseases rather than to the pneumonia per se. Fetal complications may occur, as may preterm labor. Transplacental transmission of varicella-zoster virus occurs uncommonly (<5%) but can produce limb deformities and neurologic involvement. The nonimmune pregnant woman exposed to varicella-zoster should receive prophylaxis with varicella-zoster immunoglobulin within 96 h of exposure and acyclovir if clinical disease develops. Unlike the treatment of active disease, tuberculosis prophylaxis can usually be deferred until after pregnancy, except in the case of recent exposure or skin test conversion.

When investigating and managing lower respiratory tract infections, it is important to consider effects on the fetus (i.e., radiation exposure, drug toxicities), but necessary evaluations and interventions should not be avoided inappropriately.

Acute Respiratory Distress Syndrome in Pregnancy

Epidemiology and Pathophysiology

The pregnant patient is at risk for development of ARDS from a number of pregnancy-associated problems (Table 57-4). Gastric acid aspiration is a particular risk because of the increased intraabdominal pressure, reduced lower esophageal sphincter tone, and supine position during delivery. Iatrogenic factors such as excessive fluid administration and tocolytic therapy may contribute, as may a reduced albumin level.

Clinical Features and Diagnosis

The clinical features are similar to those in the patient who is not pregnant. The diagnosis is by the usual criteria of hypoxemia in the presence of diffuse pulmonary infiltrates and in the absence of left ventricular failure. A detailed history is critical to identification of the underlying problem.

Treatment and Clinical Course

There are no major differences in the management of pregnant patients who have ARDS compared with those who are not pregnant, other than the need for continuous assessment of the fetus. When administering pharmacologic therapy, it is critical to consider the effects on both the fetus and the mother. Ventilatory management includes consideration of the normal physiologic changes of pregnancy. Adequate maternal oxygen saturation is essential for fetal well-being. Alkalosis has an adverse effect on placental perfusion and should be limited. Acidosis seems to be reasonably well tolerated by the fetus. Fetal delivery may benefit both the mother and the fetus. Epidural anesthetic may reduce the increased oxygen demand produced by uterine contractions.

Survival seems to be similar or better than that in the general population, possibly because of the young age of the patients and the reversibility of many of the predisposing conditions.

Specific causes of ARDS that pertain to pregnancy should be sought when assessing patients who have this syndrome. When women of childbearing age are seen with ARDS, they should be checked for pregnancy.

Pleural Disease

Although pleural effusions may accompany obstetric complications such as preeclampsia and choriocarcinoma, small, asymptomatic pleural effusions develop in a substantial proportion of women in the postpartum period. These result from the increased blood volume and reduced colloid osmotic pressure that occur in pregnancy, as well as from impaired lymphatic drainage caused by Valsalva maneuvers that occur during labor. Moderate-size effusions or the presence of symptoms should prompt a full clinical evaluation. Repeated expansion to total lung capacity with or without Valsalva maneuvers of labor may also cause spontaneous pneumothorax and pneumomediastinum, particularly in patients affected by predisposing conditions such as asthma. This diagnosis should be considered in patients who experience chest discomfort and dyspnea during or immediately after delivery.

Interstitial Lung Disease

Interstitial lung disease is uncommon in pregnant women, because most cases occur in women who are older than their childbearing years. When it exists in pregnant women, certain physiologic effects must be considered. A reduced diffusing capacity may lead to difficulty meeting the increased oxygen consumption requirements of pregnancy. Pulmonary hypertension carries increased risks because cardiac output increases during pregnancy. Little data exist on management and outcome of these patients, but restrictive lung disease seems reasonably well tolerated in pregnancy. Patients who have a vital capacity less than 1 L and those who have pulmonary hypertension should consider avoiding pregnancy. Lymphangioleiomyomatosis and systemic lupus erythematosus may worsen as a result of pregnancy.

Management involves careful assessment and monitoring of respiratory and cardiovascular status. Exercise intolerance is common, and patients may require supplemental oxygen early in pregnancy to avoid hypoxemic episodes, because these may be dangerous to the fetus. During labor, maternal effort should be limited and oxygen saturation must be monitored. Invasive hemodynamic monitoring may be indicated in the presence of pulmonary hypertension.

Obstructive Sleep Apnea

Pregnancy may be complicated by obstructive sleep apnea (OSA), with potential adverse effects for both the mother and fetus. Although upper airway narrowing has been documented in pregnancy, apnea and hypopnea are relatively uncommon because of the respiratory stimulatory effect of progesterone. Usually, OSA is confined to obese patients, perhaps being precipitated by pregnancy-associated airway mucosal edema and vascular congestion. OSA may worsen in late pregnancy, coupled with the development of hypertension. There is an association between OSA and preeclampsia, probably because of the generalized edema that occurs. Nocturnal hypoxemia may adversely affect the fetus, and poor fetal growth has been documented in these patients. Treatment with nasal continuous positive airway pressure is safe and effective. Snoring is not associated with fetal risk and is not a good marker for OSA in pregnant women.

Cystic Fibrosis

Advances in the management of patients who have cystic fibrosis have extended life expectancy into the childbearing age. Although fertility is impaired, contraception and planned pregnancy should be considered in the management of these patients. Available data indicate that pregnancy does not increase mortality in patients who have stable disease, but poor outcomes can occur in those affected by advanced disease.

TABLE 57-4 Causes of ARDS in Pregnancy

Pregnancy specific	Preeclampsia Amniotic fluid embolism Chorioamnionitis Placental abruption Trophoblastic embolism
Risk increased by pregnancy	Gastric acid aspiration Sepsis, particularly pyelonephritis Transfusion related acute lung injury Air embolism Pneumonia (e.g., varicella, fungal)
Nonspecific	Trauma Drugs/toxins Pancreatitis

Those with a forced vital capacity <50% predicted and pulmonary hypertension before pregnancy are at greatest risk. Perinatal mortality is increased, related largely to preterm delivery that occurs spontaneously or to maternal complications of cystic fibrosis. Management requires a multidisciplinary approach with careful attention to nutrition, glucose monitoring, and genetic counseling. Respiratory exacerbations require early aggressive therapy, with due consideration of the potential fetal toxicity of antibiotics such as aminoglycosides and quinolones, and the altered maternal pharmacokinetics.

Gastric Aspiration

Gastric acid aspiration may occur during labor because of delayed gastric emptying, reduced lower esophageal sphincter tone, and the effects of increased intraabdominal pressure. The presentation is with cough, bronchospasm, and dyspnea, which can progress to ARDS. Prophylaxis with antacids, histamine-2 receptor antagonists, or proton pump inhibitors is often given before cesarean section.

Pulmonary Vascular Disease

Pregnancy in the patient with pulmonary hypertension is associated with an extremely high mortality rate. The increased blood volume and cardiac output during pregnancy may precipitate right ventricular failure. Left ventricular filling may also be impaired as a result of ventricular interdependence. Hospitalization is recommended early in the third trimester, with close monitoring, anticoagulation, and oxygen therapy.

The cardiovascular effects of labor pose a particular risk, and hemorrhage is poorly tolerated. Invasive hemodynamic monitoring may be of value. Successful pregnancy in these patients requires a multidisciplinary team approach in a referral center.

Pulmonary arteriovenous malformations expand during pregnancy because of the increase in blood volume and venous distensibility, which increases the likelihood of bleeding. Embolization and surgical management have been performed in pregnancy.

SUGGESTED READINGS

Budev MM, Arroliga AC, Emery S: Exacerbation of underlying pulmonary disease in pregnancy. Crit Care Med 2005; 33:S313–S318.

Elkus R, Popovich J: Respiratory physiology in pregnancy. Clin Chest Med 1992; 13:555–565.

Goodnight WH, Soper DE: Pneumonia in pregnancy. Crit Care Med 2005; 33:S390–S397.

Greer IA: Prevention and management of venous thromboembolism in pregnancy. Clin Chest Med 2003; 24:123–137.

Lapinsky SE: Concise definitive reviews in critical care: Cardiopulmonary complications of pregnancy. Crit Care Med 2005; 33:1616.

Murphy VE, Gibson PG, Smith R, Clifton VL: Asthma during pregnancy: mechanisms and treatment implications. Eur Respir J 2005; 25: 731–750.

NHLBI. Managing Asthma During Pregnancy: Recommendations for Pharmacologic Treatment—Update 2004. www.nhlbi.nih.gov/health/prof/lung/asthma/astpreg.htm.

Scarsbrook AF, Evans AL, Owen AR, Gleeson FV: Diagnosis of suspected venous thromboembolic disease in pregnancy. Clin Radiol 2006; 61:1–12.

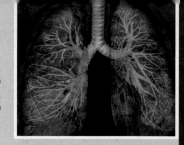

58 Pulmonary Complications of Hematopoietic Stem Cell Transplantation

JESSICA Y. CHIA • RODNEY J. FOLZ

INTRODUCTION

Hematopoietic stem cell transplantation (HSCT) refers to the transplantation of stem cells from various sources (bone marrow, growth factor–stimulated peripheral blood, and umbilical cord blood) for the treatment of malignant and nonmalignant hematologic, autoimmune, and genetic diseases.

Despite advances in HSCT, transplant recipients remain at high risk for serious and fatal complications developing as a consequence of cytoreductive conditioning regimens used before transplant, immunologic sequelae following engraftment of allogeneic lymphoid cells (which mediate graft-versus-host responses), the patient's immunosuppressed state, and infections secondary to immunosuppression. Pulmonary complications after HSCT are common and contribute considerably to the morbidity and mortality of transplant recipients, and respiratory failure is the most common cause of critical illness after HSCT.

TYPES OF HSCT

There are three types of stem cell transplantation: autologous, syngeneic, and allogeneic. In autologous transplants, the stem cells serving as a marrow graft are derived from the patient themselves; in syngeneic transplants, the stem cells are derived from a genetically identical twin; and in allogeneic transplants, the stem cells are taken from a nonidentical sibling or unrelated donor. Because autologous and syngeneic transplants involve stem cells that are immunologically identical to the recipient, reactions between graft and host are avoided. In allogeneic transplants, mismatch between donor and recipient human leukocyte antigens (HLAs) mediate graft-versus-host disease (GVHD) and graft rejection. The decision about which type of transplant to perform is based on the nature and stage of the underlying disease, on whether a suitable donor is available, and the medical condition of the recipient. The advantages to allogeneic transplantation over autologous transplantation include a higher likelihood that the stem cell product is free of tumor contamination and the presence of graft-versus-tumor activity.

INDICATIONS FOR HSCT

The main indication for HSCT is the treatment of hematologic malignancies and solid tumors, but it is also used in many nonmalignant disorders.

Nonmalignant Conditions Treated with HSCT

1. Autoimmune diseases (rheumatoid arthritis, systemic sclerosis, systemic lupus erythematosus, multiple sclerosis)
2. Amyloidosis
3. Aplastic anemia
4. Hemoglobinopathies (thalassemia and sickle cell anemia)
5. Other genetic disorders and inborn errors of metabolism (severe combined immunodeficiency, Wiskott–Aldrich syndrome)

CONDITIONING REGIMENS IN HSCT

One prerequisite for successful HSCT is conditioning therapy before transplant, which serves to ablate the bone marrow, eradicate tumor cells, and induce immunosuppression to permit engraftment and prevent rejection of the transplanted donor stem cells. These preparative regimens consist of high-dose chemotherapy with or without total body irradiation (TBI) and contribute considerably to the pulmonary complications seen after transplantation. Irradiation is generally omitted from autologous conditioning regimens because of concerns for late toxicity and secondary malignancies.

Most myeloablative regimens used before allogeneic transplantation consist of cyclophosphamide administered either with busulfan or TBI. Prophylaxis after allogeneic transplant to prevent GVHD usually involves methotrexate, cyclosporine, corticosteroids, or *in vitro* T-cell depletion of the graft before infusion.

"Minitransplantation," "nonmyeloablative," or "reduced intensity" conditioning regimens were developed in the late 1990s to reduce the toxicity profile associated with myeloablative regimens and are used primarily in older patients and those with multiple comorbidities who may not tolerate the more intense conditioning regimens. These less intense preparative regimens usually involve purine analogs like fludarabine in conjunction with immunosuppressive chemotherapeutic agents, low-dose TBI, total lymphoid irradiation, antithymocyte globulin, or other antibody preparations. In contrast to traditional myeloablative preparations, these regimens do not ablate host hematopoiesis but only immunosuppress sufficiently to allow engraftment of the donor stem cells and rely on the graft to eradicate cancer by means of the graft-versus-malignancy effect. These reduced-intensity conditioning regimens are associated with reduced transplant-associated morbidity and lower incidence of pulmonary complications after transplantation.

PULMONARY COMPLICATIONS OF HEMATOPOIETIC STEM CELL TRANSPLANTATION

Pulmonary complications after HSCT are common, with an incidence of 40–60% and with up to one third of recipients requiring intensive care after transplantation. Respiratory failure is the most common cause of critical illness, and pneumonia is the leading infectious cause of death after HSCT.

Pulmonary complications can occur early or late in the posttransplant course, can be due to infectious and noninfectious etiologies, and can present with assorted radiographic findings. The pulmonary complications of HSCT also vary depending on the indication for, type of, and preparative regimen preceding stem cell transplantation.

Key differences between pulmonary complications after autologous HSCT compared with allogeneic HSCT result from the fact that cellular interactions between graft and host cells are essentially eliminated with autologous transplantation, obviating the need for immunosuppression to prevent or treat GVHD. As such, autologous transplantation is associated with lower incidence of infection (particularly with viral pneumonias/CMV pneumonitis, invasive fungal disease, and other opportunistic infections such as *Toxoplasmosis*) and late airflow obstructive defects.

RISK FACTORS FOR DEVELOPMENT OF PULMONARY DISEASE AFTER HSCT
(Box 58-1)

Relapse status at time of transplant and donor–recipient HLA mismatching/nonidentity are risk factors for pulmonary complications and mortality after HSCT. Active phase of malignancy, age greater than 21 years, and receipt of HLA-nonidentical donor marrow are risk factors for respiratory failure after HSCT.

Abnormalities in pretransplant pulmonary function testing may be predictive of subsequent risk of pulmonary complications and mortality. Reduced diffusing capacity and increased alveolar-arterial oxygen gradient are independent risk factors for

interstitial pneumonitis and are also independently associated with increased early mortality after HSCT.

Measurement of cytokine levels in plasma and BAL fluid before transplant may also help predict patients at risk for posttransplant pulmonary complications. Patients with elevated levels of transforming growth factor (TGF)-β in plasma, TGF-α in BAL fluid, and granulocyte-macrophage colony-stimulating factor (GM-CSF) in BAL fluid seem to be at increased risk for pulmonary complications. One study showed that elevated pretransplant TGF-β levels in patients with breast cancer undergoing autologous HSCT were associated with increased posttransplant risk of pulmonary toxicity and hepatic venoocclusive disease.

Recipients of allogeneic transplantation, all of whom require administration of immunosuppressive agents after transplant to treat and prevent GVHD, have more infectious complications than recipients of autografts. This is not only due to chronic immunosuppression, but also because GVHD itself causes an immunodeficient state by affecting mucosal surfaces, the reticuloendothelial system, and bone marrow. These factors predispose allogeneic recipients to fatal viral pneumonias, multidrug-resistant bacteria, and invasive fungi. Similarly, bronchiolitis obliterans is almost exclusively seen after allogeneic HSCT.

TIME COURSE

Specific pulmonary complications associated with HSCT tend to occur in a relatively well-defined time line. The timing and intensity of cytoreductive therapies and the pattern of immune reconstitution that follows influence the duration of these intervals.

Preengraftment

The preengraftment phase (i.e., 0–30 days after transplant) is characterized by prolonged neutropenia and breaks in the mucocutaneous barrier. Accordingly, infectious complications are expected and primarily caused by bacterial and fungal infections. However, surgical lung biopsy in patients receiving HSCT with radiographic infiltrates who are receiving broad-spectrum antibiotics have shown that during this time, the prevalence of infection is low at 19% and that pulmonary complications are primarily noninfectious related to regimen-related toxicities (Box 58-2).

Early Postengraftment

The early postengraftment period spans days 30–100 after transplant and is characterized by persistent impairment in cellular and humoral immunity, in part determined by exogenous immunosuppression, GVHD, deficiency of immunoglobulins, and a loss of protective alveolar macrophages. During this period, neutropenia has usually resolved, decreasing the risk of bacterial and fungal infections. The epidemiology of infectious etiologies thus changes to involve predominantly viral infections, especially cytomegalovirus (CMV). With the routine use of antivirals for CMV prophylaxis, however, the incidence of posttransplant CMV pneumonia has decreased substantially. Noninfectious etiologies during this time include engraftment syndrome and delayed pulmonary toxicity syndrome.

Late Postengraftment

The late postengraftment period begins at day 100 after transplant. During this time, immune recovery and function are variable and depend on the type of HSCT. Autologous

---

BOX 58-1 Risk Factors for Pulmonary Disease After HSCT

Donor-recipient HLA mismatch
Relapse status
Active phase of malignancy
Age >21 y
Pretransplant pulmonary function abnormalities
  Reduced diffusing capacity
  Increased alveolar-arterial oxygen gradient
  Restrictive lung disease
  FEV$_1$ ≤80% predicted
Elevated pretransplant cytokine levels
  (TGF-β, TGF-α, GM-CSF)
Allogeneic transplantation
  GVHD and type of GVHD prophylaxis
Renal disease

BOX 58-2 Time Course of Pulmonary Complications After HSCT

Preengraftment (after transplant day 0–30)

Infections (primarily bacterial and fungal > viral and protozoal)
Pulmonary edema
Drug toxicity
Radiation toxicity
Diffuse alveolar hemorrhage
ARDS (caused by chemoradiation injury or sepsis)
Recurrent aspiration (enhanced by oral mucositis)
Pulmonary venoocclusive disease
Acute GVHD

Early postengraftment (posttransplant day 30–100)

Infections (especially viral/CMV)
Engraftment syndrome
Delayed pulmonary toxicity syndrome
Idiopathic pneumonia syndrome
Acute GVHD

Late postengraftment (posttransplant day 100+)

Infections (bacterial, fungal, viral, and protozoal)
Chronic GVHD
Drug-related pulmonary toxicity
Bronchiolitis obliterans
Restrictive/fibrotic lung disease
BOOP

BOX 58-3 Infectious Causes of Pulmonary Infiltrates After HSCT

Bacteria

Staphylococcus aureus
Streptococcus pneumoniae
Haemophilus influenzae
Pseudomonas aeruginosa
Klebsiella
Legionella
Nocardia
Mycobacteria tuberculosis
Atypical mycobacteria

Fungi

Aspergillus
Cryptococcus
Histoplasma capsulatum
Coccidioides immitis
Blastomyces
Fusarium
Zygomycetes (Mucor, Rhizopus)
Candida

Viruses

CMV
Respiratory virus (RSV, parainfluenza, influenza A and B, adenovirus)
Herpes family (HSV, VZV, HHV-6, HHV-7)
EBV

Other

Pneumocystis carinii (P. jiroveci)
Toxoplasma

---

recipients recover more rapidly than allogeneic recipients. T-cell responses to alloantigens return to normal, but immunoglobulin levels frequently remain depressed. Viral pathogens cause infections because of poor lymphocyte function, whereas inadequate cellular immunity results in bacterial and fungal pathogens. Noninfectious etiologies are primarily responsible for the pulmonary complications seen during this time, including chronic GVHD, drug-related pulmonary toxicity, bronchiolitis obliterans, restrictive/fibrotic lung disease, and BOOP.

INFECTIOUS COMPLICATIONS (Box 58-3)

The overall risk of pulmonary infection in patients receiving HSCT (see Box 58-1) depends on multiple factors, including chemotherapy and radiation-induced neutropenia, lung injury induced by the conditioning regimen, rejection in the form of GVHD, local disruption of host defenses, and intensity of pathogen exposure. In addition, HSCT recipients need to develop a functional immune system from donor-derived cells. Although the production of red blood cells, platelets, and granulocytes occur soon after HSCT, production of lymphocytes (and T cells in particular) is considerably delayed. In the first 2 years after transplant, serious infection occurs in 50% of otherwise uncomplicated transplants from histocompatible sibling donors and in 80–90% of matched unrelated donors or histocompatible recipients who have GVHD develop.

There has been a shift in the microbiology of posttransplant pneumonia over the past two decades, largely in part because of changes in supportive care in the posttransplant period. Prophylactic administration of trimethoprim/sulfamethoxazole, antivirals, antifungals, and fluoroquinolones has decreased the incidence of *Pneumocystis carinii* (*P. jiroveci*, PCP), cytomegalovirus (CMV), herpes simplex (HSV), and *Candida albicans*

BOX 58-4 Typical Prevention Strategies Against Opportunistic Infections After HSCT

Infections	Prophylaxis
Pneumocystis carinii (*jiroveci*)	Trimethoprim/sulfamethoxazole
CMV	Ganciclovir
HSV	Acyclovir
Candida sp.	Fluconazole
Aspergillus sp.	Voriconazole
Toxoplasma	Trimethoprim/sulfamethoxazole

---

infections. Resistant gram-negative and gram-positive bacteria, viruses, and other fungi remain important pathogens (Box 58-4).

Bacterial

Bacterial pneumonia is a major cause of morbidity and mortality in patients receiving HSCT. The first month after transplant is notable for pneumonias caused by usual nosocomial pathogens, with an incidence of ~15%. Bacterial pneumonia is frequently due to *Staphylococcus* and *Streptococcus* species (24% and 13%, respectively, in one series), and gram-negative organisms including *Pseudomonas, Klebsiella, Escherichia, Stenotrophomonas, Legionella, Acinetobacter, Serratia, Proteus, Enterobacter,* and *Citrobacter* species. Other organisms include

Enterococcus and rare anaerobes such as *Bacteroides* and *Fusobacterium* species. Community pathogens emerge after the immediate posttransplant period. *Haemophilus influenzae* is the most common isolate, followed by *Streptococcus pneumoniae* and *Legionella* species.

Tuberculous and atypical mycobacterial infections are quite uncommon in nonendemic areas, with an overall incidence of *M. tuberculosis* after allogeneic HSCT of only 0.1–0.25%. In a series from Hong Kong, where the prevalence of TB in the general population is 10-fold higher than that of other developed countries, the incidence of post-HSCT tuberculosis was 5.5%. Median time to infection onset is late, occurring at 150–324 days after transplant. Most patients are initially seen with fever, cough, and radiographic infiltrates, and standard treatment is highly effective. Nontuberculous mycobacterial infection is uncommon among HSCT recipients. *M. haemophilum* can be an important pulmonary pathogen after HSCT and should be suspected in patients with skin and joint findings in conjunction with pulmonary infiltrates. Another rare cause of bacterial pneumonia in allogeneic patients is *Nocardia*.

Fungal

Invasive fungal infection is a life-threatening complication of HSCT. Fungal disease should be considered in patients with persistent focal radiographic abnormalities that do not respond to empiric antibiotics and in those with nodular opacities on chest imaging, prolonged neutropenia, corticosteroid use, or a history of prior fungal infections.

Invasive aspergillosis is the leading cause of infectious death, with a mortality of 70–90% in allogeneic recipients despite treatment. The incidence of invasive aspergillosis in allogeneic recipients is 10–15%, with a bimodal distribution of cases. During the early preengraftment period that is characterized by profound neutropenia, both allogeneic and autologous recipients are at increased risk for invasive aspergillosis. Allogeneic patients experience a second period of vulnerability, however, during the postengraftment phase, coincident with the development of chronic GVHD, because of the need for augmented immunosuppression.

Most cases of invasive aspergillosis are limited to the lungs, but sinus and CNS involvement can also be seen. Common presenting symptoms include cough and dyspnea, with fever absent in up to two thirds of patients. Concomitant pleuritic chest pain and hemoptysis are clues. Radiographic findings include single or multiple nodules, cavities, and consolidation. The "air crescent sign" describes a central nodule partially or fully surrounded by air, indicting a sequestrum of necrotic lung tissue that has separated from the surrounding parenchyma. The "halo sign" on CT describes a rim of low attenuation representing edema or hemorrhage that surrounds a pulmonary nodule and is present in >90% of patients with neutropenia with invasive pulmonary aspergillosis.

Intravenous amphotericin B, voriconazole, and caspofungin are available therapies for treatment of invasive aspergillosis. Despite treatment, mortality is still high. Adjunctive surgical resection of localized disease may be beneficial in selected patients but remains controversial.

Candida, *Cryptococcus*, and *Zygomycetes* (including *Mucor* and *Rhizopus*) are also important pathogens. The prevalence of invasive zygomycotic infection is 2% and bears a similar clinical course to that of *Aspergillus*. Zygomycetes are angioinvasive, leading to thrombosis, pulmonary infarction, and hemorrhage, with radiographs showing cavitation and halo sign,

and mortality rates are high at 60–80% despite treatment with amphotericin B and surgical resection.

The endemic fungi are encountered less frequently. *Histoplasma* and *Coccidioides* usually occur as reactivation of latent infection. *Blastomyces* usually represents primary disease. Other emerging fungal pathogens reported to cause pulmonary infections include *Fusarium* and *Scedosporium* species.

Viral

Viral infections, particularly CMV pneumonia, are an important cause of morbidity and mortality in the postengraftment period. Mortality from CMV pneumonia in posttransplant patients exceeded 90% until the advent of combination therapy with ganciclovir and intravenous immunoglobulin (IVIG) that improved survival rates to up to 70%.

The use of prophylaxis has not only reduced the incidence but has also delayed the onset of disease. Previously, 35% of CMV infections occurred during the first 100 days after transplant, but now only 6% are occurring in this time frame; infection after the first 100 days has increased from 4% to 15%. Prophylaxis regimens have taken two approaches: universal prophylaxis to all high-risk patients for a defined period after engraftment, and preemptive treatment of patients only after detection of subclinical viremia by PCR assay. Both strategies reduce the risk of early CMV disease and are endorsed by published practice guidelines.

Immunosuppression and delayed reconstitution of cytotoxic T cells places patients receiving HSCT at increased risk for CMV pneumonia. Those at highest risk are seronegative patients who underwent allogeneic transplant from seropositive donors. Other risk factors include viral shedding from other sites, viremia, chronic steroid use, and GVHD. Patients with chronic GVHD are particularly susceptible to late CMV infection because of an increased need for immunosuppression and inherent immunodeficiency as part of the GVHD process.

CMV pneumonia has a nonspecific clinical presentation that includes fever, nonproductive cough, and hypoxia. Chest imaging demonstrates various abnormalities, most commonly bilateral interstitial opacities on chest X-ray, but may also have focal or diffuse consolidation, nodular opacities, and ground-glass opacities on chest CT. A definitive diagnosis relies on demonstrating viral inclusion bodies in lung tissue (which can be difficult on transbronchial biopsy specimens) or detection of virus in BAL fluid by shell vial assay, polymerase chain reaction, or viral culture (in patients with a compatible clinical presentation). Long-term sequelae include bronchiolitis obliterans organizing pneumonia and restrictive lung disease.

Community-acquired viruses such as influenza A and B, parainfluenza, respiratory syncytial virus, and adenovirus can also cause respiratory failure in HSCT recipients, and collectively these are recovered from up to 33% of patients receiving HSCT who are hospitalized with acute respiratory illness, with RSV being the most common. Parainfluenza virus infection causes both upper and lower respiratory tract symptoms and can present as laryngotracheitis, croup, bronchiolitis, or pneumonia. The incidence in allogeneic transplants is >2%, most commonly with serotype 3, which is associated with lower respiratory tract symptoms. There is no seasonal variation to infection with parainfluenza virus serotype 3. In contrast, infection with the other viruses occurs in colder months (late fall to early spring). Respiratory syncytial virus peaks between January and March and is often associated with concomitant otitis media or sinusitis. Progression to pneumonia occurs frequently, and the mortality of untreated RSV pneumonia approaches 80%. Early treatment with ribavirin and IVIG may decrease pneumonia-related mortality.

Adenovirus is an uncommon cause of pneumonia and can be isolated in 3–5% of patients after HSCT. It affects the upper and lower respiratory tracts, as well as the gastrointestinal and genitourinary systems. Infection usually develops within the first 3 months of transplantation, with a presentation that might include pharyngitis, tracheitis, bronchitis, pneumonitis, enteritis, hemorrhagic cystitis, or disseminated disease. Mortality with pulmonary involvement may exceed 50%.

Other viral infections include HSV, varicella zoster virus, and human herpesviruses 6 and 7. In the absence of prophylaxis, infection with HSV occurs in up to 18% of transplant recipients, with severe pneumonia in 10% and a mortality up to 20%. The incidence of HSV has been markedly reduced by acyclovir prophylaxis. HSV may cause a severe tracheobronchitis associated with endobronchial ulcers. Human herpes virus 6 has been associated with the idiopathic pneumonia syndrome. Epstein–Barr virus infections usually manifest as posttransplant lymphoproliferative disorder, usually as a B-cell lymphoma, thought to be related to T-cell depletion or suppression strategies. Even coronavirus pneumonia has been reported after hematopoietic stem cell transplant.

Others

The incidence of PCP pneumonia has been markedly reduced by trimethoprim-sulfamethoxazole prophylaxis. Prophylaxis is recommended from time of engraftment to 6 months after transplant in all allogeneic recipients and indefinitely for those on augmented immunosuppressive therapy and those with chronic GVHD. PCP presents approximately 60 days after transplantation with cough, dyspnea, fever, and nearly any chest X-ray finding (most commonly, bilateral interstitial and alveolar infiltrates). Diagnostic yield of BAL is near 90%. Despite trimethoprim-sulfamethoxazole, treatment, mortality can be as high as 89% for PCP infections occurring within the first 6 months after transplant versus 40% for late-onset infections.

Toxoplasma infection is uncommon with a lifetime incidence of 0.3%, but in patients with prior cat exposure and positive pretransplant serologic findings, the frequency is as much as 2%. The infection is typically associated with GVHD; develops by reactivation in the first 6 months after transplant; and affects the brain, heart, and lungs. Another rare cause of pulmonary infection in HSCT patients is *Microsporidia*.

NONINFECTIOUS COMPLICATIONS (Box 58-5)

Pulmonary Toxicity

In the immediate posttransplant period, pulmonary toxicity from prior chemoradiotherapy or the pretransplant conditioning regimen may manifest as fever, dyspnea, cough, hypoxemia, and patchy or diffuse mixed interstitial and alveolar infiltrates on chest radiography. No prospective studies document the efficacy of steroids in this setting, but in clinical practice, prednisone, 1–2 mg/kg/day, is usually used to treat lung toxicity once infection has been excluded.

Pulmonary Edema

Pulmonary edema, both cardiogenic and noncardiogenic, is the most common early posttransplant complication, usually seen in

BOX 58-5 Noninfectious Causes of Pulmonary Infiltrates After HSCT

Cardiogenic and noncardiogenic pulmonary edema
Diffuse alveolar damage (DAD) or drug toxicity
Idiopathic pneumonia syndrome (IPS)
Diffuse alveolar hemorrhage (DAH)
Engraftment syndrome
Delayed pulmonary toxicity syndrome (DPTS)
Interstitial pneumonitis or interstitial lung disease
Bronchiolitis obliterans (BO) or airflow obstruction
Pulmonary venoocclusive disease
Posttransplant lymphoproliferatirve disorder (PTLD)
Bronchiolitis obliterans organizing pneumonia (BOOP)
Respiratory failure
Interstitial fibrosis
Radiation pneumonitis
Pulmonary cytolytic thrombi
Pulmonary alveolar proteinosis
Transfusion related acute lung injury

the first month after transplant. Patients may have underlying cardiac dysfunction secondary to previous treatment with high dose cyclophosphamide, anthracycline, and chest irradiation; IV fluids (given for resuscitation, antibiotics, or maintenance therapy) can lead to cardiogenic pulmonary edema. Drug-induced pulmonary toxicity, sepsis, aspiration, blood transfusions, cytokine release during acute GVHD, and hepatic venoocclusive disease can induce noncardiogenic pulmonary edema. There are also reports of cardiac arrest immediately after infusion of autologous marrow, possibly secondary to noncardiogenic pulmonary edema.

Diffuse Alveolar Damage

Diffuse alveolar damage, as the histologic/pathologic correlate of the acute respiratory distress syndrome, can occur after HSCT, usually in the setting of sepsis or in response to treatment with agents known to cause pulmonary toxicity.

Idiopathic Pneumonia Syndrome

Idiopathic pneumonia syndrome (IPS) is a noninfectious form of acute lung injury defined as widespread alveolar injury in the absence of active lower respiratory tract infection (Box 58-6). Published series report an incidence ranging from 2% to 35%, reflecting the relative difficulty in making the diagnosis, because patients with "idiopathic" pneumonia may actually have occult infection (particularly CMV pneumonia) or pulmonary toxicity because of conditioning regimens. Some have reported a trend toward a higher IPS occurrence after allogeneic transplantation, whereas others have shown a relatively equivalent incidence in recipients of allogeneic and autologous HSCT at 7.6% and 5.7%, respectively. Among allogeneic recipients, the incidence of IPS is significantly lower after nonmyeloablative conditioning regimens than traditional high-dose regimens, consistent with the idea that IPS is the result of chemoradiotherapy. Other risk factors include older age, transplantation for malignancy other than leukemia, high-dose conditioning regimens, total body irradiation, and high-grade acute GVHD. Studies in murine models suggest that the etiology involves an alloimmune cytokine storm from myeloablative conditioning, recruitment of inflammatory and immune-effector cells to the lung, release of oxidants and proinflammatory cytokines, and resultant inflammatory lung injury.

BOX 58-6 Diagnostic Criteria for Idiopathic Pneumonia Syndrome

1. Evidence of widespread alveolar injury as evidenced by:
   a. Multilobar infiltrates on routine chest radiographs or CT scans
   b. Symptoms and signs of pneumonia, e.g., cough, dyspnea, rales
   c. Evidence of abnormal pulmonary physiology
      1. Increased alveolar to arterial oxygen gradient (compared with previous, if available).
      2. New or increased restrictive pulmonary function test abnormality.
   – AND –
2. Absence of active lower respiratory tract infection as evaluated by:
   a. Bronchoalveolar lavage or transbronchial biopsy or open lung biopsy negative for infectious pathogens (bacterial, CMV, respiratory syncytial virus, parainfluenza virus, other respiratory viruses, fungi, *Pneumocystis carinii*, and other organisms).
   b. Ideally, a second confirmatory negative test is done 2–14 days after the initial negative bronchoscopy

---

The median time to onset of IPS ranges from 21 to 50 days after transplantation. Patients are seen with fever, dyspnea, nonproductive cough, hypoxia, and diffuse pulmonary infiltrates. Patients may progress to respiratory failure within a few days. Mortality approaches 75%. Treatment is primarily supportive care. The response to pulse steroids at a dose equivalent of 1–2 mg/kg/day of intravenous methylprednisolone is generally poor and of uncertain efficacy. Novel agents such as etanercept, a TNF-α blocker, are being investigated.

Diffuse Alveolar Hemorrhage (DAH)
(Figure 58-1 and Box 58-7)

Diffuse alveolar hemorrhage (DAH) was first described in 21% of 141 consecutive patients who underwent autologous HSCT who had dyspnea, nonproductive cough, fever, hypoxemia, diffuse alveolar infiltrates, and progressively bloodier return from BAL develop. The mortality in this retrospective series was 80%. Subsequent studies reported a lower incidence at 5%, with no significant differences noted between those undergoing autologous versus allogeneic transplant. Risk factors include age >40, total body irradiation, transplantation for solid tumors, high fevers, severe mucositis, and renal insufficiency. The pathophysiology is not well understood, but infection, thrombocytopenia, and coagulopathy do not seem to be directly implicated. Autopsy specimens show diffuse alveolar damage. DAH, like IPS, is part of a spectrum of acute lung injury induced by conditioning chemotherapy, radiation, and occult infection. Rapid immune system reconstitution has also been theorized to contribute to DAH. Neutrophil influx into the lung may accentuate the injury and precipitate hemorrhage.

Patients usually are seen during the periengraftment period within the first month after transplantation, but up to 42% of patients are seen late, beyond day 30. Symptoms and radiographic findings usually progress within 48 h, and radiographic changes may precede the clinical presentation by several days. Chest X-rays show patchy interstitial or alveolar infiltrates, often with mid-lower lung predominance, which then become diffuse and widespread. Because DAH has an 80–100%

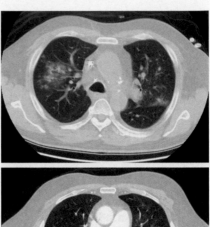
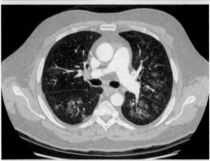
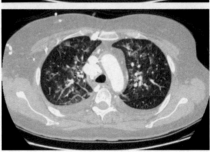

FIGURE 58-1 Representative chest CT images of three individuals who had diffuse alveolar hemorrhage develop (diagnosed by BAL) after hematopoietic stem cell transplantation. Typical findings include bilateral scattered ground-glass opacities that can coalesce with corresponding airspace disease. All microbiology studies (bacterial, fungus, viral, and AFB) were negative.

BOX 58-7 Diagnostic Criteria for Diffuse Alveolar Hemorrhage (DAH)

Evidence for widespread/diffuse alveolar injury as manifested by:
 Multilobar pulmonary infiltrates
 Abnormal pulmonary physiology with increased alveolar to arterial oxygen gradient
 Restrictive ventilatory defect
Absence of infectious etiologies compatible with the diagnosis
Bronchoalveolar lavage (BAL) showing progressively bloodier return from three separate subsegmental bronchi or the presence of blood in at least 30% of the alveolar surfaces of lung tissue

---

mortality with supportive care alone, prompt diagnosis and treatment are crucial. BAL with progressively bloodier aliquots in the return fluid is the classic diagnostic finding (Figure 58-2). Treatment is with methylprednisolone, 500–1000 mg/day for 3–4 days, followed by steroid taper. Better outcomes are associated with early presentation and autologous transplants (~30% mortality) versus those with late-onset hemorrhage or

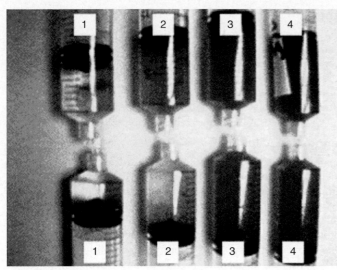

FIGURE 58-2 Bronchoalveolar lavage findings demonstrating diffuse alveolar hemorrhage. Four sequential 20-mL lavages were performed in the RML (*top syringes*) and repeated in the lingula (*bottom syringes*). Each lobe shows increasing bloody return with each sequential lavage, and these findings are consistent with a diagnosis of diffuse alveolar hemorrhage.

allogeneic transplants, in which mortality was 70%. Recombinant factor VIIa may be a useful adjunct.

Engraftment Syndrome (Box 58-8)

The engraftment syndrome is by characterized by fever, rash, and noncardiogenic pulmonary edema that occurs coincident with neutrophil recovery and engraftment. The incidence of engraftment syndrome is 7–11% and occurs most frequently after autologous HSCT. Proposed risk factors include transplantation for breast cancer, use of peripheral blood rather than bone marrow stem cells, and use of granulocyte colony-stimulating factors to mobilize marrow. The etiology is unclear; it may be attributed to increased cytokine release and neutrophil degranulation during engraftment. As in DAH,

---

BOX 58-8 Diagnostic Criteria for Engraftment Syndrome*

Major criteria

Temperature $\geq 38.3°$ C with no identifiable infectious etiology.
Erythrodermatous rash involving more than 25% of body surface area and not attributable to a medication.
Noncardiogenic pulmonary edema, manifested by diffuse pulmonary infiltrates consistent with this diagnosis, and hypoxia.

Minor criteria

Hepatic dysfunction with either total bilirubin ≥ 2 mg/dL or transaminase levels $\geq$ two times normal
Renal insufficiency (serum creatinine $\geq$ two times baseline)
Weight gain $\geq 2.5\%$ of baseline body weight
Transient encephalopathy unexplainable by other causes

---

*A diagnosis of ES is established by the presence of all three major criteria or two major criteria and one or more minor criteria. ES should occur within 96 h of engraftment (PMN $\geq 500/\mu$L for 2 consecutive days).

rapid immune system reconstitution is also theorized. Treatment is 1–2 mg/kg/day of intravenous methylprednisolone followed by a rapid taper.

Delayed Pulmonary Toxicity Syndrome

Interstitial pneumonitis and fibrosis developing after high-dose chemotherapy and autologous HSCT for breast cancer is referred to as delayed pulmonary toxicity syndrome (DPTS). This syndrome most often presents between 6 weeks to 3 months after HSCT, is generally responsive to corticosteroid therapy, and has a better prognosis than IPS. Patients are seen with dyspnea on exertion, nonproductive cough, and fever. Pulmonary function tests (PFTs) show a restrictive ventilatory defect and diminished diffusion capacity. DPTS is thought to represent a manifestation of chemotherapy-induced lung injury, because lung biopsy shows alveolar septal thickening, interstitial fibrosis, and type II pneumocyte hyperplasia, all consistent with drug toxicity. Moreover, carmustine (BCNU) and cyclophosphamide, both of which are used in the conditioning regimens that are associated with DPTS, are known to be pneumotoxic.

Interstitial Pneumonitis or Interstitial Lung Disease

Interstitial pneumonitis manifests with diminished diffusing capacity, and total lung capacity is common and can occur at virtually any time after transplantation, with many patients remaining asymptomatic. These PFT changes are usually secondary to treatment with conditioning regimens, particularly those containing carmustine.

Bronchiolitis Obliterans

Chronic airflow limitation caused by bronchiolitis obliterans is the most common late complication of allogeneic HSCT and is exceptionally rare after autologous HSCT. The incidence varies from 6% to 26%, depending on how the airflow limitation is defined. It typically occurs after the third month posttransplant and is associated with underlying chronic GVHD. Other risk factors include older age, lower pretransplant FEV_1/FVC ratio, low serum immunoglobulin levels, methotrexate use, and early posttransplant respiratory viral infections. The etiology is unclear, but its strong association with GVHD suggests an immune-mediated injury induced by donor cytotoxic T cells against host bronchial epithelium. The reported association with methotrexate suggests direct drug-related injury may also play a role.

Patients with bronchiolitis obliterans are seen with insidious onset of nonproductive cough, dyspnea, and wheezing. Chest radiographs are often normal, but high-resolution CT shows air trapping, hypoattenuation, and bronchial dilatation. PFTs show airflow limitation that progresses with time; also, the rate of progression is variable, with some having rapid progression to hypercapnic respiratory failure and death and others having a protracted course. Airflow limitation has been associated with a substantial attributable mortality: 9% and 18% at 3 and 10 years after transplant, respectively. Mortality is higher in the subpopulation of patients who have chronic GVHD (22% and 40% at 3 and 10 years, respectively). Treatment involves augmented immunosuppression and, in some cases, lung transplantation. Azithromycin has been suggested as possible therapy.

Pulmonary Venoocclusive Disease

Pulmonary venoocclusive disease (PVOD) is a rare complication of HSCT characterized by intimal proliferation and fibrosis of pulmonary venules, leading to progressive vascular obstruction and increased pulmonary capillary and arterial pressures. The process is thought to be due to an infectious or toxic injury to the endothelium. Chemotherapeutic agents most commonly associated with PVOD include carmustine, mitomycin C, and bleomycin.

Patients are seen several months after transplantation with progressive dyspnea on exertion and fatigue. They may also have pleural effusions with right upper quadrant tenderness and ascites. The presence of pulmonary arterial hypertension, pulmonary edema, and normal pulmonary artery occlusion pressure strongly suggests the diagnosis. Pulmonary vasodilators can exacerbate the pulmonary edema. Anecdotal reports describe response to high-dose corticosteroids.

Posttransplant Malignancy/ Lymphoproliferative Disorder

Posttransplant lymphoproliferative disorder (PTLD) is another uncommon complication of allogeneic HSCT. It represents an uncontrolled expansion of donor-derived, Epstein–Barr virus–infected B lymphocytes. The overall incidence is 1% but increases to 22% in patients with more than two of the following risk factors: unrelated or HLA-mismatched related donors, T cell–depleted donor stem cells, and use of antithymocyte globulin.

Patients are usually seen within the first 6 months after transplant with lymph node, liver, and spleen involvement, often with relapse with the original malignancy (especially lymphoma) or with secondary lymphomas. Lung involvement is seen in 20% of cases. PTLD is often refractory to standard chemotherapy, and treatment involves administration of anti-B–cell monoclonal antibodies and reduced immunosuppression. Survival is poor, especially for those with underlying hematologic malignancies.

Bronchiolitis Obliterans Organizing Pneumonia

Bronchiolitis obliterans organizing pneumonia (BOOP) occurs as a late complication of HSCT and can be a sequela of treated CMV pneumonitis, related to chronic GVHD, or can be idiopathic. The incidence is 1.3% in adult allogeneic recipients who have survived beyond 3 months. This is often a steroid-responsive lesion, and with treatment long-term survival is 80%.

Respiratory Failure

Respiratory failure occurs commonly after HSCT and is associated with poor outcomes. In a series of >1400 consecutive patients who underwent HSCT at the Fred Hutchinson Cancer Research Center between 1986 and 1990, 23% required mechanical ventilation and only 4% of those survived. Risk factors include older age, active malignancy at the time of transplant, and receipt of HLA-nonidentical allogeneic transplant. Later studies report survival rates of 16–26% in ventilated patients, in part because of the use of peripheral stem cell transplantation and perhaps early institution of noninvasive mechanical ventilation. Uniformly fatal outcomes are seen in patients with multisystem organ failure, especially those with hepatic and renal dysfunction.

Other

Pulmonary cytolytic thrombi (PCT) is the term describing a vasculopathy that occurs in pediatric allogeneic HSCT recipients that is characterized by an obliterative arteriopathy, occlusive vascular lesions, and hemorrhagic infarcts. This entity can resolve spontaneously without specific therapy. Pulmonary alveolar proteinosis has also been reported as a reversible cause of respiratory failure after allogeneic HSCT for acute leukemia.

Diagnostic Evaluation

The approach to evaluation should consider the time frame at which the pulmonary problem is occurring, the radiographic abnormalities, and a number of individual patient factors, such as exposure to cardiopulmonary-toxic drugs during the pretransplant conditioning regimen, a history of receiving chest radiotherapy, current and previous immunosuppression regimens, current and previous prophylaxis for infectious agents, CMV status of donor and recipient, any history of previous opportunistic invasive fungal disease, and exposure to cats, birds, mycobacteria, or endemic fungi. Pulmonary function test abnormalities can provide clues to the underlying disorder, and evidence of a restrictive ventilatory defect on PFTs should be followed by a chest CT to assess for subtle interstitial disease. Sputum examination can also be very useful in identifying certain pathogens. Invasive diagnostic procedures are usually reserved for patients who are stable enough to undergo the procedure and/or who have progressive disease despite initial therapy.

Patterns on Imaging

The chest radiograph can be normal in 15% of symptomatic patients with proven infiltrative lung disease and can miss small nodules, cavitations, radiation pneumonitis, GVHD, and bronchiolitis obliterans. Chest CT is more sensitive than the plain chest radiograph and is often used for localization to guide invasive diagnostic procedures.

Diffuse infiltrates are common and are highly nonspecific. During the preengraftment phase, pulmonary edema is the main cause. Other noninfectious processes include DAH, engraftment syndrome, and drug reactions. After engraftment, infections are the main cause of diffuse infiltrates. Typical chest radiographic findings in viral pneumonia consist of reticulonodular opacities in a peribronchial, perivascular distribution. The most common radiographic findings of CMV pneumonitis after HSCT are parenchymal opacification (90%) and multiple (<5 mm) nodules (29%), but X-rays may be normal in 10%. Noninfectious processes in the postengraftment period include pulmonary edema, DAH, IPS, NSIP, lymphangitic spread of tumor, and chemoradiation-induced pneumonitis.

Focal infiltrates usually reflect infectious processes and have a higher likelihood of yielding a specific diagnosis. Segmental or lobar infiltrates are usually caused by bacterial, fungal, or mycobacterial infections. Localized consolidation accompanied by an ipsilateral pleural effusion suggests bacterial infection. The noninfectious processes associated with focal infiltrates include hemorrhage, pulmonary emboli, acute radiation pneumonitis, and carcinoma.

Nodular infiltrates with or without cavitation are typical of fungal infections, with aspergillosis being the most common (often including the "air crescent" and "halo" signs as described previously). *Nocardia* and *Cryptococcus* also present as nodular masses, the former commonly cavitating. Invasive candidiasis may also present as disseminated nodules, and septic emboli as nodular infiltrates, with feeding pulmonary vessels and wedged-shaped subpleural lesions representing infarcts.

Pleural effusions suggest bacterial, mycobacterial, or nocardial infections. Noninfectious processes associated with pleural effusions include pulmonary edema, hepatic venoocclusive disease, pulmonary infarction, and malignancy.

PULMONARY FUNCTION TESTS

Baseline PFTs should be obtained before HSCT, after transplant in symptomatic patients, and at regularly scheduled intervals in high-risk individuals. Pretransplant abnormalities in the diffusion capacity and the alveolar-arterial oxygen difference are independent risk factors for interstitial pneumonitis and death. Reduction in pretransplant FEV_1 is a strong predictor for the subsequent development of CMV pneumonia in CMV-seropositive allogeneic HSCT recipients. After transplant, PFTs abnormalities commonly seen include decline in lung volume, diffusing capacity, and airflow. Posttransplant reduction in DL_{CO} is found in half of the patients and may be persistent from 3 months to several years. Restrictive pattern is reported in 34% of HSCT recipients. The etiology of the restrictive impairment and the reduced DL_{CO} seems to be multifactorial, including toxic effects of chemoradiation, recurrent pulmonary infections, pulmonary edema, generalized muscle weakness, idiopathic interstitial pneumonias, and BOOP.

Invasive Diagnostic Procedures

After radiographs, the next diagnostic step in a patient with a worsening clinical picture is usually an invasive test. Patients with focal infiltrates can often be given a trial of empiric antibiotics, with invasive testing performed several days later if there is no response. Additional testing is discussed in the following text.

Serologic Studies

Aspergillus is the most common invasive fungal infection in posttransplant patients, and noninvasive testing for early diagnosis can alter the posttransplant course. The galactomannan assay (which uses monoclonal antibody directed against galactomannan, a cell wall antigen) detects *Aspergillus* antigen by ELISA and is the only approved serologic marker for *Aspergillus* infection. It can be done on blood and BAL fluid. Early studies showed a sensitivity and specificity >90% with improvement in time to diagnosis. Results can be obtained in 3 h as opposed to the 4 weeks by standard culture methods. Serial monitoring increases the sensitivity and may detect the disease before development of clinical symptoms.

Determining CMV serologic status of both recipient and donor is essential in pretransplant screening, especially because CMV disease in the posttransplant period is one of the most lethal infectious complications. The serologic status of the recipient as opposed to the donor is the primary determinant for CMV conversion. A shell vial culture with monoclonal antibody to p72 requires only 48 h, and tests for antigenemia are rapid, standardized, semiquantitative, and inexpensive. Nucleic acid amplification by PCR on DNA extracted from infected leukocytes also allows rapid diagnosis (detects infection 2 weeks before viral cultures become positive and 1 week before positive antigenemia) and is highly sensitive. CMV pneumonia, once fatal to 15% of allogeneic recipients, has become markedly less common with use of these early detection techniques that allow early treatment.

PITFALLS AND CONTROVERSIES

Bronchoscopy

The efficacy of BAL is highly variable. In different retrospective series BAL had an overall diagnostic yield of 30–60%, with a 4–15% complication rate but only modified treatment in 20–35%. The additional diagnostic value of transbronchial biopsy in conjunction with BAL is likewise controversial. Transbronchial lung biopsy is superior to BAL alone for the diagnosis of malignancy and may yield lung biopsies that are consistent with pulmonary drug toxicity, DAD, or BOOP. However, transbronchial biopsy is not routinely performed in the evaluation of HSCT patients with pulmonary complications because of the attendant risks.

An NIH review on the efficacy of BAL in immunocompromised patients with pulmonary infiltrates found that the procedure was diagnostic in 55% of cases, with the most common finding being infection. The most common pulmonary complications diagnosed were DAH (5%), bacterial pneumonia (23%), RSV (19%), and *Aspergillus* (14%).

A review of 27 bronchoscopies and transbronchial biopsies in breast cancer patients who underwent HSCT found that the diagnostic yield of BAL alone was only 22%, which increased to 71% with transbronchial biopsy. The most common conditions diagnosed were pulmonary drug toxicity (47%), bacterial infection (17%), and invasive aspergillosis (11%). The NIH experience with the diagnostic yield of transbronchial lung biopsy was less positive, with nondiagnostic or negative findings in 47% and 24%, respectively.

Transthoracic Needle Aspiration

The yield of transthoracic needle aspiration (TTNA) under CT or fluoroscopic guidance has a high sensitivity (70%), with the most common findings being infection and malignancy. Pneumothorax is a common complication, however, frequently requiring chest tubes.

Surgical Lung Biopsy

If no diagnosis is made with either bronchoscopy or TTNA, surgical lung biopsy by either open thoracotomy or video-assisted thorascopic approach is considered next and is the diagnostic "gold standard" (60–83% sensitivity) in evaluating pulmonary infiltrates after HSCT. The effect of surgical lung biopsy on patient outcome and survival is still controversial, however. Some studies have shown that patients with surgical lung biopsy had poorer outcomes, that the results rarely led to a change in therapy, and that the patients frequently had complications such as pneumothorax, hemothorax, prolonged mechanical ventilation, wound hematoma and dehiscence, incisional neuritis, and tumor recurrence at chest tube site. The procedure is associated with a postoperative mortality up to 8%. Survival at 30 and 90 days may be increased in patients who have a specific diagnosis. We recommend reserving open biopsy for patients whose underlying condition has a reasonable prognosis and those in whom the results might have a good chance of changing management.

SUGGESTED READINGS

Afessa B, Peters SG: Major complications following hematopoietic stem cell transplantation. Semin Respir Crit Care Med 2006; 27:297–309.

Afessa B, Peters SG: Chronic lung disease after hematopoietic stem cell transplantation. Clin Chest Med 2005; 26:571–586.

Bhalla KS, Wilczynski SW, Abushamaa AM, *et al:* Pulmonary toxicity of induction chemotherapy prior to standard or high–dose chemotherapy with autologous hematopoietic support. Am J Respir Crit Care Med 2000; 161:17–25.

Chien JW, Madtes DK, Clark JG: Pulmonary function testing prior to hematopoietic stem cell transplantation. Bone Marrow Transplant 2005; 35:429–435.

Chien JW, Martin PJ, Gooley TA, *et al:* Airflow obstruction after myeloablative allogeneic hematopoietic stem cell transplantation. Am J Respir Crit Care Med 2003; 168:208–214.

Duncan MD, Wilkes DS: Transplant-related immunosuppression: a review of immunosuppression and pulmonary infections. Proc Am Thorac Soc 2005; 2:449–455.

Dykewicz CA: Summary for the Guidelines for Preventing Opportunistic Infections among Hematopoietic Stem Cell Transplant Recipients. Clin Infect Dis 2001; 33:139–144.

Franquet T, Muller NL, Lee KS, *et al:* High-resolution CT and pathologic findings of noninfectious pulmonary complications after hematopoietic stem cell transplantation. AJR Am J Roentgenol 2005; 184:629–637.

Fukada T, Hackman RC, Guthrie KA, *et al:* Risks and outcomes of idiopathic pneumonia syndrome after nonmyeloablative compared to conventional conditioning regimens for allogeneic hematopoietic stem cell transplantation. Blood 2003; 102:2777–2785.

Kotloff RM, Ahya VN, Crawford SW: Pulmonary complications of solid organ and hematopoietic stem cell transplantation. Am J Respir Crit Care Med 2004; 170:22–48. Epub 2004 Apr 7.

Scaglione S, Hofmeister CC, Stiff P: Evaluation of pulmonary infiltrates in patients after stem cell transplantation. Hematology 2005; 10:469–481.

Watkins TR, Chien JW, Crawford SW: Graft versus host-associated pulmonary disease and other idiopathic pulmonary complications after hematopoietic stem cell transplant. Semin Respir Crit Care Med 2005; 26:482–489.

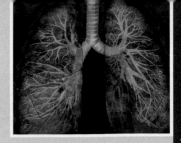

SECTION XIII

PULMONARY MANIFESTATIONS OF SYSTEMIC CONDITIONS

59 Hepatic and Biliary Disease

MICHAEL J. KROWKA

EPIDEMIOLOGY, RISK FACTORS, AND PATHOPHYSIOLOGY

The pulmonary consequences of liver disorders can be classified according to whether they predominantly affect the pleural space, the lung parenchyma, or the pulmonary circulation (Table 59-1). Unique pulmonary abnormalities occur in the setting of severe α_1-antitrypsin deficiency, primary biliary cirrhosis (PBC), and primary sclerosing cholangitis (PSC).

Hepatopulmonary syndrome (HPS) and portopulmonary hypertension (POPH) are the major pulmonary vascular problems that complicate portal hypertension from any cause. HPS, a pulmonary vascular dilatation problem leading to arterial hypoxemia, occurs in 5–15% of patients with portal hypertension. POPH, resulting from pulmonary vascular obstruction or obliteration, has been reported in 4–16.5% of patients with advanced liver disease. Pleural effusions related to the formation of ascites develop in 5–10% of patients with cirrhosis.

Pulmonary function abnormalities can be demonstrated in approximately 50% of patients with advanced liver disease. The most common abnormality is a reduced diffusing capacity for carbon monoxide (DLco). Abnormal oxygenation (measured by an increased alveolar-arterial oxygen gradient or reduced PaO_2 is frequent (40–50%). Specific reasons for such abnormalities are usually multifactorial, resulting from problems listed in Table 59-1, as well as the effects of smoking and abdominal ascites.

RISK FACTORS

Portal hypertension seems to be a prerequisite for the development of either HPS or POPH. Previous portosystemic surgical shunts have been reported in up to 30% of patients with POPH. Conditions leading to abnormal ascites usually precede the development of pleural effusions ("hepatic hydrothorax"). Smoking in the setting of ZZ or SZ antitrypsin-deficiency phenotypes leads to the greatest risk of emphysema. The Child–Pugh classification for the severity of liver diseases correlates poorly with most pulmonary consequences, with the exception of hepatic hydrothorax. The epidemic of hepatitis C disease does not seem to be related to any unique pulmonary abnormality.

PATHOPHYSIOLOGY

Circulating mediators, associated with the appropriate genetic predisposition, would seem to be the cause of HPS or POPH. Such mediators (causing vasodilatation or vasoproliferation, respectively) should arise because of the abnormal metabolism of the dysfunctional liver. In humans, such specific circulating mediators have yet to be identified. HPS is characterized by arterial hypoxemia caused by precapillary-capillary dilatations or direct arteriovenous communications. Excess perfusion for a given area of ventilation, diffusion limitation, and true anatomic shunting contribute to the degree of abnormal arterial oxygenation (Figure 59-1). Increased amounts of exhaled nitric oxide have been demonstrated in HPS; an upregulation of endothelin B receptors causing vasodilation has been found in animal models of HPS.

POPH results from vasoproliferation (endothelium and smooth muscle), along with *in situ* thrombosis, which results in increased pulmonary vascular resistance (PVR) to arterial flow. It is important to note the various pulmonary hemodynamic patterns that may exist in the setting of advanced liver disease (Table 59-2).

Hepatic hydrothorax is a transudative pleural effusion caused by the formation of ascitic fluid. A combination of negative pleural pressure and positive abdominal pressures force ascitic fluid into the pleural spaces through diaphragmatic defects and lymphatics. Rarely, the fluid may be chylous.

PBC has systemic manifestations presumably because of autoimmune phenomena. Pulmonary granulomas, lymphocytic infiltrates, and organizing pneumonia can result. Rarely, both PBC and PSC may be associated with airway inflammation, hilar, and mediastinal adenopathy (noncaseating granulomas found at biopsy).

CLINICAL FEATURES

Exertional dyspnea is the most common, nonspecific presentation of any pulmonary consequence of liver dysfunction.

Hepatopulmonary Syndrome

Clubbing, cyanosis of the digits, and spider angiomas suggest the arterial hypoxemia of HPS. The chest examination is usually unremarkable. Worsening dyspnea (platypnea) and arterial oxygenation (orthodeoxia) as one moves from the supine to the standing position is frequently noted in HPS.

Portopulmonary Hypertension

Chest pressure, syncope, and palpitations suggest later manifestations of POPH. An accentuated second heart sound (increased P2) is frequent when POPH is advanced.

Primary Biliary Cirrhosis/Primary Sclerosing Cholangitis

Inspiratory crackles may be associated with the interstitial lung problems that complicate PBC or chronic aspiration in patients with hepatic encephalopathy. Productive sputum may be

TABLE 59-1 Major Pulmonary Consequences of Portal Hypertension (with or without Cirrhosis)

Pleural space	Hepatic hydrothorax Chylothorax Thoracobiliary fistulae Elevated hemidiaphragms due to massive ascites
Pulmonary parenchyma	Bronchitis/bronchiectasis Emphysema (ZZ or SZ α_1-antitrypsin deficiency Organizing pneumonia (PBC) Lymphocytic interstitial pneumonitis (PBC) UIP or NSIP (PBC, autoimmune hepatitis/ hepatitis C virus)

Pulmonary circulation	Hepatopulmonary syndrome
	Pulmonary hypertension
	  High-flow state
	  Excess volume
	  Left ventricular dysfunction
	Portopulmonary hypertension

PBC, Primary biliary cirrhosis; *PSC*, primary sclerosing cholangitis; *UIP*, usual interstitial pneumonitis; *NSIP*, nonspecific interstitial pneumonitis.

TABLE 59-2 Pulmonary Hemodynamic Patterns Associated with Advanced Liver Disease

	MPAP	CO	PAOP	TPG	PVR
High flow, hyperdynamic circulatory state*	↑	↑↑	↓	↓	↓
Excess volume†	↑	↑	↑	↑↓	↑↓
Portopulmonary hypertension					
Normal volume‡	↑↑↑	↑→↓	↓	↑↑↑	↑↑↑
Excess volume	↑↑↑	↑→↓	↑	↑↑	↑↑

Specific data associated with these patterns can be found in Hepatology 2005; 44:555–555.

MPAP, Mean pulmonary artery pressure; *CO*, cardiac output; *PAOP*, pulmonary artery occlusion pressure (same as pulmonary capillary wedge pressure); *TPG*, transpulmonary gradient (MPAP-PAOP); *PVR*, pulmonary vascular resistance (TPG/CO).

*This pattern usually seen in HPS.
†Depending on the duration and reason for excess volume, PVR and TPG may be increased or normal.
‡As POPH worsens, PVR increases, right heart fails and CO declines.

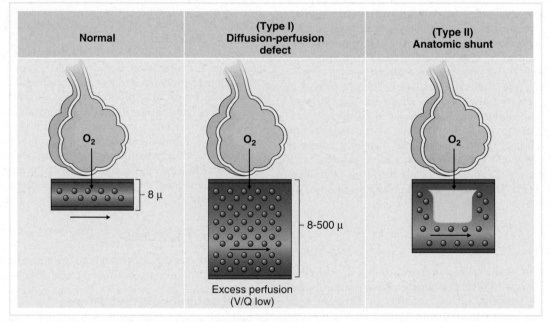

FIGURE 59-1 Two types of vascular dilatations associated with hepatopulmonary syndrome (HPS). Breathing room air, oxygen may not reach the middle of the dilated pulmonary capillary blood flow in type I HPS (the most common scenario) and hypoxemia results. Anatomic shunts (type II) are uncommon discrete structures that do not abut normal alveoli, thus breathing room air or supplemental oxygen may not interact with the capillary blood flow and hypoxemia occurs.

related to the airway abnormalities (bronchiectasis) associated with antitrypsin deficiency or PSC (bronchitis).

Hepatic Hydrothorax

Pleural effusion caused by liver dysfunction will be associated with diminished breath sounds depending on the location and extent of the pleural effusion. Egophony suggests atelectatic lung caused by compressive pleural effusions; affected patients may have significant hypoxemia. Pleuritic or chest wall pain is not a symptom of hepatic hydrothorax and suggests another diagnosis.

Alpha₁-Antitrypsin Deficiency

Signs and symptoms are similar to advanced chronic obstructive lung disease, especially emphysema. Chest radiography and CT imaging, however, suggest predominantly lower lung field distribution of emphysematous or bullous abnormality. Such changes are seen only in the severely deficient ZZ or SZ phenotypes. Approximately 50% of cirrhotic patients with ZZ or SZ phenotypes have abnormal PFTs, such as increased residual volume, and/or reduced forced expiratory volume in 1 sec.

Diagnosis

Hepatopulmonary Syndrome

This diagnosis is established by demonstrating pulmonary vascular dilatation as the cause for hypoxemia. Hypoxemia is usually defined as PaO_2 less than 70 mmHg or alveolar-arterial oxygen gradient greater than 15–20 mmHg. Two noninvasive methods are available to document abnormal pulmonary vascular dilatation. Qualitatively, a positive contrast-enhanced transthoracic echocardiogram reflects the passage of microbubbles (usually absorbed during a first pass through normal lungs) through dilated pulmonary vessels, with subsequent detection in the left atrium. Quantitatively, an abnormal brain uptake of technetium-labeled macro aggregated albumin (^{99m}Tc MAA) (uptake >6%) after lung perfusion reflects the passage of radiolabeled albumin aggregates through the lungs and subsequent uptake in the brain (Figure 59-2). Contrast echocardiography is more sensitive than ^{99m}Tc lung scanning to detect pulmonary vascular dilatation. A lung biopsy is not necessary. A practical clinical algorithm for the evaluation of suspected HPS is shown in Figure 59-3.

Portopulmonary Hypertension

Screening for pulmonary hypertension is accomplished by transthoracic Doppler echocardiography. Increased right ventricular systolic pressures greater than 50 mmHg suggest clinically significant POPH. A right heart catheterization must be accomplished to establish the diagnosis. A screening algorithm used at the Mayo Clinic is shown in Figure 59-4; clinicians may have other criteria to determine who should have a right heart catheterization. Most centers adhere to the triad of mean pulmonary artery pressure (MPAP) >25 mmHg, and PVR >240 dynes/sec/cm^{-5} as definitive criteria for POPH. A lung biopsy is not necessary or advised. Chronic pulmonary emboli should be excluded.

Hepatic Hydrothorax

This is a clinical diagnosis made on the basis of the chest radiograph showing a pleural effusion that can be right sided (70%), left sided (15%), or bilateral (15%). Thoracentesis is usually performed only when atypical symptoms (e.g., pain or fever) exist or there are suspicions of another process such as empyema or metastatic hepatocellular carcinoma. Hepatic hydrothorax may occur in the absence of clinical ascites.

Antitrypsin Deficiency

Pulmonary dysfunction in the setting of severe α_1-antitrypsin deficiency should be established by standard pulmonary testing (assess degree of expiratory airflow limitation and hyperinflation) and high-resolution computed tomography of the chest (assess for subclinical emphysema, bullae, and bronchiectasis). A combination of serum genotypes and decreased levels of α_1-antitrypsin protein confirm the diagnosis.

Treatment

Hepatopulmonary Syndrome

No pharmacologic treatments have proved efficacious in improving arterial hypoxemia caused by HPS. Liver transplantation (LT) is the treatment of choice. Rarely, coil embolization of discrete arteriovenous communications that occur in

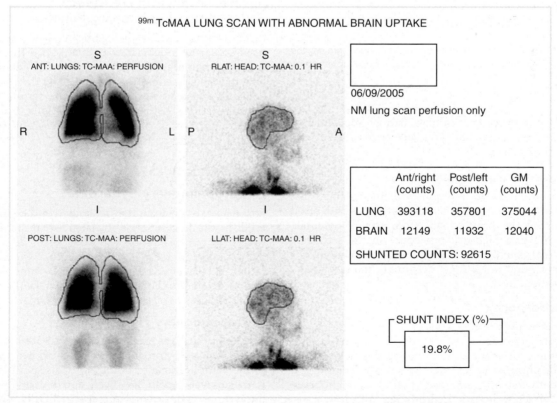

FIGURE 59-2 Lung perfusion scan with quantified technetium-99 macroaggregated albumin (MAA) abnormal uptake over the brain.

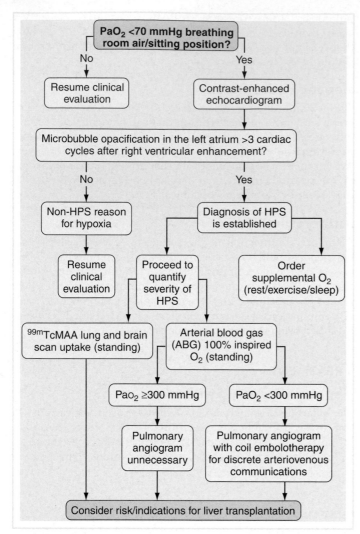

FIGURE 59-3 Current screening and diagnostic algorithm at the Mayo Clinic for patients suspected of having hepatopulmonary syndrome *(HPS)*.

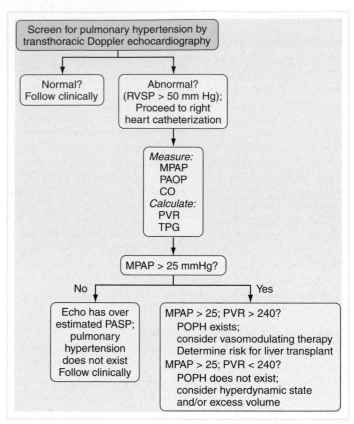

FIGURE 59-4 A screening, diagnostic, and staging algorithm followed at the Mayo Clinic in patients with portopulmonary hypertension.

HPS can result in improvement in oxygenation. Supplemental oxygen should be given depending on PaO_2 levels at rest, with exertion, and during sleep.

Portopulmonary Hypertension

Significant improvement in pulmonary hemodynamics has been reported with the long-term use of continuous 24-h intravenous infusion of the prostacyclin epoprostenol, bosentan, and sildenafil. LT is a high-risk procedure in the setting of POPH and is contraindicated if pulmonary vasomodulating therapy does not result in MPAP < 50 mmHg and satisfactory right heart function.

Hepatic Hydrothorax

Repetitive thoracentesis is not advised. Chest tube drainage with pleurodesis and video-assisted thoracoscopy rarely provide long-term improvement by obliterating the pleural space and repairing diaphragmatic defects, respectively. Transjugular intrahepatic portosystemic shunting (TIPS) is appropriate treatment for refractory hepatic hydrothorax, as is liver transplantation. Outcome of LT is not affected by the presence of hepatic hydrothorax.

Severe Antitrypsin Deficiency and Abnormal Pulmonary Function

In the setting of clinically significant liver disease and severe serum α_1-protein deficiency (<80 mg/dL), therapy to replace the α_1-protein is appropriate and safe. The goal is to minimize lung function deterioration. LT results in the phenotype of the donor liver and usually normalizes the serum α_1 level. Lung transplantation in the setting of serious liver dysfunction caused by ZZ or SZ phenotype may be problematic and must be considered on a case-by-case basis.

CLINICAL COURSE

Hepatopulmonary Syndrome

Few data exist to accurately characterize the clinical course in HPS. In the largest series to date, 5-year survival associated with liver transplantation was 76% versus 23% in those who did not undergo transplantation (Figure 59-5). Complete resolution of HPS after LT is frequent; the time to resolution is directly related to the severity and may take months. Mortality is rarely a direct consequence of hypoxemia.

Portopulmonary Hypertension

The 5-year survival ranges from 30% to 50%. Mortality is frequently caused by progressive right-sided heart failure, as well as the complications related to liver disease. No proven long-term survival benefit has been noted with 24-h continuous intravenous epoprostenol therapy in POPH. Despite pulmonary vasomodulating therapy, outcome during and after LT remains problematic and unpredictable.

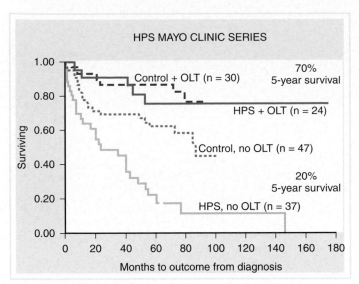

FIGURE 59-5 Survival curves demonstrating better long-term outcome when liver transplantation can be accomplished in patients with HPS. (From Swanson et al: Hepatology 2005; 41:1222–1229.)

Antitrypsin Deficiency

In those with the ZZ phenotype, long-term survival is significantly reduced in smokers. There are no data that describe the long-term outcomes in patients with ZZ phenotype, cirrhosis, and pulmonary function abnormalities.

PITFALLS AND CONTROVERSIES

Transjugular intrahepatic portosystemic shunting may or may not have a therapeutic role in the treatment of HPS. TIPS may acutely worsen pulmonary hemodynamics because of increased preload and, therefore, may be contraindicated in the setting of POPH.

The priority for LT in patients with either HPS or POPH is evolving. $Pao_2 < 60$ mmHg caused by HPS now warrants higher priority for LT. In POPH, it is hypothesized that pulmonary hemodynamic improvement with pulmonary vasodilators (goal of MPAP < 35 mmHg and PVR < 400 dynes/sec/cm^{-5}) may facilitate safe LT and improved long-term survival. The optimal medical therapy (prostacyclins, endothelin receptor antagonists, or phosphodiesterase inhibitors) for POPH has yet to be defined.

SUGGESTED READINGS

Garcia N Jr, Mihas AA: Hepatic hydrothorax: pathophysiology, diagnosis and management. J Clin Gastroenterol 2004; 38:52–58.

Hoeper MM, Halank M, Marx C, et al: Bosentan therapy for portopulmonary hypertension. Eur Respir J 2005; 25:502–508.

Kawut SM, Taichman DB, Ahya VN, et al: Hemodynamics and survival in patients with portopulmonary hypertension. Liver Transplant 2005; 11:1107–1111.

Krowka MJ, Mandell MS, Ramsay MA, et al: Hepatopulmonary syndrome and portopulmonary hypertension: A report of the multicenter liver transplant database. Liver Transplant 2004; 10:174–182.

Krowka MJ, Swanson KL, McGoon MD, et al: Portopulmonary hypertension: results of a 10-year screening algorithm. Hepatology 2006; 44:1140–1152.

Moorman J, Saad M, Kosseifi S, et al: Hepatitis C virus and the lung. Chest 2005; 128:2882–2892.

Reichenberger F, Voswinckel R, Steveling E, et al: Sildenafil treatment for portopulmonary hypertension. Eur Respir J 2006; 28:563–567.

Rodriguez-Roisin R, Fallon MB, Krowka MJ, et al: Pulmonary-hepatic vascular disorders: report of a Task Force. Eur Respir J 2004; 24:861–880.

Stoller JK, Aboussouan LS: Alpha₁ antitrypsin deficiency. Lancet 2005; 365:2225–2236.

Swanson KLM, Wiesner RH, Krowka MJ: Natural history of hepatopulmonary syndrome: impact of liver transplantation. Hepatology 2005; 41:1122–1129.

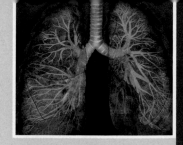

60 Inflammatory Bowel Disease

PHILIPPE CAMUS • THOMAS V. COLBY

INTRODUCTION

Several pulmonary/thoracic complications can occur before or in the course of treated or untreated inflammatory bowel disease (IBD), including ulcerative colitis (UC) and Crohn's disease (CD). These include (1) nonspecific manifestations such as thromboembolism, pulmonary edema related to low serum albumin, and opportunistic infections, for which a chance association is possible; (2) anatomic complications such as colobronchial, ileobronchial, or esophagobronchial fistulae; (3) therapy-related lung disease, including drug-induced pneumonitides and opportunistic infections; and (4) distinctive intrathoracic complications that show more than a coincidental association with the background IBD (Table 60-1). This chapter deals with the latter group of manifestations, which were reviewed recently (see "Suggested Reading").

The distinctive thoracic manifestations of UC and CD include tracheobronchial inflammation with or without suppuration, various kinds of infiltrative lung disease (InLD) nodules (pulmonary *pyoderma gangrenosum*), and serositis. Because of the unusual character of these manifestations, rigorous proof of an association is lacking. However, the suggestive clinicopathologic, endoscopic, and imaging pattern of several of these manifestations, notably airway inflammation, and their striking and exquisite response to corticosteroid therapy suggest that they are causally related to IBD.

The distinctive manifestations of IBD can occur in both UC and CD, albeit with slight differences in incidence in the two conditions (see Table 60-1). For instance, tracheobronchial inflammation occurs preferentially in UC, particularly when there is a history of colectomy; infiltrative lung disease tends to occur preferentially in patients receiving bowel disease–modifying drugs, whereas granulomatous infiltrative lung disease is seen more often in CD versus UC (see Table 60-1).

The diagnosis of these changes, particularly the group of infiltrative lung disease, is set against the background of possible pulmonary toxicity of the bowel disease–modifying drugs such as azathioprine, 6-mercaptopurine, sulfasalazine, mesalazine (5-aminosalicylate), and methotrexate in patients being exposed to these compounds, or of opportunistic pulmonary infections in patients with CD exposed to the anti-TNF agent infliximab. Careful investigation of an infectious etiology and judicious drug therapy withdrawal and corticosteroid therapy often will solve this issue.

EPIDEMIOLOGY

One hundred seventy-one cases with the association of IBD and respiratory involvement were reviewed recently. Only a few case series are available, because these cases are rare; only approximately 0.2% of patients with IBD are affected. Main groups of thoracic involvement in UC and CD included upper airway inflammation (8.8%), large airway inflammation (39.2%), small airway inflammation/fibrosis (9.8%), infiltrative lung disease (23.4%), involvement of the pulmonary vasculature (5.85%), and serosal involvement (12.9%).

Among patients with UC and airway involvement, females outnumber males, with an approximate ratio of 1.8:1, whereas the ratio ranges between 0.58 and 1.74:1 for the other manifestations.

Although the respiratory manifestations in IBD can develop at any time during the course of the disease, in approximately 80% of the cases, respiratory involvement follows the IBD by weeks to years. At the time of onset of the respiratory manifestations, the bowel disease may be active, flaring, or quiescent under the influence of bowel disease–modifying drugs or after colectomy. Indeed, patients who have had a colectomy in the past are not immune to the development of, mainly, airway involvement, which may manifest as severe airway inflammation, and destruction up to decades after surgery. It has been suggested that colectomy or coloproctectomy may be play a causal role, because, in a few patients, airway inflammation developed shortly after surgery, suggesting a shift of inflammation from the gut to the bronchial tree. Alternatively, airway inflammation may result from the abrupt discontinuation of bowel disease–modifying drugs after colectomy.

Other extraintestinal manifestations were present in association with the intrathoracic involvement in 18–52% of patients, depending on the type of intrathoracic involvement.

Smoking cigarettes may not be a risk factor for airway inflammation in IBD, because most patients with the association are nonsmokers.

The causal role of bowel disease–modifying drugs is difficult to ascertain.

1. Regarding airway inflammation in patients with IBD with a remote history of colectomy, the causal role of sulfasalazine or mesalazine is quite unlikely, because such patients do not generally receive these drugs any longer. In patients with no history of colectomy who were being exposed to bowel disease–modifying drugs, there was no improvement in airway inflammation after removal of these drugs. On the other hand, bowel disease–modifying drugs rarely improve IBD-related airway inflammation, except in rare patients with Crohn's disease, who may improve on infliximab. For these reasons, drugs are unlikely to play a causal role in IBD-related airway inflammation.

2. In patients with IBD with infiltrative lung disease, both untreated IBD and IBD exposed to drugs have been associated with the same patterns of infiltrative lung disease, and drug therapy withdrawal may not fully resolve the issue.

TABLE 60-1 Thoracic Involvement in Inflammatory Bowel Diseases

Site of Predominant Involvement*	Pattern	UC	CD	Presenting Symptoms	Imaging	Bronchoscopy/Pathology†	BAL	Treatment Option	Prognosis/Outcome
LARGE AIRWAYS									
Larynx/glottis/epiglottis	Glottic/subglottic inflammation & narrowing	++	+	Barking cough, noisy breathing, hoarseness, stridor, asphyxia	Normal/narrowing on CT/MRI	Glottic/subglottic inflammation (granulomatous in CD), inward bulging, marked stenosis. Erosion, ulceration + inflammation	ND	IV corticosteroids, laser ablation, emergent tracheostomy	Favorable
Trachea	Tracheitis (inflammation/stenosis)	++	+	Dry/productive cough, dyspnea, chronic sputum, hemoptysis	Normal/narrowing on CT/MRI	Tracheal inflammation, edema, hemorrhage with consequent stenosis. Can be impressive. Granulomas possible in CD	ND	IV/oral steroids. Occasional response to infliximab therapy in CD	Variable
Main bronchi	"Simple" chronic bronchitis	++	±	Chronic cough, slightly productive, wheeze	Normal	Mild/moderate inflammation and redness of large airways. Little or no stenosis	PMN	ICS ± short burst of oral CS	Often spectacular effect of CST
	Bronchial distention‡	+	−	Asymptomatic <−>	Airway distention on CT	ND	ND	ICS if patient symptomatic	May recover on CST
	Lone mucoid impaction	+	−	Asymptomatic	Branched, gloved-finger shadow(s) on CT	ND	ND	Watching or CSR	Good
	Disseminated endobronchial granulomas	−	+	Chronic cough	Normal or narrowing on CT/MRI	Spotted granulomas	ND	Oral ± ICS	?
	Chronic bronchial suppuration	++	+	Marked chronic cough, wheeze, copious sputum	Thickened bronchial walls "Dirty lungs"	Large airway inflammation, often severe. Deep-seated inflammatory cell infiltrate	PMN	ICS/oral CST/nebulized CS. Early treatment recommended	Variable. Residual symptoms and physiologic impairment common
	Bilateral bronchiectasis	++	+	Chronic cough & wheeze. Often, abundant sputum. Hemoptysis	Thickened/dilated bronchi. Mucoid impaction. Tree-in-bud distally	Widespread airway inflammation & narrowing. Exuberant cellular infiltrate. Lumenal exudate, metaplastic epithelium	PMN	ICS/oral CST/nebulized CS. Serial bronchial lavages with CS or resection of affected lobe rarely indicated	Variable. Residual impairment despite CST common. Refractoriness to any form of CST unusual
Small airways£	Acute neutrophil-rich or purulent bronchiolitis‡	+	+	Nonproductive cough ± dyspnea	Small irregular opacities. Mosaic on CT	ND	ND	Oral CST (+ICS?)	Variable
	Granulomatous bronchiolitis‡	−	+	Nonproductive cough ± dyspnea	Small irregular opacities. Mosaic on CT	ND	Ly	Oral CST	Favorable
	Diffuse panbronchiolitis pattern	+	−	Dyspnea ± sputum	Tree-in-bud mosaic on CT	Normal/mild inflammation	ND	Oral CST (+ICS?)	May progress to COPD
	Constrictive bronchiolitis fibrosa obliterans§	+	−	Dyspnea	ND	N	ND	ICS / oral CST	Associated with moderate-to-severe COPD

TABLE 60-1 Thoracic Involvement in Inflammatory Bowel Diseases—Cont'd

Site of Predominant Involvement*	Pattern	UC	CD	Presenting Symptoms	Imaging	Bronchoscopy/Pathology†	BAL	Treatment Option	Prognosis/Outcome
Lung parenchyma	OP	+	+	Dry cough, dyspnea, fever, ARF	Bilateral focal or diffuse infiltrates	N	Variable	Oral (IV) CST depending on severity	Usually favorable; this pattern may also be caused by drugs
	PIE	+	±	Dry cough, malaise, dyspnea ± slight fever	Bilateral focal or diffuse infiltrates	N	Eos	Oral (IV) CST depending on severity	Usually favorable; this pattern may also be caused by drugs
	NSIP-cellular	+	+	Dry cough, dyspnea	Basilar or diffuse opacities	N	Ly	Oral (IV) CST depending on severity	Usually favorable; this pattern may also be caused by drugs
	InLD, granulomatous	±	++	Dry cough, dyspnea	Diffuse shadowing	N	Ly	Oral (IV) CST depending on severity	Favorable
	InLD, desquamative	+	–	Dyspnea	Disseminated pulmonary opacities	N	ND	Oral (IV) CST depending on severity	Favorable
	Sterile necrobiotic nodules	+	–	Dyspnea, dull chest pain sometimes, cutaneous Pyoderma gangrenosum present	Multiple lung nodules/cavitation	N	ND	Oral (IV) CST depending on severity	Favorable
Pleura	Pleural effusion	+	+	Chest discomfort, pleuritic chest pain	Pleural effusion	–	–	Drainage/NSAIDs/corticosteroids	Favorable
	Pneumothorax			Stabbing chest pain, dyspnea	PNO ± PNM	–	–	Exsufflation	Favorable
Pericardium and heart	Pericarditis pericardial effusion myocarditis	+	+	Anterior chest pain, tamponade arrhythmias, heart block, heart failure	Enlarged heart	–	–	Drainage/NSAIDs/corticosteroids	Favorable; pericardial constriction unusual

ARF, Acute respiratory failure; *BAL*, bronchoalveolar lavage; *CD*, Crohn's disease; *CS*, corticosteroids; *CST*, corticosteroid therapy; *CT*, computed tomography; *Eos*, eosinophils; *ICS*, inhaled corticosteroids; *InLD*, infiltrative lung disease; *Ly*, lymphocytes; *ND*, no data available; *NSAIDs*, nonsteroidal antiinflammatory drugs; *NSIP*, nonspecific interstitial pneumonia (this pattern of InLD may also be due to the bowel disease-modifying drugs sulfasalazine or mesalazine); *OP*, organizing pneumonia also known as BOOP (this pattern of InLD may be due to the bowel disease-modifying drugs sulfasalazine or mesalazine); *PIE*, pulmonary infiltrates and eosinophilia also known as eosinophilic pneumonia (this pattern of InLD may also be due to the bowel disease-modifying drugs sulfasalazine or mesalazine); *PMN*, neutrophils; *UC*, ulcerative colitis.

*Location of airway inflammation tends to remain the same with time in a given patient (ex in upper airway, trachea, bronchi, or small airway), but may vary depending on patient and sometimes, time into the disease.

†Not all cases reach pathology.

‡Very few cases/data available for review, or unpublished; *N*, normal; *?*, unknown, unproven; *++*, quite common, suggestive; *+*, occasional; *±*, uncommon; *–*, not described, does not apply.

§Sometimes, pneumothorax or pneumomediastinum occur in association.

The issue is also complex because it can be difficult at times to differentiate IBD- and/or drug-related InLD from an opportunistic pulmonary infection. Microbiologic workup is necessary in all cases, along with prudent drug withdrawal or rechallenge and judicious use of corticosteroid therapy.

CLINICAL MANIFESTATIONS

Distinctive respiratory manifestations in patients with IBD may involve the large or small airways in the form of airway inflammation, lung parenchyma in the form of diffuse or focal InLD or necrobiotic nodules, or the serosal cavities in the form of pleural or pericardial effusion or thickening. Symptoms vary according to location of the pathologic process and include dyspnea, cough, regular production of sputum, fever, and chest pain.

Airway Inflammation

Airway inflammation is the most common and distinctive pattern of respiratory involvement in IBD, and it has a clear predilection for UC, as opposed to CD, and for patients with a history (at times remote) of colectomy. Inward bulging caused by inflammation results in airway narrowing that can be marked. These changes often are amenable to corticosteroid therapy, which will diminish or abolish them. Inflammation may predominate in:

1. The glottic/subglottic area (epiglottitis), producing narrowing and stenosis with the corresponding symptoms of dry, deep-toned cough, noisy breathing, stridor, and asphyxia. Asphyxia may develop in a few days and follow a period of subacute symptoms related to the upper airway. Urgent tracheostomy may be required
2. Large airways in the form of chronic tracheobronchitis. The condition manifests with chronic, otherwise unexplained, cough, which can be dry or productive of copious (up to a quart per day) amounts of mucopurulent sputum: Hence, the term *chronic bronchitis* or *chronic bronchial suppuration* used to name this condition. Imaging studies reveal thickened airway walls, mucus plugging in large-to-medium airways, and a tree-in-bud appearance of distal airways. These changes predominate in the lung bases. Chronic purulent sinusitis may be found on appropriate CT slices. On endoscopy, there is inflammation and narrowing, which can be marked. Inflammation may assume a granulomatous pattern in CD. Chronic uncontrolled inflammation and suppuration may lead to bronchiectasis.
3. Small airways, in the form of acute cellular or granulomatous (in CD) bronchiolitis. This pattern is distinctly uncommon as the dominant feature, although involvement of distal airways is often present on histopathologic examination in patients with involvement of proximal airways. Distal airway involvement manifests as airflow obstruction, with or without sputum production, and diffuse reticular shadows on imaging.

The preceding classification of airway inflammation is somewhat arbitrary, because overlapping features are common. Involvement of the glottis and epiglottis is often associated with tracheal inflammation. Tracheal inflammation may coexist with bronchial and small airway inflammation. Sometimes, inflammation involves the bronchial tree in its entirety, from the epiglottis or trachea down to the bronchiolar region of the lung.

Diffuse Infiltrative Lung Disease

Diffuse infiltrative lung disease manifests with moderate-to-severe breathlessness and fever, in the context of more or less symmetric focal, disseminated, or diffuse parenchymal opacities. Rarely is InLD discovered incidentally on a routine chest radiograph. In some patients, acute respiratory failure may develop. Typically, organizing pneumonia (OP) (BOOP-like pattern) manifests with bilateral ovoid elongated subpleural opacities, which may contain air bronchograms. Eosinophilic pneumonia also may assume a masslike appearance or manifests as wandering opacities. Less often, OP or eosinophilic pneumonia involves the lung diffusely. Other histopathologic patterns of diffuse infiltrative lung disease include nonspecific interstitial pneumonia and granulomatous interstitial pneumonia. The latter is almost exclusively seen in CD. Depending on pattern of involvement, bronchoalveolar lavage (BAL) shows a proportional increase in lymphocytes, neutrophils, or eosinophils. It is generally difficult to categorize the histologic pattern of InLD from the appearances on imaging or according to BAL data, except if there is eosinophilia in the BAL, which points to a diagnosis of eosinophilic pneumonia. The main difficulty in IBD-associated InLD is that this is also a common pattern of lung response to drugs, including those used to treat the IBD. Distinguishing IBD- from drug-related InLD often is difficult (see later).

Necrobiotic Nodules

Necrobiotic nodules are a distinctive but unusual pattern of involvement in IBD. Necrobiotic nodules are probably more common in UC than they are in CD, but in either case the numbers are small. Patients are seen with the rapid onset of fever, dyspnea with or without a dull pain in the chest, and multiple round, shaggy, parenchymal opacities on imaging. The nodules evolve in a roughly parallel fashion, may cavitate over a few days, diminish in size, and leave a residual scar. Deep-seated necrotic nodules may be present in the dermis in association with the lung nodules, with histopathologic features similar to those in the lung. Drug-induced injury, including that from sulfasalazine, can occasionally manifest with multiple lung nodules. However, these do not seem to undergo cavitation, and the histopathologic features of IBD-associated lung nodules are quite distinctive: suppurative with neutrophils without true granulomatous features.

Serositis

Patients with *serositis* with or without effusion are seen with dyspnea, pleuritic or anterior chest pain and, often, fever is present. Myocarditis as an associated feature is suggested by arrhythmias, heart block, or left ventricular failure. The disease usually is self-limited. Pleural effusion is a rare possibility in drug-induced injury, with or without the biologic features of drug induced *lupus*.

Pneumomediastinum

Pneumomediastinum was diagnosed in a few patients with a flare of UC. It is unclear whether this relates to colonic microfistulas or results from acute obstruction of distal airways analogous to the pneumomediastinum seen in the context of asthma attacks.

DIAGNOSIS AND MANAGEMENT OF IBD-RELATED THORACIC INVOLVEMENT

1. Two respiratory conditions require emergent management.

   • Acute upper airway (glottis, epiglottis) inflammation and obstruction may progress rapidly, causing acute chest discomfort and/or asphyxia. Diagnosis is suggested by visual inspection on endoscopy and is confirmed on biopsy of the airway mucosa. Treatment includes high-dose corticosteroids and, depending on the pattern of obstruction, laser ablation or emergent tracheostomy to restore airway patency. A single patient with CD improved within a few days of starting infliximab therapy.

   • Acute infiltrative lung disease may manifest with diffuse pulmonary infiltrates and acute respiratory failure, requiring emergent mechanical ventilation. Fiberoptic bronchoscopy is indicated to rule out an infection. In patients who receive drugs, drug therapy withdrawal is indicated. Video-assisted thoracoscopic (VATS) lung biopsy may be justified to rule out an infection, determine the exact histopathologic background, and guide corticosteroid therapy. Although this approach seems satisfactory, particularly as regards elimination of an infectious cause, there is no proof that establishing the histopathologic diagnosis of InLD in IBD improves the outcomes of these patients.

2. In other situations, the strategy for evaluating pulmonary involvement is guided by symptoms, and data on chest imaging or ultrasound, often are suggested on endoscopy, and/or confirmed on histopathologic examination.

In addition to complete blood count with differential and metabolic panel, blood work should include antineutrophil cytoplasmic antibody (ANCA) testing, because a perinuclear snowdrift, not a cytoplasmic staining pattern, can be found in a fraction of patients with IBD. Antinuclear antibodies help identify the drug-induced *lupus* syndrome. Coagulation studies are indicated in patients with IBD with a suspicion of thromboembolism.

Chest radiograph, CT, and MRI are indicated to diagnose upper airway obstruction and stenosis; however, endoscopy may be more efficient in this respect.

In patients with large airway inflammation, the chest radiograph may be normal or show a pattern of dirty lung, tram line opacities corresponding to thickened bronchial walls (Figure 60-1) or, in advanced cases, predominantly basilar bronchiectasis (Figure 60-2).

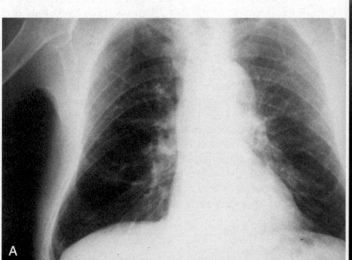
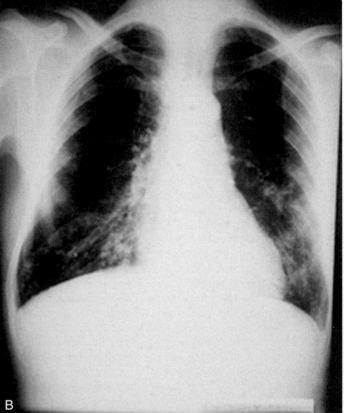

FIGURE 60-1 Involvement of large airways (glottis, trachea, mainstem bronchi) in chronic ulcerative colitis. **A,** Volume loss, increased parenchymal attenuation, small irregular opacities, and tram lines reflecting increased bronchial thickness are present in the bases bilaterally. **B,** Patients with chronic bronchitis or bronchial suppuration may progressively have bibasilar bronchiectasis develop. Bronchiectasis as opposed to early stages of the disease is less likely to show improvement after treatment with inhaled or oral corticosteroids.

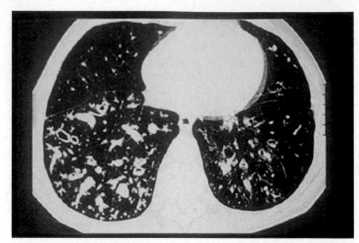

FIGURE 60-2 With time, patients with chronic airway inflammation or suppuration may have bilateral bronchiectasis develop as shown on this CT scan. Increased airway caliber, bronchial wall thickening gloved-finger branched shadows are a common finding distal to bronchiectasis (*right lower lobe, distally*) and suggest mucoid or mucopurulent impaction in the airways.

In untreated cases, CT findings include tracheal and/or bronchial wall thickening, airway filling with inspissated secretions, mucoid impaction, airway distention or dilatation, centrilobular micronodules, a tree-in-bud appearance exhibiting a branching pattern according to small airway dichotomy, and inhomogeneous lung attenuation numbers and evidence for air trapping distally. Follow-up studies indicate that these changes are less with time in patients who respond to corticosteroid therapy.

Most patients with significant airway inflammation demonstrate a mixed obstructive and restrictive disturbance on pulmonary function testing, and the obstructive component is largely uninfluenced by inhaled bronchodilators. In contrast, regular corticosteroid therapy will improve these changes, and pulmonary function tests are used to monitor the effect of antiinflammatory therapy, determine the lowest possible corticosteroid dosage, and detect relapse. Changes in pulmonary physiology correlate with the extent of involvement at endoscopy and imaging. Pulmonary function has been studied in patients with IBD without symptoms in the chest. Mild restrictive or obstructive changes, impaired diffusing capacity, and hyperinflation were found in a sizable fraction of patients with UC or CD, but there is no indication that these changes predict the development of overt airway or lung parenchymal involvement.

Endoscopy is essential to diagnose inflammation of accessible airways, from the glottis to subsegmental airways or beyond, scope size permitting. Inflammation at endoscopy ranges from redness without bulging of the bronchial walls to shiny exuberant cobblestone-like or pseudotumoral hemorrhagic inflammation reminiscent of the appearance of the colonic mucosa in IBD. These changes may severely restrict airway patency. Tracheobronchial inflammation and narrowing may impede the progression of the fiberscope. Curving may be required to cross stenotic areas. Bronchoscopy may be macroscopically normal in patients with specific involvement of the small airways and in those with InLD.

BAL typically yields an increased number of neutrophils (especially in the first fraction of BAL retrieved) in patients with large airway inflammation. An increase in lymphocytes, neutrophils, or eosinophils or a mixed BAL pattern is found in infiltrative lung disease. Studies of BAL in patients with CD with no pulmonary complaints or evidence for involvement of any kind showed an increase in lymphocytes. There is no indication that these patients may be at increased risk of overt infiltrative lung disease developing.

Histopathologic evaluation of airway or lung tissue may be required to substantiate a diagnosis of IBD-related respiratory involvement, rule out other causes, and guide treatment. In patients with large airway involvement, bronchial biopsies are easily performed, and there is evidence of a luminal exudate of neutrophils, mucosal epithelial metaplasia, and a submucosal inflammatory infiltrate composed of mononuclear cells (Figure 60-3). Involvement of the small airways can be seen in association with involvement of larger airways or occurs in isolation; in either instance, the histologic appearance of the small airway lesions may be suppurative, dominated by chronic inflammation of the airways, granulomatous, or fibrosing, with or without luminal narrowing (constrictive bronchiolitis). Occasionally, prominent interstitial foamy histiocytes are present around the respiratory bronchioles, and these changes simulate diffuse panbronchiolitis as encountered in Japan. The preceding changes in distal airways may be similar in UC and CD. When in the late stage of constrictive *bronchiolitis obliterans*, patients may have severe airflow obstruction.

Lung biopsy may be required in patients with diffuse InLD in whom diagnostic issues are not solved by less invasive methods. Patterns of InLD include nonspecific cellular interstitial pneumonia, organizing pneumonia with intraalveolar plugs of granulation tissue (BOOP-like pattern) typical for this condition regardless of the cause for it, granulomatous interstitial pneumonia (a feature more often seen in CD), eosinophilic pneumonia, and, rarely, desquamative interstitial pneumonia or a pattern of pulmonary fibrosis or IPF (Figure 60-4). Although some of these patterns may simulate sarcoidosis or hypersensitivity pneumonitis, subtle histopathologic differences may allow segregation of these entities. A pattern of diffuse reticular lung disease on imaging may also result from diffuse involvement of the distal airways, such as chronic bronchiolitis with or without nonnecrotizing granulomatous inflammation and/or acute bronchiolitis associated with a sterile neutrophil-rich bronchopneumonia.

Necrobiotic nodules (Figure 60-5) are sterile but resemble abscesses with a central fibrinous exudate with neutrophils, central necrosis of lung tissue (which accounts for the cavitation seen radiologically), a rim of histiocytes peripherally, and chronic inflammation without giant cells or nonnecrotizing granulomas as would be seen in granulomatous infections or Wegener's granulomatosis. The lesion resembles *pyoderma gangrenosum* in the skin. The main differential diagnosis is pyogenic abscesses, and special stains, cultures, and other appropriate tests are required to rule out an infection.

TREATMENT

Only corticosteroids have demonstrated efficacy in the management of IBD-related thoracic complications. These drugs can improve symptoms, pulmonary physiology, imaging, BAL, and pathology. No convincing response follows the use of immunosuppressive agents. There is anecdotal response to bowel disease–modifying drugs, infliximab, or mycophenolate.

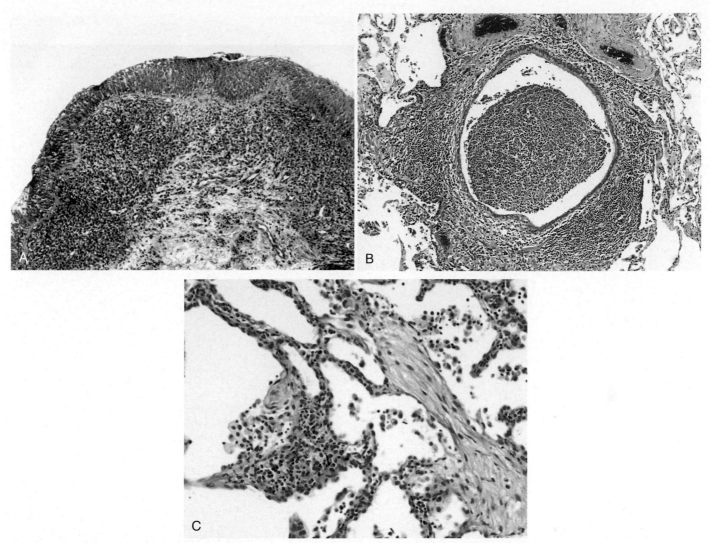

FIGURE 60-3 **A,** Marked submucosal inflammation and metaplastic mucosal epithelium in a large airway in ulcerative colitis. **B,** Bronchiolitis in chronic ulcerative colitis with luminal exudate of neutrophils and chronic inflammation in the wall of a small bronchiole. **C,** Organizing eosinophilic pneumonia in inflammatory bowel disease (ulcerative colitis in this case). Ductal organization is visible in the form of an elongated fibrous mass on the right. The cluster of interstitial cells (*lower left*) are eosinophils.

Airway Inflammation

In patients with airway inflammation, the site, extent, and degree of involvement dictate how the individual patient should be treated. The mainstay of treatment of patients with large airway inflammation is inhaled corticosteroids. The following guidelines are derived from the literature and our personal experience, because there are no data with a high level of evidence in the area. It is important to treat the inflammation early and aggressively to achieve clinical remission as quickly as possible with high-dose inhaled corticosteroids and, often, a burst of oral corticosteroid therapy for a few weeks. It is also important to monitor patients carefully by use of pulmonary function testing for possible flares of airway inflammation. These are undesirable in that they produce annoying symptoms and may prove increasingly difficult to control with time.

Large airway inflammation (trachea excepted) is the most common form of involvement in IBD and is often amenable to topical corticosteroids. A fairly high initial dosage is

recommended (e.g., 2000–2500 μg of beclomethasone, budesonide, or equivalent in divided dosages q.i.d.) until relief of symptoms is obtained and a "best" lung function is attained, to which any further measurement during tapering is compared. Dosage should be prudently tapered after 2–4 weeks to 800–1000 μg/day. Tapering must be slow and is guided by symptoms and pulmonary function. Patients should be instructed promptly to report recurrence of symptoms early, and their help is essential. Oral corticosteroids (e.g., 40–50 mg equivalent prednisolone for 4 weeks, to be tapered over an additional 4–8 weeks) may be prescribed in association with the inhaled corticosteroids with the hope of maximizing improvement in all aspects of airway and lung functions. Higher dosages may be required in patients with severe involvement, or 500–1000 μg nebulized budesonide three to four times daily is given, in conjunction with oral corticosteroids. After a response has been documented, oral steroids are maintained, and dry powder–inhaled corticosteroids can be substituted gradually for nebulized budesonide. The airway inflammation may

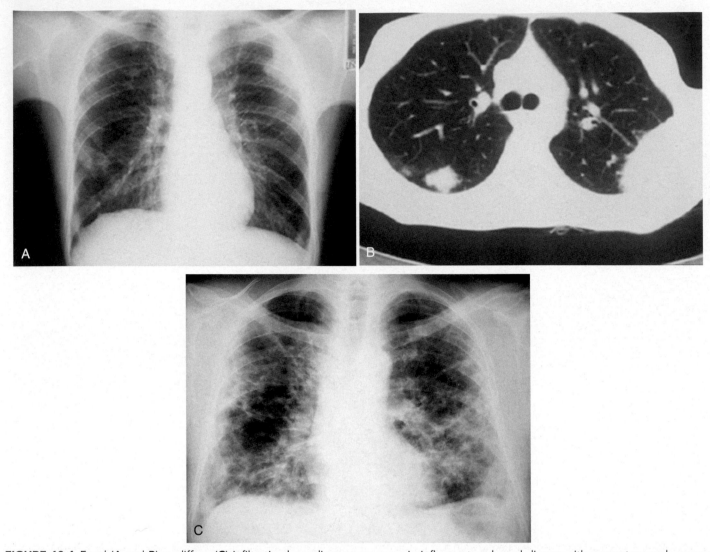

FIGURE 60-4 Focal (**A** and **B**) or diffuse (**C**) infiltrative lung disease can occur in inflammatory bowel disease either spontaneously or as a complication of therapy with drugs. **A** and **B,** Dense focal pulmonary infiltrates correspond histopathologically to organizing pneumonia or BOOP. **C,** Diffuse infiltrative lung disease (corresponding to distinct histopathologic entities such as nonspecific interstitial pneumonia, eosinophilic pneumonia, or organizing pneumonia in this case) (see Table 60-1).

be so severe and refractory to inhaled and oral corticosteroids that endoscopic administration of corticosteroids has been proposed to enhance topical drug delivery. Twice or thrice weekly instillations or bronchial lavages with methylprednisolone (40–80 mg dissolved in 50–125 mL saline) are given through the fiberoptic bronchoscope while oral and inhaled corticosteroids are continued in the meantime as previously. This may provide at least temporary improvement. Corticosteroids tapering to dosages not exposing patients to adverse effects may not be possible in patients with very severe involvement. There is no experience with macrolides, and an empiric trial is justified in any patient requiring high dosages of corticosteroids. Follow-up includes symptom reporting, pulmonary function, imaging, endoscopy, and monitoring for the development of adverse effects of corticosteroids.

Late treatment or insufficient dosages expose patients to the risk of tolerance or refractoriness and ongoing airway inflammation, leading to irreversible bronchiectasis. There is clinical evidence that corticosteroids are less efficacious in patients with advanced disease. This emphasizes the need for early recognition and treatment of IBD-related airway involvement. Nevertheless, patients with advanced disease, even those with bronchiectasis, often benefit from corticosteroid therapy.

Acute upper airway stenosis requires expeditious laser use to relieve obstruction or urgent tracheostomy in addition to high-dose intravenous corticosteroids.

Provided an infectious etiology has been carefully ruled out, patients with InLD may be observed if they have patchy infiltrates suggesting OP or if the imaging and BAL features coincide with those of eosinophilic pneumonia. In patients exposed to methotrexate, sulfasalazine, or mesalazine, drug therapy withdrawal may be followed by improvement, supporting the drug etiology. Prudent rechallenge with the two latter drugs (but *not* with methotrexate) may be attempted under close medical supervision to induce tolerance and maintain control of the IBD. When possible, labeling of infiltrative lung disease by means of VATS lung biopsy is preferred to an empiric trial of

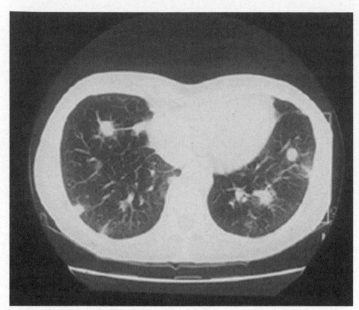

FIGURE 60-5 Necrobiotic lung nodules in a patient with ulcerative colitis and pyoderma of the skin. The nodules correspond to neutrophilic aggregates and tend to cavitate within a few days.

corticosteroid therapy. Nonspecific interstitial lung disease, eosinophilic pneumonia, and organizing pneumonia usually respond fairly well to oral or intravenous corticosteroid therapy.

Moderate pleuritis and pericarditis respond well to nonsteroidal antiinflammatory drugs or corticosteroids. Pleural drainage, pericardiocentesis, and surgical drainage may be required in patients with large effusions when these occasion compression or tamponade.

CONCLUSION

It is important that physicians are cognizant of the various patterns of respiratory involvement in IBD (see Table 60-1). Some of these manifestations occur in the setting of quiescent IBD or many years after proctocolectomy. It is essential to diagnose airway involvement in IBD early to avoid long periods of disabling symptoms and the development of bronchiectasis. Late stages of the disease are more difficult to control.

The location and extent of airway inflammation is unpredictable, as is the onset and progression of the disease. Unfortunately, some patients are refractory to any form or dosage of corticosteroid drugs and have uncontrollable airway inflammation develop. Macrolide drugs, which have shown some efficacy in diffuse panbronchiolitis, may be tried, although there is no experience yet. The role of anti-TNF-antibody therapy remains to be studied. Lung transplantation remains an option in some patients.

NOTE: *A registry of cases is kept by the authors, who are happy to discuss clinical or histopathologic data (philippe.camus@chu-dijon.fr or colby.thomas@mayo.edu). Inquiries on the possibility of drug-induced involvement are also welcome on Pneumotox.com®*

SUGGESTED READINGS

Black H, Mendoza M, Murin S: Thoracic manifestations of inflammatory bowel disease. Chest 2007; 131:524–532.

Camus P, Colby TV: Respiratory manifestations in ulcerative colitis. Eur Respir Monographs 2006; 10:168–183.

Camus P, Piard F, Ashcroft T, et al: The lung in inflammatory bowel disease. Medicine (Baltimore) 1993; 72:151–183.

Casey MB, Tazelaar HD, Myers JL, et al: Noninfectious lung pathology in patients with Crohn's disease. Am J Surg Pathol 2003; 27:213–219.

Chenivesse C, Bautin N, Wallaert B: Pulmonary manifestations in Crohn's disease. Eur Respir Monographs 2006; 10:151–167.

Colby TV, Camus P: Pathology of pulmonary involvement in inflammatory bowel disease. Eur Respir Monographs 2007; 12:199–207.

Higenbottam T, Cochrane GM, Clark TJH, et al: Bronchial disease in ulcerative colitis. Thorax 1980; 35:581–585.

http://www.pneumotox.com: Pneumotox® Website: 1997. Producers: P Foucher and Ph Camus: Last update: December, 2007.

Mahadeva R, Walsh G, Flower CD, Shneerson JM: Clinical and radiological characteristics of lung disease in inflammatory bowel disease. Eur Respir J 2000; 15:41–48.

Storch I, Sachar D, Katz S: Pulmonary manifestations of inflammatory bowel disease. Inflammatory Bowel Dis 2003; 9:104–115.

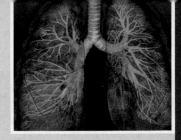

PULMONARY VASCULAR DISORDERS, VASCULITIDES, AND HEMORRHAGE

61 Pulmonary Embolism

MICHAEL P. GRUBER • TODD M. BULL

INTRODUCTION

"The philosophies of one age have become the absurdities of the next, and the foolishness of yesterday has become the wisdom of tomorrow."

William Osler

Pulmonary embolism (PE) and deep venous thrombosis (DVT) are different manifestations of the same pathologic process best grouped under the heading venous thromboembolism (VTE). VTE as a disease entity is responsible for significant morbidity and mortality while imparting great socioeconomic impact. Appropriately, much attention has been devoted to its diagnosis and treatment. Although the medical literature has, at times, presented conflicting opinions, increased numbers of better-designed trials are helping to build consensus toward the optimal approach for the management of pulmonary embolism. This is not to say that significant controversies do not still exist. As in all areas of medicine, as one question is "answered," others arise. In the course of this chapter, we will attempt to summarize the most important literature regarding the clinical approach to pulmonary embolism.

EPIDEMIOLOGY, RISK FACTORS, AND PATHOGENESIS

Epidemiology

PE is a common clinical problem. In the United States, hospital-based studies estimate the incidence of PE at 1 case per 1000 persons per year, equating to 200,000–300,000 hospital admissions per year. Estimates suggest that as many as 30,000–50,000 people die from PE annually in the United States, with an estimated 3-month disease-specific mortality rate of 10%. In nearly 20% of cases, the initial clinical manifestation is sudden death. Figures for Europe and other parts of the world are broadly similar.

Significant differences in mortality caused by pulmonary embolism by age, gender, and race have been observed. Age-adjusted PE mortality rates are as much as 50% higher among African-Americans than Caucasians. Among racial strata, PE mortality rates are 20–30% higher in men than women. African-American men have the highest reported mortality from PE, with an incidence rate of 6.0 deaths per 100,000 persons followed by African-American women at 4.8 deaths per 100,000 persons. The PE mortality for Caucasian males is 2.4 deaths per 100,000 persons and is the lowest for Caucasian females at 2.3 deaths per 100,000 persons. The incidence of PE is also age dependent, with increasing incidence of death occurring with advancing age. From 1979 to 1998, accounting for both gender and race, age-specific mortality rates doubled for each 10-year age group over 15–24 years.

Over the past 25 years, the overall mortality rate from PE has decreased. From 1979 to 1998, the annual mortality decreased by approximately 30%. The decline in PE mortality has been observed across gender and ethnic groups. The decreasing mortality rates from PE have been attributed to improved VTE risk factor modification, including improved prophylaxis of DVT, better detection and treatment of DVT, and/or enhanced PE diagnostic techniques, which has led to a decrease in disease misclassification.

Risk Factors

The risk of VTE, which includes PE and DVT, is a dynamic process resulting from synergistic interaction between acquired and genetic risk factors. Historically, Rudolph Virchow is credited as the first individual to describe the classic triad of vascular endothelial injury, hypercoagulability, and venous stasis as the combination of host factors that predispose to VTE. VTE risk factors are traditionally categorized as either genetic (inherited thrombophilia) or acquired.

Inherited Thrombophilia

The presence of a well-documented family history of VTE in one or more first-degree relatives strongly suggests the presence of a hereditary thrombophilia. An inherited thrombophilia can be identified in 24–37% of unselected patients with VTE compared with 10% in the control population. Estimates suggest that 1–2% of patients with idiopathic VTE have combined mutations. Inherited thrombophilias may result from qualitative or quantitative defects of coagulation factor inhibitors (antithrombin, protein C, protein S), increased levels or function of coagulation factors (activated protein C resistance, factor V Leiden mutation, prothrombin gene mutation, elevated factor VIII levels), hyperhomocysteinemia, defects in fibrolysis, or altered platelet function. Epidemiologic features of the common inherited thrombophilias are shown in Table 61-1.

Antithrombin Deficiency

Formerly termed *antithrombin III*, antithrombin (AT) is a single-chain vitamin K–independent glycoprotein belonging to the serine protease inhibitor superfamily. AT functions as a natural anticoagulant by binding and inactivating thrombin and activated coagulation factors IXa, Xa, XIa, and XIIa. The AT molecule also has an active heparin-binding site, which, when heparin bound, has marked affinity and function for

TABLE 61-1 Inherited Thrombophilias

Disorder	Prevalence (%) General Population	Prevalence (%) Patients with VTE	Inheritance	Relative Risk	Clinical Features
AT deficiency	0.2	1–3	AD	20	VTE, heparin resistance
Protein C deficiency	0.2–0.4	3–5	AD	10	VTE
Protein S deficiency	0.03–0.1	1–5	AD	10	VTE and ATE
Factor V Leiden	5	10–50	AD	5	VTE and ATE
Prothrombin G20210A	2–5	6–18	AD	3	VTE
Hyperhomocysteinemia	5	10	Not known	3	VTE and premature ASCVD
Elevated factor VIII	11	25	Not known	5	VTE

(Data from Franchini M, Veneri D, Salvagno GL, et al: Inherited thrombophilia. Crit Rev Clin Lab Sci 2006;43:249–290.)
AT, Antithrombin; VTE, venous thromboembolism, ATE, arterial thromboembolism, ASCVD, atherosclerotic cardiovascular disease.

binding and inactivating coagulation factors such as thrombin. The augmentation of the inhibitory activity of AT by heparin is the basis for the clinical use of heparin therapy. Mutations in AT lead to decreased ability of the molecule to inhibit the coagulation cascade, therefore leading to increased risk of thrombosis. AT deficiency is inherited as an autosomal-dominant trait affecting both males and females equally. Most affected individuals are heterozygotic for AT deficiency, because homozygotic inheritance is typically fetal lethal. Heterozygote AT deficient individuals have AT levels that are 40–70% of normal. Two different types of AT deficiency caused by more than 250 mutations have been described. Type I AT deficiency is characterized by a quantitative reduction in normally functioning AT. Type II AT deficiency is characterized by both quantitative and qualitative defects resulting in the classification of three different subtypes on the basis of the type of receptor defect: (1) abnormality of active thrombin binding site, (2) abnormality of heparin-binding site, and (3) abnormalities of both thrombin- and heparin-binding sites. These classifications are clinically relevant in that defects in the active thrombin-binding site confer a higher risk of VTE than defects that only involve the heparin-binding site or that are strictly quantitative.

Despite a low prevalence, AT deficiency is considered the most severe inherited thrombophilia, with increased risk of thrombosis as much as 20-fold over individuals without deficiency. Patients with AT deficiency typically have VTE develop during the latter part of the second or third decades of life. The most common sites of thrombosis include the lower extremity or iliofemoral veins. However, other sites including the upper extremities, mesenteric veins, vena cava, renal veins, and retinal veins have been reported. Thrombotic events in AT-deficient individuals are often precipitated by acquired thrombophilic risk factors such as surgery, trauma, pregnancy, drugs, and/or infection. Approximately 60% of individuals have recurrent thrombotic events develop, and clinical signs of PE are evident in up to 40% of these patients.

The diagnosis of AT deficiency should be determined by a functional assay of heparin cofactor activity, which is able to detect all cases of AT deficiency of clinical relevance. AT levels are not usually influenced by warfarin therapy but can be decreased during the acute phase of a thrombotic event, with disseminated intravascular coagulation, or with the concomitant use of heparin. Heparin therapy can lower AT levels by

as much as 30%. Screening for AT deficiency is recommended within at least 2 weeks of an acute thrombotic event or at least 5 days after discontinuation of heparin therapy.

Protein C Deficiency

Protein C is a vitamin K–dependent glycoprotein synthesized in the liver. Protein C is activated by the thrombin–thrombomodulin complex. Protein C circulates as an inactive precursor and exerts its anticoagulant function after activation to the serine protease, activated protein C. Once activated, protein C proteolytically degrades activated coagulation factors Va and VIIIa. More than 160 qualitative and/or quantitative mutations in protein C have been described. Protein C is inherited as an autosomal-dominant trait affecting both males and females equally. Homozygous individuals typically have more severe and earlier onset thrombophilia. Two different subtypes of inherited protein C deficiency have been identified. Type I deficiency is a quantitative disorder characterized by parallel reductions in functional and antigenic levels of protein C to 50% of normal levels. Type II deficiency is a qualitative defect with reductions in functional levels of protein C but preserved antigenic function. The prevalence of protein C deficiency is estimated at 0.2–0.4% in the general population and 3–5% in individuals with VTE. Three clinical syndromes are associated with protein C deficiency: (1) VTE in teenagers and adults, (2) neonatal purpura fulminans in homozygous or doubly heterozygous newborns, or (3) warfarin-induced skin necrosis. Acquired protein C deficiency occurs in a variety of clinical settings, including liver disease, infection, septic shock, disseminated intravascular coagulation, acute respiratory distress syndrome, postoperative states, and in association with chemotherapeutic drugs.

The diagnosis of protein C deficiency should be made by use of functional testing on the basis of activation with thrombin-thrombomodulin or snake venom. Pregnancy and oral contraceptive use can increase plasma protein C levels. Protein C levels are decreased by acute thrombotic events and therapy with warfarin. In the absence of warfarin therapy and known medical conditions that result in acquired protein C deficiency, patients with a protein C level less than 55% of normal are very likely to have a genetic abnormality, whereas levels from 55–65% normal are consistent with either a deficient state or low normal values. Thus, repeat testing and/or genetic testing is recommended in most populations.

Protein S Deficiency

Protein S is a vitamin K–dependent glycoprotein synthesized by hepatocytes, megakaryocytes, and endothelial cells. Protein S functions as a cofactor of activated protein C for the degradation of activated factors Va and VIIIa. Protein S circulates in plasma in equilibrium as a free functionally active form and an inactive form bound to a carrier protein (C4BP). The bioavailability of protein S is closely linked to the concentration of C4BP. C4BP functions as an important regulatory protein in the protein C: protein S inhibitor pathway. Three subtypes of protein S deficiency have been defined on the basis of total protein S concentrations, free protein S concentrations, and activated protein C cofactor activity. Type I protein S deficiency is associated with approximately 50% of normal protein S levels, more marked decrease in free protein S concentrations, and decreased functional activity. Type II deficiency is characterized by normal total and free protein S levels but decreased functional activity. Type III deficiency, also know as type IIa, is characterized by normal total protein levels but decreased free protein concentrations and decreased functional activity. Conditions that result in reductions in protein C levels, as mentioned in the preceding section, can similarly influence protein S levels. The prevalence of protein S deficiency in the general population is estimated to be 0.03–0.1% of the general population and 1–5% in individuals with VTE. The clinical presentation of VTE in patients with protein S deficiency is similar to that of protein C deficiency. Warfarin-induced skin necrosis has been reported with protein S deficiency.

Measurement of the free protein S concentration is the preferred screening test for protein S deficiency. Similar to protein C measurements, acute thrombosis, pregnancy, oral contraceptive use, comorbid disease, and/or use of warfarin can alter assay results. Heparin does not alter plasma protein S or protein C concentrations and thus is an acceptable antithrombotic therapy during diagnostic workup. In patients on warfarin therapy, recommendations support waiting at least 2 weeks after discontinuation to investigate for suspected protein S deficiency.

Factor V Leiden and Activated Protein C Resistance

Factor V Leiden is the most common recognized cause of inherited thrombophilia, accounting for 20–50% of new VTE cases. Factor V circulates in the plasma as an inactive cofactor. After activation by thrombin, Factor Va serves as a cofactor in the conversion of prothrombin to thrombin. In 1993, investigators in Leiden, The Netherlands, identified a single point mutation in the factor V gene in a cohort of individuals with unexplained VTE. The molecular defect is a single amino acid change (arginine[506] to glutamine) at one of the activated protein C (APC) cleavage sites, making the factor V molecule resistant to activated protein C at this site. This genetic defect, termed *factor V Leiden*, is the most common cause of inherited APC resistance, although other mutations have been identified. Factor V Leiden is a common mutation. The prevalence of factor V Leiden in the general population is estimated at 5%. Individuals who are heterozygous for the factor C Leiden mutation have approximately a fivefold increase in VTE risk compared with the general population. Individuals who are homozygous for the mutation are estimated to have an 80-fold increase in the risk of VTE over the general population.

The major clinical manifestation of thrombosis in individuals with factor V Leiden is venous. Thrombosis in the deep veins of the lower extremities is common, whereas superficial veins, portal vein, and cerebral vein thrombosis as less common. Because of the high frequency of this mutation in the general population, a synergistic effect with other inherited or acquired VTE risk factors has been observed. In addition to inherited APC resistance, acquired APC resistance has been reported. The use of third-generation oral contraceptives, individuals with malignancy, and connective tissue disease, in particular systemic lupus erythematosus and the antiphospholipid antibody syndrome, have APC resistance.

Activated partial thromboplastin time (aPTT)–based assays serve as the screening test for APC resistance. The aPTT is performed in the presence and absence of a standardized amount of APC, and the two clotting times are expressed as an APC ratio (aPTT in the presence to absence of APC). APC resistance reduces the APC ratio. The standard aPTT screening test may be influenced by a variety of factors, including inflammatory states, pregnancy, oral contraceptives, antiphospholipid antibodies, and anticoagulation. Genetic testing for the factor V Leiden mutation is also available.

Prothrombin Gene Mutation

Prothrombin (factor II), the precursor of thrombin, is a vitamin K–dependent protein synthesized in the liver. In 1996, researchers identified a single nucleotide change (guanine to adenine) at nucleotide position 20210 in the prothrombin gene as a risk factor for thrombosis. The prevalence of this mutation is 6–18% in individuals with VTE and 2–5% in the general population. Heterozygote carriers of this mutation have 30% higher plasma prothrombin levels than normal, which corresponds to a threefold higher risk of thrombosis than in the general population. Given the relatively low thrombotic risk, there remains controversy as to whether this mutation confers an increased risk of recurrent VTE. Studies have shown that the estimated risk of thrombosis associated with the prothrombin G20210A mutation is significantly increased only in those individuals with additional thrombotic risk factors. Moreover, studies have demonstrated that the prothrombin G20210A mutation is often coinherited with factor V Leiden mutation. Approximately 1–10% of symptomatic factor V Leiden carriers also have the prothrombin G20210A gene mutation. Diagnostic evaluation for the prothrombin G20210A gene mutation is best completed by direct genomic DNA analysis.

Elevated Factor VIII Levels

High levels of factor VIII are a strong independent risk factor for VTE. The prevalence of increased factor VIII levels in the general population is approximately 11%. Up to 25% of individuals initially seen with VTE have higher factor VIII levels than normal. Research has demonstrated that for each 10% increase in factor VIII levels, the risk of single and recurrent VTE increases by 10% and 24%, respectively. Elevated factor VIII levels have been shown to remain independent risk factors for VTE when controlling for inflammation, blood group antigens, and von Willebrand factor levels.

Hyperhomocysteinemia

Homocysteine is an intermediary amino acid formed by the conversion of methionine to cysteine. Hyperhomocysteinemia may result from either acquired or inherited traits. Homocysteine is metabolized by means of two pathways. The first involves cystathionine B-synthase (CBS) enzyme and requires vitamin B_6 as a cofactor. The second involves methionine synthase enzyme and requires both vitamin B_{12} and methyltetrahydrofolate reductase (MTHFR). Acquired forms of hyperhomocysteinemia may result from dietary deficiencies in vitamins B_{12}, B_6, or folate. Inherited forms may result from genetic defects in the CBS or MTHFR enzymes. Evidence suggests that hyperhomocysteinemia is a risk factor for VTE. In individuals with homocysteine levels greater than two standard deviations above normal, the odds ratio of VTE is two to three times greater than the control groups. Elevated homocysteine levels have also been associated with premature coronary artery disease and cerebrovascular disease, although debate regarding the strength of these associations continues. Screening for hyperhomocysteinemia is suggested in individuals with unexplained VTE. Sensitive laboratory assays are available for the quantification of total plasma homocysteine concentrations. If elevated plasma homocysteine levels are identified, additional laboratory evaluation may be warranted. Treatment varies with the underlying cause but typically involves supplementation with folate, vitamin B_{12}, and vitamin B_6.

Acquired Risk Factors

Acquired risk factors for VTE are far more prevalent than inherited thrombophilias. Box 61-1 lists common acquired VTE risk factors.

Surgery and Trauma. The risk of VTE among surgical patients can be stratified by patient age, type of surgery, and comorbid conditions. The incidence of VTE in surgical patients is highest in those aged 65 years or older. High-risk procedures include orthopedic surgery; neurosurgery; thoracic, abdominal, or pelvic surgery for malignancy; renal transplantation; and cardiovascular surgery. The risks from surgery may be less with neuraxial anesthesia than general anesthesia.

The association between trauma and VTE has long been recognized. As for surgical risks, the risk of VTE after trauma is related to predisposing host factors; the location, nature, and extent of injuries; and the use of prophylaxis. The risk of VTE in trauma patients is highest with advancing age. Injuries involving the lower extremities and/or pelvis confer the highest VTE risk. Other VTE risk factors associated with trauma include spinal cord injuries with paralysis, head injuries, vascular injuries, circulatory shock on admission, requirement for mechanical ventilation greater than 3 days, and the need for major surgical procedure.

Age. The incidence of VTE increases significantly with advancing age for both idiopathic and secondary VTE, suggesting that the associated risk may be due to the biology of aging and not simply an increased accumulation of VTE risk factors. In one study, the annual incidence rates for VTE increased from 17 per 100,000 persons per year for individuals age 40–49 years to 232 per 100,000 persons per year for individuals age 70–79 years.

Pregnancy. Pregnancy is associated with increased risk of VTE caused by the hypercoagulable state associated with pregnancy, as well as the increased resistance to venous return by

---

BOX 61-1 Acquired Risk Factors for Venous Thromboembolism

Age > 40 years
Smoking
Obesity (>120 kg)
Malignancy
  -Chemotherapy
Oral contraceptive use/hormone replacement therapy
Prolonged immobilization
  -Hospitalization
  -Long air travel
Surgery/Trauma
Acute inflammatory states
  -Acute infection
  -Inflammatory bowel disease
  -Connective tissue disease
Intravascular devices
  -Pacemaker or implantable cardiac defibrillator leads
  -Indwelling venous catheters
Pregnancy/Post-partum
Atherosclerotic cardiovascular disease
Congestive heart failure
Cerebrovascular accident
Previous venous thromboembolism
Varicose veins/venous stasis
Acquired hypercoaguability
  -Nephrotic syndrome
  -Lupus anticoagulant
  -Antiphospholipid antibody syndrome
  -Hyperhomocysteinemia
  -Heparin-induced thrombocytopenia

---

compression from the gravid uterus. Approximately 1 in 2000 women will have VTE develop during pregnancy. Age-adjusted estimates of the risk of VTE range from 5–50 times higher in pregnant versus nonpregnant women. The risk in the postpartum period is approximately fivefold higher than the risk during pregnancy. Prior superficial vein thrombosis is an independent risk factor for venous thrombosis during pregnancy and postpartum.

Hormone Replacement Therapy. Hormone therapy is associated with a twofold to fourfold increased risk of VTE. The risk of thrombosis increases within 4 months of the initiation of therapy and is unaffected by the duration of use. The VTE risk decreases to baseline levels within 3 months of discontinuation of hormone therapy. First- and third-generation oral contraceptives have a higher associated risk of VTE than second-generation agents. Therapy with selective estrogen receptor modulators, including tamoxifen and raloxifene, has been associated with increased rates of VTE.

Cancer. Malignancy accounts for approximately 20% of incident VTE in the community. Many primary malignancies are associated with VTE. Risk of VTE in cancer patients seems highest for those with pancreatic cancer, lymphoma, malignant brain tumors, hepatocellular carcinoma, leukemia, colorectal carcinoma, and other digestive cancers. Furthermore, the use of certain chemotherapy regimens, including thalidomide, tamoxifen, and L-asparaginase, is associated with higher VTE risks in cancer patients.

Obesity. Emerging evidence supports obesity as an independent risk factor for VTE. The relative risk of VTE in obese individuals is greater in women than men, with the greatest effect being noted younger than the age of 40 years. In addition to the independent risk of obesity and VTE, obesity is a common contributing factor for VTE in individuals undergoing long-duration air travel and in women concomitantly taking oral contraceptives or hormone replacement therapy.

Previous Venous Thromboembolism. Prior VTE is a major risk factor for recurrence. The magnitude of the risk depends on host factors. Individuals with reversible risk factors such as immobility or surgery have a lower rate of recurrence than those with nonmodifiable risk factors such as malignancy or inherited thrombophilia for example.

Heparin-Induced Thrombocytopenia. Heparin-induced thrombocytopenia (HIT) is a life-threatening disorder that follows exposure to unfractionated (UF) or (less commonly) low-molecular-weight heparin (LMWH). HIT classically presents with a low platelet count ($<150,000/mm^3$) or a relative decrease in platelet count by 50% from baseline typically within 5–10 days of the initiation of heparin or LMWH therapy. The incidence of HIT among patients treated with UF heparin is 10 times greater than those receiving LMWH. In patients with HIT, the thrombotic risk is more than 30 times the rate of the control population. The risk of thrombosis remains high for days to weeks after discontinuation of heparin, even after the platelet counts return to normal.

HIT is caused by antibodies against complexes of platelet factor 4 (PF4) and heparin. The heparin-PF4–antibody complex binds to the platelet surface, where it is recognized by circulating IgA, IgG, and IgM antibodies. Immunoglobulin recognition leads to further platelet activation and release of PF4, thus creating a positive feedback loop. The activated platelets aggregate, resulting in thrombocytopenia and thrombosis. Early-onset HIT, defined as onset within hours after initiation of heparin therapy, may be seen in approximately 30% of patients with persistent antibodies to the use of heparin therapy within the previous 3 months. Diagnosis of HIT is based on recognition of the clinical syndrome and specific serologic testing. Serologic assays can detect circulating IgG, IgA, and IgM heparin-dependent antibodies with high sensitivity (97%) but modest specificity (74–86%). Therefore, positive serologic assays must be confirmed by more specific tests, including serotonin release assays, heparin-induced platelet aggregation assays, or solid phase immunoassays.

The first intervention in a patient with suspected HIT is immediate cessation of all exposure to heparin, including heparin-bonded catheters and heparin flushes. LMWH should be avoided because it may cross-react with heparin-induced antibodies. In addition to heparin cessation, patients with suspected HIT should be started on alternative anticoagulation because of high risk of thrombosis. In patients with suspicion of HIT and/or need for alternative anticoagulation, direct thrombin inhibitors such as lepirudin or argatroban may be used. The duration of alternative anticoagulant therapy and the subsequent use of oral anticoagulants depends on whether the patient has had a thrombotic event or requires continued anticoagulation. For patients with HIT without evidence of thrombus, therapeutic doses of alternative anticoagulation should be continued until the platelet counts return to normal. Consideration should be given to continuing anticoagulation therapy with alternative anticoagulation or warfarin for 2–4 weeks after the diagnosis of HIT because of persistent high risks of thrombosis over this time. For a patient with HIT and thrombosis, therapeutic doses of alternative anticoagulation should be continued until the platelet count has normalized, then the patient should be transferred to warfarin therapy with at least a 5-day overlap until the international normalized ratio (INR) is therapeutic for at least 48 h. Skin necrosis and warfarin-induced venous gangrene of the limbs have been reported during shorter periods of overlap or shorter duration of therapeutic INR.

Pathogenesis

Between 60% and 90% of pulmonary emboli (PE) arise from the deep veins of the lower extremity and pelvis. Other sources of thrombi include the renal veins, upper extremities, or right side of the heart. Iliofemoral thrombi are the most clinically recognized sources of pulmonary emboli. Thrombi dislodge and embolize to the pulmonary arteries, where they cause hemodynamic abnormalities and impair gas exchange. The hemodynamic response to PE is determined by the embolic burden in association with the host's hemodynamic reserve and compensatory adaptive response. After traveling through the right heart, large thrombi may lodge and obstruct the main pulmonary arteries or travel distally within the pulmonary vascular tree leading to hemodynamic alterations. In addition to the physical obstruction to flow, acute PE triggers the release of vasoactive substances, resulting in further increase in pulmonary vascular resistance and right ventricular (RV) afterload. Because RV afterload increases, increased RV wall tension may lead to RV dilatation and hypokinesis with further RV dysfunction, tricuspid regurgitation, and RV failure. RV pressure overload can lead to flattening or bowing of the interventricular septum toward the left ventricle (LV) with resulting impairment of LV filling, systemic arterial hypotension, and cardiac arrest. Increased RV wall stress caused by RV pressure overload may also lead to right-sided stress-induced ischemia.

Impaired gas exchange may result from impaired ventilation-to-perfusion matching, increased alveolar dead space, and/or right-to-left shunting through a patent foramen ovale. Stimulation of pulmonary irritant receptors results in hyperventilation and contributes to the observed hypocapnia and respiratory alkalosis. The presence of hypercapnia in acute PE suggests a large amount of physiologic dead space and impaired minute ventilation that can result from massive PE.

CLINICAL FEATURES

The clinical consequences of pulmonary embolism range from incidental and clinically unimportant to circulatory collapse and sudden death. Equally challenging, the clinical signs and symptoms related to PE are diverse and nonspecific. Therefore, clinicians use a combination of history and examination findings in association with clinical prediction tools to determine appropriate diagnostic tests and the need for therapeutic interventions. The differential diagnosis of acute pulmonary embolism is listed in Table 61-2.

TABLE 61-2 Differential Diagnosis of Acute Pulmonary Embolism

Pneumonia or bronchitis	Rib fracture
Asthma or exacerbation of chronic obstructive lung disease	Pulmonary edema/ Congestive heart failure
Pleuritis	Thoracic malignancy
Pericarditis/Cardiac tamponade	Pulmonary hypertension
Pneumothorax	Myocardial infarction
Musculoskeletal pain	Aortic dissection
Costochondritis	Anxiety

TABLE 61-3 Frequency of Signs and Symptoms in Acute Pulmonary Embolism

Symptoms	Frequency (%)
Dyspnea	73
Pleuritic chest pain	66
Cough	37
Leg swelling	33
Hemoptysis	13
Wheezing	9
Chest pain	4
Signs	
Respiratory rate $\geq$20/min	70
Crackles	51
Heart rate $\geq$100/min	30
Third or fourth heart sound	26
Loud pulmonary component of second heart sound	23
Temperature $> 38.5°$ C	7
Pleural rub	3

(Data from Stein PD, Terrin ML, Hales CA, et al: Clinical, laboratory, roentgenographic, and electrocardiographic findings in patients with acute pulmonary embolism and no pre-existing cardiac or pulmonary disease. Chest 1991; 100:598–603.)

Medical History

Patients with PE often have one or more identifiable risk factors for the development of VTE at the time of clinical presentation (see previous discussion of "Risk Factors"). Details should be sought regarding the patient's personal and family history of prior VTE, coexisting medical conditions, functional status, travel history, and current medications. Major risk factors for VTE include surgery or trauma within the preceding 30 days, prolonged immobility, advanced age, malignancy, prior VTE, known thrombophilia, recent myocardial infarction or cerebrovascular accident, or indwelling venous catheter. Moderate risk factors include obesity, use of estrogen or hormone replacement therapy, or family history of VTE. Scoring systems, such as the Wells score and the Geneva Score have been devised to help assess a patient's probability of being diagnosed with a pulmonary embolism (see diagnosis of PE later in this chapter).

Symptoms and Signs

Acute pulmonary embolism may present with a wide spectrum of signs and symptoms. The most common symptom in angiographically confirmed acute pulmonary embolism is dyspnea (Table 61-3). Less frequently, patients with acute PE present with hemoptysis, wheezing, or chest pain. Frequent findings on physical examination include tachypnea (respiratory rate $\geq$ 20/min), tachycardia (heart rate $\geq$ 100/min), and crackles on lung auscultation (see Table 61-3). The presences of syncope, cyanosis, jugular venous distention, pulsatile liver, parasternal heave, accentuated pulmonic component of the second heart sound, right-sided third heart sound, and/or an audible systolic murmur at the left sternal border may reflect significant right ventricular dysfunction.

Laboratory Tests

Standard laboratory tests do not significantly contribute to the evaluation of patients with suspected pulmonary embolism. Routine laboratory findings such as increased erythrocyte sedimentation rate and/or leukocytosis are nonspecific. Common laboratory tests obtained as part of the evaluation of pulmonary embolism include arterial blood gas assessment, D-dimer, B-type natriuretic peptide (BNP), and troponin assays. Both troponin and BNP measurements have been suggested as prognostic indicators, differentiating between low risk and intermediate risk of PE-related complications, including hemodynamic collapse and death. Elevated levels of BNP and troponin have yet to become incorporated into formal PE guidelines for risk stratification and treatment, although this change is likely in

the future. Normal levels of BNP and troponin have high negative predictive values that identify patients at low risk of adverse outcome related to PE. Alternatively, in hemodynamically stable individuals with acute PE and elevated BNP and/or troponin levels, RV dysfunction is suggested and should be assessed by echocardiography. Because of their short half-lives and delay between the acute event and release of these markers into the circulation, if the duration of symptoms is less than 6 hours, a second laboratory measurement of both BNP and troponin is clinically warranted.

Arterial Blood Gas

Analysis of arterial blood gas tensions cannot accurately be used as a diagnostic tool to discriminate between individuals with and without PE. Typically, patients with acute PE are initially seen with hypocapnia and respiratory alkalosis. The partial pressure of oxygen (Po_2) may be increased, decreased, or normal in individuals with PE. The alveolar-arterial oxygen gradient (A-a gradient) is typically increased; however, this finding also lacks sufficient discriminatory characteristics to be used as a screening test. Thus, a normal Po_2 and A-a gradient do not obviate the need for further diagnostic investing in individuals with a clinical suspicion for disease.

D-Dimer

D-Dimer is a plasmin-derived fibrin degradation product most commonly measured by a quantitative enzyme-linked immunosorbent assay (ELISA). D-Dimer testing is characterized as highly sensitive with a high negative predictive value useful in the exclusion of VTE, particularly in the outpatient or emergency department setting. With most assays, a level >500 ng/mL is considered abnormal. Used in combination with a low clinical probability of disease, a negative D-dimer (value <500 ng/mL) has a 99% negative predictive value for pulmonary embolism. D-Dimer assays lack specificity (30–75%). Elevated D-dimer results are observed in individuals with inflammatory states, infection, acute coronary syndromes, malignancy, or recent surgery. Current evidence supports that a quantitative D-dimer level <500 ng/mL measured by ELISA can exclude the diagnosis of VTE in patient with low/intermediate pretest probability of disease. At present, D-dimer testing should not be used as the sole test to rule out VTE in individuals with high pretest probability for disease. Clinicians should note that D-dimer assays vary in their sensitivities and specificities. Thus, it is important to be aware of the assay used for appropriate interpretation of results.

B-Type Natriuretic Peptide

B-type natriuretic peptide (BNP) is a hormone released by ventricular myocardial cells in response to volume overload and wall stretch. Because of its lack of sensitivity and specificity, BNP is not a useful diagnostic test for PE. In the absence of RV dysfunction, BNP levels are typically normal in the setting of acute PE. However, increased levels of BNP seem to have prognostic significance in individuals with PE.

Elevated BNP levels (>90 pg/mL) obtained within 4 h of admission have a sensitivity of 85% and specificity of 75% for predicting PE-related clinical outcomes such as death, need for emergent thrombolysis, cardiopulmonary resuscitation, mechanical ventilation, vasopressor therapy, or emergency surgical embolectomy. Normal BNP values in the setting of acute PE have a 97–100% negative predictive value for in-hospital death.

Troponin

Cardiac troponins are sensitive and specific markers of myocardial cell damage. Troponin elevation in acute PE is presumed to be related to acute right heart strain with resulting myocyte ischemia and microinfarction. Troponin I and troponin T levels are elevated in 30–50% of individuals with large PE. However, these elevations are mild and short-lived compared with what is observed in acute coronary syndromes. Like BNP, troponin levels correlate with right heart dysfunction in acute PE. Normal troponin T values in the setting of acute PE have a 97–100% negative predictive value for in-hospital death.

Nonthrombotic Pulmonary Emboli

(Box 61-2)

Fat Embolism Syndrome

Fat embolism syndrome (FES) is a poorly understood complication of skeletal trauma. Although rare, FES most often

---

BOX 61-2 Causes of Nonthrombotic Pulmonary Emboli

Fat Embolism
Amniotic fluid embolism
Air Embolism
- Venous
- Arterial
Tumor embolism
Septic pulmonary embolism

---

occurs after fractures of long bones or other conditions resulting in bone marrow disruption. FES is characterized by the appearance of free fat and fatty acids in the blood, lungs, brain, kidneys, and other organs. The classic triad of respiratory insufficiency, neurologic abnormalities, and petechial rash occurs in 0.5–2.0% of solitary long bone fractures. The incidence increases to 5–10% in multiple fractures with pelvic involvement. FES is a clinical diagnosis that typically manifests within 12–72 h of initial injury. Respiratory impairment leads to hypoxemia in up to 30% of patients and, on occasion, respiratory failure and the need for mechanical ventilation. The chest radiograph often shows diffuse infiltrates but can appear normal. Cerebral symptoms may occur in 60% of patients and tend to follow the pulmonary symptoms. Neurologic findings may range from restlessness, confusion, and altered sensorium to focal deficits, seizures, and coma. The characteristic petechial rash is observed in 50% of patients and is usually found on the neck, axilla, trunk, or conjunctiva. The rash is often the last of the triad to develop and resolves within a range of hours to days. Treatment of FES includes aggressive supportive care and early ventilatory support. Steroids have been demonstrated to be efficacious as a prophylaxis for FES, although experience with steroids as a treatment remains anecdotal.

Air Embolism

Air embolism is a consequence of air entering the vascular system, resulting in mechanical obstruction, end-organ ischemia, and/or hemodynamic compromise. Air can enter the venous system when two simultaneous conditions coexist. First, there is a direct communication between the source of air and the venous system. Second, a pressure gradient favoring the passage of air into the venous system is present. Under high pressure, gas may be forced into the venous system such as with laparoscopic procedures, pressurized infusion sets, or mechanical ventilation. Conversely, generating high negative intrathoracic pressures (as in hyperventilation, exacerbation of underlying lung disease, hypovolemia, or upright positioning) may predispose patients to venous air embolism (VAE) by increasing the pressure gradient between the atmosphere and the thorax. Most VAE occurs in relation to central venous catheters (0–2% incidence). Mortality for VAE associated with central venous catheters has been reported to be as high as 32%. In humans, the lethal volume of air is estimated to be 300–500 mL. With a pressure gradient of only 5 cm water (as with normal tidal breathing), air can pass through a 14-g catheter at a rate of 100 mL/sec. The clinical symptoms of VAE are nonspecific. Care providers must maintain a high index of suspicion to consider this diagnosis in patients who have sudden cardiopulmonary and/or neurologic decompensation develop in the appropriate clinical setting. Patients may experience a gasping reflex, light-headedness, dizziness, chest pain, or sudden-onset dyspnea. If venous gas reaches the arterial circulation, evidence of myocardial or central nervous system injury may occur. Physical examination may reveal tachycardia, tachypnea, and elevated jugular venous pressure. A mill-wheel murmur produced by movement of air bubbles in the right ventricle is considered the only specific sign, but it is a rare, transient, and late finding. Wheezing or rales may occur secondary to induced bronchospasm. Transthoracic or transesophageal echocardiography is the most sensitive method for detection of venous air and may show evidence of both acute RV dilatation and pulmonary hypertension.

Indwelling pulmonary arterial (PA) catheters will show an acute increase in PA pressure. Although this finding has a sensitivity of only 45%, the presence of a PA catheter at the time of VAE can result in early therapeutic intervention. If VAE is suspected, the patient should be placed left side down in Trendelenburg position, allowing air to migrate toward the right apex of the heart, thus diminishing pulmonary outflow obstruction. Manual removal of air from an indwelling central line or pulmonary artery catheter may be attempted and is most effective at or above the right atrial junction, not in the RV or pulmonary artery outflow tract. Closed-chest cardiac massage improves survival to the same extent as does proper positioning, presumably by mechanically forcing air out of the right ventricle and pulmonary outflow tract. Patients should be administered 100% Fio_2 to increase the rate of bubble absorption. For patients with persistent cardiopulmonary or cerebrovascular deficits despite these modalities, hyperbaric oxygen therapy should be initiated.

Amniotic Fluid Embolism Syndrome

Amniotic fluid embolism syndrome (AFES) is a rare complication of pregnancy with variable manifestations and high morbidity and mortality. The reported incidence of this catastrophic syndrome ranges from 1 in 8000 to 1 in 80,000 pregnancies. Amniotic fluid is a complex mixture of both maternal and fetal components, including particulate matter such as fetal squamous cells, lanugo hairs, and variably meconium. Amniotic fluid is postulated to enter the maternal circulation through endocervical veins, through the site of placental insertion, or through uterine trauma. Once in the circulation, amniotic fluid triggers an immunologically mediated systemic inflammatory response leading to cardiovascular compromise, respiratory failure, coagulopathy, and disseminated intravascular coagulation. AFES occurs during labor but before delivery in 70% of cases, after vaginal delivery in 11%, and during cesarean section in 19%. In the patients who had AFES develop after delivery, 69% occurred within the first 5 min postpartum. AFES has also been reported to occur as early as the second trimester and as late as 36 h postpartum. AFES may occur during therapeutic abortion, abdominal trauma, amniocentesis, and labor and delivery. Factors historically associated with increased risk for AFES include advanced maternal age, multiparity, large fetal size, premature placental separation, fetal death, fetal male sex, meconium staining, and a history of allergy or atopy in the mother. The clinical presentation of AFES is often dramatic, with sudden onset respiratory distress, cyanosis, convulsions, and cardiovascular collapse classically occurring during labor and delivery. Patients may rapidly progress to asystole or pulseless electrical activity. Patients who survive the initial event later go on to have a major coagulopathy develop in 40% of cases.

The diagnosis of AFES is clinical. Early aggressive support is imperative, because most maternal deaths occur within 1 h of symptom onset. AFES is a life-threatening condition that requires prompt resuscitation, including airway and hemodynamic support in an intensive care setting. Maternal mortality for AFES ranges from 30% to 90%. The fetal survival is 40% when the fetus is *in utero* at the time of AFES onset. Furthermore, AFES is associated with significant morbidity with neurologically intact survival by some reports to be observed in only 15% of maternal survivors.

Tumor Embolism

Pulmonary tumor embolism occurs when solid tumors seed the systemic circulation with individual cells, clusters of cells, or large tumor fragments. Emboli travel to the pulmonary vasculature, causing microvasculature obstruction. Furthermore, tumor emboli may activate the coagulation system, resulting in concomitant thrombotic obstruction. The pathologic spectrum of tumor embolism varies from large tumor masses that may mimic pulmonary embolism to the more common microvessel embolism in small arterioles and capillaries that cause a subacute clinical syndrome. The incidence of tumor embolism is estimated by autopsy series to be 3–26% of patients with solid tumors. Tumor embolism seems to be more common in patients with mucin-producing adenocarcinomas such as breast, gastric, and lung carcinoma; however, this observation may be explained by the higher prevalence of these tumors within the population.

DIAGNOSIS

The diagnosis of pulmonary embolic disease can present a significant challenge. Typical presenting clinical signs of dyspnea and chest pain are nonspecific and can be confused as manfestations of other serious diseases states such as acute myocardial infarction or pneumonia. Many patients with thromboembolic disease present with atypical symptoms, and the diagnosis of PE becomes even more difficult when patients harbor diseases such as congestive heart failure (CHF) or chronic obstructive pulmonary disease (COPD) that could otherwise explain their presenting complaints. Because of the high prevalence of venous thromboembolism and the potential serious consequences of misdiagnosis, it is essential to maintain a high clinical suspicion for the possibility of PE.

Clinical Assessment

Typical clinical features of PE have been discussed earlier in this chapter. It is important to stress that clinical judgment is an essential initial step in the evaluation of thromboembolic disease and figures prominently in diagnostic algorithms. The importance of a clinician's assessment of the probability of PE was initially highlighted in the 1990 landmark PIOPED (Prospective Investigation of Pulmonary Embolism Diagnosis) study. Physicians in this study were asked to record their clinical impression (high, intermediate, or low probability) as to the likelihood of PE in patients they were treating before learning the results of the radiographic study (ventilation/perfusion [V/Q] scan or pulmonary arteriogram). The clinical impression was based on an agreed-on set of information but without standardized diagnostic algorithms. One very important finding of the PIOPED study was that diagnosis or exclusion of PE was only possible when there were clear and concordant clinical and radiographic findings. If the clinical impression did not match the findings on imaging (V/Q scan in this study), pulmonary thromboembolic disease could not be ruled in or out by that imaging study, and further investigation was necessary. Since the publication of PIOPED, there have been numerous attempts to standardize the definition of "clinical impression." This has resulted in a variety of scoring systems, assigning points to historical, physical, and laboratory features of an individual patient. Patients receive scores on the basis of inherent risk factors and presenting signs that are then used to predict likelihood of disease. Currently, the two most commonly used scoring systems are the *Wells Criteria* and the *Geneva Score* (Table 61-4). These two scoring systems and subsequent modifications have been validated in a number of studies. By themselves, scoring systems lack adequate sensitivity or specificity to diagnose or exclude disease. Their true usefulness comes in conjunction with other laboratory or imaging studies allowing the assessment of disease risk.

ECG and Chest X-Ray

Electrocardiograms and chest radiographs are frequently used in the evaluation of patients initially seen with dyspnea or chest pain. Although these studies are neither adequately sensitive nor specific to diagnose or exclude PE, they can suggest the diagnosis. ECG findings such as T-wave inversions in the anterior leads, in particular V1–V4, are typical of RV strain and should raise suspicion for pulmonary thromboembolic disease (Figure 61-1). Other typical ECG changes include a deep s-wave in lead I, a q-wave in lead III, and t-wave inversions in lead III. Rhythm and conduction abnormalities such as new onset of atrial fibrillation or right bundle branch block are occasionally noted in association with acute PE.

In the evaluation for PE, chest X-rays predominately serve to exclude other potential explanations for a patient's symptoms (i.e., a lobar infiltrate consistent with pneumonia). Occasionally, the chest X-ray will demonstrate changes suggestive of PE such as focal oligemia (Westermark's sign), a peripheral wedge-shaped density that indicates infarct (Hampton's hump) (Figure 61-2), or an enlarged right descending pulmonary artery (Palla's sign).

D-Dimer

Measurement of plasma D-dimer levels in peripheral blood has become an important screening tool to help exclude the presence of venous thromboembolism. Plasma D-dimer is a degradation product of cross-linked fibrin. After a thrombotic event, endogenous fibrinolysis results in clot dissolution and a measurable increase in plasma D-dimer levels. However, an elevated D-dimer is not specific for the presence of VTE. Numerous other conditions (e.g., trauma, inflammation, surgery) can raise plasma D-dimer levels; therefore, an abnormal laboratory result has a low positive predictive value for VTE. Laboratory tests to measure D-dimer levels in peripheral blood have been available since the mid 1980s, but their acceptance as an early screening tool in the evaluation of VTE is relatively recent. Contributing to the initial confusion regarding the usefulness of D-dimer in the assessment of VTE was the presence of significant variability between the various D-dimer assays (ELISA, quantitative latex agglutination, semiquantitative agglutination latex, and whole blood agglutination assays) in their sensitivities and specificities. ELISA assays have the highest sensitivities and, therefore, are superior in their ability to exclude the diagnosis of VTE. Numerous studies have validated the usefulness of D-dimer in the evaluation of VTE.

TABLE 61-4 Wells and Geneva Scoring Systems Used in Risk Assessment for the Diagnosis of PE*

Wells Score	Points	Geneva Score	Points
Previous VTE	1.5	Previous VTE	2
Heart Rate>100 bpm	1.5	Heart rate > 100 bpm	1
Recent surgery or immobilization	1.5	Recent surgery	3
Clinical signs of DVT	3	Age (years) 60–79 / ≥ 80	1 / 2
Alternative diagnosis less likely	3	PaCO₂ < 36 mmHg (4.8 kPa) / 36–38.9 (4.8–5.19)	2 / 1
Hemoptysis	1	PaO₂ < 48.7 mmHg (6.5 kPa) 48.7–59.9 (6.6–7.99) 60–71.2 (8–9.49) 71.3–82.4 (9.5–10.99)	
Cancer	1	Atelectasis / Elevated hemidiaphragm	1 / 1
Clinical Probability		**Clinical Probability**	
Low	0–1	Low	0–4
Intermediate	2–6	Intermediate	5–8
High	>6	High	≥9

*Both scoring systems divide patients into low, intermediate and high clinical probability for the diagnosis of PE. For the Wells score: total points of < 2 indicates a low clinical probability for PE, a score of 2–5 is intermediate, and a score of > 6 is high probability of PE. For the Geneva score: total score of < 4 indicates low probability for PE, 4–10 points indicates intermediate probability, and ≥ 11 points indicates high probability for PE. These scoring systems and their variations have been validated in prospective cohorts of patients. In aggregate, a low clinical probability score indicates a subgroup with a 10% prevalence of PE. Intermediate clinical probability indicates prevalence of approximately 30% and high clinical probability indicates > 70% prevalence of PE approximately.

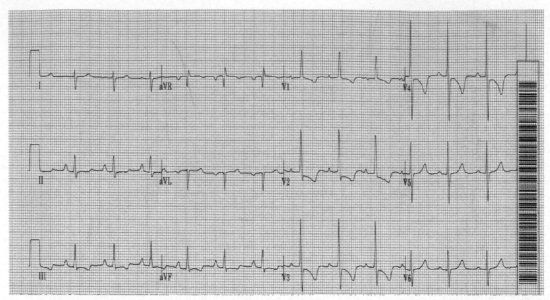

FIGURE 61-1 ECG in a patient with RV strain secondary to thromboembolic disease. Note the right axis deviation, deep S wave in lead I, inverted T wave in lead III, and RV strain pattern in V1–V4. This patient was diagnosed with chronic thromboembolic pulmonary hypertension secondary to multiple PEs.

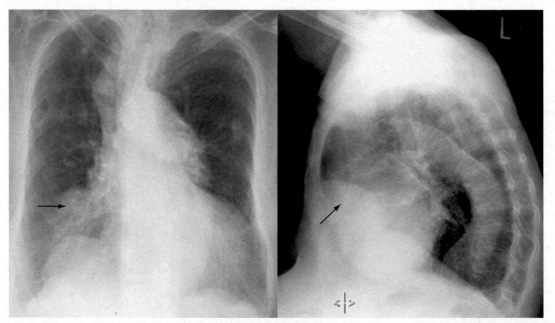

FIGURE 61-2 Chest X-ray example of a wedge-shaped pulmonary infarct (Hampton's hump) secondary to a pulmonary embolism. The infarct is located in the anterior segment of the right middle lobe (*arrows*).

A D-dimer ELISA of less than 500 ng/mL is strong evidence against pulmonary embolism in patients with a low or intermediate clinical probability score. The Christopher study investigators demonstrated that the incidence of pulmonary embolism was only 0.5% at 3 months in patients with a low probability clinical score (by use of a modified version of the Wells criteria) and a D-dimer plasma level of 500 ng/mL or less. Other VTE outcome studies have demonstrated similar results, showing the D-dimer assay to have a sensitivity of between 92% and 99% for the diagnosis of VTE. However,

as previously discussed, the specificity for this study has been reported to be as low as 25%.

Venous Compression Ultrasonography

Ultrasound of the deep venous system searching for thrombosis is frequently used to assist with the diagnosis of pulmonary embolism. This approach is pragmatic since the treatment for both DVT and PE is similar, and the first disease process begets the second. Ultrasound is frequently used when the initial tests for pulmonary embolism are nondiagnostic.

A positive test result confirms the need for anticoagulation and obviates the need for further diagnostic studies. A negative result, however, is more difficult to interpret and requires consideration of certain caveats when considering a treatment plan. In the presence of acute pulmonary embolism, DVT is detectable by compression ultrasound in only approximately 50% of cases (50% sensitivity). In patients with nondiagnostic chest imaging studies, compression ultrasound of the proximal vein detects DVT in approximately 5% of cases. Normal bilateral proximal venous ultrasounds, therefore, do not rule out PE in patients with nondiagnostic lung scans. However, they do imply a reduced probability of this event (negative likelihood ratio of approximately 0.7). Negative ultrasound studies, therefore, imply a lower short-term risk of thromboembolic disease developing or having a fatal thromboembolism if anticoagulant therapy is withheld. Some studies have recommended a follow-up serial ultrasound when anticoagulation therapy is withheld on the basis of an initial negative ultrasound. These studies, examining a variety of time frames (2 days to 2 weeks) have reported that approximately 2% of patients with an initially negative venous ultrasound will be diagnosed with a DVT by serial testing. If the ultrasound remains negative during serial examinations, there is a low risk of subsequent symptomatic venous thromboembolism, which is similar to the risk observed after a normal pulmonary angiogram (1% incidence at 6 months).

Contrast Venography

Venography was for many years the only reliable technique to confirm or exclude the possibility of a DVT. More recently, compression ultrasonography has all but replaced this more invasive approach of venography for assessment of deep venous thrombosis. Still, venography remains the "gold standard" for diagnosis of DVT with a reported sensitivity ranging from 70–100% and specificity of 60–88%. Some diagnostic algorithms advocate contrast venography in patients with a negative compression ultrasound who have a high pretest clinical probability of DVT. Another, more commonly used approach in this patient population, however, is serial ultrasonography (see earlier). Potential complications of contrast venography include nephrotoxicity (secondary to contrast dye), bleeding complications from the venous puncture, and postprocedure phlebitis.

Ventilation/Perfusion Lung Scan

For many years, the V/Q lung scan was considered the imaging study of choice to evaluate for PE (Figure 61-3). Recently, CT

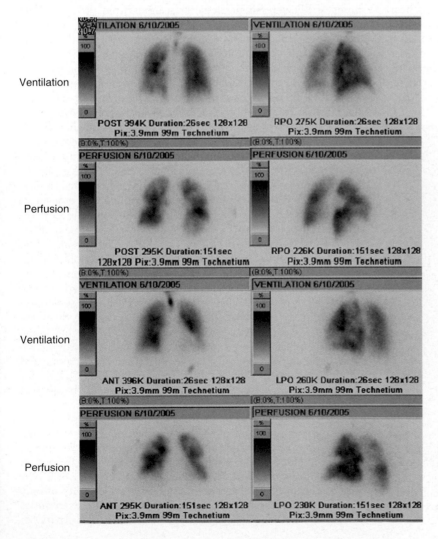

FIGURE 61-3 Ventilation/perfusion (V/Q) lung scan. Ventilation images are above their respective perfusion images. There is significant heterogeneity between the ventilation and perfusion images with multiple unmatched defects in the perfusion images consistent with thromboembolic disease.

angiography has begun to supplant the V/Q scan in many scenarios. However, the V/Q scan maintains an important place in the evaluation of patients for thromboembolic disease. As mentioned previously, the PIOPED study associated the clinical probability of a PE (high, intermediate, or low probability as assessed by history and clinical findings) with the interpretation of the V/Q scan (high, intermediate, or low probability or normal perfusion). When there is concordance of the clinical assessment and the interpretation of the V/Q scan in the high or low probability range, PE can be diagnosed or excluded with reasonable certainty. When the clinical assessment and the interpretation of the V/Q scan are discordant (i.e., high clinical probability but low probability V/Q scan or vice versa), the possibility of PE cannot be adequately assessed, and other studies are required. A normal V/Q scan essentially excludes the diagnosis of PE.

Echocardiogram

Transthoracic and transesophageal echocardiography have limited use in the diagnosis of pulmonary embolism. The sensitivity and specificity of these tests are inadequate for diagnosis, because the offending emboli are rarely proximal enough to be visualized. Echocardiography can assist in acute care management decisions for those patients too unstable to be moved from a critical care setting for more definitive imaging. Although it is rare to visualize a thrombus within the pulmonary arteries by echocardiogram, changes in RV size and function and increases in tricuspid regurgitation imply acute right heart strain. In the appropriate clinical scenario, these changes in the RV can suggest the diagnosis of acute pulmonary embolism (Figure 61-4).

Perhaps a more important use of echocardiography in the evaluation of patients with pulmonary embolism is that of risk stratification. Multiple studies have demonstrated that patients who develop RV dysfunction associated with an acute PE have increased mortality compared with those with preserved RV function. This observation is not surprising, because worsening RV function relates directly to the degree the pulmonary vascular bed is affected by the thrombus and, therefore, the size of the embolic event. Some investigators have suggested that more aggressive therapy, such as thrombolysis, is indicated in patients with RV dysfunction. This will be discussed further in the section on treatment of pulmonary embolism.

CT Angiogram

CT pulmonary angiogram (CTPA) has become a favored study for the evaluation of pulmonary embolism over the past decade (Figure 61-5, B). CTPA provides a number of potential advantages over other imaging modalities in the diagnosis of PE, including: (1) direct visualization of the embolus, (2) the ability to assess for other potential etiologies of the patient's complaints such as pneumonia, and (3) imaging algorithms that scan through the pelvis and lower extremities, as well as the chest, allow the simultaneous evaluation for PE and DVT. The ability to evaluate for other thoracic disease is of no small consequence, because studies have shown that up to two thirds of patients initially suspected to have PE eventually receive another diagnosis. Many of these diagnoses (i.e., pneumonia, thoracic aorta dissection, pneumothorax) can be visualized on CT scan. The interobserver agreement for CT is better than that for V/Q scan. The initial hardware used for assessment of PE were single detector scanners that provided high specificity for the diagnosis of PE (>90%). However, their sensitivity was unacceptable (approximately 72%) for the exclusion of this potentially life-threatening diagnosis. More recently, multidetector (4-, 8-, and 16-slice) scanners have been studied in the evaluation of PE, and even later generation (32-, 40-, and 64-slice) scanners are now being used. The very high spatial resolution of these studies allows rapid evaluation of pulmonary vessels down to the sixth order branches during a single breath hold and, therefore, increases the detection rate of segmental and subsegmental PEs. The sensitivity of the newer generation hardware and imaging algorithms is significantly improved compared with the earlier generation scanner, and a number of outcome studies have implied that a negative multidetector CTPA study in patients with low or intermediate clinical probability for VTE is adequate for the exclusion of PE (sensitivity and specificity of >90%). The recently published prospective investigation of pulmonary embolism diagnosis-II (PIOPED-II) has raised some questions regarding the positive and negative predictive power of these studies. The investigators of PIOPED-II sought to establish the sensitivity and specificity of multidetector CT scanners in the diagnosis of PE in the same fashion as the original PIOPED had done for V/Q scans. They undertook a multicenter, prospective study assessing the accuracy of multidetector CTPA alone and combined it with venous phase imaging (CTPA-CTPV) for the diagnosis of acute PE. However, in contrast to the original PIOPED study that used pulmonary angiography as the reference test to which V/Q was compared, PIOPED II used a composite reference test for VTE that was based on the V/Q lung scan, venous compression ultrasound of the lower extremities, and digital subtraction pulmonary angiography (performed in only a minority of cases). They reported the specificity of CTPA for the diagnosis of PE to be 96% but with a sensitivity of only 83%. Venous scanning of the pelvis and lower extremities improved the sensitivity of the study. The sensitivity of

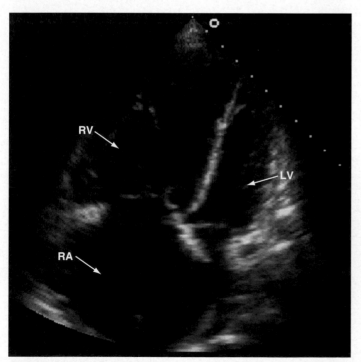

FIGURE 61-4 Echocardiogram of a patient with markedly dilated right ventricle (RV) and right atrium (RA) secondary to pulmonary thromboembolic disease. The interventricular septum is bowing into and compressing the left ventricle (LV).

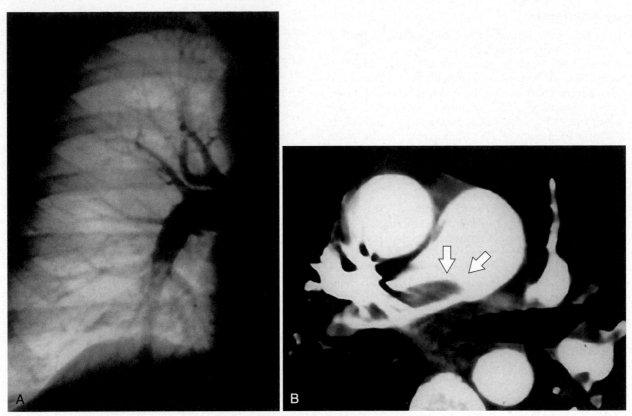

FIGURE 61-5 Pulmonary imaging for embolism. **A,** Pulmonary angiogram showing a filling defect in the right lower lobe pulmonary artery. **B,** A spiral computed tomography angiogram in another patient showing multiple filling defects (*arrows*).

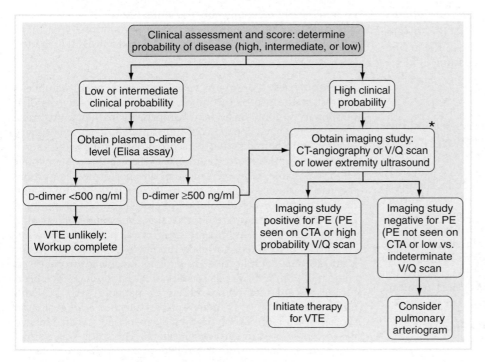

FIGURE 61-6 Diagnostic algorithm for evaluation of pulmonary embolism. *CTA CTV is becoming the initial imaging study of choice. US and V/Q scan can be used in patients in whom CTA is contraindicated (i.e., renal insufficiency) or when additional studies are needed to assist with the diagnosis.

CTPA-CTPV for the diagnosis of PE was 90% with a specificity of 95%. PIOPED-II also attempted to associate clinical probability with imaging studies to assess positive and negative predictive values. The results were reminiscent of the original PIOPED study in that positive predictive value of the CT studies was 96% with a concordantly high or low clinical probability, 92% with an intermediate clinical probability, and nondiagnostic with a discordant clinical probability. CTPA now plays the predominant role in most published diagnostic algorithms for the evaluation of PE (Figure 61-6).

Pulmonary Arteriogram

Pulmonary angiography remains the "gold standard" for the diagnosis of pulmonary embolism (see Figure 61-5, *A*). Because of its invasive nature, it is also associated with the most inherent risk. Arrhythmias, hypotension, bleeding, and nephrotoxicity from contrast dye are potential complications. The mortality associated with pulmonary angiography has been estimated at 0.5% with major nonfatal adverse events occurring with a frequency of 1%. Angiography is also more expensive than the noninvasive means of evaluating for PE and not always immediately available. As other imaging modalities, such as CT angiogram, have gained popularity in the assessment of PE, angiography has become less used. Approximately 1% of patients with a normal pulmonary angiogram will be diagnosed with a VTE at 6 months, implying the angiography was falsely negative. Although large, segmental embolic events are easily appreciated, there can be significant interobserver variability when evaluating smaller subsegmental emboli. Still, pulmonary angiography remains an important tool in the diagnosis of PE when other studies are nondiagnostic and is frequently held out as the "gold standard" against which other tests are measured.

Magnetic Resonance Imaging (MRI)

Magnetic resonance imaging (MRI) and magnetic resonance angiography (MRA) are beginning to be considered as a tool for the diagnosis of pulmonary embolism. Early results from PE studies that used MRI/MRA imaging were poor because of respiratory motion artifact and poor contrast between flowing blood and embolus. However, the development of faster hardware combined with dynamic gadolinium enhancement now permits high-resolution angiography during a single breath hold. More recent studies have reported sensitivities ranging from 75% to 100% with specificities of 70–90%. MRI/MRA has not yet gained an accepted place in the diagnosis of PE but rather remains an area of investigation.

TREATMENT

The basic approach to treatment of pulmonary embolism has not changed appreciably over the past half century. However, there have been refinements in recommendations regarding duration of therapy. Also there have been some recent additions of medications available for anticoagulation. The possibility of adding mechanical barriers to prevent further embolization to the pulmonary vasculature is now also readily available. Thrombolytics present the opportunity to rapidly dissolve the offending thrombus but with a higher incidence of bleeding complications. The discussion regarding treatment of PE can be divided into two distinct entities: (1) treatment of the acute PE, and (2) secondary prophylaxis against recurrent VTE.

Treatment of Acute Pulmonary Embolism

Anticoagulation

Heparin and Vitamin K Antagonists. The goal of the initial treatment of pulmonary embolism is to obtain adequate, rapid anticoagulation while minimizing bleeding complications. There is consensus that the initial treatment of acute nonmassive pulmonary embolism should include heparin for a period of 5 days overlapping with the initiation of a vitamin K antagonist (VKA). The VKA should be started on the first day of treatment of the PE if possible, but recommendations for 5 days of heparin therapy remain even if the desired level of VKA anticoagulation is achieved earlier. This recommendation stems from studies of patients with DVT demonstrating a higher incidence of recurrence if heparin therapy was truncated. The goal of therapy for UF heparin is an activated partial thromboplastin time (aPTT) between 1.5 and 2.0× control. An important development in the use of UF-heparin in the treatment of VTE was the implementation of weight-based dosing to rapidly obtain appropriate levels of anticoagulation. This recommendation stemmed from the frequent observation of recurrent thromboembolism in subtherapeutic heparin dosing. For many years, UF heparin was the treatment of choice for initial therapy of VTE. However, more recently, LMWH has begun to replace UF-heparin as first-line therapy. LMWH has better bioavailability and a longer half-life (t½) than UF-heparin. These features permit once- or twice-daily subcutaneous dosing without the need for coagulation monitoring in appropriate clinical populations (i.e., normal renal function). The ability to obtain a predictable and reliable level of anticoagulation through a subcutaneous route then allows for the possibility of outpatient therapy, significantly decreasing health care costs and increasing patient satisfaction. LMWH was first used in the treatment of DVT. In addition, the use of LMWH for at-home therapy of DVT was quickly shown to be both safe and effective. Its use has more recently been studied as the initial treatment of acute submassive PE, where it was also found to be efficacious and safe. These trials showed no difference in morbidity or mortality in patients treated with LMWH versus those treated with UF-heparin. A small number of patients in these studies were treated at home or were allowed to go home early receiving subcutaneous LMWH. There was no difference in outcome in the at-home population. Treatment with LMWH is less commonly associated with HIT than is UF-heparin.

Thrombolytics. For many years there has been significant interest in the use of thrombolytic agents to rapidly dissolve pulmonary emboli in hopes of improving patient outcomes. These agents have been successfully applied in acute coronary syndromes to help dissolve intracoronary thrombus and, therefore, their application to pulmonary vascular thrombus would seem reasonable. However, most studies performed examining the use of these agents in the treatment of acute PE, while demonstrating earlier dissolution of clot, improved physiologic parameters, and improvement in the appearance of imaging studies did not demonstrate improved patient mortality. As would be expected, however, there was an increase in significant bleeding complications in patients receiving thrombolysis compared with anticoagulation alone. Attention has since been turned toward identifying subsets of patients with PE who might benefit from this therapy. Jerjes-Sanchez *et al* evaluated the efficacy of thrombolytic therapy in patients with massive PE who presented in cardiogenic shock. The study was a small prospective, randomized controlled trial, enrolling a total of only eight patients before it was terminated early (a total of 40 patients had been planned for enrollment). The four patients enrolled who received thrombolytics (streptokinase in this study) followed by heparin survived, and at 2 years of follow-up demonstrated no evidence of pulmonary hypertension. The four who received heparin alone died within 1–3 h of arrival in the emergency department. It is highly unlikely this study will be repeated, and there is essentially uniform agreement that patients who have cardiogenic shock develop related to PE should receive thrombolytics unless there are major contraindications. A more controversial use of these medications is in patients with PE without hemodynamic compromise but with RV dysfunction. A number of studies have demonstrated that patients with RV dysfunction associated with PE have a significantly increased mortality. It would, therefore, seem reasonable to treat this group of patients more aggressively. Two large studies have suggested a potential benefit of thrombolytics in patients with PE and RV dysfunction or pulmonary hypertension, although both of these studies have received criticism regarding their design. The first study, Management Strategies and Prognosis of Pulmonary Embolism (MAPPET), demonstrated a survival benefit in patients with RV dysfunction who received heparin and thrombolytics (alteplase, streptokinase, or urokinase were the medications used) compared with heparin alone. The 30-day mortality for those who received thrombolysis was 4.7% versus 11.1% for those receiving heparin alone. In addition, recurrent PE was significantly less frequent in those receiving thrombolytic therapy (7.7% versus 18.7%). However, this study was not randomized, and further inspection of the results reveals that the patients who received heparin alone were significantly older than those who received thrombolysis. This is relevant in that older age is a recognized risk factor for mortality in PE. The patients who received thrombolytics plus heparin also had less underlying cardiac and pulmonary disease than those receiving heparin alone, which also may have influenced the mortality outcomes. The second study demonstrating an improvement in outcome for patients receiving thrombolytics was the Management Strategies and Prognosis of Pulmonary Embolism-3 (MAPPET-3). This was a randomized prospective study examining the use of medical thrombolysis in PE associated with RV dysfunction. The primary endpoint of this study was a combined endpoint of survival and escalation of therapy. A significant benefit in terms of this combined primary endpoint was met in patients who received thrombolytics (alteplase) and heparin versus those who received heparin alone. However, close review of this study demonstrates no survival benefit between the two groups. Rather, the difference in the primary endpoint between groups was due to a difference in escalation of therapy, and in most patients this escalation of therapy related to later thrombolysis for PE. A number of experts have cited this article as evidence of benefit of thrombolytics in patients with PE and RV dysfunction, although others are more skeptical of its use in this patient population.

Prophylaxis Against Recurrent Venous Thromboembolism (Secondary Prevention)

There is clear evidence that "early" discontinuation of anticoagulation after an acute VTE results in a substantially increased risk of symptomatic extension of the thrombus, embolization, or recurrence of clot. The difficulty, however, is defining "early." Most studies examining optimal duration of anticoagulation have found that the longer an individual receives anticoagulation after a DVT or PE, the less likely they are to have a repeat VTE. Furthermore, when anticoagulation is discontinued, the risk of VTE increases substantially and is significantly above the risk of individuals without a history of VTE.

TABLE 61-5 Recommendations for Duration of Anticoagulation in Patients Diagnosed with VTE

Indication for Anticoagulation	Duration of Therapy
1st VTE with reversible or transient risk factor	Minimum of 3 months
1st episode of idiopathic VTE	Minimum of 6–12 months, consider indefinite period
VTE associated with malignancy	LMWH for the first 3–6 months then indefinite or until the malignancy resolves
1st episode of VTE associated with hypercoaguable state	12 months, suggest indefinite
Two or more documented episodes of VTE	Indefinite

This elevation in risk is reflected in the clinical scoring systems (Wells score, Geneva Score) discussed earlier in the chapter. However, chronic anticoagulation presents its own inherent risks, cost, and requirements for lifestyle modification. The challenge then becomes balancing the inherent risk of anticoagulation with the individual patients risk of recurrent disease. The American College of Chest Physicians (ACCP) has published consensus statement recommendations regarding the duration of chronic anticoagulation to prevent recurrent VTE by considering patient risk factors and presentation (Table 61-5). These recommendations by necessity are directed at broad categories of patients. Clinicians, therefore, must consider their individual patients risk of anticoagulation when applying these standards.

Novel Anticoagulants

The traditional anticoagulants used in the treatment of VTE, warfarin and UF heparin, have been used successfully for many years. However, both medications suffer from two important limitations: (1) variable dose responses among individuals, and (2) narrow therapeutic windows of adequate anticoagulation without excessive risk of bleeding. These liabilities require close laboratory monitoring of patients receiving these medications. Another limitation of UF-heparin is its reduced ability to inactivate thrombin bound to fibrin and factor Xa bound to activated platelets. These limitations have prompted the development of new anticoagulant medications, including LMWH, factor Xa inhibitors, and direct thrombin inhibitors.

The successful application of LMWH in the treatment of PE has been discussed earlier in this chapter. Its superior bioavailability, predictable anticoagulant effect, and subcutaneous delivery route makes LMWH an attractive alternative compared with UF-heparin in the therapy of VTE. The direct thrombin inhibitors include hirudin, argatroban, and bivalirudin. These medications block the action of thrombin. Their potential advantage over heparin includes their ability to inactivate clot-bound thrombin and their resistance to circulating inhibitors released by activated platelets including PF4 and heparinase. Importantly, these agents do not cause heparin-induced thrombocytopenia (HIT) and are, in fact, approved for the treatment of this condition. Factor Xa inhibitors act by catalyzing factor Xa inhibition by antithrombin. These agents block thrombin generation, as opposed to thrombin inhibitors that block the activity of thrombin.

Factor Xa inhibitors such as fondaparinux have a relatively long half-life (17 h) and can be administered once daily subcutaneously. Fondaparinux has been studied in the treatment of PE and was found to be as efficacious as UF-heparin. It also does not induce HIT and is being evaluated for the treatment of this condition. Another factor Xa inhibitor, idraparinux is also being evaluated in the treatment of VTE. This agent has an even longer half-life (80 h) than fondaparinux and, therefore, could be administered on a weekly basis. Both fondaparinux and idraparinux are cleared by the kidney and, therefore, must be used with caution in patients with renal insufficiency. Neither agent has a specific antidote, which is a significant drawback in situations where there is bleeding or a need for urgent surgery. Recombinant factor VIIa has been reported to reverse the anticoagulant effect of fondaparinux in healthy volunteers but has not been studied in patients who are actively bleeding. Factor VIIa is also not available in all hospitals, and its cost is substantial.

Treating Pulmonary Embolism Associated with Malignancy

The pathophysiology of venous thrombosis in cancer patients is complex and is influenced by a number of variables, including tumor type, stage, and overall tumor burden. Malignancies such as renal cell carcinoma are associated with a 43% incidence of VTE. Cancer patients with DVT or PE have increased 6-month mortality over cancer patients without VTE. The CLOT (Randomized Comparison of Low-Molecular Weight Heparin vs. Oral Anticoagulant Therapy for the Prevention of VTE in Patients with Cancer) study demonstrated that LMWH (dalteparin) was more efficacious in the prevention of recurrent VTE in patients with malignancy than was warfarin. Patients with cancer complicated by acute DVT, PE, or both were randomly assigned to receive 6 months of warfarin or the LMWH dalteparin. Patients receiving dalteparin had less recurrent VTE then those receiving warfarin (9% vs 17%).

Treatment of Pulmonary Embolism in Pregnancy

Treatment of PE in pregnancy is complicated by risk to both the mother and the fetus. Warfarin is contraindicated in pregnancy because of its ability to cross the placenta and its association with both fetal hemorrhage and teratogenic effects such as central nervous system and neural developmental defects and nasal hypoplasia. Both UF-heparin and LMWH can be used in the treatment of VTE in pregnancy because neither crosses the placenta. Long-term use of UF-heparin is associated with an increased risk of osteoporosis, but the risk is lower in patients treated with LMWH. Current recommendations for the treatment of VTE in pregnancy advocate the use of LMWH because of its favorable dosing and monitoring characteristics and its lower toxicity compared with other agents. However, it is important to recognize that a women's volume of distribution increases significantly during pregnancy, and, therefore, the LMWH doses must be adjusted accordingly. Full-dose anticoagulation significantly increases the risk of hemorrhage at the time of delivery; therefore, LMWH and UF-heparin should be discontinued 24 h before planned induction of labor. If spontaneous labor occurs, consideration should be given to reversal of anticoagulation with protamine. Anticoagulation can be restarted within 12–24 h of delivery if there is no ongoing bleeding. Neither warfarin,

UF-heparin, nor LWMH is excreted in breast milk, so these medications can be administered to breastfeeding women.

Pulmonary Embolectomy

Surgical resection of acute PE is a consideration in some patients. The operation is plagued by a high reported mortality (30% in some series), caused, in part, by the critically ill, hemodynamically unstable patients that are usually considered for the operation. Patients selected to undergo emergency embolectomy for acute PE have frequently had a large PE with resulting RV dysfunction (a marker of increased mortality in itself). They often have had anticoagulation or thrombolysis fail or are not eligible for these treatments.

Chronic Thromboembolic Disease

In most patients, the usual histologic and clinical course of pulmonary embolism is complete resolution of the thrombus and restoration of normal pulmonary artery pressures, usually within 30 days of the event. However, on the basis of a prospective incidence study, Pengo and colleagues reported that up to 4% of patients who survive a symptomatic pulmonary embolism might develop a condition termed *chronic thromboembolic pulmonary hypertension (CTEPH)*. Most of these individuals are seen late in their clinical course after significant pulmonary arterial hypertension (PAH) develops; therefore, little is known about the natural history of this disease. In the currently accepted model for the pathogenesis of CTEPH, acute PE, either symptomatic or asymptomatic, serves as the initiating event, followed by disease progression. For reasons that are unknown, these emboli do not resolve but rather are eventually covered by endothelial cells, a process referred to as endothelialization, making them inaccessible to endogenous or exogenous thrombolysis. This process eventually results in remodeling and obstruction of the pulmonary vascular bed and PAH. What predisposes patients to CTEPH is unclear. Increased factor VIII levels have been detected in the peripheral blood of some of these patients, whereas an increased incidence of anticardiolipin antibodies has also been reported. The predicted 5-year survival of untreated severe CTEPH (PA mean > 50 mmHg) is poor, with some estimates as low as 10%. The treatment for CTEPH differs significantly from that of acute PE. Although these patients require anticoagulation to prevent further embolic events, the endothelialized clot is not accessible to these medications. Therapy, therefore, revolves around either removing the thrombus surgically or treating the elevation in PA pressures medically. Surgical

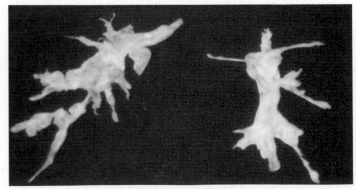

FIGURE 61-7 Thrombus removed from right and left pulmonary arteries in a patient with chronic thromboembolic pulmonary arterial hypertension.

resection, termed *pulmonary endarterectomy (PEA)*, is the treatment of choice in eligible patients (Figure 61-7). It is performed by dissecting away the endothelialized thrombus through careful separation of the thrombus from the pulmonary artery wall. This procedure is associated with significant operative and postoperative risk (5–10% mortality) and should only be performed in experienced centers. When successful, there is significant improvement of pulmonary artery pressures, right heart function, cardiac output, and functional class. However, a substantial number of patients (10–50%) with CTEPH referred for PEA are not deemed eligible because of inaccessible distal thrombus or other serious comorbidities. Furthermore, persistent PH after successful PEA is frequent with substantial small vessel occlusion or arteriopathy. For these reasons, medical therapy for CTEPH has been applied. These treatments include nonspecific therapies such as diuretics to improve fluid status, long-term oxygen therapy for hypoxemia, and digoxin to improve RV contractility. However, more recently, novel therapies more specific for the treatment of PAH and approved in the treatment of idiopathic pulmonary arterial hypertension (IPAH) have garnered attention as possible medical therapies for CTEPH. These treatments include the prostacyclin analogs (epoprostenol, treprostinil, and iloprost), endothelin receptor antagonists (bosentan), and the phosphodiesterase-5 (PDE-5) inhibitors (sildenafil). However, evidence of the success of these medications is limited to case series, retrospective studies, and prospective cohort studies. The only randomized controlled clinical trial to date that has included patients with CTEPH, as well as patients with other causes of PAH, is the Aerosolized Iloprost Randomized (AIR) study. Iloprost is an inhaled prostacyclin analog approved for the treatment of PAH. This study did not demonstrate significant beneficial effects of inhaled iloprost in the CTEPH population, however.

Prevention of Pulmonary Embolism

VTE is a major cause of morbidity and mortality. Approximately 10% of in-hospital deaths are attributed to PE. Recognition of the prevalence and consequences associated with VTE has led to recommendations regarding primary prevention or thromboprophylaxis. Thromboprophylaxis has been demonstrated to be highly efficacious in a variety of patient populations and is associated with minimal risk. Recommendations for VTE prophylaxis advocate assessing a patient's risk for thrombosis and adjusting the aggressiveness of the approach on the basis of that risk. Although means of assessing a specific individual's risk exist, these systems are cumbersome, have not been adequately validated, and are unlikely to be used routinely in clinical practice. An easier, more applicable method involves a "group-specific" approach applied routinely to all patients falling within a specific target group. A full discussion of these recommendations is reviewed in detail in the Seventh American College of Chest Physicians (ACCP) conference consensus statement on the prevention of venous thromboembolism. The statement divides patients into medical and surgical groups. The surgical patients are classified on the basis of individual risk factors, such as age, preexisting conditions, and the type of surgery planned. Recommendations are then made regarding the type of thromboprophylaxis the patient should receive. A similar approach is used for medical patients. It is important to note that most medical patients admitted to the hospital in the current era will have at least one and likely multiple risk factors for

VTE. Therefore, thromboprophylaxis is indicated in most hospitalized patients and is considered essential in the optimal approach to their care. In most cases, the agents recommended for prophylaxis are anticoagulants. These anticoagulants include subcutaneous UF-heparin or LMWH with occasional recommendations for agents such as Xa inhibitors (fondaparinux) or oral vitamin K antagonists in very high-risk groups such as those status post hip or knee surgery. There is a developing consensus discouraging the use of mechanical compressive devices in the use of thromboprophylaxis against VTE. The ACCP currently recommends that mechanical methods of thromboprophylaxis be used primarily in patients at high risk of bleeding or as an adjunct to anticoagulant-based prophylaxis. Currently, however, there are little data supporting their role as adjunctive therapy.

Inferior Vena Cava Filters

The concept of mechanically obstructing the vena cava to prevent embolization to the pulmonary vasculature is not new, being originally conceived by Trousseau in 1868. However, techniques to insert this protective barrier have been refined substantially over the years, and now the placement of inferior vena cava (IVC) filters can be achieved safely and reliably. More recently, the development of retrievable IVC filters has expanded the number of patients considered for this procedure. The two most common scenarios in which IVC filters are used include (1) inability to anticoagulate and (2) failure of adequate anticoagulation in patients with known VTE. Other scenarios meriting consideration of IVC filter placement include patients at high risk for PE even with recommended thromboprophylaxis, such as trauma patients with lower extremity or pelvic fractures and patients at high risk of death from pulmonary embolic disease and/or with severe pulmonary hypertension and a known DVT. Only one randomized trial of IVC filter in the treatment of VTE has been published. This study demonstrated a decrease in the incidence of PE in the first 12 days after placement of the device (1.1% vs 4.8%), but an increase in the incidence of DVT at 2 years after placement (11.6% vs 20%). The incidence of PE at 2 years after filter placement was only slightly decreased (3.4% vs 6.2%). All patients in this study received anticoagulation for a minimum of 3 months, and many remained on anticoagulation indefinitely. There are no randomized trials examining the incidence of PE in patients who received an IVC filter but did not receive anticoagulation. Retrievable filters are a potential option in patients who have only a transiently increased risk of VTE (Figure 61-8). The filters should be removed before epithelization of the struts occurs, which is usually with 7–21 days of placement.

CONTROVERSIES AND PITFALLS

Although great progress has been made in our understanding and approach to the clinical entity of pulmonary embolism, new developments frequently bring with them new questions and controversies.

Isolated Subsegmental Pulmonary Emboli

The development of faster, multidetector scanners has improved our ability to see the subsegments of the pulmonary vasculature on CT angiography. This ability, however, has raised an interesting conundrum. Are isolated small, subsegmental pulmonary emboli clinically meaningful? On one side of this argument are

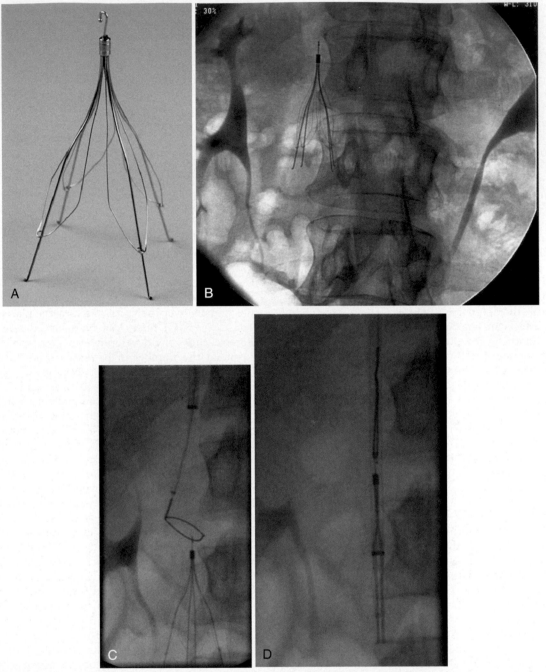

FIGURE 61-8 Images of an inferior vena cava (IVC) retrievable filter. **A,** Gunter Tulip® IVC filter. **B,** Filter status post deployment in the inferior vena cava. **C,** Preparation for retrieval of the filter. A snare is inserted percutaneously, which is used to engage the end of the filter. **D,** The filter is retracted and drawn into a sheath for percutaneous extraction.

those who believe that any thrombus in the pulmonary vasculature is pathologic, and even if a subsegmental thrombus does not have immediate clinical effects, it implies a risk of subsequent PE that, therefore, merits anticoagulation. The converse argument is that very small thrombi may intermittently occur in normal individuals, and perhaps it is the lungs' role to serve as a filter for these events, thus preventing them from migrating into the arterial circulation. This possibility, although interesting to consider, has never been substantiated. At present, there is no consensus on the appropriate clinical approach toward an isolated subsegmental PE detected by multidetector CTA and very little expert opinion published on this topic.

Outpatient Treatment of Pulmonary Emboli

As discussed earlier in this chapter, LMWH has been demonstrated to be safe and effective in the treatment of submassive pulmonary embolism. This raises the possibility of treating patients with PE at home, avoiding a hospital stay. This paradigm is well accepted in the treatment of DVT, where it has been demonstrated to be safe, cost-effective, and popular from a patient perspective. Some of the studies examining the use of LMWH for the treatment of PE have permitted small percentages of the patients enrolled to either be treated entirely as an outpatient or to be discharged early from the hospital to complete home therapy. There were no increases in adverse events in patients treated as outpatients. This possibility of home therapy raises concern, however, because patients with PE have an increased mortality compared with patients with DVT. It is possible that there is increased risk in treating them in a less monitored environment. Also, studies examining the use of LMWH in the treatment of PE have excluded patients with hemodynamically significant thromboembolic disease, a subgroup recognized to have even higher mortality. Realistically, however, more and more patients with PE are being treated as outpatients. This approach merits caution in patients who have adverse hemodynamic changes or RV dilatation or strain related to the thromboembolic event. This group of patients likely should be observed in an inpatient setting, at least initially in their treatment course.

Thrombolytic Therapy in Patients with Pulmonary Embolism without Hemodynamic Instability

There is no convincing evidence demonstrating survival advantage in hemodynamically stable patients with pulmonary emboli who are treated with thrombolytics plus anticoagulation compared with those treated with anticoagulation alone. Two studies have suggested thrombolytics improve outcomes in patients with pulmonary emboli and RV dysfunction; however, both of these have been criticized for their design. Although it is currently agreed that patients with hemodynamic collapse secondary to PE should receive thrombolysis if possible, controversy exists regarding the use of this therapy in less-affected patients.

SUGGESTED READINGS

Buller HR, Agnelli G, Hull RD, et al: Antithrombotic therapy for venous thromboembolic disease: the Seventh ACCP Conference on Antithrombotic and Thrombolytic Therapy. Chest 2004; 126:401S–428S.

Decousus H, Leizorovicz A, Parent F, et al: A clinical trial of vena caval filters in the prevention of pulmonary embolism in patients with proximal deep-vein thrombosis. Prevention du Risque d'Embolie Pulmonaire par Interruption Cave Study Group. N Engl J Med 1998; 338:409–415.

Geerts WH, Pineo GF, Heit JA, et al: Prevention of venous thromboembolism: the Seventh ACCP Conference on Antithrombotic and Thrombolytic Therapy. Chest 2004; 126:338S–400S.

Goldhaber SZ: Pulmonary embolism. Lancet 2004; 363:1295–1305.

Goldhaber SZ: Thrombolysis in pulmonary embolism: a debatable indication. Thromb Haemost 2001; 86:444–451.

Jerjes-Sanchez C, Ramirez-Rivera A, de Lourdes GM, et al: Streptokinase and heparin versus heparin alone in massive pulmonary embolism: A randomized controlled trial. J Thromb Thrombolysis 1995; 2:227–229.

Konstantinides S, Geibel A, Heusel G, et al: Heparin plus alteplase compared with heparin alone in patients with submassive pulmonary embolism. N Engl J Med 2002; 347:1143–1150.

Stein PD, Woodard PK, Weg JG, et al: Diagnostic pathways in acute pulmonary embolism: recommendations of the PIOPED II investigators. Am J Med 2006; 119:1048–1055.

The PIOPED Investigators: Value of the ventilation/perfusion scan in acute pulmonary embolism. Results of the prospective investigation of pulmonary embolism diagnosis (PIOPED). JAMA 1990; 263: 2753–2759.

van Belle A, Buller HR, Huisman MV, Huisman PM, et al: Effectiveness of managing suspected pulmonary embolism by use of an algorithm combining clinical probability, D-dimer testing, and computed tomography. JAMA 2006; 295:172–179.

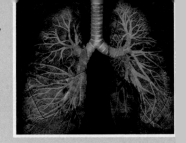

PULMONARY VASCULAR DISORDERS, VASCULITIDES, AND HEMORRHAGE

62 Pulmonary Hypertension

ANNA K. REED • TIMOTHY W. EVANS • STEPHEN J. WORT

EPIDEMIOLOGY, RISK FACTORS, AND PATHOGENESIS

Pulmonary arterial hypertension (PAH) is defined as a mean pulmonary artery pressure greater than 3.3 kPa (>25 mmHg) at rest or greater than 4 kPa (>30 mmHg) during exercise. For many years PAH was subclassified as being primary (i.e., idiopathic) or secondary (i.e., developing in association with another disease). It is now clear that despite differences in causation, different forms of PAH exhibit similarities in clinical features and response to treatment. This is not surprising, given that the histopathologic findings of the pulmonary vessel are similar in both *primary* and *secondary* forms of the disease. These terms were, therefore, discarded in 2003 by a third World Health Organization (WHO) symposium that developed a revised clinical classification on the basis of groups of diseases causing PAH (Box 62-1). This reclassification had important consequences for clinical management, because it provided a structured approach to the diagnosis and ongoing management of these patients. Advances in understanding of the cellular processes of this disease have led to the development of new targeted drug therapies. For the first time treatment can improve both quality of life and survival in this hitherto rapidly progressive and universally fatal disease.

The main aspects of the reclassification was to remove the term *primary PAH* and replace it with *idiopathic* or *familial PAH*. Second, staging of patients with PAH became based on their functional capacity rather than on their hemodynamic abnormalities (Box 62-2). The WHO also identified known risk factors for development of PAH (Box 62-3).

Idiopathic and Familial Pulmonary Arterial Hypertension

The incidence of idiopathic PAH is approximately 1–2 cases per million population. It can present at any age, but the peak incidence is in the third and fourth decades (although a recent French registry suggested that the age of peak incidence may be increasing). In childhood, the gender distribution is almost equal. In adults, however, the female/male ratio is approximately 2:1. Familial PAH accounts for 6–10% of cases of idiopathic PAH when more than 70% of cases have an abnormality in the BMPR II gene. Of the remaining "sporadic" cases, 26% have a mutation in this gene, although it remains possible that these are really as yet undiagnosed "familial" cases.

Histopathologically, pulmonary arterial hypertension is characterized by luminal obliteration of small pulmonary arteries (<500 μm in diameter). This process of vascular remodeling involves proliferation of smooth muscle cells, fibroblasts, and endothelial cells in the vessel wall. In severe cases, the formation of a neointima is observed as concentric intimal lesions.

Abnormal endothelial cell and myofibroblast proliferation results in the formation of plexiform lesions (Figure 62-1). To some extent the pathology varies according to the etiology, but more severe forms of precapillary PAH are usually pathologically indistinguishable.

The pathogenesis of most forms of PAH remains unclear. The histopathologic features suggest an imbalance between endogenous vasodilators and vasoconstrictors, growth inhibitors and mitogenic factors, and antithrombotic and prothrombotic substances (Figure 62-2). It seems that a triggering stimulus in susceptible individuals initiates a cascade of events resulting in pulmonary vascular endothelial injury with consequent vascular remodeling. Vasoconstriction seems to be important in only a minority of cases. There is increasing evidence that endothelial dysfunction plays a pivotal role in the pathogenesis of PAH (i.e., impaired production of endogenous vasoactive mediators such as prostacyclin, nitric oxide, and vasoactive intestinal peptide, in conjunction with overexpression of vasoconstrictor molecules, including thromboxane A_2, endothelin-1, and serotonin). There is also evidence of abnormalities in smooth muscle potassium channels and altered levels of apoptosis.

Conditions Associated with PAH

This group of disease shares very similar pulmonary vascular histopathologic features and has a similar, and generally poor, prognosis.

Connective Tissue Disease

PAH is most often seen in association with scleroderma. Autopsy studies indicate that up to 80% of patients have histopathologic changes consistent with PAH, although only 10–15% have clinically significant disease. Less commonly, PAH is seen in systemic lupus erythematosus, mixed connective tissue disease, rheumatoid arthritis, polymyositis, and dermatomyositis. The strongest association seems to be with disorders associated with Raynaud's disease. This occurs exclusively in women and often predates the development of PAH. The prognosis for patients with scleroderma and PAH is extremely poor.

Congenital Systemic to Pulmonary Shunts

The characteristics of systemic-to-pulmonary shunts that affect the development of PAH are the position and size of the shunt and the complexity of the anatomic defect(s) involved. Eisenmenger syndrome is defined as severe PAH associated with a large and nonrestrictive intracardiac or extracardiac shunt, which, with time, leads to reversal of flow and cyanosis. A more favorable clinical course can be anticipated in patients with Eisenmenger syndrome when the reaction is

BOX 62-1 World Health Organization Classification of PAH

Group I: Pulmonary Arterial Hypertension

Idiopathic
Previously known as primary PAH
Familial
Related conditions
Collagen vascular disease,
Congenital systemic-to-pulmonary shunts,
Portal hypertension,
HIV infection,
Drugs and toxins (e.g., anorexigens, rapeseed oil, L-tryptophan, methamphetamine and cocaine);
Other conditions: thyroid disorders, glycogen storage disease, Gaucher's disease, hereditary hemorrhagic telangiectasia, hemoglobinopathies, myeloproliferative disorders, splenectomy
Associated with significant venous or capillary involvement.
Pulmonary venoocclusive disease
Pulmonary capillary hemangiomatosis
Persistent PAH of the newborn.

Group II: Pulmonary Venous Hypertension

Left-sided atrial or ventricular heart disease
Left-sided valvular heart disease
Group III: PAH Associated with hypoxemia
Chronic obstructive pulmonary disease
Interstitial lung disease
Sleep-disordered breathing
Alveolar hypoventilation syndrome
Chronic exposure to high altitude
Developmental abnormalities

Group IV: PAH Caused by Chronic Thromboembolic Disease, Embolic Disease, or Both

Thromboembolic obstruction of proximal pulmonary arteries
Thromboembolic obstruction of distal pulmonary arteries

Group V: Miscellaneous

Sarcoidosis
Langerhans'cell histiocytosis
Lymphangiomatosis
Compression of pulmonary vessels (adenopathy, tumor, fibrosing mediastinitis)

BOX 62-2 Functional Classification of PAH–WHO 1998

Class I: Patients with PAH but without resulting limitation of physical activity. Ordinary physical activity does not cause undue dyspnea or fatigue, chest pain or near syncope.
Class II: Patients with PAH resulting in slight limitation of physical activity. They are comfortable at rest. Ordinary physical activity causes undue dyspnea or fatigue, chest pain or near syncope.
Class III: Patients with PAH resulting in marked limitation of physical activity. They are comfortable at rest. Less than ordinary activity causes undue dyspnea or fatigue, chest pain or near syncope.
Class IV: Patients with PAH with inability to carry out any physical activity without symptoms. These patients manifest signs of right heart failure. Dyspnea and/or fatigue may even be present at rest. Discomfort is increased by any physical activity.

BOX 62-3 World Health Organization Classification of Risk Factors for PAH

A. Drugs and toxins
  1. Definite
    Aminorex
    Fenfluramine
    Toxic rapeseed
  2. Very likely
    Amphetamines
    L-Tryptophan
  3. Possible
    Methamphetamines
    Cocaine
    Chemotherapeutic agents
  4. Unlikely
    Antidepressants
    Oral contraceptives
    Estrogen therapy
    Cigarette smoking
B. Demographic and medical conditions
  1. Definite
    Sex
  2. Possible
    Pregnancy
    Systemic hypertension
  3. Unlikely
    Obesity
C. Diseases
  1. Definite
    Human immunodeficiency virus infection
  2. Very likely
    Portal hypertension/liver disease
    Collagen vascular disease
    Congenital systemic–pulmonary cardiac shunts
  3. Possible
    Thyroid disorders

due to (1) the naturally occurring right-to-left shunt (sustaining systemic cardiac output, albeit at the expense of cyanosis) and (2) the right ventricular remodeling occurring over a long period of time. Despite the varied and often complex underlying cardiac anatomy and physiology, pulmonary vascular histologic changes are, however, remarkably similar to other forms of PAH. Although annual mortality rates for patients with Eisenmenger syndrome are relatively low compared with other forms of PAH, median survival is reduced by at least 20 years and is worse in patients with complex cardiac anatomy.

Portal Hypertension

PAH has been reported in 2–10% of patients with portal hypertension from hepatic cirrhosis. Ten percent of patients also have extrahepatic portal hypertension. The diagnosis of PAH is usually made within 4–7 years of the diagnosis of portal hypertension, and the risk of PAH increases with

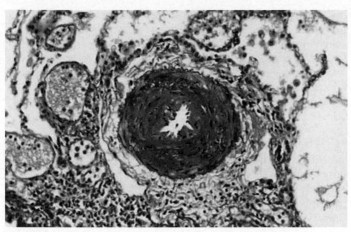

FIGURE 62-1 Pulmonary arteriole showing the medial hypertrophy and concentric intimal narrowing that occur as a result of vascular remodeling in pulmonary arterial hypertension.

the duration of portal hypertension rather than relating to the underlying hepatic disorder. Four percent of patients with end-stage liver disease undergoing assessment for liver transplant show evidence of pulmonary arterial hypertension. A putative mechanism for the development of PAH in this setting is that an endogenous or exogenous vasoconstrictor derived from the splanchnic circulation may bypass the liver and gain access to the pulmonary vasculature.

HIV Infection

In a recent large French registry, the prevalence of PAH in HIV-positive patients was 0.5%. This figure does not seem to have changed since highly active antiretroviral therapy (HAART) was widely available. The occurrence of PAH is independent of the CD4 count, but it seems to be related to the duration of HIV infection and is more common in those infected through intravenous drug abuse. No clear etiologic link has been established with either foreign body pulmonary embolus or portal hypertension related to cirrhosis from coinfection with hepatitis C or B. PAH is an independent predictor of mortality in these patients.

Drug- or Toxin-Induced PAH

PAH is associated with use of selected appetite suppressants. In the 1960s, 0.1% of patients taking Aminorex eventually had PAH develop, and in the 1990s 0.01% of patients taking fenfluramine progressed to PAH, which developed over a period of 10 years after drug administration. Interestingly, 10% of that population has been shown subsequently to have a BMPR II mutation. These medications are associated with metabolism of serotonin, a putative mediator in the pathogenesis of PAH. The ingestion of illegally marketed rapeseed oil in Spain in 1981 resulted in a multisystemic, inflammatory disorder, which was subsequently complicated by PAH in 8% of patients (although the PAH persisted in only 2% of patients). The toxin has remained unidentified.

A second inflammatory condition associated with PAH occurred after the ingestion of L-tryptophan in Mexico. Finally, solvent abuse and inhalation of crack cocaine have been associated with PAH.

Other Conditions Associated with PAH

The hemoglobinopathies, such as sickle cell disease, are associated with PAH, although the true prevalence is unknown. The underlying pathogenesis is also unclear but may be related to hemolysis and scavenging of the vasodilator nitric oxide by

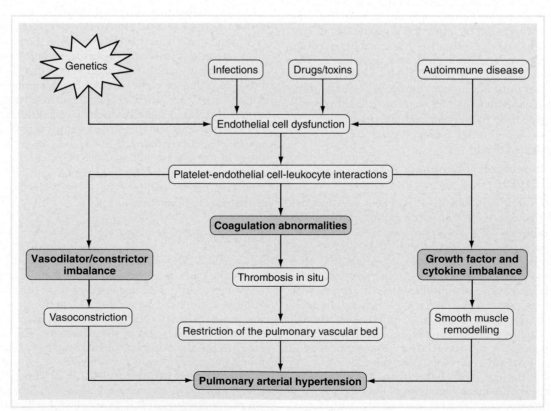

FIGURE 62-2 Proposed pathogenesis of PAH.

free hemoglobin. Thyroid disorders, glycogen storage disease, Gaucher's disease, hereditary hemorrhagic telangiectasia, myeloproliferative disorders, and splenectomy can all be complicated by PAH

Pulmonary Venoocclusive Disease (PVOD) and Pulmonary Capillary Hemangiosis (PCH)

This group of extremely rare disorders is characterized, respectively, by significant postcapillary and capillary vascular obstruction. Interestingly, PVOD has also been associated with BMPR II mutations. PVOD is extremely difficult to diagnose but should be suspected in the clinical setting of PAH associated with crackles on auscultation, digital clubbing, and pulmonary edema. The CT scan trilogy of thickened septal lines, ground-glass shadowing, and lymph node hypertrophy are highly suggestive of PVOD in the context of other features of PAH. Right heart catheterization may reveal a normal pulmonary arterial occlusion pressure. Lung biopsy is hazardous, and patients may react adversely to pulmonary arterial vasodilators. The prognosis without transplantation is extremely poor.

Pulmonary Venous Hypertension

This relates to the group of postcapillary disorders (apart from PVOD) resulting from increased left atrial pressure, with consequent pulmonary venous hypertension. Most commonly, these are conditions resulting in left ventricular systolic or diastolic dysfunction and/or mitral valvular disease.

Associations with Hypoxia/Respiratory Disease

The role of PAH in the clinical course of respiratory disorders, many of which are associated with hypoxia, remains undefined. Mild PAH would be expected in patients who are chronically hypoxemic, and it is not surprising that it occurs in the setting of diffuse parenchymal or airway disease (e.g., the interstitial lung diseases, chronic obstructive pulmonary disease [COPD], sleep-disordered breathing with alveolar hypoventilation, and acute respiratory distress syndrome, as well as a selection of conditions represented in the WHO classification as "miscellaneous"). In most pulmonary disorders, however, there are groups of patients with moderate to severe PAH that seems out of proportion to their underlying respiratory pathology.

Embolic Causes of PAH

Chronic Thromboembolic Pulmonary Arterial Hypertension (CTEPH)

The incidence of CTEPH is unknown. A recent retrospective study found the incidence after an acute pulmonary embolus to be 1% at 6 months, 3.1% at 1 year, and 3.8% at 2 years. Only 50% of cases have an identifiable history of venous thromboembolism. The average time to diagnosis after a known acute event is 2 years. CTEPH is characterized pathologically by organization of intraluminal thrombus with fibrous stenosis or complete obliteration of the pulmonary arterial lumen. Importantly, the level of pulmonary vascular resistance is higher than the calculated extent of obstruction by pulmonary angiogram as a result of vascular remodeling in obstructed and nonobstructed beds. The natural history of untreated CTEPH is poor, with fewer than 20% of patients surviving 2 years if the mean pulmonary artery pressure is >50 mmHg at presentation. Factors associated with progression to CTEPH after acute pulmonary embolism are a previous

history of PE, younger age, larger perfusion defects, idiopathic pulmonary embolus at presentation, and the presence of procoagulant factors (i.e., anticardiolipin antibodies, elevated factor VIII), chronic inflammatory disease, myeloproliferative syndromes, ventriculoatrial shunt, and splenectomy. The treatment of choice remains pulmonary endarterectomy (PTE) for proximal disease, although this is readily performed in only selected specialized centers.

Other Embolic Causes

Worldwide, parasitic diseases such as schistosomiasis are an important cause of "embolic" PAH, although, like CTEPH, a more widespread chronic underlying inflammatory condition probably exists. Other embolic causes, although rare, include tumors and amniotic fluid and air embolus.

Miscellaneous Causes of PAH

These include conditions such as sarcoidosis, Langerhans cell histiocytosis, lymphangioleiomyomatosis, and compression of pulmonary vessels by lymphadenopathy, tumors, or fibrosing mediastinitis.

PATHOPHYSIOLOGY

The normal pulmonary circulation is a high-flow, low-resistance system. Blood flow can increase threefold to fivefold, with minimal changes in pulmonary artery pressures because of recruitment and distention of the vasculature. Under physiologic conditions, the right ventricle is a thin-walled cavity that can accommodate large changes in venous return with little change in filling pressures, but it is poorly equipped to generate high systolic pressures. PAH develops as a consequence of a reduction in the cross-sectional area and the distensibility of the pulmonary vasculature, resulting in increased vascular resistance and right ventricular afterload. Initially, cardiac output may remain normal at rest through compensatory tachycardia and right ventricular hypertrophy but fails to increase appropriately with exercise (Figure 62-3). Increased heart rate and systolic pressures may compromise right ventricular myocardial blood flow, resulting in right ventricular ischemia. As right ventricular afterload increases, further cardiac output falls, even at rest. Increased right ventricular pressures can, in addition, cause septal shift and impair left ventricular filling and performance. Fluid retention occurs secondary to the low output state. Most patients will die from right ventricular failure, but sudden death occurs in approximately 7%. Common precipitating events are believed to be arrhythmias, pulmonary embolism, and infection.

GENETICS

The familial form of PAH (FPAH) accounts for 6–10% of all idiopathic cases. Approximately 100 families worldwide have been identified. Inheritance occurs in an autosomal-dominant fashion with 20% penetrance. Genetic anticipation is also shown (i.e., in affected families, each successive generation has more PAH develop at an earlier age). The first gene implicated in the development of PAH encodes type II bone morphogenic protein receptor (BMPR II, a member of the transforming growth factor-β [TGF-β] super-family) and has been localized to chromosome 2q31–32. More than 45 different mutations in BMPR II have been identified in patients with familial PAH, and more than 70% of patients with FPAH have

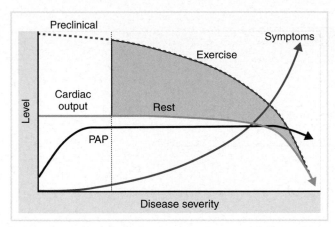

FIGURE 62-3 Pathophysiology of pulmonary arterial hypertension. In the early stages, cardiac output remains normal at rest but fails to increase appropriately with exercise. With disease progression, cardiac output falls even at rest.

mutations at this gene locus. Interestingly, 26% of patients with supposed "sporadic" idiopathic PAH also have mutations affecting this gene. It is thought that the genetic mechanism involves haploinsufficiency. Not all individuals carrying the BMPR II mutation—and consequently half of the wild-type BMPR II gene—have PAH develop, however. Accordingly, the mutation alone is not sufficient to cause PAH, and a "second hit" may be required. This theory is supported by experimental data. In mice, BMPR II heterozygote deleted animals only have PAH develop when exposed to some form of inflammatory/hypoxic stress. Finally, mutations in other genes belonging to the TGF-β superfamily have been implicated in the development of PAH, such as ALK-1 and TGF-β receptor 1.

CLINICAL FEATURES

A diagnosis of PAH should be considered in any patient presenting with breathlessness in the absence of specific cardiac or pulmonary disease, or in patients who have underlying cardiac or pulmonary disease but present with increasing breathlessness that is not explained by the underlying disease itself.

History

Early diagnosis of PAH is difficult and requires a high index of suspicion because of the nonspecific nature of the symptoms and the subtle findings on physical examination. Patients are, therefore, frequently misdiagnosed and are identified only when the later and more severe stages of the condition have been reached. In the NIH registry, the mean length of time from onset of first symptoms to diagnosis was more than 2 years. This has not changed in the past 10 years. Dyspnea is the presenting complaint in 60% of patients and is eventually reported by virtually all as the disease progresses. Breathlessness may be graded I–IV according to the WHO criteria, which reflects both the severity of the PAH and the prognosis (see Box 62-2). Fatigue is common. Angina occurs in 47% of patients and is usually caused by right ventricular ischemia. Syncope or presyncope, especially on exertion, is an ominous complaint and indicates severe limitation of cardiac output.

Physical Examination

Careful examination may alert the physician to an underlying cause for PAH. Establishing an accurate diagnosis has important implications for therapy. Physical findings caused by PAH may be few and subtle in the earliest stages of the condition. With progression, tachycardia occurs, with a low-volume pulse. Poor peripheral perfusion results in cold extremities, with associated cyanosis. Central cyanosis is common. Finger clubbing is not a feature of idiopathic PAH, and its presence should alert the examiner to consider other associated conditions. The jugular venous pressure is often raised, frequently with signs of tricuspid regurgitation. A parasternal right ventricular heave may be found, along with a palpable pulmonary component of the second heart sound (P_2). Auscultation reveals a loud, split-second heart sound. Right ventricular third and forth heart sounds are present in more severe cases. Tricuspid regurgitation is very common, and evidence may also be found for pulmonary valvular insufficiency (i.e., Graham Steell's murmur, resulting from dilatation of the pulmonary valve ring). Peripheral edema, ascites, and even scrotal edema may be detectable in severe disease.

Diagnosis

Once the suspicion of PAH is raised, subsequent investigations should aim to confirm the diagnosis, to identify the clinical category of PAH (from WHO Venice classification), and to further evaluate those with idiopathic PAH, familial PAH, and some forms of associated PAH (functional capacity and hemodynamics) to give appropriate treatment. An algorithm for the investigation of the patient suspected to have PAH is shown in Figure 62-4.

Initial Investigations to Confirm the Diagnosis

Electrocardiogram. The electrocardiogram is abnormal in 85% of patients with established PAH. Typical changes include right-axis deviation with evidence of right ventricular and/or right atrial hypertrophy and right ventricular strain. The degree of these changes does not always reflect the severity of disease, and a normal ECG does not eliminate the diagnosis of PAH.

Chest Radiography

Chest radiography shows abnormalities in more than 90% of patients with idiopathic PAH. Prominence of the main pulmonary arteries (90%), enlargement of the hilar vessels (80%), and peripheral pruning (51%) are the most common abnormalities (Figure 62-5). Of patients enrolled in the NIH registry, only 6% had a normal chest radiograph. Associated parenchymal abnormalities may also exist.

Echocardiography. Echocardiography is the screening tool of choice for PAH. It provides a noninvasive estimation of right ventricular function and pulmonary arterial pressure and can reveal other underlying cardiac abnormalities. Right ventricular and right atrial enlargement, with a normal left ventricular cavity size, are typically seen. In severe cases, interventricular septal curvature may be reversed, and the left ventricular cavity compromised. The presence of a pericardial effusion is a poor prognostic finding. Pulmonary and tricuspid regurgitation can be detected and quantified by use of Doppler techniques.

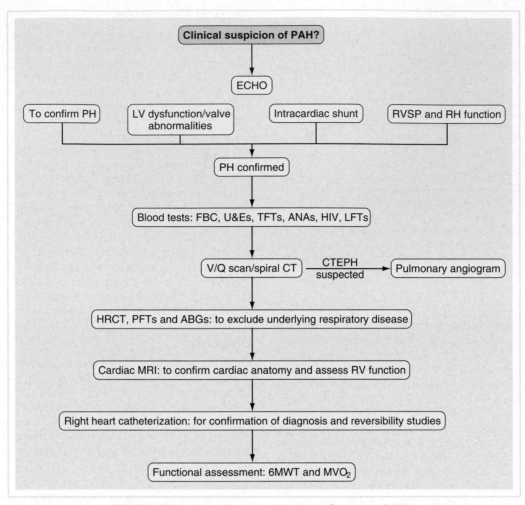

FIGURE 62-4 Approach to investigation of suspected PAH.

According to the Bernoulli equation, the pressure across the valve in question is equal to $4 \times v^2$, where v is the velocity of the regurgitant jet. An estimate of right atrial pressure can be made from inferior vena cava collapsibility with respiration. Then:

$$PASP = RVSP = (4 \times v^2) + RAP$$

where *PASP* is pulmonary artery systolic pressure, *RVSP* is right ventricular systolic pressure, *RAP* is right atrial pressure, and v is tricuspid jet velocity (PASP is assumed to equal RVSP if there is no gradient between these structures).

Echocardiography also provides an index whereby disease progression can be monitored, removing the need for repeated pulmonary artery catheterizations. When there is echocardiographic evidence of significant PH, however, a right heart catheter should *always* be undertaken at least once to provide an accurate baseline assessment of the pulmonary hemodynamics and to permit reversibility studies.

Pulmonary Function Tests and Arterial Blood Gases. The main role of lung function studies is to *exclude* parenchymal lung diseases as an underlying cause for PAH. However, mild restrictive defects and evidence of small airways dysfunction are seen in idiopathic PAH, as is impairment of gas exchange, with reduced transfer capacity of the lung for carbon monoxide (TLCO). Hypoxemia, hypocapnia secondary to alveolar hyperventilation, and an increased alveolar-arterial oxygen (PAO_2-PaO_2) difference are also characteristic. Severe hypoxemia is usually the result of intracardiac shunting.

Ventilation and Perfusion ($\dot{V}/\dot{Q}$) Lung Scanning. $\dot{V}/\dot{Q}$ scintigraphy is essential to exclude chronic thromboembolic disease. The scan is typically normal in PAH or displays only minor, patchy perfusion defects. In patients who have PAH as a result of thromboembolic disease, however, at least one, but often several, major segmental or subsegmental mismatches in $\dot{V}/\dot{Q}$ relationships are seen (Figures 62-6 and 62-7). Note that unmatched perfusion defects are also seen in PVOD. A negative or low-probability scan effectively excludes thromboembolic disease. In positive scans, it is usual to proceed to further imaging such as CT pulmonary angiography or magnetic resonance angiography. In most centers the "gold standard" still remains contrast angiography at time of catheterization to characterize the nature and extent of any thromboembolic disease.

High-Resolution Computed Tomography. High-resolution computed tomography (HRCT) scanning is required to exclude parenchymal lung disease as the cause of the PAH. HRCT is indicated in the setting of an abnormal CXR with interstitial markings in the absence of left ventricular failure. HRCT is particularly important in the diagnosis of PVOD.

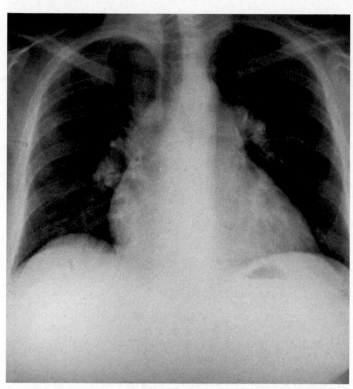

FIGURE 62-5 Chest radiograph in pulmonary arterial hypertension. Enlargement of the proximal pulmonary arteries (spurious cardiomegaly caused by poor inspiration).

Continuous Volume (Spiral) CT Pulmonary Angiography (PA).
As experience with CT-PA increases, this technique is superseding V̇/Q̇ lung scanning in some centers to exclude significant thromboembolic disease. Certainly in experienced centers resolution is adequate to the subsegmental vessels (sixth- or seventh-generation pulmonary arteries). With 64 multislice CT-PA, higher resolution is possible. In most centers, however, V̇/Q̇ scanning is still recommended in conjunction with CT-PA. CT features of chronic thromboembolic disease are complete occlusion of pulmonary arteries, irregular filling defects consistent with thrombi, recanalization, stenoses, or webs (Figure 62-8). Interpretation of spiral CT images may be highly observer dependent, however, and only sixth- or seventh-generation pulmonary arteries can be visualized with confidence. Pulmonary angiography is still considered the "gold standard" for the investigation of patients with CTEPH (Figure 62-9).

Cardiac Magnetic Resonance Imaging (MRI).
Cardiac MRI is now the most accurate means for examination of the structure and function of the right ventricle, being more accurate than echocardiography and providing accurate estimates of ventricular size and mass, as well as pulmonary blood flow. Gadolinium contrast, pulmonary angiography can be performed to at least subsegmental level. The use of noninvasive imaging, such as cardiac MRI, to monitor disease-targeted therapy is currently being evaluated.

Biomarkers.
Brain natriuretic peptide (BNP) is released from cardiac myocytes in response to increased ventricular wall tension. ProBNP (the prohormone) is cleaved into active BNP and more stable N-terminal fragment (NT)–pro-BNP. BNP and/or ProBNP has been shown to be elevated in idiopathic PAH and associated with interstitial lung disease, COPD, congenital heart disease, CTEPH, and scleroderma. NT-pro-BNP may have an advantage over BNP, because it is less affected by renal function and age. Baseline and serial changes in BNP correlate well with mortality and other markers such as pulmonary hemodynamics, WHO functional class, and 6-min walk test (6MWT). Other biomarkers under evaluation include troponin and uric acid.

Other Blood Tests. All patients should have routine hematology, biochemistry, and thyroid function tests. Antinuclear antibody testing is frequently positive in patients with PAH (29% in the NIH registry), despite the absence of connective tissue disease. These are usually of a nonspecific pattern and are present in low titers. Strongly positive serology should lead to further, more specific serologic testing to exclude PAH related to connective tissue disease. HIV testing should be considered in all patients seen with apparent PAH.

Evaluation of Functional Class and Severity of PAH

Functional class and severity of PAH determine the appropriate therapy. WHO functional class is determined from history and clinical observation (see Box 62-2). The exercise tests routinely available in most PAH centers are the 6MWT and cardiopulmonary exercise testing (CPET). A full hemodynamic profile is only possible by use of right heart catheterization.

6MWT. The role of the 6MWT in the assessment of PAH is now established. Baseline values for distance walked are known to correlate with WHO functional class, pulmonary vascular hemodynamics, CPET variables, and survival. Serial values have proven to be a useful outcome measure. It is technically simple to perform (according to published guidelines), and results are reproducible. However, it gives no indication as to the source of exercise impairment and is less discriminatory for walk distances greater than 450 m ("plateau effect"). Consequently, it is less useful for patients in functional classes I and II.

Cardiopulmonary Exercise Testing (CPET). Incremental CPET is also now standardized, although technically more difficult to perform. It allows measurement of ventilation and pulmonary gas exchange (Vo₂) during exercise and hence provides additional pathophysiologic data. CPET shows characteristic changes in PAH and can predict whether PAH is the limiting factor in patients with mixed pathology. Baseline values are predictive of disease severity. Significantly, however, this test has not proved robust for serial monitoring in drug trials.

Right Heart Catheterization. Right heart catheterization is an essential procedure to confirm the presence of and cause of PAH, the severity of hemodynamic compromise, and the vasoreactivity of the pulmonary circulation. Information gained at this procedure has important implications for treatment and prognosis. Hemodynamic variables with prognostic implication include elevation in mean right atrial pressure, high mean pulmonary artery pressure, reduced cardiac output, and low mixed venous oxygen saturation. These patients have the worst prognosis. Pulmonary artery occlusion pressure (PAOP) is, by definition, normal in PAH. An elevated PAOP

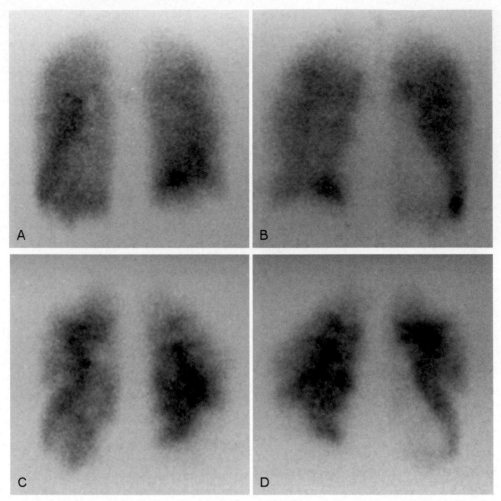

FIGURE 62-6 Typical ventilation-perfusion scans in pulmonary arterial hypertension. **A** and **B,** Normal ventilation scans. **C** and **D,** Patchy subsegmental defects on corresponding perfusion scans.

in the absence of left-sided heart disease should raise the suspicion of PVOD, although PAOP is commonly normal, given the patchy nature of this disease. Before vasoreactivity testing, a diagnosis of PVOD must be carefully excluded via thorough review of imaging and hemodynamic data.

Pulmonary vascular resistance is derived from the equation:

$$(PAPm - LAPm)/CO$$

where *PAPm* is mean pulmonary artery pressure, *LAPm* is mean left atrial pressure, and CO is cardiac output. A value of greater than 3 Woods units or 240 dyne/sec/cm^{-5} is considered abnormally high. LAPm is not always measured but can normally be replaced by PAWP or LVEDP (left ventricular end-diastolic pressure).

Pulmonary vasoreactivity studies are carried out by use of short-acting pulmonary vasodilators such as nitric oxide, adenosine, and prostacyclin (Table 62-1). A positive acute vasoreactive response is now defined as a reduction in mean pulmonary artery pressure of >10 mmHg to a value of <40 mmHg with an unchanged or improved cardiac output. Less than 10% of patients with idiopathic PAH display such a response. These "responders" have an improved survival when treated with calcium channel blockers (95%, 5-year survival). It is also important to exclude patients with suspected PVOD from vasoreactivity

studies, because it may precipitate life-threatening pulmonary edema.

Treatment

Treatment of PAH involves education, general supportive measures, and treatment of any associated contributing conditions, as well as more specific "disease-targeted" therapies. The rarity and life-threatening nature of severe PAH, as well as the complexities of therapy, suggest that patients are more likely to be optimally managed if they are referred to specialist centers that have greater experience with this condition. An algorithm for the treatment of PAH is shown in Figure 62-10.

Education

Patients are advised to engage in activities appropriate to their physical capabilities to prevent deconditioning and subsequent worsening of overall function. Excessive physical exercise is discouraged, because it may induce abrupt increases in pulmonary artery pressure and precipitate cardiac arrhythmias. Altitude, with its associated hypoxia, should be avoided. Commercial air travel is usually safe for those with mild or moderate disease, although supplementary oxygen should be available, and a fitness-to-fly test before the trip considered. Pregnancy, in particular the postpartum period, is associated

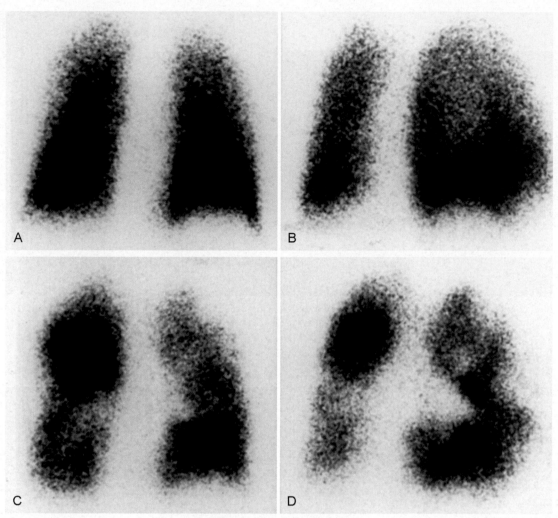

FIGURE 62-7 Chronic thromboembolic PAH. **A** and **B,** Normal ventilation scans. **C** and **D,** Multiple segmental (or larger) defects on corresponding perfusion scans.

with a high risk of accelerated deterioration and maternal death (20–50%). The WHO recommends adequate birth control and advises discussion of termination of any pregnancy. Progesterone-only preparations such as Depo-Provera and Implanon are highly effective contraceptives. The Mirena coil is also highly effective (>95% survival at 5 years), but 5% of women experience a vasovagal response during insertion, which can be potentially fatal in the setting of reduced cardiovascular reserve. Surgical sterilization is rarely used because of increased perioperative risk. Patients who become pregnant and choose to continue with their pregnancy after risk counseling should be referred to high-risk obstetric centers. Early treatment with targeted pulmonary vascular therapy and planned elective delivery with incremental anesthesia may improve the chance of maternal survival. Patients should be given general advice as how to avoid pulmonary infection with annual influenza vaccination. They should also be advised to seek the advice of their PAH center for appropriate management before undergoing any form of elective surgery.

Diuretics, Antiarrhythmics, and Anticoagulation

In recent trials looking at disease-targeted therapy, 49–70% of patients were being treated with diuretics to treat peripheral edema associated with right ventricular dysfunction. However, there are no trials that show a mortality benefit. Caution must be exercised to avoid overdiuresis, because right ventricular performance is highly dependent on preload for maintenance of adequate cardiac output and/or systemic blood pressure.

Arrhythmias, particularly atrial flutter and other tachyarrhythmias, are very poorly tolerated, indeed, and often herald worsening right ventricular function. Prognosis is improved if sinus rhythm is restored. Cardioversion may be performed electrically or chemically with amiodarone, but ablation therapy may be a better option.

The evidence base for the use of anticoagulation in patients with PAH is poor. However, most centers routinely anticoagulate patients with idiopathic PAH and CTEPH, warfarin being the agent most commonly used. The potential role of antiplatelet agents is uncertain, and trials comparing warfarin to antiplatelet therapy are needed.

Oxygen

Alveolar hypoxia causes local pulmonary vasoconstriction that can further increase vascular resistance. Current recommendations aim to maintain oxygen saturations above 90% at all times.

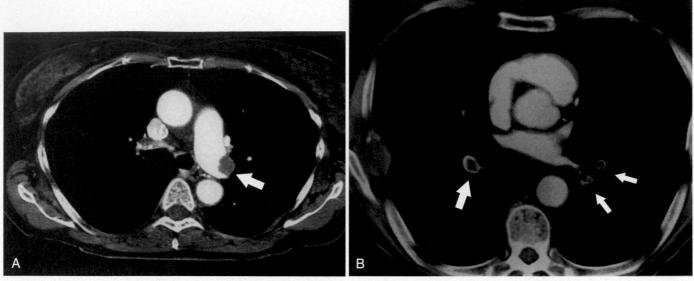

FIGURE 62-8 Spiral computed tomography with contrast. **A,** Massive filling defect in the main pulmonary artery (*arrow*). **B,** Filling defects in lobar (*large arrow*) and segmental (*small arrows*) pulmonary arteries.

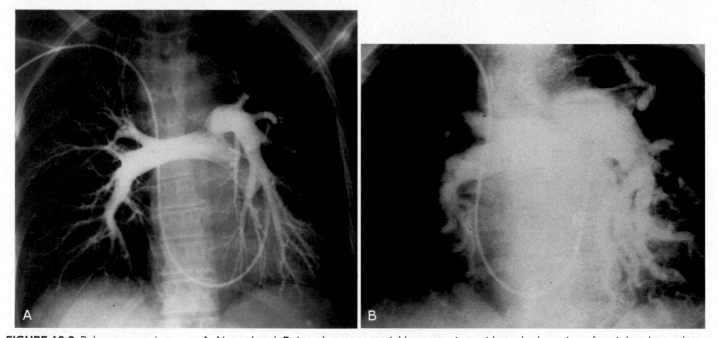

FIGURE 62-9 Pulmonary angiograms. **A,** Normal and, **B,** in pulmonary arterial hypertension, with marked pruning of peripheral vasculature.

Calcium Channel Blockers

The use of calcium channel blockers (CCB) should be restricted to patients with idiopathic PAH after a positive vasodilator trial at right heart catheterization. This group represents approximately 10% of patients undergoing the procedure. Only 5% will show benefit at 3 months. However, this group has a very favorable long-term prognosis (>95% at 5 years). CCBs are used in higher doses than for systemic hypertension or coronary artery disease, and doses are slowly increased. Thus, up to 240 mg/day of nifedipine or 900 mg/day of diltiazem can be tolerated with careful monitoring. Verapamil has significant negative inotropic effects and should be avoided. The main limitations to therapy are systemic hypotension, peripheral edema, and hypoxia caused by

increased $\dot{V}/\dot{Q}$ mismatch. More severe adverse reactions, including arrhythmias, cardiogenic shock, and death, have been reported. Abrupt withdrawal of CCBs may be associated with fatal rebound PAH and should be avoided. If there is no clinical improvement at 3 months, disease-targeted therapies should be considered.

Disease-Targeted Therapies

Recent advances in understanding the cellular mechanisms underlying the development of PAH have led to the development of specific disease-targeted therapies; specifically prostacyclin (and analogs), endothelin receptor antagonists, and phosphodiesterase inhibitors. The use of these agents has changed the clinical course of idiopathic PAH. Thus,

TABLE 62-1 Vasodilators Frequently Used in the Investigation and Management of Pulmonary Arterial Hypertension

Drug	Route	Dose Range	Half-Life
Epoprostenol*	Intravenous	2–20 ng/kg of body weight per min	3–5 min
Adenosine	Intravenous	50–200 mg/kg of body weight per min	5–10 sec
Nitric oxide	Inhaled	5–40 parts per million	15–30 sec
Bosentan	Oral	125–250 mg/day	4–5 h
Sildenafil	Oral	20–80 mg td	3–5 h
Nifedipine[†]	Oral	30–240 mg/day	2–5 h
Diltiazem[†]	Oral	120–900 mg/day	2–4.5 h

Reproduced with permission from Rubin.
*The dose range shown is for a short-term infusion; the dose range for a long-term infusion often exceeds 100–50 ng/kg/min.
[†]The half-life shown refers to conventional preparations; sustained-relief preparations may be administered once daily.

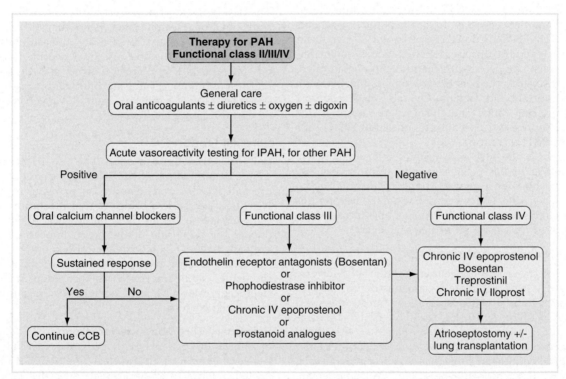

FIGURE 62-10 Algorithm for treatment of pulmonary arterial hypertension.

prostacyclin and bosentan have been shown to reduce mortality. Although the exact mechanism of benefit is not known, it is likely to involve vascular remodeling and improved right ventricular function.

Prostacyclin and Analogs

Prostacyclin (prostaglandin I_2) is produced endogenously by the vascular endothelium and is the principal product of arachidonic acid metabolism. It is a potent vasodilator and inhibitor of platelet activation and smooth muscle proliferation. The discovery that patients with idiopathic PAH have deficient production of prostacyclin led to the use of replacement therapy. Because prostacyclin has a very short circulating half-life, a continuous intravenous infusion is necessary, usually through an indwelling catheter. Intravenous infusion of synthetic prostacyclin (epoprostenol) has been shown to improve exercise capacity, quality of life, pulmonary

hemodynamics, and survival. Longer-term studies are now available demonstrating a 5-year survival in the treated group of 55% compared with only 28% of historical controls. Epoprostenol has also been shown to benefit patients with connective tissue disease–associated PAH and that associated with Eisenmenger syndrome.

At present, intravenous prostacyclin is the first-line treatment for patients with WHO class IV disease or in those with class III disease who have had treatment with other disease-targeting therapies fail.

The main drawbacks to intravenous epoprostenol therapy are mode of delivery, expense, and side effects, which include jaw pain, flushing, diarrhea, headache, backache, leg pain, and (rarely) hypotension. Catheter-related adverse effects include infection, thrombosis, pump failure, and rebound PAH. Successful management of patients with this mode of therapy requires an infrastructure probably only feasible at a specialized center.

The difficulties with intravenous prostacyclin have led to the development of more stable analogs that can be administered by alternative routes. Treprostinil is a tricyclic benzidine analog with a longer half-life than epoprostenol. As such, it can be administered as a continuous subcutaneous infusion and has been shown to significantly improve exercise capacity, quality of life, and hemodynamics in patients with idiopathic PAH and PAH associated with CTD and CHD (all in WHO functional class II, III, or IV). Improvements are greatest in patients with more severe disease and are dose related. The most common side effect is pain and inflammation at the infusion site. This occurs in a large proportion of patients and may warrant discontinuation of therapy. Trials on the intravenous and inhaled use of this drug are ongoing.

Iloprost is a stable prostacyclin analog that can be given by inhalation, orally, and intravenously. Most work has been performed by use of the inhaled (nebulized) route by which it has a relatively short duration of action and must be administered between six to nine times per day. In an RCT study of patients with PAH and CTEPH (functional class III and IV), significant improvements in exercise capacity, functional class, and hemodynamics were seen compared with placebo. An uncontrolled, long-term study suggests the benefits are long lasting, although data regarding mortality are lacking. Overall, inhaled iloprost is well tolerated, but cough and flushing are common side effects. Inhaled iloprost is licensed for treatment of WHO class II patients with PAH in Europe.

Oral beraprost is the first chemically stable, orally active prostacyclin analog. It has been shown to improve exercise capacity in two short-term clinical studies performed up to 6 months. However, this effect was not sustained beyond this time, and side effects were common. As such, beraprost is only currently approved for treatment of PAH in Japan.

Endothelin Receptor Antagonists

Endothelin-1 (ET-1) is an endogenous peptide with diverse biologic activity. It acts as a potent vasoconstrictor and promoter of smooth muscle cell proliferation, effects mediated by endothelin A and B receptors (ET-A and ET-B). ET-1 is overexpressed in the plasma and lungs of patients with PAH. Circulating levels correlate with disease severity. Until recently, the only approved endothelin antagonist was bosentan, an oral, dual ET-A and ET-B receptor antagonist. However, sitaxsentan, an ET-A receptor antagonist, has recently been approved for treatment of PAH in patients with WHO class III disease. In the BREATHE-1 trial, bosentan improved cardiopulmonary hemodynamics, exercise tolerance, dyspnea score, WHO functional class, and time to clinical worsening in patients with PAH. Long-term studies have shown bosentan therapy had persistent efficacy over time, with 1- and 2-year survival rates improved at 96% and 89%, respectively. Bosentan has also been shown to benefit patients with connective tissue disease, HIV, and Eisenmenger syndrome. The therapy is well tolerated, with asymptomatic elevation of liver function test results noted in 10% of patients. This is a dose-dependent phenomenon and is reversible after dose reduction or discontinuation of the drug. The STRIDE 1 and 2 studies have recently demonstrated a similar benefit for the ET-A receptor antagonist sitaxsentan.

Phosphodiesterase Inhibitors

Phosphodiesterases (PDEs) are the enzymes responsible for metabolism of cyclic nucleotides. Of these, type 5 PDE is found predominantly in the lung vasculature and is responsible for the actions of nitric oxide. Inhibition of type 5 PDEs with selective drugs, such as sildenafil, increase cyclic GMP and induce a fall in intracellular calcium concentration, with consequent vasodilatation (and other effects such as inhibition of vasoproliferation). A double-blind, placebo-controlled study investigating the effects of sildenafil in 278 patients with PAH enrolling patients with WHO functional classes II–IV were randomly assigned 1:1:1:1 to receive either placebo or sildenafil at doses of 20, 40, or 80 mg tds, respectively, over a 12-week period. There were significant improvements in 6MWD, functional class, and hemodynamics with no significant adverse events reported. Sildenafil is currently approved for patients with PAH in the United States (all functional classes) and in Europe (Class III only) at a dose of 20 mg tds.

Future Medical Therapies

The development of new treatments for PAH is a particularly active area of research. New agents that have been shown to have promise in animal models and translation to small series in man include vasoactive intestinal peptide (VIP) and imatinib (Gleevec™), a platelet-derived growth factor (PDGF) receptor inhibitor. Promising pilot data suggest that simvastatin and agents acting by apoptotic mechanisms may soon be useful treatment adjuncts.

Surgical Options

Balloon Atrial Septostomy. The use of atrial septostomy should be limited to patients who have signs of right heart failure and syncope and who are on maximal medical therapy. It is often viewed as a bridge to transplantation. Atrial septostomy creates a left-to-right intracardiac shunt that decompresses the right side of the heart, increases left ventricular preload, and augments systemic cardiac output. Thus, despite significant arterial oxygen desaturation, oxygen delivery to the tissues can be improved. The procedure is associated with significant mortality and should be performed only in specialized centers.

Pulmonary Thromboendarterectomy. PTE is the treatment of choice for patients with proximal CTEPH and offers a potential cure in carefully selected patients. If CTEPH is suspected, referral to an appropriate specialist center is mandatory. During PTE, organized thromboembolic material is carefully removed from the affected pulmonary arteries under hypothermic circulatory arrest, attempting to restore pulmonary hemodynamics to normal or near normal levels. Those patients with a disproportionately higher pulmonary vascular resistance than the segmental obstruction seen on imaging have a higher mortality and benefit less from PTE. With advances in both surgical technique and postoperative intensive care, the procedure-associated mortality has progressively diminished to approximately 6–8%. More than 90% of survivors return to functional class I or II. Patients with CTEPH caused by distal disease are not amenable to such treatment, and evidence is emerging for a role for both phosphodiesterase inhibitors and endothelin antagonists in this group. A randomized controlled trail to establish the safety and efficacy of bosentan in this group is currently underway.

Lung Transplantation

The advent of improved medical therapies in recent years has led to a reduction in the number of patients listed for

TABLE 62-2 Who Should Be Screened, and When?

	Prevalence	Should We Screen?
Family history	10%	Yes
Connective tissue disease	Scleroderma 10% Other <1%	Yes No
Congenital heart disease	Large ASD nonoperated 10% Large VSD nonoperated 50%	Yes Yes
HIV Infection	0.5%	No
Portal Hypertension	2.0%	No Yes if undergoing liver transplant assessment
Use of appetite suppressant drugs	0.01%	No
Previous pulmonary embolus		In all patients who have increasing dyspnea develop and routinely 8–12 weeks after the index event in any patient with massive or submassive PE

transplantation. Two recent studies demonstrated, however, that up to a quarter of patients with idiopathic PAH fail to improve on prostanoid therapy, and those who remain in functional class III or IV have a poor prognosis. Current recommendations are that patients in functional class III or above should be considered for transplantation. Those who show significant improvement on medical therapy, in particular those who move to a functional class II, can defer further assessment or listing for transplantation. There is little difference in efficacy between single lung, bilateral sequential lung, and heart lung transplantation with survival rates of 70–80% at 1 year and 50–60% at 4 years regardless of procedure. Single-lung transplantation is more complicated in the immediate postoperative period because of reperfusion edema in the transplanted lung. Because of the finite nature of available organs, heart-lung blocks are reserved for patients with coexistent left-sided heart disease or congenital heart disease with Eisenmenger's syndrome.

Clinical Course and Prevention

Without treatment, PAH is associated with an extremely poor prognosis. After the introduction of disease-targeting therapies such as prostanoids and endothelin receptor antagonists, survival has improved, although none is curative. Preliminary results from studies treating patients in WHO class II seem encouraging. Earlier diagnosis may allow more effective treatment. Disappointingly though, the mean time to diagnosis has not changed over the past 10 years. It is still unclear which patients should be screened and how to improve early clinical pickup.

Several factors are identifiable at presentation that predict poorer prognosis. These include higher pulmonary vascular resistance and pressures, absence of a favorable response to vasodilator therapy, worse WHO classification, elevated right atrial pressure (>10 mmHg), decreased cardiac output (<2.1 L/min), pulmonary arterial oxygen saturation less than 63%, and shorter distance walked in the 6-minute walking test (<332 m).

PITFALLS AND CONTROVERSIES

Combination Therapy

Combination therapy that uses drugs with different therapeutic mechanisms is an attractive option for patients who fail to improve or deteriorate with first-line treatment (monotherapy), but trials to confirm this are ongoing.

DO THE RESULTS OF TRIALS OF DISEASE-MODIFYING AGENTS IN IPAH, APAH (SCLERODERMA) TRANSLATE TO OTHER CATEGORIES OF PAH?

Evidence is emerging that bosentan is an effective treatment in Eisenmenger syndrome. Case reports suggest that bosentan and sildenafil may also be useful in patients with severe PAH associated with interstitial lung disease. Clearly, well-designed trials are needed before such treatments are routinely used in these categories.

Warfarinization Versus Antiplatelet Therapy

Anticoagulation is accepted as good practice for patients with idiopathic PAH and CTEPH. However, it is unclear whether this extends to patients with PAH associated with other conditions. In addition, there is a theoretical benefit of antiplatelet therapy in patients with PAH. Trials to determine the relative benefits are needed.

Screening Issues

Who to screen poses a difficult clinical dilemma. A possible strategy is shown in Table 62-2.

WEB RESOURCES FOR GUIDELINES OR PROTOCOLS

http://www.pha-uk.com.

SUGGESTED READINGS

Barst RJ, Rubin LJ, Long WA, et al: A comparison of continuous intravenous epoprostenol (prostacyclin) with conventional therapy for primary PAH. N Engl J Med 1996; 334:296–302.

Farber HW, Loscalzo J: Mechanisms of disease: Pulmonary arterial hypertension. N Engl J Med 2004; 351:1655–1665.

Galiè N, Beghetti M, Gatzoulis MA, et al: Bosentan therapy in patients with Eisenmenger syndrome: A multicenter, double-blind, randomized, placebo-controlled study. Circulation 2006; 114:48–54.

Galiè N, Ghofrani HA, Torbicki A, et al: Sildenafil citrate therapy for pulmonary arterial hypertension. N Engl J Med 2005; 353:2148–2157.

Galiè N, Torbicki A, Barst R, et al: Guidelines on diagnosis and treatment of pulmonary arterial hypertension. The Task Force on Diagnosis and

Treatment of Pulmonary Arterial Hypertension of the European Society of Cardiology. Eur Heart J 2004; 25:2243–2278.

Hoeper MM, Markevych I, Spiekerkoetter E, *et al*: Goal-oriented treatment and combination therapy for pulmonary arterial hypertension. Eur Respir J 2005; 26:858–863.

Humbert M, Sitbon O, Simonneau G: Treatment of pulmonary arterial hypertension. N Engl J Med 2004; 351:1425–1436.

Kawut SM, Horn EM, Berekashvili KK, *et al*: New predictors of outcome in idiopathic pulmonary arterial hypertension. Am J Cardiol 2005; 95:199–203.

Rubin LJ, Badesch DB, Barst RJ, *et al*: Bosentan therapy for pulmonary arterial hypertension. N Engl J Med 2002; 346:896–903.

Simmoneau G, Galiè N, Rubin L, *et al*: Clinical classification of PAH. J Am Coll Cardiol 2004; 43:5S–12S.

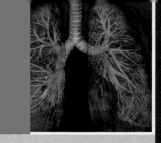
63 Pulmonary Vasculitis and Hemorrhage

MARVIN I. SCHWARZ

PULMONARY VASCULITIDES

Epidemiology, Risk Factors, Pathophysiology

The pulmonary vasculitides are a component of a group of systemic disorders (Table 63-1) that are characterized by vascular wall inflammation and destruction, leading to tissue necrosis and subsequent end-organ dysfunction. Although a pulmonary vasculitis can complicate an established autoimmune disorder (i.e., the connective tissue or collagen vascular diseases), the other conditions listed in Table 63-1 for the most part occur without a definable, underlying precipitating cause. Although vasculitis has been recognized for more than 60 years, specific etiologies, or even reliable risk factors, have not been identified. In general, the vasculitides are uncommon conditions and involve the lung with a variable frequency (see Table 63-1). It does seem, however, that the incidence, or at least the recognition, of the vasculitides is increasing, presumably as a result of widespread availability of antineutrophil cytoplasmic antibody (ANCA) testing. These antibodies are found in the serum of four of these disorders (i.e., Wegener's granulomatosis, microscopic polyangiitis, polyarteritis nodosa, and Churg–Strauss syndrome). The projected annual incidence for most of the disorders ranges from 2–13 cases per million population.

Vasculitis implies inflammation that can progress to necrosis of the vascular walls. If medium- or large-sized vessels are involved, infarction, necrosis, and end-organ dysfunction will result. When smaller vessels are affected (i.e., capillaries, arterioles, and venules), there is a loss of vascular integrity and leakage of blood into the tissue. When this small-vessel vasculitis occurs in the lung, it is referred to as *pulmonary* (or *alveolar*) *capillaritis*, resulting in the clinical syndrome of diffuse alveolar hemorrhage (DAH). When it occurs in the skin, it appears as a leukocytoclastic vasculitis and manifests as visible, raised palpable purpura, and sometimes as petechiae and ulcers. In the kidney, small vessel involvement results in a focal segmental necrotizing glomerulonephritis, which can be either subclinical (manifesting only as hematuria, red blood cell casts, crenated red blood cells, and proteinuria) or present as renal insufficiency that can lead to chronic renal insufficiency, sometimes requiring dialysis. Any organ may, however, be affected by the vasculitic process.

A granulomatous vasculitis involving small- and medium-sized vessels is the characteristic histologic feature of Wegener's granulomatosis. There is vascular inflammation and tissue necrosis, producing the characteristic feature known as geographic necrosis (Figure 63-1). An area of central necrosis is

seen, surrounded by mixed acute and chronic inflammatory cells and palisading histiocytes. The lung is involved in 75–90% of cases (Figure 63-2). Renal tissue usually shows a small-vessel vasculitis (capillaritis) appearing as focal segmental necrotizing glomerulonephritis, often with crescent formation (Figure 63-3). The renal findings are nonspecific and common to many of the systemic vasculitides and connective tissue disease.

Another systemic vasculitis that often affects the lung and causes granulomatous inflammation is the Churg–Strauss syndrome in which medium- and small-vessel inflammation, including numerous eosinophils, is associated with eosinophilic pneumonia. Giant-cell arteritis, the most common type of vasculitis, is also granulomatous in character; however, it rarely involves the lungs. Necrotizing sarcoidal granulomatosis is another example of a granulomatous vasculitis involving medium-sized vessels and has been considered to be a variant of sarcoidosis. Necrotizing sarcoidal granulomatosis only involves the lung. Takayasu arteritis is a large- and medium-sized vessel vasculitis of a granulomatous nature that infrequently can lead to major pulmonary artery occlusion.

The precipitating injury that results in vasculitis remains unknown. Exacerbations of Wegener's granulomatosis are more likely to occur in patients whose upper respiratory tract is chronically colonized by staphylococci. Similarly, some cases of polyarteritis nodosa, cryoglobulinemia, and microscopic polyangiitis are associated with chronic hepatitis B and C viral infections. Takayasu arteritis is most often seen in young women of Asian descent. Churg–Strauss syndrome follows a several-year prodrome of allergic rhinitis and asthma.

At present, two pathogenetic pathways for the development of systemic vasculitis have been suggested. The first involves development of antibodies to various neutrophil cytoplasmic components or ANCA. In Wegener's granulomatosis, more than 85% of patients demonstrate a serum antibody to a serine proteinase (i.e., proteinase 3 or c-ANCA), which is found in the cytoplasm of neutrophils and macrophages. In microscopic polyangiitis and the Churg–Strauss syndrome, 85% and 45% of patients, respectively, have antibodies directed against the neutrophil cytoplasmic myeloperoxidase (p-ANCA) develop. Approximately 10–20% of cases of polyarteritis nodosa also demonstrate serum p-ANCA; however, lung involvement is rare in this disorder. The c and p prefixes refer to the pattern of immunofluorescent staining, cytoplasmic or perinuclear.

Figure 63-4 outlines the potential role for ANCA in the pathogenesis of vasculitis. Circulating neutrophils become primed by either inflammatory cytokines or bacterial products.

TABLE 63-1 The Systemic Vasculitides and Relative Frequencies of Lung Involvement

Entity	Serum Antineutrophil Cytoplasmic Antibody	Vessels Involved	Cases/Million Per Year	Lung Involvement
Takayasu's arteritis	No	L and M	?	Uncommon
Giant cell arteritis	No	L and M	13	Rare
Behçet's syndrome	No	L, M, and S	?	Uncommon
Wegener's granulomatosis	Yes	M and S	3–9	Common
Churg–Strauss syndrome	Yes	M and S	2–3	Common
Polyarteritis nodosa	Yes	M and S	3–4	Rare
Collagen vascular disease	No	M and S	12	Common
Kawasaki's disease	No	M	?	Rare
Necrotizing sarcoid granulomatosis	No	M	?	Common
Microscopic polyangiitis	Yes	S	3	Common
Isolated pauci-immune pulmonary capillaritis	Yes/No	S	?	Common
Henoch–Schönlein purpura	No	S	?	Uncommon
Cryoglobulinemia	No	S	2–3	Rare
Goodpasture's syndrome	Yes/No	S	?	Common

The systemic vasculitides and their relative frequency of lung involvement. *L,* Large pulmonary arteries (major branches); *M,* medium-sized muscular pulmonary arteries; *S,* small pulmonary vessels (arterioles, venules, and capillaries); *ANCA,* antineutrophil cytoplasmic antibody.

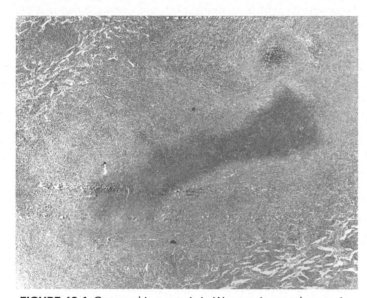

FIGURE 63-1 Geographic necrosis in Wegener's granulomatosis.

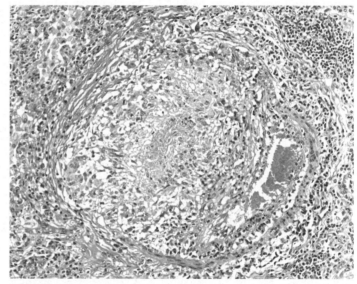

FIGURE 63-2 Wegener's granulomatosis. Inflammation and destruction of a small pulmonary vessel.

It is proposed that the primed neutrophils express proteinase 3 or myeloperoxidase on their cell surfaces, thereby allowing ANCA to bind to the target sites on the neutrophil cell membrane. The neutrophil then undergoes a respiratory burst and degranulates as it fragments and undergoes apoptosis (cell death). This results in the release of toxic oxygen radicals and cytoplasmic proteolytic enzymes into the surrounding tissue that, in turn, causes endothelial and eventually tissue matrix injury. Antineutrophil cytoplasmic antibodies also inhibit the naturally occurring antiinflammatory α_1-antiprotease inhibitor, thereby enhancing the enzymatic injury caused by the serine proteases. There is also evidence to support a role for ANCA in direct endothelial cell cytotoxicity and in the release of chemokines that are capable of attracting inflammatory cell populations. Although this pathogenetic potential role for ANCA is appealing, similar vasculitic changes can occur in patients without circulating ANCA. Moreover, ANCA levels do not necessarily correlate with clinical activity.

The second proposed pathogenetic mechanism involves immune complexes (Figure 63-5). Immune complex deposition has been found in the kidney and lungs of patients with systemic lupus erythematosus, mixed connective tissue disease, rheumatoid arthritis, Henoch–Schönlein purpura, and Goodpasture's syndrome. All of these conditions can have underlying pulmonary capillaritis and focal segmental necrotizing glomerulonephritis. Figure 63-6 shows that antigens are either acquired or derived from a tissue component from circulating antigen–antibody complexes, particularly when there

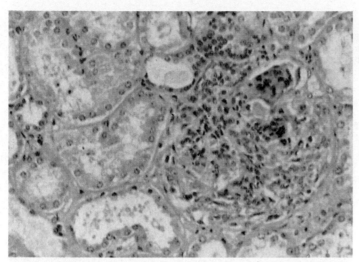

FIGURE 63-3 Renal biopsy. Focal segmental necrotizing glomerulonephritis with crescent formation.

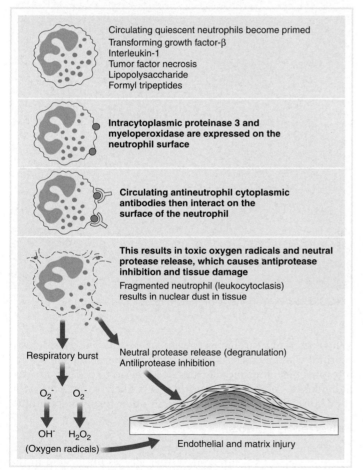

Circulating quiescent neutrophils become primed
Transforming growth factor-β
Interleukin-1
Tumor factor necrosis
Lipopolysaccharide
Formyl tripeptides

Intracytoplasmic proteinase 3 and myeloperoxidase are expressed on the neutrophil surface

Circulating antineutrophil cytoplasmic antibodies then interact on the surface of the neutrophil

This results in toxic oxygen radicals and neutral protease release, which causes antiprotease inhibition and tissue damage
Fragmented neutrophil (leukocytoclasis) results in nuclear dust in tissue

Respiratory burst

Neutral protease release (degranulation)
Antiliprotease inhibition

O_2^- O_2^-

OH^- H_2O_2
(Oxygen radicals)

Endothelial and matrix injury

FIGURE 63-4 Antineutrophil cytoplasmic antibody in the pathogenesis of vasculitis.

is antigen excess. These complexes attach to the vascular endothelium and activate complement that, in turn, results in the chemotaxis and adhesion of inflammatory cells and subsequent vascular necrosis. In Goodpasture's syndrome, a specific antibody, the antibasement membrane antibody, is found in both the lung and the kidney. This antibody is directed against an antigen found in type 4 collagen, the major component of

basement membranes. The antibody is present in the serum of most cases of Goodpasture's and stains as a linear, continuous immunofluorescence along the basement membranes in renal and lung tissue (see Figure 63-6). Immune complexes in the other aforementioned entities produce a granular, interrupted pattern of immunofluorescence, indicating immune complex formation in the circulation and deposition on tissue. In contrast, despite being ANCA positive, Wegener's granulomatosis, microscopic polyangiitis, and Churg–Strauss syndrome are not associated with tissue immune complex deposition and are referred to as pauciimmune.

Clinical Features

Patients with systemic vasculitis generally have myalgias and arthralgias. Fever, malaise, and anorexia and weight loss of varying durations are also common. With lower respiratory tract involvement, cough, dyspnea, and hemoptysis are reported. Upper respiratory tract involvement mimics chronic sinusitis, rhinitis, or otitis media.

Wegener's Granulomatosis

Wegener's granulomatosis affects the upper and lower respiratory tract early in the course of the disease, and this type of involvement may be the only manifestation (i.e., limited Wegener's granulomatosis). These patients may have chronic pansinusitis, but nose crusting, nosebleeds, and septal perforation leading to saddle nose deformity, chronic otitis media, and mastoiditis may also seen. Sinus and nasal manifestations are often the first signs of the disease. Eye involvement appears in up to 70% of patients and includes conjunctivitis, episcleritis, uveitis, and retinal artery occlusion and may have up to a 12-month delay from symptom to eventual diagnosis.

Involvement of the trachea or the major bronchi can result in tracheobronchial inflammation, ulceration, and bronchomalacia, and these can ultimately lead to stenosis with symptoms of upper airway obstruction. Airway involvement may result in permanent airflow limitation and/or atelectasis and postobstructive pneumonias resulting from endobronchial obstructions. In the lung parenchyma, the most typical lesions are single or multiple nodules that cavitate (Figure 63-7). These heal by forming scars. Another, often dramatic, presentation is hemoptysis with widespread radiographic infiltration resulting from DAH. Pulmonary capillaritis and DAH may be present singly, may appear in conjunction with typical cavitating lesions, or may occur as the opposite manifestation in a treated case that initially presented with one or the other. Recurrence of disease after remission is the rule in more than 50% of patients with Wegener's granulomatosis. In a small percentage of patients, pleural effusions or hilar lymphadenopathy may be seen.

Other systemic manifestations, which can appear initially or at a later date, include palpable purpura (leukocytoclastic vasculitis), peripheral neuropathy (mononeuritis multiplex), cranial neuropathies, and pituitary gland involvement causing diabetes insipidus. Glomerulonephritis (focal segmental necrotizing glomerulonephritis) is a common manifestation of the generalized forms of Wegener's granulomatosis and often causes substantial renal impairment that sometimes requires chronic dialysis and, eventually, renal transplantation. The glomerular lesion is not specific for Wegener's granulomatosis, because it is also seen in the glomerulonephritis associated with other systemic vasculitides, Goodpasture's syndrome, and the collagen vascular diseases.

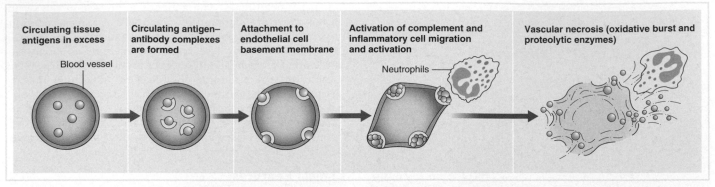

| Circulating tissue antigens in excess | Circulating antigen–antibody complexes are formed | Attachment to endothelial cell basement membrane | Activation of complement and inflammatory cell migration and activation | Vascular necrosis (oxidative burst and proteolytic enzymes) |

FIGURE 63-5 Immune complexes in the pathogenesis of vasculitis.

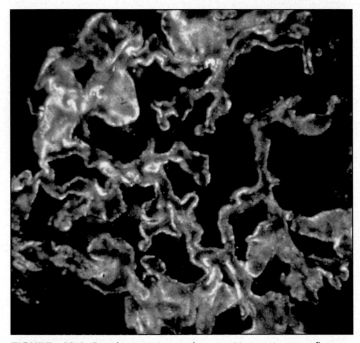

FIGURE 63-6 Goodpasture's syndrome. Linear immunofluorescence (antibody to immunoglobulin G) in a lung biopsy.

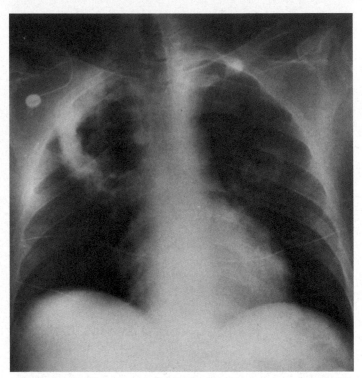

FIGURE 63-7 Wegener's granulomatosis. Two cavitating lesions.

Churg–Strauss Syndrome

The vasculitis component of the Churg–Strauss syndrome usually follows a several-year history of atopy (i.e., rhinitis, nasal polyps, asthma, peripheral eosinophilia, and sometimes chronic eosinophilic pneumonia). The vasculitis, when it appears, is recognized by tissue eosinophil infiltration, extravascular granulomas, and necrotizing vasculitis of small- and medium-sized vessels. Sinus involvement in the form of an allergic rhinitis and asthma is present in all affected individuals. Lung parenchymal infiltration, with or without a pleural effusion, is present in 66–75% of cases. Differentiating Churg–Strauss syndrome from chronic eosinophilic pneumonia is sometimes difficult, because 50% of patients with the latter also have an allergic prodrome, and chronic eosinophilic pneumonia may also lead to the development of the Churg–Strauss syndrome. Subcutaneous skin nodules occur in 66% of patients, mononeuritis multiplex is seen in 65–75%, and cardiac disease manifesting as congestive heart failure, pericardial effusion, or a restrictive cardiomyopathy is present in 50%.

When present, cardiac involvement results in considerable morbidity and increases the mortality. Abdominal pain, gastrointestinal bleeding, and diarrhea occur in up to 66% of affected individuals. Glomerulonephritis is less likely to be present in the Churg–Strauss syndrome than in other forms of vasculitis.

Polyarteritis Nodosa

Up to one third of patients with polyarteritis nodosa have evidence of hepatitis B infection. Other viruses implicated in the pathogenesis include the human immunodeficiency virus, cytomegalovirus, parvovirus B19, and hepatitis C virus. The clinical manifestations of polyarteritis nodosa are similar to the vasculitic phase of the Churg–Strauss syndrome, except that:

1. There is no atopic prodromal phase in polyarteritis nodosa.
2. There is a higher incidence of glomerulonephritis that often results in hypertension.
3. Lung parenchymal involvement is almost never seen.

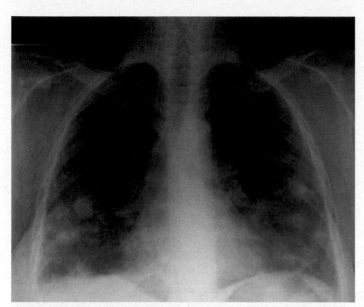

FIGURE 63-8 Necrotizing sarcoid granulomatosis. A young woman with a slight cough. Chest radiograph indicates multiple lower zone nodules. Diagnosis was proven by biopsy.

Microscopic polyangiitis, thought by some to represent a small-vessel variant of polyarteritis nodosa, is discussed with the diffuse alveolar hemorrhage syndromes in the next section.

Necrotizing Sarcoidal Granulomatosis

Necrotizing sarcoidal granulomatosis occurs in young individuals, it only affects the lung, and the pulmonary nodules are often only discovered after routine chest radiography (Figure 63-8). Although this rare entity is thought to represent a variant of sarcoidosis by some, the localization to the lung and the distinct vasculitic features help distinguish it from classical sarcoidosis.

Diagnosis

All the aforementioned vasculitic syndromes increase the peripheral blood sedimentation rate, often to levels exceeding 75 mm/h. There is also an increase the serum C-reactive protein and nonspecific elevations of serum rheumatoid factors and antinuclear antibody titers. Leukocytosis is common, and peripheral eosinophilia should suggest the Churg–Strauss syndrome. Nonspecific elevations of serum immunoglobulins can be expected, but an elevated serum immunoglobulin (Ig) E also supports the diagnosis of the Churg–Strauss syndrome. A urinalysis indicating red blood cells, red blood cell casts, and protein indicates the presence of active glomerulonephritis. Every patient should have microscopic examination of the urine.

A positive serum c-ANCA level confirmed by an enzyme-linked immunosorbent assay (ELISA) for antibodies to proteinase 3 is highly specific for Wegener's granulomatosis; however, the sensitivity of this test is lower in patients with disease limited to the respiratory tract. In these, when ANCA is negative, tissue biopsy, preferably lung by a thoracoscopic approach, is indicated. Nasal, sinus, or even endobronchial biopsy specimens often only show inflammation or necrosis, but not granulomatous vasculitis. Although a positive serum p-ANCA representing antibodies to neutrophil cytoplasmic myeloperoxidase supports the diagnosis of Churg–Strauss syndrome, polyarteritis nodosa, or microscopic polyarteritis,

it can also be positive in up to 15% of patients with Wegener's granulomatosis. Lung tissue is required to definitely establish the diagnosis of necrotizing sarcoidal granulomatosis.

Treatment and Outcome

The accepted and usually effective therapy for systemic vasculitis is a combination of systemic corticosteroids and cyclophosphamide. In most cases, oral preparations (e.g., prednisone 1 mg/kg ideal body weight/day and cyclophosphamide 2 mg/kg ideal body weight/day) are all that is required. The prednisone is tapered over a several-month period, after which it is discontinued. Full doses of cyclophosphamide are continued for 6–12 months, and then gradually tapered over the next 2–6 months. Intravenous therapy with methylprednisolone, up to 1 g daily in divided doses, and intravenous cyclophosphamide 2–4 mg/kg ideal body weight, is recommended for DAH leading to acute respiratory failure or to rapidly progressive renal failure. Cyclophosphamide occasionally seems to be necessary in the treatment of the Churg–Strauss syndrome, although its role has not been well established. Necrotizing sarcoid granulomatosis resolves in essentially all patients after treatment with corticosteroids alone, and, as opposed to what is seen with the other vasculitic syndromes, recurrences are rare.

Although adding cyclophosphamide to the treatment regimen of the vasculitides has significantly improved survival (particularly in patients with Wegener's granulomatosis, microscopic polyarteritis, and polyarteritis nodosa), the medication has a number of important complications, including sterility, alopecia, bone marrow suppression, and an increased incidence of opportunistic infections. Moreover, the development of transitional cell carcinoma of the bladder, non-Hodgkin's lymphoma, and myeloproliferative disorders are long-term complications. For this reason, after induction of remission with prednisone and cyclophosphamide, weekly oral methotrexate or daily azathioprine is now recommended for long-term immunosuppression. Newer treatments for maintenance of remission or for resistant cases are being tested. These include rituximab, mycophenolate mofetil, antithymocyte globulin, and leflunomide.

Trimethoprim-sulfamethoxazole prophylaxis is recommended to reduce the incidence of *Pneumocystis jiroveci* pneumonia when treating patients with corticosteroids, cyclophosphamide, or other immunosuppressive agents.

Clinical Course and Prevention

More than 90% of patients with Wegener's granulomatosis achieve complete remission, and up to 80% survive at least 8 years. Patients with more limited forms of the disease (i.e., no renal or central nervous system involvement) have an even better prognosis. Relapses are common, however, and monitoring of the urine, sedimentation rate, and possibly the serum c-ANCA levels is advised. There are limited data regarding the survival of patients with the Churg–Strauss syndrome. There is no known method to prevent any of these disorders.

Pitfalls and Controversies

A potentially fatal complication of cyclophosphamide therapy, particularly in older individuals, is hemorrhagic cystitis. Accordingly, monitoring of the urine sediment is important. Azathioprine or methotrexate can be substituted in those who have hemorrhagic cystitis develop. A late complication is transitional cell cancer of the bladder, particularly in those with persistent microscopic hematuria after cessation of treatment.

There is disagreement in the literature about whether an asymptomatic rise in c-ANCA necessarily portends an impending exacerbation of Wegener's granulomatosis. Accordingly, some suggest that the c-ANCA should not be routinely monitored but only measured in conjunction with clinical findings that may represent an exacerbation of the disease. In patients with Wegener's granulomatosis that is limited to the respiratory tract, trimethoprim-sulfamethoxazole alone can induce remissions. Adding trimethoprim-sulfamethoxazole to the standard therapeutic regimen of patients with systemic forms of Wegener's granulomatosis reduces relapse rates by 50%. Accordingly, there is debate about whether and when to include trimethoprim-sulfamethoxazole with corticosteroids and cyclophosphamide.

DIFFUSE ALVEOLAR HEMORRHAGE

Pathophysiology

DAH is caused by diffuse intraalveolar bleeding from the small vessels of the lungs, particularly the alveolar capillaries, but also the arterioles and venules. Intraalveolar collections of red blood cells and fibrin are seen, as well as hemosiderin-bearing macrophages and free hemosiderin, in the distal airspaces. The causes of DAH include a broad spectrum of etiologies with dissimilar underlying histologic findings (Table 63-2).

Pulmonary (alveolar) capillaritis defines a small-vessel vasculitis of the lungs, which may be isolated to the lung, but may also appear as a component of a number of systemic disorders. The distinct histologic finding is neutrophilic infiltration of the alveolar wall, with many of the cells being fragmented and appearing pyknotic. Because these cells are undergoing necrosis, nuclear dust collects in the tissue.

TABLE 63-2 Histologic and Clinical Classification of Diffuse Alveolar Hemorrhage

Histology	Frequency	Disease
Pulmonary capillaritis and glomerulonephritis (pulmonary–renal syndrome)	More common	Wegener's granulomatosis Microscopic polyangiitis **Systemic lupus erythematosus** **Goodpasture's syndrome**
	Less common	**Rheumatoid arthritis** **Mixed connective tissue disease** **Scleroderma** Henoch–Schönlein purpura IgA nephropathy Pauci-immune glomerulonephritis Drug-induced (propylthiouracil, penicillamine, diphenylhydantoin) Cryoglobulinemia Behçet's syndrome
Pulmonary capillaritis without glomerulonephritis	More common	Isolated pauci-immune/pulmonary capillaritis Acute allograft rejection
	Less common	Polymyositis Rheumatoid arthritis Mixed connective tissue disease Retinoic acid toxicity Goodpasture's syndrome Primary antiphospholipid antibody syndrome
Bland pulmonary hemorrhage	More common	Idiopathic pulmonary hemosiderosis **Goodpasture's syndrome** **Systemic lupus erythematosus**
	Less common	Coagulopathies Trimellitic anhydride exposure Mitral stenosis Drugs (amiodarone, nitrofurantoin) Subacute bacterial endocarditis
Diffuse alveolar damage (acute lung injury)	More common	Idiopathic pneumonia syndrome (bone marrow transplantation) Crack cocaine inhalation Cytotoxic drug injury Acute respiratory distress syndrome
	Less common	Acute radiation pneumonitis **Systemic lupus erythematosus**
Other histologies	More common	Lymphangioleiomyomatosis Pulmonary veno-occlusive disease
	Less common	Pulmonary capillary hemangiomatosis Fibrillary glomerulonephritis Malignancy (renal cell carcinoma, hemangioepithelioma, angiosarcoma, choriocarcinoma, Kaposi's sarcoma)

Entities with more than one underlying histology. Adapted from Schwarz MI: Diffuse alveolar hemorrhage. In Schwarz MI, King TE (eds): Interstitial Lung Disease, ed 3. Hamilton, Canada, BC Decker, 1998, pp 535–558.

The alveolar interstitium has neutrophilic infiltration, edema, and fibrinoid necrosis. It is hypothesized that the fragmented, dying neutrophils cause fibrinoid necrosis of the alveolar walls and disruption of the alveolar capillaries through their oxidative burst and the release of cytoplasmic enzymes. This leads to leakage of red blood cells, fibrin, and the fragmented neutrophils into the alveolar spaces, producing the histologic picture described (Figure 63-9).

Pulmonary capillaritis is primarily associated with a number of systemic vasculitides, as well as with the collagen vascular diseases (see Table 63-2). Other associations include pauci-immune pulmonary capillaritis, lung allograft rejection, and a variety of medications. Lung allograft rejection and the isolated pauci-immune pulmonary capillaritis are examples of lung-limited rather than a systemic disease process.

Bland alveolar hemorrhage, on the other hand, refers to a form of DAH in which there is no evidence of alveolar wall inflammation or necrosis, and the histologic appearance is that of DAH alone (Figure 63-10). This pathology implies a capillary endothelial injury without inflammation. In idiopathic pulmonary hemosiderosis and Goodpasture's syndrome, for example, disruptions in the alveolar-capillary basement membrane may be identified by electron microscopy.

Diffuse alveolar damage, the underlying histology associated with the acute respiratory distress syndrome, and other

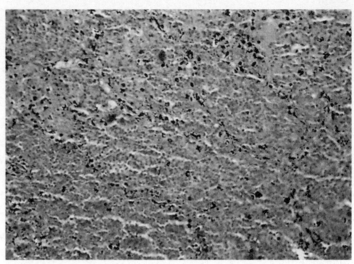

FIGURE 63-10 Goodpasture's syndrome. Bland pulmonary hemorrhage. The alveoli are filled with blood, and the alveolar walls are intact.

conditions listed in Table 63-2 can result in DAH, particularly if the insult is acute and extensive. In this setting, alveolar wall and intraalveolar edema and fibrin deposition are seen, as well as capillary congestion, capillary microthrombi, and the characteristic intraalveolar hyaline membranes. There are also a number of less common miscellaneous, but characteristic, histologic findings that present with DAH (see Table 63-2).

Clinical Features

Hemoptysis is the hallmark of DAH, but as many as 33% of patients are seen without hemoptysis. The hemoptysis may vary in amount, the frequency may range from intermittent to continuous, and it may persist from and it can last from several days to several weeks. In some instances (e.g., crack cocaine inhalation), hemoptysis may only occur for a few hours before presentation. Cough, progressive dyspnea, fatigue, and low-grade fever may accompany the hemoptysis. With extensive DAH, blood gas abnormalities can be so severe that mechanical ventilation for respiratory failure may be necessary. Other systemic symptoms, such as skin rash, visual disturbances, myalgias, and arthralgias, may also be reported, depending on the underlying etiology. Considerable intraalveolar bleeding may occur, as manifested by a falling hematocrit and a hemorrhagic bronchoalveolar lavage, without the patient experiencing hemoptysis. A sequential bronchoalveolar lavage that demonstrates bloody return and increasing red blood cell counts confirms the presence of DAH.

A prior history of hemoptysis should be sought since DAH, particularly one that occurs with the vasculitic syndromes, the collagen vascular diseases, mitral stenosis, idiopathic pulmonary hemosiderosis, and pulmonary venoocclusive disease is often recurrent. Conversely, DAH is frequently the first and only apparent manifestation of these disorders. It is important to obtain a medication history, specifically seeking use of penicillamine, crack cocaine, diphenylhydantoin, amiodarone, propylthiouracil, nitrofurantoin, and various cytotoxic drugs, because all of these have all been associated with DAH. Penicillamine, propylthiouracil, and diphenylhydantoin can produce hypersensitivity vasculitis with skin and renal involvement as well. Spontaneous DAH may occur in patients receiving

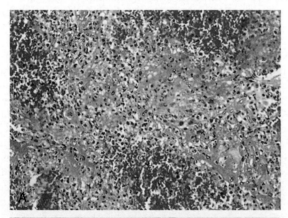

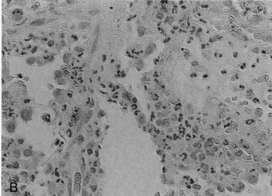

FIGURE 63-9 Pulmonary capillaritis and diffuse alveolar hemorrhage. **A,** The alveolar spaces are filled with blood in the biopsy specimen of this patient with microscopic polyangiitis. Note the marked broadening and destruction of the intervening alveolar walls. An area of fibrinoid necrosis is visible in the lower left-hand corner. **B,** Note the neutrophilic infiltration of the alveolar walls (interstitium) in this earlier stage. Some of these cells appear pyknotic and fragmented.

anticoagulant or thrombolytic agents. Although a history of prior cardiac problems may be found in patients with mitral stenosis, however, DAH may also be the first manifestation of this disorder.

Extrapulmonary physical findings are often helpful. The presence of conjunctivitis, iridocyclitis, or episcleritis points to a systemic disease, as does palpable purpura and active synovitis. Cardiac examination may disclose a heart murmur. The pulmonary examination is nonspecific.

The chest radiograph demonstrates diffuse or scattered, patchy alveolar infiltrates (Figure 63-11). Occasionally, DAH can have a more localized radiograph distribution early in its course. The cardiac silhouette and pulmonary vasculature should be examined for the possibility of mitral stenosis. In pulmonary venoocclusive disease or mitral valve disease, Kerley B lines may be seen. High-resolution computed tomographic scans of the lung offer no advantage over conventional radiography.

The urine should be evaluated for the presence of proteinuria, microscopic hematuria, or red blood cell casts, all of which are indicative of focal segmental necrotizing glomerulonephritis, a lesion common to the systemic vasculitides, the collagen vascular diseases, and Goodpasture's syndrome. The hemoglobin level is decreased (frequently with microcytic indices) and often continues to fall, and the white blood cell count may be elevated. The platelet count is either normal or increased, except in those patients with DAH secondary to bone marrow suppression as a result of the primary disease process (e.g., leukemia) or ensuing cytotoxic therapy. DAH can also complicate thrombotic thrombocytopenic purpura, idiopathic thrombocytopenic purpura, and the primary antiphospholipid antibody syndrome—conditions associated with thrombocytopenia.

Clinical Features of Selected Entities
Wegener's Granulomatosis

DAH with underlying pulmonary capillaritis is the initial manifestation of 5–10% of patients with Wegener's granulomatosis.

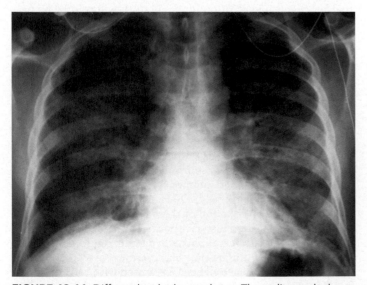

FIGURE 63-11 Diffuse alveolar hemorrhage. The radiograph shows nonspecific diffuse alveolar infiltration.

All reported cases are also associated with a focal segmental necrotizing glomerulonephritis. DAH and capillaritis may be seen in lung biopsy specimens in addition to the more typical granulomatous vasculitis. In patients whose initial manifestation is DAH, the more characteristic clinicohistologic picture may evolve months to years after the initial episode. Moreover, in patients with more classic disease, recurrences may appear in the form of acute DAH. Because of the association with glomerulonephritis, the DAH presentation in Wegener's granulomatosis mimics microscopic polyangiitis. A positive serum c-ANCA establishes the diagnosis of Wegener's granulomatosis, but a negative c-ANCA does not exclude it.

Microscopic Polyangiitis

Microscopic polyangiitis possibly represents the small vessel variant of polyarteritis nodosa. The lack of medium vessel involvement, the relatively high incidence of lung involvement in the form of DAH caused by capillaritis (33% of cases), and the absence of hypertension characterize and differentiate microscopic polyangiitis from polyarteritis nodosa. All patients with microscopic polyangiitis have focal segmental necrotizing glomerulonephritis. Additional clinical features similar to other systemic vasculitides include a dermatologic vasculitis, arthritis, myositis, gastrointestinal bleeding resulting from mucosal vasculitis, and a peripheral neuropathy. Nonspecific laboratory findings include an elevated sedimentation rate and increases in both serum rheumatoid factors and antinuclear antibodies. More specifically, antibodies to either hepatitis B or C virus are present in 33%, and serum p-ANCA is found in more than 90% of patients.

Two related entities deserve comment. The first is pauci-immune idiopathic glomerulonephritis. This histologic pattern is associated with serum p-ANCA positivity and is considered to be a localized form of renal vasculitis. In 50% of these subjects, however, DAH and other systemic manifestations evolve. It is likely that this entity initially is a localized form of microscopic polyangiitis. There is also a recently reported isolated form of alveolar capillaritis and DAH associated with p-ANCA positivity. It is not known whether these patients have a more generalized form of vasculitis develop, because follow-up data are not available.

Connective Tissue or Collagen Vascular Diseases

DAH develops in 3–4% of patients who have systemic lupus erythematosus. In a study of 15 patients, the underlying histologic finding in most was capillaritis, but bland pulmonary hemorrhage and diffuse alveolar damage were also found. Although 80–90% of the time DAH occurs in the setting of established disease, in up to 20% of patients it may be the initial manifestation. Most patients also have lupus nephritis. DAH infrequently complicates the other collagen vascular diseases. In polymyositis, rheumatoid arthritis, mixed connective tissue disease, and scleroderma DAH resulting from pulmonary capillaritis has been described, and sometimes with evidence of generalized systemic vasculitis. In these patients, and in those with systemic lupus erythematosus, granular deposition of immune complexes is often, but not always, seen. There is also a report of p-ANCA–positive DAH and glomerulonephritis in rheumatoid arthritis, but this may represent a complicating microscopic polyangiitis. Isolated DAH has also been reported in the primary antiphospholipid antibody syndrome.

Goodpasture's Syndrome

Goodpasture's syndrome (antibasement membrane antibody disease) is a distinct pulmonary-renal syndrome that causes DAH and glomerulonephritis, but without other systemic findings. Both pulmonary capillaritis and bland pulmonary hemorrhage may be responsible for the DAH. It is believed to be caused by the development of an antibody that is specific to an antigen found in the type 4 collagen of alveolar and glomerular basement membranes. This antibasement membrane antibody is also present in the serum of affected patients and is expressed in tissue as noninterrupted linear immunofluorescence with antibody to IgG and complement (see Figure 63-6). Most cases occur in the second or third decade of life, the condition is more frequent in men, and it may develop after a viral upper respiratory tract infection. In 60–80% of patients, lung and kidney manifestations appear simultaneously. In 10–30%, glomerulonephritis is the only manifestation; in 5–10%, DAH occurs without renal disease. Older affected individuals are more apt to have isolated renal disease, and active smokers in all age groups are more likely to have DAH develop alone or in combination with renal disease.

Isolated Pauci-Immune Pulmonary Capillaritis

Isolated pauci-immune pulmonary capillaritis is a newly described, small-vessel vasculitis that is confined to the lungs without serologic or clinical evidence of an accompanying collagen vascular disease or one of the systemic vasculitides listed in Table 63-2. Immunofluorescent examination of lung tissue does not reveal evidence of granular or linear immune complex deposition, and an extended follow-up of these patients failed to demonstrate the development of a systemic disease.

Henoch–Schönlein Purpura

Henoch–Schönlein purpura is a systemic vasculitis typified by circulating and tissue immune complexes consisting of IgA antibodies. Although the condition is most common in children, adults can sometimes be affected, and, in several of these, pulmonary capillaritis causing DAH has been described. Although immunoglobulin A nephropathy is a common form of glomerulonephritis in adults and includes the presence of serum and renal IgA immune complexes, DAH is a rare complication of this disorder.

Idiopathic Pulmonary Hemosiderosis and Miscellaneous Disorders

A bland, recurrent form of DAH is idiopathic pulmonary hemosiderosis (IPH). The pathogenesis of this disorder is poorly understood. More than 75% of patients have the condition develop in childhood. A review of some adult cases indicates that they are isolated pauci-immune pulmonary capillaritis, and several cases of IPH have developed a full-blown systemic vasculitis (microscopic polyangiitis) or a collagen vascular disease (systemic lupus erythematosus and rheumatoid arthritis) years after initial diagnosis. There are unexplained cases of recurrent bland pulmonary hemorrhage in adults, however, that are considered to be recurrent IPH. In addition to familial and geographic clustering, there is an association of IPH with celiac disease.

Pulmonary venoocclusive disease, another usual cause of DAH, is caused by fibrous obliteration of the postcapillary venules, leading to severe progressive pulmonary hypertension that is complicated by episodes of DAH. In some cases, a mutation in the bone morphogenesis protein receptor gene that also occurs in some cases of familial primary pulmonary hypertension has been found. Although most cases are idiopathic, pulmonary venoocclusive disease has been reported as a complication of bleomycin and carmustine therapy, thoracic radiation, human immunodeficiency virus infection, and collagen vascular disease.

Diagnosis

Establishing a diagnosis of DAH is not difficult in patients who have hemoptysis, diffuse pulmonary infiltrates, a falling hematocrit, and a sequentially hemorrhagic bronchoalveolar lavage. In those without hemoptysis, however, the bronchoalveolar lavage differentiates DAH from other acute infectious and noninfectious pulmonary processes. Table 63-3 outlines the expected findings for the more common causes of DAH.

Treatment

Treatment for the systemic vasculitides and the collagen vascular disease–associated DAH is identical to that already described for vasculitis with the addition that plasmapheresis is of use in patients with Goodpasture's syndrome and those with systemic microscopic polyangiitis and DAH. In patients with collagen vascular disease and Wegener's granulomatosis–induced DAH, the role of plasmapheresis is still questionable. For the treatment of diffuse alveolar damage–induced DAH, high-dose intravenous methylprednisolone is recommended (see previous section). Mitral stenosis causing DAH requires surgical intervention. Patients with Goodpasture's syndrome must stop smoking.

Clinical Course and Prevention

DAH occurring in the setting of a systemic vasculitis or collagen vascular disease adversely affects prognosis. More than half of these patients require mechanical ventilation, and death frequently occurs as a result of respiratory and renal failure or from superimposed infection as a complication of immunosuppressive therapy. Only 50% of patients with systemic lupus erythematosus survive the initial episode of DAH. In Wegener's granulomatosis and microscopic polyangiitis, the initial mortality is 25–30%, and the 5-year survival is also reduced (65%). The mortality and survival data are more encouraging in isolated pauci-immune pulmonary capillaritis. In Goodpasture's syndrome, the 2-year survival rate is 50%. Lower survival rates in Goodpasture's syndrome are to be expected in patients with severe renal failure and persistent DAH. An early mortality (25%) can be expected in IPH; however, 50% survive for 5 years.

The only known preventive approach that can be suggested for patients with this group of disorders is smoking cessation in patients with Goodpasture's syndrome.

Pitfalls and Controversies

In adults with isolated DAH who do not have evidence of a drug exposure, mitral stenosis, or a coagulopathy, a lung biopsy to differentiate between IPH, isolated pauciimmune pulmonary capillaritis, and Goodpasture's syndrome without renal involvement should be performed. In fact, in those patients with isolated DAH, open or thoracoscopic lung biopsy should be performed after mitral valve disease, a coagulopathy, a potential drug exposure, or conditions that can lead to diffuse alveolar damage are excluded. The clinical and

TABLE 63-3 Diagnosis of Diffuse Alveolar Hemorrhage

Disease	Glomerulo-Nephritis	Arthritis	Dermatologic Vasculitis	Anti-Nuclear Antibody	Rheumatoid Factor	Serum Complement	Antibasement Antibody Syndrome	Cytoplasmic Anti-neutrophil Cytoplasmic Antibody	Perinuclear Anti-neutrophil Cytoplasmic Antibody	Antideoxy-Ribonucleic Acid Antibody	Tissue Immuno-Complex Antibody
Wegener's granulomatosis	+	+	+	±	±	Within normal limits	−	+	±	−	−
Microscopic polyangiitis	+	+	+	±	±	Within normal limits	−	−	+	−	−
Systemic lupus erythematosus	+	+	±	+	±	Low	−	−	±	+	+ (granular)
Goodpasture's syndrome	+	−	−	−	−	Within normal limits	+	±	±	−	+ (linear)
Henoch–Schönlein purpura	+	±	+	−	−	Within normal limits	−	−	−	−	+ (IgA)
Idiopathic pauci-immune pulmonary capillaritis	−	−	−	−	−	Withinin normal limits	−	−	−	−	−
Idiopathic pulmonary hemosiderosis	−	−	−	−	−	Within normal limits	−	−	−	−	−
Pulmonary veno-occlusive disease	−	−	−	±	±	Within normal limits	−	−	−	−	Occasional

(Adapted from Schwarz MI, Cherniack RM, King TE: Diffuse alveolar hemorrhage and other rare pulmonary infiltrative disorders. In Murray J, Nadel J (eds): Textbook of Respiratory Medicine, ed 2. WB Saunders, Philadelphia, 1993, pp 1889–1912.)

radiographic features of pulmonary venoocclusive disease can be confused with mitral stenosis.

There are two potential pulmonary complications related to recurrent DAH. One is pulmonary fibrosis causing a progressive restrictive lung disease; the other is a progressive obstructive lung disease in patients with recurrent DAH resulting from pulmonary capillaritis. It is unclear why recurrent bleeding in the lung causes interstitial fibrosis. In iron-overload states such as transfusion hemosiderosis or primary hemochromatosis, pulmonary fibrosis does not occur. Obstructive lung disease is thought to be due to the development of emphysema in patients with pulmonary capillaritis because of the release of neutral proteases from destroyed neutrophils and ANCA inhibition of antiproteases.

SUGGESTED READINGS

Brown KK: Pulmonary vasculitis. Proc Am Thorac Soc 2006; 3:48–57.

D'Agati V: Antineutrophil cytoplasmic antibody and vasculitis: Much more than a disease marker. J Clin Invest 2002; 110:919–921.

Fauci AS, Haynes BF, Katz P, Wolff SM: Wegener's granulomatosis: Prospective clinical and therapeutic experience with 85 patients for 21 years. Ann Intern Med 1983; 98:76–85.

Jennette JC, Falk RJ, Andrassy K, *et al:* Nomenclature of systemic vasculitides: A proposal of an international consensus conference. Arthritis Rheum 1994; 37:187–192.

Jennings CA, King TE, Tuder R, *et al:* Diffuse alveolar hemorrhage with underlying isolated, pauciimmune pulmonary capillaritis. Am J Respir Crit Care Med 1997; 155:1101–1109.

Kelly PT, Haponik EF: Goodpasture's syndrome: Molecular and clinical advances. Medicine 1994; 73:171–185.

Schwarz MI, Brown KK: Small vessel vasculitis of the lung. Thorax 2000; 55:502–510.

Schwarz MI, Cherniack RM, King TE: Diffuse alveolar hemorrhage and other rare pulmonary infiltrative disorders. In Murray J, Nadel J, eds: Textbook of Respiratory Medicine, 3rd ed. Philadelphia: WB Saunders; 2000:1733–1756.

Specks U: Pulmonary vasculitis. In Schwarz MI, King TE, eds: Interstitial Lung Disease, 4th ed. Hamilton, Canada: BC Decker; 1998: 507–534.

Specks U: Diffuse alveolar hemorrhage syndromes. Curr Opin Rheumatol 2001; 13:12–17.

Travis WD, Hoffman GS, Leavitt RY, *et al:* Surgical pathology of the lung in Wegener's granulomatosis. Am J Surg Pathol 1991; 15:315–333.

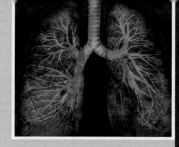

64 Silicosis and Coal Worker's Pneumoconiosis

BENOIT WALLAERT • SYLVIE LEROY

Pneumoconiosis has been defined as the nonneoplastic reaction of the lung to inhaled mineral or organic dust. The prolonged inhalation of coalmine dust may result in the development of coal worker's pneumoconiosis (CWP), silicosis, and industrial chronic bronchitis and emphysema, either singly or in various combinations. CWP is the term generally applied to interstitial disease of the lung resulting from chronic exposure to coal dust, its inhalation and deposition, and the tissue reaction of the host to its presence, whereas silicosis is due to inhalation of dust containing silica. The pneumoconioses differ in a number of ways from the acute allergic and toxic interstitial diseases, which are associated with exposure to organic dusts, principally because of their long latency periods (usually 10–20 years or more) between exposure onset and disease recognition.

SOURCES OF EXPOSURE

Coal is not a mineral of fixed composition. Coal is graded by rank, reflecting its carbon content and thus combustibility: anthracite is the highest ranked coal, with a carbon content of approximately 98%. Lower ranked coals, bituminous and sub-bituminous, have carbon contents of approximately 90–95% carbon. The rank of coal has an influence on the risk of disease: higher-rank coals entail higher risk than lower-rank coals. However, exposure to coal dust with a quartz concentration greater than 15% is associated with a high risk of a rapidly progressive form of pneumoconiosis that has the characteristics of silicosis. In open mines, dust levels rarely approach those of underground mines.

The most common form of crystalline silica is quartz. Quartz is almost pure silicone dioxide but often contains traces of other elements. Other crystalline forms of silica are cristobalite and tridymite. The importance of silica as a health hazard is due to its ubiquity (Table 64-1). Diatomite is a siliceous sedimentary rock used for filtration; for heat and sound insulation; as an adsorbent; as a filter for plastics, paper, and insecticides; and for floor coverings.

It seems that development and progression of silicosis depend on the total amount of quartz to which workers are exposed, the time over which that exposure occurs, and the presence of others minerals that may interfere with the toxicity of the quartz.

Epidemiology

CWP was first recognized in Scottish miners in 1830. In recent decades, the incidence of CWP has been declining in industrial countries because of improved dust controls, although increased mechanization in the mid-1960s led to a temporary increase in dust levels. In parallel, through the period 1950–1980, the annual UK rate for the recognition of CWP for state compensation in current and retired miners decreased from approximately 7% to 1–2%. The overall prevalence of CWP, which reflects more distant exposure and earlier incidence, declined from approximately 13% to 5%, but there were substantial regional differences. Similar regional differences and similar declines have been noted in the United States and other countries.

PATHOPHYSIOLOGY

There are three groups of factors known to influence the character and severity of lung tissue reaction to the mineral dusts. The risk of pneumoconiosis is related to the intensity and years of exposure. However, among a group of workers exposed to the same dust, only a fraction have pneumoconiosis develop because of an individual susceptibility. The nature and properties of each specific dust constitute the third factor under consideration. For each mineral, geometric and aerodynamic properties, chemistry, and surface properties have to be considered. The particles that can cause pneumoconiosis are those aerodynamically and geometrically small enough to reach the respiratory bronchioles and be deposited there—this generally means spherical particles 0.5–5 μm.

The pathogenesis of pneumoconiosis is similar to that of all interstitial lung diseases. There is a chronic inflammatory state (alveolitis) in which inflammatory cells are activated and damage the pulmonary architecture. Inorganic particles are phagocytosed by alveolar macrophages, causing activation and the release of inflammatory mediators such as cytokines and arachidonic acid metabolites. The mediators, in turn, induce the recruitment of other inflammatory cells within the alveolar wall and on the alveolar epithelial surface. The alveolitis is dominated by alveolar macrophages. Toxic oxygen derivatives and proteolytic enzymes are released by the inflammatory cells, which cause cellular damage and disruption of the extracellular matrix.

The inflammatory phase is followed by a reparative phase in which growth factors stimulate the recruitment and proliferation of mesenchymal cells and regulate neovascularization and reepithelialization of injured tissues. During this phase, abnormal, or uncontrolled, reparative mechanisms may result in the development of fibrosis. Fibrogenic particles activate proinflammatory cytokine production within the respiratory tract. Tumor necrosis factor (TNF)-α seems to play a key role in the recruitment of inflammatory cells induced by toxic dusts (Figure 64-1). In addition, neutrophils recruited in the area

TABLE 64-1 Major Industries with Silica Exposure

Occupation	Exposure
Sand blaster	Ship building, oil rig maintenance, preparing steel for painting
Miner	Surface coal mining, roof bolting, shot firing, drilling, tunneling
Miller	Silica flour
Glass maker	Polishing with sand and enamel work
Potter	Crushing flint and fettling, foundry work, mold making and cleaning, vitreous enameling, manufacture of cultured quartz crystal
Quarry and stone worker	Cutting of slate, sandstone, and granite
Abrasive worker	Inhalation of fine particles during grinding

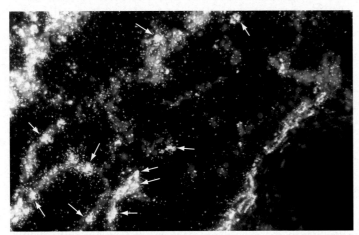

FIGURE 64-1 Expression of tumor necrosis factor-α messenger RNA. Tumor necrosis factor-α messenger RNA (by *in situ* hybridization) is expressed in alveolar macrophages *(arrows)* in lung section from a patient with coal worker's pneumoconiosis.

of inflammation may contribute to the alveolitis, and respiratory and endothelial cells may play a further role by releasing various chemokines such as interleukin (IL)-8. Last, growth factors such as platelet-derived growth factor, insulin-like growth factor, fibroblast growth factor, and transforming growth factor-β are involved in the pathogenesis of lung fibrosis and in the proliferative response of type II epithelial cells, which occurs in progressive massive fibrosis.

GENETICS

More recently, associations of polymorphisms in genes coding for inflammatory cytokines like TNF-α, IL-6, IL-18, and their receptors have been reported with CWP incidence, prevalence, and progression. In silicosis, a significant association was found between disease severity and the TNF-α-238 variant. Irrespective of disease severity, the TNF-α-308 and IL-1RA + 2018 variants conferred an increased risk for the presence of disease. The TNF-α polymorphisms in positions 238, 376, and 308 of the promoter region were also found associated with severe silicosis in South African miners. In French coalminers differentially exposed to coal dust and cigarette smoke, the TNF-α-308 SNP showed an interaction

with erythrocyte GSH-Px activity in individuals with high occupational exposure, whereas the lymphotoxin-α (LTA) *Nco*I polymorphism was associated with CWP prevalence in miners with low blood catalase activity. An understanding of genetic variability and environmental factors is crucial to the identification of high-risk individuals and prevention and treatment of CWP.

PATHOLOGY

The lesions of CWP are focal. Simple CWP is associated with the macular and nodular lesions, whereas complicated CWP is associated with progressive massive fibrosis (PMF) and the lesions of rheumatoid pneumoconiosis (Caplan syndrome).

The initial lesions in the lung are the coal dust macules, which correspond macroscopically to focal areas of black pigmentation. Microscopically, the macule is composed of coal dust–laden macrophages within the walls of the respiratory bronchioles and adjacent alveoli (Figure 64-2). Focal emphysema around the coal dust macule is common and is considered an integral part of the lesion of simple CWP.

The histologic hallmark of simple CWP is the nodule. The nodules are rounded lesions with collagenous centers. Microscopically, the nodule can be divided into three zones: a central zone composed of whorls of dense, hyalinized fibrous tissue; a middle zone made up of concentrically arranged collagen fibers (onion skinning); and a peripheral zone of more randomly oriented collagen fibers mixed with dust-laden macrophages and lymphoid cells (Figure 64-3). "Old" inactive nodules are often relatively acellular. Particles of silica may be demonstrated in the nodules as birefringent particles under polarized light. Nodules represent a form of mixed dust fibrosis (i.e., coal dust plus silica exposure), are usually found in association with macules, and in some instances may develop from preexisting macules. They are not confined to the respiratory bronchioles but are also seen in the subpleural and peribronchial connective tissues. There is a tendency for nodules to cluster and eventually coalesce to produce PMF. Degenerative changes are commonly observed in the nodular lesions, including calcification, cholesterol clefts, and cavitation. In severe silicosis, there may be structural alterations of the pulmonary vasculature resulting from the accumulation of

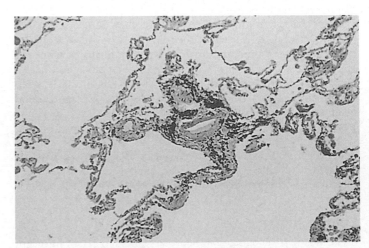

FIGURE 64-2 Macular lesion of coal worker's pneumoconiosis. This coal macule consists of collections of macrophages that are laded with coal dust and extend into the connective tissue surrounding the respiratory bronchioles.

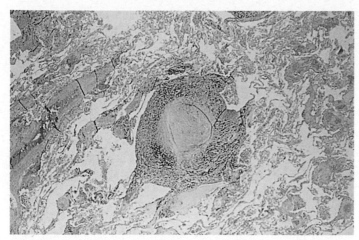

FIGURE 64-3 Coal nodule. Coal nodule is a rounded lesion with a collagenous center and a peripheral anthracotic pigmented area. This nodule shows a smooth, sharp border, dust-laden macrophages, and laminated collagen deposition within the interstitium of the lung. The small central area is pale and rich in collagen, and the periphery contains a varying amount of fibrogenic dust.

dust in the adventitia of large vessels and involvement of the smaller blood vessels by silicotic nodules.

PMF is defined as an opacity or fibrotic pneumoconiotic lesion of 1 cm in diameter or greater. PMF lesions appear as black fibrotic masses that may be round, oval, or irregular in shape. The lung and bronchovascular rays become markedly distorted. Microscopically, the lesions are composed of bundles of haphazardly arranged hyalinized collagen fibers and/or reticulin fibers and coal dust. Dust particles near the periphery of the lesion are mainly found within macrophages, whereas in the center, the dust tends to lie free in clefts and cavities. Areas of liquefactive necrosis containing fragments of degenerating collagen as well as cholesterol crystals are frequently observed.

The pathology of acute silicosis is quite different from the chronic form. There is infiltration of the alveolar walls with plasma cells, lymphocytes, and fibroblasts with some collagenation. The alveoli are filled with an eosinophilic coagulum (Figure 64-4). Electron microscopy shows widening of alveolar walls with some collagen and clusters of type II cells; the

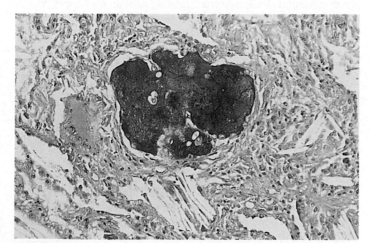

FIGURE 64-4 Acute silicosis. Infiltration of the alveolar walls by plasma cells and lymphocytes. Note the alveoli filled with an eosinophilic coagulum.

alveolar spaces contain degenerating cells that are probably type II alveolar cells and macrophages. Silica particles may be demonstrated in the lungs and lymph nodes; silicotic nodules are few or absent.

CLINICAL FEATURES AND DIAGNOSIS

Coal worker's pneumoconiosis and silicosis are generally first recognized from the plain chest radiograph, which is also critical in evaluating disease progression. Requirements for the diagnosis include a history of significant exposure, radiographic features consistent with these illnesses, and the absence of illnesses that may mimic these diseases (primarily infections with a predominantly miliary radiographic pattern, such as tuberculosis, fungal infections, or sarcoidosis). The radiographic appearances are most usefully described by the coding system devised for standard films of pneumoconiosis under the auspices of the International Labour Office (ILO) (Table 64-2). In clinical practice, simple CWP is characterized by small rounded opacities (nodules) rather than small irregular opacities, although the latter may be seen in much lesser profusion (profusion categories [0–3] are the number of small opacities apparent on the chest radiograph). When large opacities occurred, the term *progressive massive fibrosis (PMF)* or *complicated CWP* is in common use.

Clinical Features

Simple CWP and category A–complicated CWP are not associated with respiratory symptoms. As in most populations engaged in manual work, breathlessness and cough in coal miners are usually a consequence of cigarette smoking. However, coalmine dust may itself cause chronic bronchitis and chronic obstructive pulmonary disease, which together are known as *industrial bronchitis*. The evidence that coal dust

TABLE 64-2 International Labour Organization Radiographic Classification of Pneumoconioses

Small Opacities*	Regular	Irregular
< 1.5 mm in diameter	p	s
> 1.5 mm but < 3 mm in diameter	q	t
> 3 mm but < 10 mm in diameter	r	u

*Small opacities are defined by their average size and profusion.

Profusion: 0–3†

Large opacities (PMF or complicated CWP)‡

> 10 mm in diameter

Category
A - sum of diameters of lesions is not more than 50 mm
B - total area occupied by lesions is not greater than the area of the right upper zone
C - total area occupied by lesions is greater than the area of the right upper zone
†Profusion categories (0–3) refer to the concentration (density) of small opacities apparent on the radiograph: category 0, small opacities are absent or less profuse than category 1; 1, few in number; 2, numerous; 3, opacities are very numerous and obscure the normal radiographic markings.
‡Complicated pneumoconiosis or progressive massive fibrosis is divided into categories based on the size of the large opacities. To be classified as progressive massive fibrosis, at least one nodule should be 1 cm or greater.

exposure is associated with the development of significant respiratory impairment has led to it becoming a compensable disease despite the absence of CWP.

By contrast, complicated pneumoconiosis (PMF) at categories B and C may present with undue breathlessness and productive cough. Melanoptysis is the result of necrosis within the conglomerate, coal-containing lesions that characterize PMF. Progressive, undue exertional dyspnea is usually the dominant symptom, but rarely there may be breathlessness at rest.

There are no specific abnormal physical signs in CWP. Finger clubbing and fine inspiratory crackles are not features of the disease, and, if these are present, another explanation should be sought. Only in a small proportion of severe cases of complicated disease does CWP evolve to produce chronic respiratory failure and cor pulmonale.

Irrespective of PMF, there are a number of other disorders with which CWP may be associated—most notably the autoimmune disorders of rheumatoid disease and progressive systemic sclerosis. The association of rheumatoid disease with CWP is known as Caplan syndrome (Figure 64-5). The diagnosis is suggested by the association of coal dust exposure, rheumatoid arthritis, and multiple well-defined large, rounded opacities (nodules with >10 mm diameter) on the chest radiograph. Spontaneous disappearance is common, with or without initial cavitation, and new nodules commonly emerge in different locations. The Caplan nodule is also more likely to cavitate, thereby producing a concentric ring pattern, and so is also known as a necrobiotic nodule. Central necrosis is rare in nodules of CWP, although it may occur in conglomerate lesions.

CWP has also been linked with a number of specific infections, the most prominent of which has been tuberculosis. In contrast to silicosis, however, CWP does not increase significantly the risk for infection with *Mycobacterium tuberculosis*. Nontuberculous mycobacteria, on the other hand, may infect lungs damaged by CWP and other types of pneumoconiosis with greater than usual frequency, and so CWP does seem to increase the risk for infection with opportunistic organisms. *Mycobacterium avium* is probably the most important of these and is poorly sensitive to antibiotic agents. *Mycobacterium kansasii* and *Mycobacterium malmoense* may also be pathogenic in

this setting. It may similarly be difficult to attribute change in the radiographic appearances to advancing infection or progressive PMF. Experimental studies also suggest that mycobacterial infection is a factor that helps explain the progression from simple to complicated pneumoconiosis.

Other opportunistic infections reported in association with CWP have included nocardiosis, sporotrichosis, and cryptococcosis; *Aspergillus* spp. have been noted to colonize cavities in conglomerate lesions of complicated CWP.

A further association with complicated CWP, if manifested by bullous emphysema, is spontaneous pneumothorax. The advanced stages of complicated CWP are also associated with recurrent episodes of acute and subacute bronchitis. Persistent productive cough is common in coal miners in the absence of CWP. There is no evidence of a causal relationship between silicosis and carcinoma of the lung, although association is consistent for silicotics and limited nonsilicotic workers. The available data leave open the issue as to whether silica per se materially increases lung cancer risk in absence of silicosis. In 1997, the International Agency for Research on Cancer (IARC) classified crystalline silica dust exposure as a known human carcinogen, group 1. Currently, CWP and silicosis should be considered conditions that predispose workers to an increased risk of lung cancer.

Accelerated silicosis is rare and is clinically identical to the classic forms of silicosis, except that the time from initial exposure to the onset of disease is shorter and the rate of progression of disease is dramatically faster.

Acute silicosis is rare. Symptoms begin with cough, weight loss, and fatigue; there may be rapid progression to fulminant respiratory failure over several months. Chest auscultation reveals diffuse crackles, and workers with this clinical picture rapidly have cor pulmonale develop and progress to a respiratory death. Survival after the onset of symptoms is often less than 2 years. Diffuse alveolar filling, most apparent at the bases, is the most prominent finding on the chest X-ray (Figure 64-6). Although serial chest X-rays from workers with this illness have been infrequently reported, it seems that the bibasilar filling pattern progresses into large opacities located in the middle zones rather than the upper zones.

Chest Radiology

The radiographic pattern of simple CWP is typically one of small rounded opacities that appear first in the upper zones (Figure 64-7). The middle and lower zones become involved as the number of opacities increases. The nodules increase in profusion with increasing dust exposure; a change in profusion after dust exposure has ceased is very unusual. Calcification of the nodules may occur (10–20% of cases).

Complicated pneumoconiosis is defined as a lesion of 1 cm or greater in longest diameter. The large opacities are usually predominant in the upper lobes, may be unilateral or bilateral, and are symmetrically or asymmetrically distributed. The pattern of change in size is variable and unpredictable. Most PMF occurs on a background of simple pneumoconiosis, but this is not invariably so, and it may occur after dust exposure has ceased. Cavitation can develop within a PMF lesion (Figure 64-8), and occasionally there is a dense peripheral arc or rim at its lower pole that represents calcification. Dense calcification with the lesion is also sometimes seen. PMF is often associated with bullous emphysema and fibrotic scarring, leading to distortion of the lung and shift of the trachea and mediastinum to the affected side. Irregular, mainly basal, opacities

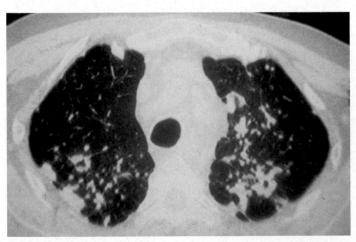

FIGURE 64-5 Caplan syndrome. High-resolution computed tomography scan obtained at the level of the upper lobes showing bilateral parenchymal micronodules and coalescence in the right upper lobe. Note the cavitation of the nodule in the left upper lobe.

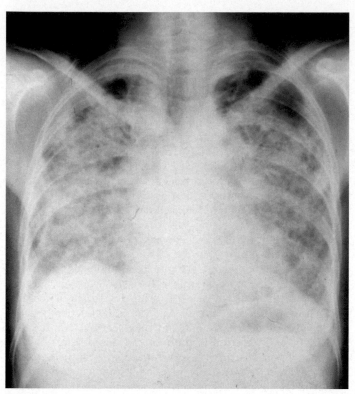

FIGURE 64-6 Chest X-ray showing alveolar filling in acute silicosis. A 28-year-old woman inhaled fine particles of silica from abrasive powder. The disease that has developed was rapidly progressive silicosis, which was typically fatal over the next several years.

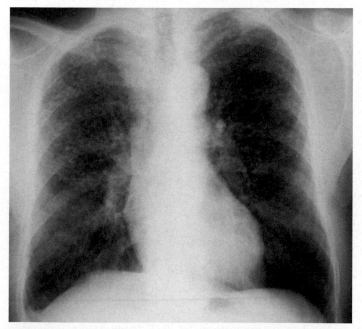

FIGURE 64-7 Chest X-ray of simple coal worker's pneumoconiosis. Simple coal worker's pneumoconiosis in a 55-year-old man who had worked for 18 years in an underground coal mine. He was a nonsmoker with a chronic cough and normal lung function. The X-ray shows a diffuse distribution of small rounded opacities, more prominent in the upper zones than the lower zones.

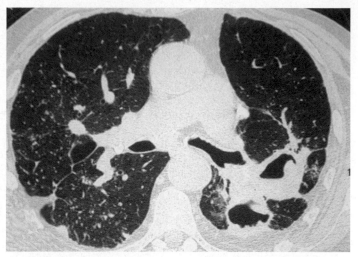

FIGURE 64-8 Cavitation within progressive massive fibrosis lesion. High-resolution computed tomography showing cavitation of the left masses. Note the diffuse micronodulation and associated emphysema.

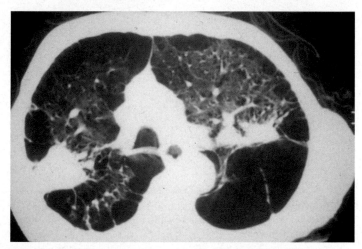

FIGURE 64-9 Progressive massive fibrosis. High-resolution computed tomography scan showing bilateral masses consistent with progressive massive fibrosis. There is a background of nodules associated with bullous changes around progressive massive fibrosis lesions referred to as paracicatricial emphysema.

may also be seen on standard radiographs. Eggshell calcification is uncommon in CWP but may occur in intrapulmonary, hilar, or mediastinal lymph nodes, possibly because of concomitant exposure to silica. Pleural effusion is uncommon in CWP. Its presence may be related to an associated infection or an interaction with a systemic collagen vascular disease.

In simple CWP, CT shows parenchymal lesions that can be detected in miners with normal chest radiographs. There is thus greater sensitivity compared with plain radiographs in detecting simple CWP, but less obvious benefit for complicated pneumoconiosis. There is a posterior and right-sided predominance in the upper zones.

Nodules are usually observed against a background of parenchymal micronodules and are generally associated with subpleural micronodules. Two categories of lesions can be observed in PMF: lesions with irregular borders that are associated with disruption of the pulmonary parenchyma and lead to typical scar emphysema (Figure 64-9) and lesions with regular borders that are unassociated with scar emphysema. When the lesions are >4 cm in diameter, irregular areas of aseptic necrosis can be observed with or without cavitation (Figure 64-10).

Two major forms of emphysema occurring in coal workers can be detected on CT: bullous changes around PMF lesions (see Figure 64-9), referred to as paracicatricial or scar emphysema, whereas nonbullous emphysematous lesions are defined as irregular emphysema (Figure 64-11). Lesions of diffuse pulmonary fibrosis can be detected on high-resolution CT as honeycombing or areas of ground-glass attenuation. Two specific etiologies of fibrosis of coal miners should be considered: a direct effect of deposited coal or silica particles and an indirect effect resulting from an association with scleroderma. In addition, the extent of air trapping on expiratory thin-section CT scans may assess obstructive abnormalities.

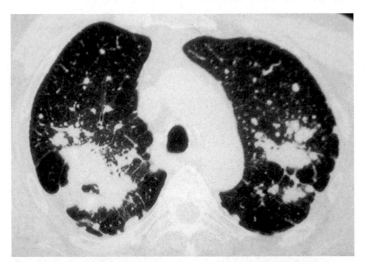

FIGURE 64-10 Aseptic necrosis. Computed tomography scan showing bilateral masses with necrosis of the right upper lobe mass and bilateral emphysema.

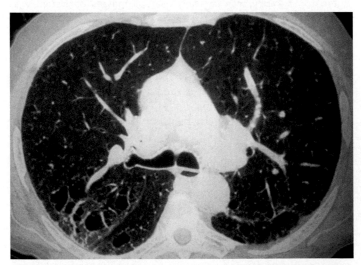

FIGURE 64-11 Nonbullous emphysema. High-resolution computed tomography scan showing small bullae and low attenuation, without progressive massive fibrosis lesions, defined as centrilobular or nonparacicatricial emphysema.

Lung Function

In all studies about lung function of patients with pneumoconiosis, account should be taken of a number of different and confounding influences; the effects of smoking need to be considered. It can be stated that simple CWP has no important effect on spirometric measures when prior dust exposure is taken into account and when smoking habits are also considered. Similarly, simple silicosis has no appreciable effect on lung function. In more advanced disease, slight reduction in volumes, compliance, and gas transfer can be present; there is a predominantly restrictive pattern. Slight reduction in arterial oxygen tension on effort may be observed in advanced disease. Oxygen desaturation is not present at rest or on moderate effort in the nonconglomerate stages of disease. As in the case of radiographic progression, the changes in pulmonary function are more likely to occur in workers who have had intense exposure to dust. In addition, it must be pointed out that miners who did not have CWP on chest radiography exhibited lower forced expiratory volume in 1 sec than controls, suggesting the frequent presence of coal dust–induced chronic obstructive pulmonary disease. In PMF, lung function depends on the extent of the lesions and of associated emphysema. Studies of lung function in the more advanced stages of PMF have shown an obstructive and restrictive pattern; therefore, diffusing capacity is usually reduced. Compliance is usually somewhat decreased. Ultimately, hypoxemic respiratory failure may occur.

Serologic and Immunologic Features

There are no specific biologic features of pneumoconiosis. However, immunologic abnormalities are now well described: positive circulating antinuclear antibodies or rheumatoid factor. Serum immunoglobulins A and G have significantly raised levels in miners with pneumoconiosis. Finally, increased serum angiotensin-converting enzyme level was observed in 45% of pneumoconiotic coal miners, whatever the radiologic classification of pneumoconiosis.

Bronchoalveolar Lavage

There was no change in differential cell count, in contrast to a number of other interstitial disorders of the lung. Alveolar inflammatory cells from patients with CWP, especially those with PMF, released spontaneously more superoxide anions, proinflammatory cytokines, and profibrotic mediators than did those from control subjects.

CLINICAL COURSE, TREATMENT, AND PREVENTION

Prognosis

Simple CWP is not associated with premature mortality, but approximately 4% of deaths in coal miners are due directly to complicated pneumoconiosis. In categories 1, 2, and 3 of simple CWP and category A of complicated CWP, life expectancy is the same as that among the general population without pneumoconiosis.

The rate of progression to PMF seems to be influenced chiefly by the age at which the miner begins to show radiographic changes of CWP; the earlier the diagnosis, the more likely there is to be progression reflecting individual susceptibility and the level of cumulative exposure.

Management

No specific treatment affects the course of CWP, although treatment options are available for complications such as tuberculosis, pneumothorax, and chronic hypoxemia.

When a miner is found to have CWP, further dust exposure should be excluded. Simple pneumoconiosis does not necessarily imply complete exclusion from mining, whereas when PMF is detected, all further dusty work should be prevented. Additional information is given from pulmonary function tests, because the development of an obstructive ventilatory defect (resulting from dust exposure) may occur in the absence of CWP. In all smoking patients, advice and support of smoking cessation should be given. If a physician concludes there is disability from CWP, he or she should be able to direct the patient toward whatever mechanism exists for compensation.

Prevention

The prevention of pneumoconiosis depends on controlling exposure concentrations of ambient dust to levels known to be associated with minimal and acceptable risk. Dust control is affected primarily by ventilation, although water sprayed at points of dust generation is a useful measure of dust suppression. The effectiveness of such measures should be monitored by regular measurement of dust concentrations and by regular clinical and radiologic surveillance of the workforce. Surveillance allows early recognition of workers with simple pneumoconiosis, who are likely to be those with greatest susceptibility, so that ongoing exposure can be restricted (perhaps by transfer to jobs with lower exposure) and the risk of future disablement from PMF reduced.

Variability of individual susceptibility is likely to be an important determinant for CWP, as it is for most occupational disorders, and a number of predictive factors may be useful in identifying miners with higher than average risk: initial presence of expiratory wheezes, obstructive pattern of lung function, and more micronodules on CT scan. An alternative approach for the future might involve genetic screening evaluating polymorphism in the promoter of various mediators.

In any event, control of exposure levels alone is likely to prevent most cases of disabling PMF, and it has been predicted that an exposure concentration over 35 working years that does not exceed an average of 4.3 mg/m^3 is associated with a probability for the development of category 2 or more CWP of no more than 3.4%. This represents a dramatic reduction in risk over the past 50 years.

SUGGESTED READINGS

Attfield MD, Seixas NS: Prevalence of pneumoconiosis and its relationship to dust exposure in a cohort of U.S. bituminous coal miners and exminers. Am J Ind Med 1995; 27:137–151.

Begin R, Cantin A, Massé S: Recent advances in the pathogenesis and clinical assessment of mineral dust pneumoconioses: Asbestosis, silicosis and coal pneumoconiosis. Eur Respir J 1989; 2:988–1001.

Goldsmith DF: Research and policy implications of IARC's Classification of silica as a Group 1 carcinogen. Indoor and Built Environment 1999; 8:136–142.

International Agency for Research on Cancer: http://www.iarc.fr/

Piguet PF, Collart MA, Grau GE, et al: Requirement of tumour necrosis factor for development of silica-induced pulmonary fibrosis. Nature 1990; 344:245–247.

Remy-Jardin M, Remy J, Farre I, Marquette CH: Computed tomography evaluation of silicosis and coal worker's pneumoconiosis. Radiol Clin North Am 1992; 30:1155–1176.

Rom WN, Bitterman PB, Rennard SI, et al: Characterization of the lower respiratory tract inflammation of nonsmoking individuals with interstitial lung disease associated with chronic inhalation of inorganic dust. Am Rev Respir Dis 1987; 136:1429–1434.

Vanhee D, Gosset P, Boitelle A, et al: Cytokines and cytokine network in silicosis and coal workers' pneumoconiosis. Eur Respir J 1995; 8:1–9.

Wouters EFM, Jorna THJM, Westenend M: Respiratory effects of coal dust exposure: Clinical effects and diagnosis. Exp Lung Res 1994; 20:385–394.

Yu It, Tse LA: Exploring the join effects of silicosis and smoking on lung cancer risks. Int J Cancer 2007; 120:133–139.

Yucesoy B, Luster MI: Genetic susceptibility in pneumoconiosis. Toxicol Lett 2007; 168:249–254.

Zhai R, Jetten M, Schins RP, et al: Polymorphisms in the promoter of the tumor necrosis factor alpha in coal miners. Ann J Ind Med 1998; 34:318–324.

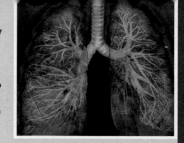

65 Asbestosis

LEE S. NEWMAN • E. BRIGITTE GOTTSCHALL

Inhalational exposure to asbestos produces both malignant and nonmalignant diseases of the chest. In this chapter, the focus is on the two major categories of nonmalignant disease—asbestosis and asbestos-related pleural disorders, presented in Table 65-1. These conditions have received a great deal of attention from the scientific and medical communities because of the ubiquitous use of asbestos in modern society and its diverse and pernicious toxicities. Despite major progress in the awareness and control of exposure, a large burden of asbestos-related disease will continue because of ongoing exposure and because of disease latency.

EPIDEMIOLOGY, RISK FACTORS, AND PATHOLOGY

Epidemiology

The first well-documented cases of asbestosis were reported in 1906 among asbestos textile workers. Through the 1920s and 1930s, reports emerged of asbestosis, pleural thickening, pleural calcification, and right ventricular failure in asbestos-exposed workers. Radiographic studies that began in the 1930s documented an asbestosis prevalence of 25–55% in these workers, especially among those who have greater cumulative exposure. With thousands of commercial applications and the mineral's resistance to degradation, asbestos remains ubiquitous. Between 1940 and 1979, more than 20 million people had potential exposure in the United States alone. Given the long latency required before asbestosis becomes clinically apparent, past and current asbestos workers must all be considered to be at risk of this fibrosing lung disorder. Disability and mortality from asbestosis will continue well into the 21st century.

Etiology and Risk Factors

The minerals referred to herein as asbestos are a family of naturally occurring, flexible, fibrous hydrous silicates found in soil worldwide. Mined asbestos fibers are categorized as either long and curly (serpentine) or straight and rodlike (amphibole). The serpentine fiber, chrysotile, accounts for most of the commercially used asbestos, favored for its properties of heat resistance, flexibility, and ease of spinning for textiles. There are five categories of amphiboles—crocidolite, amosite, anthophyllite, tremolite, and actinolite. These more rigid fibers are less commonly used but are still pathogenic. All major commercial forms have been associated with nonmalignant respiratory disorders and with lung cancer and mesothelioma, as discussed in Chapters 47 and 70.

Asbestosis is the result of either direct or bystander exposure to asbestos-containing materials. Major sources of exposure are summarized in Table 65-2. During the first half of the 20th century, high exposures to asbestos dust occurred in the manufacturing of asbestos textiles and construction materials and in the construction and shipbuilding trades. Potential exposures still occur in the construction trades and in the process of asbestos abatement. Although the use of asbestos has been curtailed in many developed nations since the 1970s, in less-developed countries this inexpensive but hazardous material continues to be used widely. High cumulative, occupational exposures in these settings are still commonplace.

Environmental exposure to asbestiform fibers is also well described as the cause of nonmalignant and malignant asbestos-related lung disease in countries such as Turkey, Greece, Japan, China, and New Caledonia. Exposure in these settings usually occurs when villagers in rural areas disturb natural soil deposits while working in fields or when applying whitewash prepared from these outcrops to their dwellings. In the United States, asbestos-related lung disease caused by nonoccupational exposures is a recently recognized problem, mostly in current and former residents of Libby, Montana. Amphibole asbestos–contaminated vermiculite was mined, milled, and processed near this small town for many years. Personal and commercial use of the contaminated mineral was widespread among residents. During a health screening in 2000/2001, nearly 18% of 6668 participants were noted to have pleural thickening on chest radiographs. Less than 1% had findings compatible with asbestosis.

A clear dose-response relationship exists between asbestos exposure and asbestosis, although controversy remains concerning risks at low-level exposure. Risk for asbestosis varies widely among industries, with more disease seen in textile and construction workers than with those in mining. Development of the disease is associated with factors such as how respirable the fiber type is, the cumulative dose of exposure, the capacity of the lung to clear the fibers, and the biopersistence of the asbestos. In general, the relative risk of asbestosis developing for asbestos workers increases in proportion to the asbestos exposure levels in the workplace. More severe disease has been associated with higher retention of asbestos fiber in the lungs. Typical asbestos fibers found in the lungs are 20–50-μm long, and are initially deposited at the bifurcations of conducting airways. Thin fibers, of diameters <3 μm, translocate readily into the alveolar space, interstitium, and pleural space. Thicker fibers tend to be incompletely phagocytosed by alveolar macrophages and are retained in the

TABLE 65-1 Nonmalignant Asbestos-Related Diseases

Condition	Pathologic Effect	Description
Asbestosis	Parenchymal effect	Interstitial pulmonary fibrosis
Benign nodules	Parenchymal effect	Lymphoid or fibrotic nodular scars
Benign pleural effusion	Pleural effect	Exudative, transient effusion
Pleural plaques	Pleural effect	Collagenous, hyalinized masses; circumscribed, avascular, usually affecting the parietal pleura
Diffuse pleural thickening	Pleural effect	Collagenous, hyalinized masses; diffuse, avascular, affecting the parietal and visceral pleura, and interlobular space
Rounded atelectasis	Combined pleural and parenchymal effects	Scarring of pleura and adjacent lung tissue, resulting in retraction, entrapment, and local partial collapse of lung

The nonmalignant diseases caused by asbestos. Categorization is based on the effects on the lung parenchyma and pleura.

TABLE 65-2 Major Asbestos Uses and Sources of Exposure

Environment	Type of Exposure	Source of Exposure
Occupational	Asbestos-cement products	Construction industry (sheeting used in roofing and cladding of structural materials, molded into roof tiles, pipes, gutters; filler for wall cracks, cement, joint compound, adhesive, caulking putty)
	Floor tiling	Filler and reinforcing agent in asphalt flooring, vinyl tile, adhesive
	Insulation, fireproofing	Insulators, pipefitters
		Construction industry (pipes, boiler covers, ship bulkheads, sprayed on walls and ceilings as fireproofing, soundproofing)
	Textiles	Fireproof textiles used in clothing, blankets
	Paper products	Roofing felt, wall coverings, mill board, insulating paper
	Friction materials	Brake linings
	Rubber, plastic manufacture	Filler in rubber and plastics
	Building trades, secondhand exposure	Building maintenance activities, pipefitting, electrical repair, boiler tending and repair, boiler tending and repair, power station maintenance
		Carpenters, plumbers, welders
Domestic	"Fouling the nest"	Carrying home asbestos in hair and clothes of exposed workers results in exposure to family members
	Secondhand exposure	Residential remodeling, removal, handling of frayed, friable asbestos in homes can cause environmental exposure
General	Contaminated buildings	Found in low levels in buildings under normal use
		Elevated exposures from remodeling, renovation, asbestos removal, disturbance of contaminated materials such as acoustic ceiling tiles, vinyl floor tiles, paints, plaster, pipes, boilers, steel beams
	Geologic exposure	Living near asbestos mines or cement factories, or in geographic areas in which naturally occurring asbestos is found in ambient air
	Urban environment	Ambient air levels slightly higher in cities, perhaps because of automotive brakes, and high concentration of industry and construction

The major enviromental and occupation sources of asbestos exposure. Categorization is based on exposures in the workplace, home, or general environment.

lung, where they can trigger the inflammatory events that lead to fibrosis, as discussed in the following section.

Pathology

Asbestosis is defined pathologically as bilateral, diffuse interstitial fibrosis of the lungs caused by the inhalation of asbestos fibers (Figure 65-1). Gray streaks of fibrosis can be seen in the parenchyma along interlobar and interlobular septa. Later, the pleural surface becomes more nodular in appearance, and the parenchyma loses volume and elasticity and forms more fibrotic scars and honeycombing. The gross pathologic appearance is most obvious in the lower lung zones bilaterally, with the worst disease nearest to the pleura. The pathology

definition remains unclear. The College of American Pathologists has defined four grades of severity:

- Grade 1—fibrosis that involves the wall of a respiratory bronchiole
- Grade 2—Grade 1 plus involvement of alveolar ducts and adjacent alveoli, but with some nonfibrotic adjacent alveolar septae
- Grade 3—Grade 2 fibrosis, but with coalescence, such that all alveoli between two adjacent bronchi show fibrotic septa, with some complete obliteration
- Grade 4—Grade 3 fibrosis plus honeycombing

A supplementary scoring system has been developed to describe the degree of airway involvement.

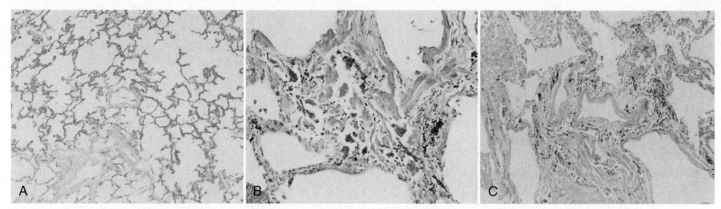

FIGURE 65-1 Histology of asbestosis. **A,** In this grade 1 lesion, fibrosis is limited to the peribronchiolar tissue and the walls of the respiratory bronchioles (hematoxylin and eosin). **B,** Enlargement of a grade 1 lesion illustrates presence of asbestos bodies (hematoxylin and eosin). **C,** In this grade 3 lesion, fibrosis extends into the interstitial space between the respiratory units and into the alveolar ducts (hematoxylin and eosin). (Courtesy of Dr. Val Vallythan, National Institute for Occupational Safety and Health, Morgantown, West Virginia.)

Although histologic evidence of pulmonary fibrosis may occasionally be obtained in the course of clinical evaluation, routine lung biopsy and lavage are not recommended, and microscopic evidence is rarely required to diagnose asbestosis.

Occasionally, the determination of asbestos fibers in lung tissue, bronchoalveolar lavage, or sputum may be used to document past exposure, although these measurements are neither usually relied on nor required for the clinical diagnosis of asbestosis. Under light microscopy or by use of transmission electron microscopy, uncoated fibers or fibers coated with proteinaceous material may be detected. These latter so-called asbestos bodies or ferruginous bodies are nonspecific, because they can be found in occupationally unexposed individuals, in occupationally exposed individuals who have no asbestos-related lung disease, and in workers who have asbestosis. Generally, the most exposed and most severely affected individuals have higher asbestos fiber counts, but a significant interlaboratory variability is found in these measures.

Pathogenesis

Some of the major events thought to be involved in the pathogenesis of asbestosis are summarized in Figure 65-2. Within minutes after asbestos fibers have been inhaled, a local tissue response is initiated at the bifurcations of terminal bronchioles and alveolar ducts. The first changes occur in epithelial cells and then in alveolar macrophages as they attempt to engulf and are pierced by the fibers. In addition to cell death, which leads to the release of macrophage contents, asbestos-activated macrophages release reactive oxygen species that directly damage the tissue through peroxidation and direct cytotoxicity. Asbestos can also induce toxicity by mechanisms independent of its ability to promote reactive oxygen species.

Increasing numbers of alveolar macrophages accumulate within 48 h of first exposure. With chronic inhalation, a localized fibrosing alveolitis in the peribronchiolar region develops, followed by diffuse fibrotic scarring. Increasing the dose of asbestos increases the cellular response. A cascade of events ensues, in which the macrophages and neutrophils release various cytokines (such as interleukin-8 and gamma-interferon), chemokines, oxidants, and growth factors (such as fibronectin, platelet-derived growth factor, insulin-like growth factor, transforming growth factor-β, tumor necrosis factor-α, and fibroblast growth factor). These attract and alter the function of other inflammatory cells and resident cells, and thus promote inflammation and fibrosis. The response of fibroblasts to these signals is to proliferate and produce the constituents of extracellular matrix (e.g., collagen, proteoglycans) in the pulmonary interstitium. Resident cells themselves are both targets and perpetrators of the fibrotic response. The pathogenesis of the chronic fibrotic response remains sketchy. However, it is clear that this chronic response is progressive and that, apart from macrophage, neutrophil, and epithelial cells, a number of other cell types, such as lymphocytes and mast cells, contribute to the cycle of lung remodeling and fibrosis. Multiple, functionally overlapping, redundant inflammatory events occur in the lung simultaneously during the period of fibrogenesis. The consequence is an irreversible alteration in the structure and function of the lung.

Genetics

Asbestos exposure is the principal risk factor for the development of nonmalignant asbestos-related disorders. The genetic contribution to this risk is uncertain. A small number of cross-sectional, candidate gene studies have examined the possible contribution of genetic determinants of susceptibility to asbestosis. The glutathione-S-transferases (GST) and N-acetyltransferases (NAT) are enzymes that aid in the detoxification of hazardous agents. Several small studies examined GST null (deletion) polymorphisms and NAT2 slow-acetylator genotype in workers with and without asbestosis. Results from these studies, although somewhat contradictory, suggest that individuals who have a constitutional, homozygous deletion in the GSTM1 gene that codes for GST class mu, and who are NAT2 slow-acetylators, may be at higher risk for asbestosis if exposed to sufficiently high levels of asbestos. On the basis of the premise that asbestos causes DNA damage and alters DNA repair, Zhao and colleagues demonstrated an association between polymorphisms of the DNA repair gene XRCC1 and the *in vitro* extent of asbestos-induced DNA damage in Chinese asbestosis cases versus nonasbestosis cases. In Spain, asbestosis cases were more likely than exposed controls to be heterozygous for the α_1-antitrypsin polymorphism Pi*Z.

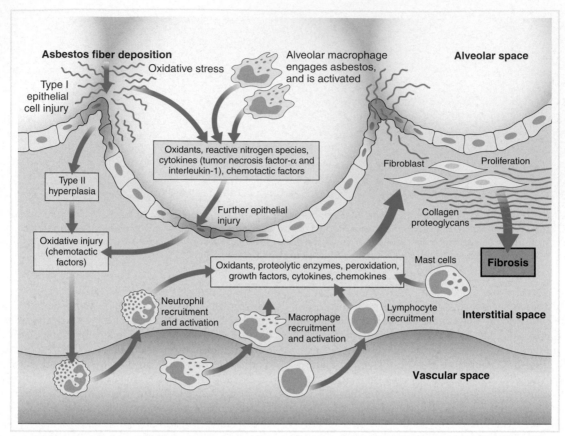

FIGURE 65-2 Proposed pathogenesis of asbestosis. Asbestos fibers deposit at branch points in the distal airways and alveolar ducts, which prompts an inflammatory cascade characterized by cellular activation, recruitment, and injury. The result is fibroblast proliferation and extracellular matrix deposition in the interstitial space.

CLINICAL FEATURES

Asbestosis is the pulmonary fibrotic disease that results from asbestos exposure. It affects the lungs symmetrically and is typically diagnosed on the basis of a consistent occupational or environmental history of asbestos exposure plus evidence of pulmonary fibrosis, usually by chest radiography. The latency period from first exposure to clinical disease is 10–20 years, but can be up to 40 years or more, with shorter latency and more severe disease seen in those workers who have the highest inhalational exposures. In some situations, the exposure history may be difficult to document. If needed, further evidence of occupational exposure can be verified by identifying high numbers of asbestos bodies in bronchoalveolar lavage fluid, sputum, or lung tissue, as discussed previously. Evidence of bilateral pleural plaques is pathognomonic for previous asbestos exposure. The radiographic finding of bilateral interstitial markings in the lower lung zone is sufficient radiographic evidence of asbestosis, although (as discussed in the following section) other tools such as computed tomography and measures of lung physiology also aid diagnosis.

The most common symptoms of asbestosis are the insidious onset of dyspnea on exertion (and eventually at rest), dry cough that can be paroxysmal, and fatigue. Hemoptysis, chest pain, and weight loss are not common and should raise suspicion of asbestos-related malignancy. Although physical abnormalities are uncommon at the early stages of asbestosis, over time these patients may have dry, bilateral basilar rales develop at end inspiration, digital clubbing cyanosis, and signs of cor pulmonale.

Radiologic Findings

Radiographically, asbestosis typically presents in the lower lobes with irregular "reticular" markings toward the lung periphery and costophrenic angles (Figure 65-3). Linear opacities that resemble extensions of vascular markings may assume a netlike appearance. In early or less severe disease, the middle and upper lung zones may appear relatively spared. With progression, the linear and irregular opacities thicken and spread to the midlung zones, but rarely to the apex. The International Labour Organization (ILO) International Classification of Radiographs characterizes each type of irregular opacity on the basis of increasing size and thickness as either *s*, *t*, or *u*, and on a scale of profusion (number) of opacities from normal profusion (0/−, 0/0, 0/1) to severe (3/2, 3/3, 3/+; see Chapter 64, Table 64-2 for classification details). When irregular opacities are seen on the chest radiograph in conjunction with pleural thickening, the radiograph can be considered virtually pathognomonic for asbestosis. However, the chest radiograph lacks sensitivity, because 15–20% of symptomatic, biopsy-proven cases have normal chest radiographs. Focal masses are uncommon except those caused by rounded atelectasis.

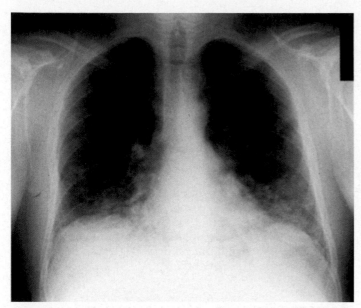

FIGURE 65-3 Chest radiograph illustrating parenchymal abnormalities in asbestosis. Descriptive terms from the International Labour Organization's classification for the radiographic appearance of pneumoconioses are used here (see Chapter 64, Table 64-2). Coarse "u" and "t" reticular opacities can be seen in the lower lung zones. In this advanced case, the profusion of small opacities is 3/3.

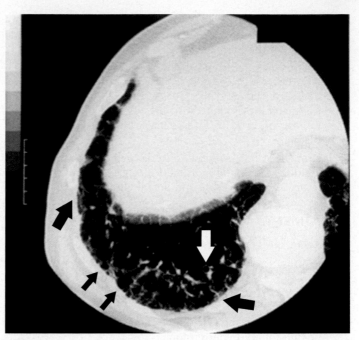

FIGURE 65-4 Asbestosis. High-resolution computed tomography of an asbestos-exposed worker who has asbestosis and mild pleural thickening. Patchy subpleural accentuation of interstitial markings (*thick arrows*) with honeycombing (*thin arrows*) and traction bronchiectasis (*white arrow*) are classic for the computed tomography appearance of advanced asbestosis.

Computed Tomography

As a result of the limited sensitivity of the radiograph, computed tomography has been thoroughly investigated. High-resolution computed tomography (HRCT), obtaining 1- to 3-mm slices, has sensitivity superior to the plain chest radiograph in detection of the fine reticular opacities in this disease. Of asbestos-exposed workers who have normal chest radiographs, 10–30% have HRCT scans that suggest underlying interstitial disease. Thus, the HRCT can prove useful when the clinical index of suspicion for asbestosis is high, but the chest radiograph appears normal. The most common HRCT findings in asbestosis are short, peripheral septal lines, subpleural curvilinear lines, peripheral cystic lesions (honeycombing), parenchymal bands adjacent to areas of pleural thickening, and bronchiolar thickening (Figure 65-4). The density of interstitial abnormalities found on HRCT has been shown to correlate with the symptoms and with physiologic and inflammatory indicators of asbestosis, although, in general, both the chest radiograph and the HRCT show only a limited correlation with disease severity measured physiologically.

Pulmonary Physiology

The earliest physiologic changes include small airway dysfunction (e.g., decreased forced expiratory flow). As the disease progresses, restriction (diminished total lung capacity and forced vital capacity) is observed, as is worsening gas exchange as measured by diffusing capacity and by exercise- and rest-associated arterial blood gas partial pressures. These parameters do not necessarily show the same degree of abnormality. Measures of gas exchange are generally more sensitive than are measures of lung volumes in this disorder. Isolated, severe,

obstructive airway disease is usually not attributable to asbestosis alone, although airflow obstruction can be observed with or without restriction, and occurs even in asbestos-exposed workers who were nonsmokers.

DIAGNOSIS

The long latency between asbestos exposure and development of asbestosis and the gradually progressive nature of the symptoms mean that this disease has a tendency to remain undetected until fairly late in its course. Efforts to conduct workplace surveillance by use of the chest radiograph and ILO readings of these films have improved disease detection. The diagnosis is based on a consistent history of exposure to asbestos, with sufficient latency, and evidence of interstitial fibrosis. A careful work and environmental history holds the key to determining that past exposure has occurred. As discussed previously, the presence of bilateral pleural plaques or demonstration of asbestos bodies in lavage or on biopsy can also aid in the assessment of exposure. Although most algorithms for diagnosis of asbestosis suggest that the combination of histologic material plus mineralogic assessment is the most sensitive and specific method of diagnosis, frequently such biopsy material is unavailable and unnecessary in making a probable determination of disease. Even the lung pathology should be considered in context with clinical data. The main considerations in the histologic differential diagnosis include the other pneumoconioses and other causes of pulmonary fibrosis such as pharmaceutic drugs, metal dusts, infectious agents, autoimmune disorders, and idiopathic pulmonary fibrosis.

In the absence of lung histologic and mineralogic analysis, the clinical diagnosis of asbestosis can be made with reasonable confidence on the basis of:

- History of significant asbestos exposure
- Appropriate time interval between exposure and disease detection (latency)
- Radiographic evidence of bilateral lung fibrosis by chest radiograph or HRCT (especially with co-existing pleural plaques)

Helpful, but less essential, criteria include evidence of restrictive lung function, abnormalities of gas exchange, bilateral inspiratory crackles (rales), and digital clubbing.

TREATMENT

At present, no cure exists for asbestosis, and no benefit from the use of corticosteroids or other immunosuppressive therapy has been documented. After exposure and early disease have occurred, no prophylactic measures are available.

Medical management in cases of asbestosis focuses on:

- Supplemental oxygen therapy in the face of hypoxemia or pulmonary hypertension
- Treatment of intercurrent infections
- Treatment of right ventricular failure in advanced disease
- Immunization for influenza and pneumococcal infections
- Appropriate medical documentation of the degree of physical impairment and appropriate advice to the patient to apply for workers' compensation benefits if exposure was occupational
- Education on the signs and symptoms of lung cancer and mesothelioma
- Assistance in smoking cessation among current smokers who have asbestosis to help reduce the risk of lung cancer
- Cessation of ongoing asbestos exposure is advisable, because it may slow disease progression, on the basis of experimental evidence.

CLINICAL COURSE

The prognosis for patients with asbestosis varies widely. It is dependent, in part, on the magnitude of exposure. In 1906, the disease was almost uniformly fatal by the third decade of life. However, with fewer exposures and lower exposure times, and with superior detection and supportive care, few patients demonstrate such severe progression of their disease. After removal from exposure, progression is usually slow and occurs in 5–40% of patients over approximately a decade of follow-up. Thus, if clinical deterioration occurs over a period of days or weeks, the clinician must look first for other explanations, such as infection or malignancy. Many patients may remain mildly symptomatic for many years and show little or no objective signs of disease progression, whereas others show steady, inexorable decline in lung function, gas exchange, worsening symptoms, development of end-stage respiratory insufficiency, and cor pulmonale with right ventricular failure.

Patients who have asbestosis are at increased risk of intercurrent lung infections and lung cancer. The best prognosis is found in those workers who have the lowest ILO profusion scores (i.e., chest radiographs that show the fewest irregular opacities) at time of termination of exposure. Tobacco smoking contributes to radiographic evidence of disease severity. Greater age at time of diagnosis is a strong predictor of

progression; both smoking and duration of exposure contribute relatively smaller, yet significant, effects as well. Multiple studies demonstrate that those with the greatest average and cumulative dust exposures tend to have the higher initial profusions of small opacities on chest radiographs and more rapid disease progression.

On the basis of National Center for Health Statistics data through 1992, for U.S. residents the age-adjusted mortality rate attributable to asbestosis began to plateau in the 1990s, but only after having risen from an age-adjusted mortality rate of 0.44 per 1,000,000 population in 1968 to 3.01 per 1,000,000 in 1990. Mortality rates are much higher among men than among women, and the age at which people die of asbestosis has risen from a median of 60 years in 1968 to approximately 74 years in 1992. In 1992, asbestosis resulted in nearly 12,000 years of potential life lost to life expectancy. Lung cancer is a significant contributing cause of increased mortality in asbestosis patients.

ASBESTOS-RELATED, NONMALIGNANT PLEURAL DISORDERS

The most common pleural changes caused by asbestos are pleural plaques, with or without pleural calcification and diffuse pleural thickening. Presence of pleural thickening is a marker of exposure. Pleural changes are now known to contribute to the lung function abnormalities seen in asbestos-exposed workers. Both types of pleural alteration contribute independently to restrictive lung physiology (reduced vital capacity), reduced lung compliance, and diminished diffusing capacity. Of asbestos-exposed construction workers, 20–60% demonstrate chest radiographic evidence of pleural disease, which is remarkable in light of the insensitivity of the radiograph.

Circumscribed pleural plaques that involve the parietal pleura are usually symmetric and bilateral, most commonly between the fifth and eighth ribs toward the posterolateral aspects of the thorax (Figure 65-5); they also frequently involve the diaphragmatic pleura (Figure 65-6). These lesions remain discrete. Thus, if radiographic evidence of more diffuse thickening is found, either mesothelioma or diffuse pleural thickening must be considered. Histologically, pleural plaques are hyalinized, acellular, avascular masses, and they rarely contain asbestos bodies. They have a tendency to calcify, which can be mistaken for nodular infiltrates on the chest radiograph. Although the ILO classification system has an elaborate section devoted to characterization of pleural abnormalities on the chest radiograph, interreader agreement is relatively low. Because HRCT is more sensitive than chest radiography in the detection of pleural plaques, it helps to determine past asbestos inhalation because these plaques are pathognomonic for that exposure. Also, HRCT helps to differentiate plaques from extrapleural fat pads. Asbestosis can occur in the absence of pleural disease and, inversely, pleural disease can occur without underlying pulmonary fibrosis, although autopsy studies suggest that when pleural changes are seen, there is often histologic evidence of asbestosis even if the radiograph is normal. Pleural plaques rarely, if ever, undergo malignant transformation.

Diffuse pleural thickening involves both parietal and visceral pleura and is strongly associated with prior, benign asbestos pleural effusions. It may also develop when subpleural

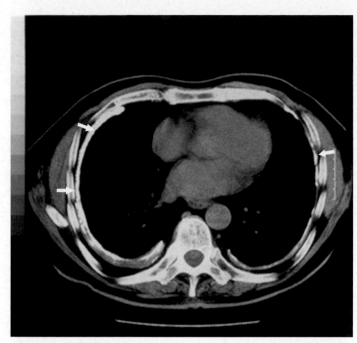

FIGURE 65-5 Pleural plaque. A conventional computed tomography scan of an asbestos worker shows extensive bilateral pleural calcifications (*arrows*).

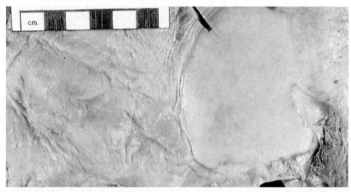

FIGURE 65-6 The gross pathologic appearance of a pleural plaque adjacent to the diaphragm of a construction worker. The benign pleural plaques that form as a consequence of asbestos inhalation have a smooth, shiny appearance and are usually well circumscribed.

parenchymal fibrosis extends to the visceral pleura. Diffuse pleural thickening is most commonly located in the lower thorax, can blunt the costophrenic angles, and may be either unilateral or bilateral. Because it is so diffuse, this form of pleural thickening can produce dyspnea on exertion and dry cough, as well as loss of lung function. Other conditions that can induce similar diffuse thickening include past tuberculosis, thoracic surgery, chest trauma with hemorrhage, adverse drug reactions, and infection.

After direct contact of asbestos fibers and the pleural space, an inflammatory, exudative, and often hemorrhagic effusion can develop. It is asymptomatic in two thirds of cases but can be associated with acute chest pain with or without fever. It can occur in the presence or absence of asbestosis. Its incidence in asbestos-exposed workers has been estimated to be <5%. Although it can be the first manifestation of

asbestos-related disease, the mean latency for benign, asbestos-related pleural effusions is 30 years. These effusions often resolve spontaneously, but recur in approximately one third of cases. The regression may be associated with pain. The consequences include not only diffuse pleural thickening, but also the formation of adhesive fibrothorax. Benign pleural effusion is considered a diagnosis of exclusion.

Rounded atelectasis, although uncommon, is important to recognize because of its tendency to mimic lung tumors. It is thought to occur when visceral pleural thickening invaginates and folds on the lung parenchyma, resulting in atelectasis; computed tomography is the preferred method of detecting its typical cicatricial pattern. Malignancy has only rarely been described in areas of rounded atelectasis. A positron emission tomography scan is usually negative in rounded atelectasis and may help differentiate the lesion from a lung cancer.

PITFALLS AND CONTROVERSIES

The threshold of asbestos exposure below which asbestosis will not occur is unclear, so any asbestos exposure carries some potential risk of asbestos-related disease. Prevention is superior to treatment of disease because there is no cure. The best preventive measure is to eliminate inhalational exposure by:

- Not working with asbestos
- Not disturbing asbestos in buildings or other locations where it has been used in the past
- Encapsulating exposed areas of friable asbestos
- Having asbestos removed by those experienced in asbestos abatement technologies

Substitute materials that have less toxicity must be considered in industrial applications. When asbestos substitutes are not available, appropriately designed and maintained engineering controls must be used, such as local exhaust ventilation systems. Personal respiratory protection is appropriate for short periods of exposure or when other controls are not feasible. Such respirators must be appropriately fitted to the individual and tested for the degree of protection they afford the worker by quantitative fit testing. Showering and changing of work clothes at the end of work shifts help to eliminate take-home exposures. Workers must be educated about the combined risks of asbestos exposure and smoking for lung cancer and must be counseled to avoid future asbestos exposure. Companies that use asbestos must strictly comply with government regulations as to the permissible exposure limits and appropriate medical surveillance of workers.

SUGGESTED READINGS

American Thoracic Society Documents: Diagnosis and initial management of nonmalignant diseases related to asbestos. Am J Respir Crit Care Med 2004; 170:691–715.
Burgess WA: Asbestos products. In Burgess WA, Ed. Recognition of Health Hazards in Industry. New York: John Wiley & Sons; 1995: 443–451.
Craighead JE, Abraham JL, Churg A, et al: The pathology of asbestos-associated disease of the lung and pleural cavities: Diagnostic criteria and proposed grading scheme. Arch Pathol Lab Invest 1982; 106:544–595.
Division of Respiratory Disease Studies, National Institute for Occupational Safety and Health (NIOSH) Work-related Lung Disease Surveillance Report 2002 (DHHS [NIOSH] Publication No. 2003–2111). Washington, DC: U.S. Government Printing Office.

Hillerdal G: Rounded atelectasis: clinical experience with 74 patients. Chest 1989; 9:836–841.

International Labor Office: International classification of radiographs of pneumoconiosis. Geneva, Switzerland: International Labor Organization; 2003.

Kamp DW, Weitzman SA: The molecular basis of asbestos induced lung injury. Thorax 1999; 54:638–652.

Peipins LA, Lewin M, Campolucci S, *et al:* Radiographic abnormalities and exposure to asbestos-contaminated vermiculite in the community of Libby, Montana, USA. Environ Health Perspectives 2003; 111: 1753–1759.

Tossavainen A: International expert meeting on new advances in the radiology and screening of asbestos-related diseases. Scand J Work Environ Health 2000; 26:449–454.

Yamamoto S: Histopathological features of pulmonary asbestosis with particular emphasis on the comparison with those of usual interstitial pneumonia. Osaka City Med J 1997; 43:225–242.

Zhao XH, Jia G, Liu YQ, *et al:* Association between polymorphisms of DNA repair gene XRCC1 and DNA damage in asbestos-exposed workers. Biomed Environ Sci 2006; 19:232–238.

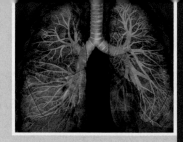

66 Occupational Asthma

MOIRA CHAN-YEUNG • JEAN-LUC MALO

There has been a growing interest in occupational asthma (OA) recently for several reasons:

- The frequency of asthma has increased progressively during the past two decades with a recent plateau, and occupational exposure may be a contributing factor.
- The list of agents that can cause OA is steadily lengthening (www.asmanet.com; www.asthme.csst.qc.ca).
- OA, together with diseases related to exposure to asbestos dust, has become the most prevalent occupational lung disease in many developed countries, resulting in an increased burden to society.
- OA is an excellent model to study the epidemiology, pathophysiology, genetics, and other aspects of asthma in humans.

OA is defined as a disease characterized by variable airflow limitation and/or bronchial hyperresponsiveness and/or airway inflammation because of causes and conditions attributable to a particular working environment and not to stimuli encountered outside the workplace. OA can be classified according to the pathogenic mechanisms: immunologically or nonimmunologically mediated. Immunologically mediated OA is characterized by a latency period that is necessary for acquiring sensitization, whereas nonimmunologically mediated OA has no latency period.

EPIDEMIOLOGY AND RISK FACTORS

It has been estimated that 5–15% of adult-onset asthmatic subjects relate that their workplace makes their asthma worse, although it can be suspected that the workplace causes asthma in only a portion of them. Several types of studies have been used to estimate the frequency of immunologic OA: population based–surveys, cross-sectional surveys in high-risk workplaces, registry on the basis of physician reporting, and medicolegal statistics. Some results of these approaches are summarized in Table 66-1. In general, the prevalence of OA caused by high-molecular-weight agents is <5% and 5–10% by low-molecular-weight agents. Reactive airways dysfunction syndrome (RADS) or irritant-induced asthma accounted for nearly 10–20% of all cases of OA. This is the most common form of nonimmunologically induced asthma.

The degree of exposure is the most important determinant of OA. Exposure-response relationships may be affected by individual susceptibility and timing of exposure. Levels of exposure at a critical point may be more relevant to the development of OA than cumulative doses of exposure or current levels of exposure. It is now possible to measure levels of exposure by personal sampling by use of direct chemical analytic method or, in the case of protein-derived allergens, by

immunologic methods. Some agents seem to be more potent in inducing sensitization than others. Gautrin and co-workers found that laboratory animals caused the onset of sensitization more often than latex and flour.

PATHOPHYSIOLOGY

The development of OA results from a complex interaction between environmental factors and individual susceptibility. Asthma is a multifactorial disease and seems to be genetically heterogeneous. Most reported genetic studies of OA have investigated the importance of HLA class II polymorphisms in increasing or decreasing the risk of developing sensitization and OA. Glutathione-S-transferase (GST) is an important protector of cells from oxidative stress products. The polymorphic GST seems to play an important role in OA because of isocyanates.

Overwhelming evidence now exists of a dose-response relationship between the level of exposure to occupational agents and the development of sensitization and/or work-related symptoms.

OA induced by immunologic mechanisms is characterized by a latency period. Only a small proportion of the exposed subjects are affected, and exposure to a minute quantity of the offending agent can lead to a severe asthmatic reaction. Although some agents induce asthma through the production of specific IgE antibodies, in others, the immunologic mechanism(s) responsible has not yet been identified.

Immunologic, Immunoglobulin E (IgE) Mediated

High-molecular-weight occupational agents act as complete antigens and induce specific IgE antibody production. The best examples are laboratory animals and flour. Some low-molecular-weight occupational agents, including platinum salts, trimellitic anhydride, and other acid anhydrides, also induce specific IgE antibodies, and some others, specific IgG antibodies. They probably act as haptens and bind with proteins to form complete antigens and are recognized by antigen-presenting cells and mount a $CD4^+$ response with production of specific IgE antibodies by B cells stimulated by interleukin-4 (IL-4) to IL-13.

Quantitative structure-activity relationship models have recently contributed to characterize further the structural and physicochemical properties that determine the potential for inducing respiratory sensitization. Reactions between specific IgE and antigens lead to a cascade of events that result in the release of inflammatory mediators and influx of cells in the airway, resulting in airway inflammation and development of airway hyperresponsiveness as in asthma because of common allergens. Although other classes of antibodies have

TABLE 66-1 Frequency of Occupational Asthma

Survey Type	Population	Number of Subjects	Participation (%)	Prevalence
Population-based	Spain	2646	61	5.0–7.7%
	New Zealand	1609	64	1.9–3.1%
Registry based on voluntary reporting	United Kingdom	554	Not relevant	22/million per year
	Quebec	287	Not relevant	60/million per year
	British Columbia	124	Not relevant	92/million per year
	Sweden	1010	Not relevant	80/million per year
Survey in high-risk workplaces	**Prevalence data**			
	Agents of high molecular weight			
	Snow-crab processors	303	97	15%
	Clam/shrimp	57	93	4%
	Psyllium (pharmacists)	130	93	4%
	Psyllium (nurses)	194	91	4%
	Guar gum	151	96	3%
	Agents of low molecular weight			
	Isocyanates	51	100	12%
	Spiramycin	51	100	8%
	White cedar	31	94	10%
Incidence data	Animal-handlers	395	>85%	7.9% per person-year
	Pastry making	186	>60%	4.2% per person-year
	Dental hygiene (latex)	109	>80%	2.5% per person-year
Medicolegal	Quebec	c. 60/year	Not relevant	c. 20/million per year
	Finland	352	Not relevant	c. 156/million per year

been postulated to have a role in asthma, evidence for their participation is not available. In the case of isocyanates, it is possible that there are mechanisms of allergic sensitization that are independent of IgE antibody. There are no apparent differences in the pathogenetic mechanisms between OA induced by high-molecular-weight occupational agents and those of allergic nonoccupational asthma.

Immunologic, Non-IgE Mediated

Many low-molecular-weight agents, including isocyanates and plicatic acid (responsible for red cedar asthma), have been shown to cause OA, and yet specific IgE antibodies cannot be found or are found in only a small percentage of the affected subjects. Specific IgG antibodies are also found and have been discovered to be significantly associated with the development of OA. The significance of IgE and IgG antibodies in the pathogenesis of asthma is not clear.

Bronchial biopsy specimens from subjects with OA obtained at the time of diagnosis have shown activation of T lymphocytes, suggesting that T lymphocytes may play a direct role in mediating airway inflammation. This hypothesis has been substantiated by the finding of proliferation of peripheral blood lymphocytes when stimulated with the appropriate antigen in a proportion of affected subjects with nickel-induced asthma and Western red cedar asthma. In isocyanate-induced asthma, an increase of CD8$^+$ cells and eosinophils were found in the peripheral blood of subjects during a late asthmatic reaction induced by exposure testing. Cloning of T cells from bronchial biopsy specimens of these subjects showed that most of the clones exhibited CD8$^+$ phenotype that produced IL-5, with very few clones producing IL-4. This finding provides supportive evidence that CD8$^+$ cells may play a direct role in OA without the necessity of producing IgE antibodies. Early asthmatic reactions induced by occupational allergens are probably associated with

smooth muscle contraction and edema induced by inflammatory mediators such as histamine and leukotrienes but not cellular infiltration. Late asthmatic reactions are associated with influx of inflammatory cells. Although asthma and OA have both been identified as diseases in which eosinophilic inflammation plays a key role, the role of neutrophils has recently been examined. Induced sputum is a noninvasive means to assess cell profiles and is currently more often used as an interesting investigative tool. Eosinophilic and neutrophilic variants of OA have been found in the case of OA because of low-molecular-weight agents, especially isocyanates. Some low-molecular-weight agents have pharmacologic properties that cause bronchoconstriction. For example, isocyanates may block the β_2-adrenergic receptor. Isocyanates and other occupational agents may also stimulate sensory nerves to release substance P and other peptides that have been shown to inhibit neutral endopeptidases necessary for the inactivation of neuropeptides. Neuropeptides affect many cells in the airways and may participate in airway inflammation by causing smooth muscle contraction, mucus production, and recruitment and activation of inflammatory cells. Thus, low-molecular-weight occupational agents such as isocyanates may have a variety of proinflammatory effects and induce asthma through more than one mechanism. An autopsy study of the lung of a subject with isocyanate-induced asthma who died after reexposure showed denudation of airway epithelium, subepithelial fibrosis, infiltration of the lamina propria by leukocytes (mainly eosinophils) and diffuse mucus plugging of the bronchioles, similar to those who died from non-OA. Bronchial biopsy specimens of 18 subjects with proven OA have also shown extensive epithelial desquamation, ciliary abnormalities of the epithelial cells, smooth muscle hyperplasia, and subepithelial fibrosis (Figure 66-1). The total cell count, eosinophils, and lymphocytes were increased compared with healthy controls.

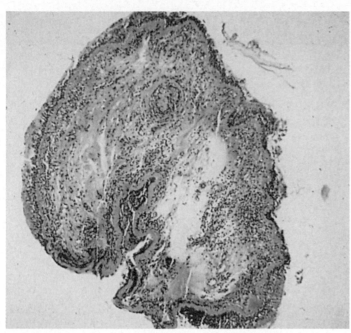

FIGURE 66-1 Bronchial biopsy specimen of a patient who had occupational asthma caused by toluene diisocyanates. After removal from exposure, partial desquamation of the epithelium, thickened basement membrane, and some cellular infiltration were found.

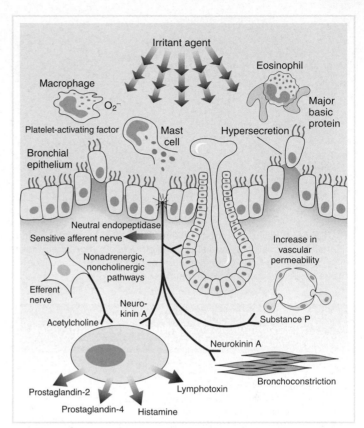

FIGURE 66-2 Proposed pathophysiology of reactive airways dysfunction syndrome.

Nonimmunologic

OA resulting from nonimmunologic mechanisms is characterized by the absence of latency. The underlying mechanism of RADS is not known. It has been postulated that the extensive denudation of the epithelium in these conditions leads to airway inflammation and airway hyperresponsiveness for several reasons, including loss of the epithelial-derived relaxing factors, exposure of the nerve endings leading to neurogenic inflammation, and nonspecific activation of mast cells with release of inflammatory mediators and cytokines (Figure 66-2). Secretion of growth factors for epithelial cells, smooth muscle, and fibroblasts may lead to airway remodeling. Sequential changes in the airways of a subject with RADS or irritant-induced asthma have been described. In the acute phase of RADS, there is rapid denudation of the mucosa with fibrinohemorrhagic exudate in the submucosa; this was followed by regeneration of the epithelium with proliferation of basal and parabasal cells and subepithelial edema (Figure 66-3). In the chronic phase of RADS, there is marked thickening of the airway wall (Figure 66-4). In a study of irritant-induced asthma caused by multiple exposures to an irritant, inflammatory infiltrate with eosinophils and lymphocytes and diffuse deposition with collagen fibers were found.

CLINICAL FEATURES

Many agents can cause OA. Agents that cause immunologically mediated OA include a broad spectrum of protein-derived and natural and synthetic chemicals used in various workplaces. Extensive lists of causative agents and workplaces have been published in databases on web sites (www.asmanet.com/asmapro, www.asthme.csst.qc.ca) and have been made available by professional agencies. The most common workplaces

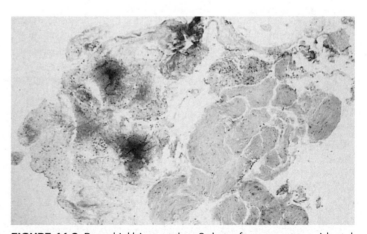

FIGURE 66-3 Bronchial biopsy taken 3 days after an acute accidental inhalation of a high concentration of chlorine. This shows almost complete desquamation of bronchial mucosa with fibrinohemorrhagic deposit (Weigert–Masson stain).

and agents causing immunologically mediated OA are listed in Table 66-2. These agents can be classified according to their molecular weight: high (MW > 5000 daltons) and low (MW < 5000 daltons).

Box 66-1 shows some of the agents reported to have given rise to RADS. All agents in exceedingly high concentrations can theoretically cause OA through nonimmunologic mechanisms, especially for agents occurring in vapor or gaseous form such as chlorine and ammonia.

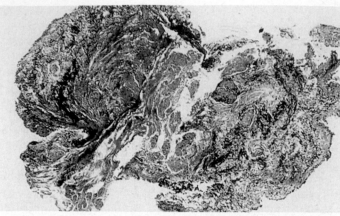

FIGURE 66-4 Bronchial biopsy taken 2 years after an acute accidental inhalation of chlorine, showing severe desquamation of epithelial cells. Smooth muscle cells are surrounded by reticulocollagenic fibrous tissue (Weigert–Masson stain).

BOX 66-1 Agents Responsible for Reactive Airways Dysfunction Syndrome

Acetic acid	Diesel exhaust	Spray paint
Sulfuric acid	Diethylaminoethanol	Sulfur dioxide
Chloridric acid	Epichlorohydrin	Gas (chlorine, mustard, phosgene, etc.)
Heated acid	Ethylene oxide	Fire/smoke
Ammonia	Isocyanates	Floor sealant
Bleaching agent	Metal remover	Formol-Zenkear
Chlorine	Oxide (calcium)	Cleaning mist
Chloropicrin	Paints (heated)	Hydrazine
Cleaning agents	Phthalic anhydride	

Agents responsible for reactive airway dysfunction syndrome. (Reproduced with permission from Lemiere C, Malo JL, Gautrin D: Nonsensitizing causes of occupational asthma. Med Clin North Am 80:749–774, 1996.)

TABLE 66-2 Common Agents That Cause Immunologically Mediated Occupational Asthma and At Risk Occupations

Agent	Workers at Risk
High Molecular Weight	
Cereals	Bakers, millers
Animal-derived allergents	Animal handlers, Detergent users, pharmaceutical workers
Enzymes	Bakers
Gums	Carpet makers, pharmaceutical workers
Latex	Health professionals
Seafoods	Seafood processors
Low Molecular Weight	
Isocyanates	Spray painters, insulation installers, manufactures of plastics, rubbers, foam
Wood dusts	Forest workers, carpenters, cabinet makers
Anhydrides	Users of plastics, epoxy resins
Amines	Shellac and lacquer handlers, solderers
Fluxes	Electronics workers
Chloramine-T	Janitors, cleaners
Dyes	Textile workers
Persulfate	Hairdressers
Formaldehyde, glutaraldehyde	Hospital staff
Acrylate	Adhesive handlers
Drugs	Pharmaceutical workers, health professionals
Metals	Solderers, refiners

Common agents that cause immounologically mediated occupational asthma and at-risk occupations. (Reproduced from Chan-Yeung M, Malo J-L: Occupational asthma. N Engl J Med 333:107–112, 1995. ©1995 Massachusetts Medical Society. All rights reserved.)

The clinical signs and symptoms of OA are similar to those of other types of asthma. However, symptoms of rhinitis are generally more important in the case of high-molecular-weight agents, and rhinitis may occur before the onset of asthma. At the onset of the illness, many workers present with cough, wheeze, and shortness of breath after their work shift with improvement after. Their symptoms improve whenever they are away from work and recur when they return to work. As they continue to be exposed, symptoms tend to occur earlier during the shift. In some individuals, symptoms may develop immediately on exposure to the causative agent. At this stage, there is no remission of symptoms during weekends; a much longer period is necessary for improvement to take place.

There are differences in the clinical presentation of subjects with OA caused by IgE- and non-IgE–mediated causes. The latency period is longer for high-molecular-weight than for low-molecular-weight agents. The temporal pattern of bronchial reactions on specific inhalation challenges in the laboratory is different. Immediate or dual reactions occur more frequently for high-molecular-weight agents, whereas isolated late or atypical reactions develop for low-molecular-weight agents.

The presence of sensitization to occupational agents can be detected either by skin tests or by RAST or ELISA tests. In subjects with a compatible clinical history of OA and bronchial hyperresponsiveness, a positive skin or RAST test probably has a diagnostic accuracy close to 80% in the case of high-molecular-weight agents. Unfortunately, there are very few standardized commercially available materials for skin tests or for RAST tests in OA, and for most low-molecular-weight agents, an IgE-mediated mechanism has not been confirmed. Stimulation production of monocyte chemoattractant protein-1 (MCP-1) *in vitro* from peripheral blood mononuclear cells by diisocyanates conjugated with human serum albumin has been shown to have sensitivity and specificity of 79% and 91%, respectively, in the diagnosis of isocyanate-induced asthma. Further studies are necessary to extend this test to other low-molecular-weight agents. Atopic subjects are more prone to have sensitization to high-molecular-weight agents develop. Smoking predisposes workers to sensitization to some agents, including platinum salts. On the other hand, nonatopic subjects and nonsmokers are more often affected in OA caused by agents that induce asthma though non-IgE–mediated mechanisms. Certain HLA class II antigens have been reported to confer susceptibility, whereas others provide protection from OA caused by low-molecular-weight compounds. The reactive airway dysfunction syndrome originally described by Brooks and colleagues in 1985 is due to acute airway injury from accidental exposure to a high dose of irritants. The typical clinical presentation is the development of symptoms of asthma within a few hours, but sometimes with a longer interval of acute exposure in a subject without history of any respiratory symptoms. The symptoms of asthma usually last for more than 3 months associated with nonallergic bronchial hyperresponsiveness.

DIAGNOSIS

It is necessary to confirm the diagnosis of OA with objective means for several reasons. The diagnosis of OA has considerable socioeconomic implication to the worker and his family; it usually means a change of job in most instances with its financial consequences. Asthma is a common disease, affecting 6–8% of the adult population in Canada and greater in other parts of the world. Having asthma and working in an environment with an agent known to give rise to OA does not make the diagnosis of OA.

An occupational cause should be suspected for all new cases of adult-onset asthma, especially those subjects who report worsening of their asthma symptoms at work (see "Epidemiology and Risk Factors"). A detailed occupational history on past and current exposure to possible causal agents in the workplace, work processes, and specific job duties should be obtained. In addition, the intensity, frequency, and peak concentrations of exposure in the workplace should be assessed qualitatively. Information can be requested from the worksite, including material safety data sheets, although in some instances, the information is incomplete on all constituents of the product, especially those constituents with concentrations <1%. Computerized databases and published lists of agents and workplaces are useful. Walk-through visits of the workplace may be necessary. Industrial hygiene data and employee health records can be obtained.

Open medical questionnaires should be regarded as fairly sensitive, but not specific, tools for diagnostic purposes. Temporal associations are not sufficient to diagnose work-related asthma. Ocular and nasal symptoms often accompany respiratory symptoms and are associated with OA. They are more frequent in OA because of high-molecular-weight than low-molecular-weight agents.

An individual with suspected OA would be best assessed by a specialist in this area. The role of this specialist is to confirm the diagnosis of OA by objective means if possible and to assess impairment/disability. A delay in referral may jeopardize the chance of confirming the diagnosis with objective measurements, because the subject may have left the workplace and have recovered or the working condition may have changed. However, in cases of OA, inhalation challenges with a specific agent generally remain positive even 2 years or more after cessation of exposure.

An algorithm for the clinical investigation of OA is shown in Figure 66-5. The advantages and pitfalls of the various tools in confirming the diagnosis of OA are listed in Table 66-3. For high-molecular-weight agents, skin tests to detect immediate reactivity and/or measurements of specific IgE antibodies are important tools. Although having immediate skin reactivity to an inhalant only reflects immunologic "sensitization" and not necessarily the disease, it has been shown that having both immediate skin reactivity and increased bronchial hyperresponsiveness results in an 80% likelihood of an asthmatic attack developing on laboratory exposure to this agent. Unfortunately, reagents used for skin and *in vitro* testings are not standardized and are generally prepared from occupational agents in individual laboratories.

The absence of nonallergic bronchial hyperresponsiveness in a subject at the end of 2 weeks of working under the usual conditions virtually excludes the diagnosis of asthma and OA. If there is nonallergic bronchial hyperresponsiveness, further

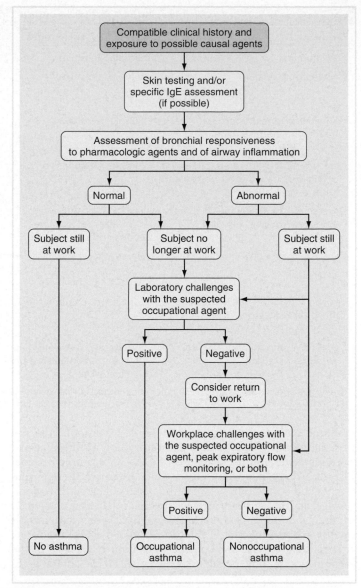

FIGURE 66-5 Clinical investigation of occupational asthma. (Reproduced from Chan-Yeung M, Malo J-L: Occupational asthma. N Engl J Med 1995; 333:107–112. Copyright Massachusetts Medical Society)

testing is required. Measuring spirometry before and after a work shift has not been found to be sensitive or specific. Two options can be considered for objective confirmation, depending on availability (see Figure 66-5). Exposure to the suspected agent under control conditions in a hospital laboratory can be done as originally described by Pepys and Hutchcroft in 1975. Attempts have been made to improve specific challenge tests by exposing subjects in the laboratory to low and stable levels of dry or wet aerosols and vapors to avoid nonspecific reactions. However, these tests can be falsely negative if an incorrect agent is used for testing or if the subject has been away from work for too long, although such occurrences are rare. If this is the case, the subject should be instructed to return to the workplace, if feasible, and specific laboratory or worksite challenges should be repeated at a later time.

TABLE 66-3 Advantages and Disadvantages of Diagnostic Methods in Occupational Asthma

Method	Advantages	Disadvantages
Questionaire	Simple, sensitive	Low specificity
Immunologic testing	Simple, sensitive	Only for agents of high molecular weight and for some of low molecular weight; identifies sensitization, not disease; no "standardized" and commercially available agents
Bronchial responsiveness to methacholine/histamine	Simple, sensitive	Not specific for asthma or occupational asthma; occupational asthma not ruled out by a negative test if workers are no longer exposed
Measurement of forced expiratory volume in 1 sec (FEV_1) before and after a work shift	Simple, inexpensive	Low sensitivity and specificity
Assessment of airway inflammation (induced sputum, exhaled NO)	Addresses the physiopathology of asthma; identifies eosinophilic bronchitis	Not specific for occupational asthma; reserved to specialized centers
Peak expiratory flow monitoring	Relatively simple, inexpensive	Requires patient's cooperation and honesty; not as sensitive as FEV_1 or a computerized method to assess airway caliber to interpret changes
Specific inhalation challenges in a hospital laboratory	If positive, confirmatory	Diagnosis not ruled out by a negative confirmatory test; (e.g., if wrong agent or subject no longer at work); expensive; few referral centers
Serial FEV_1 measurement at work under supervision	If negative, rules out diagnosis when patient tested under usual work	A positive test may be result from conditions of irritation; requires collaboration of employer

Advantages and disadvantages of diagonostic methods in occupational asthma. (Reproduced from Chan-Yeung M, Malo J-L: Occupational asthma. N Engl J Med 333:107–112, 1995. ©1995 Massachusetts Medical Society. All rights reserved.)

Burge and co-workers were the first to propose the use of serial measurement of peak expiratory flow (PEF) by use of portable devices in the diagnosis of OA. An example of serial PEF recording is shown in Figure 66-6. Although there is relatively good correlation between the results of serial PEF monitoring and OA as confirmed by specific inhalation challenges in the laboratory, there are several limitations and pitfalls in PEF monitoring (see Table 66-3). When PEF monitoring is suggestive of OA and specific inhalation challenges in the laboratory are not possible or negative, it is advisable to confirm OA by sending a technician to the workplace and record spirometry serially throughout a work shift. The use of computerized peak flowmeters is very helpful in overcoming some of the problems of PEF monitoring. Computerized programs to assess changes in PEF are currently available (OASYS). Combining PEF monitoring with serial assessments of nonallergic bronchial responsiveness can provide further objective evidence, although this does not add to the sensitivity and specificity of PEF monitoring alone. Finally, assessment of airway inflammation (% eosinophils) in induced sputum has

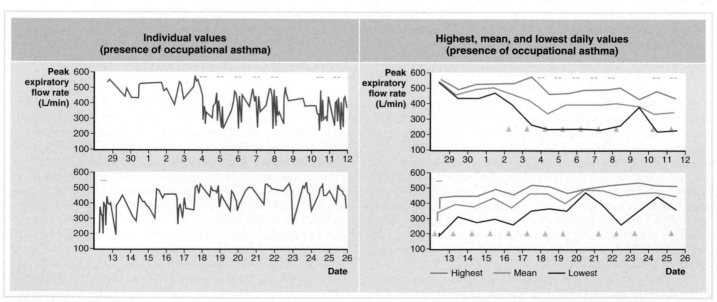

FIGURE 66-6 Pattern of changes in peak expiratory flows that suggest occupational asthma. The horizontal lines show the periods at work; the triangles illustrate the need for an inhaled bronchodilator. (Reproduced from Malo JL, Cote J, Cartier A, *et al*: How many times per day should peak expiratory flow rates be assessed when investigating occupational asthma? Thorax 1993; 48:1211–1217.)

recently been found to be sensitive and specific in the diagnosis of OA. They improve the sensitivity and specificity of PEF monitoring.

TREATMENT

The ideal treatment for patients with OA is removal from the causal exposure permanently, with retraining for alternative employment if necessary. Larger companies may be able to relocate the affected worker to another job in the same plant or another plant with no exposure; they may also be able to improve ventilation and/or change work practices to eliminate or reduce exposure. This is usually not possible for smaller companies. Any subject with OA who remains in the same job should have respiratory protection and have close medical follow-up. Worsening of asthma should lead to immediate removal from exposure. Pharmacologic treatment of patients with OA is similar to other types of asthma. Although removal from exposure generally results in improvement, patients generally (~75% of time) continue to require medication and have airflow limitation or nonallergic bronchial hyperresponsiveness or airway inflammation.

After the diagnosis is made, physicians should counsel patients concerning compensation; the specifics vary from country to country. The appropriate public health authority should be notified. Such agencies should initiate surveillance programs when sentinel cases have been identified. Patients should also be referred to compensation boards or similar agencies when appropriate. Patients should be evaluated for temporary impairment when their asthma is under control. Evaluation for permanent impairment and disability should take place when improvement is maximal, which may take 1–2 years. The guidelines for assessment of impairment and disability for patients with chronic irreversible lung diseases are inappropriate for patients with asthma. The American Thoracic Society guidelines endorsed by the American Medical Association attempt to take into account all the special features of asthma. In addition to measurements of lung function, assessment of impairment includes the degree of nonallergic bronchial hyperresponsiveness or airway reversibility, the minimum amount of medication required for maintaining control of asthma, and the effects of asthma on the quality of life. When there is a change in clinical status, reassessment is recommended.

CLINICAL COURSE

Subjects with OA deteriorate if they continue in the same job without protection. Fatalities in workers who continue to be exposed have been reported. A scheme of the progressive natural history of OA is shown in Figure 66-7.

Most patients with OA improve but do not recover completely even several years after removal from exposure. Table 66-4 shows some of the studies. The proportion of subjects followed up in these studies is high, suggesting that the high rate of persistence of asthma is not due to bias (i.e., "sick" ones came for the follow-up examination). Follow-up studies of patients with various types of OA have shown that subjects who became asymptomatic after leaving exposure had higher lung function and lower degree of nonallergic bronchial hyperresponsiveness at the time of diagnosis and a shorter duration of exposure after the onset of symptoms. These findings suggest that they were diagnosed at an earlier stage of the disease. Early diagnosis and removal from exposure are essential in ensuring recovery.

Although symptoms and lung function improve within 1 year of leaving exposure, improvement in nonallergic bronchial hyperresponsiveness depends on the length of interval from cessation of exposure. Specific IgE antibodies decrease even more slowly, with no plateau after 5 years as shown in subjects with snow crab–induced asthma. It has been recommended that assessment of permanent respiratory impairment/disability take place after at least 2 years of cessation of exposure.

The rate of decline in lung function of subjects with OA with continuous exposure is greater than subjects without asthma. Moreover, specific bronchial reactivity to the offending occupational agents often persists after the subject has left exposure for 2 or more years. Thus, it is not advisable for these patients to return to the same job after they became asymptomatic.

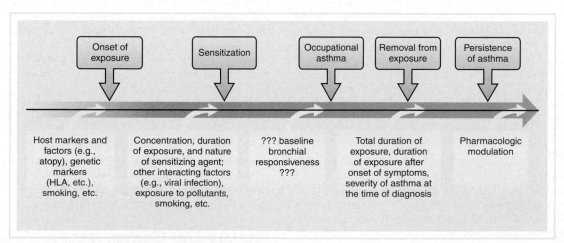

FIGURE 66-7 Natural history of asthma and occupational asthma. The boxes illustrate the steps, whereas the modifying factors before each step are listed under the horizontal line. (Reproduced from Malo JL, Ghezzo H, D'Aguino C, et al: Natural history of occupational asthma: Relevance of type of agent and other factors in the rate of development of symptoms in affected subjects. J Allergy Clin Immunol 1992; 90:937–943.)

TABLE 66-4 Retrospective Evidence for the Persistence of Symptoms and Bronchial Hyperresponsiveness after Removal from the Offending Agent

Agent	Number of Cases	Duration of Follow-up (years)	Persistence of Symptoms (%)	Nonspecific Bronchial Hyperreactivity	
				Number	Percentage
Red cedar	38	0.5–4.0	29	38/38	100
	75	1–9	49	25/33	76
Colophony	20	1.3–3.8	90	7/20	35
Snow-crab	31	0.5–2.0	61	28/31	90
	31	4.8–6.0	100	26/31	84
Various	32	0.5–4.0	93	31/32	97
Isocyanates	12	1–3	66	7/12	58
	50	>4	82	12/19	63
	20	0.5–4.0	50	9/12	75
	22	1	77	17/22	77
Various	28	4–11	100	25/26	96

Retrospective evidence for the persistence of symptoms and bronchial hyperresponsiveness after removal of the offending agent. (Reproduced from Chan-Yeung and Malo by courtesy of Marcel Dekker Inc. Chan-Yeung M, Malo JL: Natural history of occupational asthma: In Bernstein IL, Chan-Yeung M, Malo JL, Bernstein D (eds): Asthma in the Workplace. New York, Marcel Dekker, 1993, pp 299–322.)

There is a histologic basis to the persistence of symptoms and nonallergic bronchial hyperresponsiveness in patients with OA. Higher total cell count and eosinophils in bronchoalveolar lavage fluid were found in subjects with Western red cedar asthma who did not recover compared with those who recovered completely after removal from exposure. Saetta and co-workers in 1992 have documented improvement in airway wall remodeling (thickness of subepithelial fibrosis and number of subepithelial fibroblasts) in patients with TDI-induced asthma 6 months after the cessation of exposure, but there was no improvement in bronchial inflammation and in the degree of nonallergic bronchial hyperresponsiveness. Signs of airway inflammation and remodeling may persist for intervals of 10 years or more after the cessation of exposure. The reasons for the persistence of symptoms, nonallergic bronchial hyperresponsiveness, as well as of airway inflammation and remodeling after removal from exposure are not known.

Some researchers have explored the possibility of "curing" subjects with OA with inhaled steroids to reduce the degree of airway inflammation after the patients have been removed from the workplace. Although some improvement in various clinical and functional parameters was found, no case of cure from asthma was documented.

Because most cases of RADS occur in isolation, it is difficult to study the natural history involving a series of such patients. However, improvement and cure in the first 2–3 years after the inhalational accident have been described in approximately 25% of subjects.

PREVENTION

Primary prevention programs should be implemented for OA in high-risk industries. The most important measure is to reduce the level of exposure. For example, the introduction of powder-free gloves with reduced protein levels and education about natural rubber latex (NRL) allergies in health care facilities led to a decline in the number of suspected cases of occupational allergies and asthma caused by enzymes and to natural latex. Other measures may include the use of alternative nonsensitizing agents, improved ventilation, and the use

of appropriate ventilators. Permissible exposure limits should be established for all high-risk agents for OA as for flour. It should be noted that once a person is sensitized, he or she might react to a much lower level of exposure. Another method is to identify susceptible subjects at the time of preemployment examination and exclude them from employment. Unfortunately, there are no reliable markers of susceptibility. Atopy is one of the predisposing factors for sensitization in OA because of high-molecular-weight compounds; however, atopy has a low predictive value for the development of asthma. Moreover, 40–50% of young adults are atopic; thus atopic subjects should not be excluded from high-risk workplaces. Genetic studies are, for the moment, at a very early stage, and genetic markers should not be used in surveillance programs.

Secondary prevention by early detection of workers with OA and removal from exposure before development of irreversible airflow obstruction has been found to be effective in isocyanate workers and platinum refinery workers. Secondary prevention requires the institution of a medical surveillance program that includes a preemployment medical questionnaire followed by a periodic questionnaire every 6–12 months in high-risk industries. Some surveillance programs include periodic skin tests if the sensitizing agent is a high-molecular-weight compound or for some chemical sensitizers such as platinum salts or measurement of specific IgE, whereas others include periodic spirometry.

Tertiary prevention is aimed at limiting respiratory impairment among those with established OA. For workers with occupational allergen–induced asthma, complete avoidance of the responsible agent in addition to standard asthma treatment are recommended. For those with irritant-induced asthma, early treatment with oral corticosteroids may improve long-term outcome; regular treatment for asthma should be given to those with persistent symptoms.

PITFALLS AND CONTROVERSIES

It is important to have objective evidence that the patient's asthma is due to occupational exposure. There are many pitfalls in confirming the diagnosis of OA. Although lists of agents causing OA found in published articles and databases are useful to alert the physician, the absence of an agent on such lists does not exclude the possibility of OA, because new chemicals are constantly being introduced into the market. Patients are often asked to leave the job when the diagnosis is suspected. However, one of the objective tests is to ask the patient to do serial monitoring of PEF for a period at work and a period away from work. Unless the patient has severe symptoms, it is best to obtain objective evidence first before asking the patient to resign from his or her job. PEF monitoring also has limitations as discussed previously. It should be done properly according to a protocol and by use of a logged device or together with serial measurement of nonallergic bronchial hyperresponsiveness and airway inflammation. Specific challenge tests have been said to be the "gold standard" in diagnosing OA, but it is not without pitfalls, because there are both false-positive and false-negative results. When a new agent is suspected, investigators often use several methods to confirm the diagnosis.

Although most people include RADS as a form of OA, others think that it is an entirely different condition because of differences in pathologic features. There is still considerable controversy as to whether exposure to a low level of irritant gases or fumes in the workplace or in the environment can actually induce asthma *de novo*. The long-term outcome of RADS has yet to be studied.

Despite a great deal that has been learned about OA over the past few years, there are still many gaps in our knowledge. Future research priorities should include further improvement in diagnostic, surveillance methods, and control of exposures to prevent the development of the disease and the psychosocioeconomic impact.

SUGGESTED READINGS

Becklake MR, Chan-Yeung M, Malo JL: Epidemiological Approaches in Occupational Asthma. In Bernstein IL Chan-Yeung M, Malo JL, Bernstein DI, eds: Asthma in the Workplace, 3rd ed. New York, NY: Taylor & Francis; 2006:37–85.

Bernstein IL, Chan-Yeung M, Malo JL, Berstein DI: Asthma in the Workplace, 3rd ed. New York, NY: Taylor & Francis; 2006.

Burge PS, Moscato G, Johnson A, Chan-Yeung M: Physiological assessment: Serial measurements of lung function and bronchial responsiveness. In Bernstein IL Chan-Yeung M, Malo JL, Bernstein DI, eds: Asthma in the Workplace, 3rd ed. New York NY: Taylor & Francis; 2006:199–226.

Gautrin D, Bernstein IL, Brooks SM, Henneberger PK: Reactive airways dysfunction syndrome and irritant-induced asthma. In Bernstein IL Chan-Yeung M, Malo JL, Bernstein DI, eds: Asthma in the Workplace, 3rd ed. New York NY: Taylor & Francis; 2006:579–627.

Maestrelli P, Fabbri LM, Mapp CE: Pathophysiology. In Bernstein IL Chan-Yeung M, Malo JL, Bernstein DI, eds: Asthma in the Workplace, 3rd ed. New York: Taylor & Francis; 2006:109–140.

Malo JL, Chan-Yeung M: Agents causing occupational asthma with key references. In Bernstein IL Chan-Yeung M, Malo JL, Bernstein DI, eds: Asthma in the Workplace, 3rd ed. New York: Taylor & Francis; 2006:825–866.

Malo JL, Yeung M Chan: Occupational asthma. J Allergy Clin Immunol 2001; 108:317–328.

Mapp CE, Boschetto P, Maestrelli P, Fabbri LM: Occupational asthma. Am J Respir Crit Care Med 2005; 172:280–305.

Newman-Taylor AJ, Yucesov B: Genetics and occupational asthma. In Bernstein IL Chan-Yeung M, Malo JL, Bernstein DI, eds: Asthma in the Workplace, 3rd ed. New York, NY: Taylor & Francis; 2006:87–108.

Vandenplas O, Malo JL: Inhalation challenges with agents causing occupational asthma. Eur Respir J 1997; 10:2612–2629.

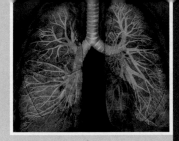

67 Toxic Inhalational Lung Injury

LEE S. NEWMAN • KAYLAN E. STINSON

A variety of chemicals when liberated into the atmosphere as gases, fumes, or mist can cause irritant lung injury or asphyxiation. As summarized in Table 67-1, any level of the respiratory tract can be the target for toxins, which produce a wide range of disorders from tracheitis and bronchitis to pulmonary edema.

EPIDEMIOLOGY, RISK FACTORS, AND PATHOLOGY

Epidemiology

Smoke inhalation is common among the general population. The use of potentially toxic chemicals in industry continues to rise, and accidental spills, explosions, and fires can result in complex exposures for which little is known of the health consequences. It is challenging to estimate the potential magnitude of the health effects produced by inhaled toxins. For example, in the United States alone, more than 500,000 workers are at risk of exposure to ammonia (NH_3) and other gases such as sulfur dioxide (SO_2). More than 100,000 individuals have potential exposure to hydrogen sulfide (H_2S). Tens of thousands risk smoke inhalation from household fires. The number of people environmentally exposed to potentially hazardous levels of air pollutants such as ozone can be estimated in the tens of millions. As a consequence of the World Trade Center collapse, it is now clear that firefighters and other rescue workers who respond to emergencies form an additional class of individuals at risk from exposures to complex mixtures of dust, fumes, and gas.

Etiology and Risk Factors

Major risk factors for inhalational exposure and injury are related to the environment and not to the host. Exposures occur randomly in the general environment, such as when a chemical spill occurs on a highway or railroad, carbon monoxide (CO) leaks in a home, or a person incorrectly mixes household chemicals together and releases a gas or aerosol. Smoke that comprises the pyrolysis products of synthetic materials is a common cause of injury to the respiratory tract, as well as a cause of pulmonary insufficiency and death from fires.

Occupational injuries are more common and occur especially when workers handle chemicals, work in areas that are inadequately ventilated, or enter exposed areas with improper protective equipment. Sources of occupational exposure to major chemical causes of irritant lung injury and asphyxiation are given in Table 67-2.

Factors that influence the acute effects of toxic chemicals include solubility, particle size, concentration, duration of exposure, chemical properties, and host factors such as minute ventilation of the exposed individual. The more water-soluble compounds dissolve in the upper respiratory tract and airways, whereas the less water-soluble agents tend to bypass the upper airway and affect peripheral airways and pulmonary parenchyma, as summarized in Figure 67-1.

Pathology

In general, the upper airway can be affected by most inhaled toxins, which result in edema of the nasal passage, posterior oropharynx, and larynx. In severe cases, mucous membrane ulceration and hemorrhage can ensue. Toxins of low water solubility may reach the lung parenchyma without necessarily producing upper airway lesions. If breath-holding, laryngospasm, and normal "scrubbing" activities of the nasopharynx fail to contain the exposure, lesions develop in the trachea and bronchi (e.g., paralysis of cilia, increased mucus production, goblet cell hyperplasia, injury to airway epithelium, epithelial denudation, exudation, submucosal hemorrhage, and edema). Pseudomembranes may form along the trachea and bronchi. The consequences may include various degrees of bronchiolitis, bronchiolitis obliterans (Figure 67-2), and organizing pneumonia (Figure 67-3). Bronchiolitis has been associated with exposures to nitrogen oxides (nitric oxide [NO]; nitrogen dioxide [NO_2], and nitrogen peroxide [N_2O_4]); sulfur dioxide; ammonia; chlorine [Cl_2]; phosgene; fly ash that contains trichloroethylene [C_2HCl_3]; ozone [O_3]; hydrogen sulfide; hydrogen fluoride [HF]; metal oxide fumes; dusts such as asbestos, silica, talc, and grain dust; free-base cocaine; tobacco smoke; and fire smoke.

Parenchymal injury is less common than airway damage. When alveolar or interstitial injury occurs, both epithelial and endothelial damage are observed. Injury typically results in alveolar-capillary leak, and the pathologic changes of acute respiratory distress syndrome (ARDS). Diffuse alveolar damage is a common histologic pattern in acute interstitial lung disease caused by inhaled toxins. It is characterized by widespread, diffuse edema, epithelial necrosis and cell sloughing (with exudates that fill the alveolar spaces), and formation of hyaline membranes (Figure 67-4). Later, diffuse alveolar damage may organize, which leads to proliferation of type II pneumonocytes, resorption of the hyaline membranes and exudates, and fibroblast proliferation. Long-term survivors of such parenchymal injury may fully recover or be left with various degrees of permanent interstitial fibrosis.

Pathogenesis

Asphyxiants, such as methane (CH_4) and carbon dioxide (CO_2), displace oxygen (O_2) from the air or, in the case of carbon monoxide, interfere with normal oxidative metabolism and oxygen transport. Typically, the more soluble gases

TABLE 67-1 Range of Toxicity Produced by Inhaled Agents

Example of Toxins	Effect
Carbon monoxide, cyanide, hydrogen sulfide	Asphyxiation
Ammonia	Mucous membrane irritation and sloughing
Ammonia, phosgene, hydrogen sulfide	Laryngeal edema and obstruction
Hydrogen chloride, chlorine	Tracheobronchitis
Ammonia	Bronchiectasis
Sulfur dioxide, hydrogen chloride, oxides of nitrogen, ozone	Bronchoconstricition, airway edema, asthma
Oxides of nitrogen, sulfur oxides	Bronchiolitis obliterans
Hydrongen fluoride, mustard gas	Chemical pneumonitis
Chlorine, phosgene	Acute respiratory distress syndrome
Hydrogen sulfide	Bacterial pneumonia
Ammonia	Pulmonary interstitial fibrosis
Hydrofluoric acid	Systemic effects, hypocalcemia, hypomagnesemia
Nitric oxide	Systemic effects, methemoglobinemia

produce greater injury in the upper airway, whereas less-soluble gases injure distal airways and parenchyma. Some of the irritant gases produce direct cellular injury because they are alkalis (e.g., ammonia) or acids (e.g., phosgene). Others, such as ozone and oxides of nitrogen, form oxygen-free radicals that cause respiratory tract injury. These gases may also produce smooth muscle bronchoconstriction and stimulate afferent parasympathetic receptors, which explain some of their ability to induce airway hyperreactivity and bronchoconstriction. Chronic lower-level exposures to various toxic gases, such as sulfur dioxide and chlorine, can induce copious mucus secretion, cough, bronchoconstriction, and bronchitis as a physiologic response to the inhalational exposure. Chronic bronchitis is common among workers exposed to relatively low levels of irritants and may increase their risk for development of chronic airflow obstruction and accelerated longitudinal decline in forced expiratory volume in 1 sec (FEV_1). In some instances, nonspecific airway hyperreactivity is induced by persistent, nonspecific irritant exposures.

CLINICAL FEATURES AND DIAGNOSIS

Initial efforts at diagnosis focus on the nature of the compound inhaled, approximating the probable circumstances of exposure (including the magnitude and duration of exposure), determining the water solubility of the inhaled agent, and determining whether the individual was exposed to multiple irritants and asphyxiants simultaneously, as occurs in firefighters or others subjected to smoke inhalation. Inhalational injury is suspected in those who have facial burns or inflamed nares. Headache and dizziness, along with chest pains and emesis, suggest systemic poisons, such as cyanide or hydrogen sulfide. Unconscious victims found in confined spaces are assumed to have received longer inhalational exposures than conscious ones because of the unprotected airways and concentrated exposures. Evidence of hoarseness, upper airway stridor, wheezing or rales, cough, and sputum production is assessed. Chest radiographs may show pulmonary edema, atelectasis, or infiltrates (Figure 67-5), although they are often negative early after exposure. Flow-volume loops are the most sensitive noninvasive indicators of upper and lower airway obstruction. Hypoxemia in the face of a normal arterial partial pressure of oxygen suggests carbon monoxide toxicity. Carboxyhemoglobin levels are obtained for all fire and explosion victims. Metabolic acidosis may indicate cyanide or hydrogen sulfide intoxication.

In individuals who have persistent symptoms months after exposure, bronchial provocation tests with methacholine may help assess whether the individual has reactive airway dysfunction syndrome. Computed tomography may help determine whether permanent fibrotic changes have developed.

TABLE 67-2 Sources of Exposure to Inhalational Toxins

Toxin	Sources of Exposure
Ammonia	Agriculture, explosives, plastics
Hydrogen chloride	Fertilizers, textiles, dyes, rubber, manufacture
Hydrofluoric acid	Fertilizers, insecticides, glass and ceramic etching, masonry, metal working, pharmaceuticals, chemical manufacture
Sulfur dioxide	Air pollution, smelting, power plants, chemical manufacture, paper manufacture, food preparation
Chlorine	Household cleaners, paper, textiles, sewage treatment, swimming pools
Oxides of nitrogen	Air pollution, welding, hockey rinks, chemical and dye manufacture, agriculture
Phosgene	Firefighters; paint strippers; chemical, pharmaceutical, and dye manufacturing; and chemical warfare
Mustard gas	Chemical welfare
Ozone	Welding, air pollution, high altitude, chemical manufacture
Carbon monoxide	Firefighters, smoke inhalation, smelters, miners, transportation, home furnaces
Hydrogen cyanide	Metallurgy, electroplating, plastics, polyurethane manufacture
Hydrogen sulfide	Metallurgy, chemical manufacture, wastewater treatment, natural gas and oil drilling, paper mills, coke ovens, rayon manufacture, rubber vulcanization

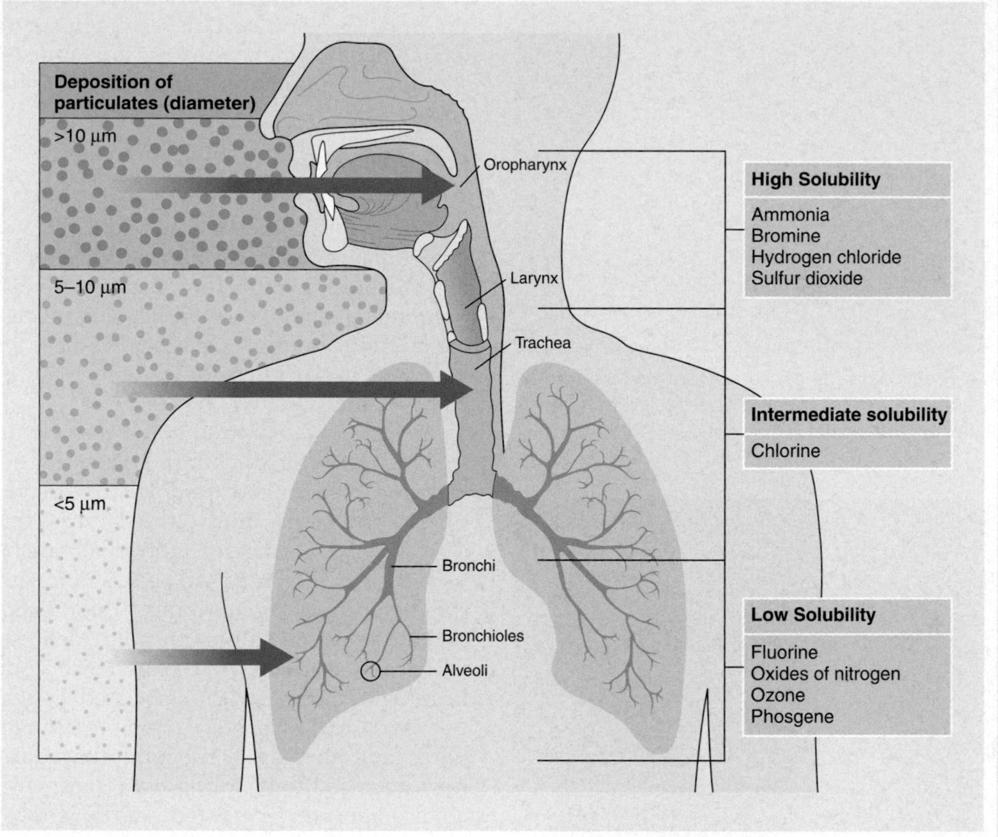

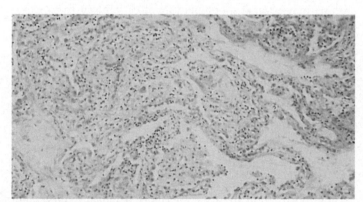

FIGURE 67-1 Distribution of gases and particulate matter in the respiratory tract influences the site of toxic injury.

FIGURE 67-2 Bronchiolitis obliterans organizing pneumonia caused by inhalation of oxides of nitrogen in a silo filler.

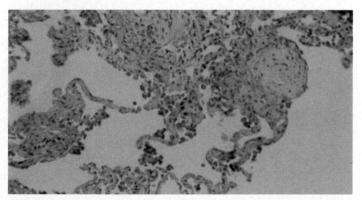

FIGURE 67-3 Organizing pneumonia after sulfur dioxide intoxication.

Chemical Irritants

Ammonia

Ammonia is a colorless, water-soluble, alkaline gas with a pungent odor. Because it is usually transported as a liquid, many accidents occur when it is being transferred from tanks to farm equipment. When it comes in contact with the mucosa, ammonia reacts with water to form a strong alkali, ammonium hydroxide (NH_4OH). Acute irritation of mucous membranes can be followed within hours by sloughing of the upper airway mucosa, edema, and obstruction. Laryngeal edema can present without other obvious clinical signs of burns, but if skin burns are present, inhalational injury is likely. Unusual complications include pneumonia and ARDS, which occur within hours to a few days of exposure. Long-term consequences include persistent bronchitis, bronchiectasis, airflow obstruction, interstitial fibrosis, and impaired gas exchange. Treatment is supportive—bronchodilators, oxygen therapy, and observation for need for airway protection. Early intubation may be required to defend the airway from acute laryngeal obstruction.

Hydrogen Chloride

Hydrogen chloride (HCl) is highly water soluble and injures the mucosa of the upper airways because of its acidity. Typically encountered in the manufacture of fertilizers, textiles,

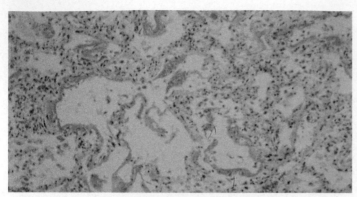

FIGURE 67-4 Diffuse alveolar damage caused by anhydrous ammonia inhalation. An agricultural worker inhaled the gas when a hose broke during the transfer of this fertilizing agent.

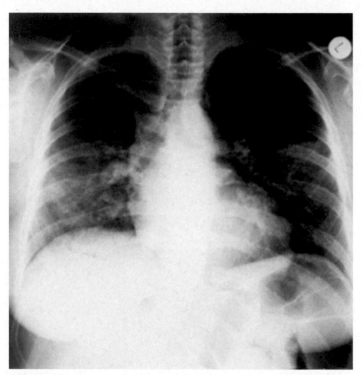

FIGURE 67-5 Radiographic changes produced by diffuse alveolar damage. Chest radiograph of the same patient as in Figure 67-4 shows acute, diffuse alveolar and interstitial infiltrates.

rubber, and dyes, acute exposure causes mucous membrane irritation of the eyes and airways at levels as low at 5–10 parts per million (ppm). Acute higher levels of exposure can cause acute airflow obstruction and gas exchange abnormalities. Meat wrappers become exposed to hydrogen chloride when they heat polyvinyl chloride film.

Hydrofluoric Acid

Hydrofluoric (HF) acid is highly corrosive, and most of the health effects from hydrofluoric acid involve dermal injury to the hands. HF acid releases free hydrogen ions that penetrate and corrode the skin, potentially down to bone, and even produce bone demineralization and necrosis. The respiratory effects parallel those of the skin, except that in the lungs the effects have a very rapid onset and patients are initially seen with acute respiratory distress. HF acid

is water soluble and thus exerts its predominant effects on the upper airways, which results in the rapid onset of tissue damage and bronchoconstriction, and sometimes even leads to chemical pneumonitis, delayed-onset pulmonary edema, and death.

Sulfur Dioxide

Sulfur dioxide and sulfuric acid (H_2SO_4) aerosols are produced by fossil fuel combustion. They are encountered in power plants and in various industrial processes such as smelting, chemical manufacture, paper manufacture, food preservation, metal and ore refining, and refrigeration. Past sulfur dioxide air pollution catastrophes have been associated with increased death rates for patients with chronic lung disease and the elderly.

As little as 0.5 ppm of sulfur dioxide can be detected in air from its characteristic odor. At levels of 6–10 ppm, immediate irritation of eyes and nasopharynx are reported. High exposures (≥ 50 ppm) injure the larynx, trachea, bronchi, and alveoli. A wide range of individual variability in the response to this substance is found, but atopic and asthmatic subjects show the most susceptibility. Prior exposure to ozone may potentiate the effect of sulfur dioxide in subjects with asthma. Classically, patients first experience a burning of the eyes, nose, and throat (with associated cough, chest pain, chest tightness, and dyspnea), along with conjunctivitis, corneal burns, and pharyngeal edema, followed hours later by pulmonary edema. Bronchiolitis obliterans can develop 2–3 weeks after exposure. Persistent airflow obstruction has been observed in smelter workers up to 4 years after overexposure, probably because of bronchiolitis obliterans.

Treatment is symptomatic. Systemic corticosteroids may be beneficial in acute toxicity. Bronchospasm in patients with asthma may reverse spontaneously after removal from exposure or may require administration of bronchodilators and inhaled corticosteroids.

Chlorine

Chlorine is of intermediate solubility and liberates hydrogen chloride and oxygen free radicals when it contacts water. The result is dose-dependent epithelial cell injury. At low levels of exposure, the upper airways and eyes are irritated. Increasing levels of exposure injure the nasopharynx and larynx. Higher exposures result in pulmonary edema within 6–24 h. Pulmonary function tests typically show airflow obstruction and air trapping. Long-term consequences include persistent airflow obstruction in some survivors. Clinical management is supportive. Even symptomatic individuals who have negative physical examinations and laboratory tests must be observed for at least 6 h because of the potential for a delay in the onset of significant airway toxicity. If symptoms persist, corticosteroids may improve outcome.

Oxides of Nitrogen

The oxides of nitrogen (NO, NO_2, N_2O_4) can produce fatal respiratory injury for some of the millions of workers who come into contact with these gases. Occupations at risk include coal miners after firing of explosives, welders who work with acetylene torches in confined spaces, hockey rink workers, and chemical workers who may be exposed to by-product fumes in the manufacture of dyes, lacquers, and nitric acid (HNO_3). "Silo-filler's disease" is caused by inhalation of nitrogen dioxide that forms when corn or alfalfa stored in a silo ferments. The risk is greatest in the first few weeks after the silo is filled. Because the oxides of nitrogen have low water solubility, the lower respiratory tract can be exposed to these potent oxidizers with little warning. Nitrogen dioxide reacts with water in the lung to form nitric and nitrous (HNO_2) acids. The oxides dissociate into oxygen free radicals, nitrates, and nitrites, which cause tissue inflammation, lipid peroxidation, and impairment of surfactant activity (among other cellular changes). Notably, nitric oxide has a high affinity for hemoglobin and so causes methemoglobinemia.

With exposures of 15–25 ppm, acute mucous membrane irritation affects the eyes and throat. At exposure levels of 25–100 ppm, toxic pneumonitis and bronchiolitis can develop, often with a smothering sensation and dyspnea. Exposures greater than 150 ppm are often fatal and are associated with bronchiolitis obliterans, chemical pneumonitis, and pulmonary edema. Nitrogen oxide and nitrogen dioxide produce the greatest degree of toxicity, which includes pulmonary edema and subsequent bronchiolitis obliterans. Symptom onset may be delayed, and patients are also cautioned that relapses can occur 3–6 weeks after initial exposure, with symptoms of cough, chills, fever, and shortness of breath. In some individuals, persistent obstructive lung disease and chronic bronchitis develop. Case reports suggest improvement after corticosteroids in those who manifest bronchiolar inflammation.

Phosgene

Also called carbonyl chloride, phosgene replaced chlorine as the preferred chemical weapon of World War I and resulted in most gas attack fatalities. Phosgene is an intermediate product in the manufacture of isocyanates, pesticides, dyes, and pharmaceuticals. It has a low odor threshold at 1 ppm and produces a characteristic smell of musty hay. As a result of its poor water solubility, phosgene causes only mild upper airway and eye irritant symptoms and deposits distally in the lung where it hydrolyzes to form hydrochloric acid (aqueous HCl) and carbon dioxide. At high levels of exposure, dyspnea, chest tightness, and cough occur. Acute exposure produces necrosis and sloughing of tracheal, bronchial, and bronchiolar mucosa with associated edema, hemorrhage, and atelectasis. Progressive respiratory failure and ARDS may follow.

Mustard Gas

Sulfur mustard gas was first used as a chemical warfare agent in Europe in 1917. Mustard agents are not gases but liquids at environmental temperatures. They are volatile, enter vapor phase at ambient temperatures, and have low water solubility. Exposure to sulfur mustard produces eye irritation and swelling within 2–3 h. With higher exposure, blurred vision, conjunctival edema, and iritis can occur, with potential for corneal ulceration. The skin itches, becomes pruritic and erythematous, and, 4–16 h later, forms blisters. Acute respiratory damage in this setting may be evident within a few hours or, more commonly, several days later. Chemical pneumonitis and pulmonary edema can also occur, with upper airway irritation, sneezing, hoarseness, epistaxis, cough, and dyspnea. Acute injury includes edema, inflammation, and destruction of the airway epithelium, with pseudomembranes developing that are similar to those seen with diphtheria. Secondary complications include infection and airway stenosis. The long-term effects include death caused by respiratory infections, chronic bronchitis, and accelerated longitudinal decline in airflow.

Ozone

Ozone is a light blue gas with an acrid "electric" odor. It occurs naturally in the stratosphere, where it is produced by the interaction between oxygen and ultraviolet light. In the troposphere, it is produced as a result of photochemical reactions between oxides of nitrogen and volatile organic compounds. Ozone is a major component of environmental air pollution and remains a serious pollutant for urban populations worldwide. Its low water solubility means that ozone principally affects the lower respiratory tract. In healthy individuals exposed to low concentrations of ozone, acute increases in airway resistance and decreases in FEV_1 and forced vital capacity have been reported, probably through a neural reflex mechanism. With acute exposures to low concentrations, patients can experience chest pain, dyspnea, and cough. Exposure to concentrations as low as 0.08 ppm for 6 h with intermittent exercise has been shown to cause lung function and inflammatory changes. Exposure to 0.12 ppm for 1 h is the U.S. Environmental Protection Agency Air Quality Standard.

Chemical Asphyxiants

Nitrous oxide, carbon monoxide, hydrogen cyanide (HCN), and hydrogen sulfide interfere with oxygen delivery, which results in asphyxiation. Others, such as methane, ethane (C_2H_6), argon (Ar), and helium (He_2), are more innocuous at low concentrations, but at high exposure levels can displace oxygen or block the reaction of cytochrome oxidase or hemoglobin, impairing cellular respiratory and oxygen transport. Several important asphyxiants are discussed in the following sections.

Carbon Monoxide

Carbon monoxide is colorless, tasteless, and odorless and is the major cause of death by poisoning in the United States and most industrialized countries. Exposure results from incomplete combustion of carbon-containing materials such as gasoline, coal, and wood. Home exposures occur from furnace gas leaks or fire smoke inhalation. Methylene chloride (CH_2Cl_2), which is used in paint strippers and as a household solvent, metabolizes into carbon monoxide and can be deadly if handled in poorly ventilated areas.

Severe forms of carbon monoxide poisoning are characterized by unconsciousness, seizures, syncope, coma, neurologic deficits, pulmonary edema, myocardial ischemia, and metabolic acidosis. Lower exposures produce symptoms of headache, nausea, weakness, giddiness, and tinnitus. Confusion typically occurs at carboxyhemoglobin levels greater than 30%, with coma ensuing at 35–45% and death at 50%. In addition to acute toxic effects, victims are at risk for delayed neuropsychologic effects. Carboxyhemoglobin levels correlate poorly with the clinical severity of neurologic sequelae. Carbon monoxide half-life in individuals at rest is approximately 4 h and can be reduced to 60–90 min by breathing 100% oxygen by face mask or to less than 60 min with oxygen administered by manual bag–assisted ventilation.

Nonrandomized studies have found that hyperbaric oxygen reverses the acute effects of carbon monoxide poisoning and is the most rapid means of reversing acute poisoning. Additional treatments may improve acute neurologic defects. Results of controlled trials are unclear as to the efficacy of hyperbaric oxygen as a treatment for the delayed neuropsychological symptoms. Cardiac monitoring is warranted for individuals who have carboxyhemoglobin levels greater than 25% because of the risk of arrhythmias and myocardial infarction.

Hydrogen Cyanide

Individuals exposed to smoke generated by the combustion or pyrolysis of plastics and polyurethanes are at particular risk of hydrogen cyanide toxicity. The fumes are absorbed through the skin and respiratory tract. By binding to the cytochrome A–cytochrome A$_3$ subcomplex, hydrogen cyanide blocks oxidative phosphorylation and mitochondrial oxygen use, which results in lactic acidosis.

Symptoms produced by exposures to 50 ppm of cyanide gas include headache, tachycardia, tachypnea, and dizziness. Exposures greater than 100 ppm can cause confusion, apnea, and seizures. The patient may emit a bitter almond odor, but this is not a reliable or consistent marker of exposure. The key to diagnosis rests with the occupational and environmental history. Venous blood appears hyperoxygenated, and the patient may have a distinctive red appearance before respiratory insufficiency, although, as in carbon monoxide poisoning, this is not a reliable clinical sign. Carboxyhemoglobin levels are measured to help separate cyanide intoxication from carbon monoxide poisoning. Treatment focuses on life support measures and detoxification. Early mechanical ventilation, hyperoxygenation, and treatment of metabolic acidosis are critical. Both amyl nitrate and sodium nitrite are recommended. Amyl nitrate and sodium nitrite form methemoglobin.

Hydrogen Sulfide

Hydrogen sulfide is both a respiratory irritant and asphyxiant. As a colorless, naturally occurring gas, it is found in marshes and sulfur springs, and as a decay product of organic matter. It is known for its typical "rotten egg" odor. Occupational exposure occurs in the manufacture of chemicals and metals, and in petroleum refineries, natural gas plants, coke ovens, paper mills, rubber vulcanization, rayon manufacture, and tanneries. Heavier than air, hydrogen sulfide accumulates in low-lying areas; it causes poisoning during oil drilling and wastewater treatment and as a result of natural gas field leaks. The hydrogen sulfide reaction with metalloenzymes, such as cytochrome oxidase, accounts for much of its toxicity in humans.

The odor threshold for this gas is low (0.13 ppm). At concentrations of 50 ppm, hydrogen sulfide is a mucous membrane irritant. Above 100 ppm, the gas fatigues the sense of olfaction, which makes individuals insensitive to its continued presence. When inhaled, it preferentially affects the lower respiratory tract. At concentrations of 250 ppm, pulmonary edema can occur. At 500 ppm, systemic and neurologic effects develop, with sudden loss of consciousness seen above 700 ppm. Above 1000 ppm, the gas produces hyperpnea and apnea, which paralyze respiratory drive centers. Thus, death caused by asphyxia can result at 1000 ppm or above.

Prolonged low-level (50 ppm) exposures can cause respiratory tract inflammation and drying; typical symptoms of cough, sore throat, hoarseness, rhinitis, and chest tightness occur between 50 and 250 ppm. At higher acute exposure levels, such symptoms may not manifest because of the rapid absorption of the gas through the lung into the bloodstream.

Management is generally supportive, with prompt endotracheal intubation and mechanical ventilation for severe cases of intoxication. Oxygen enhances sulfide metabolism and benefits hypoxic tissue. Because the mechanism of toxicity is similar to that of cyanide, induction of methemoglobinemia with infusion of 3% sodium nitrite or inhalation of amyl nitrate is recommended. Hyperbaric oxygen therapy may be beneficial.

Complex Exposures

In practice, individuals who incur inhalational injuries are frequently exposed to complex mixtures of toxic compounds rather than a single agent. Such mixtures may be poorly characterized but can contain admixtures of combustion products, pyrolysis products, metals, particulates, and gas. Recent studies illustrate the ability of such mixtures to produce a range of airway and diffuse interstitial lung lesions. Most notably are those studies done on rescue workers after the World Trade Center collapse.

World Trade Center Health Effects

As a consequence of exposures immediately after the World Trade Center collapse on September 11, 2001, pulmonary function decline, reactive airways dysfunction syndrome (RADS), asthma, reactive upper airways dysfunction syndrome (RUDS), sinus complaints, gastroesophageal reflux disease (GERD), and cases of inflammatory pulmonary parenchymal diseases such as sarcoidosis have been documented among rescue and recovery workers and volunteers. Specifically, among rescue workers with a high level of exposure, 8% experienced new onset of cough, 95% had symptoms of dyspnea, 87% had GERD, 54% had nasal congestion, and 23% of workers were identified as having bronchial hyperreactivity at 6 months after the collapse. Sixteen percent of rescue workers met the diagnosis criteria for RADS 1 year after the collapse. In a longitudinal study of pulmonary function in rescue workers before and after exposure, the average adjusted FEV$_1$ fell 372 mL during the year after September 11, which translates to an estimated 12 years of aging-related FEV$_1$ decline.

Factors such as dust alkalinity may have contributed to some of these conditions, although, as is often the case in acute situations, detailed information about the inhalational exposures in those workers is limited. Detailed qualitative and quantitative analyses of airborne pollutants with their changing composition during initial rescue/recovery and subsequent cleanup have been published; however, incomplete air quality monitoring during and early after the structural collapse make full individual assessment of this exposure problematic.

PITFALLS AND CONTROVERSIES

Many of the uncertainties in this arena of pulmonary medicine pertain to the management and treatment of inhalational injury, for which a few general comments apply. In cases of severe inhalational injury, intubation may be required for airway protection. Careful observation, preferably in an intensive care setting, is recommended for suspected cases of significant inhalational injury. Direct laryngoscopy or fiberoptic bronchoscopy is advocated by some investigators to assess for laryngeal edema. However, no clear guidelines are available to direct clinicians as to when intubation, laryngoscopy, or bronchoscopy is warranted. Although many clinicians may empirically prescribe corticosteroids, such medications have not proved efficacious. We depend on case reports and small case series to justify the use of corticosteroids.

A common clinical pitfall is to dismiss patients prematurely who may be at risk for delayed-onset respiratory disorders such as asthma, bronchiolitis obliterans, chemical pneumonitis, or pulmonary edema. Given sufficient dose and solubility, most acutely inhaled substances pose a risk for immediate or delayed-onset pulmonary edema, which warrants careful observation. Even those toxin victims who are thought to be stable and ready for discharge from the emergency department must be given detailed instructions about the warning signs of delayed-onset respiratory tract injury.

Routine performance of spirometry in groups that are considered to be at high risk for acute inhalational exposures may be warranted on the basis of the exposures of New York City firefighter and rescue worker clinics.

SUGGESTED READINGS

Amshel CE, Fealk MH, Phillips BJ, Caruso DM: Anhydrous ammonia burns: Case report and review of the literature. Burns 2000; 26: 493–497.

Banauch GL, Dhala A, Prezant DJ: Pulmonary disease in rescue workers at the World Trade Center site. Curr Opin Pulm Med 2005; 11:160–168.

Banauch GL, Hall C, Weiden M, *et al*: Pulmonary function after Exposure to the World Trade Center collapse in the New York City Fire Department. Am J Respir Crit Care Med 2006; 174:312–319.

Das R, Blanc PD: Chlorine gas exposure and the lung: A review. Toxicol Ind Health 1993; 9:439–455.

Douglas WW, Hepper NGG, Colby TV: Silo-filler's disease. Mayo Clin Proc 1989; 64:291–304.

Hnizdo E, Sullivan PA, Bang KM, Wagner G: Association between chronic obstructive pulmonary disease and employment by industry and occupation in the US population: A study of data from the Third National Health and Nutrition Examination Survey. Am J Epidemiol 2002; 156:738–746.

Mapp CE, Boschetto P, Maestrelli P, Fabbri LM: Occupational asthma. Am J Respir Crit Care Med 2005; 172:280–305.

Miller K, Chang A: Acute inhalation injury. Emerg Med Clin North Am 2003; 21:533–557.

Newman LS: Current concepts: Occupational illness. N Engl J Med 1995; 333:1128–1134.

Perkner JJ, Fennelly KP, Balkissoon R, *et al*: Irritant-associated vocal cord dysfunction. J Occup Environ Med 1998; 40:136–143.

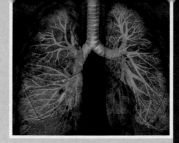

SECTION XV
OCCUPATIONAL AND ENVIRONMENTAL LUNG DISEASE

68 Air Pollution

CHRISTOPHER CARLSTEN • JOEL D. KAUFMAN

INTRODUCTION

Air pollution is a global problem with an impact on respiratory morbidity and mortality. Although exposures in developed countries have declined because of a variety of exposure controls and regulations, health effects are still substantial at current concentrations, and levels remain high in less-developed countries. We consider "air pollution" and associated respiratory (and some related cardiovascular) disease broadly but will focus on the agents and outcomes of greatest concern.

BACKGROUND

History

Air pollution has posed a threat to human health since the advent of fire. Products of combustion brought exposure to soot, and air pollution exposures accelerated dramatically with the industrial revolution, widespread use of fossil fuels, and dense urban growth. Only in the past century (particularly the past few decades), however, have the health impacts of air pollution been described in detail. In the mid-20th century, coal burning and industrial pollution combined with air stagnation to produce tragic episodes resulting in dozens of deaths clearly associated with acute pollution increases, such as in the Meuse Valley of Belgium (1930) and in Donora, PA (1948). With the 1952 London episode, when thousands of deaths resulted from a smog (Figure 68-1), fueled largely by coal-burning and held in place by a temperature inversion, recognition of the problem deepened. Furthermore, the episode gave early warning of the tight relation between pulmonary and cardiovascular complications of air pollution. Since that time, our understanding of air pollution–attributable disease has expanded greatly, most notably in its demonstration of chronic effects (including lung cancer, worsening of cystic fibrosis, and probably progression of atherosclerosis), and in teasing out the mechanisms and effects associated with specific air pollution sources and components. Importantly, the diversity of exposure and effects suggests that essentially all individuals, except perhaps the most isolated, are at risk for some air pollution–related toxicity. Furthermore, massive short-lived exposures, such as that associated with the destruction of the World Trade Center towers in New York City in 2001, still occur.

Concepts

Air pollution refers to any airborne substance unexpected in a "pristine" environment. Most commonly within the medical literature, however, the term refers to products of fossil fuel and biomass burning, industrial processes, and vehicular traffic. The focus of this chapter is on the air pollutants with the most evidence of ongoing and widespread threat to public health, but it should be noted that other federally regulated airborne toxins not covered here (e.g., lead and several "air toxics" such as benzene) are the products of diverse industrial processes. Still other air pollutants, such as environmental tobacco smoke, plant antigens, and windblown agricultural dusts, are primarily addressed in other chapters.

Urban air pollution is a complex mixture of particles and gases, and its composition varies considerably by both season and region. These variations are largely caused by differences in sources of pollutants, meteorology, and effects of physical geography. For example, sulfur dioxide (SO_2) and particulate sulfate is a concern in the Northeastern United States, largely because of regional transport of atmospherically transformed pollutants originating from coal-burning power plants, but less so in the Western United States. The Los Angeles basin has typically struggled to attain safe levels of ozone and particulate more so than other U.S. regions because of the combination of intense traffic sources of pollution, plentiful ultraviolet rays resulting in ozone and secondary particulate formation, and winds and mountains conspiring to promote air stagnation. Outside the developed world, exposures are complicated by fewer environmental controls, resulting in high pollutant concentrations in both cities (typically from vehicular and/or coal-burning sources) and in rural areas (because of the pronounced use of biomass fuel, including animal dung) for heating and cooking.

The chemistry, state, and size of a pollutant influence the resulting health effects (Figure 68-2). For example, deposition of particulate matter (PM) in the respiratory tract, the essential portal of entry, varies considerably by its size (Figure 68-3), with larger particles impacting in the more proximal airways, whereas finer particles achieve the greatest distal deposition (Figure 68-4). For other pollutants (especially gases), solubility is the primary determinant of effective dose, with more soluble substances, such as SO_2, being better absorbed by proximal mucosa. Furthermore, although most particulate matter health effects are attributed to a simple mass measurement in the air, particle composition is probably important in determining toxicity.

Air pollution remains an area of intense investigation, in which effects are increasingly documented, understood, and related to public health policy. Respiratory clinicians need to be aware of current standards for the air pollutants regulated under the Clean Air Act by the U.S. Environmental Protection Agency (EPA; Table 68-1). Notably, several states, such as California, have taken the lead in legislating lower standards than those promulgated by the EPA and have legislated limits on additional "air toxics" such as hydrogen sulfide and vinyl chloride (http://www.arb.ca.gov/toxics/id/taclist.htm). Many agencies and local organizations now have web- or e-mail–based

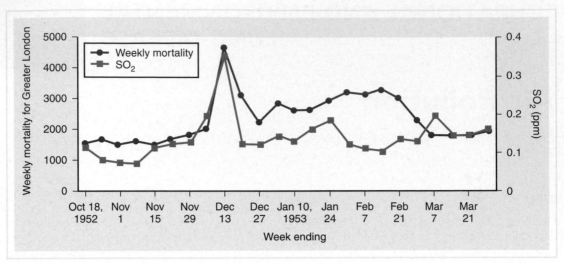

FIGURE 68-1 Weekly mortality in greater London, October 1951–March 1952. (Adapted from Bell ML, Davis DL: Reassessment of the lethal London fog of 1952: Novel indicators of acute and chronic consequences of acute exposure to air pollution. Environ Health Perspect 2001; 109 Suppl 3:389–94.)

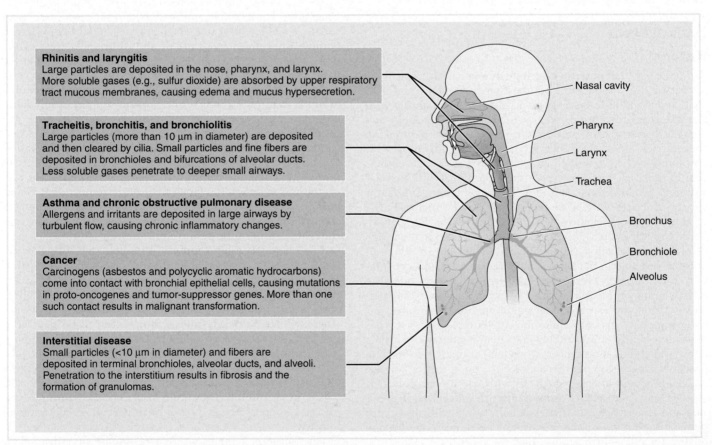

FIGURE 68-2 Physicochemical dynamics of air pollution deposition within airways. (Adapted from Beckett WS: Occupational respiratory diseases. N Engl J Med 2000; 342:406–13.)

air quality surveillance data, alerting systems, or at least an air quality index (AQI, a standardized index calibrating major air pollutants' levels to a common scale). These are available for easy access by the public (e.g., www.airnow. gov), and such data are often summarized and/or forecast in local newspapers as well. Most such systems indicate recommended actions, targeted to vulnerable populations (e.g., persons with asthma, elderly individuals), for given air quality circumstances, as exemplified in Table 68-2. Such recommendations regarding activity level and whether or not to stay indoors may be further discussed with one's personal physician. However, advice is complicated by an unclear

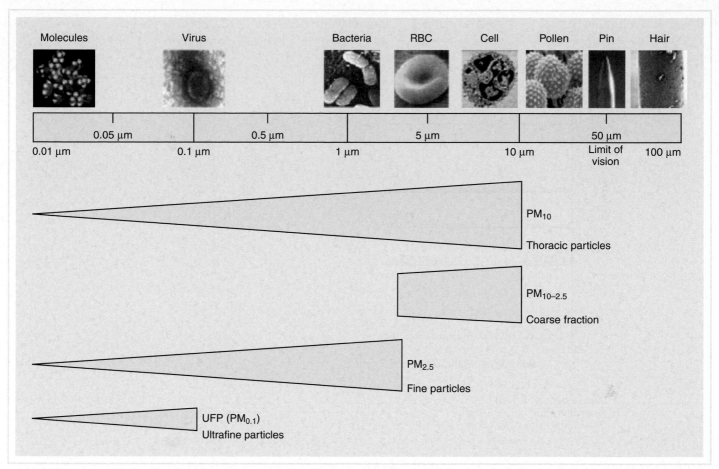

FIGURE 68-3 Size classification of particulate matter with reference to common structures. (Adapted from Brook RD, Franklin B, Cascio W, et al: Air pollution and cardiovascular disease: a statement for healthcare professionals from the Expert Panel on Population and Prevention Science of the American Heart Association. Circulation 2004; 109:2655–2671.)

understanding of the efficiency of indoor penetration of pollutants (e.g., relatively higher for particulate matter than for ozone); because the AQI is nonspecific with regard to pollutant, a recommendation to stay indoors may be falsely reassuring in a situation with high AQI driven mainly by PM. Further challenging is consideration of long-term trends in local air quality, as worried members of the population consider relocating to a "cleaner" environment in the face of minimal scientific guidance on the basis of scientific consensus.

KEY AGENTS OF CONCERN

Particulate Matter

PM refers to a wide range of particles, organic and nonorganic, but predominantly the product of combustion processes that are traditionally subdivided into size categories (see Figure 68-3) for the purposes of research and regulation. For example, diesel exhaust PM, a major contributor to total PM in urban environments, consists of a carbonaceous core and many organic and inorganic substances, including metals. It is important to consider the complex interplay between particle size and the chemical composition of context-specific PM in resultant cardiopulmonary toxicity. At present, only PM mass in $\mu g/m^3$ (in two size fractions, see Figure 68-3 and Table 68-1) is formally regulated, but there is increasing appreciation that this is an imperfect metric.

The global burden of disease attributable to PM is considerable, with $PM_{2.5}$ alone estimated to be responsible for 3% of cardiopulmonary mortality and up to 5% of airway cancer mortality, amounting to more than 1% of premature deaths, worldwide. Early evidence for mortality associated with chronic exposure to PM was demonstrated by the Six Cities Study, in which citizens of six U.S. cities (representing a range of air pollution severity) were studied as a prospective cohort. Fine particles were associated with an increased risk of mortality (rate ratio 1.26 for the most polluted vs the least polluted city; Figure 68-5). The American Cancer Society study, by use of a much larger cohort, again documented increased cardiopulmonary mortality risk associated with fine PM and, in addition, demonstrated increased lung cancer risk. Increased lung cancer risk has also been shown to be associated with PM_{10} in a distinctly nonsmoking cohort of Seventh Day Adventists. Recent epidemiologic approaches have demonstrated, among women, a dramatic 76% increase in cardiovascular deaths associated with a $10 \, \mu g/m^3$ increase in $PM_{2.5}$. Annual PM exposure averages have been associated with increased pulmonary exacerbations in those with cystic fibrosis.

Studies of acute effects of PM (Figure 68-6) have shown increases in asthma symptoms, emergency room visits, and hospitalizations (adults and/or children); COPD exacerbations and admissions; upper respiratory infections; and a range of cardiovascular outcomes, including myocardial infarction events, admissions, and deaths. Overall, acute PM exposure

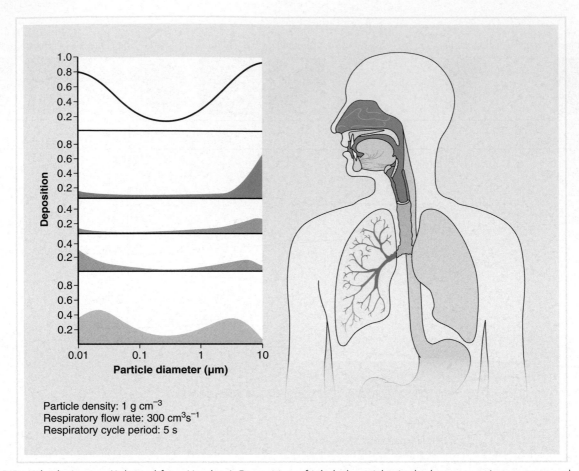

FIGURE 68-4 Particle dosimetry. (Adapted from Heyder J: Deposition of inhaled particles in the human respiratory tract and consequences for regional targeting in respiratory drug delivery. Proc Am Thorac Soc 2004; 1:315–320.)

TABLE 68-1 U.S. National Ambient Air Quality Standards (Primary Standards Only)

Pollutant	Standard	Averaging Time
Carbon monoxide	9 ppm (10 mg/m^3)	8-h
Lead	1.5 µg/m^3	Quarterly average
Nitrogen dioxide	0.053 ppm (100 µg/m^3)	Annual (arithmetic mean)
Particulate matter (PM$_{10}$)	150 µg/m^3	24-h
Particulate matter (PM$_{2.5}$)	15.0 µg/m^3	Annual (arithmetic mean)
	35 µg/m^3	24-h
Ozone	0.08 ppm	8-h
	0.12 ppm (applies only in limited high-ozone areas)	1-h
Sulfur oxides	0.03 ppm	Annual (arithmetic mean)
	0.14 ppm	24-h

From http://epa.gov/air/criteria.html.

TABLE 68-2 Air Quality Index for 8-Hour Ozone and Associated Recommendations

AQI Index Values	Health Categories	Cautionary Statements for 8-h Ozone
0–50	Good	None
51–100	Moderate	Unusually sensitive people should consider limiting prolonged outdoor exertion.
101–150	Unhealthy for sensitive groups	Active children and adults and people with respiratory disease, such as asthma, should limit prolonged outdoor exertion.
151–200	Unhealthy	Active children and adults and people with respiratory disease, such as asthma, should avoid prolonged outdoor exertion; everyone else, especially children, should limit prolonged outdoor exertion.
201–300	Very unhealthy	Active children and adults and people with respiratory disease, such as asthma, should avoid all outdoor exertion; everyone else especially children, should limit outdoor exertion.
301–500	Hazardous	Everyone should avoid all outdoor exertion.

From www.airnow.gov.

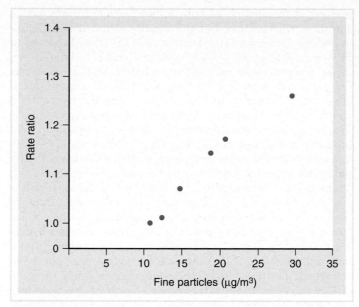

FIGURE 68-5 Association of fine particulate concentration and mortality rate ratio from Harvard Six Cities Study. (Adapted from Dockery DW, Pope CA, Xu X, *et al*: An association between air pollution and mortality in six U.S. cities. N Engl J Med 1993; 329:1753–1759.)

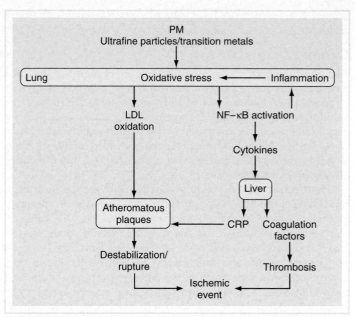

FIGURE 68-7 Proposed mechanistic pathways describing lung mediation of cardiovascular events. (Adapted from Donaldson K, Stone V, Seaton A, *et al*: Ambient particle inhalation and the cardiovascular system: Potential mechanisms. Environ Health Perspect 2001; 109 Suppl 4:523–527.)

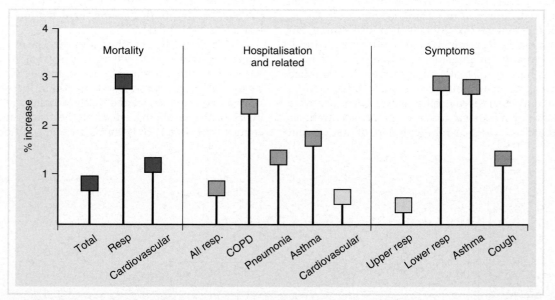

FIGURE 68-6 The percentage increase in mortality, morbidity, and symptoms associated with an acute 10 μg/m³ increase in PM_{10}, average of more than 100 studies. (Adapted from Donaldson K, Mills N, Macnee W, *et al*: Role of inflammation in cardiopulmonary health effects of PM. Toxicol Appl Pharmacol 2005; 207[2 Suppl]:483–488.)

studies suggest an approximately 1% increase in mortality associated with each 10 μg/m³ increase in PM_{10}. On a population basis, this implies significant adverse public health impact.

The mechanism by which fine PM might cause cardiovascular disease is not known. Although it has been proposed that small particles can translocate directly from the lung into the vasculature, preliminary observations to support this have not been consistently replicated. It may be that subtle inflammatory changes in the lung initiate a cascade of events leading to downstream vascular effects (Figure 68-7).

At present, there is great interest in the ultrafine (<0.1 μm in aerodynamic diameter) subset of fine PM; given the relatively high surface area of ultrafine PM and the belief that surface area may be a key metric of toxicity, this particle fraction may be subject to more attention and controls in the future, but routine monitoring is not now undertaken. Conversely, for specific disorders such as COPD, others have argued for an increased toxicity of coarse particles (particle diameter between 2.5 and 10 µm).

Ozone

Although several occupational settings are recognized for focal ozone production, ground-level ozone (O_3) is largely the result of tropospheric photolysis of nitrogen oxides (the product of vehicular and industrial combustion processes) and volatile organic compounds, catalyzed by ultraviolet radiation. In contrast to other air pollutants, O_3 levels are often higher far from heavily trafficked areas where traffic-derived nitric oxides effectively scavenge O_3.

There is evidence for ozone-related cardiovascular mortality, but not as compelling support for ozone-associated respiratory mortality on an epidemiologic basis. However, O_3-induced respiratory morbidity has been studied and documented extensively and includes decreases in lung function (in both normal and asthmatic individuals) and increases in rhinitis, airway inflammation, asthmatic emergency room visits and hospitalization, COPD admissions, and several respiratory symptoms. Most of these associations are strongest in vulnerable populations, such as children and the elderly. In children, increases in asthma incidence have also been noted at levels below the current standards; the evidence is mixed regarding blunted lung function growth. As a result, many have recommended lowering the 0.08 ppm 8-h federal standard, which is currently up for review and is commonly exceeded in some parts of the United States (Figure 68-8). There is evidence that further lowering of O_3 levels can result in substantial reduction in asthma events.

The mechanism of ozone toxicity is likely multifactorial, but the primary functional effect is thought to be a decrease in inspiratory capacity. Airway inflammation, particularly in persons with asthma, has been consistently demonstrated in controlled exposures; increased neutrophils, eosinophils, inflammatory cytokines, and epithelial permeability have been noted in bronchoalveolar fluid in response to variable O_3 concentrations. In addition, there is evidence for depletion of antioxidant

reserves in the airways of both asthmatics and healthy adults and those with asthma, but the severity of this deficit (worse in persons with asthma) did not predict O_3-related changes in FEV_1 or neutrophilia (Figure 68-9). In children, limited evidence suggests that antioxidant supplementation abrogates O_3-associated decreases in lung function. Oxidant-induced effects occur through activation of the transcription factor NFκB and its nuclear translocation. Decreased inspiratory capacity may be mediated neurogenically by means of arachidonic acid products' stimulation of C (pain) fibers in the lung.

Coexposures to ozone and allergens interact to considerably potentiate bronchial hyperreactivity, and it is likely that this interaction is augmented by exposure to endotoxin, which is common. Moreover, ozone interacts with other air pollutants, such as PM, to augment lung inflammation, and such copollutant dynamics may compound the severity of bronchial hyperreactivity even further, although the relationship between lung inflammation and pulmonary function has not been consistent. Further complicating our understanding of these effects, it has been shown that repeated exposure to high-dose O_3 (400 ppm) results in tolerance (e.g., attenuation of lung function decrements).

Sulfur Dioxide

Sulfur dioxide (SO_2) is derived primarily from combustion of sulfur-containing fuels, particularly at power plants and oil refineries. It is used in several industrial settings, including chemical manufacturing, paper manufacturing, and food preservation, and in these contexts is subject to a significantly higher 8-h standard (2 ppm) than the regulated limit for ambient air levels (see Table 68-1).

SO_2 is efficiently absorbed into the mucosa of the eyes and upper respiratory tract, where it is a strong irritant, but more distal effects are facilitated by adsorption of SO_2 onto carbonaceous PM. Furthermore, oral breathing, particularly at high ventilatory rates associated with exercise, at least partially bypasses the scrubbing effect of the nasal mucosa. When in contact with water, SO_2 forms an acid solution that includes

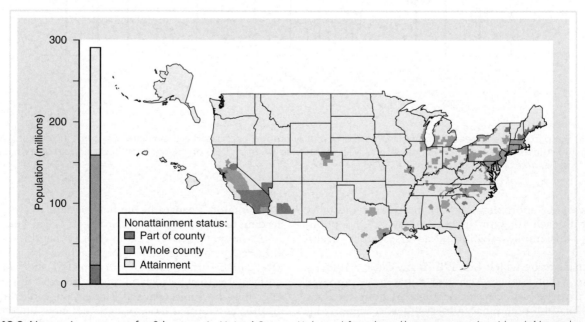

FIGURE 68-8 Nonattainment map for 8-h ozone in United States. (Adapted from http://www.epa.gov/oar/data/. November 2, 2005.)

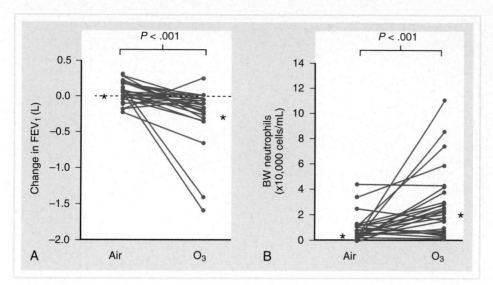

FIGURE 68-9 Changes in airflow and bronchial wash neutrophils associated with 2-h exposure to 0.2 ppm ozone. (Adapted from Mudway IS, Stenfors N, Blomberg A, et al: Differences in basal airway antioxidant concentrations are not predictive of individual responsiveness to ozone: A comparison of healthy and mild asthmatic subjects. Free Radic Biol Med 2001; 31:962–974; as noted in text of this chapter, but not in figure, relationship not altered by antioxidant status.)

sulfuric acid, thought to be responsible for at least some of the inflammation and cellular damage noted in animal and human studies.

Lung function in healthy individuals is relatively resistant to the effects of considerable doses of SO_2 (5 ppm), but even lower doses (e.g., <1 ppm) elicit acute and substantial bronchoconstriction in asthmatics, an effect that is intensified with exercise and cold or dry air. Recovery from the insult generally occurs within a few hours, and there is some evidence for attenuated effect with repeated exposure (like ozone) and for blunting of effect with mast cell–stabilizing agents or theophylline. Although SO_2-specific lung function changes have been consistently shown, these have not been demonstrated with sulfuric acid aerosol exposure in persons with asthma. Furthermore, there are inconsistent reports on whether SO_2 induces an increased sensitivity to nonspecific agents such as methacholine, and there is no consistent relationship between one's baseline sensitivity to methacholine and one's sensitivity to SO_2. The effects of SO_2 on bronchial hyperresponsiveness are accentuated with preceding ozone exposure, and SO_2 may enhance responsiveness to allergens. SO_2 does not seem to be independently responsible for air pollution–related mortality or carcinogenicity.

The hypothesized mechanisms of SO_2-induced bronchoconstriction include increased resistance because of vascular distention with consequent mucosal edema, smooth muscle contraction, intra-airway secretions, and airway cholinergic nerve stimulation promoting cough and/or "neurogenic inflammation."

Nitrogen Dioxide

NO_2 is formed during the combustion of fossil fuels, predominantly at power plants and in vehicles and, therefore, may contribute, along with PM, to the overall toxicity of vehicle-derived combustion products, such as diesel exhaust. Indoor production of NO_2 can also be significant, through the use of gas or kerosene cooking stoves or heaters, in closed settings such as mining (through diesel exhaust combustion), and in ice skating arenas.

Although also an oxidant, NO_2 does not seem to have as significant a bronchoconstricting effect as ozone. High concentrations found in silos (often >10 ppm) can cause the acute

and severe pulmonary edema (silo-filler's disease), and the Air Pollution and Health: A European Approach (APHEA) project has shown that peak ambient NO_2 levels correlate with asthma admissions. Moreover, subclinical deficits in lung development in healthy adolescents, with presumed potential for clinical implications in adults, were noted in a prospective cohort (Figure 68-10). Typical ice arena levels, in the 200-ppb range, seem not to cause adverse effects beyond upper respiratory symptoms. However, as with other air pollutants, NO_2 is likely to be harmful by acting in synergy with other agents. For example, modest short-term NO_2 levels (20 ppb), in conjunction with a viral respiratory infection, led to more severe symptoms and decreased peak flows in a study of children; a similar design has not yet been replicated in adults. Furthermore, realistic domestic concentrations of NO_2 (400 ppb), in combination with house dust mite allergen but not alone, have been shown to significantly decrease FEV_1 in adults with asthma. Much higher levels (3 ppm as an 8-h time-weighted average) are considered tolerable according to occupational standards, although animal studies show significant damage to bronchial epithelium at similar levels and peak ice arena levels (2–3 ppm) have been associated with cases of severe pneumonitis.

NO_2, like O_3, seems to be potently proinflammatory (e.g., increased IL-8 and neutrophils) but has less oxidative potential. NO_2-induced airway inflammation may occur more proximally, relative to ozone, although their solubilities are similar. In addition, NO_2 seems to impair the function of alveolar macrophages and epithelial cells, which may explain its interaction with infectious agents.

Products of Biomass Burning

Intentional or unintentional burning of wood, agricultural crops, and other biomass produces a complex mixture of gases and particles (including NO_2, SO_2, PM, and polyaromatic hydrocarbons). In certain regions of the United States, including episodically in the Pacific Northwest, and perennially in much of the rural developing world, biomass smoke may be the predominant contributor to PM and may produce PM levels that exceed federal standards by an order of magnitude. Biomass smoke has been associated with a range of health effects, including COPD and asthma exacerbations and hospitalizations, lung function declines, and circulating neutrophils.

FIGURE 68-10 Association between average NO_2 and average growth in FEV_1 in girls and boys approaching adulthood over a 8-year period. (Adapted from Gauderman WJ, Avol E, Gilliland F, et al: The effect of air pollution on lung development from 10 to 18 years of age. N Engl J Med 2004; 351:1057–1067.)

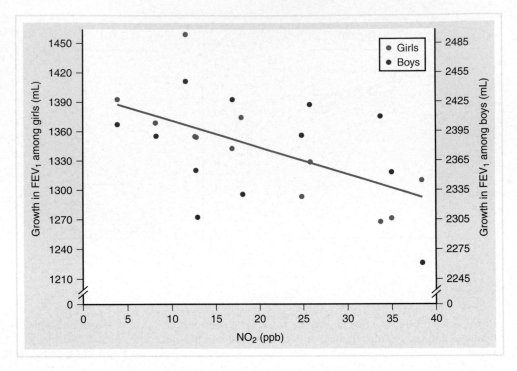

Dramatic short-term increases in biomass burning (i.e., forest fires) are associated with increased mortality, and up to 2 million deaths annually are attributed to biomass exposures.

Traffic-Related Air Pollution

Several studies consider proximity to traffic, with mixed emissions of particulate matter and several noxious gases (e.g., oxides of nitrogen [NO_x]), as the fundamental exposure metric. Overall mortality and respiratory and cardiac morbidity have all been associated with proximity to traffic, even after controlling for possible socioeconomic confounders. Recently, proximity to freeways has also been associated with blunted lung function development in children entering adulthood. Allergens seem to exacerbate upper respiratory inflammatory phenomena because of traffic-derived PM, such as diesel exhaust (DE), but such an effect has not yet been clearly demonstrated in the lung. DE, the prototypical traffic-based source of ultrafine particulate matter, is currently of great interest, given significant toxicity potentially driven by the very high surface area-to-mass ratio of ultrafine PM relative to other PM.

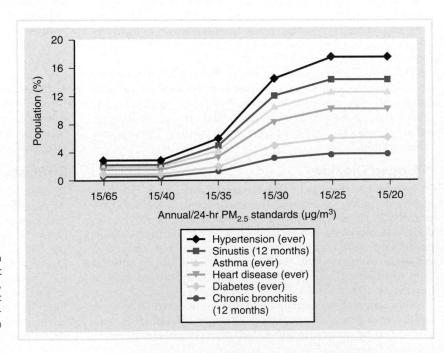

FIGURE 68-11 Hypothetical benefits of reductions in annual $PM_{2.5}$ standards (y-axis refers to percent expected to benefit). (Adapted from Johnston RS, Graham JJ: Fine Particulate Matter National Ambient Air Quality Standards: Public Health Impact on Populations in the Northeastern United States. Environ Health Perspect 2005; 113:1140–1147.)

CURRENT RESEARCH FRONTIERS AND CHALLENGES AND CLOSING COMMENTS

Unanswered questions are suggested by the uncertainties described previously, and a few major topics require some discussion.

Global warming, now accepted as an active phenomenon by all but a diminishing minority of scientists, is likely to impact air pollution patterns and associated morbidity and mortality through effects on tropospheric reactions, fossil fuel use for air conditioning, and increased stress on vulnerable populations. Some scientists believe that climate change will significantly increase the number of summer days that exceed air-quality standards, but the ultimate effect of this trend is highly debated.

Genetic variation, and the impact of specific genetic polymorphisms on air pollution–mediated health effects, is of increasing interest. For example, genes for quinone- and glutathione-metabolizing enzymes have been shown to modulate ozone-associated changes in lung function and PM-associated changes in heart rate variability. Further insight may lead to effective interventions and further understanding of mechanisms.

Oxidative stress seems to be a common underlying mechanism in air pollution's respiratory effects, but capitalizing on this understanding with preventive or therapeutic antioxidant strategies remains largely theoretical.

The interaction between pulmonary and cardiac effects of air pollution remains poorly understood. As noted previously, a seminal controversy in this regard is the extent to which particles directly cross the alveolar–capillary border. If this does not occur, it remains uncertain how major cardiovascular complications occur in the absence of a more dramatic pulmonary reaction, although mediation by soluble mediators or the autonomic nervous system is proposed.

Safe thresholds, particularly for PM, have not been demonstrated. Regardless, reductions in $PM_{2.5}$ commensurate with recently tightened standards (from 65 to 35 μg/m^3 by 24-hour average) are projected to generate tangible gains in respiratory health end points (Figure 68-11).

SUGGESTED READINGS

Atkinson RW, Anderson HR, Sunyer J, et al: APHEA 2 project. Air Pollution and Health: a European Approach. Am J Respir Crit Care Med 2001; 164:1860–1866.

Brook RD, Franklin B, Cascio W, et al: Air pollution and cardiovascular disease: a statement for healthcare professionals from the Expert Panel on Population and Prevention Science of the American Heart Association. Circulation 2004; 109:2655–2671.

Brunekreef B, Holgate ST: Air pollution and health. Lancet 2002; 360:1233–1242.

D'Amato G: Outdoor air pollution, climatic changes and allergic bronchial asthma. ERJ 2002; 20:763–776.

Dockery DW, Pope CA, Xu X, et al: An association between air pollution and mortality in six U.S. cities. N Engl J Med 1993; 329:1753–1759.

Ezzati M, Kammen DM: The health impacts of exposure to indoor air pollution from solid fuels in developing countries: knowledge, gaps, and data needs. Environ Health Perspect 2002; 110:1057–1068.

McConnell R, Berhane K, Gilliland F, et al: Asthma in exercising children exposed to ozone: a cohort study. Lancet 2002; 359:386–391.

Miller KA, Siskovick DS, Sheppard L, et al: Long–term exposure to air pollution and incidence of cardiovascular events in women. N Engl J Med 2007; 356:447–458.

Naeher LP, Brauer M, Lipsett M, et al: Woodsmoke health effects: a review. Inhalation Toxicol 2006; 19:67–106.

Pope CA, Burnett RT, Thun MJ, et al: Lung cancer, cardiopulmonary mortality, and long-term exposure to fine particulate air pollution. JAMA 2002; 287:1132–1141.

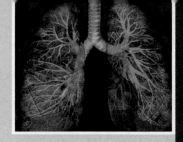

69 Pleural Effusion, Empyema, and Pneumothorax

HELEN E. DAVIES • Y.C. GARY LEE

PLEURAL EFFUSION

Pleural effusions, defined as the accumulation of fluid in the pleural space, are common and affect more than 3000 people per million population each year. Pleural effusions occur when the rate of pleural fluid formation exceeds that of absorption and may occur with pleural, pulmonary, or systemic disease. A systematic approach is required to explain the underlying cause.

EPIDEMIOLOGY AND PATHOPHYSIOLOGY

Epidemiology

There are more than 55 documented causes of pleural effusions. The relative incidences of different types of effusion vary according to patient demographics and geographic areas. Heart failure is responsible for approximately one third of all pleural effusions (Table 69-1), with pleural infection and malignancy accounting for most exudative effusions.

Pathophysiology

In the healthy person, the pleural cavity contains a small amount of physiologic pleural fluid (<10 mL in a 70-kg man) in part to facilitate smooth gliding of the lung over chest wall during respiration. The rate of normal fluid production is approximately 17 mL/day, with the estimated maximal absorptive capacity 0.2–0.3 mL/kg/h into lymphatic channels.

Transudative effusions accumulate because of an increase in hydrostatic pressure and/or a reduction in plasma oncotic pressure; the pleura usually remain normal. In contrast, development of exudative effusions is usually a result of various pleural pathologic conditions, resulting in increased vascular permeability and/or impaired fluid resorption (e.g., lymphatic obstruction).

Pleural fluid can accumulate from extrapleural sources. Transdiaphragmatic migration of peritoneal fluid is well recognized. Abnormal communications between the pleural cavity and the thoracic duct (chylothorax), esophagus, pancreas, renal tract (urinothorax), dura mater, etc. can also cause pleural effusions.

CLINICAL FEATURES

Patients may be asymptomatic but often present with dyspnea, chest pain, or features of underlying disease. Dyspnea is a result of altered diaphragmatic and chest wall mechanics and compression of the lung. Pleuritic chest pain indicates disease involvement of the parietal pleura. Physical examination reveals a stony dull percussion note with decreased fremitus and absent breath sounds over the effusion. Note that such signs are not distinguishable from those of an elevated diaphragm.

DIAGNOSIS

In most cases, the underlying diagnosis can be established from a detailed history, physical examination, radiologic imaging, and pleural fluid/tissue analysis.

Imaging

Most pleural effusions can be recognized on posteroanterior or lateral chest radiographs. Large effusions may produce contralateral mediastinal shift. Blunting of the costophrenic angle may be the only sign for a small effusion but may also represent pleural thickening. The role of decubitus X-ray has been largely replaced by ultrasonography, which can detect pleural fluid with a sensitivity approaching 100%. Ultrasound also enables differentiation of fluid, consolidated lung, and pleural thickening and is sensitive in detecting fluid loculations (Figure 69-1). Computed tomography (CT) with pleural-phase contrast enhancement provides better detection of pleural abnormalities and aids discrimination of benign and malignant disease (Figure 69-2). To date, magnetic resonance imaging (MRI) has a limited clinical role in the management of pleural diseases. The roles of positron emission tomography (PET) and PET/CT scanning are under investigation.

Diagnostic Approach

Investigation of a pleural effusion should be performed with a stepwise approach (Figure 69-3). Thoracentesis should be the initial investigation in all pleural effusions of uncertain origin. Small effusions should be aspirated under radiologic guidance. Thoracentesis is generally safe. Complications are uncommon but include vasovagal syncope (0.6%), pneumothorax, infection, and bleeding. Removal of large amounts of fluid may precipitate reexpansion pulmonary edema, and, if patients develop a cough or chest pain, the procedure should be discontinued. Pleural manometry has been advocated but is not widely available.

If initial pleural fluid analysis is inconclusive, repeat thoracentesis and obtaining pleural tissue (e.g., by thoracoscopy or percutaneously) for histologic examination should be considered. (See Chapter 13.)

TABLE 69-1 Approximate Annual Incidence of Various Types of Pleural Effusions in the United States

Etiology	Number	Percentage	Percentage of Noncardiac Effusions
Congestive heart failure	500,000	37.4	
Other causes		62.6	
Pneumonia	400,000		48.0
Malignant disease	200,000		24.0
Pulmonary embolism	150,000		18.0
Cirrhosis with ascites	50,000		6.0
Gastrointestinal disease	25,000		3.0
Collagen vascular disease	6000		0.7
Tuberculosis	2500		0.3
Asbestos pleuritis	2000		0.25
Mesothelioma	1500		0.2
Total	1,337,000	100.0	100.0

Adapted with permission from Light RW, ed: Pleural Diseases. 4th ed. Philadelphia: Lippincott Williams & Wilkins; 2001.

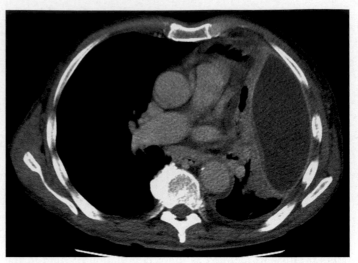

FIGURE 69-2 A contrast-enhanced computed tomography image of a pleural empyema. The "split pleura" sign is demonstrated with enhancement of both the visceral and the parietal pleural surfaces evident. (Courtesy of Dr Rachel Benamore, Oxford, UK.)

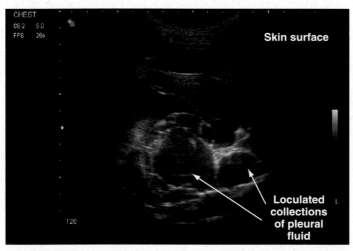

FIGURE 69-1 Pleural ultrasound is valuable in detecting pleural fluid and septations within an effusion.

Pleural Fluid Analysis

Pleural fluid analysis can help determine the diagnosis or direct further investigations. Large numbers of tests are now available. Understanding the indications and limitations of the individual tests is essential for the clinicians to provide an efficient and cost-effective service (Table 69-2).

Bedside Examination of the Fluid. Most pleural fluids are straw colored (serous), serosanguineous (blood stained), or hemorrhagic. A genuine hemothorax is characterized by fluid hematocrit of greater than 50% of blood hematocrit.

Appearance of the fluid may reveal the diagnosis: presence of pus confirms empyema; food particles in the fluid suggest esophageal perforation; and chyle is diagnostic of chylothorax

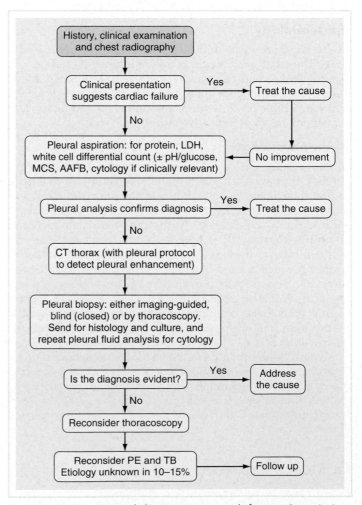

FIGURE 69-3 Suggested diagnostic approach for a unilateral pleural effusion. (Investigations requested should correlate with clinical suspicion.)

TABLE 69-2 Investigative Parameters of Pleural Effusion

Obligatory	For Specific Purposes	
	Assay	Suspected Pathology
Appearance/smell	Glucose/pH	Pleural infection
Total protein/LDH	Microbiology:	Pleural infection/TB
White cell differential count	Gram staining	
	Bacteriology	
	AAFB/tubercle bacilli	
	Fungi, parasites	
	Cytology	Malignancy
	Amylase	Pancreatitis
	Hematocrit	Hemothorax
	Cholesterol/triglycerides	Chylothorax/pseudochylothorax
	Adenosine deaminase (ADA)	TB
	Bilirubin	Bilothorax
	Creatinine	Urinothorax

LDH, Lactate dehydrogenase; *TB,* tuberculosis; *AAFB,* acid and alcohol fast bacilli.

or pseudochylothorax. Pleural fluid that appears milky should be centrifuged: in empyema, a clear supernatant is seen, whereas chyle remains cloudy. The smell of ammonia is often the diagnostic hint for urinothorax.

Separation of Exudates and Transudates. Exudative pleural effusions are most commonly defined by Light's criteria (Box 69-1), by use of the fluid/serum ratio of protein and lactate dehydrogenase, which have an accuracy of 96%. Numerous other markers and criteria have been tested (including measurement of pleural fluid cholesterol values), but none has proved superior. Distinguishing exudates from transudates narrows the range of differential diagnoses and helps streamline further investigations.

Differential Leukocyte Count. The cellular portion of physiologic pleural fluid consists predominantly of macrophages/monocytes. In disease states, the differential cell count of the pleural fluid may be helpful in determining the etiology (Table 69-3). Acute pleural inflammation or injury generates increased levels of chemotaxins, such as interleukin-8, which attract neutrophils to the pleural space. Therefore, a neutrophil-predominant effusion is seen with acute bacterial pneumonia or pulmonary infarction. A lymphocyte-rich fluid is more common in disease of insidious onset such as tuberculosis or malignancy. However, up to 10% of tuberculous effusions may be neutrophilic. An increased eosinophil count (>10% of total leukocytes) may be found in various diseases (e.g., Churg–Strauss syndrome or drug-induced pleural effusions) but is often nonspecific.

pH and Glucose. Pleural fluid pH (or glucose) can add useful information for management. Low glucose levels are associated with a similar spectrum of diseases that give rise to low pH effusions (e.g., infection and connective tissue diseases) (Box 69-2) and are equally informative except in patients with hyperglycemia.

TABLE 69-3 Pleural Fluid Differential Cell Count

	Common Causes
Lymphocytic effusion (>85% total nucleated cells)	Tuberculosis Malignancy including lymphoma Rheumatoid effusion Sarcoidosis Yellow nail syndrome Chylothorax
Eosinophilic effusion (>10% eosinophils)	Pneumothorax Hemothorax Drug-induced pleurisy Infection (tuberculosis/fungal/parasitic) Benign asbestos pleural effusion Churg-Strauss syndrome Malignancy Early post CABG
Neutrophilic effusion	Acute pleural injury/inflammation Parapneumonic Pulmonary embolism

BOX 69-1 Light's Criteria

A pleural fluid is an *exudate* if any of the following criteria are met:
1. Pleural fluid to serum protein ratio >0.5
2. Pleural fluid to serum lactate dehydrogenase (LDH) >0.6
3. Pleural fluid LDH more than two thirds the upper limit of normal serum LDH

Caveat: False positive results may occur in patients taking diuretic therapy resulting in a pleural/serum protein ratio >0.5. Clinical judgment and calculation of the serum-pleural fluid protein gradient (>3.1 g/dL) will define a true transudate.

BOX 69-2 Conditions Commonly Associated with Low pH (<7.3) and Low Glucose (<3.3 mmol/L [60 mg/dL]) Pleural Effusions

Empyema
Complicated parapneumonic effusion
Malignant effusion
Rheumatoid pleuritis
Tuberculosis
Lupus pleurisy
Esophageal rupture
Urinothorax (transudate)

Physiologic pleural fluid pH is approximately 7.6 and reflects bicarbonate accumulation within the pleural cavity. Pleural fluid pH is best measured by use of an arterial blood gas analyzer. Values <7.3, with a normal blood pH, arise secondary to hydrogen ion accumulation and increased anaerobic metabolism of leukocytes, bacteria, or tumor cells.

In malignant pleural effusions, a low pH correlates with more extensive tumor involvement of the pleura, a higher chance of positive cytologic examination, a lower success rate of pleurodesis, and a poorer prognosis.

Tests for Specific Diseases. The diagnosis of malignant effusions should be established only by histocytopathologic confirmation of malignant cells in the pleural fluid or tissue. Pleural fluid cytologic examination is the first line of investigation in suspected cases and has a sensitivity up to 60% (dependent on tumor type, extent, and experience of the cytologist). Tumor markers, cytokine, and cytogenetic assessment in pleural fluid are neither sensitive nor specific enough for clinical use. Cytogenetic evaluation may be a helpful addition to characterize chromosomal markers of hematolymphoid and mesenchymal malignancies. Flow cytometry of the pleural aspirate should be considered if lymphoma is a possibility.

Gram staining and culture of pleural fluid should be performed whenever pleural infection is suspected. A significant pleural fluid neutrophilia, low pH (or glucose), in an appropriate clinical setting should raise the index of suspicion. Collection of fluid in blood culture bottles and preparation of cellblocks for Gram staining may improve yield. In cases of frank pus, the diagnosis of empyema is secured, but Gram staining and culture may help to identify the causative organism(s) and guide therapy.

Testing for TB should be conducted if clinically indicated, and if the fluid is lymphocyte-predominant (>50% of total leukocytes are lymphocytes). Direct smears (<20%) and culture of the aspirate and pleural tissues all have low sensitivities (<50%) because of the low mycobacterial load in the pleural cavity. Most cases are confirmed by demonstration of caseating granulomata in pleural tissue. Considerable debate exists regarding the role of adenosine deaminase (ADA), interferon, and polymerase chain reaction (PCR) techniques in diagnosing tuberculous pleuritis. At present, ADA is commonly used in endemic countries, and a high ADA level suggests tuberculous effusions. False-positive results do exist (especially empyema, rheumatoid effusions, lymphomas, etc.). Hence, routine ADA measurements are not encouraged in non-endemic areas. Assays for the isoenzyme ADA_2 which predominates in tuberculous effusions, are not widely available.

Routine measurements of pleural fluid amylase levels are not justified. However, a raised amylase in the appropriate clinical setting can help confirm effusions from esophageal rupture and pancreatic diseases (acute pancreatitis or pseudocyst). Isoenzyme analysis may further differentiate the source of amylase (salivary or pancreatic) but is rarely needed. A raised amylase is present in some malignant (usually adenocarcinomas) effusions.

In suspected cases of chylothorax, lipoprotein electrophoresis for chylomicrons or a triglyceride concentration >1.24 mmol/L (110 mg/dL) confirm the diagnosis. The presence of cholesterol crystals at microscopy with a pleural fluid cholesterol level >5.18 mmol/L (200 mg/dL) is diagnostic of a pseudochylothorax. Chylomicrons are not found in pseudochylothoraces.

Pleural fluid levels of rheumatoid factor and antinuclear antibody mirror serum values and add little to clinical management of rheumatoid or systemic lupus erythematosus related pleuritis. Complement levels can be reduced but are of little clinical value. Very low pleural fluid glucose levels are typically seen in patients with a rheumatoid effusion, and differentiation from empyema fluid may be difficult.

β_2-transferrin is found in cerebrospinal fluid, and its presence in pleural fluid confirms a duropleural fistula. Raised creatinine values are seen in urinothorax.

Pleural Biopsy

Histologic examination (with or without culture) of pleural tissue can aid the diagnosis of specific pleural diseases. Tissue can be collected percutaneously (by "blinded" or imaging-guided biopsy) or under direct vision (by thoracoscopy or thoracotomy), each with its pros and cons. (See chapters by Spiro and Cassivi.)

Percutaneous Biopsy

"Blind" biopsy (with Cope's or Abrams' needle) can be performed by the bedside and is valuable in establishing the diagnosis in diseases with diffuse involvement of the pleura (e.g., granulomatous [especially TB] pleuritis). The procedure is less useful in diseases with patchy pleural involvement (e.g., early malignancy). The risk of lacerating vital structures (e.g., intercostal artery or lung) is higher in blind biopsy than in imaging- or thoracoscopic-guided ones.

In patients with detectable pleural abnormalities on CT or ultrasound, imaging-guided pleural biopsies, targeting focal areas of pleural nodularity (especially in malignant pleural disease), has been shown to be more sensitive than blind biopsies.

Thoracoscopy

Thoracoscopy is indicated in patients with undiagnosed exudative pleural effusions despite thoracentesis with or without pleural biopsy (up to 25% of effusions). Thoracoscopy, preferably video assisted, is traditionally performed by surgeons with the patient under general anesthesia. This is increasingly replaced by thoracoscopy performed under conscious sedation by physicians. Thoracoscopy allows direct visualization (with or without biopsy) of almost the entire pleural surface (Figure 69-4), drainage of fluid, and pleurodesis by talc poudrage in the same procedure. Diagnostic sensitivity approaches 95% in malignant pleural diseases and almost 100% in tuberculous pleurisy. Complications are few and mortality rates low (<0.01% of cases). (For details of the technique, refer to Chapter 17.)

Thoracotomy

Open biopsy with thoracotomy is seldom indicated now. It is a more invasive procedure with a higher morbidity, especially post-thoracotomy pain.

TREATMENT

Therapeutic objectives in patients with a pleural effusion include treatment of underlying disease, palliation of symptoms, and prevention of fluid recurrence.

Management of the Underlying Cause

Optimizing the management of the underlying cause (e.g., appropriate diuretic therapy in patients with congestive

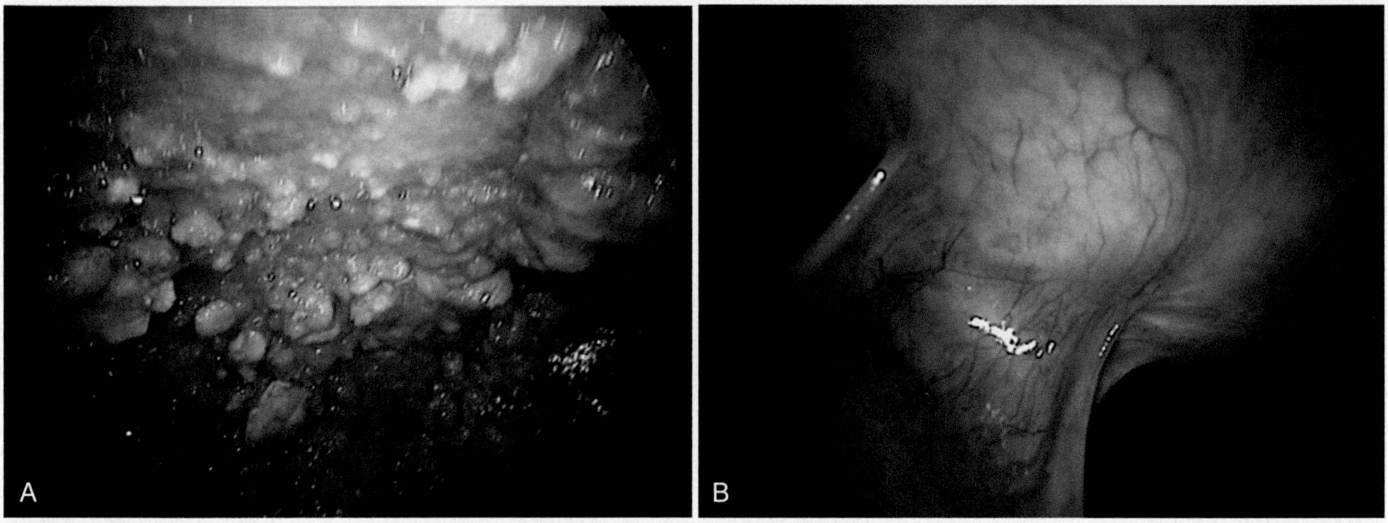

FIGURE 69-4 A, Thoracoscopic view into the right pleural cavity showing multiple tumor nodules covering the parietal pleura. **B,** Thoracoscopy allows identification and biopsy of pleural abnormalities under direct vision while avoiding potentially hazardous structures (e.g., highly vascularized adhesion).

cardiac failure) is adequate for some effusions. In others (e.g., malignant effusions), the underlying cause may not be treatable, and other strategies to prevent reaccumulation of pleural effusions are needed.

Symptom Control

Thoracentesis

Therapeutic pleural aspiration can be performed at the bedside to relieve breathlessness. For recurrent effusions (e.g., malignant pleural effusions), a definitive procedure to stop fluid reaccumulation, such as pleurodesis, should be considered. If this fails, repeat thoracenteses may be necessary for palliation of breathlessness.

Indwelling Catheters

The insertion of a long-term indwelling tunnelled pleural catheter allows outpatient management of refractory malignant pleural effusions. The ambulatory catheters can be inserted as a day case, averting hospital admission. Its presence induces a complete or partial pleurodesis in up to 70% of patients, and the patient (or caregiver) can drain the effusion as guided by symptoms, avoiding hospitalization. Implantation of an indwelling catheter is also indicated in patients with a symptomatic effusion and underlying "trapped lung." The catheters are usually well tolerated by patients, but complications include local tumor invasion at the insertion site, pleural infection, and catheter displacement. A randomized trial is underway to evaluate their use as first-line therapy in malignant effusions.

Insertion of a pleuroperitoneal shunt is another alternative if pleurodesis fails; potential complications include infection and shunt occlusion (approximately 10%).

Noninvasive Palliation

In terminally ill patients with symptomatic effusions, opiates and oxygen therapy to alleviate breathlessness may be appropriate.

Prevent Fluid Reaccumulation

Pleurodesis

The aim of pleurodesis is to achieve fusion between the visceral and parietal pleurae and prevent reaccumulation of pleural fluid (or air). It is indicated in symptomatic malignant pleural effusions and occasionally for recurrent benign effusions when other treatments fail. Dyspnea in patients with malignant effusions is often multifactorial. Only patients with symptomatic improvement from evacuation of effusion should be considered for pleurodesis.

To achieve successful pleural symphysis, pleural fluid is drained to allow apposition of the pleural layers. Pleurodesis, by mechanical abrasion or by chemical agents, aims to induce damage to the pleurae. The resultant acute pleural inflammation, if sufficiently intense, will progress to chronic inflammation and development of adhesion and pleural fibrosis. Pain and fever are common, secondary to the inflammatory process. In animal studies, dampening of this inflammatory process with corticosteroids inhibits pleurodesis. Whether this applies to humans remains untested.

Pleurodesis is not indicated if close contact of the pleural layers cannot be achieved. The presence of a "trapped lung," when lung expansion is restricted either by visceral pleura tumor encasement or by endobronchial obstruction, prohibits effective pleurodesis (Figure 69-5).

Talc is the most commonly used pleurodesis agent worldwide and is more effective than comparative agents in most published studies. Talc can be insufflated as a dry powder (poudrage) during thoracoscopy or instilled through a chest tube as a slurry with similar efficacy. Although talc is effective, adverse effects are common (e.g., pain and fever) and can be serious. The incidence of talc-induced adult respiratory distress syndrome ranged from 0–9% in the literature, and its mechanism remains poorly understood. Particle size, presence of contaminants, reexpansion lung edema, etc. have all been implicated. A randomized, controlled trial has confirmed that talc preparations with "small" particle size ($<20 \mu m$ median

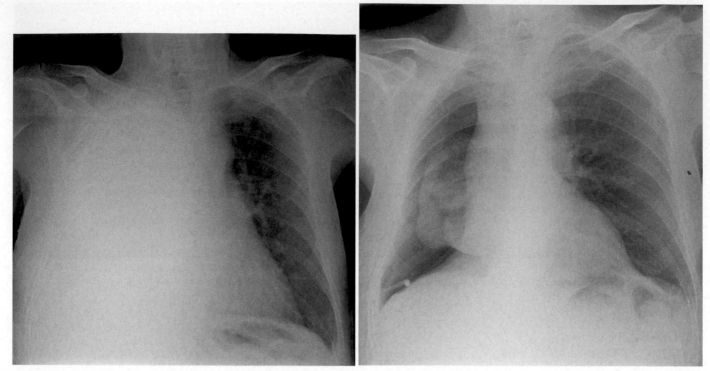

FIGURE 69-5 Radiograph of a patient with trapped lung. This patient had bronchogenic adenocarcinoma and was initially seen with a massive right-sided pleural effusion causing mediastinal shift. After pleural drainage (intercostal drain *in situ*), his lung failed to reexpand. Recognizing the presence of trapped lung is important, because pleurodesis is unlikely to be successful but may induce visceral fibrosis, causing further restriction of the underlying lung.

diameter) led to more systemic and pulmonary inflammation with resultant hypoxemia. In patients with pre-existing respiratory compromise, alternative agents (e.g., tetracycline, doxycycline, bleomycin) should be considered.

SPECIFIC ENTITIES ASSOCIATED WITH PLEURAL EFFUSION

Conditions Associated with Transudative Effusions

Congestive Cardiac Failure

Effusions from congestive cardiac failure account for most transudative effusions worldwide. It is also the most common cause of pleural effusions in acute medical hospital admissions, and as many as 50–75% of these patients will have pleural effusions, commonly bilateral. It is believed that these effusions arise from transpleural migration of pulmonary interstitial fluid accumulated from elevated pulmonary capillary pressure.

Clinical history and physical examination usually secure the diagnosis. Chest radiography commonly reveals bilateral effusions, cardiomegaly, and venous congestion.

Management is of the underlying congestive cardiac failure. Pleurodesis has been performed in refractory cases with variable success. If the patient fails to respond, or there are other atypical features (i.e., unilateral effusion, massive pleural effusion, or fever), further investigation is warranted.

Occasionally, the pleural fluid may be classified as an exudate by use of Light's criteria, probably because of differential drainage of fluid over protein molecules from the pleural space as a result of diuretic therapy. A plasma-to-effusion protein gradient of >3.1 g/dL indicates the fluid was originally formed as a transudate.

In patients with bilateral transudative pleural effusions with pulmonary hypertension and normal left ventricular function, pulmonary veno-occlusive disease (PVOD) should be considered.

Hepatic Hydrothorax

Hepatic hydrothorax occurs in approximately 5% of patients with liver cirrhosis and portal hypertension. Pleural effusions accumulate from transdiaphragmatic migration of ascitic fluid. Fluid also accumulates from the decreased oncotic pressure associated with secondary hypoalbuminemia, and extremely rarely from hemorrhage of congested collateral veins. Most hepatic hydrothoraces are right sided, and concomitant ascites is frequent but not a prerequisite. The diagnosis is based on the presence of cirrhotic liver disease, ascites, and a transudative fluid on thoracentesis. Spontaneous bacterial empyema may occur and, even with prompt recognition, carries a mortality rate of up to 20%.

Management should be directed at treating portal hypertension and reducing ascites with diuretic therapy and sodium restriction. This frequently fails, and therapeutic thoracenteses are indicated for symptomatic relief. Loss of electrolytes and protein is a concern. Pleurodesis may be tried in therapy-resistant cases and repair of any diaphragmatic defects attempted at thoracoscopy. Use of concomitant continuous positive airways pressure (CPAP) ventilation to reverse the peritoneal-pleural gradient has been successful in case reports but remains experimental at present. Transjugular intrahepatic portosystemic shunting (TIPS) can relieve symptomatic hepatic hydrothorax, but liver transplantation, in selected patients, is the only definitive therapy.

Renal Effusions

Pleural effusions may arise after nephrotic syndrome, acute glomerulonephritis, and peritoneal dialysis. Transdiaphragmatic migration of peritoneal dialysate often results in a right-sided effusion chemically resembling the dialysis fluid.

Urinothorax is rare but should be considered whenever encountering a low pH transudative effusion. It arises secondary to renal obstruction with resultant retroperitoneal urine collection and transfer into the ipsilateral pleural cavity. An ammonic smell is diagnostic and increased fluid > serum creatinine levels confirmatory.

Conditions Associated with Exudative Effusions

Parapneumonic Effusion and Empyema

Pleural effusions occur in up to 57% of patients with pneumonia. They may be sterile "simple" parapneumonic effusions reflecting hyperpermeability from pleural inflammation secondary to the underlying pneumonia. "Complicated" parapneumonic effusions are characterized by neutrophilia, low pH, and often fibrinous loculations. Current belief is that the complicated pleural effusion, although culture negative, represents one end of the spectrum of pleural infection and should be treated as such. At the other end of the spectrum is empyema, characterized usually by frank pus in the pleural space.

Differentiation between these categories is important, because rapid pleural drainage is usually required with complicated parapneumonic effusions and empyema. Approximately 10% of simple parapneumonic effusions may evolve into complicated effusions or empyemas.

Parapneumonic effusion should be suspected in all patients with pneumonia and, if detected, should be investigated especially if the patient demonstrates symptoms or signs of ongoing infection. Patients with diabetes mellitus, alcohol or substance abuse, co-existing chronic lung disease, immunosuppression, or rheumatoid arthritis have a higher incidence of pleural infection. Poor dental hygiene is more prevalent in those with anaerobic infection. Recent novel genetic studies also suggest that a variant of the protein tyrosine phosphatase (PTPN22 Trp620) is associated with susceptibility to invasive pneumococcal disease and gram-positive empyema. Primary empyema, in the absence of pneumonia, is responsible for 4% of pleural infection cases.

Chest radiography usually identifies the pleural collection and concomitant bronchopneumonia. Ultrasonography is more sensitive and allows exact localization of fluid with identification of septations and loculations. This can guide thoracentesis. Contrast-enhanced CT scanning provides detailed information and discriminates between empyema and lung abscess. Empyemas are usually lenticular in shape with compression of surrounding lung parenchyma. The "split pleura" sign, with enhanced parietal and visceral pleural tissue visible as the surfaces are separated by the pleural collection, is characteristic. Pleural thickening is seen in 86–100% of empyemas.

Frankly purulent or malodorous fluid confirms an empyema. If not macroscopically purulent, the fluid should be assessed for its pH. A pH <7.2, or reduced fluid glucose, indicates a complicated parapneumonic effusion. Positive Gram staining and/or fluid culture confirm pleural infection and

can guide antibiotic choice. In most series, culture of infected fluids was negative in approximately half of the patients. Polymerase chain reaction (PCR) techniques are being investigated to improve organism identification.

Treatment of parapneumonic effusions or empyema includes appropriate antimicrobial therapy, optimal nutritional support, and evacuation of the infected pleural fluid (by chest tube or surgery).

Bacteriology

It is important to differentiate between community and hospital-acquired pleural infection: the bacteriology and prognosis differ. Hospital-acquired cases are often iatrogenic or secondary to hospital-acquired pneumonia and carry a mortality rate several times higher than community-acquired cases. The microbiology also varies geographically. In the UK, gram-positive Streptococci such as *Streptococcus milleri* account for most community-acquired cases of pleural infection. *Staphylococcus aureus* is isolated in 11%. Anaerobic pathogens alone are present in 16%, and mixed infections are occasionally seen. Methicillin-resistant *Staphylococcus aureus* (MRSA), however, is responsible for more than a quarter of hospital-acquired pleural infection with other staphylococci accountable for 22%. *Enterococci* and *Enterobacteriae* both cause approximately 15% of cases.

Antibiotics

All patients should receive antibiotic therapy. Empirical treatment should be initiated while awaiting bacterial culture results and must take into account where the infection was acquired (hospital or community), patient co-morbidity, and local bacterial resistance patterns. Therapy may be modified in the light of positive culture and sensitivity results.

Drainage

Simple parapneumonic effusions generally do not require drainage, but drainage of complicated effusions and empyema is key to their management.

Loculation is common in pleural infection, and imaging-guided insertion of chest drains can ensure optimal placement. Although large drains are conventionally advocated, clinical outcome of patients with different size chest drains has not been compared in randomized studies.

Instillation of intrapleural fibrinolytic agents for complex parapneumonic effusions or empyema can disrupt fibrinous septations and potentially improve drainage. However, a large multicenter study failed to demonstrate a benefit on mortality, need for surgery, or duration of hospital stay for patients who received intrapleural streptokinase. Further trials with alternative intrapleural adjunct therapies such as DNase are ongoing.

Early referral for surgical drainage is indicated if there is no significant clinical improvement or if fever and inflammatory markers fail to settle. Secondary pleural thickening (fibrothorax) is seen in <10%; however, residual pleural thickening and lung function impairment always improve with time and are not indications for surgery. Video-assisted thoracoscopic surgery (VATS) is preferred, but more invasive procedures (e.g., thoracotomy or rib resection with open drainage) are sometimes needed.

Use of VATS as first-line treatment of empyema has only been tested in one randomized trial ($n = 20$) of adults and one of pediatric empyemas patients; the results did not show convincing advantage over conservative medical management.

Mortality rates for empyema vary between 7% and 33% at 1 year but exceed 50% in patients with significant co-morbidity.

Pleural Infection in Children

Significant differences exist between pleural infection in children and in adults in their clinical course and prognosis; the reasons for the differences remain unclear. Pediatric empyema has an incidence of 3.3 per 100,000, and evidence suggests this is rising in many countries. Most cases are secondary to underlying bacterial pneumonia, and *Streptococcus pneumoniae* (predominantly serotype 1) accounts for most childhood empyema, although many are culture negative.

The diagnosis is based on clinical findings and chest radiography and/or ultrasonography confirming a pleural collection. Thoracentesis and thoracostomy drainage may be difficult in babies and young children and may require anesthetics. Management with adequate fluid therapy, intravenous antibiotics, and antipyretics is sufficient in many cases, and liaison with a tertiary pediatric respiratory unit is recommended. Advocates of early surgical intervention suggest that if a child is undergoing general anesthesia for chest drain insertion, a definitive, effective procedure such as VATS debridement should be performed; however, no consensus decision exists. The prognosis in children with empyema is significantly better than in adults.

Tuberculous Pleural Effusions

Tuberculous pleural effusions represent either primary pleural mycobacterial infection or reactivation of latent infection. Most cases of TB pleuritis develop as a result of a delayed hypersensitivity reaction to the mycobacterial protein rather than mycobacterial invasion. The number of organisms within the pleural space is often low.

Acute clinical presentation with pleuritic chest pain and fever is uncommon, and, more typically, symptoms develop insidiously with dyspnea and constitutional features. Chest radiographs reveal a pleural effusion with or without parenchymal infiltrates. The pleural fluid is lymphocytic in more than 90% of cases and may be associated with a low glucose and pH. Samples should be sent for staining for acid-fast bacilli and TB culture, although the diagnostic yield is usually low. Obtaining tissue for culture and a histologic diagnosis is important. Because involvement of the pleura in TB is commonly generalized, percutaneous pleural biopsy is sensitive, although thoracoscopy may further increase yield.

Adenosine deaminase (ADA) levels have a high sensitivity and specificity and are routinely used in many countries where TB is endemic. Low ADA concentrations make tuberculous pleuritis unlikely. High levels also occur in empyema, malignancy (e.g., lymphoma), and collagen vascular diseases.

Spontaneous resolution is frequently seen in tuberculous effusions irrespective of anti-mycobacterial chemotherapy. However, left untreated, approximately 60% of patients will have clinically overt tuberculosis develop elsewhere within 5 years. Mycobacterial resistance patterns in cases of tuberculous pleuritis are usually similar to the local resistance patterns of pulmonary tuberculosis cases. The treatment of tuberculosis is covered in Chapter 31. Thoracentesis may aid symptom relief, and steroids may help to reduce fluid volume, but neither alters the long-term outcome nor the incidence of fibrothorax.

Pleural Effusions Secondary to Other Organisms

Viruses, Legionnaires' disease, *Mycoplasma*, and *Rickettsia* spp. may be associated with pleural effusion in approximately 20% of cases. The diagnosis is made clinically, with serologic tests, urinary antigen detection (Legionnaires' disease), or positive culture results providing confirmation. Pleural fluid is commonly lymphocytic, although neutrophils may initially predominate.

Pulmonary nocardiosis may be complicated by empyema in up to a quarter of cases, and empyema is frequently seen in patients with pulmonary actinomycosis.

Mycotic lung disease accounts for <1% of all pleural effusions and usually occurs in immunocompromised hosts. *Candida albicans* is the most common pathogen in fungal empyema, and prompt treatment with systemic antifungal agents and pleural drainage is required. In approximately 4% of patients with human blastomycosis and 20% with respiratory coccidioidomycosis, pleural effusions are observed. These generally resolve spontaneously without specific treatment. *Pneumocystis jirovecii* infection is rarely associated with pleural effusion in the immunocompromised host.

Amebic lung disease can result in empyema, hepatobronchial fistulae, or a pleural effusion secondary to perforation of an amebic liver abscess. Pleural effusions related to other parasitic infections are extremely rare.

Malignant Pleural Effusions (MPEs)

MPEs are common and affect 660 patients per million population per year. They account for 22% of all pleural effusions and in 20% of patients are the first presentation of malignancy. The most common cytologic diagnoses in developed countries are metastatic breast or lung carcinoma, lymphoma, and mesothelioma. Most malignant tumors can metastasize to the pleura. Up to 50% of patients with breast cancer, a quarter of those with bronchogenic carcinoma, and more than 95% of patients with mesothelioma will develop a pleural effusion during their disease course. Symptoms with MPE can be severe, and its successful control can make significant improvement to the quality of life for the patients.

Pleural fluid accumulates as a result of increased fluid formation and/or reduced lymphatic drainage (from malignant involvement of parietal lymphatic channels or mediastinal lymphadenopathy). In some patients with underlying malignancy, a pleural effusion may exist without direct pleural involvement. These "para-malignant" effusions may be caused by pulmonary embolism, pneumonia, secondary atelectasis, pericardial tumor involvement, hypoproteinemia, or radiotherapy induced inflammation. Although distinction is important in cases in which curative resection is considered, some studies have shown that patients with a para-malignant effusion have a similar prognosis to those with frank malignant effusions.

Positive histocytologic confirmation is required for diagnosis. Pleural fluid cytologic examination establishes proof in approximately 60%, and, if negative, thoracoscopy or CT-guided pleural biopsy (if focal pleural abnormality is evident on CT) is the logical next step.

Except for a small number of chemotherapy-sensitive tumors (e.g., lymphoma), cure of the underlying malignancy is usually not possible once the cancer has metastasized to the pleura. Management is, therefore, directed toward improving symptom control and quality of life. Various options are available (see "Treatment"); the most appropriate one depends on the patients' symptoms, performance status, and expected survival.

Connective Tissue Disease

Rheumatoid Arthritis. Pleural effusions are the most common thoracic manifestation of rheumatoid arthritis and occur in up to 5% of patients, more frequently men (70%). Often the effusions develop several years after the original diagnosis and in 30% arise concomitantly with interstitial lung disease or rheumatoid lung nodules. The effusion may persist for years, although spontaneous resorption is occasionally observed. Symptomatic recurrent effusions are rare and may respond to systemic corticosteroid therapy.

Distinguishing rheumatoid effusions from empyema or pseudochylothorax is important but can be difficult. Pleural fluid from rheumatoid effusion is characterized by leukocytosis, a low glucose, low pH, and increased LDH—features indistinguishable from pleural infection. Low complement and elevated pleural fluid rheumatoid factor levels are not diagnostic.

Systemic Lupus Erythematosus (SLE). Fifty percent of patients with SLE will have a pleural effusion, often bilateral and typically exudative (occasionally hemorrhagic) with a lymphocytosis (if chronic). Non-steroidal anti-inflammatory medication may relief pleuritic chest pain, and corticosteroid treatment results in a swift clinical response if the patient remains symptomatic. Pleural effusions as a consequence of drug-induced lupus erythematosus are rare.

Others. Wegener's granulomatosis is associated with pleural effusion in approximately 30% of patients and responds to treatment of the underlying condition with immunosuppressant therapy. Pleural effusion may occur in up to 30% of those with Churg–Strauss syndrome; typically, the fluid is rich in eosinophils. The effusions are not usually of any clinical consequence and most resolve with corticosteroids.

Effusion from Vascular Causes

Pleural effusions occur in approximately 50% of patients with pulmonary embolism. This diagnosis is often overlooked and should be considered in any undiagnosed pleural effusion. The pathophysiology remains debated, and no specific diagnostic features exist; diagnosis is made by exclusion of other etiologies. Effusions are usually small and can be blood stained. Standard treatment of pulmonary emboli should be initiated. The pleural effusion seldom needs drainage and will resolve with time.

Effusions after coronary bypass graft surgery are common, and most settle spontaneously within 6 months. Post-cardiac injury syndrome (Dressler's syndrome) after myocardial infarction or bypass surgery can result in small bilateral effusions and seldom requires intervention. Sickle cell anemia related acute chest syndrome results in pleural effusion in 30–35% of cases.

Drug-Induced Pleural Effusions

Drug-induced pleural effusions do occur, and its diagnosis requires high clinical awareness from the clinicians. Prescribed medications, including amiodarone, nitrofurantoin, methotrexate, bromocriptine, or phenytoin, may result in exudative pleural effusions and eventual pleural fibrosis. Withdrawal of the offending drug and, if needed, use of corticosteroid is sufficient in many cases. Decortication has been attempted but has no established benefits.

Ovarian hyperstimulation syndrome (OHSS) is an iatrogenic complication occurring in approximately 3% of women undergoing therapeutic ovarian stimulation. It is becoming increasingly recognized as higher numbers of women undergo assisted reproductive techniques, and the exact pathogenesis remains unclear. OHSS is characterized by ovarian enlargement and rapid fluid shifts secondary to increased capillary permeability, which result in intravascular volume depletion. In severe cases, massive ascites with hydrothoraces can arise. The treatment is primarily supportive, but fatal cases have been reported.

Effusions Related to Abdominal Diseases

Pleural effusions occur in approximately 20% of those with acute pancreatitis; two thirds are left sided, and pleural fluid amylase concentrations exceed serum values. Pancreatic pseudocyst, pancreatic-pleural fistula, or abscess formation must be considered if the effusion persists. Effusions also accompany subphrenic abscess in more than 50% of patients. Cholohemothorax secondary to gallstone perforation into the pleural cavity is extremely rare and results in a bilious effusion.

Effusions arising after abdominal surgery are common, and investigation is rarely required, provided secondary infection is excluded.

Meigs' syndrome refers to the combination of benign ovarian tumors and co-existing pleural effusion and ascites. These resolve after tumor resection.

Hemothorax

Hemothorax is characterized by pleural fluid hematocrit values >50% of peripheral blood. The main causes are trauma, iatrogenic (most commonly after thoracic surgery), malignancy, anticoagulation therapy, pulmonary infarction, and aortic rupture. Complications include empyema (1–4% of traumatic hemothoraces), pleural effusion, trapped lung, and fibrothorax. Treatment is guided by the clinical scenario, but tube thoracostomy to enable evacuation of the blood and assessment of the extent of hemorrhage is advised. Surgical intervention (preferably VATS) is indicated if the bleeding rate is more than 200 mL/h. Prophylactic antibiotics are usually administered, although literature evidence to support this practice is scarce.

Chylothorax

Chylothorax develops when there is disruption of the thoracic duct, resulting in passage of chyle (lymph rich in chylomicrons) into the pleural cavity. The pleural fluid is characteristically milky, except in patients starved. Chylothoraces must be differentiated from pseudochylothoraces and empyema fluid (see "Pleural Fluid Analysis").

Trauma is the most common cause of chylothorax predominantly iatrogenic secondary to thoracic duct damage during cardiothoracic surgery (e.g., esophagectomy). Non-traumatic causes include malignancy, especially lymphoma. Congenital chylothorax arises from thoracic duct malformation, and repair of congenital diaphragmatic defects may cause chylothoraces. Lymphangioleiomyomatosis and non-surgical trauma rarely produce chylothoraces. Idiopathic chylothoraces occur in 15%. CT scanning should be performed to exclude lymphoma (and other causes) in patients without a history of trauma.

Management of chylothorax aims to optimize nutrition, relieve symptoms, and close the thoracic duct defect. Malnourishment secondary to chyle loss can be disabling. Total parenteral nutrition, or a low-fat diet with medium-chain fatty acids, should be adopted to reduce chyle flow. If the patient is symptomatic with dyspnea, fluid can be removed by thoracentesis or chest tube drainage. Pleuroperitoneal shunts have been recommended if there is no co-existing chyloascites. Pleurodesis has been attempted in refractory cases. In traumatic chylothoraces, the defect frequently closes spontaneously. Octreotide, a somatostatin analog, has also been reported, mainly in pediatric-based case series, to enhance thoracic duct closure. Percutaneous thoracic duct embolization under radiologic guidance can be attempted before consideration of surgical thoracic duct ligation by VATS or thoracotomy. This was initially described in 1998 and offers a minimally invasive treatment strategy for those patients who are unable to tolerate surgical intervention. Catheterization of the thoracic duct is a prerequisite for its use, and anatomic obstruction of the cisterna chyli or retroperitoneal lymphatic chain obviates its use. In those with underlying lymphoma, radiotherapy or systemic chemotherapy may control the chylothorax.

Pseudochylothorax

Pseudochylothorax, or cholesterol pleurisy, is very rare. It results from the accumulation of cholesterol or lecithin–globulin complexes within long-standing (usually years) pleural effusions enveloped by thickened fibrotic, often calcified, pleura. The main causes are tuberculous pleurisy and rheumatoid pleuritis. The pleural fluid has a very high cholesterol content and no chylomicrons. Demonstration of cholesterol crystals is diagnostic. Treatment of pseudochylothoraces is seldom indicated. Dyspnea is more likely a result of the pleural fibrosis and is seldom improved by thoracentesis. Respiratory insufficiency, infection, and bronchopleural or pleurocutaneous fistulas are rare complications.

Asbestos-Related Pleural Diseases

Asbestos fibers have a predilection to the pleura. Injury to the pleura can result in mesothelioma (see Chapter 70), as well as a range of benign pleural diseases, namely pleural plaques, diffuse pleural thickening, benign asbestos pleural effusions, and round atelectasis.

Circumscribed pleural thickening—pleural plaques—are seen in up to 50% of asbestos-exposed subjects. Plaques occur in the parietal pleura and are of no physiologic consequence. Benign asbestos effusions are typically small and unilateral. Their occurrence is dose-related to asbestos exposure, with a shorter latency period (within two decades of asbestos exposure) than other asbestos-related pleural disease. The effusion is an exudate, often blood-stained, and may precede the development of diffuse pleural thickening. The diagnosis depends on exclusion of other causes. Prolonged observation is required to exclude mesothelioma. Round atelectasis represents invagination of the visceral pleura and can be diagnosed radiologically by the "comet tail" sign on CT. In the absence of classical radiographic features, round atelectasis can mimic lung tumors, and differentiation can be difficult at times.

Diffuse pleural thickening may occur with asbestos exposure (<5%), especially in those with heavy asbestos contact. Significant restrictive lung function changes, and resultant dyspnea can occur.

Fibrothorax and Pleural Thickening

Diffuse pleural thickening (fibrothorax) can develop secondary to empyema or hemothorax, tuberculous pleurisy, asbestos exposure, collagen vascular disease, and drug-induced pleuritis (e.g., ergot derivatives, such as bromocriptine, pergolide, and methylsergide). Pleural fibrosis and thickening is also a result of pleurodesis to therapeutically obliterate the pleural space.

Patients with fibrothorax may be asymptomatic or complain of dyspnea. The chest radiograph typically shows concentric pleural thickening, occasionally with evidence of the predisposing cause. Reduction in the size of the hemithorax with an elevated hemidiaphragm suggests chronic fibrosis. Pulmonary function testing usually demonstrates a restrictive pattern. Likewise, long-term survivors of pleurodesis often have radiologic pleural thickening and mild restrictive physiologic changes.

Treatment should be aimed at the underlying cause, with removal of offending agents if possible. Corticosteroids are often administered, and surgical decortication is sometimes attempted; effectiveness of neither approach is established.

Other Etiologies

Rarely, exudative effusions may be associated with sarcoidosis, radiotherapy, yellow nail syndrome, familial Mediterranean fever, and amyloidosis.

Approximately 15% of pleural effusions remain undiagnosed despite thorough investigation. Close follow-up may elicit those with occult malignancy; however, most are benign and resolve spontaneously. It has been postulated, but not proven, that viral infection may be responsible.

Pitfalls and Controversies

Pleural effusions are common. However, pleural effusions are often considered a "side issue" to the underlying systemic or pulmonary disorders causing the effusion. This often results in significant delay in recognition, investigation, and management of the effusion, contributing to morbidity. For example, late recognition of parapneumonic effusions remains commonplace; better awareness and early intervention would have prevented many cases of empyema.

Advances in imaging will play an increasing role in diagnosis and investigation of pleural disease. High-quality clinical trial data are lacking in pleural disease, and management is often governed by anecdotal experiences.

There are several current controversies in pleural disease management. The use of streptokinase as a first-line therapy for empyema has not been supported by two randomized controlled trials. However, the role of fibrinolytics in pleural infection remains a topic of controversy and active research. The pros and cons of medical thoracoscopy continue to be debated. The belief that thoracoscopic talc pleurodesis is superior has not been supported by randomized controlled trials. The size of chest tube and appropriate insertion skills (surgical, radiologic, or chest physician) remain controversial.

PNEUMOTHORAX

Introduction

A pneumothorax exists when air is present within the pleural space and may be classified as spontaneous or traumatic. Traumatic pneumothoraces occur as a result of direct or indirect trauma and may be iatrogenic secondary to procedures such as transbronchial or pleural biopsies, thoracentesis, and central venous catheterization.

Spontaneous pneumothoraces are divided into primary or secondary. Primary spontaneous pneumothoraces (PSPs) arise in apparently healthy individuals, whereas secondary spontaneous pneumothoraces are associated with underlying pulmonary pathology, most commonly chronic obstructive pulmonary disease (COPD). Differentiation between these groups is important, because management and prognosis differ (Table 69-4).

Primary Spontaneous Pneumothorax

Primary pneumothoraces usually occur in young male smokers between 20 and 40 years of age. The reported incidence is 18–28 per 100,000 for men and 1.2–6.0 per 100,000 for women (male/female ratio 5:1). Cigarette smoking is a major risk factor increasing the lifetime risk of pneumothorax in healthy males from 0.1% in non-smokers up to 12% in smokers. The risk is dose related with relative risk seven times higher in light smokers (1–12 cigarettes/day), 21 times higher in moderate smokers, and 102 times higher in those smoking more than 22 cigarettes daily. This trend is less marked in women. The chronic effects of marijuana smoking and its association with bullous lung disease are now recognized as an independent risk factor for pneumothorax.

Mortality rates of primary pneumothoraces are extremely low.

Pathophysiology

Pneumothoraces are attributed to the rupture of early emphysematous-like changes (ELCs) (i.e., blebs and bulla), which are demonstrated in most patients with primary pneumothoraces despite the absence of underlying clinical disease. Pulmonary blebs are air-filled spaces between the lung parenchyma and the visceral pleura, visible in more than 75% of patients undergoing thoracoscopic treatment for primary pneumothorax. Patients with primary pneumothoraces also tend to be taller

and thinner than controls with an increased pressure gradient from lung base to apex. This creates a greater distending pressure on apical alveoli increasing the likelihood of rupture. However, ELCs are present in up to 25% of control subjects and are not always predictive of pneumothorax.

Fluorescein-enhanced autofluorescence thoracoscopy techniques have identified areas of increased visceral porosity in the absence of other visible abnormality. It is hypothesized that air leakage from these areas may be integral to the formation of primary pneumothoraces. Smoking-induced distal airway inflammation, disturbance of collateral ventilation, congenital anatomic, and morphometric abnormalities may contribute to these changes.

A tendency toward primary pneumothorax is rarely inherited, and the Birt–Hogg–Dube syndrome (autosomal-dominant condition, chromosome 17p11.2) is associated with primary pneumothorax, benign skin tumors, and renal tumors. Patients with Marfan's syndrome and homocystinuria also have an increased incidence of pneumothorax.

Clinical Features

Primary pneumothoraces may be asymptomatic, but sudden-onset pleuritic chest pain localized to the side of the pneumothorax and/or dyspnea is the most common symptom.

On examination, a hyper-resonant percussion note, absent tactile fremitus, and reduced breath sounds on the affected side may be evident. Tracheal deviation away from the affected side is seen with large, or tension, pneumothoraces. Signs of hemodynamic compromise (hypotension, severe tachycardia, and cyanosis) suggest a tension pneumothorax. Hamman's sign, an audible clicking sound synchronous with the heart sounds, can be heard with a left-sided pneumothorax, and subcutaneous emphysema may be palpable.

Diagnosis

Chest radiographs usually confirm the diagnosis. Expiratory films are no more sensitive than standard films, although lateral decubitus films facilitate the diagnosis of tiny pneumothoraces. Fifteen percent of cases have a small ipsilateral pleural effusion, and mediastinal displacement away from the pneumothorax, subcutaneous emphysema and pneumomediastinum may also exist. CT scanning is rarely necessary acutely in primary pneumothorax and is only recommended if concern exists regarding underlying complex cystic disease or to differentiate between a bulla and pneumothorax.

Pneumothoraces are best quantified as volume of hemithorax occupied and can be estimated by use of Light's index: %PNX = $100 - [100 \times$ diameter of deflated lung^3/diameter of hemithorax^3].

Arterial blood gas measurements may show a reduced arterial Pa_{O_2} and an increase in the alveolar-arterial (A-a) gradient.

Management

The management of primary spontaneous pneumothoraces varies widely with the approach to the patient determined by the clinical presentation. Supplemental high-flow oxygen is advocated by some centers because it can theoretically accelerate pleural air resorption by reducing the partial pressure of nitrogen in the blood. Observation alone may be adequate for patients with very small primary pneumothoraces, minimal symptoms, and stable cardiorespiratory status. The rate of spontaneous pleural air resorption is slow (1.25% each 24 h), and this should be anticipated.

TABLE 69-4 Causes of Pneumothoraces

Spontaneous	Iatrogenic
Primary (most common in young men)	Penetrating chest wounds
Secondary	Iatrogenic—including chest aspiration, intercostal tube insertion, transbronchial needle biopsy, needle aspiration lung biopsy, intercostal nerve block, central venous cannulation, positive pressure ventilation, pacemaker insertion
Chronic obstructive airways disease	
Asthma	
Cystic fibrosis	
Congenital cysts and bullae	
Pleural malignancy	
Interstitial lung disease	
Bacterial pneumonia	Chest compression injury—including external cardiac massage
Pneumocystis jiroveci pneumonia	
Tuberculosis	
Whooping cough	
Langerhans cell histiocytosis (LCH)	
Tuberous sclerosis	
Lymphangioleiomyomatosis (LAM)	
Marfan's syndrome	
Sarcoidosis	
Esophageal rupture	

Otherwise, treatment aims to remove air from the pleural space and decrease the risk of recurrence. The former may be achieved by simple aspiration or intercostal tube drainage with or without one-way (e.g., Heimlich) valve insertion. Prevention of recurrence involves removal of risk factors (e.g., smoking cessation) and induction of pleurodesis by means of chemical pleurodesis, thoracoscopy (usually VATS), or rarely open thoracotomy. The latter two allow identification and resection of abnormal areas (ELC treatment [e.g., bullectomy]) with or without pleurodesis, pleural abrasion, or partial pleurectomy (Figure 69-6).

Simple aspiration is the accepted treatment in patients with large or symptomatic small primary pneumothoraces. This succeeds in approximately 60% of patients. If the first attempt fails, repeat aspiration should be considered, especially if <2.5 L was obtained on the initial aspirate. If complete reexpansion is not achieved but symptoms are relieved, outpatient follow-up is appropriate. Alternatively, a Heimlich flutter valve (thoracic vent) may be inserted and the patient safely discharged with outpatient review.

Intercostal tube drainage is indicated if pleural aspiration fails to control symptoms. Small (10–14F) drains are usually adequate. Once the lung is reexpanded and the drain ceased bubbling for 24 h, it should be removed. Suction may aid reexpansion but should not be applied before 48 h to lessen the risk of reexpansion pulmonary edema. Clamping of the chest drain before removal is a contentious issue. A slow air leak may only become apparent after the drain has been clamped for several hours, hence avoiding premature removal.

Surgical Treatment

Surgery is indicated in cases of persistent air leak despite adequate tube drainage. Surgery is also indicated in patients with recurrent ipsilateral or first contralateral pneumothorax, synchronous pneumothoraces, or a spontaneous hemothorax, as well as those with job restrictions (e.g., divers and airline staff).

Minimally invasive video-assisted thoracic surgery (VATS) allows stapling of blebs and bullae by use of an Endostapler, laser ablation, or electrocoagulation. Pleurodesis can be induced mechanically with pleural abrasion or partial pleurectomy or chemically (talc poudrage). Recurrence rates after VATS are <5% and associated with shorter hospital stays and recovery time than open surgery. The emergence of fluorescein-enhanced autofluorescence thoracoscopy may help identify parenchymal abnormalities not visible on routine thoracoscopy.

Thoracotomy and transaxillary mini-thoracotomy are indicated only if VATS is unavailable. Recurrence rates are <0.5%, but potential morbidity is greater than with minimally invasive procedures.

Strategies for Avoiding Recurrence

The risk of recurrence after a primary spontaneous pneumothorax is approximately 30% (16–54%) and is greatest in the first few months. Recurrence rates increase with successive pneumothoraces—50% after one recurrence and up to 80% after a third pneumothorax. The risk of contralateral pneumothorax is approximately 15% after a primary event.

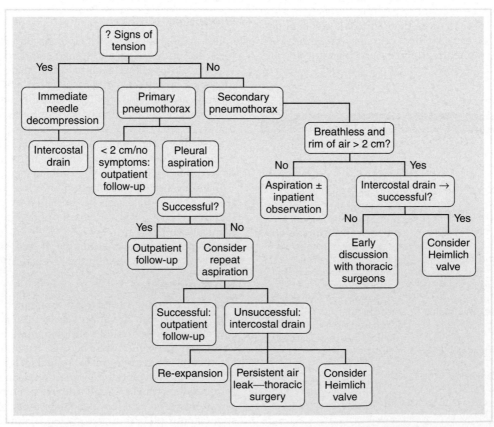

FIGURE 69-6 Diagnostic approach for initial management of a pneumothorax.

The recurrence rate is higher in taller patients, smokers, and those with greater number of subpleural blebs or bullae.

Definitive surgical intervention either by means of VATS or open thoracotomy achieves recurrence rates superior to those after instillation of a pleurodesing agent (usually sterile talc) by means of the intercostal tube. However, if the patient is unwilling or too frail to undergo surgery, or if thoracoscopy is unavailable, bedside pleurodesis may be appropriate.

Secondary Spontaneous Pneumothorax

Secondary pneumothoraces occur in patients with underlying lung disease, often with impaired respiratory reserve. The reported incidence is similar to that of primary spontaneous pneumothorax, and men older than 75 years of age have the highest rate (60/100,000 per year). COPD exists in 60% of patients. *Pneumocystis jiroveci* (PCP) infection in patients with AIDS is another risk factor. Other associated conditions are outlined in Table 69-4.

Secondary pneumothorax carries a mortality rate of up to 10%, often indicative of the severity of the underlying lung disease.

Clinical Features

The symptoms of secondary pneumothorax are similar but often more severe than those associated with primary pneumothorax. Clinical deterioration may be rapid and appear disproportionate to the pneumothorax size.

On physical examination, contralateral differences may not be readily apparent in patients with hyperexpanded lungs secondary to COPD.

Diagnosis

Chest radiography confirms the diagnosis in most cases. However, in patients with underlying lung disease, the typical appearance of a pneumothorax may be altered and careful distinction between hyperlucent bullous areas and a pneumothorax must be made. If in doubt, additional imaging (e.g., CT) should be used before attempting aspiration.

Arterial blood gases commonly show hypoxia proportional to the extent of underlying disease and pneumothorax size. Acute hypercapnic respiratory failure may be seen and resolve after treatment.

Management

Secondary pneumothoraces must be recognized and treated promptly. The evacuation of even a small pneumothorax can rapidly improve symptoms in these patients.

The initial treatment for most patients is intercostal tube insertion. Observation alone is inappropriate except in asymptomatic patients with tiny apical pneumothoraces, and aspiration should only be considered in minimally symptomatic patients with small pneumothoraces.

Because air leaks are more common in secondary pneumothoraces, the lung remains unexpanded in approximately 20% at 7 days. The median time for lung expansion is 5 days compared with 1 day for primary pneumothoraces. Suction can be applied if the lung fails to spontaneously reinflate.

Surgical Treatment

Early surgical intervention is recommended in patients with a persistent air leak or failure of re-expansion after 72 h. VATS is well tolerated by most patients and may supersede more invasive techniques (e.g., open thoracotomy). In those at high anesthetic risk, chemical pleurodesis by means of the intercostal tube can be performed.

In other patients in whom tube thoracostomy has failed and surgery is not appropriate, a Heimlich flutter valve can be inserted. Success rates of up to 100% have been reported in patients with advanced AIDS and *Pneumocystis jiroveci* pneumonia (see later).

Strategies for Avoiding Recurrence

Attempts to prevent recurrence should be considered for all patients after their first secondary pneumothorax, because approximately 45% of this group will have recurrent episodes.

Open thoracotomy and pleurectomy has the lowest recurrence rate after pneumothorax, but VATS with pleural abrasion or surgical talc pleurodesis is usually a preferred alternative. Many patients, however, will not be suitable candidates for surgical intervention, and chemical pleurodesis by means of the chest drain may be appropriate.

The effect of pleurodesing agents on future lung transplantation must be considered in selected patients. Although not an absolute contraindication, pleurodesis makes transplant technically more difficult, thereby prolonging the period of donor organ ischemia. Excessive bleeding is also more common. Close liaison with the local transplant unit is advised in all possible future transplant candidates in whom pleurodesis is contemplated (see Chapter 78).

Discharge and Follow-up

Any patient discharged with a residual pneumothorax should have a repeat chest radiograph to ensure complete lung re-expansion. Those who have undergone successful aspiration can be discharged unless there is concern about underlying lung abnormality, when CT imaging may be indicated.

All patients should be cautioned against flying until chest radiography confirms pneumothorax resolution, and air travel conventionally is not advised for 6 weeks. There is no definitive supporting evidence for this interval, and other guidelines have suggested a shorter period. The risk of recurrence is greatest within the first year, and those with secondary pneumothoraces may wish to avoid flying for a longer period.

Diving should be permanently avoided unless a definitive surgical procedure such as surgical pleurectomy has been performed. Smoking cessation should be strongly encouraged.

Specific Situations

Iatrogenic Pneumothorax

Iatrogenic pneumothorax is probably more common than primary and secondary pneumothoraces combined, and the incidence is escalating with increasing use of invasive procedures (e.g., transbronchial or percutaneous lung biopsy). Transthoracic needle aspiration accounts for up to one quarter of all cases, especially if the patient has underlying emphysema or aerated lung is traversed during biopsy.

Suspicion should be high in any patient who becomes breathless after a procedure associated with risk of a pneumothorax, and in patients being mechanically ventilated who deteriorate suddenly. The diagnosis is confirmed on a chest radiograph.

Most patients can be managed with observation and oxygen administration alone. However, if the patient is more than minimally symptomatic, simple aspiration is recommended. Chest tube drainage should be initiated should symptoms persist or if the patient has underlying lung disease. Surgical intervention is occasionally required if the air leak persists (e.g., >72 h). Pneumothorax recurrence is not an issue in those with iatrogenic pneumothoraces unless concomitant lung disease exists.

Tension Pneumothorax

Tension pneumothorax is a medical emergency. A defect in the visceral pleural surface acts as a one-way valve, so that air is drawn into the pleural space with inspiration and is unable to leave on expiration. The resulting increase in intra-pleural pressure impairs venous return, leading to reduced cardiac output and hypoxemia. Clinically, acute respiratory distress with sweating, tachycardia, and hypotension develops, and, if unrecognized, a pulseless electrical activity (PEA) cardiac arrest may ensue. Tension pneumothorax should be considered when sudden decline occurs in mechanically ventilated patients.

If suspected, there should be no delay in treatment; awaiting confirmation on chest X-ray increases mortality. The patient should receive high-flow oxygen, and a large-bore catheter needle should be inserted into the second intercostal space in the mid-clavicular line. An audible hiss may be heard. Once enough air has been aspirated to relieve symptoms, an intercostal chest drain should be sited, and a chest radiograph then performed.

Surgical/Subcutaneous Emphysema

Surgical emphysema arises as air, under pressure from the pleural space, dissects subcutaneous tissue (Figure 69-7). This may result from a misplaced drain with air holes positioned out of the pleural cavity, if the drain is blocked, or if a large air leak is present.

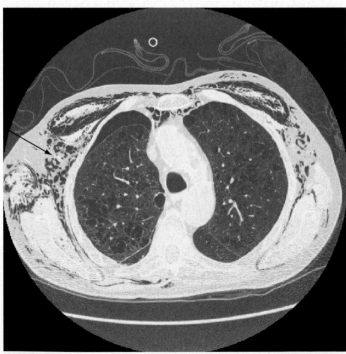

FIGURE 69-7 Subcutaneous emphysema (*arrow*) complicating a COPD-related secondary pneumothorax.

In most cases, no action is required for the surgical emphysema; correction of the drainage problem to prevent further air accumulation in the subcutaneous tissue is adequate. Rarely, acute airway obstruction may develop with secondary respiratory compromise. Tracheostomy is required to secure the airway and high-flow oxygen applied (if no contraindications). Skin incision decompression and subcutaneous drains have also been tried.

Catamenial Pneumothorax

Catamenial pneumothoraces typically develop within 48 h of menstrual flow and tend to recur. The diagnosis should be considered in women who are seen with recurrent pneumothoraces, with or without a history of endometriosis. This diagnosis is often overlooked, and patients have, on average, five episodes before diagnosis.

The pathogenesis is not fully understood. Most pneumothoraces occur on the right, supporting the hypothesis that air originates from abdominal organs (e.g., endometriosis involvement of gastrointestinal or uterine tracts) and passes into the pleural cavity through diaphragmatic defects. Pleural or diaphragmatic endometriosis may be involved in creating these defects. Alternatively, air may have originated from endometriosis in the lungs.

Treatment of endometriosis with hormonal manipulation is effective in some patients. Alternative therapeutic options include thoracoscopy for pleurodesis and closure of diaphragmatic defects.

Pneumothorax and AIDS

Pneumothoraces occur in 2–5% of patients with AIDS. *Pneumocystis jiroveci* pneumonia (PCP) induces a subpleural necrotizing alveolitis responsible for the high frequency and recurrence rate in these patients. Approximately 5% of those who use prophylactic pentamidine will also have spontaneous pneumothoraces.

Management of AIDS-related pneumothoraces is notoriously difficult. Early tube thoracostomy and talc pleurodesis or referral for VATS should be considered. Ambulatory drainage with Heimlich valves has been successfully used.

Pneumothorax in Cystic Lung Diseases
Cystic Fibrosis

Development of pneumothorax in patients with CF carries an important prognostic implication; median survival after pneumothorax is 30 months. The pneumothorax itself is not the cause of demise but is a surrogate marker of end-stage lung disease, because patients with an FEV_1 <30% predicted are most at risk. Occurrence of pneumothorax is usually unrelated to acute respiratory illness. However, the standard guidelines for management should be adhered to with concomitant antibiotic use to avoid secondary infection. Pleurodesis to prevent recurrence of pneumothorax is important, because recurrence rates are approximately 50%. Early liaison with the transplant team is appropriate if surgical input is required.

Pulmonary Langerhans' Cell Histiocytosis (LCH)

Spontaneous pneumothorax may be the presenting feature in up to 25% of patients. Treatment options are those discussed previously for pneumothoraces, together with management of the underlying LCH (see Chapter 54).

Lymphangioleiomyomatosis (LAM)

In addition to chylothorax, patients with LAM are at risk of pneumothoraces that are common (affecting up to 80%) and may be the presenting feature of the underlying LAM. Recurrent pneumothoraces occur in two thirds of patients, and early definitive intervention is recommended to reduce recurrence rates. Recent evidence suggests surgery and chemical pleurodesis are equally effective and, although increasing the rate of perioperative bleeding, do not preclude successful future lung transplantation (see Chapter 54).

Pitfalls and Controversies

The cause of pneumothorax remains poorly understood. Only a small proportion of subjects with CT evidence of blebs or cystic lung changes actually develop a pneumothorax. Advances in diagnostic technologies (e.g., fluorescein-enhanced autofluorescence thoracoscopy [FEAT]) may shed light on the pathogenesis of pneumothorax. Early evidence already casts doubts on whether air leaks truly originate from blebs (as per conventional teachings) or from other abnormal areas identified on FEAT.

The optimal management of pneumothoraces remains debatable. The use of suction early in the course of treatment and clamping of the intercostal drain remain controversial topics. Management strategies that use less invasive drainage (e.g., simple aspiration) and early ambulatory drainage with one-way valves are increasingly adopted by some clinicians. On the other hand, widespread acceptance of minimally invasive thoracoscopic surgery may prompt earlier referral in the future and even first-line thoracoscopic treatment. The best management of pneumothoraces in potential future lung transplant candidates is unclear, and further investigation is needed on optimal timing for flying in patients with recent pneumothorax.

SUGGESTED READINGS

British Thoracic Society Standards of Care Committee: BTS guidelines for the management of pleural disease. Thorax 2003; 58(Supp II):1–59.

First Multicenter Intrapleural Sepsis Trial (MIST1) Group: UK Controlled Trial of Intrapleural Streptokinase for Pleural Infection. N Engl J Med 2005; 352:865–874.

Light RW Lee YCG, eds: Textbook of Pleural Diseases. London: Arnold; 2003.

Maskell NA, Gleeson FV, Davies RJO: Standard pleural biopsy versus CT-guided cutting-needle biopsy for diagnosis of pleural malignancy in pleural effusions: a randomised controlled trial. Lancet 2003; 361: 1326–1331.

Noppen N, Dekeukeleire T, Hanon S, et al: Fluorescein-enhanced autofluorescence thoracoscopy in patients with spontaneous pneumothorax and normal subjects. Am J Resp Crit Care Med 2006; 174(1):26–30.

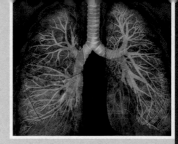

70   Malignant Pleural Mesothelioma

JAMES R. JETT • MARIE CHRISTINE AUBRY

Malignant mesothelioma originates from the lining cells (mesothelium) of the pleural and peritoneal cavities, as well as the pericardium and the tunica vaginalis. The tumor may be restricted to a small area or involve the lining cells in a multifocal or continuous manner. One of the first epidemiologic studies to link malignant mesothelioma and asbestos was reported by Wagner and colleagues by use of data collected in the 1960s among South African mine workers. This association has been confirmed by subsequent studies. The delay between exposure and development of disease is generally 20–40 years.

EPIDEMIOLOGY, RISK FACTORS, AND PATHOLOGY

Epidemiology

There are an estimated 2000–3000 cases per year in the United States. The estimates for mesothelioma mortality in Great Britain are similar, with a peak in about the year 2020 of 2700–3300 deaths. The Surveillance Epidemiology and End Result (SEER) database in the United States reports an incidence rate of approximately 2 per 100,000 of the population for men and 0.4 per 100,000 for women in 2003. The highest incidence rate by age is in 70- to 80-year-old individuals. Following the peak of mesothelioma rates in the United States and Western Europe, the numbers of cases will drop because of legislation that has decreased the exposure to asbestos in the workplace and ambient environment. That has not been the case in many developing countries.

Etiology and Risk Factors

Asbestos is a naturally occurring fibrous silicate that is present in the soil. The main asbestos mineral groups are serpentine fibers (long and curly) or amphibole fibers (straight and rod-like). Chrysotile (white asbestos), the only serpentine fiber, accounts for 95% of the asbestos used commercially. The distinction between the serpentine group and amphibole group is important, because the serpentine fiber shape is more easily cleared from the respiratory tract. Fibers with the greatest length/diameter ratios have been shown to be the most carcinogenic. Epidemiologic data suggest that the amphibole, crocidolite (blue asbestos), is associated with the highest risk of malignant mesothelioma and that chrysotile has the lowest risk. Whether or not pure chrysotile causes mesothelioma is a topic of considerable debate. Another amphibole, amosite (brown asbestos), carries an immediate risk. Environmental asbestos exposure has been associated with mesothelioma in central Turkey, where tremolite is a natural component of the soil and has been used in building construction as whitewash or stucco. A nonasbestos mineral, erionite (a fibrous zeolite), has also been identified in three villages in Cappadocia (central Turkey), and in these villages mesothelioma is reported to be responsible for nearly 50% of the deaths. Erionite has a greater carcinogenic potential than asbestos.

Roggli and colleagues quantified the number of asbestos bodies in the lung tissue of: (1) patients who died with asbestosis (fibrosis of the lung resulting from asbestos) without malignant pleural mesothelioma (MPM), (2) a group of patients with MPM without asbestosis, and (3) 50 patients who died of other causes. The lungs of patients with asbestosis without MPM had the highest fiber counts, and those with MPM, but without asbestosis, had an intermediate number of fibers. Some of the MPM patients had fiber counts that overlapped with the 50 patients who died of other causes. It is, therefore, uncertain whether there is a threshold of exposure to asbestos below which there is no risk of MPM or whether some individuals are predisposed to the disease because of inherited or acquired genetic mutations.

Asbestos, especially the amphiboles, is the main cause of MPM but does not account for all cases. Asbestos exposure is documented in only 50–70% of cases in most series. In asbestos-related cases, the disease is diagnosed 20–40 years after the first exposure, and the incidence of MPM increases with greater exposure. Among a population of asbestos insulation workers from North America, 8% of deaths were due to mesothelioma. There is also an increased incidence of MPM among the wives of asbestos workers. Presumably, this was due to asbestos that was brought home on the hair or clothing of the spouse exposed to asbestos. To avoid this risk, work practices have been put in place since 1972 in the United States that state that asbestos workers must shower and change their clothing before leaving work. Since 1990, there have been more than 30 lawsuits filed in the United States because of mesotheliomas in household members of asbestos-exposed workers. Cases of MPM with no history of asbestos exposure are common. The most notable other causal factor is thought to be radiation exposure. In one series of five cases of MPM in patients with a prior history of treated Hodgkin's disease, the average interval from radiotherapy to diagnosis of MPM was 15 years. The role of simian virus (SV40) in the etiology of MPM is controversial. SV40 has been shown to cause malignant mesotheliomas in 100% of hamsters when it is injected intrapleurally. By use of polymerase chain reaction analysis, SV40 DNA sequences have been documented in 60–80% of human MPM samples. Mesotheliomas from some countries such as Finland, Austria, and Turkey have tested negative for SV40.

Genetics

Asbestos has been shown to cause chromosomal aberrations with loss of genetic material occurring commonly. There has been documented loss of genetic material on the short arms of chromosomes 1, 3, and 9 and long arms of chromosomes 6, 15, and 22. Some of these regions contain known suppressor genes. The exact genetic alterations or signal pathways involved in the development of MPM remain to be determined. It is believed that the large T antigen (Tag) of SV40 infection is capable of inducing chromosomal alterations. Tag has been shown to cause inactivation of tumor suppressor genes such as p53 and retinoblastoma gene. The general consensus is that SV40 alone does not cause mesothelioma but may act as a cocarcinogen with asbestos. Epidemiologic data from Turkey suggest that genetic predisposition may play a role in determining individual susceptibility. No specific gene or genetic alteration that identifies the susceptible individual has been identified to date.

Pathology

Gross Features

Diffuse MPM grows on the pleural surface and, according to the stage of disease, forms multiple small tumor nodules, plaquelike masses, or large confluent sheets with near complete encasement of the lung. With advancing disease, complete obliteration of the pleural space and invasion into adjacent structures (lung, chest wall, diaphragm, mediastinum) occurs. Metastatic disease or other primary pleural malignancies can display a similar growth pattern. Occasionally, MPM can form a large bulky mass mimicking lung cancer and referred to as localized MPM.

Histologic Features

The only accurate diagnostic method is microscopic examination, and routine hematoxylin and eosin (H&E) stain is the mainstay of the diagnosis. Immunohistochemistry and electron microscopy are adjunctive techniques that are applied to confirm or inform a diagnosis on the basis of the H&E.

MPM are broadly divided into three main categories: epithelial; sarcomatous, which includes desmoplastic mesothelioma; and biphasic. A large number of less common patterns have been described, including deciduoid, lymphohistiocytoid, small cell, clear cell, pleomorphic MPM, and heterologous elements such as chondrosarcoma, osteosarcoma, and rhabdomyosarcoma can be present in otherwise typical MPM. The importance of classification lies in its prognostic significance and as such, separating epithelial MPM from sarcomatous is important, because survival is distinctively different. Further subclassification in other patterns does not seem to convey further prognostic information; however, for the pathologists, these patterns raise a wide differential diagnosis.

Epithelial MPM comprise a mixture of tubules, papillae, or solid sheets of cells. The mesothelial cells may be short cuboidal to large polygonal, contain clear to dense eosinophilic cytoplasm, and show mild to marked pleomorphism. Sarcomatous MPM usually consist of spindle cells that may also take on different appearances. Desmoplastic MPM is a variant of sarcomatous MPM and is characterized by a paucicellular, densely collagenized lesion, with cells showing no cytologic atypia. This variant is difficult to separate from a reactive process, such as fibrosing pleuritis, and requires identification of features such as invasion, necrosis, or overt sarcomatous area. Biphasic MPM represents a combination of epithelial and sarcomatous patterns, with at least 10% of each.

MPM also needs to be distinguished from benign mesothelial epithelial and spindled (fibrous pleurisy/fibrosing pleuritis) proliferation. As a rule, MPM shows complex growth pattern, dense cellularity with nodular expansion of stroma, stromal invasion, absence of zonation, storiform pattern, increased cytologic atypia, lack of capillaries, and necrosis. Stromal invasion represents the single most important and reliable feature of malignancy.

Histochemistry

MPM often produces intracellular and extracellular hyaluronic acid (Alcian blue positive removed by hyaluronidase). Only very rarely have focal intracellular neutral mucin (diastase-resistant periodic acid–Schiff [PAS-d] and mucicarmine [hyaluronidase-resistant]) been identified. In contrast, adenocarcinomas usually show intracellular neutral mucin.

Immunohistochemical Stains

A huge variety of immunostains have been studied for the diagnosis of MPM (Table 70-1). This is an area that is constantly changing with the emergence of new stains or reevaluations of old ones. This has led to many conflicting results because of use of different methods, antibodies, or types of analysis. Also, the application of immunohistochemical studies depends on the type of MPM (epithelial vs sarcomatous) and the differential diagnosis (carcinoma, including its type [i.e., lung vs ovary vs other, or sarcoma]).

The main role of immunohistochemical studies is in the differential between epithelial MPM and adenocarcinoma. Because no single marker is entirely specific or sensitive, studies usually agree that a panel of so-called positive and negative mesothelial markers should be used. Studies diverge on the exact nature of the panel, but in general, one to two positive markers, such as calretinin, WT-1, and/or CK5/6, and one to two negative markers, such as MOC31, BG8, CEA, and/or BerEp4, have been recommended. Promising positive markers include D2–40 and podoplanin, but more studies are needed before their routine use. If the differential diagnosis is with lung adenocarcinoma, adding TTF-1 is useful. For serous carcinoma of the ovary or peritoneum, WT-1 has no value, whereas ER/PR proves useful. Squamous cell carcinoma may enter the differential diagnosis and create difficulties, because it does express mesothelioma-positive markers such as CK5/6. For this differential diagnosis, a panel composed of WT-1, MOC31, and p63 has been suggested. These different panels are not helpful in the differential diagnosis of sarcomatous MPM with sarcoma, because calretinin is positive in less than half of sarcomatous MPM and CK5/6 in less than a third, whereas calretinin can be expressed in sarcomas. In this scenario, broad-spectrum keratin will prove most informative, being usually diffusely and strongly positive in MPM while negative in most sarcomas. Immunohistochemical studies do not play a significant role in the differential diagnosis between benign reactive mesothelial proliferations and MPM, except keratin in demonstrating invasion.

Electron Microscopy

Ultrastructural evidence of long, thin, bush surface microvilli is found in epithelioid mesothelioma, whereas short blunt microvilli are seen in adenocarcinomas. A length/diameter ratio of microvilli greater than 15 should be considered strongly supportive of the diagnosis of epithelioid MPM. Electron microscopy is less effective in diagnosing poorly differentiated epithelioid mesothelioma or in distinguishing sarcomatous mesothelioma from sarcoma.

TABLE 70-1 Immunohistochemistry Staining Results for Malignant Pleural Mesothelioma Histologic Types and Adenocarcinomas (Results in %- summary of several studies)

	MPM epithelial	MPM sarcomatous	Adenocarcinoma Lung	Adenocarcinoma Ovary/Peritoneum
Keratin (AE1/AE3 and CAM5.2)	100	95	100	100
D2-40	86–100	–	0	15–65
Podoplanin	85–100	–	0	0–13
Mesothelin	65–100	0	39	84
Calretinin	85–100	39–50	6–10	0–38
WT-1	90	34	0	88–100
CK5/6	64–100	26–29	0–19	22–50
Thrombomodulin	34–100	31	5–77	4
MOC31	5–10	0	90–100	95–100
BG8	3–7	–	88–96	73
CD15	0–32	10	70–95	30–60
BerEP4	0–29	0	32–100	95–100
CEA	0	4	80–97	0–16
B72.3	0–3	6	35–100	73–87
TTF-1	0	0	58–97	0
ER	0	–	5	93

Partly because of its rarity, the histologic diagnosis of MPM is difficult, and there is considerable variation in the diagnosis arrived at by different observers, which is as high as 50% in some studies. Pathology panels have been formed in a number of countries to address this problem and for purposes of referral. The members of the North American mesothelioma panel reached a consensus of 75% or more on 70% of the referral material sent to them. It is obvious, therefore, that even the experts do not always agree.

CLINICAL FEATURES

MPM is primarily a disease of adults and presents when the patient is in the fifth to seventh decade (median age, 60 years). Those diagnosed between ages 20 and 40 years usually have a history of childhood exposure. Children have rarely been reported to have this disease develop. Men account for 70–80% of cases. The most common presentations are dyspnea, nonpleuritic chest pain, or both. Table 70-2 outlines the initial presentation of 90 cases of MPM in our previously reported series and does not differ substantially from the results that have appeared in other publications. The physical examination is usually unremarkable, except for dullness to percussion at the base of one lung caused by pleural effusion and tumor infiltrating the pleura. Palpable metastatic lymph nodes may occasionally be present, and digital clubbing is observed occasionally.

The tumor originates mainly on the parietal pleura and progressively spreads to encase the lung surfaces and individual lobes by tracking along fissures. The tumor may reach several centimeters in thickness. It can penetrate into the chest wall, along needle tracts, infiltrate the diaphragm, invade mediastinal structures, and encase the heart and pericardium. Peritoneal involvement is found in approximately one third of cases at autopsy. Localized malignant mesotheliomas, sessile or pedunculated, can occur.

TABLE 70-2 Initial Symptoms in 90 Cases of Malignant Pleural Mesothelioma

Symptom	Number of Cases	%
Pain	62	69
Nonpleuritic	56	–
Pleuritic	6	–
Shortness of breath	53	59
Fever, chills, or sweats	30	33
Weakness, fatigue, or malaise	30	33
Cough	24	27
Weight loss	22	24
Anorexia	10	11
Sensation of heaviness or fullness in chest	6	7
Hoarseness	3	3

Symptoms at initial presentation in 90 evaluable cases of malignant pleural mesothelioma. Modified with permission from Adams et al: Cancer 58:1540–1551, 1986.

RADIOLOGIC FINDINGS

At the time of diagnosis, approximately 75% of patients will have a pleural effusion. In one series of 37 patients with pleural effusion, the effusion was greater than one third of the hemithorax in 19 (51%). The next most frequent abnormality on the chest radiograph is nodular thickening of the pleura with or without irregular thickening of the interlobar fissure (Figure 70-1). A localized mass may be the only radiologic abnormality in 5–10% of individuals. When the disease is more advanced, diffuse thickening of the pleura can produce decreased volume of the affected hemithorax (Figure 70-2). Calcified or noncalcified plaques may also be identified. Pleural

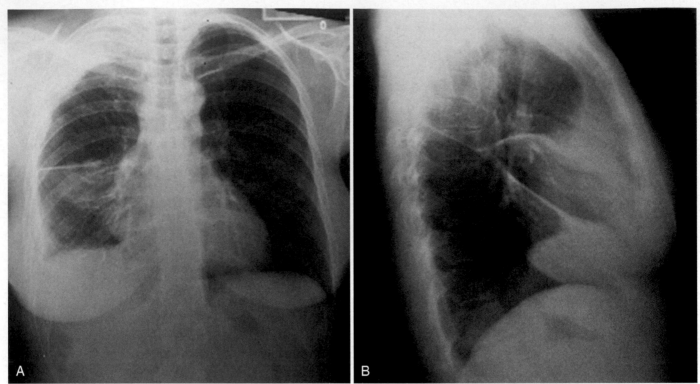

FIGURE 70-1 A, Posteroanterior and, **B,** lateral chest radiographs of a patient with malignant pleural mesothelioma. Thickening of the pleura of the major fissure is most clearly visible on the lateral view.

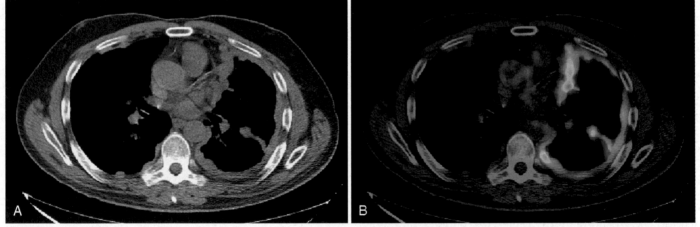

FIGURE 70-2 A, Cross-sectional CT scan and **(B)** PET-CT of a patient with MPM that demonstrates thickening of the entire circumferential pleura and invasion of the fissure. This is the same patient whose gross specimen is shown in Figure 70-4.

plaques are a sign of asbestos exposure but are not a precursor to MPM. A prospective series followed more than 1500 Swedish men with pleural plaques for 16,000 plus person-years and observed a risk of MPM of 1 in 1800 per person-year. Nevertheless, there are no convincing prospective trials that demonstrate a mortality benefit to screening high-risk individuals with CT or serum markers for mesothelioma.

Computed Tomography

Computed tomography (CT) provides more information on the extent of disease. CT examination of 50 patients with MPM showed pleural thickening that varied in extent and nodularity in 92% of patients. Thickening of the interlobar fissure was observed in 86% of cases and pleural effusion in 74%. Calcified pleural plaques were seen in 10 patients (20%) and were assimilated into the mesothelioma in six cases. There was contraction of the involved hemithorax in 42% of patients, but a mediastinal shift was present in only seven (14%). Extension of the tumor into the chest wall and abdomen, as well as involvement of the mediastinal pleura, pericardium, and lymph nodes, was documented in some cases. Magnetic resonance imaging of the thorax with the use of multidimensional planes is superior to CT scans for evaluating the relationship of the tumor to the great vessels if surgery is being considered. In one large, prospective study of 65 patients comparing CT and magnetic resonance imaging, the latter was significantly better at demonstrating invasion of the diaphragm and chest wall. With the new multislice CT scanners, the advantage of CT over MRI has diminished.

Positron Emission Tomography

Positron emission tomography (PET) is increasingly used in the evaluation of suspected and proven MPM. PET is better than CT at differentiating malignant from benign disease and can be used for evaluation of worrisome pleural lesions. A positive PET result must be pathologically confirmed, but a negative PET is reassuring and justifies careful observation without biopsy in many cases. Pretreatment evaluation with PET is increasingly being used. PET has been shown to identify distant disease in patients being considered for extrapleural pneumonectomy. In one series from The M. D. Anderson Cancer Center, integrated CT-PET was performed in 29 patients who were candidates for extrapleural pneumonectomy after clinical and conventional radiologic evaluation. Integrated CT-PET provided additional information in 11 of 29 patients that precluded surgery. Extrathoracic metastases were identified in seven individuals. The PET/CT scan in Figure 70-3 shows the extent of the disease in the hemithorax. The coronal and saggital image show the disease extending into the major fissure and into the extreme mediastinal-phrenic recess, thus clearly demonstrating the technical difficulty of achieving a complete resection with extrapleural pneumonectomy. Early reports of PET standard uptake values (SUV) have suggested that SUV may have predictive value, with higher SUV correlating with poorer survival. PET is also being investigated for its potential to detect earlier response or lack thereof to systemic treatment.

DIAGNOSIS

The initial diagnosis can be difficult and is frequently delayed. Pleural fluid cytologic examination is positive for malignant cells in one third of cases, but it is uncommon for the pathologist to make a definitive diagnosis of MPM on cytologic study alone. Percutaneous or closed-needle biopsy of the pleura yields adequate tissue for diagnosis in approximately one third of cases. Thoracoscopy with direct visualization of the pleura yields diagnostic tissue in more than 90% of samples. Before thoracoscopy, open pleural biopsy had been the "gold standard" for diagnosis, but even this method is not absolutely definitive in all cases because of problems encountered both with sampling and with pathologic interpretations. The typical visual appearance at thoracoscopy or open biopsy is that of multiple pleural nodules or masses. The nodules are usually larger and more numerous on the parietal pleura, but frequently involve the visceral pleura. A dominant mass surrounded by numerous scattered smaller nodules may occur. Pleural effusion with pleural thickening may be the only finding, and pleural symphysis with obliteration of the pleural space is encountered occasionally.

Because initial pleural fluid examination is often inconclusive, cytologic examination, in general, is an unsatisfactory technique for diagnosing this type of tumor. Closed pleural biopsy with an Abrams needle is technically difficult, because the pleura is often very thick and fibrous. In general, a core of tissue is required. Physicians may be reluctant to insert a large needle through the chest wall because of the high risk of tumor growing out along the tract formed, thus producing a painful mass. CT-guided core biopsies give a fair diagnostic yield, and thoracoscopy is the procedure of choice when the diagnosis is in doubt.

Two tumor markers have been reported recently. Mesothelin is a surface glycoprotein that is present on normal mesothelial cells and on some cancers, including mesothelioma

and ovarian and pancreatic cancers. Soluble mesothelin-related protein has been identified in the serum of 84% of patients with MPM and only 2% of individuals with other malignant or benign pulmonary diseases. More than 60% of patients have elevated soluble mesothelin at the time of diagnosis, and the levels increase with disease progression. Mesothelin may prove to be useful to monitor response to disease treatment. Mesothelin levels have been elevated in the serum of some asbestos-exposed individuals from 1–6 years before the diagnosis of MPM. However, at this time the exact sensitivity and specificity of mesothelin as a screening test is not known. Osteopontin is a glycoprotein that is overexpressed in a number of cancers. One study has reported that serum osteopontin levels were significantly higher in patients with MPM than in a group with exposure to asbestos but no MPM. The sensitivity and specificity at diagnosis with a value of 48 ng/mL were 78% and 86%, respectively The efficacy of this marker as a screening test is under investigation but currently unknown.

Staging

The International Mesothelioma Interest Group proposed a modified staging system (Table 70-3 and Table 70-4) that reconciles and updates previous systems. In 2002, this system was adopted by the International Union Against Cancer and the American Joint Committee on Cancer. These staging categories have been validated on a series of 131 patients from Memorial Sloan-Kettering Cancer Center and 48 patients from a National Cancer Institute series. Most patients have an advanced stage at diagnosis. In the National Cancer Institute series, 4 patients had stage I, 4 had stage II, 38 had stage III, and 2 had stage IV disease. In the surgical staging series of 131 patients from Memorial Sloan-Kettering, 12% were stage I, 15% stage II, 44% stage III, and 29% stage IV. In most reported series, very few patients have stage IA or IB disease at diagnosis. In The M. D. Anderson series, with CT-PET staging, only one patient had stage I and two had stage II. The remaining 26 patients had stage III and IV disease.

TREATMENT

The beneficial effects of treatment for MPM of the pleura are controversial. Perhaps the major area of debate about treatment is the role of surgery. It is estimated that 50% or fewer of all patients with MPM are potentially resectable. Two large retrospective series concluded that patients undergoing either decortication/pleurectomy or extrapleuropneumonectomy did not show improved survival compared with other treatments or with simply the best supportive care. However, a number of recent reports have suggested that surgery as part of a trimodality therapeutic approach may have an effect on survival. Sugarbaker and associates performed extrapleural pneumonectomy in 183 selected patients, who were then treated with adjuvant chemotherapy and ipsilateral hemithoracic irradiation. The overall median survival was 19 months, with 38% alive at 2 years and 15% at 5 years. Epithelioid histologic examination was associated with a better survival (median, 26 months, 21% 5-year survival). In those patients with mixed or sarcomatoid histologic findings, only 2 of 72 patients were alive at 3 years. In addition, none of the patients with N2 or N3 lymph node involvement survived for 3 years. From 1980–2000, 328 extrapleural pneumonectomies were performed with an operative mortality of 3.4% by this highly experienced group. Sixty percent had minor or major complications,

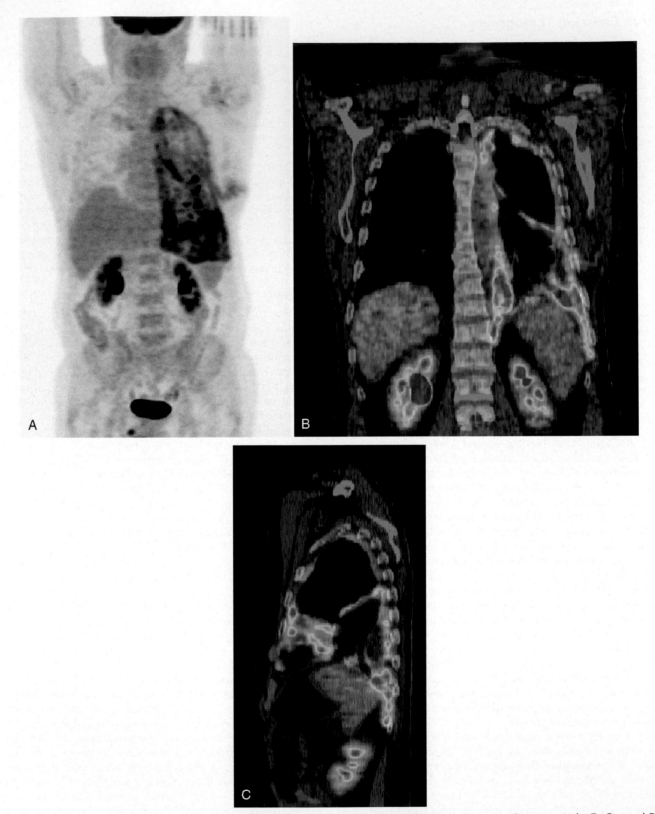

FIGURE 70-3 A, Maximum intensity projection image of the PET data in a patient with MPM. Image is taken anteriorly. **B,** Coronal PET-CT image showing tumor extending into the extreme pleural recesses. **C,** Sagittal PET-CT image showing tumor involvement of extreme costophrenic recess, posteriorly, and involvement of the major fissure.

TABLE 70-3 Tumor Nodes Metastasis (TNM) Staging System for Malignant Pleural Mesothelioma

Primary Tumor (T)

TX	Primary tumor cannot be assessed
T0	No evidence of primary tumor
T1	Tumor involves ipsilateral parietal pleura, with or without focal involvement of visceral pleura
T1a	Tumor involves ipsilateral parietal (mediastinal, diaphragmatic) pleura. No involvement of visceral pleura
T2	Tumor involves any of the ipsilateral pleural surfaces with at least one of the following: • confluent visceral pleural tumor (including fissure) • invasion of diaphragmatic muscle • invasion of lung parenchyma
T3*	Tumor involves any of the ipsilateral pleural surfaces with at least one of the following: • invasion of the endothoracic fascia • invasion into mediastinal fat • solitary focus of tumor invading the soft tissues of the chest wall • non-transmural involvement of the pericardium
T4†	Tumor involves any of the ipsilateral pleural surfaces with at least one of the following: • diffuse or multifocal invasion of soft tissues of the chest wall • any involvement of the rib • invasion through the diphragm to the peritoneum • invasion of any mediastinal organ(s) • direct extension to the contralateral pleura • invasion into the spine • extension to the internal surface of the pericardium • pericardial effusion with positive cytology • invasion of the myocardium • invasion of the brachial plexus

Regional lymph nodes (N)

NX	Regional lymph nodes cannot be assessed
N0	No regional lymph node metastases
N1	Metastases in the ipsilateral bronchopulmonary and/or hilar nodes
N2	Metastases in the subcarinal lymph node(s) and/or the ipsilateral internal mammary or mediastinal nodes
N3	Metastases in the contralateral mediastinal, internal mammary, or hilar lymph node(s) and/or the ipsilateral or contralateral supra-clavicular or scale lymph node(s)

Distant metastases (M)

MX	Distant metastases cannot be assessed
M0	No distant metastases
M1	Distant metastases

*Describes locally advanced, but potentially resectable tumor.
†Describes locally advanced, technically unresectable tumor.
Tumor-nodes-metastasis staging system for malignant pleural mesothelioma. This system was developed by the International Mesothelioma Interest Group to reconcile and update previous systems. In 2002, it was accepted by the International Union Against Cancer and the American Joint Committee on Cancer.

TABLE 70-4 Stage Grouping for Diffuse MPM

Stage I	T1	N0	M0
Stage IA	T1a	N0	M0
Stage IB	T1b	N0	M0
Stage II	T2	N0	M0
Stage III	T1, T2	N1	M0
	T1, T2	N2	M0
	T3	N0, N1, N2	M0
Stage IV	T4	Any N	M0
	Any T	N3	M0
	Any T	Any N	M1

Staging system for diffuse malignant pleural mesothelioma. Stage groupings are based on tumor-nodes-metastasis categories as defined in Table 70-3.

including atrial fibrillation (44%), prolonged intubation (8%), vocal cord paralysis (7%), deep vein thrombosis (6%), technical complications (6%), tamponade (4%), acute respiratory distress syndrome (ARDS) (4%), and others less common. Figure 70-4 shows the gross specimen of the lung from an extrapleural pneumonectomy. In a series from Memorial Sloan-Kettering Cancer Center, 88 patients were operated with extrapleuralpneumonectomies ($n = 62$), pleurectomy/decortications ($n = 5$), or exploration only ($n = 21$). Adjuvant hemithoracic radiotherapy of 54 Gy was given to those undergoing resection. The median survival was 17 months with a 27% 3-year survival. In both of these series, the patients with stage I/II disease had a much better survival (median, 24–33 months) than did patients with stage III disease (median, 10 months). More recent trials have used preoperative chemotherapy, followed by extrapleural pneumonectomy and postoperative adjuvant hemithoracic radiotherapy. A Swiss group has recently reported the results of a phase II trial with 63 patients where trimodality therapy with preoperative chemotherapy was used. Extrapleural pneumonectomy was performed in 45 participants. Only 36 patients received postoperative radiotherapy. The median survival time was 19.8 months, and the 1-year survival was 69%. Long-term survival has not been reported yet.

Radiotherapy

Radiotherapy causes occasional regression of disease, but does not alter survival compared with supportive care alone. If radiotherapy is to be used, treatment of the entire hemithorax and ipsilateral pleura is necessary. A systemic review of four noncomparative studies has shown that hemithoracic irradiation alone resulted in significant toxicity, including radiation-induced pulmonary fibrosis, radiation pneumonitis, and bronchopleural fistula, without survival benefit. However, short courses of 20 Gy in 5 fractions or 30 Gy in 10 fractions may be effective for palliating symptoms. Radiation has been reported to prevent seeding of biopsy tracts and surgical wounds. Boutin and colleagues gave 7 Gy/fraction for 3 consecutive days to 20 patients and observed no local recurrences after needle biopsy, chest tube, or thoracoscopy. In contrast, 8 of 20 patients not treated had entry tract metastasis develop. However, a pooled analysis of three small, randomized trials found no significant reduction in the frequency

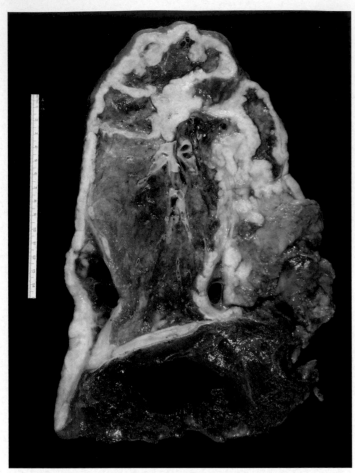

FIGURE 70-4 Gross specimen of the left lung from an extrapleural pneumonectomy. This shows extensive encasement of the lung by MPM, epithelioid type, with involvement of the fissures. This is the same person whose images are shown in Figure 70-2.

of procedure tract metastases, so this remains unsettled. Radiotherapy may be more effective when treating microscopic diseases compared with gross disease. In a series from Memorial Sloan-Kettering Cancer Center, 57 patients received hemithoracic radiotherapy (54 Gy) after extrapleural pneumonectomy. Locoregional recurrences occurred in 7 patients and distant metastases only occurred in 30 patients. This suggests that hemithoracic radiation after extrapleural pneumonectomy decreases the rate of local recurrences. A Swiss group is evaluating whether high-dose hemithoracic radiotherapy after neoadjuvant chemotherapy and extrapleural pneumonectomy will improve local disease-free survival.

Chemotherapy

There is no single drug or combination chemotherapy regimen that would be considered standard therapy for MPM. No drug has consistently produced a partial response in more than 20% of cases, and complete clinical remissions are rare. Active single agents include doxorubicin, epirubicin, mitomycin, cyclophosphamide, ifosfamide, cisplatin, carboplatin, vinorelbine, pemetrexed, and raltitrexed. Pooled response rates from phase II trials suggest that response rates with combination chemotherapy are higher than with single agents. A recent phase III international trial randomly assigned patients with unresectable MPM to chemotherapy with cisplatin and pemetrexed versus cisplatin alone. The response rate was twice as high

with the combination treatment (41% vs 17%), and survival was significantly better (median survival time, 12.1 vs 9.3 months). Another prospective phase III trial randomly assigned patients to treatment with cisplatin with or without raltitrexed. The response rates were 24% and 14%, respectively. The median survival (11.4 vs 8.8 months) and the 1-year survival (46% vs 40%) favored the combination ($P = .048$). At this time, the combination of pemetrexed and cisplatin is standard therapy in North America, provided the patient's performance status permits a platinum-based chemotherapy. Because current therapy is not curative, there are many prospective therapeutic trials underway to evaluate new and novel agents. Ideally, patients with MPM should be offered treatment on prospective clinical trials to advance our understanding of this disease.

Control of Pleural Effusion

In many patients, no specific therapy to reduce the tumor mass will be offered. Patients frequently present with large pleural effusions causing troublesome breathlessness. Although pleural effusions can be aspirated repeatedly, this may fail to relieve symptoms for long. With repeated thoracentesis, the pleural fluid may undergo loculation and be difficult to drain. If a clinically significant pleural effusion is present, it may be most effective to treat the patient initially with either thoracoscopy and talc pleurodesis or chest tube drainage and talc pleurodesis. In recent years, tunnelled pleural catheters with daily drainage by the patient or caregiver into disposable bottles have been popularized. These catheters do not require the intrapleural use of talc and the associated potential complications caused by it. Pleurodesis is frequently accomplished over time with subsequent removal of the catheter. In a recent series from Canada of 250 tunnelled pleural catheters for malignant pleural effusion, symptoms improved in 89% and pleurodesis was achieved in 43% of patients. Catheters stayed in place a median of 56 days. At present, this is our most common method of treatment of malignant pleural effusion.

A risk of thoracoscopy or tube drainage is that on emptying the pleural cavity, the lung may be encased by tumor and not able to fully expand (trapped lung) to obliterate the pleural space, thus making pleurodesis impossible. Should the pleural space be obliterated after drainage, intrapleural talc may be instilled. However, when the space persists, drainage of pleural fluid into an indwelling pleural catheter with external drainage can be extremely effective for many months. Control of the pleural fluid, if effective, is likely to bring significant symptom relief. The primary tumor does not usually metastasize outside the involved hemithorax until later in the clinical course, and local symptoms are the immediate priority.

Prognosis and Survival

The enumeration of prognostic factors has varied in different series. Histologic type has been identified as important in numerous reports, with epithelioid histology patients surviving longer than others. The Cancer and Leukemia Group B and the European Organization for Research and Treatment of Cancer each performed multivariate analyses of large numbers of patients enrolled in treatment trials for MPM through their cooperative groups. The following are the poor prognostic factors identified in one or both of these reports:

- Nonepithelioid histology
- Poor performance score
- Chest pain

TABLE 70-5 Necropsy Findings in 92 Patients with Malignant Pleural Mesothelioma

Site	Number of Patients	%
Local extension		
Mediastinum	58	63
Pericardium	45	49
Diaphragm	60	65
Lung	51	55
Opposite pleura	34	37
Chest wall	32	35
Peritoneum	36	39
Lymph node involvement		
Mediastinum	37	40
Retroperitoneum	19	21
Metastases	45	49
Liver	28	30
Contralateral lung	15	
Adrenal(s)	11	
Kidney(s)	12	
Bone	9	
Pancreas	5	
Brain	3	
Spleen	4	
Skin	4	
Thyroid	4	

Necropsy findings in 92 patients with malignant pleural mesothelioma. Other sites of metastasis occurred in two or fewer cases. Modified with permission from Ruffie et al: J Clin Oncol 7:1157–1168, 1989.

- Age older than 75 years
- Male gender
- White blood cell count $8.3 \times \tau\sigma \ 10^9/L$ or greater
- Platelets greater than 400,000 μL
- LDH greater than 500 IU/L

The median survival time varies from 8–12 months, and fewer than 20% of patients survive beyond 2 years. Most of those who survive for 2 years have epithelioid histology. Patients generally die of respiratory failure because of local extension of the disease. Some deaths are caused by pericardial constriction, congestive heart failure, or cardiac arrhythmias. Ascites and small-bowel obstruction can occur as a result of intraabdominal extension of the tumor. The sites of tumor involvement in a necropsy series of 92 patients are listed in Table 70-5.

PITFALLS AND CONTROVERSIES

It is important that MPM be considered part of the differential diagnosis of any new pleural effusion, especially in men, and, more particularly, in those with a significant history of occupational exposure to asbestos. To determine exposure, a careful occupational history is required, including information about occupations and exposures that date back 30–40 years to the individual's initial employment or hobbies. Exposure history should include questions about occupations during military service. In 30–50% of cases, there may be no significant history of asbestos exposure.

Cytologic evaluation of pleural effusion is notoriously insensitive. A negative cytologic examination or closed pleural biopsy should not, therefore, dissuade the physician from pursuing a definitive diagnosis. If the etiology of the pleural effusion is still uncertain after adequate attempts at closed biopsy, thoracoscopy should be considered as a further means of investigation to obtain a definitive histologic diagnosis.

Occasionally, the pleural fluid cytology will yield malignant cells without further definition. In such cases, additional tissue should be obtained by closed biopsy or thoracoscopy. If the physician is obviously dealing with a malignancy at the time of thoracoscopy, it may be beneficial to proceed with talc pleurodesis after obtaining the appropriate biopsy samples. The difficulties with definitive histologic diagnosis of MPM were described previously. It is important to distinguish metastatic disease to the pleura from MPM. It is especially important to rule out cancers of other sites that have a good chance of responding to therapy, such as carcinoma of the breast, ovary, prostate, or a germ cell tumor. Immunohistochemical staining of tissue is helpful in distinguishing the primary source of the malignancy. Because of the relative infrequency of MPM, the histologic specimen should be reviewed by one or more pathologist with expertise in the disease.

Treatment of MPM is controversial. No single modality or combination of therapies promises prolonged survival. Recent reports suggest that surgery may benefit patients with early-stage disease, especially if they have epithelioid histology and if lymph node metastases (N2 or N3) are absent. If surgery is planned, it should be part of a trimodality treatment program. Chemotherapy with pemetrexed or raltitrexed in combination with cisplatin has been shown to be superior to cisplatin alone. New agents or modalities of therapy are needed to combat this recalcitrant disease. Progress in discovering these new agents or modalities will be made only if we treat MPM patients in controlled clinical trials. Investigators have recently demonstrated the ability to conduct randomized phase III trials with national or international cooperation to answer important treatment questions.

SUGGESTED READINGS

Churg A, Cagle PT, Roggli VL: Tumors of the serosal membranes. AFIP atlas of tumor pathology, 4th Series, fascicle 3. Washington, DC: American Registry of Pathology, 2004.

Ellis P, Davies AM, Evans WK, et al, and the Lung Cancer Disease Site Group of Cancer Care Ontario's Program in Evidence-based Care: The use of chemotherapy in patients with advanced malignant pleural mesothelioma: A systematic review and practice guideline. J Thorac Oncol 2006; 1:591–601.

Erasmus JJ, Truong MT, Smythe WR, et al: Integrated computed tomography-positron emission tomography in patients with potentially resectable malignant pleural mesothelioma: Staging implications. J Thorac Cardiovasc Surg 2005; 129:1364–1370.

Ordonez NG: Immunohistochemical diagnosis of epithelial mesothelioma: An update. Arch Pathol Lab Med 2005; 129:1407–1414.

Pisick E, Salgia R: Molecular biology of malignant mesothelioma: A review. Hematol Oncol Clin North Am 2005; 19:997–1023.

Robinson BWS, Lake RA: Advances in malignant mesothelioma. N Engl J Med 2005; 353:1591–1603.

Sterman DH, Albelda SM: Advances in the diagnosis, evaluation and management of malignant pleural mesothelioma. Respirology 2005; 10:266–283.

Sugarbaker DJ, Jaklitsch MT, Bueno R, et al: Prevention, early detection, and management of complications after 328 consecutive extrapleural pneumonectomies. J Thorac Cadiovasc Surg 2004; 128:137–146.

Ung YC, Yu E, Falkson C, et al: and the Lung Cancer Disease Site Group of Cancer Care Ontario's Program in Evidence-based Care: The role of radiation therapy in malignant pleural mesothelioma: A systematic review. Radiother and Oncol 2006; 80:13–18.

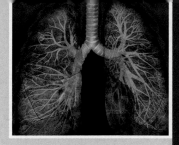

71 Acute Respiratory Distress Syndrome

MARGARET J. NEFF • LEONARD D. HUDSON

INTRODUCTION

The acute respiratory disease syndrome (ARDS) is a disease of modern medicine made possible by the development of critical care medicine. Acute diffuse alveolar damage, the pathology of ARDS, is virtually always secondary to some other acute severe injury or illness, and the syndrome was not well recognized until patients with those underlying conditions putting them at risk for ARDS survived long enough to have the condition develop. The term ARDS was first introduced in 1967 to describe a common clinical, pathophysiologic, and pathologic picture that occurred after a variety of insults. Originally called the adult respiratory distress syndrome to call attention to many features that were similar to infant respiratory distress syndrome that occurred in premature newborns, the word adult was later changed to acute, in part to acknowledge that children and adolescents can have ARDS develop.

Because no sensitive and specific biomarker has been identified to allow recognition of this lung injury syndrome, ARDS has been defined by clinical criteria, including an oxygenation abnormality, an abnormal chest radiograph picture, and the exclusion of cardiogenic pulmonary edema as the primary cause. Some definitions have included the presence of a clinical risk factor for the syndrome and/or abnormal total respiratory compliance (i.e., increased lung stiffness). In 1994, a group of clinical investigators and critical care physicians convened the American-European Consensus Conference (AECC) and developed a new definition and introduced the term acute lung injury (ALI), which differed from ARDS only by the oxygenation criterion (i.e., PaO_2/F_IO_2 of ≤ 300 for ALI and ≤ 200 for ARDS). The term ALI is commonly misused to refer to those patients meeting ALI criterion but excluding patients with ARDS. Throughout this chapter the terms ALI, ARDS, and ALI without ARDS will refer to the AECC definitions unless otherwise specified (see "Diagnosis").

EPIDEMIOLOGY, RISK FACTORS, AND PATHOGENESIS

Incidence

The incidence of ARDS varies geographically and is affected by several factors, including the prevalence and type of predisposing risk factors or conditions in the population, access to medical care (especially intensive care), the comorbidities in the population, and, likely, genetic influences in the population being studied. The incidence is greatly affected by the specific definition of

ARDS or ALI being used. Previous incidence studies resulted in figures ranging from 1.5–20 cases per 100,000 population per year, but all previous studies were limited by the use of obsolete (and often much more severe or restrictive) definitions, not being truly population-based (i.e., not having an accurate denominator), absence of procedures to ensure reliable case identification, use of administrative coding that is known to be inaccurate, and extrapolation from less than a full year of observation or from only a subset of hospitals in the region under study.

A recent study performed in King County (the county in which Seattle, Washington, is located and that includes both urban and rural areas) was designed to avoid these limitations. Identification was accomplished by a validated screening protocol and did not rely on physicians' subjective diagnoses. Observation was for a full year in every hospital in the county and the largest hospitals in neighboring counties to which King County residents might be admitted and ventilated. The AECC definitions for ALI and ARDS were used. In this study, the incidence of ALI was found to be 78.9 cases per 100,000 population/year, an order of magnitude higher than most previous estimates but similar to another study that attempted to provide an incidence figure for the entire United States. The incidence of ALI increased with increasing age. This incidence and the number of deaths per year on the basis of the overall mortality rate of 38.5% in the study and extrapolated by use of the U.S. population, makes this syndrome a major public health problem, with an estimated 190,600 cases and 74,500 deaths per year in the United States. This mortality is comparable to the number of adult deaths a year resulting from breast cancer or HIV disease in 1999 and is considerably greater than the number of deaths from prostate cancer. One possible limitation of this estimate is that the regional characteristics of King County may not reflect the United States as a whole; however, data suggest that the population in King County is younger, of higher socioeconomic status, and with fewer blacks in the racial distribution, all which would bias the study toward underestimating the true incidence and mortality.

Risk Factors

ALI and ARDS are essentially always associated with an underlying severe illness or injury. These conditions may lead to lung injury, either by a direct insult such as aspiration of gastric contents through the airways or an indirect insult through the bloodstream as occurs with sepsis or nonthoracic trauma (i.e., pulmonary vs extrapulmonary forms). Specific lung diseases such as Goodpasture's syndrome (antibasement membrane antibody disease) may have a similar clinical picture but were excluded from the definition of ALI/ARDS by the AECC.

The risk factors or risk conditions have generally been identified retrospectively. A few prospective studies, however, have defined risk factors or conditions, identified patients with those conditions, and then followed them for development of ARDS, allowing some sense of the incidence of ARDS with any given risk condition. Common associated risk conditions are shown in Box 71-1.

Sepsis or sepsis syndrome has been the most common risk factor associated with ARDS studies done in North America, Europe, South America, Asia, and India, although the causative organisms may differ (e.g., leptospirosis and malaria in some series). Severe bacterial or viral pneumonia is another common risk condition, although nearly all patients with pneumonia who have ALI develop also meet criteria for sepsis. Pneumonia can lead to diffuse lung injury from contiguous spread of infection through the airways or by blood-borne injury from inflammatory mediators that have entered the bloodstream. Miliary tuberculosis is a rare infectious cause of ARDS.

Trauma is another major risk condition and can be direct (i.e., thoracic trauma resulting in lung contusion) or, more commonly, indirect through blood-borne mediators of inflammation. Aspiration of gastric contents (usually massive) is another common cause of ARDS. Experimental studies have shown that both the acid content and presence of gastric enzymes contribute to the pathophysiology. Aspiration of partially digested food with neutral pH and without significant quantities of gastric enzymes may present with diffuse infiltrates and severe hypoxemia, but lung injury does not develop, and the hypoxemia and infiltrates rapidly resolve.

Massive transfusion of blood products has been identified as a risk condition in trauma subjects but was also found to have the same incidence in nontrauma patients experiencing severe gastrointestinal bleeding, usually from esophageal varices (i.e., ~25% when 12 or more units were transfused). In trauma patients, it is unclear whether the blood plays a specific pathogenic role, if the requirement for such large quantities of transfused blood is simply a marker of more severe injury, carrying a higher risk for systemic inflammation-related lung injury, or whether both contribute. Recent evidence suggests that the incidence of ALI increases with the duration of

storage of the transfused blood. Even small quantities of transfused blood or blood products can precipitate acute lung injury in patients, so-called transfusion-related acute lung injury or TRALI. TRALI has been associated with all plasma-containing blood products but most commonly involves whole blood, packed RBCs, fresh-frozen plasma, and platelets. TRALI can occur in patients with no other known risk for ALI but also may occur in patients with other underlying risk conditions, including trauma and sepsis, raising speculation that this may represent a so-called two-hit phenomenon, with the first hit being the underlying risk condition. What the specific pathogenic blood product–related mechanism of the second hit is remains somewhat controversial, but the most prevalent theory implicates passively transfused antibodies, functioning as leukoagglutinins that may attach to antigens on the recipients' white blood cells releasing products that injure. Alternately, these antibodies might be to the pulmonary endothelium or monocytes.

Long bone fractures represent a risk in trauma patients and are associated with fat embolism syndrome. Fat embolism presents with the features of ALI but most often is relatively mild and self-limited. Severe pancreatitis is a well-recognized but relatively uncommon cause of ARDS, presumably related to the entry of enzymes and inflammatory mediators into the blood.

Less common risk conditions but ones often associated with a high incidence of ALI development are near drowning and inhalation of toxic gases. Near drowning with ALI can result from aspirating fresh or saltwater, presumably with differing mechanisms of osmotic injury to the alveolar-capillary membrane of the lung. Studies in animal models indicate that a large amount of fluid has to be aspirated as a result of near drowning to result in ALI and that saltwater aspiration is associated with a larger degree of pulmonary edema than freshwater aspiration because of the osmotic effect (i.e., approximately three times the osmolality of normal body fluids). Aspiration of freshwater, on the other hand, is more likely to cause greater damage to the alveolar-capillary membrane. Differences between the two can be demonstrated in animal models, with freshwater causing transient hemodilution and hemolysis. These findings are rarely seen in humans, however, perhaps because the findings are no longer detectable after even relatively short transport times to a medical facility or because patients with enough aspiration of water to cause these abnormalities may not survive.

Whether patients with toxic gas inhalation have ALI/ARDS develop depends on the toxicity of the gas and the concentrations inhaled, as well as the water solubility of the gas. Gases with high water solubility tend to precipitate out in the upper airway causing irritation that, in turn, causes the victim to try to escape the exposure. Gases with lower water solubility may reach higher concentrations in the lower airways and alveoli and cause greater damage there. When high concentrations of carbon monoxide are inhaled in the gas mixture such as commonly occurs in fire victims, the effects of the carbon monoxide dominate the clinical picture. Immediate ARDS (as opposed to late ARDS related to burns and sepsis) is relatively uncommon in fire victims, presumably because they die from carbon monoxide intoxication before adequate concentrations of any toxic gases in the inhaled smoke can substantially injure the lower lung.

Patients with ALI/ARDS nearly always have one of the preceding risk factors occurring before, or simultaneously with, the

---

BOX 71-1   Risk Conditions for the Development of ALI/ARDS

Common
Sepsis
Pneumonia
Trauma (risk factors include massive blood transfusion, lung contusion, and multiple fractures)
Aspiration of gastric contents
Multiple transfusions

Less common
Pancreatitis
Near drowning
Fat embolism
Smoke or toxic gas inhalation
Drug overdose
Subarachnoid hemorrhage
Radiation
Miliary tuberculosis
Hanging with asphyxiation

onset of ALI. If no such risk condition can be identified and if infection with sepsis has been ruled out, rare causes such as military tuberculosis should be considered. If those diagnoses seem unlikely, several lung conditions that can mimic the appearance of ARDS should also be considered. This is of particular import, because these disease processes may be treatable with antiinflammatory agents that would *not* be routinely used in the treatment of most patients with ARDS. These conditions are listed in Box 71-2 and include acute interstitial pneumonia, acute eosinophilic pneumonia, acute bronchiolitis obliterans organizing pneumonia (BOOP), diffuse alveolar hemorrhage, and acute hypersensitivity pneumonitis.

A history of chronic alcohol abuse significantly increases the risk of ARDS developing in patients with septic shock, perhaps because it reduces glutathione concentrations. Conversely, a history of diabetes mellitus is associated with a lower incidence of ARDS in patients with septic shock, perhaps because diabetes decreases the ability of neutrophils to migrate into the lungs and produce oxidant damage.

Pathogenesis

Although a number of clinical risk factors associated with the development of ALI have been defined, there is still no biomarker that can either reliably identify patients at risk or predict outcome. Alveolar and systemic markers of injury and inflammation have been identified, but their exact roles in the pathogenesis have not been clearly delineated. What is well known, however, is that ALI is associated with acute inflammation in the lungs, with injury to the alveolar epithelium and the vascular endothelium that results in capillary leakage.

Markers of lung inflammation (e.g., interleukin [IL]-6 and IL-8) can be found both in the plasma and the alveolar space. A study of low versus high tidal volumes done by investigators composing the ARDS Network in the United States found that levels of IL-6 and IL-8 were associated with increased morbidity and mortality, that the severity of the inflammation was related to the type of ALI risk, and that the low tidal volume strategy attenuated the inflammatory response. This finding suggests that inflammation and lung stretch are linked and

may act synergistically. Inflammation is only one part of the lung's response to an insult such as trauma or sepsis. Damage to the airway epithelium can also be identified and tracked through biomarkers such as surfactant proteins. Injury to the endothelium is identified through biomarkers such as von Willebrand factor antigen, soluble intercellular adhesion molecule-1 (sICAM-1), and E/P-selectins.

Where to look for these biomarkers is an important consideration. Although it is easier to study cytokines and other mediators in the plasma, markers in the systemic compartment are nonspecific. Whether these and other cytokines leak from the lung into the systemic circulation or are produced in the systemic circulation in response to toxins from the lung is not well described. Another way to study these markers is through sampling of the airways—either of the upper airways by collecting edema fluid or the lower airways by way of bronchoscopy and bronchoalveolar lavage. Obtaining edema fluid is relatively noninvasive, and it is readily accessible but is only present for approximately the first 24 h after intubation. Bronchoscopy and lavage can yield samples at any point during lung injury, but the procedure requires trained personnel, and it can only be done in relatively stable patients. Previous studies of alveolar fluid, though, have shown that sustained inflammation (e.g., elevated neutrophil count in the lavage fluid) in the airways is associated with a poorer prognosis and increased mortality. This type of sampling more directly associates lung inflammation and injury with outcomes, whereas systemic markers could reflect the body's response to any of a number of insults potentially having nothing to do with lung injury.

GENETICS

A common experience for intensivists is the revelation that two patients with what seems to be the same insult (i.e., trauma, pneumonia, aspiration) can have entirely different responses to that insult. One may have severe ALI develop, whereas the other may never even require intubation. Similarly, even among those who have ALI develop from apparently the same cause, patients will vary widely in their clinical course and overall outcome. It is intuitive to think that there must be some inherent differences among these patients that lead some to have a mild course and others to have a more severe course, and this sense of presumed genetic predisposition has led to applications of genetic epidemiology to the study of ARDS/ALI. Such research has proven fruitful in other fields such as oncology, where genetic testing can identify high-risk patients and guide clinicians toward different therapeutic options.

Traditional genetic approaches that use family linkage mapping really are not feasible for the study of ALI, because it occurs sporadically and the time and type of insult is unpredictable. Also complicating genetic studies in ALI is the need for a well-defined phenotype. At present, ALI is defined entirely clinically, and variability in how that definition is applied will significantly alter the relevance of genotypes identified. The advantage of genetic testing, however, is the stability of the signal. Unlike biomarkers (e.g., cytokine levels), a person's genotype is stable throughout the course of the disease, decreasing the variability in the measurements considerably. In addition, blood is easier to obtain and to test than alveolar fluid. Also, if an association between a gene and ALI risk or outcome is identified, causation is clearer, because the patient's genotype clearly predated the lung injury.

The most common approach used in studying the genetic epidemiology of ALI has been the candidate gene approach. Unlike whole-genome scanning, the candidate-gene approach focuses on specific genes whose products and function are well understood. The study of these genes, because their function is known, is hypothesis driven. Once a candidate gene has been identified, the investigation of its relevance to disease development and/or outcomes can be evaluated either directly (e.g., is ALI associated with a specific single-nucleotide polymorphism [SNP]) or indirectly (evaluate all SNPs within a gene). For either approach, the clear identification of the phenotype (i.e., identification of ALI) is critical. In addition, factoring in the effect of race is critical as is the identification of an appropriate control group and the effect of the environment. The application of genetic epidemiology to the study of ALI and ARDS is still in its infancy. Initially, the hope is to find genetic markers that can predict the development of ALI (either with or without a secondary insult) and then to predict the severity and outcome if ALI develops. Gene therapy, an approach pursued in some other diseases, is perhaps less likely to be a therapeutic option for ALI, because it is more likely that multiple genes, rather than a single gene mutation, would be involved with ALI. This is, in part, because of the multiple biochemical effects known to have genetic counterparts: inflammatory responses, immune responses, cell proliferation, chemotaxis, and blood coagulation.

CLINICAL FEATURES

Clinical features in a patient with ALI/ARDS relate to the underlying condition (or of diseases predisposing to the risk condition such as in sepsis), the lung injury, and/or the other organ failures that may occur simultaneous with or subsequent to ALI. Manifestations of lung injury include symptoms of dyspnea and respiratory distress. Signs may include tachypnea, pink frothy edema fluid suctioned from the trachea, and evidence of increased work of breathing, including flaring of the nostrils, use of accessory muscles, and paradoxical breathing (abdomen and chest moving in opposite directions). Laboratory findings include severe hypoxemia that is largely refractory to oxygen therapy, evidence of lung stiffness (measurement of decreased respiratory system compliance), and imaging of bilateral alveolar filling and collapse with bilateral infiltrates compatible with pulmonary edema on frontal chest radiograph and diffuse alveolar filling and collapse on chest CT, especially in the dependent lung regions.

DIAGNOSIS

Unlike the situation with ischemic cardiac injury, there is no "troponin I" for ALI/ARDS. A definitive diagnosis would require lung biopsy showing diffuse alveolar damage (Figure 71-1). Because biopsy is impractical and inappropriate in most cases, the syndrome

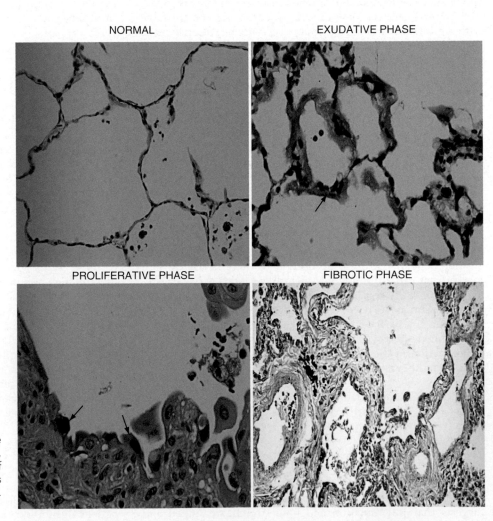

FIGURE 71-1 Lung biopsy showing acute diffuse alveolar damage. (From Penuelas O, Aramburu JA, Frutos-Vivar F: Pathology of acute lung injury and acute respiratory distress syndrome: a clinical-pathological correlation. Clin Chest Med 2006; 26:571–578.)

TABLE 71-1 American European Consensus Conference (AECC) Definition of ALI and ARDS

	Pao_2/Fio_2*	CXR	Pulmonary Artery Wedge Pressure (PAWP)
ALI	≤300 mmHg	Bilateral infiltrates seen on frontal chest radiograph	≤18 mmHg when measured or no clinical evidence of left atrial hypertension
ARDS	≤200 mmHg		

*Regardless of level of PEEP.

must be identified clinically, as standardized by the AECC (Table 71-1). Before development of the AECC definition, clinical care and research studies were being conducted by use of widely varying definitions, making it difficult to compare one trial to another or to track the disease process and outcomes over time. Despite the clear benefits of having an internationally accepted definition, a number of limitations remain (Table 71-2):

1. The oxygenation criterion does not take positive end-expiratory pressure (PEEP) into account. Patients could exceed the P/F ratio of 300 by being on high PEEP and lower F_IO_2 while still likely having lung injury. Although some centers try to extrapolate the P/F criteria to oxygen saturations, the AECC definition depends on an arterial blood gas (ABG) for P/F criterion. Finally, the P/F ratio is a less reliable measure of shunt fraction at lower inhaled oxygen fractions (F_IO_2) ranges.

2. The adequacy and accuracy of the film can be markedly affected by overlying equipment, low lung volumes, effusions, etc. (Figure 71-2). Interobserver variability in studies has resulted in ranges of 36–71% of radiographs with agreement on whether the chest X-ray (CXR) met criteria for ALI (although agreement can improve with intensive training). Finally, in the age of computed tomography (CT), how, if at all, should CT be incorporated in the definition? Some patients considered to have ARDS have diffuse airspace filling on CT, whereas others may only have lower lobe consolidation and atelectasis that appears as bilateral infiltrates on standard chest X-rays. Should patients with these two types of roentgenographic presentations be grouped together?

TABLE 71-2 Problems Affecting the Reliability of the AECC Definition for ALI

Variable	AECC Definition	Problems that Affect Reliability of the Variable
Chest radiograph	Bilateral infiltrates seen on frontal chest radiograph	Pleural effusions Low lung volumes Interobserver variability Disagreement with CT results
Hypoxemia	Pao_2/F_IO_2 ≤300, regardless of level of PEEP	No adjustment for PEEP or mean airway pressure Affected by frequency of ABG use, which ABG is chosen, and whether an ABG or oxygen saturation is available Pao_2/F_IO_2 ratio is unstable and does not reflect shunt fraction well at levels of F_IO_2 <0.5
Left atrial hypertension	PAWP ≤18 when measured or no clinical evidence of left atrial hypertension	Using a PAWP >18 excludes patients with a combination of ALI and cardiogenic edema Interobserver variability in reading PAWP PAWP may poorly reflect transmural pressures under certain conditions, for instance, high intrathoracic pressures caused by high PEEP

PAWP, Pulmonary artery wedge pressure; PEEP, positive end-expiratory pressure.

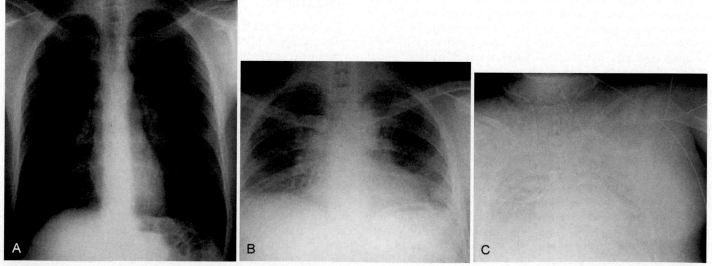

FIGURE 71-2 A, Overexposure and suggestion of chronic underlying disease (hyperinflation, small heart suggesting emphysema). **B,** Low lung volumes. **C,** Underexposed and affected by excessive soft tissue mass.

FIGURE 71-3 Chest radiograph suggests bilateral edema, but chest CT shows opacities because of effusions with normal parenchyma. CXR is consistent with ALI; CT is not.

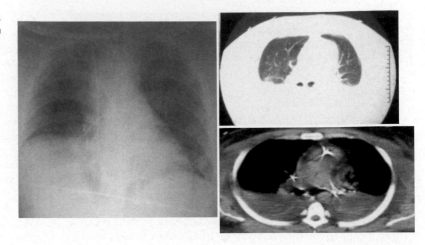

What should be done if the CXR and CT show discordant findings (Figure 71-3)?

3. Last, the criterion for "No evidence of left atrial hypertension (LAH)" is intended to exclude patients who have pulmonary edema as a result of cardiogenic (hydrostatic) problems and can arbitrarily exclude patients who have noncardiogenic edema. The pulmonary artery occlusion pressure (PAOP) may be artificially elevated because of thoracic pressures (e.g., PEEP, low chest wall compliance, or abdominal compartment syndrome). In one study, one third of patients with an initial PAOP >18 mmHg subsequently dropped their PAOP to <18 mmHg and still met criteria for ALI. In another, more than half of ALI patients had a PAOP >18 mmHg at some time during their course of lung disease. Added to this is the interobserver variability noted with PAOP readings (although this can be improved by incorporating the use of airway pressure tracings to identify the point in the respiratory cycle at which to read the PAOP).

In the absence of a pulmonary artery catheter, the onus is on the clinician (with no generally accepted protocol) to determine clinically whether there is any evidence of left atrial hypertension. Although different arbitrary criteria can result in different percentages of patients being labeled as having LAH, the recent ARDS Network study of pulmonary artery catheter versus central venous catheter use (i.e., the FACTT study) actually provided an opportunity to explore how well clinicians were identifying patients with heart failure or volume overload. Although nearly one third of patients who were thought clinically *not* to have LAH actually had an initial PAOP >18 mmHg, less than 3% of these patients had a high PAOP *and* a low cardiac index, thereby providing reassurance that clinicians' "gut instinct" of LAH is quite good.

The AECC definitions do not include the presence of a risk factor for ALI/ARDS. Up to 20% of patients with defined ALI do not have a previously identified risk factor, but the extent to which these patients have been evaluated for other conditions that might present as, or mimic, ALI/ARDS (see Box 71-2) has varied. Although clinical assessment and management can currently be on the basis of a more generalized definition of the syndrome, more rigorous definitions, hopefully that use biomarkers and/or genetic markers, can only help but improve the quality of research studies in the future.

Because a collagen vascular disease may present with an acute pneumonitis in which the lung is the only apparent organ involvement, a careful search for systemic involvement is indicated, including examining the urine for red cells, red cell casts, and protein and screening serologic testing. Bronchoalveolar lavage (BAL) should be performed in these patients seeking evidence of selected infectious agents (e.g., tuberculosis, Hanta virus), red blood cells suggesting the possibility of capillaritis or other conditions associated with alveolar hemorrhage, and for eosinophils or lymphocytes. In early ALI/ARDS associated with the risk conditions noted previously, BAL neutrophilia is present. With resolution and over time, alveolar macrophages predominate. BAL eosinophilia establishes the diagnosis of acute eosinophilic pneumonia (peripheral eosinophilia is usually absent). BAL lymphocytosis without an elevation of neutrophils suggests acute hypersensitivity pneumonitis or acute BOOP (although neutrophilia may also occur in acute interstitial pneumonia and acute BOOP). If the BAL results are nonspecific or inconclusive, and if no underlying disease or risk factor has been identified, surgical biopsy should be considered, with the risk/benefit of this procedure carefully weighed. A definitive diagnosis is particularly important when diseases requiring high-dose corticosteroids and possibly other immunosuppressive agents are in the differential diagnosis. Lung biopsy with immunofluorescent staining may be particularly indicated when diffuse alveolar hemorrhage is present.

TREATMENT

Treatment of ALI/ARDS includes: (1) treating the underlying risk condition; (2) treating the lung injury; and (3) supportive treatment of the critically ill patient. Treatment of many of the underlying disease processes is largely supportive. The obvious exception is sepsis, where treatment with antibiotics and treatment of the source of the infection, including possible drainage of abscesses, is critical.

Treatment of ALI starts with making the diagnosis. The large community and population-based epidemiologic study in which screening for ALI was not dependent on physicians found that nearly half of patients meeting criteria for ALI did not show evidence on chart review that the attending physician was aware of the diagnosis. One solution would be to allow therapists or nurses to screen for the blood gas criterion and, if that was met, to either screen the last chest roentgenograph or the radiologist's report for the presence of bilateral infiltrates that would be compatible with pulmonary edema and if so, alerting the physician that ALI criteria might be present, or prompting the physician to review the chest X-ray and consider whether left atrial hypertension might be present and whether other diagnostic considerations should be entertained. This strategy was part of a multipronged intervention that resulted in increased use of lung-protective ventilation in patients with ALI.

Lung-Protective Ventilation

Lung-protective ventilation has become the most important element in the management of patients with ALI after control of the underlying cause. In the first two decades of ARDS management, relatively large tidal volumes (i.e., 12–15 mL/kg body weight) were generally used to improve oxygenation and counteract the known diffuse microatelectasis that is part of the pathophysiology. Over time, studies in a variety of animal models suggested that high ventilating volumes could injure normal lung and could propagate injury in already injured lungs, but because many of these experiments used tidal volumes or pressures that exceeded those used clinically, the relevance of ventilator-induced lung injury (VILI) to patients with ALI was unclear. Luciano Gattinoni called attention to the fact that much of the lung was consolidated on chest CT scans of patients with ARDS, and only part of this consolidated (either fluid filled or atelectatic) lung was recruitable by use of high volumes or pressures. He reasoned that the tidal volume was being delivered to only a fraction of the alveolar volume of the normal lung (i.e., the "baby lung"), thereby increasing the possibility that overdistension of some lung regions could occur with resulting injury. Other investigators demonstrated that patients with ARDS receiving tidal volumes as low as 7 mL/kg body weight showed evidence of possible overdistention from pressure-volume (P-V) curves of the respiratory system (i.e., tidal volumes exceeding the upper inflection point of the P-V curve; see Figures 71-4 and 71-5). An uncontrolled series of patients with ARDS from New Zealand treated with limited tidal volume (i.e., "permissive hypercapnia") showed a lower mortality than an historical comparison group and sparked new interest in attempts to avoid VILI.

Although a number of relatively small studies of various lung protective strategies in patients with, or at risk for, ALI gave mixed results, the landmark study of the ARDS Clinical Trials Network (ARDSnet) provided evidence that a lung-

protective ventilatory strategy could save lives. In this prospective, randomized, controlled trial, all patients were ventilated by use of a volume-regulated mode of mechanical ventilation, and the level of PEEP and the F_{IO_2} were adjusted with a predetermined PEEP/F_{IO_2} "ladder" on the basis of keeping the PaO_2 or the SpO_2 in a desired range (Figure 71-6). Patients were randomly assigned to receive a tidal volume (V_T) of either 6 mL/kg predicted body weight (PBW; on the basis of a formula that uses the patient's height and gender; see Box 71-3) or 12 mL/kg PBW. If the plateau pressure (P_{plat}, i.e., the airway pressure under no flow condition required to maintain the delivered V_T) exceeded 30 cm H_2O in the patients receiving 6 mL/kg PBW, V_T was lowered to 5 mL/kg PBW. If the P_{plat} still exceeded 30, V_T was furthered lowered to a minimum value of 4 mL/kg PBW. Patients receiving the higher V_T (12 mL/kg PBW) had significantly better oxygenation for the first 4 days but those in the lower V_T group had a lower mortality (40 vs 31%, a relative reduction in mortality of 22%; $P = 0.007$).

Previous studies indicated that only approximately 15% of deaths in patients with ARDS were a result of respiratory failure (i.e., unsupportable hypoxemia or respiratory academia) and that most died of multiple organ failure. A small trial of a lung-protective strategy in patients with ARDS found that BAL and blood neutrophils and inflammatory cytokines were lower in patients treated with lung-protective ventilation after 3 days compared with those treated with what was considered to be the conventional ventilatory strategy at the time. These findings are compatible with the hypotheses that VILI may result in production of inflammatory mediators in the lung that then enter the systemic circulation and cause distal organ injury, and that a lung protective ventilatory strategy can ameliorate this risk. The ARDSnet study found lower levels of plasma IL-6 and IL-8 in the group ventilated with lower V_T.

We recommend use of the ARDSnet lung-protective ventilation (LPV) protocol in patients with ALI/ARDS, while recognizing that alternative therapies have credible and reasonable proponents and that some controversy still exists (see later). We base this recommendation on the observation that the ARDSnet LPV study is the only multicenter RCT demonstrating a survival benefit in patients with ALI and that the criticisms offered by others have largely been dealt with. Although further refinements in ventilatory strategies will undoubtedly occur, particularly with respect to treating individual patients, the ARDSnet LPV protocol is supported by the best evidence that a particular ventilatory strategy can save lives.

A recent Canadian Critical Care Trials Group study of 1000 patients, the Lung Open Ventilation Study (LOVS), compared the ARDSnet protocol to a regimen that used pressure control ventilation, recruitment maneuvers, and levels of PEEP that were approximately 5–7 cm H_2O higher for any given F_{IO_2} than what was used in the ARDSnet trial. Although survival was marginally better in the intervention arm, this was not statistically significant ($P = .3$). One interpretation of these results is the major lung-protective effect is gained by limiting V_T and P_{plat} and that pressure control ventilation, higher PEEP, and recruitment maneuvers have little or no additional effect. On the other hand, they had no clear adverse effect suggesting that some aspects of the ventilatory strategy for patients with ARDS/ALI can be left to the choice of the clinician.

Knowledge transfer (i.e., the process of translating evidence-based information on patient care into actual practice) is a relatively new area of research focus in academic and health care institutions. The process is often slow in all areas of medicine

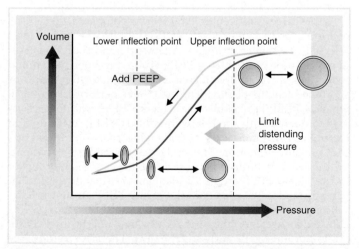

FIGURE 71-4 Pressure-volume curve of the respiratory system in patients with ALI. LIP, Lower inflection point; UIP, upper inflection point. The upper (*yellow*) curve reflects the hysteresis occurring after the lungs are fully inflated.

FIGURE 71-5 Percent of patients with ARDS with plateau pressure (P_{plat}) exceeding the upper inflection point (UIP) of the pressure volume curve (see Figure 71-4) by tidal volume. (Adapted from Roupie E, et al: Am J Respir Crit Care Med 1995; 152:121–128.)

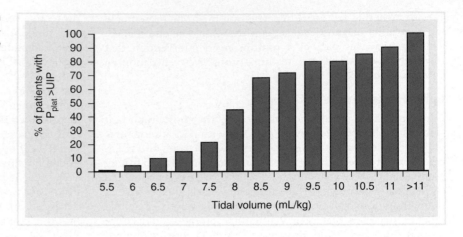

FIGURE 71-6 NIH ARDS Clinical Trials Network (ARDSnet) Fio_2/PEEP "ladder." Fio_2 and PEEP are set at one of the fixed combinations above to meet the arterial oxygenation goals. If the oxygenation falls below the goals, then the Fio_2/PEEP combination selected moves to the right. If oxygenation is above the target goals, then a combination to the left is selected.

Fio_2	.3	.4	.4	.5	.5	.6	.7	.7	.7	.8	.9	.9	.9	1.0
PEEP	5	5	8	8	10	10	10	12	14	14	14	16	18	18–24

Target arterial oxygenation: Spo_2 = 88–95%
Pao_2 = 55–80 mm Hg

BOX 71-3   Formula for Calculating Predicted Body Weight (Used for Tidal Volume Selection in the ARDSnet Study)

Male: 50 + 0.91 (cm of height − 152.4)
Female: 45.4 + 0.91 (cm of height − 152.4)

---

and might be especially so in critical care, where any evidence base demonstrating patient-centered benefits is very recent. Education alone is not sufficient to effect substantial change in practice. One study has demonstrated that a multifaceted strategy, including education of physicians, nurses, and respiratory therapists, screening and prompting by nurses and therapists, and use of a protocol with physician oversight and the ability to override protocol-driven instructions, can improve compliance with LPV in patients with ALI.

Positive End-Expiratory Pressure (PEEP)

Striking improvement in oxygenation in ARDS was first demonstrated in 1967 in the article describing and naming the syndrome. Despite considerable research, the optimal level of PEEP for any given patient is not certain. Animal model studies of VILI demonstrated partial protection of the resulting lung injury when PEEP was applied, even if high distending volumes and pressures were maintained. This observation, and other supporting evidence, led to the hypothesis that VILI resulted in part from repetitive opening and closing of small airways or alveoli with each breath. As a corollary to this hypothesis, the notion developed that maintaining the PEEP at a level that would prevent cyclic airspace opening and closing would diminish the risk of VILI. One strategy to accomplish this involves describing the P-V curve for an individual patient and then using a level of PEEP that is approximately 2 cm H_2O above the lower inflection point (LIP) of the P-V curve (see Figure 71-4), the point taken to represent the opening point of most of the alveoli.

Several problems prevented this strategy from gaining widespread acceptance including: (1) an LIP is not identifiable on all P-V curves in patients with ALI/ARDS; (2) when an LIP is present, variability exists among observers with regard to the actual PEEP level (because it represents a change in slope rather than an actual point); (3) constructing the P-V curve is somewhat difficult requiring a trained technician (although newer generation ventilators now have more ability to generate a P-V curve); and (4) the P-V curve reflects the overall behavior of the respiratory system and does not reflect regional differences; thus, when some areas of previously collapsed lung are opening, other areas are already overdistended. For example, it has been demonstrated that opening of alveolar units continues well above the LIP of the P-V curve.

Three large multicenter RCTs have compared the effects of lower versus higher levels of PEEP, with the higher level selected by different strategies. All have demonstrated increases in oxygenation in the higher PEEP group, but none have found reductions in mortality, increases in ventilator-free days, or shortened lengths of stay. The ARDSnet performed a trial in which a PEEP/Fio_2 ladder with higher PEEP and lower $F_{I}O_2$ was compared with the relatively modest PEEP levels used in the original ARDSnet LPV trial studying tidal volume and plateau pressure limitation. The study was stopped at 549 patients on the basis of futility, because mortality was slightly higher in the higher PEEP group. Subsequent analysis disclosed that patients randomly assigned to the higher PEEP group were significantly older than those in the lower PEEP group; when adjusted for age, mortality was slightly higher in the lower PEEP group but not significantly so ($P = .47$). The LOVS study (see earlier) had similar mean differences in PEEP between the two study groups ($\sim$5–7 cm H_2O, depending on the study day) to those seen in the ARDSnet trial. Mortality was slightly lower in the higher PEEP group but again not significantly so.

The EXPRESS study conducted in France used a different strategy to individualize PEEP, resulting in considerably higher PEEP in one arm with similar results to the other trials.

Several possibilities exist for interpreting these results including (1) the modest PEEP levels used in the original ARDSnet PEEP/$F_{I}O_2$ ladder are adequate in most patients to prevent VILI, (2) higher PEEP levels may open more collapsed lung units (as suggested by the higher $PaO_2/F_{I}O_2$ ratio), but this benefit may be counteracted by more overdistention of other areas of lung; (3) most of the lung protection may already have been gained by limiting V_T and P_{plat}. Data have been published suggesting that determining the degree of lung recruitability (i.e., the capacity for previously closed alveoli to be opened with high distending pressures; see Figure 71-7) might predict which patients would benefit from higher PEEP. In patients with relatively low recruitability, higher PEEP might only result in overdistention and reduction in cardiac output. Including such patients in a randomized trial with one arm receiving higher PEEP might negate the possibility of recognizing a survival benefit in those patients with a high degree of recruitable lung. This hypothesis has not yet been tested in a clinical trial as of this writing. Until further data are available, use of the ARDSnet PEEP/$F_{I}O_2$ ladder seems reasonable, but other acceptable options include use of any of the higher PEEP strategies from the preceding three trials or a strategy of individualizing PEEP. What seems apparent from animal model work is that some degree of PEEP is important in VILI prevention.

Alternate Ventilatory Modes

Alternate modes of ventilation include pressure control ventilation (PCV), high-frequency oscillating ventilation (HFOV), and airway pressure–release ventilation (APRV). No convincing data have been generated showing that PCV is superior to AMV, although it is a reasonable alternate approach.

HFOV has theoretical reasons suggesting that it may be the best way to deliver LPV, because the tidal volumes used are so small (i.e., considerably less than the dead space). These small volumes delivered at high frequency facilitate gas diffusion but must be used at some baseline distending volume and pressure. Accordingly, the mean airway pressure may be higher, lower, or the same as "conventional" LPV, and this may determine whether HFOV has any survival benefit or morbidity reduction compared with ARDSnet LPV. A multicenter randomized controlled trial studying HFOV organized by the Canadian Critical Care Trials Group is ongoing.

APRV is continuous positive airway pressure (CPAP) with an intermittent pressure release phase. It is a pressure-limited, time-cycled ventilatory mode with the principal potential advantage being that it allows spontaneous ventilation (at the relatively high distending pressure or CPAP) throughout the ventilatory cycle. The possible disadvantage of this approach is that the spontaneous breath increases inhaled volume, raising the possibility that the pressure limits set by the CPAP level may be misleading and that overdistention can occur during the spontaneous breaths. No large trials comparing APRV to conventional ventilation and none to ARDSnet LPV have been performed.

Noninvasive Ventilation

No randomized trials of noninvasive ventilation (NIV) limited to patients with ALI/ARDS have been reported. An earlier randomized trial with CPAP delivered by a face mask found that CPAP, despite early physiologic improvement, did not reduce the need for intubation or improve outcomes in patients with ALI. A recent multicenter observational survey of experience with NIV in patients with early ARDS reported experience in approximately one third of patients with ARDS admitted to three ICUs in Italy and Spain (the remaining two thirds were already intubated). Approximately half of the patients treated with NIV did not require intubation, and these patients had less ventilator-associated pneumonia and a lower mortality. This series suggests that NIV for patients with ALI/ARDS is feasible, and it may have some advantages, but, because this was not an RCT, no definitive conclusions can be reached. Accordingly, NIV may be considered for patients with ALI of lesser severity, but no consensus currently exists regarding its indications and efficacy.

Prone Ventilation

Ventilation of patients with ARDS in the prone compared with the supine position improves oxygenation in two thirds to three fourths of patients. The key question is whether it improves patient-centered outcomes. Proning results in physiologic changes that have the potential to protect against VILI, raising the possibility that it might improve outcome independent of (or in addition to) the improvement in oxygenation. Acute lung injury greatly exaggerates the normal pleural pressure gradient from the top to the bottom of the lung, potentially predisposing to overdistention of alveoli in the nondependent aspect of the lung and collapse of alveoli in the dependent area. The pleural pressure gradient with lung injury is greatly reduced with a change from the supine to the prone position, providing a rationale by which proning may be lung protective (Figure 71-8).

A large multicenter RCT from Italy compared patients with ARDS nursed in the supine position with patients turned prone for 6 h/day. Oxygenation was improved while prone, and this effect was noted on each of the 10 days of observation. No survival benefit was seen. Post hoc subgroup analysis suggested that the sickest patients might have had improved survival. Because the experience from other post hoc subgroup analyses in intervention studies of critically ill patients has not been confirmed on subsequent prospective testing, this finding requires such confirmation before it can be accepted. The major criticisms of this study were the limited period of proning per day and the fact that patients were enrolled rather late in the course of their ARDS. The study did demonstrate that use of the prone position in patients with ARDS is both feasible and safe. A smaller study from Spain that attempted to maintain the prone position for 18 h/day was stopped at 140 patients because enrollment was difficult as a result of competing studies resulting in the study being underpowered for the primary end point of mortality. Analysis revealed a trend toward improved survival in the prone group compared with the supine group (25% improvement, $P = .1$). These results, although inconclusive, were encouraging and supported further study. Because both of these studies were designed before the ARDSnet LPV trial results were known, a specified LPV strategy was not part of the study design. A repeat multicenter study is underway in Italy in which the prone position is maintained for most of the day in the intervention arm and ARDSnet LPV is mandated in all patients.

Our current use of the prone position is limited to patients with severe oxygenation abnormality. We recommend considering proning if an $F_{I}O_2$ of 0.7–0.8 or greater is required to achieve adequate arterial oxygenation, particularly if the

FIGURE 71-7 Chest CT scans in patients with ARDS showing degree of recruitability. (Adapted from Gattinoni L, Caironi P, Cressoni M, et al: Lung recruitment in patients with the acute respiratory distress syndrome. N Engl J Med 2006; 354:1775–1786.)

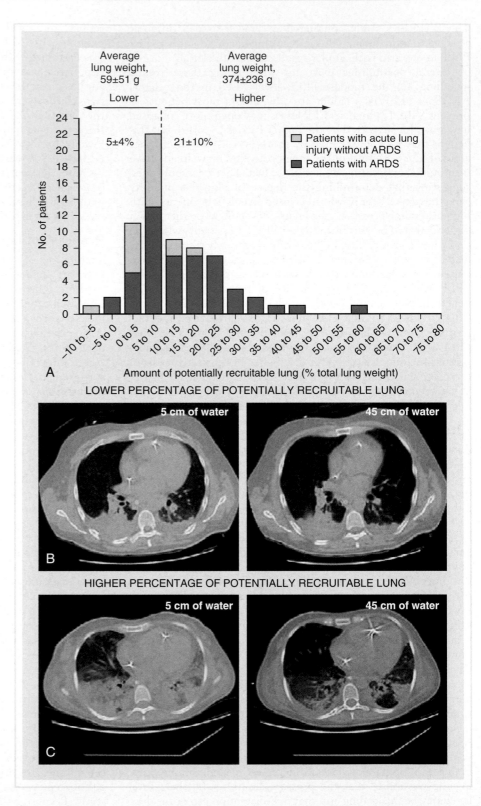

patient has adverse effects from high levels of PEEP being used to maintain adequate oxygenation. The patient should be maintained prone nearly all of each day, turning them supine only when nursing care activities or procedures are required. Proning should be continued until the patient's status is clearly improving and there is no longer a substantial oxygenation advantage of the prone compared with the supine position. It is important to recognize that this approach is not yet based on any firm evidence and that outcome benefit may not be predicted by improvement in oxygenation. We generally use a special bed designed for proning, but this is not required. We have found that initial nursing resistance to proning is minimal with greater experience with the technique.

Inhaled Nitric Oxide (NO)

The administration of small amounts of inhaled NO (iNO) improves oxygenation in many patients with ARDS. iNO is a potent vasodilator, as well as a bronchodilator. Administration

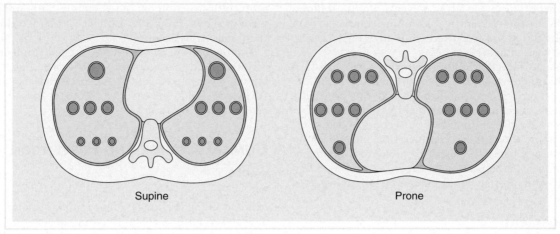

Supine   Prone

FIGURE 71-8 Drawing of the lungs illustrating the effect of position on alveolar size. The pleural pressure gradient from the nondependent to the dependent parts of the lung is considerably greater in the supine than the prone position. Because of this, there is a tendency in the supine position for alveolar units to be larger (and more susceptible to overdistention) at the top of the lung and smaller (and more susceptible to compression) at the bottom of the lung. This is ameliorated to some degree in the prone position (exaggerated in the figure). This is the basis of the hypothesis that the prone position may help prevent against ventilator-induced lung injury.

by the inhaled route dilates vessels supplying areas that are being ventilated, leading to improvement in ventilation/perfusion matching. iNO has no other recognized effects on the pathophysiology of ARDS (e.g., protection against VILI or antiinflammatory effect). Most studies have demonstrated a modest improvement in oxygenation that is lost after 1 or 2 days (although individual patients may continue to show improved oxygenation for weeks), but none have demonstrated any benefits of iNO on outcomes. We generally relegate inhaled NO use to those patients with extreme oxygenation abnormalities (e.g., when arterial oxygenation is inadequate or borderline on an F_{IO_2} of 1.0). Our practice is to use prone ventilation, when feasible, before considering iNO. Others prefer a trial of HFOV or nebulized prostacyclin before iNO is used.

Surfactant

The quality and quantity of surfactant are abnormal in patients with ALI/ARDS. Surfactant administration produced promising results in animal models of lung injury, but studies in humans have been disappointing, with no outcome benefits found to date. The optimal composition of glycoprotein and method of delivery (i.e., direct intratracheal administration, nebulization, and lung lavage) have been difficult to determine. Surfactant administration is not currently recommended for patients with ALI.

Partial or Full Liquid Ventilation

Perflubron is a dense liquid with oxygen-carrying capacity. Oxygenation can be maintained in animals with normal or injured lungs when their lungs are partially or nearly fully filled with perflubron and then ventilated mechanically. Studies showing antiinflammatory properties and demonstrating feasibility in patients with lung injury raised hopes for this therapy, but a randomized controlled trial showed higher mortality in the treatment arm, resulting in abandonment of active investigation in ALI. Interest remains in the use of perflubron as a delivery vehicle for gene therapy in the lungs.

Corticosteroids

The use of corticosteroids to treat ALI/ARDS has been controversial since the syndrome was first described. The inflammatory

nature of the lung injury provides a strong rationale for antiinflammatory therapy. Data have also been generated showing a reduction in proinflammatory cytokines in BAL and blood compared with controls when corticosteroids are administered. The first report of corticosteroid use in ARDS was in the article that first described the syndrome. Early studies tested high doses given early in the course of the disease for 1 or 2 days and found no demonstrable benefit and, in some instances, more infections and a higher mortality. Accordingly, the practice of giving steroids in this fashion was largely abandoned. A new approach emerged when several uncontrolled series reported use of a prolonged course of a moderate dose (usually as methylprednisolone intravenously 500 mg/day or greater in divided doses for approximately 2 weeks or until extubation, followed by a gradual tapering) in patients with severe, persistent disease that was usually of 1–2 weeks duration. Overall survival was higher than expected compared with a pooled survival from all series of 76%. A subsequent small trial of 24 patients who were randomly assigned 2:1 to receive methylprednisolone or placebo found a greater reduction in Lung Injury Score in those receiving steroids. Intention-to-treat analysis showed a significant decrease in mortality for steroid-treated patients compared with placebo; four placebo patients, however, were crossed over to the steroid arm within the time window of study eligibility. When analyzed by treatment actually received, the survival benefit was no longer significant. Criticisms of the study have included the small size for a mortality end point, the 2:1 randomization scheme, the unusual study design regarding time of analyses (a sequential trial with nonconstant inspection intervals on the basis of the number of deaths observed, i.e., after three and five deaths), and the crossover design complicating the survival analysis.

The ARDSnet performed a randomized controlled trial in patients with ARDS of at least 1-week duration by use of a similar dose of methylprednisolone as noted previously but with a shorter tapering interval. Oxygenation and lung compliance improved more, and ventilator-free days and ICU-free days were greater in the steroid-treated group, but more patients had to be returned to mechanical ventilation, and 60-day mortality was no different between the two arms (29.2% vs 28.6% for steroids vs placebo). Concern about possible toxicity was raised by nine reported severe adverse events of critical illness neuromyopathy in the steroid-treated group compared with none in the placebo group (reported while investigators were blinded to study assignment).

The physiologic and clinical improvements seen with steroids suggest that there might be a role for their use in ARDS, but the lack of proven survival benefit and the possibility of complications including neuromyopathy indicate further research is necessary before they can be recommended. Current research approaches under consideration include better selection of patients likely to benefit from steroid treatment, use of lower doses, perhaps a longer taper, and more extensive prospective monitoring for development of unexpected adverse effects.

Fluid Management

Appropriate fluid management is another longstanding controversy in the management of patients with ARDS. The rationale for conservative fluid management is that in the injured lungs, any excessive fluid leak will cause more pulmonary edema, potentially worsening outcomes. Advocates of liberal fluid management suggest that the amount of lung water is not closely associated with outcomes and that limiting fluid administration increases the risk of renal failure, which, in combination with respiratory failure, *is* associated with worse survival. In essence, the argument has been whether you attempt to protect the lungs at risk of the kidneys failing or protect the kidneys and accept worse pulmonary function and status. Until recently, the evidence supporting either stance has been flawed. Accordingly, the ARDSnet undertook a study to determine outcomes when patients are managed by use of a conservative versus a liberal fluid strategy. The study design used a 2×2 factorial design to also evaluate whether a pulmonary artery catheter (PAC) used to assist with fluid management offered any risks or benefits over central venous catheters (CVC). Vascular filling pressures (determined by CVC or PAC) were assessed every 4 h along with circulation status (i.e., measuring cardiac index in those with PACs or capillary refill time of the fingers, urinary output, and blood pressure in those with CVCs). The targets of therapy were a CVP or pulmonary arterial occlusion pressure <4 or <8 mmHg, respectively, in the conservative fluid group, or 10–14 or 14–18 mmHg, respectively, in the liberal fluid group. If the patient entered a state of shock, instructions were superseded by the patient's clinician.

No difference in 60-day mortality was observed in the patients managed with PACs versus CVCs (27.4% vs 26.3%, respectively, $P = .69$). The fluid-liberal group had a mean positive cumulative fluid balance of ~7 L over 7 days, almost identical to what had previously been observed in other ARDSnet trials in which fluid management was not protocolized. Patients in the conservative fluid strategy group did have more ventilator-free days (14.6 vs 12.1 days, $P < .001$) and more ICU-free days (13.4 vs 11.2 days, $P < .001$), but no mortality difference was observed (28.4% in the fluid liberal group vs 25.5% in the fluid conservative group, $P = .30$). Although the conservative strategy was associated with a slightly higher blood urea nitrogen level, the creatinine level, the number of days without renal failure, the need for dialysis, and the incidence and prevalence of shock were similar in the two groups.

It is important to note that these results do not relate to initial fluid resuscitation or fluid management of patients in shock. The time from admission to the ICU until the first fluid protocol instruction exceeded 40 h in both groups. If patients were in shock, fluid management was left to the judgment of the treating physician.

On the basis of these results, it seems prudent to use a conservative fluid management strategy once initial fluid resuscitation is completed and if the patient is not in shock. The ARDSnet fluid conservative protocol has been simplified and is shown in Table 71-3.

CLINICAL COURSE AND PREVENTION

Acute

The acute presentation of ALI is the result of inflammatory exudate filling the lungs. Hypoxemia (because of shunt from atelectasis and/or alveolar flooding) occurs early, along with a reduction in compliance (because of alveolar filling and the effects on surfactant). Patients also have ineffective hypoxic pulmonary vasoconstriction. The abnormal gas change causes dyspnea, tachypnea, and the need for endotracheal intubation.

The characteristics change when patients have persistent lung injury lasting more than 3–7 days. The initial exudative phase transitions to a fibroproliferative phase in which hyaline membranes development is followed by collagen, deposition, and fibrosis. This process is manifested by worsening compliance and increasing dead space (ineffective ventilation), both of which can persist even if oxygenation is improving. This destruction can extend into the delicate pulmonary capillaries leading to microthrombi that, in combination with the fibrosis of the alveoli, can cause mild to moderate pulmonary hypertension and even right heart dysfunction or failure.

Mortality

The mortality in patients with ALI and ARDS remains high, but it seems to have improved over the past two decades, even before any specific interventions were implemented as a result of randomized controlled trials. Single-center registries allow historical comparisons, adjusted for age, risk factor, and severity of illness. In one center in the United States, mortality decreased from the 60–70% range in the early to mid-1980s to approximately 40% in the mid-1990s, results that were subsequently confirmed in additional studies. Although the cause(s) of this improvement is not known, one possible factor is maturation of the relatively young field of critical care medicine with the culmination of many small advances in the processes of care. The community population-based study described previously (see "Incidence") found an overall mortality of 38.5% in all patients with ALI in all 17 hospitals in a US county over a full year of observation.

After the term ALI was coined and defined by the AECC, initial reports comparing mortality in patients with ALI without ARDS (PaO_2/F_IO_2 of 200–300) with those with ARDS (PaO_2/F_IO_2 <200) failed to find a substantial difference. Subsequent studies have found a modestly higher mortality in those with ARDS; however, it seems that the PaO_2/F_IO_2 at onset of ALI/ARDS does not have a major effect on mortality until it is quite low (e.g., <100). Several recent trials have reported significant improvements in oxygenation that were not associated with reductions in mortality.

Factors associated with increased risk of death in patients with ALI/ARDS include: increasing age; underlying risk condition (medical patients with a greater risk than trauma patients,

TABLE 71-3 ARDSnet Conservative Fluid Management Algorithm

This fluid protocol captures the primary positive outcome of the FACTT trial on increasing ventilator-free days. This protocol should be initiated after initial fluid resuscitation has been achieved and the patient does not meet criteria for shock. In the study the protocol was continued until UAB or study day 7, whichever occurred first.

1. Discontinue maintenance fluids.
2. Continue medications and nutrition.
3. Manage electrolytes and blood products per usual practice.
4. For shock, use any combination of fluid boluses* and vasopressor(s) to achieve MAP ≥60 mmHg as fast as possible. Wean vasopressors as quickly as tolerated beginning 4 h after blood pressure has stabilized.

		MAP ≥60 mmHg AND Off Vasopressors for ≥12 h	
CVP (Recommended)	PAOP (Optional)	Average Urine Output <0.5 ml/kg/h	Average Urine Output ≥0.5 ml/kg/h
> 8	>12	Furosemide‡ Reassess in 1 h	Furosemide‡ Reassess in 4 h
4–8	8–12	Give fluid bolus as fast as possible* Reassess in 1 h	Furosemide‡ Reassess in 4 h
< 4	< 8	Give fluid bolus as fast as possible* Reassess in 1 h	No intervention Reassess in 4 h

*Recommended fluid bolus = 15 mL/kg crystalloid (round to nearest 250 mL) or 1 Unit packed red cells or 25 g albumin.
†Recommended Furosemide dosing = begin with 20 mg bolus or 3 mg/h infusion or last known effective dose. Double each subsequent dose until goal achieved (oliguria reversal or intravascular pressure target) or maximum infusion rate of 24 mg/h or 160 mg bolus reached. Do not exceed 620 mg/day. Also, if patient has heart failure, consider treatment with dobutamine.
‡Renal failure: Dialysis dependence, OR oliguria with serum creatinine >3 mEq/dL, OR serum oliguria with creatinine 0–3 mEq/dL with urinary indices indicative of acute renal failure.
FACTT = The NHLBI Acute Respiratory Distress Syndrome Clinical Trials Network. Comparison of two fluid-management strategies in acute lung injury. N Engl J Med 2006; 354:2564–2575.

those with sepsis having a greater risk than those with other contributing conditions); number of organs failing (particularly liver failure or chronic liver disease); an increased number of comorbid conditions; increased severity of illness as measured by scoring systems such as SAPS II or the acute physiologic score (APS) portion of the APACHE score; and having a direct (i.e., a pulmonary) cause of ALI/ARDS compared with an indirect (i.e., a nonpulmonary) cause. The mortality rate from ARDS is higher for men, African-Americans, and especially African-American men.

Long-Term Outcomes

Survival in patients who have survived an episode of ALI/ARDS and have been discharged from the hospital depends on the underlying risk condition and predisposing comorbidities. In a cohort of survivors of ARDS with either trauma or

sepsis as their risk condition who were matched for hospital survivors of trauma and sepsis of similar severity but without ARDS, survival after hospital discharge was not influenced by whether or not ARDS was present (see Figure 71-9). Subsequent fatalities in the trauma cohort were rare, whereas sepsis survivors had considerable subsequent mortality (30–40% over the next three and a half years), similar to other series of patients surviving an episode of sepsis, but not different between those with ARDS compared with those without.

Long-term sequelae in survivors of ARDS have received increasing attention over the past decade, as mortality rates have improved. Recent studies indicate that survivors of ARDS can have considerable morbidity in several realms or domains. The first indication of this came from studies of health-related quality of life (HRQL), which found decrements in ARDS survivors compared with both population

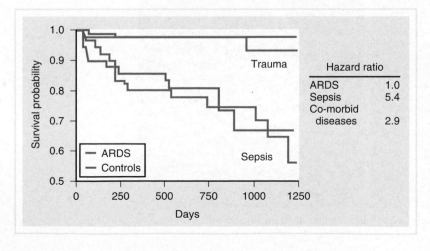

FIGURE 71-9 Effect of an episode of ARDS on subsequent long-term survival. Survivors to hospital discharge of an ARDS episode with trauma or sepsis as their risk condition for development of ARDS are compared with patients with trauma and sepsis matched for severity of illness or injury (by Injury Severity Score for trauma and APACHE II for sepsis) but without development of ARDS. The episode of ARDS has no effect on survival compared with the controls. Patients with sepsis have continuing mortality after hospital discharge compared with trauma patients. (Adapted from Davidson TA, et al: Am J Respir Crit Care Med 1999; 160:1838.)

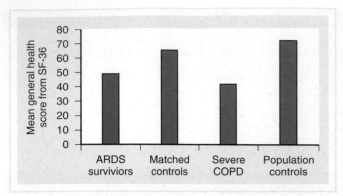

FIGURE 71-10 Health-related quality of life (HRQL) as determined by the SF-36 questionnaire in ARDS survivors with sepsis or trauma as their risk condition for ARDS development, compared with **(A)** matched controls with sepsis or trauma but without ARDS, **(B)** patients with severe COPD, and **(C)** normal subjects (population controls). (Adapted from Davidson TA, et al: JAMA 1999; 281:354.)

controls and with survivors of sepsis and trauma who had similar severities of illness or injury at ICU admission but who did not have ARDS develop (see Figure 71-10). Studies in survivors of ARDS show remarkably similar degrees of decrease in quality of life, even with different clinical settings. Initially, it was assumed that this decrement in HRQL was related to continuing pulmonary abnormalities, but studies of serial pulmonary function found that although an occasional patient had moderate to severe pulmonary dysfunction, most had normal or near normal function, with only mild abnormalities in diffusing capacity. Subsequent studies began to report other types of abnormalities in this patient population with psychological, neurocognitive, and especially neuromuscular abnormalities prevailing.

Neurocognitive abnormalities (i.e., defects of memory, concentration, or attention) are consistently found in most survivors at 1 year and can be very disconcerting to the patients, but these are generally mild in severity and improve to some degree over time. Psychologic abnormalities in ARDS survivors include depression, anxiety, and posttraumatic stress disorder (PTSD). A correlation was reported between recollection of adverse events from the ICU stay and PTSD. Another study has found that patients with "real" memories from the ICU stay had lower levels of PTSD compared with those with "delusional" memories. The first report of PTSD in ARDS survivors presented information on the level of sedation during their ICU stay; all patients with subsequent PTSD were deeply sedated until the time of extubation. These same investigators later reported a retrospective analysis suggesting that patients treated with corticosteroids tended to have a lower rate of PTSD.

A landmark study from the University of Toronto followed patients surviving ARDS for 1 year. All subjects reported poor function and attributed this to loss of muscle bulk, proximal weakness, and fatigue (Figure 71-11). A decrease in 6-min walk distance was consistent with the clinical reports of muscle dysfunction and fatigue. The authors speculated that the cause of the muscle wasting and weakness was likely multifactorial, with the exact contributing factors remaining to be explained, but with possible factors including corticosteroid-induced myopathy and critical illness myopathy. Whether the findings are specific for patients with ARDS or represent residua from any severe critical illness remains unclear. Quality of life testing in survivors in this study showed abnormalities, especially in the physical role and physical functioning domains, similar to reports from other studies, with improvement in these areas over the year of follow-up. It seems likely that the abnormal muscle findings are a major contributor to the impaired HRQL. Approximately half of the patients in this cohort had not returned to work after 1 year from hospital discharge.

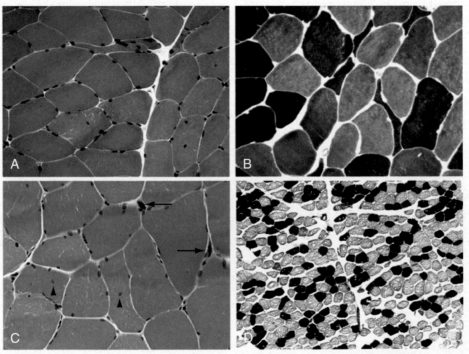

FIGURE 71-11 Muscle biopsy 18 months after ARDS showing type II muscle fiber atrophy and myofibrillary disarray. (Courtesy of Margaret Herridge, MD, MSc, MPH.)

Prevention

Many investigators studying ALI/ARDS believe the syndrome is the result of a "two-hit" phenomenon in which an initial insult such as trauma or a biologic predisposition combines with a second injury such as overstretching with mechanical ventilation resulting in the condition. Accordingly, attempts at prevention can follow a variety of approaches. Trauma is a major risk factor for ALI/ARDS, and public health programs aimed at reducing the risk of trauma (e.g., requiring seatbelts and helmets, bicycle safety programs, fall prevention programs) can have a significant effect. Expanding access to preventative medicine (e.g., influenza and pneumococcal vaccine programs) can play a role. Once hospitalized, efforts should be targeted at avoiding additional risk factors: Aspiration can be reduced by keeping the head of the bed elevated >30 degrees; ventilator-associated pneumonia can be reduced by use of LPV, and catheter-related infections can be reduced by use of full-barrier precautions at the time of insertion.

For those patients who do have ALI/ARDS develop, outcomes might be improved by triaging them to centers caring for a large volume of these types of patients, similar to what is done for victims of trauma or burns. Recent data suggest that better ICU outcomes are related to the volume of patients treated in the ICU, a finding remarkably similar to that previously reported for a number of surgical procedures.

PITFALLS AND CONTROVERSIES

Lung Protective Ventilation

The appropriate form and use of LPV remains controversial years after the ARDSnet study on limiting tidal volume and pressure showed survival benefit. Some of the controversy emanates from criticism of the trial itself, some from concern about the use of protocols, and some from a desire to be able to individualize a ventilation strategy to each patient's characteristics and needs. The major criticisms of the trial were that the study design was flawed and should have included a "usual management" or "wild-type" control group in which management was left to each treating physician (such that the "positive" results were not the result of the lower tidal volume reducing mortality but that those receiving a higher tidal volume had a higher mortality, or that the values of 6 and 12 mL/kg theoretically might represent the ends of a U-shaped curve and that some intermediate V_T might be associated with lower mortality than either "extreme") and that a V_T of 6 mL/kg PBW might be too hard to use, requiring higher doses of sedatives and neuromuscular blocking agents, which could have an adverse effect.

Including a "usual management" control group might be appropriate when the variation in usual practice can be explained by guiding principles. The range in practice of V_T selection was large at the time of the ARDSnet trial, and no guiding principles directing V_T selection were apparent. Interpretation is made more difficult by the various approaches used to adjust for weight (e.g., predicted body weight, which in North America is on average 20% lower than measured body weight). A V_T of 12 mL/kg PBW is thus roughly equivalent to one of 10.5 mL measured body weight, a value that fell roughly in the middle of the range of V_T used when ventilating patients with ARDS at the time the ARDSnet study was designed. Two independent "blue ribbon panels" asked to adjudicate this issue unanimously agreed that the V_Ts used in the

ARDSnet study were appropriate and that the study design was ethical.

Two previous studies of the effect of V_T on mortality in ARDS were negative, but the control V_T was 10 mL/kg of measured body weight in one case and of an estimated body weight in the other. When all studies are adjusted for PBW (on the basis of height and gender), the control V_t in the ARDSnet study was similar to that used in the other two studies. In addition, the mortality in the 12 mL/kg PBW group of ARDSnet was similar to that of the control groups in the other two studies, and the mortality of the intervention arm (6 mL/kg PBW) was considerably lower than any other study group (Figure 71-12). Three subsequent ARDSnet studies that used the lower V_T strategy in both arms found comparable or lower mortalities to that of the lower V_T arm of the initial ARDSnet trial.

Although there is certainly a theoretical possibility that the relationship between V_T and mortality could be U-shaped, all the available evidence suggests the opposite; that the lower the plateau pressure, the lower the mortality. Although this may be due, in part, to the possibility that patients who can be ventilated with lower plateau pressures might be less sick, nothing supports that patients receiving lower V_T have a higher or even an intermediate mortality.

Doses of sedatives were not recorded in the ARDSnet study, but reports from three of the centers found no differences in doses in the two groups.

Use of protocols is an issue that applies to many practices in the ICU and continues to be controversial. The major concerns are that protocolized care is "cookbook" medicine that is not adjusted to the individual patient. This concern is based on the assumption that caregivers can recognize differences in patients and their presentations, and that altering treatment in response to these perceived differences improves care. Neither assumption can be solidly supported by existing literature, and, in fact, the opposite seems to be the case. A well-designed protocol includes adjustment to the characteristics of the individual patient. Its use should be under the oversight of a physician who decides whether the patient's condition meets the assumption(s) on which the protocol is based, whether some other characteristic of the patient requires a modification, and whether any given protocol instruction should be rejected. Widespread evaluation of several different types of protocols used in the ICU indicates that between 5 and 10% of the instructions generated by a protocol are rejected with rationale for the rejection given. Many ICU protocols have been tested and found to reduce length of stay or improve a variety of other morbidities. Whether there are some patients who could have even better outcomes if identified and treated separately by individual physicians remains to be determined. Until we know how better to achieve that goal, it seems prudent to use standardized protocols for patients meeting the entry criteria into studies that have demonstrated global effectiveness.

Another controversy is whether the ARDSnet LPV protocol should be applied to *other* patients being mechanically ventilated, especially those *at risk* for ARDS. A recent retrospective study of patients with known risk factors for ALI but not yet meeting ALI criteria found that the range of tidal volume used was the single factor best correlating with subsequent ALI development, with patients receiving larger tidal volumes having a higher incidence of ALI development. Although there are no prospective data on this issue, it seems reasonable to use this LPV strategy in patients with known risk conditions for

FIGURE 71-12 Comparison of mortality in studies of lung protective strategies and other therapies in patients with ALI. The yellow bars represent mortality in the control arms of the cited studies. The blue bars show data from three ARDSnet studies that used a lung protective ventilation strategy, including the intervention arm of the ARMA trial and data for all patients in the ALVEOLI and FACTT trials. PBW, Predicted body weight. Brochard (Brochard L, et al: Am J Respir Crit Care Med 1998; 158:1831–1838). Stewart (Stewart TE, et al: N Engl J Med 1998; 338: 355–361). Brower (Brower RG, et al: Crit Care Med 1999; 27:1492–1498). Exosurf (Anzueto A, et al: N Engl J Med 1996; 334:1417–1421). ARMA (The Acute Respiratory Distress Syndrome Network: N Engl J Med 2000; 342:1301–1308). ALVEOLI (The NHLBI ARDS Clinical Trials Network: N Engl J Med 2004; 351:327–336). FACTT (The NHLBI ARDS Clinical Trials Network: N Engl J Med 2006; 354:2564–2575).

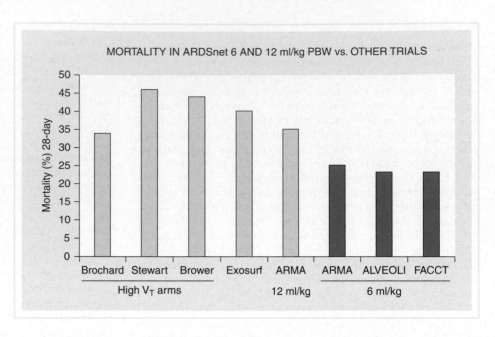

ALI, given the proven feasibility and safety of the ARDSnet protocol. We know of no compelling reasons why the protocol should be mandatory for other ventilated patients not known to be at risk for ALI development.

Transfer of ALI/ARDS Patients to Regional Centers

Recently, published data show that a correlation exists between hospital volume and ICU outcomes, similar to what has previously been recognized with respect to various surgical procedures. This finding provides some rationale for transferring patients with ALI/ARDS from small hospitals in rural or small town settings to larger regional centers where personnel have more experience managing patients with ALI/ARDS.

SUGGESTED READINGS

The Acute Respiratory Distress Syndrome Network: Ventilation with lower tidal volumes compared with traditional tidal volumes for acute lung injury and the acute respiratory distress syndrome. N Engl J Med 2000; 342:1301–1308.

Gong MN: Genetic epidemiology of acute respiratory distress syndrome: implications for future prevention and treatment. Clin Chest Med 2006; 27:705–724.

Herridge MS, Cheung AM, Tansey CM, et al: One-year outcomes in survivors of the acute respiratory distress syndrome. N Engl J Med 2003; 348:683–693.

The National Heart, Lung and Blood Institute Acute Respiratory Distress Syndrome (ARDS) Clinical Trials Network: Comparison of two fluid-management strategies in acute lung injury. N Engl J Med 2006; 354:2564–2575.

Penuelas O, Aramburu JA, Frutos-Vivar F, et al: Pathology of acute lung injury and acute respiratory distress syndrome: a clinical-pathological correlation. Clin Chest Med 2006; 27:571–578.

Rubenfeld GD, Caldwell E, Peabody E, et al: Incidence and outcomes of acute lung injury. N Engl J Med 2005; 353:1685–1693.

Schwarz MI, Albert RK: "Imitators" of the ARDS. Implications for diagnosis and treatment. Chest 2004; 125:1530–1535.

Wheeler AP, Bernard GR: Acute lung injury and the acute respiratory distress syndrome: a clinical review. Lancet 2007; 369:1553–1564.

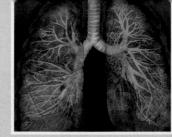

72 Scoliosis and Kyphoscoliosis

ANITA K. SIMONDS

INTRODUCTION

Scoliosis describes lateral curvature of the spine (Figure 72-1) and was described by Hippocrates as early as 500 BC. Kyphosis indicates backward and lordosis forward curvature in an anteroposterior (median) plane. Many patients who have a thoracic scoliosis are mistakenly described as having a kyphoscoliosis, because the rib angle prominence is misinterpreted as a kyphotic component. In fact, most idiopathic thoracic scolioses incorporate a lordotic and rotatory element. The degree of lateral curvature is expressed by the Cobb angle, which is calculated from a radiograph as shown in Figure 72-2.

EPIDEMIOLOGY, RISK FACTORS, AND PATHOPHYSIOLOGY

Spinal curvature is the most common cause of chest wall deformity. The causes of chest wall deformity are shown in Table 72-1. By far, the most frequently found scoliosis is the idiopathic variety, which accounts for approximately 80% of cases. Whereas idiopathic scoliosis is defined as lateral curvature for which no cause can be identified, congenital scolioses are related to a developmental abnormality of the spine (e.g., failure of segmentation [partial or fused vertebrae], failure of formation [hemivertebrae], or genetic syndromes such as spondylocostal dysostosis, Klippel Feil, and Goldenhar's syndrome).

Scoliotic curves of more than 35 degrees affect 1 in 1000 of the population, and those that exceed 70 degrees are estimated to occur at a rate of 0.1 in 1000; females are at greater risk of severe curves than are males. It has been estimated that there are approximately 500,00 individuals with a scoliosis >30 degrees in the United States. Approximately 3 or 4 children per 1000 will require specialist supervision for their spinal curvature, and a third of these will require intervention (e.g., corrective surgery or bracing). Idiopathic scoliosis occurs more often with increasing maternal age and in higher socioeconomic groups, but there is no association between the incidence of scoliosis and birth order or season of birth. A subclassification of idiopathic scoliosis is based on age of onset of the curve—infantile (birth to age 3 years), juvenile (3–11 years), and adolescent (11 years and older).

Marfan syndrome affects 1 in 5000 of the population, and approximately 63% of affected individuals have a spinal deformity develop. Diagnosis can be confirmed by linkage to the Marfan's syndrome gene MFS1, which produces fibrillin. Related syndromes may result from mutations in microfibrils that interact with fibrillin in the extracellular matrix. Congenital contractual arachnodactyly (Beals' syndrome), in which scoliosis is common, has also been shown to be caused by fibrillin deficiency.

GENETICS

The genetic basis of idiopathic scoliosis remains unclear, and causation may be multifactorial, in that particular growth patterns may exacerbate a genetic predisposition. Support for an underlying genetic cause comes from data showing as incidence of idiopathic scoliosis in 6.94%, 3.69%, and 1.55%, respectively, in first-, second-, and third-degree relatives of 114 affected individuals, findings that are consistent with either an autosomal-dominant or multifactorial mode of inheritance. A large family with autosomal-dominant idiopathic scoliosis has been identified with a locus on chromosome 17p11. By contrast, congenital scoliosis is relatively common among congenital malformations and is associated with congenital heart and renal tract anomalies. An autosomal-recessive form of congenital scoliosis has been found in male and female sibship of consanguineous parents, associated with lack of vertebral segmentation and fused ribs. Mouse models for idiopathic scoliosis have been developed, and the list of candidate genes continues to grow, indicating the underlying complexity of etiology and probable interaction of genetic, environmental, and developmental factors.

Spinal curvature is acquired in neuromuscular disorders (Figure 72-3) that involve the chest wall and thoracic musculature before skeletal maturity occurs. More than 50% of boys who have Duchenne muscular dystrophy have a scoliosis develop, and spinal curvature is common in many of the other congenital muscular dystrophies, myopathies, and conditions such as types I and II spinal muscular atrophy. A scoliosis often develops after a thoracotomy carried out in childhood or young adulthood.

Kyphosis

Idiopathic kyphosis is rare. An increase in thoracic kyphosis occurs with age and is exacerbated by factors that increase a tendency to osteoporosis such as oral corticosteroid therapy. Pott's tuberculosis (TB) of the spine is still a common cause of acquired kyphosis.

Effects of Chest Wall Deformity on Respiratory and Cardiac Function

Chest wall disorders affect respiratory function and cause a restrictive ventilatory defect. Any significant scoliosis or kyphosis results in a loss of height, so that arm span is used to predict normal lung volumes. As a rule of thumb, patients who have a

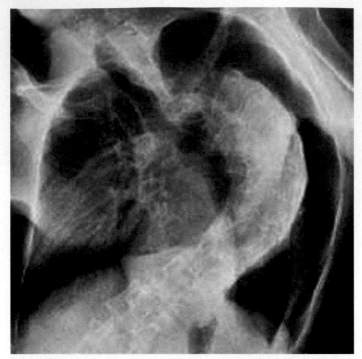

FIGURE 72-1 Radiograph of patient with congenital idiopathic scoliosis.

TABLE 72-1 **Classification of Spinal Deformity**	
Idiopathic deformities	**Associated with neuromuscular disease**
Idiopathic scoliosis	Cerebral palsy
Idiopathic kyphosis	Poliomyelitis
Congenital deformities	Muscular dystrophies
Bone	Myopathies
Scoliosis	Hereditary sensory motor
Kyphosis	neuropathies
Cord	Friedreich's ataxia
Myelodysplasia	Syringomyelia
Syndromes in which scoliosis is common	**Acquired deformity caused by**
Neurofibromatosis	Surgery/trauma
Marfan syndrome	Infection
Osteogenesis imperfecta	Pyogenic
Klippel–Feil syndrome	Tuberculosis (Pott's kyphosis)
Mucopolysaccharidoses	Radiotherapy
Treacher Collins syndrome	Tumor
Goldenhar's syndrome	Neuroblastoma
Apert's syndrome	Osteoma
Ehlers-Danlos syndrome	Hemangioma
Vertebral and epiphyseal dysplasias	Chordoma
	Eosinophilic granuloma
Arthrogryposis	

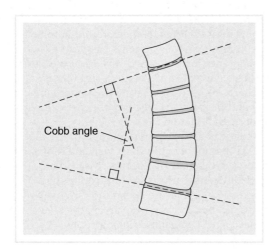

FIGURE 72-2 Method of calculating Cobb angle.

thoracic curve >70 degrees are subject to significant ventilatory limitation.

Lung Volumes. Although both scoliosis and kyphosis diminish lung volumes, which results in a restrictive ventilatory defect, lateral curvature has a more profound effect on chest wall mechanics. Total lung capacity is reduced in all chest wall disorders. In a pure scoliosis, both vital capacity (VC) and expiratory reserve volume are decreased with relative preservation of residual volume (Table 72-2). An obstructive ventilatory defect is rare in scoliosis and kyphosis, unless the individual is a smoker, has coexistent asthma, or the scoliosis results in bronchial torsion.

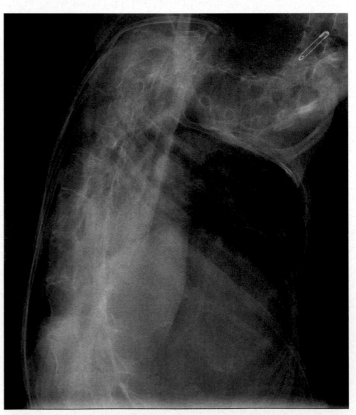

FIGURE 72-3 Radiograph of an extensive severe neuromuscular scoliosis in a patient with type II spinal muscular atrophy.

TABLE 72-2 Typical Pulmonary Function Results in Idiopathic Thoracic Scoliosis

Parameter	Effect
Forced expiratory volume in 1 s (FEV$_1$)	Reduced
Forced vital capacity (FVC)	Reduced
FEV$_1$/FVC	Normal
Residual volume	Normal
Total lung capacity	Reduced
Transfer factor for carbon monoxide (DL$_{CO}$)	Reduced
Transfer coefficient (DL$_{CO}$/accessible alveolar volume; K$_{CO}$)	Supranormal*

*Transfer co-efficient is usually supranormal, but it is reduced in the presence of pulmonary hypertension.

The relationship between pulmonary impairment and the deformity is complex and cannot be predicted accurately from the Cobb angle alone. The four major determinants of a reduced VC are the number of vertebrae involved in the curve, cephalad position of the curve, Cobb angle, and the degree of loss of normal thoracic kyphosis.

In paralytic scoliosis, lung volumes are reduced not only by chest wall restriction but also by inspiratory muscle weakness.

Chest Wall Mechanics. Chest wall compliance (C$_{CW}$) is an important determinant of lung volumes and the work of breathing. Individuals with a Cobb angle of <50 degrees experience a minimal reduction in C$_{CW}$, whereas C$_{CW}$ is likely to be significantly reduced if the Cobb angle is >100 degrees. A direct relationship between Cobb angle and C$_{CW}$ is not seen in patients who have neuromuscular disorders, because respiratory muscle weakness contributes independently to chest wall stiffness. Alteration in chest wall properties cannot solely be attributed to the mechanical deformity of scoliosis, because a decrease in CCW has been found in patients affected by chronic respiratory muscle weakness in the absence of a scoliosis.

Lung Compliance. Although lung expansion is compromised by chest wall properties, primary pulmonary pathology is unusual in patients who have idiopathic scoliosis. However, lung compliance is reduced because of a shift in the pressure-volume curve to the right. These changes in pulmonary characteristics largely arise from an alteration in alveolar forces caused by chronic hypoventilation. In patients with neuromuscular disease, microatelectasis and macroatelectasis may complicate the picture. Microatelectasis seems relatively rare, however, because fine-section CT scans have shown areas of atelectasis in only a minority of patients affected by respiratory muscle weakness. Recurrent pneumonia may occur in patients with neuromuscular disease who have bulbar weakness or an ineffectual cough. Pulmonary fibrosis is also seen in patients who have old TB, and these individuals may have areas of bronchiectasis. Cystic lung changes affect some individuals with neurofibromatosis.

Gas transfer coefficient tends to be raised in patients with scoliosis in the presence of a low transfer factor (see Table 72-2), because extrathoracic compression squeezes more air than blood out of the lungs, and thereby decreases accessible alveolar volume.

Respiratory Muscles/Thoracic Pump during Sleep

Impaired respiratory muscle function might be expected in idiopathic scoliosis, because the respiratory muscles work at a mechanical disadvantage when chest wall shape is altered. A reduction in transdiaphragmatic pressure and static respiratory mouth pressures have been demonstrated in patients who have scoliosis or a thoracoplasty. These findings tend to support the contention that the efficiency of the respiratory muscles may be affected by relatively small degrees of chest wall deformity. Respiratory muscle action is further reduced by the loss of intercostal muscle tone during rapid eye movement (REM) sleep and a reduced ability to compensate for added respiratory load. This explains why early features of ventilatory failure during sleep predate the development of daytime ventilatory failure.

Control of Breathing. Impaired hypercapnic ventilatory drive is usually secondary to chronic CO_2 retention in patients with scoliosis. However, primary drive disorders may complicate some neuromuscular conditions (e.g., myotonic dystrophy) and may be acquired in patients who have poliomyelitis that affects brainstem control mechanisms. Generally, however, ventilatory drive is increased in patients with neuromuscular disease to compensate for respiratory muscle insufficiency.

Pulmonary and Cardiac Hemodynamics. Cor pulmonale is the end-stage result of severe, untreated chest wall deformity. Pulmonary artery pressure becomes elevated at rest with an inverse correlation between pulmonary artery pressure and arterial oxygen tension. In some patients with severe scoliosis, a disproportionate rise in pulmonary artery pressure on exercise can be seen in the absence of hypoxemia, because the restricted thorax is unable to accommodate the increase in cardiac output on exertion.

An additional stress on hemodynamics is the effect of nocturnal hypoventilation on pulmonary artery pressure. The exact level of nocturnal hypoxemia that generates pulmonary hypertension is unknown, but severe, nocturnal arterial blood gas disturbances inevitably lead to daytime problems if untreated.

CLINICAL FEATURES

Spinal abnormalities are best understood by describing the age of onset, etiology, and location of the curve (e.g., adolescent onset, idiopathic thoracic scoliosis). During physical examination, accompanying features should be sought, such as café-au-lait spots and neurofibromata. Marfan's syndrome is a clinical diagnosis that requires the involvement of two of three main systems (ocular, cardiac, and skeletal). A careful search for cardiac lesions is mandatory in early-onset scoliosis, which is associated with an increased incidence of congenital heart disease. Lesions demonstrated radiologically, such as hemivertebrae and rib fusion, suggest the presence of a congenital scoliosis.

Patients are observed in the standing position and viewed bending forward to obtain an indication of the degree of lateral rib hump deformity. Assessment of shoulder and pelvic asymmetry, leg length, and gait is helpful. The lower back should be examined for hairy tufts and other cutaneous stigmata of spinal dysraphism, and a full neurological examination should be carried out.

Progression of Curvature

Only one in five curves that are <20 degrees progress. Detailed studies of the natural history of untreated idiopathic scoliosis are rare, but the younger the age at presentation, the greater the potential for progression because more of the growth spurt needs to be accommodated, and spinal growth continues until at least the age of 25 years. High and low thoracic curves together with thoracolumbar curves seem to be more unstable than lumbar deformities. Curves most likely to progress include those caused by congenital failure of segmentation, infantile idiopathic scoliosis, the angular curve of neurofibromatosis, pronounced paralytic curves, and scoliosis associated with progressive childhood neuromuscular conditions.

DIAGNOSIS

Cardiopulmonary Decompensation—Identification of High-Risk Cases

Most patients who have a thoracic spinal curvature do not have cardiorespiratory problems develop and, therefore, do not require long-term respiratory follow-up. However, it is important to be able to identify the minority at risk of problems so that appropriate monitoring and therapeutic intervention is carried out.

Cor pulmonale was the primary cause of death in a series of 102 untreated patients with idiopathic thoracic scoliosis. Age at onset of the scoliosis is crucial. Branthwaite showed that in patients who had cardiorespiratory problems attributable to their scoliosis develop, 90% had an early-onset curvature (i.e., onset before the age of 5 years).

A VC of 50% predicted is an important cutoff figure, because those with a VC <50% predicted at presentation are much more likely to have respiratory decompensation develop than those who have larger lung volumes.

The mean age of patients in respiratory failure who presented for ventilatory support was 49 years in idiopathic scoliosis patients, 51 years in patients who had previous poliomyelitis, and 62 years in those who had sequelae of pulmonary TB. Pehrsson *et al* followed lung function over a period of 20 years in patients with idiopathic scoliosis. Respiratory failure occurred in 25%, all of whom had a VC <45% predicted and a thoracic Cobb angle >110 degrees.

Monitoring High-Risk Patients

Monitoring high-risk patients should include the following:

- Assessment of breathlessness, exercise tolerance and what limits this, symptoms of nocturnal hypoventilation
- Clinical examination
- Pulmonary function tests
- Arterial blood gas tensions
- Measurement of respiratory muscle strength (e.g., mouth pressures, sniff inspiratory pressure)
- Spinal and chest radiology
- MRI scanning may be required to delineate spinal cord and vertebral anomalies, and computed tomography may be needed to investigate abnormalities such as pulmonary hypoplasia or bronchial torsion
- Echocardiography (ECG) is mandatory in all patients with congenital/early-onset scoliosis

A fall in VC >15% predicted on assuming the supine position indicates significant diaphragm weakness. Daytime

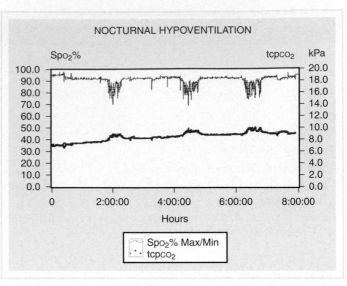

FIGURE 72-4 Overnight traces of oximetry and transcutaneous carbon dioxide tension in a patient with early-onset scoliosis, who was initially seen with sleep disturbance and morning headaches showing three periods of dips in SaO_2 and peaks of $TcCO_2$ in rapid eye movement sleep.

hypercapnia is associated with an inspiratory mouth pressure <30% predicted.

As well as inquiries about breathlessness and exercise tolerance, patients should be asked about symptoms of nocturnal hypoventilation (morning headache, poor sleep quality, frequent arousals, nocturnal confusion, and morning anorexia), and if any are present, the patient should undergo monitoring of respiration during sleep. A characteristic picture of nocturnal hypoventilation is usually found with episodes of desaturation and CO_2 retention most pronounced in REM sleep (Figure 72-4).

TREATMENT

Management of Spinal Deformity

Conservative Management

The success of a conservative approach depends on the age of the patient, the curve size at presentation, and its propensity to progression. For example, an infantile idiopathic scoliosis may spontaneously regress, whereas a juvenile-onset scoliosis is more likely to progress.

Bracing

Devices such as the Milwaukee and Cotrell braces have been used extensively. The mechanical aim of the brace is to recreate a normal thoracic kyphosis, hyperextend the spine, and limit forward flexion, all of which will act to derotate the scoliosis. Bracing probably works more effectively in a kyphosis than a scoliosis. In paralytic disorders, a circumferential brace can support the trunk and make sitting more comfortable. Vital capacity should always be measured with and without the brace in place.

Surgery for Scoliosis

In general, surgery is performed to correct unacceptable deformity and prevent progression. It is not carried out to improve ventilatory function.

Thoracic scolioses >45 degrees are usually judged unacceptable. However, a lesser curve associated with a greater degree of rotation may create a rib hump, which is just as concerning to the patient. It is a surgical maxim that even the best operative technique does not completely straighten a spine. Approximately a 50% correction of the Cobb angle in smaller curves can be expected from an instrumental procedure. The best guide to a successful result is the initial amount of spinal flexibility. Also, the greater the degree of rotation, the greater the inflexibility of the curve.

Spinal fusion followed by casting has now been superseded in many situations by rod instrumentation (Figure 72-5). The system provides distraction to the concave side of the spine and compression to the convex side, which enhances stabilization and reduces any rotational tendency. Instrumentation is used to stabilize the curve and spinal fusion to prevent growth. A posterior approach is used, but if there is a severe deformity or very rigid curvature, an anterior approach may be required to release the disk space. The combined anterior and posterior approach carries greater anesthetic and surgical risk. Preoperative assessment should include the investigations listed previously. In individuals with a VC less than 50% predicted, a sleep study should be considered. If there is evidence of nocturnal hypoventilation, use of noninvasive ventilation (NIV) in the perioperative period may be helpful. A recent consensus conference of scoliosis surgery in patients with Duchenne muscular dystrophy (DMD) highlighted the fact that scoliosis surgery should be carried out in centers with full access to multidisciplinary respiratory and cardiac input. The key aim of scoliosis surgery in these neuromuscular conditions is *not* to improve lung function, because most studies show no major impact on lung volumes after surgery, but to prevent further progression of the curve and improve comfort and sitting position in a wheelchair. Surgery should optimally be performed in DMD and other neuromuscular conditions when pulmonary function is not too compromised (FVC >30% predicted) but has been carried out safely in those with VC between 20% and 30% predicted as supportive care such as NIV in postoperative period and cough assistance with cough in-exsufflator has become available. All patients with DMD are at risk of cardiomyopathy, and left ventricular function and ECG should be monitored closely. Risks of surgery are likely to increase markedly if left ventricular fractional shortening is <25%, and these risks should be carefully balanced against the overall prognosis.

Ventilatory Impairment

Optimization of Respiratory Function

Patients must be advised about the adverse effect of smoking and obesity. The influenza and pneumococcal vaccine are recommended for those who have ventilatory limitation.

Biphosphonate therapy reduces the risk of osteoporosis in postmenopausal women and also in men. Care should be taken not to miss the reactivation of TB in patients with a thoracoplasty. Patients who have Marfan's syndrome may require β-adrenergic blocker therapy to reduce the risk of aortic dissection.

Exercise should be encouraged, apart from those in the group with pulmonary hypertension and those who have Marfan's syndrome. Pulmonary rehabilitation programs suggest that exercise and a reduction in deconditioning is just as valuable in restrictive disorders as in chronic obstructive pulmonary disease.

Ventilatory Failure

The evidence now clearly shows that ventilatory failure in patients who have chest wall disease can be successfully treated by use of noninvasive ventilation at night. Negative pressure devices are effective but have been largely supplanted by noninvasive positive-pressure ventilation (NIV). In patients with scoliosis who receive NIV, 5-year survival is approximately 80%, with 100% in patients with previous poliomyelitis, and more than 90% in those with posttuberculous conditions. It seems increasingly likely that individuals who have nonprogressive disorders may live a normal or near-normal life span, provided NIV is introduced before the development of intractable pulmonary hypertension. Patients report good quality of life by use of NIV, and many are able to return to work. It should be noted that NIV produces a more favorable outcome than long-term oxygen therapy (LTOT) in patients with scoliosis. In a retrospective analysis of consecutive patients with kyphoscoliosis who started LTOT alone or NIV in Belgium, 1-year survival was higher in the NIV group (100 vs 66%), and NIV patients demonstrated a greater improvement in PaO_2 and $PaCO_2$. More recently, these results have been confirmed in a larger Swedish cohort that showed survival rate was three times greater in NIV users than in those receiving LTOT alone, and this was unrelated to baseline arterial blood gas tensions, gender, or respiratory comorbidity. In general, oxygen is usually combined with NIV at night if mean SaO_2 on NIV alone is not >90%, despite adequate control of $PaCO_2$. There is no evidence that any one type of ventilator is superior in patients with scoliosis, although some patients with congenital or idiopathic scoliosis may require relatively high inflation pressures.

NIV can be also used to palliate symptoms of breathlessness and cor pulmonale in patients who have progressive disorders

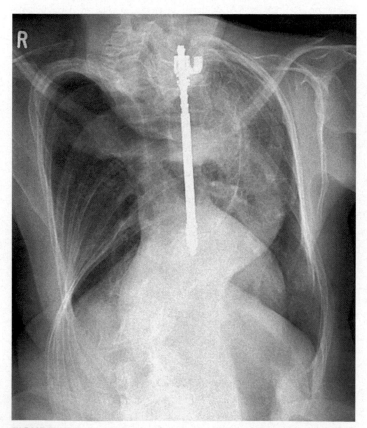

FIGURE 72-5 Radiograph of patient with scoliosis treated with a Harrington rod.

and will alter the natural history of these conditions. A 5-year survival as high as 73% can be achieved in Duchenne muscular dystrophy.

PITFALLS AND CONTROVERSIES

Clinical Signs in Scoliosis

In patients who have severe scoliosis and who have asthma develop, importantly a characteristic wheeze may not be heard because of low airflow. Measurement of spirometry and home peak-flow monitoring is useful in these cases. An isolated unifocal wheeze may indicate bronchial torsion or kinking that can occur in patients with severe scoliosis and may be associated with bronchiectasis or hyperinflation in the distal lung lobe. Bronchial stenting has been successfully used in this situation. In the case shown in Figure 72-6, the right bronchus

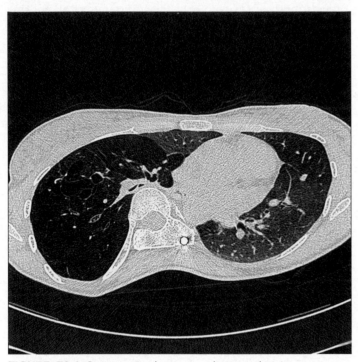

FIGURE 72-6 Computerized tomograph scan showing compression of right bronchial tree and hyperinflated right lower lobe with cystic change. (Courtesy of P. Rafferty.)

intermedius was partially obstructed by torsion and compression against the spine. The patient had a staphylococcal pneumonia and cystic change develop affecting the right lower lobe.

Pregnancy and Scoliosis

A successful outcome from pregnancy is usual in most patients who have adolescent-onset idiopathic scoliosis. In a survey of 118 pregnancies in 64 women who had thoracic scoliosis, no serious medical problems were encountered, with a cesarean rate of 17% for obstetric reasons. However, cardiorespiratory complications can be expected in those with a VC <1.25 L. Stable curves are unlikely to progress during pregnancy. Prepregnancy counseling and assessment is sensible in patients with scoliosis, particularly those with congenital or early-onset curves or a VC <50% predicted. Assessment should include full pulmonary and cardiologic evaluation and genetic counseling. Pregnancy is contraindicated in the presence of pulmonary hypertension and hypoxemia. If ventilatory problems arise in pregnancy, the situation may be successfully managed by use of noninvasive ventilation.

SUGGESTED READINGS

Bergofsky EH: Thoracic deformities. In Roussos C, ed, The Thorax; Part C: Disease. New York: Marcel Dekker, Inc; 1995:1915–1949.

Branthwaite MA: Cardiorespiratory consequences of unfused idiopathic scoliosis. Br J Dis Chest 1986; 80:360–369.

Buyse B, Meersseman W, Demedts M: Treatment of chronic respiratory failure in kyphoscoliosis: oxygen or ventilation. Eur Respir J 2003; 22:525–528.

Giampietro PF, Blank RD, Raggio CL, et al: Congenital and idiopathic scoliosis: clinical and genetic aspects. Clin Med Res 2003; 1:125–136.

Gustafson T, Franklin KA, Midgren B, et al: Survival of patients with kyphoscoliosis receiving mechanical ventilation or oxygen at home. Chest 2006; 130:1828–1833.

Leatherman KD, Dickson RA: Basic principles. In Leatherman KD, Dickson RA, eds: The Management of Spinal Deformities. Oxford: Butterworth-Heinemann; 1988:1–27.

Lowe TG, Edgar M, Margulies JY, et al: Etiology of idiopathic scoliosis: Current trends in research. J Bone Joint Surg 2000; 82A:1157–1168.

Pehrsson K, Bake B, Larsson S, Nachemson A: Lung function in adult idiopathic scoliosis: A 20 year follow up. Thorax 1991; 46:474–478.

Simonds AK: Domiciliary non-invasive ventilation in restrictive disorders and stable neuromuscular disease. In Simonds AK, ed. Non-invasive Respiratory Support: A Practical Handbook. London: Arnold; 2001: 133–145.

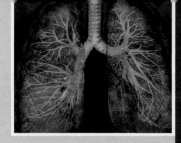

73 Diseases of the Thoracic Cage and Respiratory Muscles

JEAN-WILLIAM FITTING

EPIDEMIOLOGY, GENETICS, AND CLINICAL FEATURES

A variety of neurologic disorders can affect respiration. The most important are presented here according to the anatomic level of the lesion. They are classified as acute or chronic, but some acute disorders have permanent consequences, and some chronic disorders may manifest with acute respiratory failure. Table 73-1 summarizes the main disorders, their site, type of damage, and respiratory outcome.

Central Nervous System

Acute Disorders

Head and Spinal Cord Injury. Traumatic injury to the brain and the spinal cord may result in total or subtotal loss of respiratory muscle function and a number of resulting acute complications. Patients with brain injury develop early arterial hypoxemia related to ventilation-perfusion inequality. Neurogenic pulmonary edema is frequent and is believed to result from massive α-adrenergic discharge, pulmonary vasoconstriction, systemic hypertension, and capillary disruption. Other early complications include pulmonary embolism, hypersecretion of tenacious bronchial mucus, and pneumonia. Tetraplegia results from cervical spinal cord trauma, spinal artery infarction, or compression by tumor. The function of intercostal and abdominal muscles is partially or completely lost, and the only remaining expiratory muscle is the clavicular portion of the pectoralis major. This results in a profound impairment in expiratory force and cough efficacy. The degree of inspiratory muscle impairment depends on the level of the lesion with respect to the innervation of the trapezius (C1–C4), sternocleidomastoid (C2–C4), scalene (C3–C8), diaphragm (C3–C5), and intercostal muscles (T1–T11). Diaphragmatic function is intact in patients with lower cervical lesions. Inspiratory function is, however, impaired by a paradoxical movement of the upper rib cage that occurs because of the intercostal muscle paralysis. In contrast, high cervical lesions induce a paradoxical movement of the abdomen because of diaphragmatic paralysis. Pulmonary function and ventilatory autonomy improve after the initial phase of spinal shock in these patients. Higher cord injuries result in a nearly complete loss of respiratory muscle function, which necessitates immediate and long-term ventilatory assistance.

Stroke. Hemispheric strokes affect the voluntary pathway of respiration, with elevation and decreased voluntary activation of the contralateral hemidiaphragm. Cheyne–Stokes breathing may develop, particularly in patients with bilateral hemispheric lesions. These alterations have only modest clinical consequences, however, because the automatic pathway is preserved. Brainstem strokes may affect respiratory rhythm in various ways. Lesions of the dorsolateral medulla result in fatal apnea. In contrast, injuries that spare the dorsolateral medulla do not impair automatic respiratory rhythm, even when the strokes are extensive and patients are left with the locked-in syndrome. Lateral medullary strokes that result from occlusion of a distal vertebral artery induce the loss of automatic breathing, or Ondine's curse. Although breathing is maintained during wakefulness, potentially fatal hypoventilation and central apnea develop during sleep. This must be differentiated from obstructive apnea, which may also be associated with lateral medullary strokes and which results from paralysis of pharyngeal muscles.

Tetanus. After disruption of the skin barrier, tetanus toxin produced by *Clostridium tetani* reaches the central nervous system by means of retrograde axonal transport and blocks the synaptic release of inhibitory transmitters. Localized or generalized spasms develop through loss of central inhibition, and death results from respiratory failure because of laryngospasm or generalized spasms of the respiratory muscles. Specific therapy includes antibiotics, human tetanus immune globulin, muscle relaxants or neuromuscular blockade, sedation, and intubation and mechanical ventilation.

Chronic Disorders

Multiple Sclerosis. Multiple sclerosis is an inflammatory, demyelinating disease that can affect almost any area of the central nervous system. Different types of respiratory abnormalities may develop, depending on the location of the lesion, and occasionally these can be life threatening. Respiratory control can be affected by loss of automatic breathing, loss of voluntary breathing, or both. Bulbar dysfunction increases the risk of respiratory failure from aspiration and pneumonia. Respiratory muscle weakness is usually moderate in degree but may become severe and include diaphragmatic paralysis during relapses of the disease. Patients are particularly at risk of acute respiratory failure when infection and fever accompany an exacerbation. In these circumstances, severe respiratory muscle weakness can occur acutely because of a conduction block of demyelinated fibers.

Extrapyramidal Diseases. Parkinson's disease is associated with frequent respiratory complications, including pneumonia, which is the most common cause of death in these patients. Abnormal control of breathing is frequently present, with tachypnea accompanied by dyspnea. Respiratory muscle

TABLE 73-1 Disorders Causing Respiratory Insufficiency: Their Site, Damage, and Effect on the Respiratory System

Disorder	Site of Lesion	Type of Damage	Respiratory Outcome
Central nervous system			
Head and spinal cord injury	Brain and spinal cord	Trauma, infarction, compression	Neurogenic pulmonary edema Ventilatory failure
Stroke	Cerebral hemispheres, brainstem	Infarction	Cheyne-Stokes breathing, central apnea, loss of automatic breathing
Tetanus	Inhibitory neurons	Synaptic block by *Clostridium tetani* toxin	Ventilatory failure by laryngeal and respiratory muscle spasms
Multiple sclerosis	Central nervous system	Inflammatory demyelinating disease	Aspiration, ventilatory failure, loss of automatic or voluntary breathing
Parkinson's disease	Substantia nigra	Neuronal degeneration	Tachypnea, upper airway obstruction, impaired cough
Shy-Drager syndrome	Multiple	Neuronal degeneration	Irregular breathing, vocal cord abductor paralysis
Anterior horn cells			
Paralytic poliomyelitis	Bulbar and anterior horn motor neurons	Inflammation and degeneration induced by poliovirus	Upper airway obstruction, aspiration, ventilatory failure
Postpoliomyelitis syndrome	Anterior horn motor neurons	Late degeneration of reinnervated motor units	Ventilatory failure
Rabies	Central nervous system, spinal cord	Inflammation induced by rabies virus	Laryngeal spasms, ventilatory failure
Flavivirus encephalomyelitis	Central nervous system, spinal cord	Inflammation induced by a tick-borne flavivirus	Ventilatory failure
Amyotrophic lateral sclerosis	Upper and lower motor neurons	Neuronal degeneration	Impaired cough, ventilatory failure
Spinal muscular atrophies	Anterior horn motor neurons	Neuronal degeneration	Intercostal muscle paralysis, ventilatory failure
Peripheral nerves			
Guillain-Barré syndrome	Motor, sensory, and autonomic neurons	Acute demyelinating polyneuropathy	Aspiration, ventilatory failure
Critical illness polyneuropathy and myopathy	Motor and sensory neurons, skeletal muscles	Axonal degeneration, myopathic changes	Prolonged ventilator dependency
Diphtheria	Motor, sensory, and autonomic neurons	Acute demyelinating polyneuropathy	Ventilatory failure
Herpes zoster	Phrenic nerve	Acute demyelinating neuropathy	Hemidiaphragm paralysis
Neuralgic amyotrophy	Cervical roots	Acute axonal degeneration	Diaphragmatic paralysis
Phrenic nerve injury	Phrenic nerve	Trauma, tumor, infection	Hemidiaphragm paralysis
Hereditary neuropathies	Motor and sensory neurons	Chronic demyelinating neuropathy	Rarely diaphragmatic paralysis
Neuromuscular junction			
Botulism	Presynaptic cholinergic nerve terminals	Blockade of acetylcholine release by *Clostridium botulinum* exotoxin	Ventilatory failure
Snake and tick paralysis	Presynaptic cholinergic nerve terminals	Blockade of acetylcholine release	Ventilatory failure
Organophosphate poisoning	Postsynaptic nerve endings	Inhibition of cholinesterase	Ventilatory failure
Myasthenia gravis	Postsynaptic nerve endings	Antibodies against acetylcholine receptors	Aspiration, stridor, ventilatory failure
Diseases of muscles			
Acute corticosteroid myopathy	Skeletal muscles	Muscle necrosis and atrophy	Prolonged ventilator dependency
Duchenne muscular dystrophy	Skeletal muscles and myocardium	Absence of dystrophin, muscle atrophy	Impaired cough, ventilatory failure

TABLE 73-1 Disorders Causing Respiratory Insufficiency: Their Site, Damage, and Effect on the Respiratory System—Cont'd

Disorder	Site of Lesion	Type of Damage	Respiratory Outcome
Diseases of muscles—cont'd			
Myotonic dystrophy	Skeletal muscles	Myotonia and muscle atrophy	Central hypoventilation, aspiration, impaired cough, ventilatory failure
Facioscapulohumeral muscular dystrophy	Face and arm muscles	Progressive muscle atrophy	Rarely ventilatory failure
Limb girdle dystrophies	Proximal muscles of upper and lower limbs	Progressive muscle atrophy	Rarely ventilatory failure
Congenital myopathies	Skeletal muscles	Unique anomalies of various types	Variable: mild impairment to ventilatory failure
Pompe disease	Skeletal muscles	Acid maltase deficiency + organ glycogen accumulation	Ventilatory failure in infant and child Diaphragm weakness in adult
Mitochondrial myopathies	Skeletal muscles	Anomalies of mitochondrial DNA	Ventilatory failure
Dermatomyositis, polymyositis, inclusion body myositis	Skeletal muscles	Various types of muscle inflammation	Respiratory muscle weakness, nonspecific interstitial pneumonia
Systemic lupus erythematosus	Diaphragm	Muscle atrophy and fibrosis	Shrinking lung syndrome

weakness manifests by reduced lung volumes, impaired ability to clear secretions, and a delay in achieving peak expiratory flow. Finally, some patients with Parkinson's disease have dynamic instability of upper airway patency, which can be recognized as manifesting a sawtooth pattern on both the inspiratory and expiratory limbs of a flow-volume curve. Respiratory dysfunction can also be induced by L-dopa therapy in patients with Parkinson's disease. Some patients have dyskinesias develop associated with tachypnea and dyspnea within 1 h of drug administration as a result of choreiform movements and rigidity-akinesis of the respiratory muscles.

Shy–Drager syndrome is a multiple system atrophy that manifests by parkinsonism and autonomic failure. It is often associated with abnormal control of breathing, including irregular respiratory rate and tidal volume, central apneas, Cheyne-Stokes breathing, apneustic breathing, or central hypoventilation. The most dangerous anomaly is bilateral vocal cord abductor paralysis, which manifests by stridor and can result in obstructive sleep apnea and death.

Anterior Horn Cells

Acute Disorders

Paralytic Poliomyelitis. Before the advent of poliovirus vaccines, poliomyelitis was the most frequent neuromuscular disorder causing respiratory failure. It is now rare and usually attributed to live, attenuated polio vaccines. The acute infection has few symptoms, with fever and myalgia occurring in adults and upper airway infection in children. Only a minority of infected persons have paralysis develop, which is widely and asymmetrically distributed. Respiratory complications include irregular breathing and apneas, upper airway obstruction, aspiration, and respiratory muscle weakness or paralysis. Approximately 25% of patients require ventilatory assistance during the acute infection, but ventilatory autonomy is often recovered within months through reinnervation of denervated fibers.

Rabies. Rabies is usually transmitted to humans by animal bites and is an almost universally fatal disorder. The virus is transported along the peripheral nerves and enters the central nervous system, where it induces inflammation. In 20% of cases, the inflammation predominates in the spinal cord and manifests as paralytic rabies with progressive, ascending paralysis that may lead to respiratory muscle weakness and eventual respiratory arrest in a fashion that may be indistinguishable from the Guillain–Barré syndrome (GBS). Immediate local treatment of wounds and postexposure prophylaxis is mandatory for subjects likely to be exposed to rabies and consists of human rabies immune globulin and rabies vaccine.

Flavivirus Encephalomyelitis. Tickborne encephalitis is caused by a flavivirus and is endemic in Central Europe. In a minority of patients, acute myelitis develops in which paralysis and areflexia predominate in upper limbs. Severe weakness of respiratory muscles may develop, requiring prolonged mechanical ventilation.

Chronic Disorders

Amyotrophic Lateral Sclerosis. Amyotrophic lateral sclerosis (ALS) is a progressive degenerative disorder characterized by loss of both upper and lower motor neurons. With an incidence of 1–2 per 100,000 persons, ALS is the most frequently occurring motor neuron disorder in developed countries. It affects predominantly middle-aged to older subjects, with a male/female ratio of 2:1. The cause is unknown, but 5–10% of cases are familial, usually with autosomal-dominant transmission, caused by a defect localized in chromosome 21. ALS has a very poor prognosis, with 50% of patients dying within 3 years and 80% within 5 years, usually of respiratory failure.

The clinical features are not uniform, however. Loss of lower motor neurons often predominates, resulting in fasciculations, amyotrophy, and weakness, whereas loss of upper motor neurons manifests with spasticity and hyperreflexia. In most cases, weakness initially develops in the extremities; in a minority, the bulbar lesions are most prominent. Similarly, respiratory muscle dysfunction is quite variable during the course of ALS. In some patients, respiratory muscle strength and lung volumes are relatively preserved even when peripheral muscle weakness has progressed to the point where the patients are wheelchair bound. Abdominal muscle dysfunction usually occurs before diaphragmatic dysfunction, leading to expiratory muscle weakness. In rare cases, however, the initial manifestation may be severe respiratory weakness from phrenic motor neuron lesions. Ultimately, most patients have alveolar hypoventilation develop unless ventilatory support is initiated. Death most commonly occurs as a result of acute respiratory failure that develops as a result of aspiration pneumonia.

Spinal Muscular Atrophies. The spinal muscular atrophies (SMAs) have an autosomal-recessive inheritance pattern and arise from an anomaly of chromosome 5. All are characterized by weakness and amyotrophy, which predominates in the proximal muscles and begins in the lower limbs. Respiratory muscle weakness is caused by paralysis of intercostal muscles, whereas the diaphragm is preserved. The SMAs are classified into three types according to the age of onset; types I and II are also termed *Werdnig–Hoffmann disease*, and type III is *Kugelberg–Welander disease*. Type I SMA begins before the age of 6 months and results in respiratory failure before the age of 2 years. Type II begins before the age of 18 months, progresses more slowly, and leads to respiratory failure in late childhood as a result of both respiratory muscle weakness and scoliosis. Type III begins after 18 months and is associated with late respiratory complications resulting mainly from kyphoscoliosis.

Postpoliomyelitis Muscular Atrophy. Approximately 25% of patients with previous poliomyelitis have further muscular weakness as a result of degeneration of reinnervated motor units 20–40 years after the initial episode. In patients with respiratory muscle sequelae and kyphoscoliosis, further dysfunction of respiratory muscles may induce alveolar hypoventilation. The loss of muscle strength is gradual, however, and can be detected by appropriate tests before respiratory failure develops.

Peripheral Nerves
Acute Disorders

Guillain–Barré Syndrome. An acute, multifocal, demyelinating polyradiculoneuropathy, GBS is of uncertain pathogenesis. Infection is the most common predisposing factor: *Campylobacter jejuni, cytomegalovirus, Epstein–Barr virus, Mycoplasma pneumoniae*. The condition has also been reported to occur after surgery and in the setting of concurrent malignancy. Cerebrospinal fluid is characterized by elevated proteins and usually a cell count of 10 or fewer mononuclear leukocytes per cubic millimeter. Muscle weakness and paralysis commonly begin in the lower extremities and progress in an ascending pattern to include the respiratory muscles. Maximum weakness is attained within 2 weeks in 50% of cases and within 4 weeks in 90%. Respiratory failure develops as a result of both respiratory muscle weakness and pulmonary infections caused by aspiration and requires mechanical ventilation in 15–30% of patients. Sensory impairment is minor, but autonomic dysfunction may be severe and include arrhythmias and hypertension or hypotension. Specific therapy is based on repeated plasma exchange or on high-dose immunoglobulin therapy, which may limit progression of the disease and accelerate recovery when given early. Corticosteroids are ineffective and may be harmful. Most patients recover fully from GBS, but 15% manifest residual weakness, and 5% develop a chronic form with relapsing episodes of demyelination.

Critical Illness Polyneuropathy and Myopathy. Adult patients staying in the intensive care unit and who have sepsis and failure of two or more organs are at high risk for critical illness polyneuropathy and myopathy developing. This is an acute, reversible axonal neuropathy manifested by symmetric and predominantly distal weakness or paralysis. Cerebrospinal fluid is unremarkable, in contrast to GBS. Electrophysiologic examination shows normal nerve conduction velocities but low or absent action potential amplitudes. Neural biopsy specimens show axonal degeneration without inflammation. Muscle biopsy samples show denervation atrophy but also myopathic changes. The resulting respiratory muscle weakness is a frequent cause of prolonged and difficult weaning from mechanical ventilation. Complete recovery can occur, but rehabilitation is often needed for persistent functional disability.

Diphtheria. Diphtheria, caused by *Corynebacterium diphtheriae*, is characterized by a pharyngeal and tracheal inflammatory membrane. In 20% of cases, an exotoxin provokes cardiac and neurologic complications, beginning with palatal paralysis. A demyelinating polyneuropathy develops 6 weeks after the initial infection and can result in respiratory failure if the respiratory muscles are involved. Neurologic symptoms progress over 1–2 weeks, then stabilize and regress over several months. Antitoxin is the only specific therapy and must be administered as early as possible.

Herpes Zoster. Herpes zoster is caused by reactivation of varicella-zoster infections and generally affects sensory nerves, causing a unilateral vesicular eruption involving a single dermatome. Motor neurons may occasionally be affected, with resultant flaccid paralysis. The phrenic nerve may be involved in midcervical lesions, and this can result in complete and permanent hemidiaphragmatic paralysis—a cause of dyspnea, but not of respiratory failure. Because herpes zoster is not invariably accompanied by a cutaneous eruption, it may remain undetected in cases of unexplained, usually unilateral, diaphragmatic paralysis.

Neuralgic Amyotrophy. Neuralgic amyotrophy (Parsonage–Turner syndrome) is an acute neuritis that affects cervical roots and is manifested by sudden onset of neck and shoulder pain, followed by sensory and motor impairment with prominent weakness and amyotrophy of the shoulder and arm muscles. A recent history of viral infection or immunization is present in a minority of patients. Diaphragmatic paralysis, commonly bilateral, may ensue and induce dyspnea and orthopnea (see Table 73-1). Slow and partial recovery of diaphragmatic function occurs in most patients over a period of 2–3 years.

Phrenic Nerve Injury. Damage to or compression of the phrenic nerves induces unilateral or bilateral diaphragmatic paralysis. Such injury can be caused by trauma to the neck, neck or intrathoracic surgery, mediastinal tumors, pleural space infections, or forceful manipulation of the neck. Diaphragmatic paralysis is a common complication of open-heart surgery and results from cold- or stretch-induced injury to the nerve. This dysfunction is reversible, with recovery of 80% of cases within 6 months and 90% within 1 year. Spontaneous phrenic nerve paralysis has a much worse prognosis for recovery.

Metabolic and Toxic Causes. Acute intermittent porphyria causes an axonal neuropathy, which may be severe enough to induce respiratory failure. Acute hyperkalemic paralysis, commonly triggered by drugs in patients with acute or chronic renal failure or, less commonly, with adrenal insufficiency, may be complicated by respiratory failure. Other causes of acute neuropathy that result in respiratory muscle paralysis include poisoning with ciguatoxin (produced by protozoan algae and transmitted by fish), saxitoxin (transmitted by shellfish), tetrodotoxin (elaborated by the puffer fish), and thallium.

Chronic Disorders

Hereditary Motor and Sensory Neuropathies. Hereditary motor and sensory neuropathies (Charcot–Marie–Tooth disease) represent a group of inherited, autosomal-dominant or recessive disorders that are characterized by chronic degeneration of the peripheral nerves and roots, leading to muscle weakness of the extremities. Phrenic nerve involvement is frequent, but diaphragmatic paralysis is relatively uncommon and late.

Neuromuscular Junction

Acute Disorders

Botulism. Botulism is caused by an exotoxin elaborated by *Clostridium botulinum*, a gram-positive, spore-forming anaerobe widely present in soil. The disease can be acquired three ways: foodborne organisms can be acquired from the consumption of improperly cooked food that contains the spores and toxin; infantile botulism can be acquired by colonization of the gastrointestinal tract in the first 6 months of life; and wound botulism can be acquired from entry of the organism through breaks in the skin or from injectable drugs, given either intravenously or subcutaneously. The toxin is hematogenously disseminated, enters the neurons by endocytosis, binds irreversibly to calcium channels, and blocks acetylcholine release at the neuromuscular junction and at postganglionic parasympathetic nerve terminals. The incubation period lasts hours to days in foodborne disease and days to 2 weeks in wound botulism. Gastrointestinal symptoms appear first, with nausea and vomiting, followed by blurred vision, diplopia, and a descending paralysis, which includes the respiratory muscles. Mortality is less than 10% with the use of mechanical ventilation, but support may be required for up to 3 months in severe cases. Respiratory muscles seem to recover more slowly than other muscle groups. The diagnosis is made by isolating the toxin or the organism in food remnants or from gastric aspirate, stools, or serum in foodborne botulism, and in serum and wound tissue in wound botulism. Specific therapy includes enemas and gastric lavage, surgical débridement of wounds, high-dose penicillin, and antitoxin within the first days.

Organophosphate Poisoning. Poisoning occurs with ingestion, inhalation, or absorption by mucous membranes of organophosphate insecticides. These compounds are anticholinesterases, which induce a cholinergic crisis and skeletal muscle weakness from dysfunction of postsynaptic neuromuscular junctions. The acute intoxication presents as a potentially fatal cholinergic crisis. An intermediate form may develop 1–4 days after intoxication and manifest with cranial and proximal muscle weakness and respiratory failure. Specific therapy includes atropine and the cholinesterase reactivator pralidoxime.

Snake Bite and Tick Paralysis. Snake neurotoxins act by preventing the release of acetylcholine at the neuromuscular junction. Paralysis develops 6–12 h after the bite, with ptosis, diplopia, blurred vision, dysphagia, proximal muscle paralysis, and respiratory failure. After mechanical ventilation is initiated, paralysis usually regresses in 2–3 days. Specific therapy includes monovalent or polyvalent antivenom.

Tick paralysis is also caused by a neurotoxin that blocks the release of acetylcholine. After a 5-day latent period, a rapidly ascending paralysis develops and leads to respiratory failure. Removal of the tick rapidly reverses the process.

Chronic Disorders

Myasthenia Gravis. Myasthenia gravis is the most common disorder of the neuromuscular junction and is mediated by antibodies against acetylcholine receptors. Muscle weakness, which is exacerbated by exercise, is due to a reduction of available acetylcholine receptors. The onset of the disease is usually insidious but may be abrupt. Weakness most commonly affects the extraocular muscles (causing ptosis and/or diplopia) but also affects facial muscles (causing weakness or paralysis), bulbar muscles (causing aspiration), laryngeal muscles (causing stridor), and truncal and limb muscles. Exacerbations may occur with exertion, infection, surgery, or a variety of drugs (most commonly the neuromuscular blocking agents, aminoglycosides, fluoroquinolones, β-blockers, procainamide, corticosteroids, penicillamine, lithium, and phenytoin). Treatment includes cholinesterase inhibitors, immunosuppression, thymectomy, and plasmapheresis.

Acute respiratory failure may develop during a myasthenic crisis, defined as a rapid worsening of symptoms caused by a triggering factor, like surgery, infection, stress, or drugs. A cholinergic crisis results from an excess of anticholinesterase agents. Weakness worsens because of a cholinergic blockade and is associated with muscarinic symptoms, which include hypersalivation, increased bronchial secretions, bradycardia, nausea, and vomiting. A mixed or brittle crisis causes both myasthenic and cholinergic symptoms. Because the respiratory muscles are usually affected less severely, they may suffer cholinergic block when other muscles require more anticholinesterase agents. Apart from mechanical ventilation, the treatment of acute respiratory failure includes plasmapheresis and temporary discontinuation of anticholinesterase medication. Corticosteroids are started after crisis recovery, because they may worsen symptoms during the first days. An insidious form of respiratory failure may develop in those who have long-standing, generalized muscle weakness.

Of patients with the Lambert–Eaton myasthenic syndrome, 50% have small-cell carcinoma of the lung. Weakness is caused by a reduction of acetylcholine release and predominates in the pelvic girdle and thigh muscles. Some respiratory muscle weakness is frequent, but respiratory failure is rare. It can precede the presentation of the tumor by several months.

Diseases of Muscle

Acute Disorders

Acute Corticosteroid Myopathy. Severe generalized weakness may develop in critically ill patients treated with high-dose corticosteroids and neuromuscular blocking agents. Great care should be taken to reduce or stop the drug in patients given high-dose steroids for urgent conditions such as cerebral metastases once treatment has been completed.

Rhabdomyolysis can be detected by increased serum creatine kinase levels and myoglobinuria. Histologic changes are found, with widespread muscle necrosis and atrophy and loss of myosin filaments. This syndrome may be observed in patients with acute severe asthma treated by mechanical ventilation, and severe respiratory muscle weakness may prolong weaning, or even necessitate long-term ventilatory support.

Electrolyte Disorders. Hypophosphatemia is common in chronic alcoholism, diabetic ketoacidosis, and gram-negative infections and induces generalized weakness, hypotonia, and areflexia. Acute respiratory failure can occur in patients with hypophosphatemia as a result of respiratory muscle weakness, but this is rapidly reversed by phosphate administration. Severe hypokalemia is another cause of respiratory muscle weakness. Respiratory failure can result from acute hypokalemic paralysis (as a complication of treatment for diabetic ketoacidosis), barium sulfide poisoning, or ureterosigmoidostomy.

Chronic Disorders

Duchenne's Muscular Dystrophy. Duchenne's muscular dystrophy (DMD) is an X-linked recessive disorder that is caused by a variety of mutations of the gene for the protein dystrophin, with an incidence of 1 in 3000 male births. Weakness, clumsiness, and waddling gait are observed in early childhood. With progressive muscle weakness, most patients are wheelchair dependent by the age of 12 years. Absolute values of vital capacity increase until age 10–12 years, then plateau, and inexorably diminish. From age 10–12 on, the ventilatory decline is further aggravated by the development of scoliosis. Patients with DMD may remain clinically stable despite considerable loss of lung volume. Eventually, nocturnal hypoxemia and hypercapnia develop, and they commonly die of acute respiratory failure secondary to pulmonary infection at 20–25 years of age. Congestive heart failure may also occur as a result of left ventricular fibrosis. Surgical correction of the scoliosis improves comfort but not the lung volumes. Noninvasive or invasive home mechanical ventilation, as well as assisted cough techniques, should be considered before the stage of terminal respiratory failure. Oral corticosteroids may delay muscle loss, but their use is controversial.

Myotonic Dystrophies. Type 1 myotonic dystrophy (Steinert's disease) is the most common muscle dystrophy in adults, with a prevalence of 1 in 8000. It is inherited in an autosomal-dominant pattern and results from expansion of an unstable repeat sequence in chromosome 19q. It is characterized by myotonia (delayed muscular relaxation), progressive muscle weakness, cardiac conduction defects, endocrine abnormalities, cataracts, ptosis, frontal baldness, and temporal wasting. Respiratory failure is frequent because of respiratory muscle weakness. Aggravating factors include central or obstructive sleep apnea and pharyngeal and laryngeal dysfunction that predisposes to aspiration. Rarely, severe dyspnea may result from myotonia of the respiratory muscles; this can be alleviated by antimyotonic therapy. Patients affected by myotonic dystrophy have an increased sensitivity to anesthetic agents and respiratory depressants. When surgery is needed, close postoperative monitoring is mandatory for at least 24 h. Type 1 myotonic dystrophy has an earlier onset and a more severe course in subsequent generations (phenomenon of anticipation). Type 2 myotonic dystrophy is also inherited on an autosomal-dominant pattern and results from expansion of an unstable repeat sequence in chromosome 3q. Weakness

appears later and is predominantly proximal. Respiratory failure seems infrequent. Congenital myotonic dystrophy occurs in the offspring of 15% of affected mothers. It is manifested by hypotonia, severe facial weakness, and frequent respiratory failure that necessitate mechanical ventilation.

Other Adult Muscular Dystrophies. Facioscapulohumeral muscular dystrophy is an autosomal-dominant condition associated with deletions in chromosome 4. It progresses slowly and affects the face and arm muscles. The trunk muscles are involved in 20% of patients, and in these patients respiratory failure may ensue. The limb girdle dystrophies are a heterogeneous group of autosomal and recessive conditions characterized by weakness of proximal muscles of upper and lower limbs. Some of them involve the diaphragm and can lead to respiratory failure.

Congenital Myopathies. Congenital myopathies are characterized by unique abnormalities on muscle biopsy. Nemaline myopathies are characterized by accumulation of rodlike bodies in muscle fibers and are inherited either in an autosomal-dominant or in a recessive manner. The most common form develops in infancy or childhood with generalized muscle weakness and respiratory failure. Central core disease is characterized by amorphous areas located centrally in type I fibers and is transmitted in an autosomal-dominant manner. The disease develops in infancy with generalized weakness but most often sparing the diaphragm. Centronuclear myopathy is characterized by numerous nuclei located centrally in muscle fibers and surrounded by a halo with reduced oxidative capacity. The X-linked recessive form (myotubular myopathy) develops at birth and often requires mechanical ventilation. The autosomal-dominant form develops in childhood and adulthood and rarely leads to respiratory failure. The autosomal-recessive form is intermediate, ranging from mild to severe weakness.

Metabolic Myopathies. Acid maltase deficiency (Pompe disease) is a glycogen storage disease. In the infantile form, all organs accumulate glycogen, and death ensues from cardiorespiratory failure by the age of 2 years. In the childhood form, organomegaly is variable, and respiratory failure is common because of severe muscle weakness. In the adult form, organomegaly is rare, and nocturnal hypoxemia and respiratory failure are frequent and caused by predominant dysfunction of the diaphragm.

Mitochondrial myopathies represent a group of systemic diseases resulting from a variety of anomalies of mitochondrial DNA. The following mitochondrial myopathies are associated with respiratory failure, either initial or precipitated by anesthesia or respiratory depressants: Kearns–Sayre syndrome, mitochondrial DNA depletion, myoclonic epilepsy and ragged-red fibers (MERRF), mitochondrial myopathy, encephalopathy, lactic acidosis, and strokelike episodes (MELAS).

Depressed ventilatory response to hypoxia and hypercapnia may occur independently of respiratory muscle weakness.

Inflammatory Myopathies. Inflammatory myopathies encompass dermatomyositis, polymyositis, and inclusion body myositis. Dermatomyositis is characterized by perifascicular muscle atrophy with CD4 cell infiltrates. In contrast, CD8 cell infiltrates predominate in polymyositis and in inclusion body myositis, the latter form being characterized by vacuoles and amyloid deposits. Respiratory muscle weakness is frequent, but ventilatory failure is relatively rare. Interstitial lung disease is often associated with polymyositis and dermatomyositis, usually in the form of nonspecific interstitial pneumonia (NSIP). In 30% of patients this is associated with antibodies to histidyl-transfer RNA synthetase (Jo-1 antigen). Systemic lupus erythematosus (SLE) is frequently associated with respiratory muscle weakness without signs of generalized muscle involvement. The shrinking lung syndrome observed in patients who have SLE results from dysfunction and elevation of the diaphragm, caused by both muscle atrophy and fibrosis.

PATHOPHYSIOLOGY

Neuromuscular disorders often affect the ventilatory pump that extends from the central nervous system to the chest wall and whose engines are the respiratory muscles. A variety of neuromuscular disorders may affect the ventilatory pump at different sites (Figure 73-1). When severe, acute neuromuscular disorders result in respiratory failure. Chronic neuromuscular disorders manifest with progressive respiratory insufficiency, but they may also have acute respiratory failure as the initial manifestation, an intercurrent complication, or the terminal event. With few exceptions, these disorders induce respiratory muscle weakness, which itself results in alveolar hypoventilation and impaired cough.

Lung Volumes

Inspiratory and expiratory muscle weakness reduces the vital capacity (VC) and its components. The end-expiratory lung volume, or functional residual capacity (FRC), is decreased, whereas residual volume (RV) may be normal or increased (Figure 73-2). As a consequence of the sigmoidal shape of the pressure-volume relationship of the respiratory system, large changes in inspiratory pressure exerted near total lung capacity (TLC), or large changes in expiratory pressure exerted near RV produce only small changes in lung volume (Figure 73-3). Nevertheless, the actual loss of lung volume is always higher than expected for a given loss of muscle strength

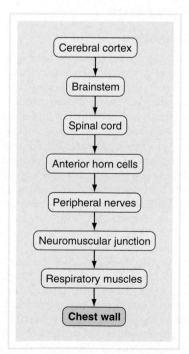

FIGURE 73-1 Components of the ventilatory pump.

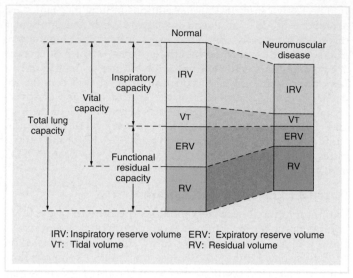

FIGURE 73-2 Modification of lung volumes in neuromuscular diseases.

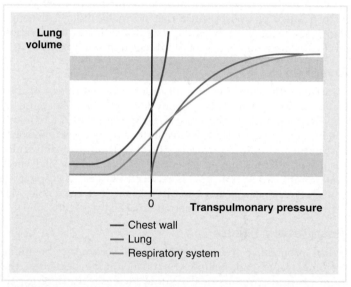

FIGURE 73-3 Minimal changes in lung volume occur with marked changes in transpulmonary pressure near total lung capacity or residual volume (*shaded areas*).

in neuromuscular disorders because of alterations of lung and chest wall mechanics, which occur even in the absence of associated scoliosis.

Lung and Chest Wall Mechanics

Acute respiratory muscle weakness results in loss of lung volume without change in compliance. In contrast, long-standing respiratory muscle weakness is associated with a number of modifications of the lung pressure-volume relationship, including the following:

1. Lung elastic recoil pressure is lower than normal at TLC (which is itself reduced).
2. Lung elastic recoil is higher than normal at any absolute lung volume.
3. Lung compliance is reduced.
4. Chest wall compliance is lower than normal.

The likely causes of these alterations in lung mechanics are a reduced number of alveoli in patients with neuromuscular disorders from early childhood and a stiffening of lung elastic fibers induced by shallow breathing. Areas of microatelectasis are an additional contributing factor but are present in only a minority of patients. The reduction in chest wall compliance occurs because of stiffening of the costosternal and costovertebral joints, tendons, and ligaments. The stiffening of the lung and chest wall is responsible for the lower level of the equilibrium position of the respiratory system (i.e., FRC) and contributes with respiratory muscle weakness to the drop in TLC and VC.

Forced Expiration and Cough

Expiratory muscle weakness modifies the contour of the flow-volume curve during a forced expiration, with a slower rise of flow, a lower peak expiratory flow, and an abrupt cessation of flow at end expiration. Because maximum expiratory flow requires only a low driving pressure, over most of VC, however, the ratio of forced expiratory volume in 1 sec to forced VC (FEV_1/FVC) is usually normal (or may be supranormal) despite expiratory muscle weakness. In contrast, cough is generally inefficient, because expiratory muscles are unable to produce the high positive pleural pressure that normally induces dynamic compression of the central airways and transient acceleration of flow. This problem leads to frequent pulmonary infections.

Dyspnea

Patients with neuromuscular disorders may complain of dyspnea despite having reduced physical activity. The cause of the dyspnea may be the increased respiratory effort required when the ratio between tidal inspiratory pressure and maximal inspiratory pressure increases (PI/PI_{max}). In neuromuscular disorders, PI may increase because of lower lung and chest wall compliances, and PI_{max} is reduced because of inspiratory muscle weakness. When muscle weakness is reversible, the sensation of dyspnea may fluctuate markedly (Figure 73-4).

Respiratory Failure

With progressive respiratory muscle weakness, breathing becomes rapid and shallow. As tidal volume decreases, the ratio of dead space to tidal volume increases, causing hypercapnia and ultimately hypoxemia as alveolar ventilation falls. The prevalence of hypercapnic respiratory failure increases with the degree of respiratory muscle weakness, being more common when respiratory muscle strength is less than 30% of normal. Considerable individual variability occurs, however, and the risk of respiratory failure cannot be predicted with certainty from measurement of VC or PI_{max}.

Part of this variability can be explained by the respiratory problems that occur during sleep. Nocturnal studies show that alveolar hypoventilation develops initially at night, particularly during rapid eye movement (REM) sleep. This sleep stage is normally characterized by shallow breathing and inhibition of the intercostal muscles. In patients with neuromuscular disorders, REM sleep is often associated with transient hypercapnia and profound desaturation. These nocturnal anomalies precede and predispose to diurnal respiratory failure.

DIAGNOSIS

History

The cause of respiratory failure is often a previously diagnosed, long-standing neuromuscular disorder. If no such disorder is present, evidence of trauma, wounds, infection, and exposure to insects, drugs, or toxic agents is sought. Clues to an underlying neuromuscular disorder may include a history of fatigability on repetitive tasks, difficulty standing up from a chair or in performing tasks with the arms elevated, difficulty with speech or swallowing liquids, tracheal aspiration, or impaired cough.

Dyspnea is a common symptom of respiratory insufficiency, although obviously not specific. Typically, dyspnea occurs on exertion but may be masked in patients whose exercise capacity is severely restricted by limb weakness. Dyspnea at rest is an alarm signal for imminent acute respiratory failure. Bilateral diaphragmatic paralysis causes orthopnea, and this problem can be severe enough to prevent normal sleep and necessitate nocturnal ventilatory support. Nocturnal hypoventilation commonly develops before the onset of diurnal hypercapnia and may be recognized by the presence of early morning headache and daytime sleepiness.

Physical Examination

Patients who complain of dyspnea of unexplained origin, or those for whom a neuromuscular disorder is suspected, are given a detailed neurologic examination. This includes assessment of the presence and distribution of muscle atrophy and weakness, fasciculation, spasticity, and abnormal tendon reflexes.

The clinical examination is often unremarkable when weakness is mild or even moderate. Rapid, shallow breathing typically accompanies more severe involvement. Signs of diaphragmatic paralysis are sought with the patient in the supine position—elevation of respiratory rate, prominent contraction of the sternocleidomastoid and scalene muscles, and abdominal paradox (i.e., an indrawing of abdominal wall during inspiration, instead of the normal synchronized outward movement of both rib cage and abdomen [Figure 73-5]). The signs of spinal cord injury vary according to the level of lesion. Patients injured above the C3–C5 level are extremely dyspneic and tachypneic, have clear use of the inspiratory neck muscles, and show abdominal paradox. Diaphragmatic function is preserved in lesions below C5. During inspiration, these patients show a normal expansion of the abdomen but often a paradoxical inward movement of the upper rib cage because of paralysis of the inspiratory rib cage muscles (see Figure 73-5).

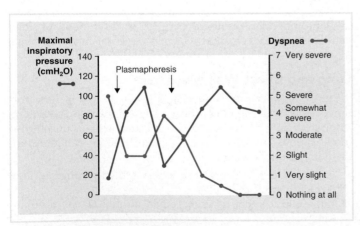

FIGURE 73-4 Dyspnea caused by respiratory muscle weakness in a patient who has myasthenia gravis.

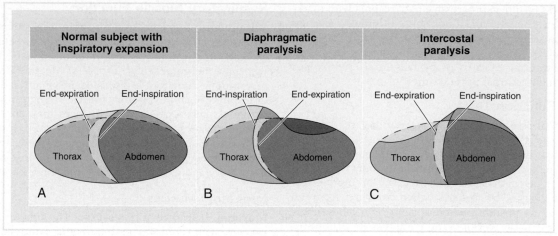

FIGURE 73-5 Different forms of chest wall paradox in neuromuscular disorders. **A,** Normal subject with inspiratory expansion of both the thorax and abdomen. **B,** Diaphragmatic paralysis with marked expansion of the thorax and paradoxical motion of the diaphragm and abdomen. Abdominal paradox should be looked for in the supine position. **C,** Intercostal muscle paralysis with paradoxical motion of the rib cage and normal diaphragmatic contraction.

Imaging

Chest radiographs showing elevation of one hemidiaphragm suggest paralysis on that side, but other causes, such as atelectasis and subpulmonary pleural effusion, must be eliminated. Elevation of both hemidiaphragms is compatible with diaphragmatic paralysis but can also result from inadequate inspiration or diffuse interstitial lung disease, or extensive intraabdominal pathology such as ascites or intestinal obstruction. Comparison with previous radiographs is most helpful (Figure 73-6). Examination of diaphragmatic movements under fluoroscopy with the patient in the supine position may be useful. During sniffing, both hemidiaphragms normally show a brisk caudad displacement. In hemidiaphragmatic paralysis, the corresponding side shows a paradoxical cephalad movement. In bilateral paralysis, both hemidiaphragms show this paradoxical shift. The hemidiaphragmatic movement can also be seen with ultrasound.

Arterial Blood Gas Tensions

The hallmarks of severe respiratory muscle weakness are hypercapnia and hypoxemia. Diaphragmatic paralysis does not cause hypercapnia, unless it is associated with an increased load caused by a lung or chest wall problem. When caused by respiratory muscle weakness, hypercapnia is a late sign and usually develops only when respiratory muscle strength is markedly reduced. In chronic disorders, global respiratory

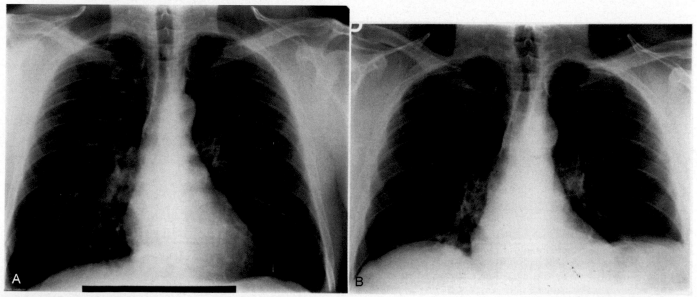

FIGURE 73-6 Bilateral diaphragmatic paralysis. **A,** Normal diaphragmatic location. **B,** In the same patient, chest radiograph during acute neuralgic amyotrophy with elevation of both hemidiaphragms.

muscle weakness results in progressive hypercapnia with markedly elevated bicarbonates and a normal pH. Initially, alveolar hypoventilation develops only during the night, in particular during REM sleep. Such episodes can be detected by transcutaneous monitoring of P_{CO_2} or by falls in arterial oxygen saturation during nocturnal pulse oximetry.

Pulmonary Function Tests

In the absence of associated lung or skeletal disease, a reduction of VC suggests respiratory muscle weakness. However, this simple test is not sensitive in mild neuromuscular disorders, because the VC falls significantly only when respiratory muscle strength is reduced by 50% or more. Normally, VC decreases by 5–10% when moving from an upright to a supine position, whereas a 30–50% fall strongly suggests diaphragmatic weakness or paralysis. In neuromuscular disorders, FRC is normal or decreased, RV is normal or increased, and TLC is decreased. The RV/TLC ratio is increased but does not reflect obstructive lung disease in this setting.

The flow-volume loop may show several anomalies: a delay in reaching peak expiratory flow, a truncation of peak expiratory and peak inspiratory flow, and/or an abrupt drop of expiratory flow at the end of expiration. In contrast to normal subjects, the forced *inspiratory* volume in 1 sec is often smaller than FEV_1 because of muscle weakness and/or bulbar involvement with upper airway obstruction.

The diffusing capacity for carbon monoxide (D_{LCO}) is reduced with respiratory muscle weakness, but less so than the lung volumes. The gas transfer coefficient (K_{CO}, or D_{LCO}/VA) is typically raised, as would be seen during a voluntary, incomplete inspiration in a normal subject.

Respiratory Muscle Function

Because loss of lung volume is neither a sensitive nor a specific test for respiratory muscle weakness, the direct measurement of respiratory muscle strength is often needed in patients who have neuromuscular disorders. Measurement of respiratory muscle function is discussed in Chapter 8. The decline of inspiratory and expiratory muscle strength may not be synchronous, and separate consequences may ensue. Inspiratory muscle weakness is a major determinant of dyspnea and hypercapnia. Expiratory muscle weakness leads to impaired cough and pulmonary infection. Hence, it is important to test *both* inspiratory and expiratory muscles in these patients.

Inspiratory Muscles

Maximal Inspiratory Pressure. The maximal inspiratory pressure (PI_{max}) developed during a volitional effort from FRC or RV is the test most commonly used to assess inspiratory muscle strength. A PI_{max} lower than 30% of normal value is a predictor of hypercapnia in patients with neuromuscular disorders. The main limitation of PI_{max} is its difficulty for the subject. As a consequence, low values are difficult to interpret, because, although they reflect true muscle weakness, they can also be found in normal subjects. Moreover, PI_{max} often cannot be interpreted in neuromuscular disorders because of air leaks around the mouthpiece caused by orofacial muscle weakness.

Sniff Nasal Inspiratory Pressure. The nasal sniff test is not hampered by orofacial muscle weakness, and it is, therefore, particularly useful for patients with neuromuscular disorders (Figure 73-7). Normal values are similar or slightly higher than for PI_{max} (Table 73-2). The sniff nasal inspiratory pressure

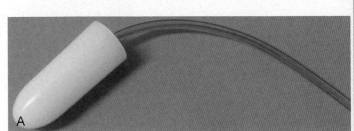
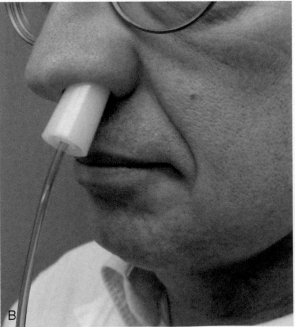

FIGURE 73-7 Method for performing sniff nasal inspiratory pressure. **A,** Nasal plug with catheter. **B,** The plug is inserted into one nostril, which enables the measurement of sniff nasal inspiratory pressure while the subject performs a maximal sniff through the contralateral nostril.

TABLE 73-2	Sniff Nasal Inspiratory Pressure (SNIP)	
Gender	Age (Years)	SNIP (cmH_2O)
Male	6–17	110 (60–160)
	20–65	110 (70–150)
	66–80	90 (50–130)
Female	6–17	95 (50–140)
	20–65	85 (50–120)
	66–80	75 (50–100)

(SNIP) declines linearly in patients with ALS and is a good predictor of hypercapnia when it falls below 30% of normal value (Figure 73-8).

Sniff Transdiaphragmatic Pressure. The formal evaluation of diaphragmatic strength requires specialized equipment (see Chapter 8). A maximum transdiaphragmatic pressure generated during a sniff less than 30 cmH_2O accurately predicts hypercapnia in patients with ALS.

Expiratory Muscles

Maximal Expiratory Pressure. A normal value of maximal expiratory pressure (PE_{max}) is useful to exclude expiratory muscle weakness in neuromuscular disorders. Low values are more difficult to interpret because of possible air leaks with orofacial weakness. Unfortunately, the loss of cough function cannot be reliably predicted from PE_{max} alone.

Cough Tests. The measurement of cough gastric pressure (cough Pga) is more invasive but is also more relevant than PE_{max} in neuromuscular disorders. Values of cough Pga below 50 cmH_2O are associated with an impaired cough function. A simple and noninvasive test consists of measuring peak expiratory flow during a maximal cough effort (cough peak flow). Whereas the normal cough peak flow ranges between 360 and 1200 L/min, values below 160 L/min are associated with the inability to clear secretions from central airways.

If the diaphragmatic function is to be specifically assessed because of concern about a suspected neuromuscular disease,

TABLE 73-3	Respiratory Assessment in Neuromuscular Disorders
Type	Notes
Clinical assessment	History—dyspnea, orthopnea, difficulty in coughing or swallowing, early morning headache, daytime somnolence
	Examination—tachypnea, cyanosis, abdominal or rib cage paradox, contraction abdominal or neck muscles, amyotrophy
Imaging	Static—chest radiography
	Dynamic—fluoroscopy, ultrasound
Functional assessment	Simple tests
	Sitting and supine vital capacities
	Lung volumes
	Flow-volume loop
	Arterial blood gases
	Nocturnal oximetry
	Maximal inspiratory and expiratory pressures
	Sniff nasal inspiratory pressure
	Cough peak flow
	Specialized tests
	Sniff transdiaphragmatic pressure
	Cough gastric pressure
	Phrenic nerve stimulation
	Twitch transdiaphragmatic pressure
	Twitch mouth pressure
	Conduction time

often the patient should be referred to a specialized laboratory for testing (Table 73-3). Simple and noninvasive tests of lung function and respiratory muscle strength are preferred to monitor the evolution over time, however.

TREATMENT

Indications for Mechanical Ventilation

Whenever possible, specific treatment of the causal neurologic process is applied. This is not possible for some of the neuromuscular disorders and is often not adequate to prevent

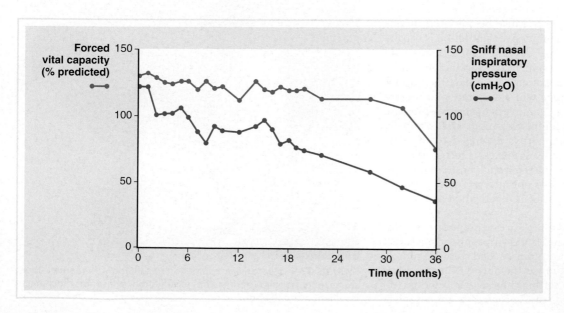

FIGURE 73-8 Evolution of a patient with amyotrophic lateral sclerosis (ALS). In this case, forced vital capacity (VC) remains initially stable and drops after 30 months. In contrast, sniff nasal inspiratory pressure falls early, heralding progression of the disease.

respiratory failure in many others. In many cases, the primary therapeutic option is ventilatory support. The methods of invasive and noninvasive mechanical ventilation are described in Chapters 18 and 19.

Mechanical ventilation is indicated when patients have severe dyspnea, tachypnea, and acute CO_2 retention develop from acute pulmonary infections. Endotracheal intubation is mandatory if the patient cannot protect the airway, if retention of secretions occurs despite assisted cough, or if any associated acute dysfunction is present. Otherwise, noninvasive mechanical ventilation may be tried if the patient is cooperative. In other patients, chronic respiratory failure develops with no or only few symptoms and is detected during scheduled periodic assessments.

Mechanical Ventilation in Specific Disorders

Acute Respiratory Failure

In spinal cord injury, the degree of ventilator dependence is mainly determined by the level of the lesion with respect to phrenic nerve roots. Endotracheal mechanical ventilation is initiated after the acute injury, but weaning or transfer to noninvasive mechanical ventilation is often possible later because of partial neurologic recovery, conditioning of the diaphragm, and/or decreased flaccidity of the chest wall. Long-term ventilatory support is required for patients with injuries above the C5 level but is often not necessary below this level.

Patients with GBS are intubated when their VC falls below 20 mL/kg or their PI_{max} below 30 cmH_2O, and they can be weaned when these values are exceeded during recovery. Intubation may be necessary earlier to protect the airway. Prolonged mechanical ventilation is common, and tracheostomy should be considered early, but virtually all patients eventually can be weaned from the ventilator. Myasthenia gravis can lead to acute respiratory failure. Intubation is often indicated, especially because of pharyngeal muscle dysfunction, but the duration of mechanical ventilation is usually short and tracheostomy is often not necessary.

Chronic Respiratory Failure

Patients with muscular dystrophies or progressive myopathies have chronic respiratory insufficiency develop at some point, starting with nocturnal hypoventilation and hypoxemia. The time at which ventilatory support must be initiated in this setting is not clear. Nocturnal noninvasive ventilation is usually started with the occurrence of daytime hypercapnia and symptoms of hypoventilation. Noninvasive ventilation can be considered earlier because most patients with daytime normocapnia and nocturnal hypercapnia will deteriorate and require this therapy within 1–2 years. Noninvasive positive-pressure ventilation is the preferred mode of treatment and is initially used only during the night. Support is extended to the daytime when mandated by progressive weakness. During daytime, the technique of mouthpiece intermittent positive-pressure ventilation can be used, which does not interfere with eating or speaking. Tracheostomy should be considered when noninvasive ventilation is no longer feasible.

In ALS, noninvasive positive-pressure ventilation can prolong survival and relieve dyspnea and symptoms of nocturnal hypoventilation. When the respiratory and bulbar muscle weakness progresses, tracheostomy is the only way of providing mechanical ventilation in this setting. Invasive ventilation will prolong survival while the disease progresses to complete paralysis, and this option must be discussed in advance to allow the patient to make a considered choice.

Diaphragmatic Pacing

Patients who are ventilator dependent because of a high cervical cord lesion or central alveolar hypoventilation are potential candidates for diaphragmatic pacing. This technique consists of stimulation of the phrenic nerves by intrathoracic implanted electrodes, the receiver being activated by radiofrequency waves generated by an external power source. Diaphragmatic pacing is an effective method of supporting ventilation in patients who have good phrenic nerve and diaphragmatic function, but its use is limited by high costs and the required specialized skills.

Assisted Cough

The most common cause of acute respiratory failure in patients with chronic neuromuscular disorders is ineffective cough during saliva aspiration and airway infections. This is manifested by a fall of oxygen saturation below 95% that cannot be reverted by noninvasive ventilation. Assisted cough techniques must be introduced to prevent this potentially lethal complication. If bulbar function is preserved, patients can be taught air stacking. The patient receives consecutive volumes of air delivered through a volume-cycled ventilator or a manual resuscitator and holds the air in with a closed glottis until maximal lung expansion has occurred. Coughing is then manually assisted by a chest squeeze or an abdominal thrust timed to glottic opening. Alternately, mechanical insufflation-exsufflation can be used: a positive-pressure deep insufflation is provided through a facemask, followed by an abrupt negative pressure. When combined with a manually assisted cough, this technique is highly efficient for the clearing of airway secretions in patients with severe respiratory muscle weakness (Figure 73-9). Assisted cough techniques must be introduced when history suggests difficulty in airway clearance or when cough peak flow is less than 200 L/min.

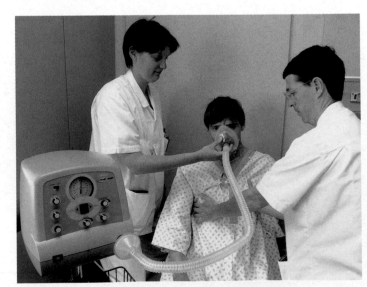

FIGURE 73-9 Mechanical insufflation-exsufflation. A manual chest squeeze is applied during the exsufflation phase of mechanical insufflation-exsufflation.

Respiratory Muscle Training

The potential benefits and adverse effects of muscle training are controversial in neuromuscular disorders. Data suggest that inspiratory muscle training may improve respiratory muscle strength and endurance in Duchenne's muscular dystrophy and in spinal muscular atrophy but only in case of moderately reduced muscle strength. The clinical significance of these findings is unclear, and, at present, respiratory muscle training cannot be recommended in neuromuscular disorders.

PITFALLS AND CONTROVERSIES

In the presence of a neuromuscular disorder, the main omission is to miss the diagnosis and fail to appreciate the likelihood of impending respiratory failure. This frequently occurs as a result of mistakenly attributing symptoms to other, more common conditions. Accordingly, in the absence of evidence of cardiac or pulmonary disease, dyspnea should not automatically be attributed to a psychogenic cause. Orthopnea is a frequent symptom of left-sided heart failure, but it may also herald diaphragmatic paralysis. Unexplained fatigue and lack of concentration should not be attributed simply to age, but should raise the suspicion of alveolar hypoventilation.

The physical examination of the respiratory system should not be performed with the patient only in the sitting position; abdominal paradox, which accompanies diaphragmatic paresis or paralysis, can be recognized only when the patient is supine. On the chest radiograph, small but normal lungs may not reflect poor inspiratory effort, but true inspiratory muscle weakness. Hypercapnia should not always be ascribed to chronic obstructive pulmonary disease, even with a positive smoking history or a mild degree of airflow limitation.

In summary, the main danger is failure to consider respiratory muscle dysfunction and to take the appropriate measurements. Respiratory muscle weakness can be diagnosed only if it is measured. The second danger is to minimize or ignore the risk of acute respiratory failure. In a patient who has a neuromuscular disorder, hypercapnia should be sought and must be considered a sign of imminent ventilatory failure. Techniques of assisted cough must also be introduced early enough to prevent dangerous consequences of saliva aspiration and minor airway infections.

WEB RESOURCES

http://www.afm-france.org
http://www.enmc.org
http://www.muscle.ca
http://www.worldmuscleforum.org

SUGGESTED READINGS

American Thoracic Society/European Respiratory Society: ATS/ERS Statement on respiratory muscle testing. Am J Respir Crit Care Med 2002; 166:518–624.

American Thoracic Society: Respiratory care of the patient with Duchenne muscular dystrophy. ATS Consensus Statement. Am J Respir Crit Care Med 2004; 170:456–465.

Baer AN: Differential diagnosis of idiopathic inflammatory myopathies. Current Rheum Reports 2006; 8:178–187.

Bruno C, Minetti C: Congenital myopathies. Current Neurol Neurosci Reports 2004; 4:68–73.

Chatwin M, Ross E, Hart N, et al: Cough augmentation with mechanical insufflation/exsufflation in patients with neuromuscular weakness. Eur Respir J 2003; 21:502–508.

Green DM: Weakness in the ICU. Guillain-Barré syndrome, myasthenia gravis, and critical illness polyneuropathy/myopathy. Neurologist 2005; 11:338–347.

Heffernan C, Jenkinson C, Holmes T, et al: Management of respiration in MND/ALS patients: An evidence based review. Amyotrophic Lateral Sclerosis 2006; 7:5–15.

Machuca-Tzili L, Brook D, Hilton-Jones D: Clinical and molecular aspects of the myotonic dystrophies: A review. Muscle Nerve 2005; 32:1–18.

Visser LH: Critical illness polyneuropathy and myopathy: clinical features, risk factors and prognosis. Eur J Neurol 2006; 13:1203–1212.

Wallgren-Pettersson C, Bushby K, Mellies U, Simonds A: 117th ENMC Workshop: Ventilatory support in congenital neuromuscular disorders—congenital myopathies, congenital muscular dystrophies, congenital myotonic dystrophy and SMA (II). Neuromusc Dis 2004; 14:56–69.

Ward S, Chatwin M, Heather S, Simonds AK: Randomised controlled trial of non-invasive ventilation (NIV) for nocturnal hypoventilation in neuromuscular and chest wall disease patients with daytime normocapnia. Thorax 2005; 60:1019–1024.

Winslow C, Rozovsky J: Effect of spinal cord injury on the respiratory system. Am J Phys Med Rehabil 2003; 82:803–814.

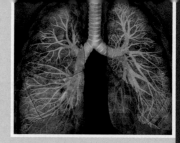

74 Obesity

BRIAN K. GEHLBACH • JESSE B. HALL

Physicians are caring for an increasing number of patients with one or more medical complications of obesity. This chapter describes the adverse effects of obesity on the respiratory system. Sleep apnea is discussed in detail in Chapter 75.

EPIDEMIOLOGY, RISK FACTORS, AND PATHOGENESIS

Obesity is typically defined by the body mass index (BMI, the ratio of body weight, measured in kilograms to height measured in meters). This easily calculable index correlates well with body fat composition in most middle-aged adults. The World Health Organization and the National Institutes of Health have proposed the following scale: BMI >25 kg/m^2 = overweight; BMI >30 kg/m^2 = obese; and BMI >40 kg/m^2 = morbidly obese. Under these definitions, data from the National Health, and Nutrition Examination Survey show an increasing prevalence of obesity in the United States over the past 15 years to the point that currently one third of all adults are obese. With more than 1 billion overweight or obese individuals worldwide, the medical and financial implications of the obesity epidemic are global in scale.

This rapid increase in the prevalence of obesity worldwide certainly indicates that environmental factors play a role in driving the epidemic. Compared with 20 years ago, the members of most societies spend more time engaged in relatively sedentary activities, both at work and during leisure time, while the typical diet has changed to one that is high in processed foods and refined sugars and low in fruits and vegetables. Still, most individuals experience very little fluctuation in weight over long periods of time, demonstrating that caloric intake and energy expenditure are tightly regulated by a variety of neurohormonal pathways. Thus, it is likely that additional factors contribute to the development of obesity in susceptible individuals. One example of such a factor is sleep deprivation, which has recently been shown to cause insulin resistance and may lead to weight gain in susceptible individuals. A number of genetic factors may also influence an individual's susceptibility to fat accumulation and weight gain.

GENETICS

The genetic contribution to obesity and body weight is well established and is responsible for between 30 and 80% of weight variation. A small percentage of all cases of obesity are caused by single-gene mutations. The disorders associated with these single-gene defects ("monogenic obesity") typically present early in life and are characterized by severe obesity and hyperphagia. The Prader-Willi syndrome, characterized by mental retardation, hyperphagia, hypogonadism, and short stature, is one well-known example of such a disorder. The study of these rare disorders has identified multiple single-gene mutations affecting the leptin and the melanocortin pathways involved in controlling food intake and energy expenditure.

In most cases, however, obesity is "polygenic," reflecting an interaction between multiple different susceptibility genes and the environment. Progress in understanding the genetic determinants of adult-onset obesity has been hindered by the large number of candidate genes and the diverse and complex environment that interacts with such genes. To date, investigators have identified more than 50 different candidate genes involved in a variety of functions related to food intake and metabolism. These diverse genetic polymorphisms have been associated with a number of different obesity phenotypes related to feeding behavior, susceptibility to different obesigenic influences, and responsiveness to weight-loss interventions. Unfortunately, the progress made to date in understanding how these gene–environment interactions lead to obesity have not resulted in practical clinical applications.

CLINICAL FEATURES

Pathophysiology

During normal inhalation, the diaphragm contracts and descends, pushing abdominal contents caudally. In obese patients, the increased weight of the abdomen reduces respiratory system compliance, shifting the pressure-volume curve for the chest wall downward and to the right (see Figures 74-1 and 74-2). Some patients also have reduced lung compliance, probably because of a reduction in functional residual capacity (FRC). In certain individuals the FRC may fall below the closing volume, particularly when supine, resulting in small airway closure in the dependent regions of the lung. An increased alveolar-to-arterial oxygen difference and hypoxemia may result. Both increased airway resistance and reduced mid- to late-expiratory flow have been described, probably as a result of reduced small airway caliber. The clinical significance of this finding is unclear.

Interestingly, although the severity of the restrictive pulmonary disease and abnormal gas exchange tend to correlate, the relationship is not strong, and there are significant interindividual differences that probably relate to differences in the distribution of body fat and respiratory muscle strength. Thus, patients with more centrally located body fat are more severely affected, and others, particularly those with obesity hypoventilation syndrome (OHS), have reduced respiratory muscle strength (at least relative to the load imposed on the respiratory muscle pump).

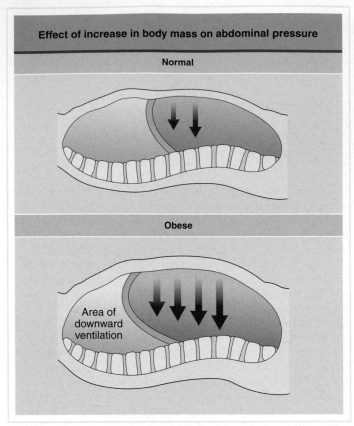

Effect of increase in body mass on abdominal pressure

Normal

Obese

Area of
downward
ventilation

FIGURE 74-1 Effect of the increase in body mass on abdominal (liquid) pressure. In turn, this effect adversely affects the dorsal lung regions, which causes a reduction in ventilation.

Respiratory drive is normal in patients in simple (uncomplicated) obesity. In contrast, patients with OHS have reduced ventilatory drive in response to carbon dioxide as assessed both by mouth occlusion pressure ($P_{0.1}$) and by diaphragm electrical activity. The risk for obstructive sleep apnea is considerably increased in obesity (see Chapter 75).

Clinical Implications

Obese patients frequently complain of dyspnea on exertion and reduced exercise tolerance. Although these symptoms are caused by cardiovascular disease in some, in many the cause is the restrictive pulmonary disease described previously. Mild to moderate hypoxemia may be present, particularly when the FRC is below closing volume and in conjunction with OHS with the accompanying alveolar hypoventilation.

In normal subjects, the oxygen cost of breathing (V_{O2RESP}) represents only a small fraction of the total oxygen consumption (i.e., 3–5%). In morbidly obese subjects, the V_{O2RESP} can be as much as 16% of total body oxygen consumption. In such patients, the neuromuscular competence of the respiratory system is adequate for the baseline load imposed on it, but there is very little reserve to accommodate increased loads such as would occur with exercise, surgery, or critical illness. Similar to patients with emphysema, who also have an increased V_{O2RESP} at rest, seemingly trivial insults may result in respiratory failure. This is particularly so in the postoperative setting (see later). Box 74-1 summarizes the pulmonary complications of obesity.

DIAGNOSIS

The evaluation of obesity-related pulmonary impairment requires pulmonary function testing. The most common abnormality on such tests is a decreased expiratory reserve volume because of cephalad displacement of the diaphragm by the abdomen. Forced vital capacity and total lung capacity (TLC) are typically preserved, except in severely obese individuals (e.g., those with a BMI >45 kg/m²) and those with the OHS. The residual volume may be elevated relative to TLC because of small airway closure and gas trapping. The diffusing capacity for carbon monoxide is typically normal. Arterial blood gases may demonstrate mild to moderate hypoxemia that worsens in the supine position. In patients with the OHS, hypercapnia and hypoxemia will be present but with a normal alveolar-to-arterial O₂ difference.

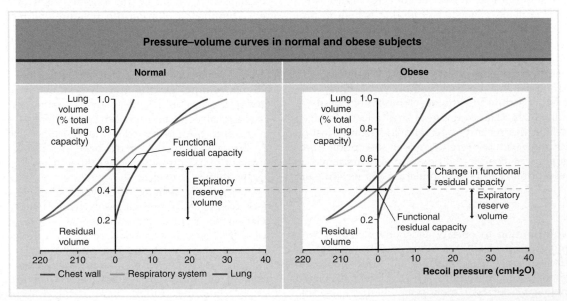

Pressure–volume curves in normal and obese subjects

Normal

Lung volume (% total lung capacity)
1.0
0.8
Functional residual capacity
0.4
0.2
Residual volume
Expiratory reserve volume
220 210 0 10 20 30 40
— Chest wall   — Respiratory system   — Lung

Obese

Lung volume (% total lung capacity)
1.0
0.8
0.6
0.2
Residual volume
Functional residual capacity
Change in functional residual capacity
Expiratory reserve volume
220 210 0 10 20 30 40
Recoil pressure (cmH₂O)

FIGURE 74-2 Lung, chest wall, and respiratory system pressure-volume curves in normal and obese subjects. Note the effect of the rightward shift in the chest wall curve on the respiratory system pressure-volume curve and on the functional residual capacity and the expiratory reserve volume (as the residual volume is unchanged).

Depending on the clinical setting, additional investigations may be warranted. Polysomnography should be performed if sleep-disordered breathing is suspected. Imaging of the chest may be limited with respect to interpretation or, in the case of computed tomography, precluded by the patient's body habitus, but may suggest pulmonary hypertension and/or other unsuspected parenchymal disorders.

Echocardiography is frequently helpful given the increased prevalence of heart disease in obese patients. Left ventricular hypertrophy and diastolic dysfunction may result from obesity-related hypertension, whereas systolic dysfunction may be caused by coronary artery disease, longstanding hypertension, or obesity-related cardiomyopathy. It is important to recognize that pulmonary hypertension, when caused by obstructive sleep apnea (OSA) *alone*, is typically mild in severity. The presence of moderate to severe pulmonary hypertension usually implicates coexisting left heart failure or daytime (in addition to nocturnal) hypoxemia, the latter usually being caused by OHS or coexisting obstructive lung disease.

TREATMENT

General Issues

Irrespective of whether obesity-related pulmonary impairment is confirmed, all obese patients should have counseling with respect to attaining weight loss by limiting caloric intake and increasing exercise. Referral to a nutritionist or weight loss expert may be appropriate. Any coexisting sleep-disordered breathing should be treated and supplemental oxygen should be provided for patients with daytime hypoxemia.

Pharmacotherapy may be appropriate for some, but medication should be used in combination with lifestyle modifications. Available agents include sibutramine, which increases satiation and decreases food intake, and orlistat, which blocks digestion and absorption of dietary fat.

Bariatric surgery is the most effective means of achieving substantial weight loss, with most studies indicating long-term loss of greater than 30% of preoperative weight. Hypertension, hyperlipidemia, diabetes, and obstructive sleep apnea frequently improve substantially or even resolve in many patients. Operative mortality is <1% in experienced centers, but it can be much higher in patients with additional comorbidities. Appropriate candidates are those with morbid obesity (i.e., BMI >35 kg/m^2) plus at least one severe obesity-related medical complication or a BMI >40 with a low likelihood of achieving successful weight loss through nonsurgical approaches. Patients >60 years of age experience less benefit and have a greater morbidity and mortality, and the decision to offer surgery to such patients should be carefully considered.

Evaluation and Management of Respiratory Failure

Morbidly obese patients are susceptible to respiratory failure from seemingly trivial insults. Unfortunately, the cause of a patient's deterioration may be difficult to diagnose. The physical examination is often unrevealing, and chest radiography is frequently insensitive to the presence of edema or subtle infiltrates. Although computed tomography yields more information, it may not be possible if the patient's weight or girth exceeds the capacity of the examination table. Echocardiography and invasive monitoring may also be limited by technical issues (e.g., poor visualization of the right ventricle).

Patients with OHS may present with an altered mental status, respiratory failure, and fluid retention. Such patients are frequently resistant to diuretic therapy until adequate oxygenation and ventilation are achieved. Most can be managed with noninvasive ventilation with the inspiratory pressure set at 10–15 cmH$_2$O and the expiratory pressure set at 5–10 cmH$_2$O. A minority of patients will not be stabilized with this approach and will require intubation. Great care should be taken at the time of intubation in those with severe pulmonary hypertension, because cardiovascular collapse may occur when switching from spontaneous (i.e., negative-pressure) to positive-pressure ventilation. Good venous access should be in place, and normal saline should be immediately available for infusion. Vasoactive drugs such as norepinephrine should also be available, but the hypotension occurring in this setting is frequently a problem of preload reduction rather than peripheral vasodilation.

Common to all intubated morbidly obese patients is the requirement for increased levels of positive end-expiratory pressure (PEEP) to avoid atelectasis and ameliorate hypoxemia. Frequently, PEEP between 8 and 15 cmH$_2$O is necessary to counter the airway collapse that occurs as a result of obesity when patients are positioned supine. An additional measure aimed at countering this pathophysiology is to nurse the patients in the reverse Trendelenburg position.

Acute Lung Injury

Lung-protective ventilation has been shown to reduce mortality in patients with acute lung injury (see Chapter 71). Unfortunately, making this diagnosis can be difficult in morbidly obese patients because of limitations in the interpretation of the chest radiograph, and many morbidly obese patients have baseline gas exchange abnormalities that increase with atelectasis that follows sedation. When in doubt, we recommend that the clinician err on the side of administering lung-protective ventilation (that sets tidal volume at 6 mL/kg of *ideal*, not measured, body weight).

Adjusting tidal volume to limit alveolar overdistension may be difficult in obese patients, because they may have a large disparity between end-inspiratory (i.e., plateau) pressures and transpulmonary pressures as a result of the decreased thoracic compliance. Accordingly, tidal volumes of 6 mL/kg *ideal body weight* may result in an end-inspiratory pressure well in excess of 30 cmH_2O in some patients, yet not be associated with alveolar overdistension, and reducing tidal volumes to achieve an end-inspiratory pressure <30 cmH_2O may result in unnecessary alveolar hypoventilation. Unfortunately, there is no clinically practicable way to know this at the bedside. We recommend first placing the patient in the reverse Trendelenburg position to minimize the effects of increased intraabdominal pressure on the assessment of respiratory mechanics. If the end-inspiratory pressure still exceeds 30 cmH_2O, a chest X-ray should be obtained. If lung volumes are small, global airspace overdistension is not occurring, and the increased end-inspiratory pressure is the result of the abnormal respiratory system mechanics (regional overdistension cannot be excluded, however).

Discontinuation of Mechanical Ventilation

Determining the obese patient's readiness to resume spontaneous breathing can be extremely challenging, irrespective of the cause of the respiratory failure. Many patients would never be extubated if the clinician waited for conventional "weaning criteria"—PEEP $\leq$ 5 and $F_{IO_2} \leq$ 0.5—to be satisfied. Such targets are frequently unrealistic because of the presence of baseline gas exchange abnormalities, as well as the amount of atelectasis than can develop in intubated, supine patients. If the disease or condition that provoked respiratory failure has been adequately treated, the patient should be given the benefit of the doubt and extubated. Noninvasive ventilation may be applied after extubation in an effort to smooth the transition to spontaneous breathing, although firm data supporting this approach are lacking. In some patients, tracheostomy should be considered early, particularly if they have a history of severe sleep-disordered breathing and the clinical course is expected to be prolonged. See Chapter 75 regarding the treatment of patients with OSA.

CLINICAL COURSE AND PREVENTION

Obesity is associated with an increased mortality, particularly from cardiovascular disease. Whether obesity independently influences the outcome of critically ill patients is presently unclear. More certain is the susceptibility of morbidly obese patients to respiratory failure. This susceptibility is particularly acute in the postoperative setting. Atelectasis, delayed clearance of sedatives and analgesics, increased susceptibility of patients with OHS to the effects of narcotics on respiratory drive, and exacerbation of underlying sleep-disordered breathing may all lead to respiratory failure. Early mobilization, the judicious use of narcotics, nursing in the reverse Trendelenburg, and, in some patients, noninvasive ventilation may be preventive.

Preventing obesity is difficult, but many can be charged with the task; the critical issue is to begin preventive measures in the early stages of obesity, which, in many, means during childhood or adolescence.

PITFALLS AND CONTROVERSIES

Both venous thromboembolism and cardiovascular disease should be included in the differential diagnosis of the obese patient with dyspnea. Heart disease is particularly common and diastolic dysfunction may exist without causing abnormal clinical findings.

Moderate to severe pulmonary hypertension can mistakenly be attributed to OSA alone. Frequently, the etiology of pulmonary hypertension is multifactorial, because it can occur as a result of OHS, pulmonary emboli, obstructive lung disease, and/or left ventricular dysfunction. In such patients, polysomnography, pulmonary function testing, echocardiograms, and/or right heart catheterization may be needed.

Obese patients are at increased risk for venous thromboembolism. Unfortunately, this diagnosis may be more difficult to establish because of the inability to obtain CT angiograms in severely obese patients. In some patients, empiric anticoagulation may be justified, particularly when an alternative diagnosis is deemed unlikely.

WEB RESOURCES FOR GUIDELINES/PROTOCOLS

National Center for Health Statistics NHANES IV Report. Available at: http://www.cdc.gov/nchs/products/pubs/pubd/hestats/obese03_04/overwght_adult_03.htm

Department of Health and Human Services and the Department of Agriculture. Dietary guidelines for America. Available at: http://www.healthierus.gov/dietaryguidelines/

SUGGESTED READINGS

Brolin RE: Bariatric surgery and long-term control of morbid obesity. JAMA 2002; 288:2793–2796.

Buchwald H, Avidor Y, Braunwald E, et al: Bariatric surgery: a systematic review and meta-analysis. JAMA 2004; 292:1724–1737.

Clément K: Genetics of human obesity: C.R. Biologies 2006; 329:608–622.

Douglas FG, Chong PY: Influence of obesity on peripheral airways patency. J Appl Physiol 1972; 33:559–563.

Farooqi IS, O'Rahilly S: Genetics of obesity in humans. Endocrine Rev 2006; 27:710–718.

Flegal KM, Carroll MD, Ogden CL, Johnson CL: Prevalence and trends in obesity among US adults, 1999–2000. JAMA 2002; 288:1723–1727.

Kaufman BJ, Ferguson MH, Cherniack RM: Hypoventilation in obesity. J Clin Invest 1959; 38:500–507.

Kress JP, Pohlman AS, Alverdy J, Hall JB: The impact of morbid obesity on oxygen cost of breathing at rest. Am J Respir Crit Care Med 1999; 160:883–886.

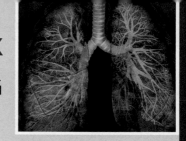

75 Obstructive Sleep Apnea

NEIL J. DOUGLAS

Sleep apnea is one of the most important respiratory conditions identified in the past 50 years. The more common form, the obstructive sleep apnea/hypopnea syndrome (OSAHS), is a major cause of morbidity and a significant cause of mortality and is the most common medical cause of daytime sleepiness. Central sleep apnea is relatively rare and is often a consequence of vascular disease.

EPIDEMIOLOGY

The frequency of OSAHS—defined as the coexistence of sleepiness or at least two other major symptoms (Box 75-1) with at least five obstructed breathing events/hour of sleep—is in the range of 2–4% of the middle-aged male population and approximately half as common in women. The syndrome also occurs in childhood, when it is usually associated with tonsil or adenoidal enlargement, and in the elderly, but the frequency is perhaps slightly lower in old age.

Irregular breathing during sleep *without sleepiness* is very much more common, occurring in perhaps 30% of the middle-aged male population. However, because these individuals are asymptomatic, by definition they do not have OSAH syndrome. There is as yet no evidence that these events are harmful in individuals who are symptom free.

RISK FACTORS

Narrowing of the pharynx is the main factor predisposing to OSAHS. This may result (Figure 75-1) from obesity—approximately 50% of OSAHS patients have a BMI >30 kg/m^2 in Western populations—or from shortening of the mandible and/or maxilla. The abnormality in jaw shape may be subtle and can be familial. Other factors that may predispose to OSAHS include hypothyroidism and acromegaly, possibly by narrowing the upper airway with tissue infiltration. Other predisposing factors for OSAHS include male gender and middle age, myotonic dystrophy, some neurologic conditions, and perhaps also smoking.

PATHOGENESIS

Apneas and hypopneas result from the airway being sucked closed on inspiration. During sleep, the upper airway dilating muscles—like all striated muscles—relax in everyone, and in OSAHS patients the dilating muscles can no longer successfully oppose the negative pressure within the airway during inspiration. The primary defect is not in the upper airway dilating muscles. Patients with OSAHS have narrow upper airways when awake, and while awake, their airway dilating muscles have increased activity that counters this and ensures airway patency. When they fall asleep, muscle tone falls, and so the airway narrows and snoring may commence; with further narrowing the airway occludes and apneas result (Figure 75-2). Apneas and hypopneas terminate when the subject arouses—wakens briefly—from sleep. This arousal is sometimes too subtle to be seen on the electroencephalogram but may be detected by cardioacceleration, blood pressure rise, or sympathetic tone increase. The arousal results in an abrupt rise in upper airway dilating muscle tone, and airway patency returns.

GENETICS

OSAHS is familial caused not only by the familial nature of obesity but also by familial jaw structure. These polygenic tendencies are being investigated. Currently, apolipoprotein E is a major focus of attention. It is particularly associated with OSA in younger subjects, and the increased risk of individuals with this allele aged less than 65 years having Apnea Hypopnea Index (AHI) of more than 15 episodes/h is 3.1.

CLINICAL FEATURES

Randomized controlled treatment trials have shown that OSAHS causes sleepiness and impairment of vigilance, cognitive performance, driving and quality of life, raised blood pressure, depression, and disturbed sleep. The main symptom of OSAHS is daytime sleepiness that may range from mild drowsiness to irresistible sleep attacks, indistinguishable from those in narcolepsy. The somnolence may result in marked impairment of work performance and may inhibit social life and damage relationships. The sleepiness is dangerous when driving (Figure 75-3), with a threefold to sixfold risk of road accidents, or when operating machinery. Experiments in normal subjects repeatedly aroused from sleep indicate that the sleepiness results, at least in part, from the repetitive sleep disruption associated with the breathing abnormality, although the recurrent hypoxemia could also contribute.

Other symptoms (see Box 75-1) include difficulty concentrating, unrefreshing nocturnal sleep, nocturnal choking, nocturia, and decreased libido. Partners report nightly loud snoring in all postures that may be punctuated by the silence of apneas. The snoring is so loud that it is often reported by those sleeping in other rooms or even by neighbors. The loud snoring often causes such embarrassment that vacations can be ruined or avoided.

BOX 75-1 Symptoms of OSAHS

Sleepiness
Difficulty concentrating
Daytime fatigue
Unrefreshing sleep
Nocturia
Depression
Nocturnal choking
Decreased libido

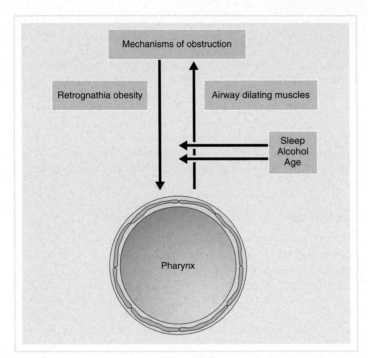

FIGURE 75-1 Factors predisposing to upper airway occlusion in OSAHS.

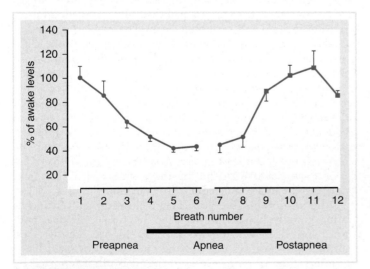

FIGURE 75-2 Genioglossal tone in the three breaths before, and the first three inspiratory attempts after apneas, followed by the last three efforts of the apneas and first three postanoxic breaths. Data (adapted from Surratt: Am Rev Respir Dis 1988; 137:889–894 with permission) show the decline in genioglossal tone immediately before and during apneas, rising with arousal at apnea termination.

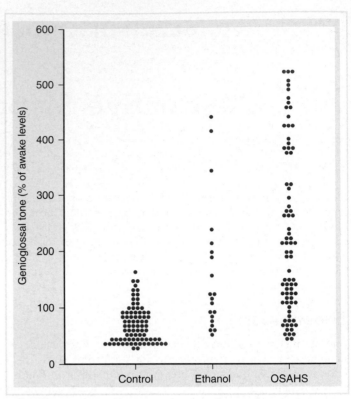

FIGURE 75-3 Steering error on a driving simulator in patients with OSAHS and controls matched for gender and driving experience. The controls were studied both sober and with a mean blood alcohol of 95 mg%. The sober patients with OSAHS drove worse than the drunk (or sober) normals. (Adapted from George: Am J Resp Crit Care Med 1996; 154:175–181 with permission.)

Associated Conditions

Cardiovascular and Cerebrovascular Disease

OSAHS raises mean 24-h blood pressure. The increase is greater in those with recurrent nocturnal hypoxemia and is at least 4–5 mmHg in those with >20 4% desaturations per hour of sleep and possibly as high as 10 mmHg in patients with severe disease who comply fully with treatment. The blood pressure rise probably results from a combination of the sympathetically mediated surges in blood pressure (Figure 75-4) accompanying each arousal from sleep that end each apnea or hypopnea and from the associated 24-h increases in sympathetic tone in patients with OSAHS.

Epidemiologic studies in normal populations indicate that this rise in blood pressure would increase the risk of myocardial infarction by approximately 20% and stroke by approximately 40%. Although there are no long-term randomized controlled trials in patients with OSAHS to indicate whether this is true in OSAHS—and such studies would not be ethically defensible—uncontrolled studies suggest an increase in the risk of myocardial infarction and stroke in untreated OSAHS (Figure 75-5). Furthermore, epidemiologic studies suggest—but cannot prove—increased vascular risk in normal subjects with raised apneas and hypopneas during sleep.

Apneas and hypopneas during sleep are common in patients with recent stroke. These seem largely to be a consequence, not a cause, of the stroke and decline over the weeks after the vascular event. Treating the apneas and hypopneas after

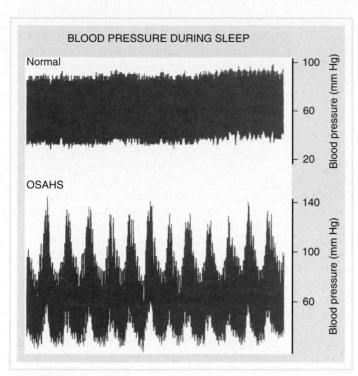

FIGURE 75-4 Beat-by-beat blood pressure during sleep in normal subject and in a patient with OSAHS with recurrent arousals. (Adapted from Davies: Thorax 1994; 49:335–339 with permission.)

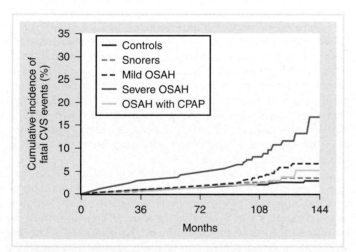

FIGURE 75-5 Cumulative incidence of fatal cardiovascular events in patients with OSAHS compared with controls. (From Marin: Lancet 2005; 365:1046–1053.)

stroke is difficult, and there is no evidence that such treatment improves stroke outcome, although only small studies have been performed.

There has been debate for decades whether OSAHS is an adult form of the sudden infant death syndrome, but no firm linkage has been established. Although earlier studies showed no increase in sudden nocturnal deaths in OSAHS, a recent large study reported excess nocturnal deaths in those previously shown to have apneas and hypopneas during sleep.

Diabetes

OSAHS and diabetes mellitus are associated and not just because obesity is common in both. Recent data suggest that increased apneas and hypopneas during sleep are associated with insulin resistance independent of obesity. In addition, uncontrolled trials indicate treatment of OSAHS in patients who also have diabetes decreases their insulin requirements, suggesting OSAHS can aggravate diabetes.

Liver

Hepatic dysfunction has been associated with irregular breathing during sleep. Subjects with apneas and hypopneas during sleep who denied alcohol consumption have been found to have raised liver enzymes and more steatosis and fibrosis on liver biopsy independent of body weight.

DIAGNOSIS

Differential Diagnosis

Causes of sleepiness that may need to be distinguished include the following:

Insufficient sleep—This can usually be diagnosed on an adequate sleep history.

Shift work—A major cause of sleepiness, especially in those older than 40 years old who are on either rotating shift or night shift work patterns.

Psychologic/psychiatric causes—Particularly depression that is a major cause of sleepiness.

Drugs—Both stimulants—by suppressing sleep—and sedatives can produce sleepiness.

Narcolepsy—That is approximately 50 times less common than OSAHS, is usually evident from childhood or teens, and associated with cataplexy (Table 75-1).

Idiopathic hypersomnolence—An ill-defined condition typified by long sleep duration and sleepiness (see Table 75-1).

Phase alteration syndromes—Both the phase-delay and the less common phase-advancement syndromes are characterized by sleepiness at the characteristic time of day.

TABLE 75-1	Clinical Indicators in the Sleepy Patient		
	OSAHS	**Narcolepsy**	**IHS**
Age of onset (y)	35–60	10–30	10–30
Cataplexy	No	Yes	No
Night sleep			
Duration	Normal	Normal	Long
Awakenings	Occasional	Frequent	Rare
Snoring	Yes, Loud	Occasional	Occasional
Morning drunkenness	Occasional	Occasional	Common
Daytime naps			
Frequency	Usually few	Many	Few
Time of day	Afternoon/ evening	Afternoon/ evening	Morning
Duration	<1 h	<1 h	>1 h

Features suggesting obstructive sleep apnea/hypopnea syndrome (OSAHS); narcolepsy or idiopathic hypersomnolence (IHS).

Recent evidence indicates that, despite their appearance on most differential diagnosis lists, periodic limb movements probably do not cause sleepiness.

Who to Refer for Diagnosis

Anyone with troublesome sleepiness that is not readily explained and rectified by taking a good sleep history (Table 75-2) and considering the preceding differential diagnosis should be referred to a sleep specialist. My threshold for troublesome sleepiness is either an Epworth Sleepiness Score >11 (Box 75-2) or problems with work or driving because of

TABLE 75-2	What to Asssess in a Sleep History
General Problem Area	**Particular Difficulties**
Daytime sleepiness	Sleep at work or other inappropriate times or places
	Difficulty driving a car because of sleepiness
	Daytime napping
Bed habits and behaviors	Bedtime—restlessness throughout night
	Out-of-bed time—can be substantial
	Number of awakenings
	Insomnia
Snoring and apneas	Patient history of snoring and apneas given by partner
	Patient awakenings with choking, gasping, or dyspnea
Habits	Alcohol / Cigaretes / Caffeine — all worsen obstructive sleep apnea
Other medical history	Hypertension / Cardiopulmonary disorders / Cerebrovascular disease — may be made worse by obstructive sleep apnea

BOX 75-2 Epworth Sleepiness Score

How often are you likely to doze off or fall asleep in the following situations, in contrast to feeling just tired? This refers to your usual way of life in recent times. Even if you have not done some of these things recently, try to work out how they would have affected you. Use the following scale to choose the *most appropriate number* for each situation:

0 = would *never* doze
1 = *slight* chance of dozing
2 = *moderate* chance of dozing
3 = *high* chance of dozing

Sitting and reading _____.
Watching TV _____.
Sitting, inactive in a public place
    (e.g., a theatre or a meeting) _____.
As a passenger in a car for an hour without
    a break _____.
Lying down to rest in the afternoon when
    circumstances permit _____.
Sitting and talking to someone _____.
Sitting quietly after lunch without alcohol _____.
In a car, while stopped for a few minutes in
    traffic _____.

TOTAL   ex 24 _____.

Epworth Sleepiness Score from Johns MW: Sleep 1991; 14:540–545.

sleepiness. The Epworth Score alone is insufficient. Many whose life is troubled by frequently fighting sleepiness but do not actually doze will rightly score themselves as having a low Epworth Score. The patient and their partner often give divergent scores for the patient's sleepiness, and I use the higher of the two scores.

Diagnosis

OSAHS requires lifelong treatment, and so the diagnosis needs to be made or excluded with certainty by a sleep specialist. This will hinge on obtaining a good sleep history and completed sleep questionnaires including the Epworth Sleepiness Scale (see Box 75-2) from both the patient and partner. Physical examination should include assessment of obesity, jaw structure, the upper airway with Mallampati grading (Figure 75-6) and for tonsillar enlargement (Figure 75-7), blood pressure, and consideration of possible predisposing causes, including hypothyroidism and acromegaly.

In adults, apneas are defined as breathing pauses lasting 10 sec and hypopneas as 10-sec events with continued breathing when ventilation is reduced by at least 50% from the previous baseline during sleep (Figure 75-8). In those with appropriate clinical features, the diagnostic test must be able to demonstrate or exclude recurrent breathing pauses during sleep. This test may be a full polysomnography with recording of multiple respiratory and neurophysiologic signals overnight (Figure 75-9) and full sleep scoring. Increasingly, and especially outside the United States, most diagnostic tests are "limited studies"—recording respiratory and/or oxygenation patterns overnight without neurophysiologic recording. Limited studies range from oximetry alone, which can be diagnostic in expert hands in patients with severe disease but cannot exclude OSAHS, to multichannel recording (Figure 75-10) of breathing pattern—from respiratory pressure and thoracoabdominal movement—snoring, oxygen saturation, and body posture, and any combination in between. Limited studies are often carried out at home to minimize patient inconvenience and cost. Such approaches in expert hands produce good patient outcomes and are cost-effective. It is important that sleep studies are scored by a trained individual; most—perhaps all—current automatic scores are highly inaccurate. It is the expertise of the scorer and clinician that is critical; the choice of the device is less vital.

It is sensible to use such limited sleep studies as the first-line diagnostic test and allow positively diagnosed patients to proceed directly to treatment. However, patients with troublesome sleepiness and a negative limited sleep study must be investigated further to establish an explanation or provide reassurance. A reasonable conservative approach at present is for patients with severe sleepiness but negative limited studies to proceed to polysomnography to exclude or confirm OSAHS (Figure 75-11).

As a syndrome is the association of a clinical picture with specific abnormalities on investigation, asymptomatic individuals with abnormal breathing during sleep should not be labeled as having OSAHS.

TREATMENT

How to Treat

Patients diagnosed with OSAHS must have the condition and its significance explained to them and their partner. This should be accompanied by written and/or web-based information

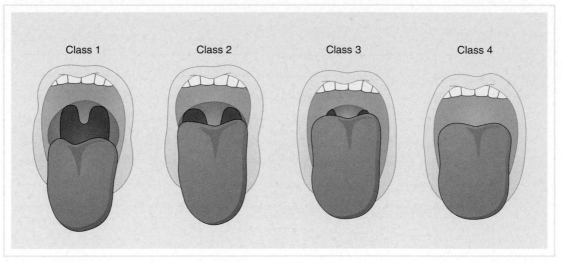

FIGURE 75-6 Mallampati grading of upper airway characteristics. (From Mallampati: Can Anesth Soc J 1985; 32:429–434.)

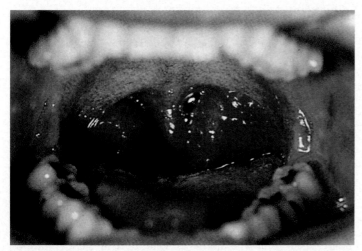

FIGURE 75-7 Enlarged tonsils can predispose to OSAHS and are particularly significant in children.

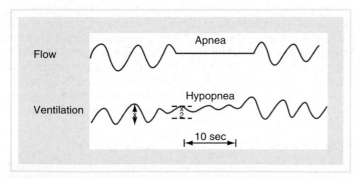

FIGURE 75-8 Schematic of apneas and hypopneas. Apneas are 10-sec cessations of airflow and hypopneas 10-sec periods when ventilation or thoracoabdominal movement is reduced by at least 50%.

for reenforcement and a discussion of the implications of the local regulations for driving. Rectifiable predispositions should be discussed, and this often includes weight loss and sometimes reduction of alcohol consumption for the twin reasons of calorie reduction and because alcohol acutely decreases upper airway dilating muscle tone, thus predisposing to obstructed breathing. For the latter reasons, sedative drugs should be carefully withdrawn, where at all possible.

CPAP

Continuous positive airway pressure therapy works by blowing the airway open during sleep (Figure 75-12), usually with pressures of 5–15 cmH$_2$O. CPAP has been shown in randomized placebo controlled trials to improve breathing during sleep, sleep quality, sleepiness, blood pressure, vigilance, cognition, driving ability, mood, and quality of life in patients with OSAHS. However, this is obtrusive therapy, and patients and their partners must be helped to understand the need for long-term treatment. All patients on CPAP must receive intensive support, including access to telephone help and regular follow-up. Initiation should include finding the most comfortable mask from the ranges of several manufacturers and trying the system for at least 30 min during the daytime to prepare for overnight use. An overnight monitored trial of CPAP is usually used to identify the pressure required to keep the patient's airway patent—a CPAP titration study—although this can be done in the patient's home. The development of intelligent CPAP machines, which vary the applied pressure depending on the patency of the airway, may make a CPAP titration night redundant, but treatment must always be initiated after education and in a supportive environment. Patients can then be treated long term either with fixed-pressure CPAP machines set at the determined pressure or by an intelligent CPAP device. The main side effect of CPAP is airway drying, often resulting from mouth leak, which can be countered by use of an integral heated humidifier or a full-face mask. CPAP use, like that of all therapies, is imperfect but on objective monitoring, approximately 94% of those with severe OSAHS are still using their therapy after 5 years (Figure 75-13).

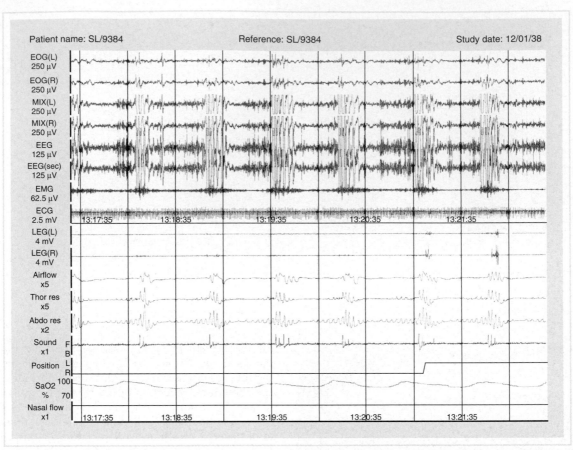

FIGURE 75-9 Polysomnography recording showing a 5-min period with seven obstructive apneas each associated with snoring and an arousal.

Mandibular Repositioning Splints (MRSs)

Mandibular repositioning splints (MRSs; also called oral devices, mandibular advancement devices) work by holding the lower jaw, and thus tongue, forward so widening the pharyngeal airway(Figure 75-14). MRSs have been shown in randomized placebo-controlled trials to improve breathing during sleep, sleepiness, symptoms, and blood pressure in OSAHS. Because there are many different devices of differing design with untested relative efficacy, these results cannot be generalized to all MRSs. Self-reports of the use of devices long term suggests high dropout rates and, unfortunately, there is as yet no method for objectively determining MRS use.

Surgery

Although it must be borne in mind that these patients have a raised perioperative risk, four forms of surgery have a role in OSAHS. Bariatric surgery can be curative in the morbidly obese. Tracheostomy is curative but rarely used because of the associated morbidity; nevertheless, it should not be overlooked in extremis. Jaw advancement surgery—particularly mandibulomaxillary osteotomy—is effective in those with retrognathia and is most useful in younger and thinner patients. Tonsillectomy can be highly effective in children, but rarely in adults. There is no robust evidence that any other form of pharyngeal surgery, whether by scalpel, laser, or thermal techniques, helps OSAHS.

Drugs

Unfortunately, no drugs are clinically useful in the prevention or reduction of apneas and hypopneas. A marginal improvement in sleepiness in patients who remain sleepy, despite CPAP, can be produced by modafinil, but the clinical value is debatable and the financial cost significant.

Choice of Treatment

CPAP and MRSs are the two most widely used and best evidence-based therapies. Direct comparisons in randomized controlled trials indicate better outcomes with CPAP in terms of apneas and hypopneas, nocturnal oxygenation, symptoms, quality of life, mood, and vigilance. Taking this in conjunction with the evidence that CPAP use is generally better and the firm evidence that CPAP improves driving, whereas there are no such data on MRSs, CPAP is the current treatment of choice. However, MRSs are evidence-based second-line therapy in those who have CPAP fail despite intensive support. In younger, thinner patients, mandibulomaxillary advancement should be considered.

Who to Treat

There is robust evidence from randomized controlled trials (RCT) for patients who have an Epworth score >11 or troublesome sleepiness driving or working and >15 apneas + hypopneas/h slept that treatment improves symptoms, sleepiness, driving, cognition, mood, quality of life, and blood pressure.

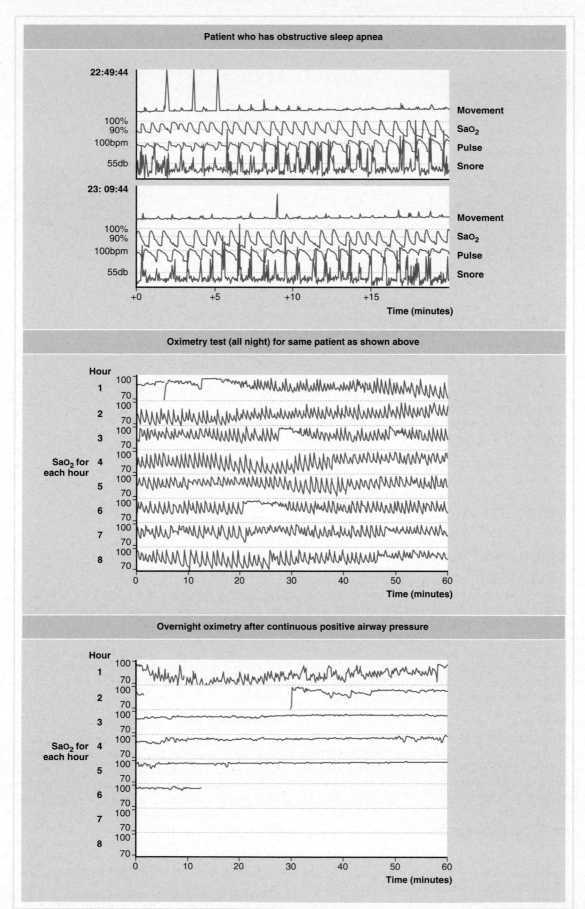

FIGURE 75-10 Limited sleep study results. *Top,* Recording of body movement (movement), oximetry (Sao₂), heart rate (pulse), and snoring (snore, in decibels) that clearly shows obstructive sleep apnea (OSA). *Middle,* The same patient's oximetry trace is shown for the entire night with desaturation throughout the night (i.e., severe OSA). *Bottom,* Oximetry for 4 h after commencement of continuous positive airway pressure (CPAP) (after a 1-h period of observation), with complete control of the OSA.

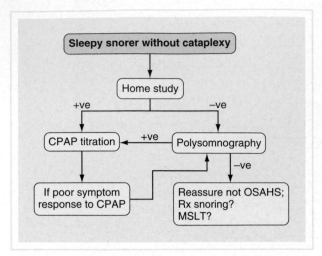

FIGURE 75-11 Flow diagram of investigation of patient with possible OSAHS. *MSLT,* Multiple sleep latency test (where subjects lie in a quiet room for up to 40 minutes with the EEG being recorded to detect whether sleep onset occurs.

For those with similar degrees of sleepiness and 5–15 events/h of sleep, RCTs indicate improvements in symptoms, including subjective sleepiness, with less compelling evidence indicating gains in cognition and quality of life, but there is no evidence of blood pressure improvements in this group.

There is no evidence that treating nonsleepy individuals with high-event frequencies improves their symptoms, function, or blood pressure. Thus, treatment cannot be advocated for this large group.

CLINICAL COURSE AND PREVENTION

Nonrandomized studies indicate that untreated patients with OSAHS are at increased cardiovascular and cerebrovascular risk with increased overall mortality. However, patients with severe OSAHS have many other risks for vascular disease, usually including obesity, hypertension, and diabetes, so definitive apportionment of risk to OSAHS is not possible.

Most patients treated with CPAP or MRS for moderate or severe OSAHS will require lifelong therapy. In a few, significant and sustained weight loss may make treatment unnecessary.

Health Resources

Untreated patients with OSAHS are heavy users of health care, dangerous drivers, and work beneath their potential. Treatment of OSAHS with CPAP is cost-effective in terms of reducing health care costs of associated illness and reducing the costs of associated accidents.

PITFALLS AND CONTROVERSIES

Diagnosis

Expertise in interpreting test results in the patient's clinical context is critical. Clinicians must be aware of the limits of the tests they use and of the differential diagnosis. Pulmonary physicians must always consider the full differential diagnosis when managing sleepy patients and not see the question as "is this, or is this not, OSAHS?" Confusion has arisen from the term "upper airways resistance syndrome"—an ill-defined

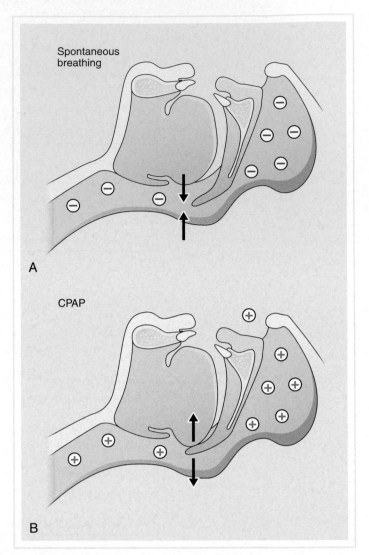

FIGURE 75-12 Schematic diagram of suction causing apneas **(A)** and CPAP blowing the upper airway open **(B)**.

condition, most "cases" of which result from the use of inappropriate technology and would otherwise be diagnosed as OSAHS.

Anesthetic Risk

Patients with OSAHS are at increased risk perioperatively, because their upper airway may obstruct during the recovery period or as a consequence of sedation. Patients who anesthesiologists find difficult to intubate are much more likely to have irregular breathing during sleep. Anesthesiologists should thus take sleep histories on all patients preoperatively and take the appropriate precautions with those who might have OSAHS. This should include referring all suspected of having OSAHS for investigation, and some operations may need to be delayed until the OSAHS is treated.

OSAHS Coexisting with Other Respiratory Diseases

The prevalence of OSAHS in patients with respiratory disease is similar to that in the general population, 2–4% in men and 1–2% in women. These patients typically have the classical

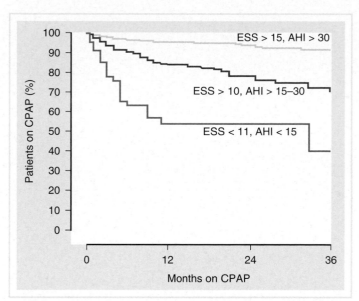

FIGURE 75-13 Effect of sleepiness (Epworth sleepiness score [ESS]) and AHI on the percentage of patients continuing to use CPAP. (Adapted from McArdle: Am J Resp Crit Care Med 1999; 159: 1108–1114 with permission.)

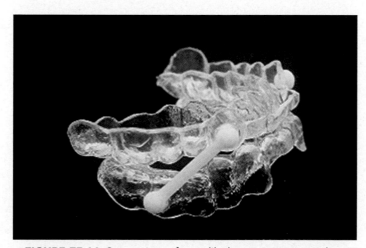

FIGURE 75-14 One variety of mandibular repositioning splint.

symptoms of OSAHS, and when they do, should be investigated and treated as previously with the following warnings. First, patients who are hypoxemic when awake will desaturate during sleep, especially during REM sleep, thus oximetry alone cannot be used to diagnose OSAHS in such patients—some measure of breathing pattern must be recorded. Second, there is no evidence that patients found to desaturate markedly during sleep but do not have OSAHS should be treated differently than others with the same daytime blood gas tensions. Third, there is some evidence that patients with symptomatic OSAHS plus COPD who are hypoxemic during sleep improve their pulmonary arterial pressure more when their OSAHS is treated than when they receive oxygen therapy alone. For this reason, as well as for the relief of OSAHS symptoms, it is vital to check a sleep history in all hypoxemic patients.

OSAHS Coexisting with Heart Failure

Central sleep apnea has received more attention than OSAHS in heart failure. However, several recent studies have suggested that OSAHS is a more common association and that treatment of the coexisting OSAHS may benefit cardiac function and quality of life. Although the magnitude of this benefit is not yet clear, sleep histories should be taken in this group, and treatment for OSAHS considered when appropriate.

WEB RESOURCES FOR GUIDELINES/PROTOCOLS

Management of obstructive sleep apnea/hypopnea syndrome. Guideline No.73 www.sign.ac.uk/guidelines/fulltext/73/index.html.

SUGGESTED READINGS

Babu AR, Herdegen J, Fogelfeld L, *et al*: Type 2 diabetes, glycemic control, and continuous positive airway pressure in obstructive sleep apnea. Arch Intern Med 2005; 165:447–452.

Barbe F, Mayoralas LR, Duran J, *et al*: Treatment with continuous positive airway pressure is not effective in patients with sleep apnea but no daytime sleepiness: a randomized, controlled trial. Ann Intern Med 2001; 134:1015–1023.

Cross M, Vennelle M, Engleman HM, *et al*: Comparison of CPAP titration at home or the sleep laboratory in the sleep apnea hypopnea syndrome. Sleep 2006; 29:1451–1455.

Douglas NJ: Clinicians' guide to sleep medicine. London: Arnold; 2002.

Douglas NJ: Home diagnosis of the obstructive sleep apnoea/hypopnoea syndrome. Sleep Med Rev 2003; 7:53–59.

Engleman HM, McDonald JP, Graham D, *et al*: Randomized crossover trial of two treatments for sleep apnea/hypopnea syndrome: continuous positive airway pressure and mandibular repositioning splint. Am J Respir Crit Care Med 2002; 165:855–859.

Gotsopoulos H, Kelly JJ, Cistulli PA: Oral appliance therapy reduces blood pressure in obstructive sleep apnea: a randomized, controlled trial. Sleep 2004; 24:934–941.

Marin JM, Carrizo SJ, Vicente E, *et al*: Long-term cardiovascular outcomes in men with obstructive sleep apnoea/hypopnoea with or without treatment with continuous positive airway pressure: an observational study. Lancet 2005; 365:1046–1053.

Sundaram S, Bridgman SA, Lim J, *et al*: Surgery for obstructive sleep apnoea. Cochrane Database Syst Rev CD001004, 2005.

Yaggi HK, Concato J, Kernan WN, *et al*: Obstructive sleep apnea as a risk factor for stroke and death. N Engl J Med 2005; 353:2034–2041.

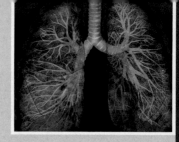

76 Central Sleep Apnea and Other Forms of Sleep-Disordered Breathing

PATRICK J. STROLLO, JR • CHARLES W. ATWOOD, JR

EPIDEMIOLOGY

Central sleep apnea occurs in between 5 and 10% of all patients who have sleep-disordered breathing (SDB). The primary or idiopathic form of central sleep apnea is less common than secondary causes such as congestive heart failure or neurologic conditions such as cerebrovascular disease. Central sleep apnea has been reported to occur in approximately 40–50% of patients with advanced heart failure.

RISK FACTORS

Risk factors include congestive heart failure, neurologic disease, chronic opioid therapy (in particular methadone), and ascent to high altitude (particularly in individuals who have spent little previous time at altitudes higher than 2500 m). In patients with congestive heart failure, male gender, atrial fibrillation, hypocapnia, and advancing age all increase the risk of central sleep apnea.

PATHOPHYSIOLOGY

Transient withdrawal of central respiratory drive to respiratory muscles results in central sleep apnea; this mechanism occurs in a number of ways (Table 76-1). In considering the pathophysiology of central sleep apnea, three subtypes can be described: hypercapnic central sleep apnea, hypocapnic central sleep apnea, and sleep-onset apnea.

Hypercapnic Central Sleep Apnea

Hypercapnic central sleep apnea results from central hypoventilation in which breathing during wakefulness is usually normal, although daytime hypercapnia can occur. Neuromuscular diseases such as postpolio syndrome, muscular and myotonic dystrophies, acid maltase deficiency, and amyotrophic lateral sclerosis are included in this category.

Patients receiving chronic pain medication or methadone maintenance for heroin addiction are at risk from this form of central sleep apnea. These patients may exhibit a central apneic breathing pattern that differs from the characteristic Cheyne–Stokes respiration seen in hypocapnic central sleep apnea associated with congestive heart failure (Figure 76-1).

Hypocapnic Central Sleep Apnea

Hypocapnic central sleep apnea can be idiopathic as well as associated with congestive heart failure and neurologic disease.

As for other forms of central sleep apnea, pathophysiologic mechanisms are not clearly understood, but it is highly dependent on a decreased arterial partial pressure of carbon dioxide ($Paco_2$). Intrinsic properties of the respiratory control system are the most important factors in predisposition to central sleep apnea. Central sleep apnea associated with congestive heart failure is characterized by a crescendo-decrescendo pattern of breathing referred to as Cheyne–Stokes respiration (Figure 76-1).

Sleep-Onset Apnea

A third form of central sleep apnea is that seen at the time of sleep onset in normal humans. Central apneas may arise during the transition between wakefulness and sleep because of transient instabilities in respiratory drive in normal subjects. The mechanism of this form of central sleep apnea is similar to that of the hypocapnic form associated with congestive heart failure. The level of $Paco_2$ is the main determinant for respiratory drive in the sleeping human.

Finally, the sensitivity of the arousal mechanism in central sleep apnea is important. In all forms of central sleep apnea, if an arousal does not occur, the cycle of apneas and arousals is broken. In sleep-onset central sleep apnea associated with insomnia, sedative medications may be useful in increasing the arousal threshold and decreasing sleep-onset arousal. The role of such medications in practice is unclear because of the potential for dependence, concern about precipitating falls in a frail population, and the potential for worsening any underlying obstructive sleep apnea (OSA).

CLINICAL FEATURES

Hypercapnia associated with central sleep apnea is usually the result of a central hypoventilation disorder, chronic opioid use, or neuromuscular respiratory disease. Affected patients may have a diminished sensation of dyspnea associated with respiratory insufficiency and hypercapnia, although patients who have neuromuscular respiratory disease may complain of dyspnea as the condition progresses. Restless sleep, daytime somnolence, and morning headache may be seen in all forms of hypercapnic central sleep apnea. Right-sided heart failure and secondary polycythemia may develop at an advanced stage. Overt respiratory failure that requires mechanical ventilation is occasionally the presenting complaint and usually occurs after another medical problem, such as bronchitis or pneumonia, has

TABLE 76-1 Mechanisms of Central Sleep Apnea	
Mechanism	**Clinical Example**
Central hypoventilation	Primary central hypoventilation Brainstem infarction Encephalitis Arnold–Chiari malformation Chronic opioid treatment
Neuromuscular respiratory dysfunction	Muscular dystrophy Spinal atrophy Amyotrophic lateral sclerosis Acid maltase deficiency
Instability of central respiratory drive	Sleep onset (transient instability) Hyperventilation-induced hypocapnia Hypoxia (pulmonary disease, high altitude) Congestive heart failure Disorders of the central nervous system Chronic opioid treatment

disrupted the existing physiologic homeostasis. The symptoms of central sleep apnea and OSA may differ (Table 76-2).

Patients who have eucapnic or hypocapnic forms of central sleep apnea are typically older, have a more normal body weight, and have coexistent cardiac or neurologic diseases. This holds true for the idiopathic form and secondary forms associated with congestive heart failure. Affected patients tend to hyperventilate during wakefulness, and, therefore, the $PaCO_2$ is lower than that in patients who have congestive heart failure without central sleep apnea. Symptoms of insomnia, nocturnal dyspnea, and daytime sleepiness (because of sleep fragmentation and frequent arousals) are common, although daytime hypersomnia is less frequent in this group of patients.

DIAGNOSIS

Regardless of the type of central sleep apnea, a high clinical suspicion is essential for its diagnosis. Objective assessment of the breathing pattern during sleep with polysomnography can confirm the diagnosis (see Figure 76-1). Central apneas are distinguished from obstructive apneas by the lack of respiratory effort during the apnea. Examples of central sleep apnea associated with sleep onset and Cheyne–Stokes respirations are shown in Figure 76-1. The potential for underlying cardiovascular and cerebrovascular disease must be assessed. An approach to the diagnostic evaluation and management is outlined in Figure 76-2.

TREATMENT

Treatment options for central sleep apnea include supplemental oxygen, nasal continuous positive airway pressure (CPAP), bilevel positive airway pressure (BPAP), respiratory stimulant medications, and a combination of these.

If the hypercapnic central sleep apnea results from central hypoventilation or neuromuscular respiratory conditions, the patient benefits most from nocturnal ventilatory assistance, which may be carried out through a tracheostomy or non-invasively by mask ventilation. Patients should avoid benzo-diazepines, narcotics, and other sedatives that may suppress respiratory drive.

Supplemental oxygen is useful for alleviating nocturnal hypoxemia, provided it does not induce hypercapnia. This may be of particular concern in central sleep apnea associated with neuromuscular disease. The optimal treatment for non-hypercapnic central sleep apnea has not been defined. Treatment of the underlying cause (e.g., congestive heart failure) is the first step. Therapy can also include supplemental oxygen, respiratory stimulants, and positive-pressure therapy. At present, supplemental oxygen therapy is the mainstay of therapy, because it "stabilizes" the respiratory control centers, although the mechanisms by which this is accomplished are not clear. Acetazolamide has been used successfully to alleviate abnormal respiratory patterns in altitude sickness. Its mechanism of action is to induce a mild degree of metabolic acidosis and increase respiratory drive by inducing a bicarbonate diuresis.

Clinically important improvements in left ventricular function have resulted from CPAP in patients with congestive heart failure, but the number of such patients treated successfully with CPAP is small. In one study, the benefit of CPAP therapy was limited to the group of patients who had higher (>1.6 kPa [>12 mmHg]) pulmonary capillary wedge pressures (PCWPs). By contrast, the lower PCWP group (<1.6 kPa [<12 mmHg]) showed a reduction in cardiac index. The mechanism by which CPAP improves central sleep apnea seems related to its improvement in oxygen saturation and a slight elevation in $PaCO_2$, which moves arterial $PaCO_2$ away from the apnea threshold.

CLINICAL COURSE

When central sleep apnea results from another condition, such as congestive heart failure, the clinical outcome is in part related to the severity of the underlying disorder. It is currently unclear whether central sleep apnea–Cheyne–Stokes respiration (CSA/CSR) is merely a marker of inadequately treated congestive heart failure or is an independent risk factor for mortality. Regardless, the finding of central sleep apnea–Cheyne–Stokes respiration has been associated with an increased mortality risk. A recent prospective randomized trial failed to demonstrate a survival advantage in patients with CSA/CSR treated with CPAP.

In most cases, treatment of central sleep apnea, whether with positive-pressure ventilation, respiratory stimulants, supplemental oxygen, or a combination of these therapies, improves clinical symptoms. If severely fragmented sleep can be consolidated and nocturnal dyspnea prevented, the patient almost certainly benefits from the therapy.

PITFALLS AND CONTROVERSIES

Compared with OSA, primary (idiopathic) central sleep apnea is uncommon. Central sleep apnea–Cheyne–Stokes respiration is frequently encountered in patients with advanced congestive heart failure. In advanced congestive heart failure, both OSA and central sleep apnea are frequently not considered. The current data suggest that treatment with CPAP improves symptoms but not survival in patients with advanced heart failure and central sleep apnea–Cheyne–Stokes respiration. Patients who are chronically treated with opioids are at risk for central sleep apnea. One recent report suggests that up to 30% of patients in methadone maintenance programs may be affected. Acid maltase deficiency (Pompe's disease) is one of the few

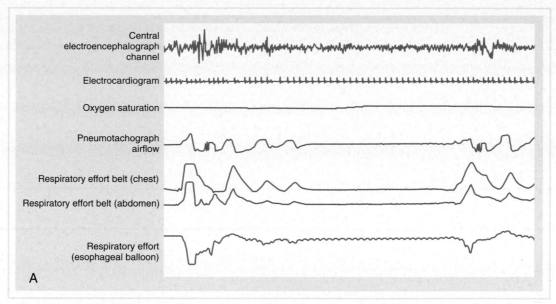

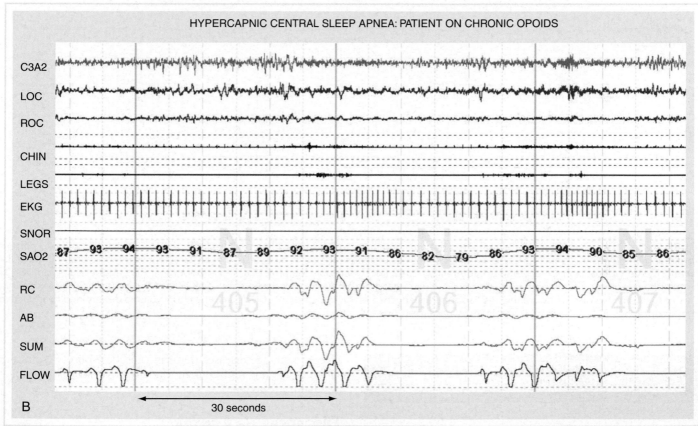

FIGURE 76-1 A, Example of central sleep apnea polysomnography. The sleep epoch shown is 30 sec. The patient is awake at the beginning of the tracing. A sleep-onset central apnea, characterized by absence of airflow and respiratory effort, occurs as stage 1 sleep is entered. An arousal at the end of the epoch ends the apnea. **B,** Hypercapnic central sleep apnea in a patient receiving chronic opioids. Note the lack of airflow associated with no effort in the inductance plethysmography channels (RC, AB, and SUM).

(Continued)

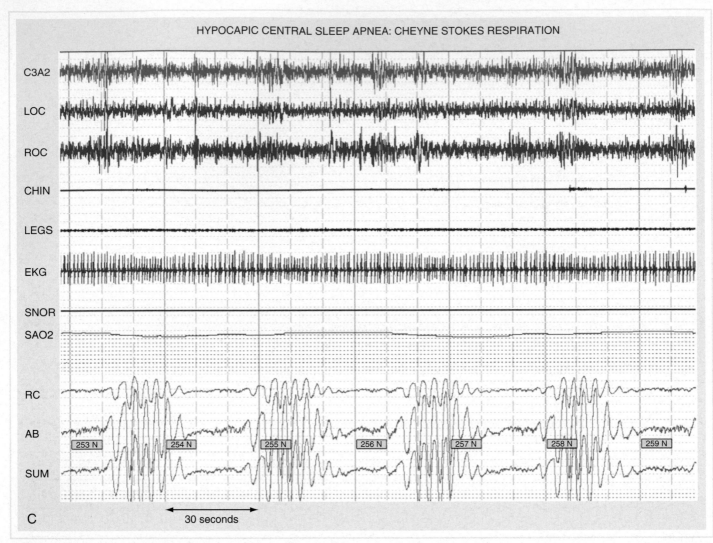

FIGURE 76-1 cont'd, C, Hypocapnic central sleep apnea in a patient with advanced heart failure Note the crescendo-decrescendo pattern of breathing in the effort channels (RC, AB, and SUM). Periods of central apnea are seen after these characteristic periodic breathing events. In **B** and **C,** the type of signals recorded are identified: C3A2 (electroencephalogram), LOC (left oculogram), ROC (right oculogram, CHIN (chin electromyogram), LEGS (right and left tibialis electromyogram), EKG (electrocardiogram), SNOR (snoring sensor), SAO₂ (oximetry), RC (rib cage inductive plethysmography), AB (abdominal inductive plethysmography), SUM (qualitative tidal volume determined by inductive plethysmography), FLOW (airflow determined by nasal pressure—**B** only).

TABLE 76-2 Signs and Symptoms of Central Sleep Apnea Versus Obstructive Sleep Apnea

Sign or Symptom	Central Sleep Apnea	Obstructive Sleep Apnea
Daytime sleepiness	Variable	Yes
Restless sleep	Yes	Yes
Snoring	No	Yes
Nocturnal choking	No	Yes
Nocural dyspnea	Variable	Variable
Morning headache	Variable	Variable
Insomnia	Yes	Variable
Nocturnal desaturation	Yes	Yes
Hypercapnia	Variable	Variable

glycogen storage diseases that can cause late-onset respiratory failure. Enzyme replacement therapy may favorably impact ventilatory function.

DISORDERS OF CENTRAL HYPOVENTILATION

Disorders of central hypoventilation constitute a heterogeneous and uncommon group of disorders characterized by the inability of the central respiratory centers to provide adequate output to the respiratory pump. The hallmark of this disorder is hypercapnia. Effective treatment involves ventilatory support to optimize gas exchange and improve quality of life.

Epidemiology and Risk Factors

Table 76-3 lists the conditions associated with central hypoventilation.

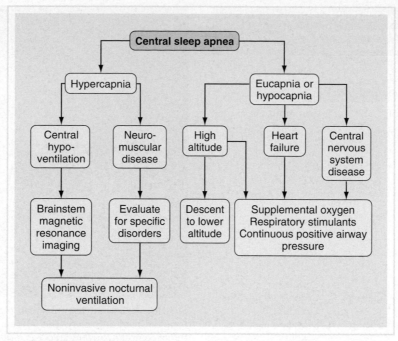

FIGURE 76-2 Evaluation and management of central sleep apnea.

TABLE 76-3	Classification of Disorders of Central Hypoventilation
Types of Neuron	**Disorder**
Brainstem motoneurons	Primary central hypoventilation
	Congenital malformations (Chiari malformations; syringomyelia)
	Trauma
	Infarction
	Encephalitis
	Tumors
	Chronic metabolic alkalosis
	Multiple sclerosis
	Sarcoidosis
Spinal neurons	Poliomyelitis
	High cervical cord trauma

Trauma accounts for most spinal cord injuries and is the leading cause of central hypoventilation, with approximately 10,000 new cervical spinal injuries occurring each year in the United States. In addition, the prevalence of this disorder is approximately 1 in 400,000.

Although no longer a public health or important clinical problem in the developed world, poliomyelitis continues to be a significant public health problem in developing nations. Patients who have chronic ventilatory failure from the polio epidemics in the 1950s still require treatment. Syringomyelia with or without Chiari malformations (types I and II) is an example of a congenital brain lesion that may result in central hypoventilation. Brain injury and neuronal loss from acute encephalitis, multiple sclerosis, and multiple system atrophy (Shy–Drager syndrome) are examples of rare acquired disorders that may lead to central hypoventilation. Structural lesions caused by brainstem infarctions or neoplasms or after encephalitis are rare but are the most common nontraumatic causes. These conditions result in severe clinical sequelae,

and the outcomes tend to be poor. Neurologic conditions, such as multiple sclerosis, multiple system atrophy, or demyelinating disorders, can result in clinically significant hypoventilation, but respiratory failure is rare.

Pathophysiology

Central hypoventilation can occur as a congenital disorder in the first several hours of life or as an acquired disorder in adulthood, usually as the result of significant brainstem injury. The basic defect is the inability to transduce afferent input from central and/or peripheral chemoreceptors into the efferent limb of the respiratory system. Flat or very decreased respiratory responses to respiratory chemostimuli, such as hypercapnia and hypoxia, may occur. The sleeping state, characterized by the transition from the behavioral control of ventilation to the metabolic control of ventilation, results in more profound gas exchange abnormalities.

Clinical Features

Hypercapnia and hypoxemia are the hallmark signs of central hypoventilation syndromes, regardless of the cause. Hypercapnia can range from mild ($P_{CO_2} < 6.6$ kPa [<50 mmHg]) to severe ($P_{CO_2} > 8.5$ kPa [>65 mmHg]). Symptoms may also include progressive lethargy and easy fatigability, daytime hypersomnia, and headache. Dyspnea is variable but is generally not a prominent complaint in central hypoventilation. The symptom of dyspnea may help differentiate patients with central hypoventilation from those with hypoventilation caused by neuromuscular disease (Table 76-4).

Diagnosis

The diagnosis of central hypoventilation is made after other possible explanations, such as neuromuscular respiratory failure, have been excluded by history, physical examination, and/or additional physiologic tests. Patients affected by central hypoventilation have impaired ventilatory responses to hypoxia and hypercapnia.

TABLE 76-4 Comparison of Clinical Features of Central Hypoventilation and Neuromuscular Disease

Clinical Feature	Central Hypoventilation	Neuromuscular Respiratory Disease
Frequency	Uncommon	Common
Ages affected	Infants through adults	Primarily adults
Hypercapnia	Yes	Yes
Hypoxia	Yes	Yes
Dyspnea	No	Yes
Respiratory mechanics	Normal	Impaired
Ability to hyperventilate	Normal	Impaired
Therapy	Oxygen Chronic ventilatory support Diaphragm pacing	Oxygen Chronic ventilatory support Disease-modifying drugs

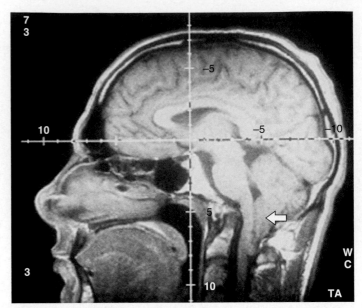

FIGURE 76-3 Contrast-enhanced magnetic resonance image of an Arnold–Chiari deformity. This 21-year-old man has progressive, nocturnal central hypoventilation as a result of the Chiari type 1 malformation demonstrated. Note the cerebellar tonsil descent into the spinal canal with impingement of brainstem structures (arrow).

Physiologic Tests

By measuring ventilatory sensitivity to hypercapnia and hypoxic ventilatory sensitivity, respiratory rate, tidal volume, minute ventilation, inspiratory flow rates, and mouth occlusion pressures in the first 0.1 sec of inspiratory activity (P0.1) can be plotted against progressively higher levels of carbon dioxide or progressively lower oxygen saturation over time. Increases in respiratory rate and minute ventilation occur in response to the ventilatory stimulus given, but the variability in these measurements in normal subjects is considerable. If a response curve with a markedly shallow slope is found, insensitivity to ventilatory stimulants is determined, and central hypoventilation must be considered.

Voluntary Hyperventilation

To distinguish between central and peripheral causes of hypoventilation, the ability to hyperventilate voluntarily and decrease carbon dioxide by 1.3 kPa (10 mmHg) or more can be measured. In central hypoventilation, maximal voluntary hyperventilation is accomplished easily for short periods of time, because the respiratory pump is not affected. If the cause of hypoventilation is peripheral (e.g., respiratory muscle weakness), the patient may be unable to lower the carbon dioxide by voluntary hyperpnea.

Imaging Studies

Magnetic resonance imaging (MRI) is the procedure of choice for imaging the brainstem and upper spinal cord. Contrast enhancement may be necessary to detect arteriovenous malformations or other small, critically placed lesions. Congenital malformations, such as Chiari malformations or a syrinx, are shown very well by MRI (Figure 76-3).

Treatment

Treatment of central hypoventilation depends on its severity, degree of impairment of other systems (e.g., level of mental status, degree of muscle paralysis), and the patient's willingness to use what may be lifelong supportive therapy, such as home ventilation or diaphragmatic pacing.

Treatment for milder cases includes ventilatory stimulants, such as progesterone and methylxanthines, which may successfully delay progression of ventilatory insufficiency. Supplemental oxygen therapy is important for all patients who have documented hypoxemia and may reduce the severity of complications such as secondary polycythemia, pulmonary hypertension, and heart failure and retard progression in respiratory insufficiency.

The rationale for diaphragmatic pacing is that electric stimulation of the muscle, either directly or by the phrenic nerve, substitutes for the intrinsic respiratory-center output. Newer approaches involve laparoscopic implantation of the pacemaker (Figure 76-4). However, an intact phrenic nerve and a tracheostomy are required to offset upper airway obstruction during sleep. Considerable commitment from the patient and medical team is required for this approach to work optimally. However, the estimated savings of diaphragm pacing compared with chronic mechanical ventilation is projected to be $13,000 (U.S. dollars) per month. One such device is now approved by the US Food and Drug Administration (FDA) for implantation. Full FDA approval is expected in the next year. Ideal candidates are patients with respiratory failure because of high cervical spinal cord injuries. Trials are underway in amyotrophic lateral sclerosis (ALS) as an intervention to slow progression of respiratory failure by conditioning the diaphragm with electrical stimulation. The preliminary data in patients with ALS is promising.

Nocturnal Ventilation

Nocturnal ventilation augments gas exchange during sleep, a time of increased vulnerability of the respiratory system because of the normal hypoventilation associated with sleep. Nocturnal

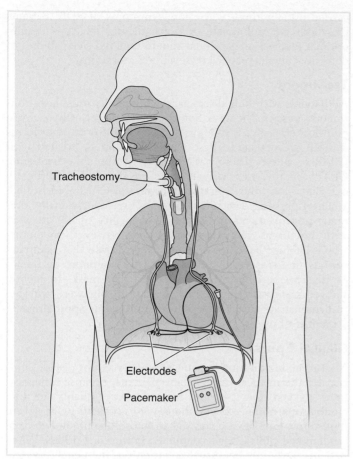

FIGURE 76-4 Diaphragmatic pacemaker. Note that electrodes placed on the phrenic nerve motor points on both leaflets of the diaphragm. Older diaphragm pacemakers involved placing bilateral leads on the neck to capture the phrenic nerves. A tracheostomy is required to offset the possibility of upper airway obstruction because of dyssynchrony of the diaphragm and upper airway dilator muscles.

ventilation can be invasive or noninvasive, and the aims are to rest ventilatory muscles and to improve gas exchange.

Invasive Ventilation

Invasive nocturnal ventilation requires a tracheostomy. Before the development of noninvasive ventilation techniques that use facemasks, invasive ventilation was standard treatment. Because effective noninvasive techniques are now available, the need for a permanent tracheostomy in the management of chronic ventilatory insufficiency has decreased.

Noninvasive Ventilation

Ventilation of patients without the need for a surgical airway can be accomplished by use of either a negative- or positive-pressure system. Negative-pressure systems, such as an iron lung or a cuirass, were the first type of noninvasive ventilators, and their main advantage over positive-pressure ventilators is that a nasal or oronasal mask, which some patients find uncomfortable, is not needed. Many disadvantages exist, however. Negative-pressure ventilators are usually uncomfortable, bulky, and cumbersome, and assistance climbing in and out of them is also sometimes required. The most important

problem is that such ventilators tend to induce upper airway collapse and thus cause OSA.

Positive-pressure, noninvasive ventilators are now the mainstay of nocturnal ventilation. They are small, easily portable, and relatively inexpensive. Both pressure-cycled and volume-cycled versions are available. Which type of positive-pressure ventilator to choose is less important than the ability of the patient to learn to successfully use it.

Noninvasive nocturnal positive-pressure ventilation may improve daytime hypersomnia, daytime gas exchange, and secondary polycythemia. It may delay the need for a tracheostomy in patients who have progressive hypoventilation disorders, and it eliminates the need for tracheostomy in patients who have stable forms of hypoventilation, depending on other factors such as secretion control. Swallowing and speech are preserved, which enhances quality of life.

Long-Term Ventilatory Support

In patients with severely compromised ventilatory function and in those who have difficulty clearing secretions, supplemental ventilatory support may be required long term if the patient desires to live with his or her disease. In cases of encephalitis, brainstem infarction, or arteriovenous malformations that affect the brainstem respiratory centers, nocturnal ventilation alone may not be a viable option; permanent, continuous ventilatory support may be needed. Permanent tracheostomy with mechanical ventilatory support is indicated here. Patients who receive continuous ventilator therapy at home require extensive support from family and outside caregivers. Nonetheless, reasonable quality of life can be achieved for motivated patients and their families.

Clinical Course

The clinical course is variable and depends on the cause and severity of the hypoventilation, its complications, and other comorbidities. The age of onset of primary central hypoventilation ranges from infancy in congenital cases to the seventh decade of life. The average age of onset is about the third to fourth decade. In one case series, half of the 30 cases were acquired. Causes include encephalitis, meningitis, Parkinsonism, syringomyelia, vascular malformation, and mental retardation.

Congenital brainstem abnormalities, such as Chiari malformations (see Figure 76-3), have a prognosis that depends on the degree of neurologic damage associated with the descent of cerebellar tissue into the upper spinal canal, the degree of medullary and spinal cord compression, and associated neurologic conditions such as hydrocephalus or meningocele. These may be detected in infancy or adulthood. Central apnea occurs as a result of impingement of the brainstem respiratory centers at the foramen magnum.

Secondary Causes of Central Hypoventilation

Only a minority of patients who have poliomyelitis have the paralytic form develop. Survivors of the outbreaks in the 1950s are still alive, and some require permanent home-ventilator support. The postpolio syndrome is a late complication that is manifested by progressive muscle weakness, fatigue, and joint pain after 20–40 years of stability. How often this leads to respiratory muscle dysfunction is not known, but a heightened index of suspicion for this late complication must be maintained.

In a population-based sample of 358 patients with spinal cord injuries, the case fatality rate was less than 4%. Of patients with cervical cord injuries, 36% experienced neurologic improvement compared with the initial severity of injury, and more than 95% of all patients who had spinal cord injury were discharged home. Unfortunately, respiratory dysfunction remains a significant problem for most patients with cervical cord injury, despite improvement in other areas of function.

The outcome after other central nervous system (CNS) injuries, such as severe encephalitis, infarctions that involve the brainstem respiratory centers, and CNS neoplasms, is usually poor. Involvement of the reticular activating system may result in permanent coma, and patients with such disorders and their family members must be involved in discussions about therapy, because often the only therapy is support with chronic mechanical ventilation.

Complications of Central Hypoventilation

Complications of central hypoventilation include pulmonary hypertension, secondary polycythemia, right- and left-sided heart failure, and respiratory failure. Complications related to treatment of this disorder, such as ventilator-associated lung and bronchial infections, must be considered as well.

Pitfalls and Controversies

Disorders of central hypoventilation are rare and easily missed, and their pathophysiology is poorly understood. Central hypoventilation may be primary and/or congenital or secondary and/or acquired. Development of these disorders typically occurs after a serious brain injury, a severe encephalitis, a neoplasm, or an infarction of the area of the respiratory centers of the medulla. Congenital cases of pure central hypoventilation may also occur, albeit rarely. The prognosis associated with these conditions is poor. Nonetheless, successful clinical management with either noninvasive ventilation or ventilation through a permanent tracheostomy is possible.

Sleep-Disordered Breathing in Chronic Lung Disease

Epidemiology

Poor sleep is a common complaint with chronic obstructive pulmonary disease (COPD). Most patients do not have OSA, but a fraction have oxygen desaturations less than 85%. The size of the subpopulation of these patients who have nocturnal desaturation is unknown, because measurements of nocturnal oxygen saturation are not routinely carried out.

Risk Factors

Risk factors for nocturnal hypoxemia include severity and type of pulmonary disease, amount of rapid eye movement sleep over the course of a night, and body weight. Patients who have obstructive airway disease seem to be at greater risk of nocturnal desaturation than patients with interstitial disease. If thoracic wall or neuromuscular disease or diaphragmatic paralysis is also present, nocturnal hypoxemia is likely to be worse for a given degree of COPD.

Diagnosis

Detection of SDB in patients who have COPD and other forms of lung disease is important, and sleep studies must be carried out for those who show symptoms of SDB. Patients in whom cor pulmonale or polycythemia develops despite optimal medical management should undergo sleep studies to detect occult sleep apnea or severe desaturations.

Treatment

All patients with lung disease and who qualify must have continuous oxygen therapy. Some centers empirically increase liter flow by 1 or 2 L/min during sleep. If OSA or other forms of SDB are detected, these patients should be treated with CPAP or BPAP. These patients may not be able to tolerate CPAP therapy, especially if the OSA is mild. If difficulty exhaling against the expiratory pressures of CPAP is identified, a bilevel pressure device may be an option. Occasionally, dramatic improvements in dyspnea and quality of life are seen with nocturnal ventilatory assistance; however, predicting who is likely to benefit is difficult. Clinical trials that examined various methods of nocturnal ventilatory support by use of positive-pressure breathing delivered by mask frequently showed positive results in the short term but were not able to demonstrate sustained positive results after approximately 3 months of use.

Clinical Course

Nocturnal desaturation in patients who have lung disease complicates the medical care of these patients, because it necessitates oxygen therapy and may decrease quality of life. Continuous home oxygen therapy for patients with severe hypoxemic lung disease was shown to prolong life in two large randomized clinical trials conducted in the early 1980s. When patients have only nocturnal desaturation, the benefit of oxygen therapy is less clear. One study compared survival over an average of 70 months between two groups of patients with COPD, one of which had less than the expected amount of nocturnal desaturation, whereas the other had greater than the expected amount of nocturnal desaturation. No major differences in survival were detected.

The combination of OSA and COPD can be debilitating and has been termed the *overlap syndrome*. Cor pulmonale, chronic respiratory insufficiency, and secondary polycythemia characterize this syndrome. Treatment is directed at both disorders, with the chief aim being to maintain normal oxygen saturation. Noninvasive ventilation is considered not only for treatment of OSA, but also for treatment of respiratory insufficiency and hypercapnia. Without therapy, affected patients are expected to have a high degree of morbidity and early mortality.

Pitfalls and Controversies

The greatest management error is the failure to consider sleep-related breathing disturbance in patients with COPD. In overlap patients, treatment of OSA can improve pulmonary hypertension, and favorably affect nighttime and daytime arterial blood gases and right-sided heart failure. Controversy exists whether low-flow oxygen prolongs survival in patients who only experience nocturnal desaturation.

SUGGESTED READINGS

Botelho RV, Bittencourt LR, Rotta JM, et al: Adult Chiari malformation and sleep apnoea. Neurosurg Rev 2005; 28:169–176.
Bradley TD, Logan AG, Kimoff RJ, et al: Continuous positive airway pressure for central sleep apnea and heart failure. N Engl J Med 2005; 353:2025–2033.

DiMarco AF: Restoration of respiratory muscle function following spinal cord injury. Review of electrical and magnetic stimulation techniques. Respir Physiol Neurobiol 2005; 147:273–287.

Pellegrini N, Laforet P, Orlikowski D, *et al*: Respiratory insufficiency and limb muscle weakness in adults with Pompe's disease. Eur Respir J 2005; 26:1024–1031.

Simonds AK: Recent advances in respiratory care for neuromuscular disease. Chest 2006; 130:1879–1886.

Wang D, Teichtahl H, Drummer O, *et al*: Central sleep apnea in stable methadone maintenance treatment patients. Chest 2005; 128: 1348–1356.

Weitzenblum E, Chaouat A: Sleep and chronic obstructive pulmonary disease. [see comment]. Sleep Med Rev 2004; 8:281–294.

White DP: Pathogenesis of obstructive and central sleep apnea. Am J Respir Crit Care Med 2005; 172:1363–1370.

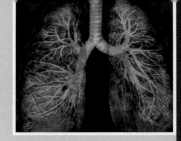

77 Drugs and the Lungs

PHILIPPE CAMUS • DOROTHY A. WHITE

Many drugs can cause adverse reactions in the respiratory system, including the lung, upper and/or lower airways, pulmonary circulation, mediastinum, pleural cavities, neuromuscular system and the hemoglobin carrier, causing distinct clinical-imaging-pathologic pictures. Drugs can also cause systemic conditions, for example, the drug-induced *lupus* or vasculitis, which may also involve the lung.

Underlying mechanisms involved include:

1. Drug—drug reactive metabolite (including reactive oxygen species)—and drug + protein (hapten)-induced inflammation of lung, airway, or pleura with consequent edema and driving of inflammatory cells toward the corresponding tissue
2. Changes in endothelial permeability, with consequent efflux of fluid ± proteins in lung tissues
3. Smooth muscle contraction, with consequent bronchospasm
4. Switching on mechanisms for fibrogenesis and/or remodeling in lung, airways, and pulmonary vasculature, leading to pulmonary fibrosis, *bronchiolitis obliterans*, pulmonary hypertension, or pulmonary venoocclusive disease, respectively
5. Abnormal deposition of fat
6. Uncontrolled bleeding

The list of causal drugs grows longer as complications are linked to novel antineoplastic agents (e.g., gefitinib), monoclonal antibody therapy against TNF-α (e.g., infliximab), soluble TNF-α receptors (e.g., etanercept), receptors on neoplastic cells (e.g., imatinib against the CD20 epitope), platelet glycoprotein IIb/IIIa receptors (e.g., abciximab), and vascular endothelial growth factor receptor (i.e., bevacizumab). Therefore, patients with a background of solid tumors or hematologic malignancies, rheumatoid arthritis, autoimmune conditions, and heart disease are particularly at risk.

The level of evidence for the iatrogenic etiology varies with drug, patient, and clinical context. Strong evidence may exist in simple case reports when there is a characteristic temporal association with exposure to the drug or relapse occurs after rechallenge. Evidence is strengthened in the absence of a basic condition that may involve the lung. Strong evidence may also come from randomized studies, when the incidence of pneumonitis is greater in exposed versus unexposed subjects. Occasionally, the histopathologic appearances of the lung are distinctive enough to suggest the drug etiology, as for instance in amiodarone pulmonary toxicity or exogenous lipoid pneumonia.

Recognition that a pulmonary problem has been caused by administration of a drug is of importance for several reasons. First, unnecessary invasive evaluation and treatment for other conditions can usually be avoided, pending results of a dechallenge test. Second, further damage can usually be prevented if use of the offending agent is stopped early and, in some cases, if corticosteroid therapy is offered. Finally, measures should be taken to not reexpose the patient to the suspect drug. Diagnosing drug-induced respiratory disease is difficult because (1) drug reactions often are against the background of possible pulmonary involvement from the underlying condition for which the drug was being administered, and pulmonary involvement from the underlying disease can mimic drug-induced disease and vice versa. (2) Not uncommonly, patients are exposed to several drugs that may all cause lung disease, and causality must be assessed for each specific agent. (3) Patients treated with immune suppressants may have an opportunistic pulmonary infection develop, with no real discriminator with drug-induced pneumonitis, and an infection must be ruled out in every patient before a diagnosis of drug-induced lung disease is entertained.

It is also important to diagnose drug-induced respiratory disease *reliably*, because inappropriate drug therapy withdrawal, for instance of amiodarone in severe cardiac arrhythmias or of antineoplastic chemotherapy in patients with solid tumors or hematologic malignancies, may negatively impact the outcomes of these basic conditions.

The list of drugs causing respiratory disease includes nearly 400 distinct compounds, and almost any route of administration may expose to the risk. Discussion of each drug is beyond the scope of this chapter. Here, the focus is on general patterns of drug-induced respiratory injury and on selected drugs that produce distinctive pulmonary toxicity. The particulars or radiation-induced lung injury can be found elsewhere.

PATTERNS OF PRESENTATION

Parenchymal Patterns

Classic Interstitial Pneumonitis— "Hypersensitivity Pneumonitis"

This group of conditions can be caused by numerous drugs, including fludarabine, gold, imatinib, methotrexate, nitrofurantoin, and sirolimus. Drug-induced interstitial pneumonia is characterized by an acute (e.g., methotrexate, gold) or subacute (e.g., nitrofurantoin, sirolimus) presentation. Systemic symptoms, such as fever, fatigue, myalgias, and arthralgias, can be present as early manifestations of the disease, followed by dry cough and shortness of breath. Chest radiographs and high-resolution computed tomography (HRCT) (Figures 77-1 and 77-2) typically show disseminated linear interlobular or intralobular shadows and ground-glass or mosaic opacities.

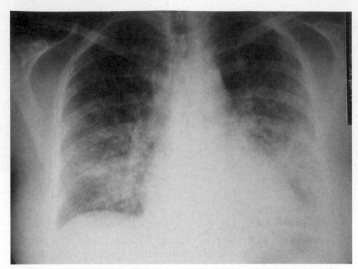

FIGURE 77-1 In drug-induced interstitial pneumonitis (also known as drug-induced hypersensitivity pneumonitis), diffuse symmetric interstitial linear or, less often, micronodular opacities are present. These changes usually develop in conjunction with exposure to the drug, rather than after completion of treatment with the causal agent. The BAL usually shows marked lymphocytosis. An infection must be ruled out in every case. A list of drugs that induce interstitial lung disease is available at www.pneumotox.com.

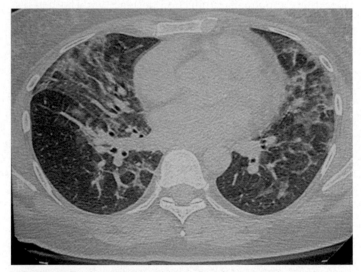

FIGURE 77-2 On HRCT in drug-induced interstitial pneumonitis, opacities are roughly symmetric and are in the form of septal thickening, ground-glass opacities, or a mosaic pattern. Pleural effusions may be present in severe cases. It is generally not possible to separate drug-induced lung disease from an infection on imaging, and appropriate tests are needed to rule out an infection.

In acute or in more advanced cases, airspace opacities and air bronchograms may develop, which may assume a focal, lobar, or diffuse distribution. The bronchoalveolar lavage (BAL) commonly shows a CD4$^+$ or CD8$^+$ predominant lymphocytosis, depending on drug, patient, and timing of BAL, and whether the patient has received corticosteroid therapy. However, the most important role of BAL is an exclusionary one, because this test is used to rule out an infection, the most important differential in drug-induced lung disease. It is particularly important to rule out an infection in patients who are immunosuppressed under the influence of their

background condition (e.g., neoplastic disease) or therapy with immune suppressants, or both (e.g., rheumatoid arthritis), because there is no reliable clinical or imaging discriminator between drug-induced and opportunistic pneumonia. Diagnosis of drug-induced interstitial pneumonia is mainly by exclusion and rests on the temporal relationship of exposure to the drug and time course of the lung disease. Not many patients will undergo a confirmatory lung biopsy, and a risk-benefit evaluation is not available. Histopathologic appearances are those of nonspecific cellular interstitial pneumonia (NSIP), including interstitial inflammation with edema and a rich cellular infiltrate of mononuclear cells infiltrating the interstitium with little or no interstitial fibrosis. Outcomes in this form of drug-induced interstitial lung disease are mostly good, with resolution of symptoms after cessation of exposure to the causal agent. A reduction in sirolimus dosage may be all that is required to improve symptoms and radiographic abnormalities. Corticosteroids are reserved for cases with respiratory failure or those who fail to improve after drug therapy withdrawal. A replica of the disease with, sometimes, increased severity or death may follow rechallenge with the culprit drug, particularly methotrexate. Therefore, deliberate reexposure is contraindicated and is contemplated only if continuing treatment is essential to control a life-threatening underlying condition.

Eosinophilic Pneumonia

Eosinophilic pneumonia is a classic and not infrequent complication of treatments with antibiotics (mainly minocycline), nonsteroidal antiinflammatory drugs (NSAIDs), antidepressants, including venlafaxine, sulfa drugs, and several other agents. Eosinophilic pneumonia is characterized by eosinophilia in blood and lung tissue. The latter feature is suggested by an increased proportion of eosinophils over lymphocytes and neutrophils in the BAL. Accordingly, the lung biopsy is rarely required to diagnose this condition. Fever, arthralgias, and a skin rash can be present at onset of the disease. The peripheral predominance of pulmonary infiltrates on imaging is suggestive, but this is not a consistent or reliable finding, and eosinophilic pneumonia often is difficult to separate from other interstitial pneumonias on imaging (Figures 77-3 and 77-4). Patients taking minocycline or a few other drugs may be seen acutely with marked dyspnea, diffuse pulmonary infiltrates, pleural effusions, and acute respiratory failure requiring emergent management. Pathologically, there is interstitial inflammation with edema and a eosinophilic interstitial infiltrate. Sometimes, overlapping features of eosinophilic and organizing pneumonia are present on the same lung specimen. Outcomes of eosinophilic pneumonia are generally good, with corticosteroid therapy or mechanical ventilation indicated in a few patients with severe presentations. Rechallenge almost invariably results in return of fever, eosinophilia, and the pulmonary infiltrates. A few patients with minocycline- or anticonvulsant-induced eosinophilic pneumonia have an extensive cutaneous rash develop along with internal organ involvement in conjunction with pulmonary infiltrates and peripheral eosinophilia. This constellation of symptoms is known as DRESS for "drug rash and eosinophilia with systemic symptoms" or "anticonvulsant syndrome," because several drugs used to treat epilepsy (e.g., carbamazepine, phenytoin) also produce the syndrome. DRESS is a severe condition, which may follow a hectic and unpredictable course despite drug therapy withdrawal and institution of corticosteroid therapy.

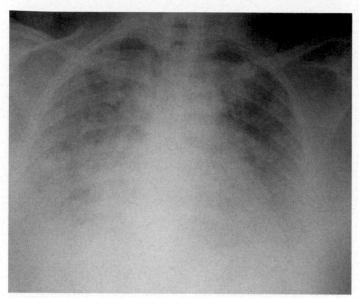

FIGURE 77-3 Drug-induced eosinophilic pneumonia. The severity of drug-induced eosinophilic pneumonia ranges from mild to severe, as in this case of acute drug-induced eosinophilic pneumonia with consequent acute respiratory failure. The diagnosis of eosinophilic pneumonia rests on the finding of elevated numbers of eosinophils in the BAL, with exclusion of other causes and abatement of symptoms on drug withdrawal. A list of drugs that induce this pattern is available on the web (www.pneumotox.com).

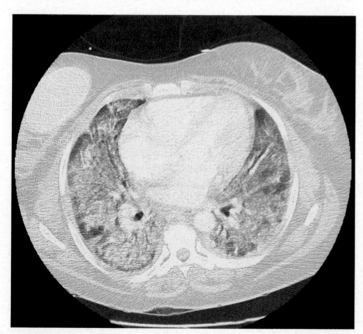

FIGURE 77-4 HRCT in drug-induced eosinophilic pneumonia; the infiltrates may be localized or diffuse. In cases with an acute presentation, eosinophilic pleural effusions may be present.

Granulomatous Infiltrative Lung Disease

Granulomatous interstitial lung disease is an uncommon pattern of involvement that may be caused by BCG therapy, etanercept, interferon-α or β, methotrexate, and sirolimus. The condition manifests in the form of diffuse micronodular or linear infiltrates, with or without hilar and/or mediastinal lymphadenopathy. Treatments with interferons may mimic thoracic sarcoidosis with or without the extrathoracic features of authentic sarcoidosis. In granulomatous interstitial lung disease, there is lymphocytosis in the BAL and a rise in serum angiotensin-converting enzyme. The diagnosis is confirmed by transbronchial or video-assisted thoracic surgery (VATS) lung biopsy or biopsy of extrapulmonary sites (e.g., the skin). The granulomas in methotrexate pulmonary toxicity are generally loosely formed as opposed to the well-formed granulomas of interferon-induced disease.

Organizing Pneumonia

Organizing pneumonia (OP), formerly known as bronchiolitis obliterans organizing pneumonia (BOOP), has been described after treatments with amiodarone, bleomycin, interferon-α/β, nitrofurantoin, and statins, as well as a complication of radiation therapy to the breast. The disease is in the form of diffuse or focal pulmonary infiltrates, migratory alveolar opacities, or dense nodules with or without air bronchograms. Organizing pneumonia induced by drugs expresses itself in a manner similar to organizing pneumonia from other causes or that occurs idiopathically. On histologic examination, buds of connective tissue populate the distal airways and alveoli. Organizing pneumonia responds well to drug therapy withdrawal and corticosteroid therapy, but the condition may relapse if corticosteroids are tapered too early or too swiftly, or if the causal drug is inappropriately continued.

Diffuse Alveolar Damage

Diffuse alveolar damage (DAD) is a subacute or acute lung reaction, which complicates treatments with antineoplastic agents, especially when grouped in a multiagent chemotherapy regimen as opposed to therapy with a solo agent or if given at high dosages or in conjunction with oxygen or radiation therapy. The condition is also known as chemotherapy lung. Drugs causing this pattern include antineoplastic antibiotics (bleomycin, mitomycin C), alkylating agents (busulfan, cyclophosphamide, chlorambucil, melphalan), antimetabolites (azathioprine, aracytine, gemcitabine, fludarabine, 6-mercaptopurine, methotrexate), nitrosamines (bischloroethyl nitrosourea [BCNU], chloroethyl-cyclohexyl nitrosourea [CCNU] and novel nitrosoureas), podophyllotoxins (etoposide), the taxanes (paclitaxel and docetaxel), tyrosine kinase inhibitors (erlotinib, gefitinib, imatinib), irinotecan, and granulocyte-monocyte colony-stimulating factors (Figure 77-5). Recipients of bone marrow or stem cell transplant and patients treated for solid tumors or hematologic malignancies are at risk, especially after the first course of chemotherapy in patients with a high tumor burden (mainly hematologic malignancies), where lysis of tumor cells can produce diffuse alveolar damage and multiple organ dysfunction, including acute renal failure. The condition is known as the tumor lysis syndrome. In early stages, DAD manifests with dyspnea, a dry cough, and diffuse pulmonary infiltrates, which range in density from a barely visible diffuse haze or ground glass to widespread densification with volume loss and severe hypoxemia or an acute respiratory distress syndrome (ARDS) picture with diffuse whiteout of the lungs. On HRCT, there is linear interlobular or intralobular thickening and/or areas of ground-glass attenuation. DAD may resemble, and is difficult to separate from, other conditions that can occur in patients with neoplastic conditions, including drug-induced cardiogenic and overload pulmonary edema, transfusion-related lung injury, alveolar hemorrhage, and opportunistic infections with bacterial, viral, or fungal agents or parasites. On histologic examination, there are varying amounts of cellular inflammation,

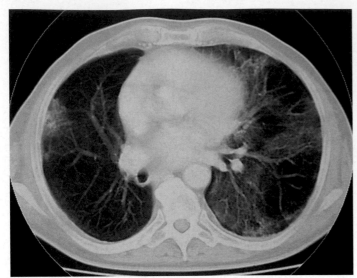

FIGURE 77-5 In drug-induced diffuse alveolar damage, the severity may range from a diffuse haze (as in the present case where DAD was caused by mitomycin C) to a pattern of dense diffuse opacities with acute respiratory failure. Early cases may respond to drug withdrawal and corticosteroid therapy. Later cases may evolve to a life-threatening ARDS picture.

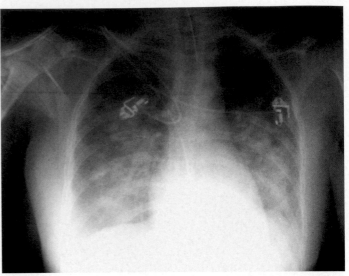

FIGURE 77-6 In drug-induced pulmonary edema, there are diffuse alveolar opacities that, usually, predominate in the lung bases and may resolve with drug therapy withdrawal.

interstitial and alveolar edema, hyaline membranes (the hallmark of DAD), reactive type II cells, alveolar deposition of fibrin and desquamated cells, organizing pneumonia, and interstitial fibrosis. A confirmatory lung biopsy rarely is requested, because patients often are too ill to undergo the procedure and, although DAD is a distinct histopathologic pattern of involvement, histopathologic examination may not be able to pinpoint the exact cause for it. The response of DAD to corticosteroid therapy is difficult to predict. Cases with moderate involvement are more likely to respond. A fraction of cases progress to an ARDS picture as the terminal event.

Pulmonary Edema

Noncardiac pulmonary edema (NCPE) results from acute drug-induced changes in pulmonary capillary permeability. Less commonly, pulmonary edema results from drug-induced deterioration of left ventricular function. NCPE generally develops during or a few hours after treatment with antineoplastic drugs (e.g., docetaxel, gemcitabine), salicylate, interleukin-2, hydrochlorothiazide, all-trans-retinoic acid (ATRA) or arsenic trioxide (As_2O_3), opiates, high-dose intravenous β-agonists, or transfusion of blood or blood products (the transfusion-related acute lung injury [TRALI]). Hydrochlorothiazide produces a form of "allergic pulmonary edema" characterized by scattered pulmonary infiltrates that closely follow administration of as little as one tablet of the drug. Glitazones can produce a mild form of interstitial pulmonary edema. Rapid deliberate or accidental administration of higher-than-normal doses of many drugs may also cause NCPE. Clinically, NCPE manifests with respiratory distress and hypoxemia. In rare cases, frothy sputum is present at the mouth. Imaging appearances include diffuse alveolar filling infiltrates with, usually, no cardiomegaly or pleural effusions (Figure 77-6). On histologic examination, there is interstitial edema and alveolar flooding with proteinaceous material with little, if any, interstitial inflammation. Prognosis of NCPE is generally good if administration of the

offending agent is stopped and supportive care, including mechanical ventilation, is given. However, a few cases progress to fatal pulmonary failure. Treatment of NCPE with diuretics is controversial, because patients may present with an unstable hemodynamic status, owing to fluid loss resulting from generalized increase in vascular permeability caused by the drug.

Diffuse Alveolar Hemorrhage

Diffuse alveolar hemorrhage (DAH) consists of diffuse bleeding into the alveoli, with or without histologically demonstrable capillaritis. DAH may occur:

1. In isolation, in the form of "bland" AH, with the use of abciximab, oral anticoagulants, or intoxication with rodenticide anticoagulants known as "superwarfarins," ATRA, clopidogrel, fibrinolytic agents, dermal injection of silicone, sirolimus, or tirofiban
2. As a secondary complication of drug-induced thrombocytopenia (e.g., with abciximab or quinidine)
3. As a manifestation of drug-induced pneumorenal syndrome or micropolyangiitis, with or without a positive ANCA serology (with the use of hydralazine, penicillamine, or propyl-thiouracil)
4. In the context of recent bone marrow or hematopoietic stem cell transplantation
5. Rarely, DAH occurs at the peak of hyperacute pneumonia from gold, methotrexate, or nitrofurantoin, or in conjunction with drug-induced acute NCPE.

Drug-induced DAH manifests with shortness of breath, anemia, and bilateral alveolar infiltrates, which may assume a butterfly or batwing pattern. Hemoptysis is not a constant feature, even though significant alveolar bleeding has occurred. An increase in the diffusing capacity for carbon monoxide suggesting free hemoglobin in the airspaces is a classic feature in DAH, regardless of its cause, but this is not a reliable finding. There is increased blood staining in serial aliquots of BAL and, microscopically, the BAL shows red cells. Hemosiderin-laden macrophages in BAL characterize those cases with subacute or resolving bleeding before full-blown DAH. A lung biopsy seldom is indicated, because this may only show the predictable changes of alveolar hemorrhage, and evidencing capillaritis on histopathology may not change the treatment approach substantially. DAH requires expeditious management, because clotting may occur in the distal airspaces causing irreversible respiratory failure or in the central airways causing fatal airway obstruction. Management includes drug therapy withdrawal, supportive care, and, depending on context, vitamin K, fresh frozen plasma, activated factor VII, corticosteroids, immune suppressants, or plasma exchange, in a manner similar to DAH of other causes.

Pulmonary Fibrosis

Pulmonary fibrosis is a delayed complication of treatments with antineoplastic chemotherapy (bleomycin, busulfan, chlorambucil, cyclophosphamide, the nitrosoureas BCNU and CCNU) or amiodarone. There is limited and circumstantial evidence for the implication of a few other drugs. Radiation therapy to the chest produces localized pulmonary fibrosis, which follows the path of the radiation beam(s). Drug-induced pulmonary fibrosis may develop acutely in the form of accelerated pulmonary fibrosis during or shortly after termination of treatment or up to many years later in a more indolent fashion (sometimes called the "delayed pulmonary toxicity syndrome"), being at times difficult to separate from idiopathic pulmonary fibrosis (Figures 77-7 and 77-8). Drug-induced pulmonary fibrosis manifests with dyspnea, a dry cough, basilar crackles, and weight loss. On the chest radiograph, there is basilar or diffuse, linear, or streaky shadowing and volume loss. On HRCT, coarse reticular perilobular and/or subpleural thickening and traction bronchiectasis predominate in the lung bases, except in the rare patient with late nitrosourea- or cyclophosphamide-induced pulmonary fibrosis, in whom the changes may display a predilection for the apices, causing retraction and secondary platythorax. Drug therapy withdrawal is indicated in all cases but is rarely followed by improvement. The response to corticosteroid therapy often is limited, and this form of treatment

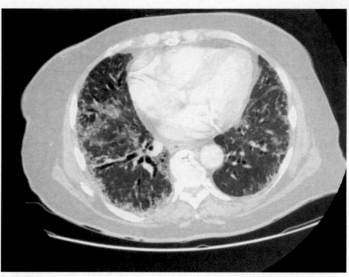

FIGURE 77-8 On HRCT in drug-induced pulmonary fibrosis, linear opacities are present along with evidence for architectural distortion.

may not halt the progression of pulmonary fibrosis. Lung transplantation has been an option for a few patients.

Airway Patterns
Upper Airway Obstruction

Treatments with angiotensin-converting enzyme inhibitors (ACEI) can produce angioedema, with consequent severe upper airway obstruction. This complication may occur shortly after the first few administrations of the ACEI or unexpectedly later at almost any time into treatment. ACEI-induced angioedema is annunciated by a sore throat and drooling of saliva, followed by the rapid development of edema of the mouth floor, tongue, and/or glottic region, causing a hindrance to breathing. A similar pattern of acute upper airway obstruction may develop with anaphylaxis, along with other signs and symptoms of the condition, which include wheezing, bronchospasm, abdominal pain, cramping, diarrhea, shock, seizures, and loss of consciousness. Management includes early recognition, securing the airway, which may quickly become difficult, if not impossible, to identify once significant edema has developed. Delaying identification of the airway might lead to fatal asphyxia before tracheostomy can eventually be performed. Drug withdrawal, corticosteroid therapy, antihistamines, and supportive care are indicated, but the efficacy of these drugs is unclear.

Less common causes of upper airway obstruction include compression of the airway by laryngeal or peritracheal hematoma in patients exposed to oral anticoagulants long term.

Acute Bronchospasm

Sudden severe bronchospasm can be induced by several drugs, most commonly aspirin or other NSAIDs, β-blockers, and a stream of inhaled drugs. Recently, inhaled heroin was recognized as a cause for acute bronchospasm requiring emergent admission. Although acute bronchospasm sometimes develops with no warning signs in subjects without a history of asthma, most of the time this complication occurs in patients who have underlying even mild asthma and/or chronic obstructive airways disease. Consequently, many of these drugs are

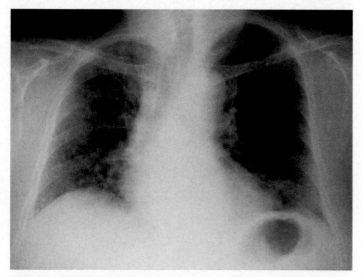

FIGURE 77-7 Drug-induced pulmonary fibrosis is a relatively uncommon pattern of lung response to antineoplastic chemotherapy or amiodarone (as in the present case). The pulmonary opacities in drug-induced fibrosis are generally disseminated and symmetric. Radiation-induced pulmonary fibrosis localizes along the radiation beams. Drug withdrawal is indicated. The condition responds poorly to corticosteroid therapy.

contraindicated in patients with these conditions. Aspirin sensitivity and intolerance to NSAIDs do not usually result from acquired sensitization but rather are intrinsic to the patient, who may exhibit the triad of recalcitrant nasal polyps and intermittent watery nasal discharge, difficult-to-treat asthma, and intolerance to NSAIDs and aspirin. Nasal symptoms and severe bronchospasm are precipitated by exposure to aspirin or NSAIDs. Bronchospasm occurs minutes to a few hours after ingestion of the offending drug. Avoidance of aspirin and NSAIDs is recommended if possible. Otherwise, induction of tolerance by use of increasing doses of the causal drug has been successful, but continued exposure is required for maintenance of tolerance.

Beta-blocker–induced asthma may be catastrophic and difficult to treat, because β-blockade blunts the response to β$_2$-agonists used to reverse bronchospasm. Patients may die from airway obstruction, acute respiratory failure, or consequent hypoxic brain damage.

A hypersensitivity reaction with bronchospasm occurs in a fraction of patients receiving vinca alkaloids or the taxanes, but this reaction can be quenched or ameliorated in most cases by premedication with antihistamines and steroids.

Cough

ACEI can cause chronic, annoying cough in up to 30% of patients. The cough develops with no identifiable reasons and occurs in women more frequently than in men, usually after 1–2 months of treatment, but occasionally later. All ACEI can induce chronic cough, but the direct angiotensin receptor II antagonists seem to do so less often. Patients with preexisting asthma are not at increased risk. Although bradykinin-induced airway irritation and bronchoconstriction are possible mechanisms, the exact cause for the cough is unclear. Drug withdrawal results in improvement within a few days or weeks. Relapse will follow rechallenge with the drug and may relapse with another ACEI as well.

Obliterative Bronchiolitis

Obliterative bronchiolitis is a very rare complication of drug therapy and has been described almost exclusively in conjunction with penicillamine use in patients with rheumatoid arthritis or in recipients of bone marrow or stem cell transplant. Patients experience increasing dyspnea and cough. Physical examination may be normal, or squeaks and crackles may be present. Chest radiographs may show hyperinflation. Expiratory chest CT shows air trapping and a mosaic pattern. Pathologically, obliteration of the small conducting airways by concentric luminal narrowing occurs because of a lymphocytic infiltration or mural or luminal fibrosis.

Pleural Patterns (see also Drug-Induced Lupus)

Several drugs can cause a free-flowing pleural effusion with or without eosinophilia in pleural fluid and tissue. A serous or, less often, serosanguineous pleural exudate may accompany the pulmonary toxicity of amiodarone, methotrexate, nitrofurantoin, or ergot drugs. Drug therapy withdrawal is followed by slow resolution of the effusion.

Long-term exposure to ergolines or ergot drugs (e.g., bromocriptine, cabergoline, ergotamine, nicergoline, or methysergide) may induce bilateral pleural thickening and disabling fibrothorax. Previous exposure to asbestos may increase the

risk. Complaints include dyspnea, chest pain, and a dull sensation in the chest. Sometimes, a friction rub is audible, or even is heard by the patient. Congestive heart failure is sometimes present. These changes develop insidiously over months to years. On imaging, pleural thickening (up to 1 inch) extends from the apices to the bases, and there are underlying areas of folded lung and rounded atelectasis. The latter changes and the thickening are best visualized on CT, which may also evidence pericardial thickening and/or effusion (Figures 77-9 and 77-10). Pulmonary function tests show varying degrees of usually severe restriction with, sometimes, hypoxemia and

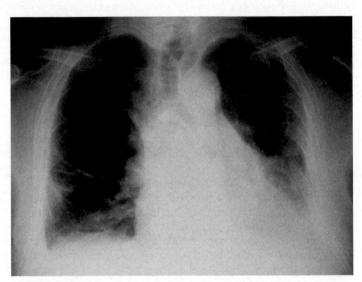

FIGURE 77-9 Long-term exposure to ergot drugs can produce a striking pattern of bilateral pleural thickening (as in the present case) or, less often, a unilateral or bilateral pleural exudate. These changes resolve very slowly after discontinuation of the agent.

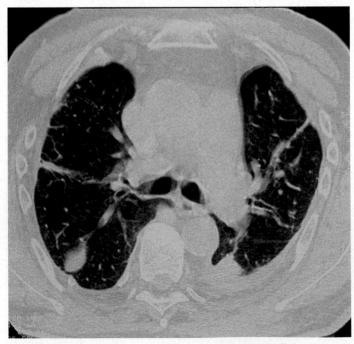

FIGURE 77-10 On CT in ergot-induced disease, there is pleural thickening, and areas of rounded atelectasis are present beneath the thickened pleura.

hypercarbia. Drug withdrawal is followed by slow and often incomplete resolution.

Some of the tyrosine kinase inhibitors, most notably dasatinib, have been associated with the development of pleural effusions in up to a third of the cases. These often have pleural fluid and tissue lymphocytosis, suggesting an inflammatory/immune-based mechanism rather than fluid retention. The effusions usually resolve with interruption of the drug and use of a lower dose.

Pulmonary Circulation Patterns (see also DAH Syndrome)

Pulmonary hypertension is the most classic pattern of drug-induced involvement of the pulmonary circulation. Drugs producing this condition include the now old-fashioned anorectic aminorex. Newer anorectics of the 1980s (e.g., fenfluramine-dexfenfluramine) produce pulmonary hypertension (PHT) in a manner similar to the older agent. Outcomes of drug-induced PHT resemble those of idiopathic PHT.

Lipiodol-laden acrylate glue administered to obliterate brain or other systemic arteriovenous fistulas may overspill and lodge distally in the pulmonary circulation. This complication manifests in the form of dyspnea, chest pain, and multiple small metallic densities with a branched pattern on the chest radiograph. Methacrylate cement injected under pressure to stabilize the vertebral body in patients with involvement from multiple myeloma, metastasis, or osteopenia may produce distal or massive life-threatening proximal pulmonary embolism and can be fatal.

Pulmonary hypertension in long-term illicit drug users results from self-injection of crushed tablets intended for oral use. This is followed by obliterative vasculopathy in reaction to the talc, starch, and/or silica filling that lodged in distal pulmonary arterioles.

Pulmonary venoocclusive disease is a rare condition of unknown etiology. It is characterized by fibrous occlusion of the pulmonary venules, which leads to pulmonary hypertension. The usual presenting sign is dyspnea of insidious development. Chest radiographs may show Kerley's B lines in the absence of cardiomegaly. Pulmonary venoocclusive disease has been reported to occur with several cytotoxic drugs or radiation therapy or in the context of marrow transplantation. Prognosis is poor.

Injection of silicone in transsexuals for the purpose of breast augmentation or altering body shape may cause acute pulmonary vascular damage, which manifests as pulmonary infiltrates and diffuse alveolar hemorrhage.

Bevacizumab is an angiogenesis inhibitor targeting vascular endothelial cells. Significant hemoptysis, which can be life threatening, has occurred in some patients with central cavitary pulmonary lesions or lesions that cavitate during treatment. This drug likely inhibits the ability of endovascular cells to recover after chemotherapy.

Mediastinal Patterns

Long-term corticosteroid therapy can lead to mediastinal lipomatosis, a radiographic curiosity in most patients and a cause for cough or mediastinal hemorrhage in a few.

Mediastinal lymphadenopathy may be present in drug-induced (e.g., interferon) "sarcoidosis" or in the anticonvulsant syndrome.

Oral anticoagulants may produce mediastinal hematomas, which can compress the trachea or esophagus.

Desiccated drug tablets or enteral nutrition may accumulate and obstruct the esophageal lumen in the form of a bezoar, causing compression of the posterior membranous tracheal wall and tracheal stenosis. Esophagoscopy with fragmentation and lavage of the condensed material is indicated.

Systemic Patterns

Some drugs cause a lupuslike syndrome. The incidence of renal and neurologic complications is low, but that of pleuro-pulmonary complications is high with the drug-induced, as opposed to idiopathic, lupus. The disease is suspected when lancinating or acute chest pain develops during treatment with an eligible drug. The drugs that most commonly cause this syndrome are hydralazine, procainamide, quinidine, isoniazid, and diphenylhydantoin. Interferon and novel TNF-α antibody therapy may also cause the syndrome.

A few drugs may cause Wegener's-like disease or polyangiitis with pulmonary or diffuse involvement (see DAH).

Neurologic Disorders

Many drugs, including aminosides, curares, corticosteroids, neuroleptics, and opiates, can inhibit neural drive, cause peripheral neuropathy, block neuromuscular functions, or produce myopathy. This may manifest as restrictive physiology and/or hypercarbic respiratory failure with clear lung fields on imaging.

SPECIFIC DRUGS

(Drugs not listed in the following, either because they produce one of the patterns listed previously or have a low incidence of toxicity, are available on Pneumotox®.)

Noncytotoxic Drugs

Amiodarone

Amiodarone is used to prevent or treat serious ventricular arrhythmias and refractory supraventricular arrhythmias. Its use is often limited by toxicity, which can be ophthalmic, cutaneous, hepatic, thyroid related, or pulmonary, and pulmonary toxicity is a major reason for adverse event–related drug discontinuance during chronic treatments with the drug. The incidence of pulmonary toxicity is 5–15% and is increased in those patients who receive more than 400 mg/day, particularly those on elevated dosages of intravenous amiodarone after cardiopulmonary surgery. Five forms of pulmonary toxicity are found, of which interstitial pneumonitis is the most common. Presenting signs and symptoms of interstitial pneumonitis develop over weeks to months and include cough, dyspnea, pleuritic chest pain, fatigue, and weight loss. The second pattern is that of acute reversible pneumonia, in which patients have the acute-to-subacute onset of fever, cough and chest pain, and tend to display lymphocytosis in the BAL more often than do patients with classic pneumonitis. In both types, the erythrocyte sedimentation rate (ESR) is elevated, and a peripheral leukocytosis occurs. An acute, severe and life-threatening form of amiodarone pulmonary toxicity (APT) with, sometimes, the features of ARDS has been described as a serious third type of toxicity and may occur after cardiac and noncardiac surgery, including pneumonectomy. A connection with use of mechanical ventilation and/or high inspired concentrations of oxygen during surgery is possible. The fourth pattern is irreversible pulmonary fibrosis, which may develop after an episode of classic APT or occurs as a *de novo* phenomenon. The fifth pattern is in the form of focal segmental or lobar infiltrates, pulmonary masses or nodules, or migratory opacities corresponding to organizing pneumonia.

Chest radiographs show scattered or diffuse, often asymmetric, interstitial pulmonary opacities in the chronic pneumonitis pattern (Figures 77-11 to 77-14). The infiltrates may localize in any area of the lung. Sometimes, there is an increased density of the involved lung and also of the liver or thyroid. This results from the sequestration of amiodarone and metabolite that are high in iodine in these tissues, where toxicity exactly develops. In acute pneumonia, there is mixture of interstitial and fluffy alveolar infiltrates, and diffuse opacification is seen with acute postoperative APT. Gallium scans are positive with amiodarone toxicity. Pulmonary physiology in APT discloses mild-to-moderate restriction, often significant hypoxemia, and a low diffusing capacity. A normal diffusing capacity virtually eliminates the diagnosis. There is no speci-

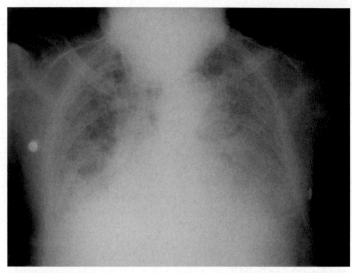

FIGURE 77-11 Exposure to amiodarone for at least a few weeks, and more commonly a few months or up to a few years, can produce localized or diffuse pulmonary changes, which are characterized by dyslipidosis and interstitial lung disease. These changes are suggestive of amiodarone pulmonary toxicity. APT is reversible in most cases on cessation of exposure. Often, corticosteroids are required to accelerate recovery.

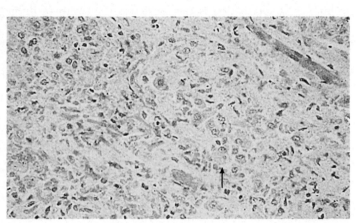

FIGURE 77-13 Lung histology associated with amiodarone pulmonary toxicity. An interstitial inflammatory infiltrate is seen with vacuolated macrophages. These "foamy" macrophages contain a large amount of abundant, pale cytoplasm of foamy appearance. The foaminess results from amiodarone-induced impaired phospholipid catabolism. Foamy macrophages can be retrieved by BAL. Although such macrophages are characteristically seen with amiodarone use, they do not mean toxicity has occurred, unless characteristic changes of interstitial lung disease are present in association.

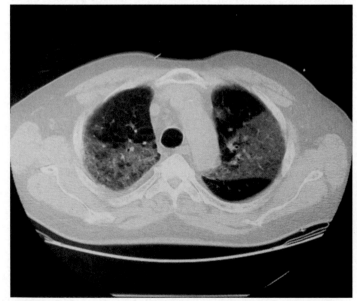

FIGURE 77-12 On HRCT, amiodarone pulmonary toxicity is characterized by interstitial and alveolar changes including interlobular and intralobular septal thickening, ground-glass opacities, or a mosaic pattern. These changes may display increased attenuation numbers because of the high iodine in amiodarone sequestered in the area of amiodarone pneumonitis.

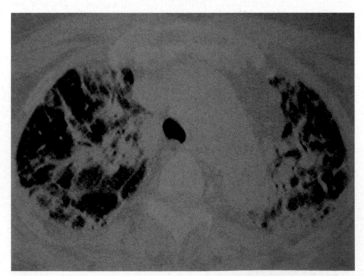

FIGURE 77-14 Nitrofurantoin pulmonary toxicity. The changes associated with subacute nitrofurantoin toxicity often have a predilection for the bronchovascular bundles, where most of the opacities localize. Most, but not all, cases show resolution after drug withdrawal and corticosteroid therapy.

fic BAL pattern in APT. Dyslipidotic alveolar macrophages indicate exposure to, not necessarily toxicity from, amiodarone.

The distinctive features of APT on imaging usually enable its distinction from cardiac pulmonary edema, pulmonary infarction, or an infection. Where needed, contrast-enhanced CT, BAL, and forced diuresis will help separate APT from these entities. Pathologically, there is interstitial and alveolar inflammation and varied amounts of fibrosis. Macrophages of foamy appearance are present in lung tissue and alveolar spaces. The foaminess results from cytoplasmic phospholipid accumulation, because amiodarone inhibits phospholipases. With acute postoperative APT, interstitial edema, hyaline membranes, foamy intraalveolar macrophages, a reactive epithelium, and intraalveolar hemorrhage can be present. The features of organizing pneumonia along with more classic features of APT can be present in patients with amiodarone-induced wandering opacities.

Once reasonable evidence for APT is obtained, treatment consists of discontinuation of the drug (underlying cardiac condition permitting), which is rarely sufficient in itself to ensure resolution of the disease, because the half-life of the drug is long (up to 60 days or more). Corticosteroids are often given at a dose of 40–60 mg/day, because spontaneous resolution after drug withdrawal can take some time. Corticosteroids should be given for several months with a slow taper, otherwise APT may "relapse" because of the long retention time of the drug in lung. In cases in which the drug cannot be stopped, a lower dose and concomitant corticosteroids may be useful. Overall mortality is approximately 10%. High doses of oxygen must be avoided in patients on amiodarone who undergo major surgery and a substitute drug used if possible. Routine use of amiodarone for the prevention of arrhythmias after pulmonary surgery is not recommended.

Aspirin

Salicylates are associated with acute noncardiogenic edema and exacerbation of bronchospasm (see "Drug-Induced Bronchospasm"). Pulmonary edema usually occurs when salicylate levels are greater than 40 mg/dL and may be accompanied by acid–base disturbances and neurologic symptoms. Salicylate-induced pulmonary edema may remain undiagnosed for as long as 72 h after admission, especially if salicylate blood levels are not measured at admittance. Two groups of patients with this complication have been noted. The first consists of younger patients who have attempted suicide by means of planned overdoses of aspirin. The second group consists of older individuals with multiple medical problems, who become accidentally intoxicated while ingesting salicylate for pain control and/or associated medical illnesses. The clinical presentation includes confusion, focal neurologic findings, tachypnea, inspiratory crackles, proteinuria, primary respiratory alkalosis, metabolic acidosis, and respiratory distress or an ARDS picture. The neurologic findings may lead to a delay in obtaining a history of aspirin ingestion. Treatment is with forced alkaline diuresis and supportive care. Salicylate-induced pulmonary edema resolves concomitant with a decline in serum salicylate levels. Prognosis is good if the diagnosis is made promptly. Delayed diagnosis is associated with higher mortality.

Blood and Blood Products

TRALI is a form of acute lung injury that occurs a few hours after transfusion of blood or blood products. In most cases,

the mechanism for TRALI is immunologic, with an antibody present in one donor that leads to cell activation, endothelial cell damage, and acute lung injury. The donor should be tracked, and all blood should be quarantined until the culprit donor, usually a multiparous woman, is identified. The responsible donor is usually deferred from further blood donation.

Gold

Gold was used to treat rheumatoid arthritis and other rheumatic diseases, and both parenteral gold sodium thiomalate and oral gold (auranofin) can cause pulmonary toxicity. The most common manifestation is an acute hypersensitivity pneumonitis, but occasionally organizing pneumonia and possibly OB may be seen. The incidence of gold toxicity is less than 1%, and a genetic predisposition to its development is possible. It typically occurs within 6 months of therapy. Patients experience cough, dyspnea, and a rash, and approximately 40% have mild peripheral eosinophilia. Radiographs show diffuse reticular infiltrates. Pathologically, interstitial inflammation is seen. BAL studies show increased lymphocytes with a predominance of suppressor or cytotoxic cells. Prognosis is good with discontinuation of the agent and treatment with corticosteroids. Gold-induced lung disease is likely to disappear as treatment with gold falls into disuse.

Nitrofurantoin

The potential for pulmonary toxicity from nitrofurantoin used for urinary suppression has been recognized for 50 years. The incidence is less than 1%, but the drug is widely used and regains interest. Nitrofurantoin causes both a hypersensitivity pneumonitis and, less commonly, a chronic pneumonitis/fibrosis. The hypersensitivity pneumonitis is characterized by systemic symptoms of fever, arthralgias, chest pain, and a maculopapular rash that occurs with pulmonary symptoms of cough and dyspnea. The syndrome usually occurs within the first few week(s) of administration of the drug. Mild peripheral eosinophilia is present in most cases. Alveolar filling and interstitial infiltrates are seen, and small pleural effusions can occur. In some symptomatic cases, radiographs are near normal. Pathologically, vasculitis, edema, and interstitial inflammation, particularly by eosinophils, are seen. Chronic toxicity may occur after months to years of therapy and is not an acute sequela. Dyspnea and cough are seen, and systemic symptoms are less common, although fatigue and weight loss may occur. Chest radiographs show interstitial infiltrates with, sometimes, a dense patchy peribronchovascular distribution. Peripheral eosinophilia can occur but is much less common than with acute toxicity. Positive antinuclear antibodies, rheumatoid factors, and elevated immunoglobulins are often found, and the disease may share features with the drug lupus. Biopsies show interstitial inflammation and fibrosis. A toxic reaction to drug metabolites or reactive oxygen species is considered a probable cause. In most cases, a diagnosis is made clinically. The prognosis is good for the hypersensitivity pneumonitis if administration of the drug is discontinued. With chronic toxicity the outcome is less favorable; in approximately 70% of cases, no improvement occurs or some abnormalities persist. Corticosteroids are used, but a beneficial effect is not seen in all cases.

D-Penicillamine

D-Penicillamine, which was once used in the treatment of rheumatic disorders and Wilson's disease, has been associated with obliterative bronchiolitis (almost exclusively in patients who have rheumatoid arthritis) and (rarely) a pulmonary renal syndrome similar to Goodpasture's syndrome. Hypersensitivity pneumonitis is very rare. Patients who have OB have severe dyspnea develop, as well as cough associated with obstructive and restrictive lung function abnormalities. Lung biopsy specimens show infiltration of bronchiolar walls with inflammation and concentric luminal narrowing. The prognosis of patients with OB is poor; little response occurs with use of bronchodilators and corticosteroids. Patients with the pulmonary renal syndrome have acute respiratory distress, DAH, and hemoptysis, similar to Goodpasture's syndrome but without, generally, the presence of antiglomerular basement membrane antibody. Patients are treated with immunosuppression, including cyclophosphamide and azathioprine, in addition to corticosteroids and plasmapheresis. Most of these complications are of historical interest, because the use of D-penicillamine is now relatively uncommon.

Paraffin

Long-term exposure to liquid paraffin to combat constipation can produce exogenous lipoid pneumonia, especially in the elderly with chronic aspiration. The condition is often missed at history taking. Other contexts of exposure include nasal or pharyngeal application of mineral oil and compulsive use of lipsticks. Nondegradable mineral oil accumulates in alveoli, where it elicits a pulmonary reaction with fibrosis. Exogenous lipoid pneumonia has a predilection for the lung bases, or it can be diffuse shadowing, which, on HRCT, assumes a ground-glass or crazy-paving appearance. The opacities exhibit low attenuation numbers and may exhibit the "spontaneous angiogram" sign. The BAL surface has an oily appearance to the naked eye and, microscopically, it contains increased numbers of lymphocytes and/or neutrophils in addition to characteristic vacuolated lipid-laden macrophages. Diagnosis of exogenous lipoid pneumonia rests on history taking and examination of sputum or BAL, which show lipid-laden cells and free-floating oil that stain positive for oil-red-O and Sudan black. A lung biopsy is not indicated for the diagnosis of this condition, except perhaps to diagnose paraffinoma, a solitary mass of exogenous lipoid pneumonia that can be mistaken for lung cancer. Not every patient with exogenous lipoid pneumonia will improve after discontinuance of oil and corticosteroid therapy. Some patients have recurrent pneumonia develop, superinfection with mycobacteria or *Aspergillus*, pulmonary fibrosis, or lung cancer.

TNF-α Antibody Therapy

The humanized monoclonal antibodies infliximab and etanercept have been developed to quench the cascade of inflammatory reactions elicited by excess production of TNF, which is central in the pathogenesis and clinical expression of inflammatory diseases such as rheumatoid arthritis and Crohn's disease. Both drugs expose to the risk of reactivation of infection with intracellular agents, mainly tuberculosis and, in specific countries, histoplasmosis. Tuberculosis with these agents occurs within weeks or months of starting the drug, suggesting reactivation rather than acquired disease; has a propensity for extrapulmonary involvement; and may be severe and difficult to treat. Tailored evaluation of tuberculosis risk is warranted in any patient who is a candidate for treatment with these agents. This includes ethnicity, a history for possible tuberculosis, or environmental exposure to

mycobacterial agents, chest imaging, and tuberculous skin testing (TST). TST is likely to be negative and is impractical in patients with rheumatoid arthritis and a history of corticosteroid therapy. Alternative tests such as the γ-interferon release assay are currently evaluated in an attempt to segregate patients with and without a history of exposure. Comparative assessment of the risk of tuberculosis and of antituberculous agent–related liver complications will dictate whether chemoprophylaxis with isoniazid or rifampin + isoniazid versus observation is required.

Several reports of accelerated pulmonary fibrosis, nonnecrotizing granulomatous lung disease, or ARDS have been described in patients with rheumatoid arthritis a few weeks or months after being switched to anti-TNF antibody therapy, but firm epidemiologic proof of an association is not currently available.

Cytotoxic Drugs
Bleomycin

Bleomycin is known to induce pulmonary fibrosis both in animal models and in patients who receive regimens containing the drug for a variety of hematologic malignancies. The incidence of clinically significant toxicity is 4%; subclinical toxicity detected through routine HRCT or pulmonary function tests has been found in 25% of cases. In most cases, interstitial pneumonitis or fibrosis is present, but acute pneumonia and hypersensitivity pneumonitis are also occasionally seen. Several risk factors have been identified for toxicity: age greater than 70 years, rapid versus slow continuous infusion, total dose received, previous radiation to the chest, use of supplemental oxygen, presence of renal insufficiency, and use of multidrug regimens. Studies suggest that although toxicity can occur even at very low doses of bleomycin, the incidence increases significantly at doses greater than 400 units. Mortality is approximately 10%, but cases that occur at higher doses are associated with increased mortality. The synergistic effect of both radiation and high inspired concentrations of oxygen has been documented in both animal models and clinical studies. No safe threshold dose of supplemental oxygen exists, and its use must be avoided or minimized in all patients who receive bleomycin or have signs of toxicity, even during short periods, such as, for instance, a surgical procedure. Patients typically have dyspnea and dry cough or chest pain of subacute to insidious onset. The physical examination characteristically shows bibasilar crackles, and chest radiographs initially show infiltrates at the bases peripherally (Figure 77-15). With more advanced disease, diffuse interstitial infiltrates and small lung fields are seen. Chest CT may reveal subpleural septal thickening and interstitial changes earlier than radiography (Figure 77-16). Acinar infiltrates can be seen and are more common when hypersensitivity pneumonitis or acute pneumonia is present. Focal infiltrates and nodular densities have also been described and correspond to organizing pneumonia histopathologically. Pathologically, atypical type II pneumocytes, alveolar and interstitial infiltration, and varying degrees of fibrosis are seen (Figure 77-17). BAL studies in animal models and some human cases have shown increased polymorphonuclear cells. Concerns have been raised that use of granulocyte colony-stimulating factor in those receiving the drug might increase the risk of toxicity, but this has not been found to be the case in all studies. Pulmonary function tests in patients who have bleomycin pulmonary

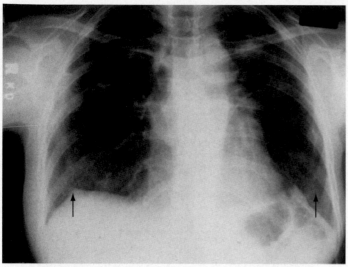

FIGURE 77-15 Chest radiograph in bleomycin toxicity. Fine bibasilar infiltrates are shown *(arrows)*, suggestive of drug toxicity.

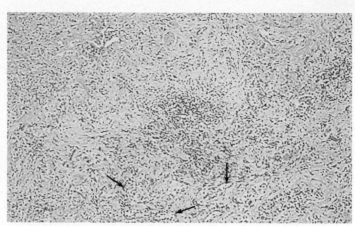

FIGURE 77-17 Atypical type II pneumocytes. This lung biopsy specimen from a patient with bleomycin toxicity shows extensive fibrosis and inflammatory cell infiltrates. The alveoli are lined by hyperplastic cuboidal cells that protrude into the lumen. These bizarre cells are consistent with drug-induced injury.

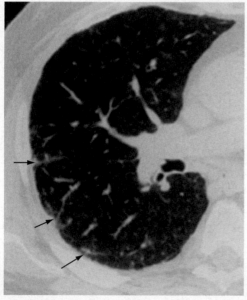

FIGURE 77-16 Bleomycin toxicity. In a patient receiving bleomycin who had a large decrease in the diffusing capacity for CO, the CT scan showed early changes of septal thickening and increased markings in the subpleural area *(arrows)*. These changes are suggestive of drug toxicity

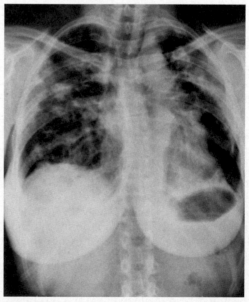

FIGURE 77-18 Cyclophosphamide toxicity. This patient received high-dose cyclophosphamide for lymphoma and a progressive restrictive disease associated with volume loss on chest radiography and patchy areas of fibrosis developed over several years. She ultimately required a lung transplant. Pathology of the native lung was consistent with a cytotoxically induced injury.

toxicity show a decreased diffusing capacity and, in more advanced cases, a restrictive defect and hypoxemia. Attempts have been made to use pulmonary function tests for screening, but no clear documentation of efficacy has been established. Such tests continue to be used clinically because of the serious nature of bleomycin toxicity. A significant decrease in diffusing capacity during treatment does not indicate definite toxicity but is a cause of concern, and further investigation with imaging and BAL may be required to exclude that possibility. Treatment of bleomycin toxicity involves discontinuation of the drug, avoidance of supplemental oxygen and of chest radiation therapy, and use of corticosteroid therapy in severe cases. Although clinical improvement often occurs, residual lung function abnormalities and respiratory symptoms are often

seen. Mortality can be as high as 50% in those who have severe pneumonitis.

Cyclophosphamide

The alkylating agent cyclophosphamide is widely used to treat a variety of malignancies and autoimmune conditions. Toxicity is rare, and the usual pattern of pulmonary toxicity is interstitial pneumonitis or fibrosis. The presentation of toxicity is usually insidious and may develop slowly after years of use. A more acute-to-subacute form of toxicity can occur after high-dose therapy. Risk factors have not been identified, partly because cyclophosphamide is almost always used in multidrug regimens with other known pulmonary toxins. Patients have progressive dyspnea. Chest radiographs show patchy areas of fibrosis (Figure 77-18). Pathologically, findings are similar to those seen with other cytotoxic drugs, including interstitial edema, diffuse alveolar damage, a reactive epithelium, and fibrosis. The prognosis is generally poor, although some improvement of symptoms can be found with corticosteroids; the fibrosis tends to be progressive. Some patients with late cyclophosphamide toxicity have debilitating upper lobe fibrosis, pleural thickening, and platythorax develop, and the course can be complicated by pneumothoraces, which are difficult to treat as the underlying fibrotic may not reexpand well.

Gefitinib

Gefitinib (Iressa) is a selective inhibitor of the epidermal growth factor-receptor (EGFR) tyrosine kinase. It has activity in patients with non-small-cell lung cancer, particularly adenocarcinomas. The drug, which is given orally, is well tolerated. The major side effects are diarrhea and skin rash, usually mild. Gefitinib has been in use in Japan, where cases of interstitial pneumonitis have been reported in 1–2% of patients, a significantly higher incidence than in unexposed controls. In some patients, concomitant radiotherapy had been given, so the exact frequency of this toxicity is uncertain. Cases manifested as either acute lung injury with patchy diffuse infiltrates or as interstitial pneumonitis. Improvement has occurred in some patients with corticosteroid treatment, but deaths have been attributed to pulmonary toxicity. The incidence of toxicity is less in Caucasians. A few cases of interstitial lung disease have been reported with the use of the other EGFR tyrosine kinase inhibitor erlotinib.

Gemcitabine

Gemcitabine is a purine-analog antimetabolite with activity in non-small-cell lung cancer, pancreatic cancer, and cancers of the bladder, ovary, and breast. It is increasingly being given because of its broad activity and very favorable toxicity profile, which allows its use in elderly or impaired patients. Myelosuppression is the major dose-limiting toxicity. Pulmonary toxicity ranges from less than 1–13% of patients in various studies. Patients typically have dyspnea of insidious development, and the clinical picture may culminate with acute respiratory failure or ARDS. Radiographs show interstitial infiltrates, which may be reticulonodular, or a diffuse ground-glass appearance consistent with noncardiac pulmonary edema. At times, the findings are subtle on radiography and can be seen only on chest CT. Peripheral edema is present in some patients and is believed to be the result of increased vascular permeability. This may be the mechanism that leads to the pulmonary toxicity. Most cases respond to treatment with corticosteroids and discontinuation of the drug. Corticosteroids may quench the pulmonary reaction after subsequent administration of the drug. Some cases of pulmonary toxicity have been severe and sudden with ARDS, and fatalities have been reported.

Methotrexate

The antimetabolite methotrexate is used in treatment of leukemia, lymphoma, osteogenic sarcoma, breast cancer, and a variety of inflammatory diseases, mainly rheumatoid arthritis. Methotrexate has caused a variety of pulmonary complications. The most common is hypersensitivity pneumonitis with or without granuloma formation, but pulmonary fibrosis, noncardiogenic pulmonary edema, and pleuritis have also been

described, although this is uncommon. The frequency of toxicity depends, in part, on how the drug is used in multidrug regimens, with some combinations reported to have rates of toxicity of up to 40%. Other risk factors are adrenalectomy, corticosteroid tapering, and more frequent administration of methotrexate. Typically, methotrexate toxicity manifests as a subacute illness over several weeks, with malaise, myalgias, fever, chills, dyspnea, and a dry cough. A skin rash has been noted in some cases. The chest radiograph shows diffuse, bilateral, reticular, reticulonodular, nodular, or patchy alveolar filling infiltrates (Figures 77-19 and 77-20). Peripheral eosinophilia is present in up to 40% of cases. Occasionally, interstitial fibrosis or noncardiogenic edema develops. Pathologically,

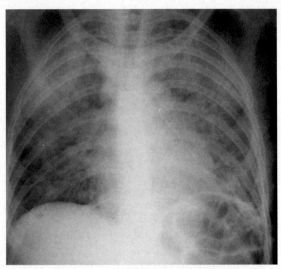

FIGURE 77-19 Acute methotrexate pneumonitis with diffuse acinar opacities and volume loss. The disease responds well to drug discontinuation. In severe cases, therapy with corticosteroids is indicated. Rechallenge with methotrexate is contraindicated, because relapse with increased severity may develop shortly after readministration of the drug.

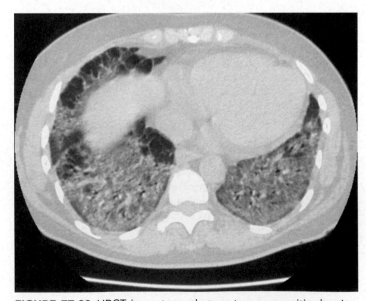

FIGURE 77-20 HRCT in acute methotrexate pneumonitis showing disseminated interstitial and alveolar opacities.

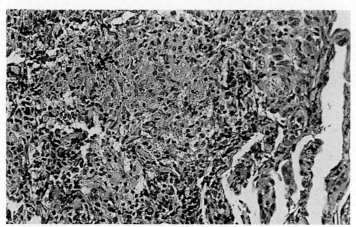

FIGURE 77-21 Histopathology of methotrexate toxicity. This biopsy from a patient who had methotrexate pneumonitis shows extensive infiltration with lymphocytes and also loosely formed granulomas. Atypical type II pneumocytes were not seen in this case and are generally absent in methotrexate lung.

lung biopsy specimens show prominent mononuclear cell infiltration with lymphocytes as the predominating cells. A loosely formed granulomatous reaction may also be seen (Figure 77-21). Overall prognosis is good, and often the response to corticosteroid therapy is dramatic. Occasionally, the syndrome resolves spontaneously. Rare patients have pulmonary fibrosis develop. Overall mortality is approximately 10%. The presence of systemic symptoms and eosinophilia and the response to corticosteroids suggest that the disorder is immunologically mediated; this theory is also supported by lavage findings that show a lymphocytic predominance with helper cells in some cases and suppressor cells in others. Occasionally, however, a lack of recurrence on rechallenge is reported. Rechallenge may also result in fatal relapse of the pneumonitis and is discouraged.

Mitomycin

Although not as well studied as bleomycin, mitomycin causes serious pulmonary toxicity in approximately 4% of cases. Three patterns of toxicity occur:

- An acute pneumonitis and DAD (most common), seen when mitomycin is used with vinca alkaloids
- Interstitial pneumonitis or fibrosis, similar to that seen with bleomycin use
- Pulmonary infiltrates (rare), associated with microangiopathic hemolytic anemia and uremia, which can be delayed several months after drug administration

In the mitomycin–vinca alkaloid reaction, patients have severe episodes of respiratory distress develop usually several hours after they receive a dose of the vinca alkaloid. In some cases, the respiratory failure requires intubation. Radiographs show new bilateral interstitial infiltrates. With supportive care and, in most cases, corticosteroids, improvement occurs over several days. Unfortunately, approximately 50% of cases have residual pulmonary impairment similar to that seen with mitomycin-induced pulmonary fibrosis. Lung histologic findings show fibrosis and a mononuclear cell infiltration. No clear risk factors are identified, and the mechanism of toxicity is

unknown. The interstitial pneumonitis or fibrosis syndrome manifests similar to toxicity with other antineoplastic agents, with the insidious onset of dyspnea. Chest radiographs show interstitial disease. In many cases, the response to corticosteroids is good. The rare entity of mitomycin-induced, microangiopathic hemolytic anemia occurs with pulmonary hemorrhage, which manifests with diffuse pulmonary infiltrates, pulmonary hypertension, and, sometimes, respiratory failure. Prognosis is poor. Treatment with corticosteroids and possibly plasmapheresis must be attempted. The incidence of mitomycin toxicity should decrease, because the drug is now used less frequently to treat lung cancer.

Nitrosoureas

The nitrosoureas, carmustine (BCNU) and lomustine, are frequently used for treatment of brain tumors because of their penetration into the central nervous system. They have also been used in high doses as part of conditioning regimens before autologous marrow or peripheral stem-cell transplantation. Most, if not all, nitrosoureas are pneumotoxic. Two patterns of injury have been noted, namely, interstitial pneumonitis or fibrosis and acute pneumonia. The first pattern has been described after treatment of brain tumors, and toxicity may not appear for months to years after treatment. In children, respiratory failure may develop up to 10 years later. Several risk factors have been identified: high dose (a relationship exists between increasing dose and risk of toxicity, particularly at doses above 1500 mg/m^2), preexisting pulmonary disease, and use in multidrug regimens.

Patients have dyspnea and dry cough of insidious onset. Physical examination reveals bibasilar crackles and occasionally rhonchi. Signs of consolidation have also been reported. Chest radiography can show a variety of findings, which include interstitial opacities, lower lobe infiltrates, patchy infiltrates, bilateral alveolar filling infiltrates, upper-lobe infiltration, and nodular densities. Cystic changes in adolescents treated for brain tumor in childhood and pneumothorax have also been reported. Lung function tests show restriction and occasionally obstruction. Pathologic findings are similar to those found with other cytotoxic agents. Often, however, fibrosis is patchy, and little inflammation is present. Treatment with corticosteroids is usually not very effective, and discontinuation of the drug is the mainstay of treatment. Prognosis is poor, with a reported mortality of up to 90% in severe cases.

An acute pneumonia-like pattern with the development of diffuse interstitial or alveolar infiltrates can occur several weeks after the use of high-dose carmustine. This form of toxicity is usually responsive to corticosteroids. In some cases in which lung function was monitored after high-dose chemotherapy, marked decreases in the diffusing capacity were noted, presumably because of carmustine toxicity; this improved with time and corticosteroid treatment.

Taxanes

The taxanes are important new antineoplastic drugs widely used for carcinomas of the lung, breast, ovary, head and neck, and melanoma. They include paclitaxel and docetaxel. A hypersensitivity reaction with dyspnea, bronchospasm, urticaria, erythematous rash, and hypotension occurred initially in up to a third of the patients. Premedication with corticosteroids, antihistamines, and H$_2$-blocker has reduced the incidence to approximately 1%, and the reactions are milder. Transient infiltrates occurring while the patient is on therapy and a syndrome of acute pneumonia have also been noted. Response to corticosteroids has been reported, and the prognosis has been generally good. However, more serious toxicity has occurred when the drugs are combined with radiation therapy. Radiation-recall phenomenon has also been described.

DIAGNOSIS

The diagnosis of drug toxicity is often difficult to confirm and is essentially made clinically (Box 77-1). Rechallenge with recurrence is the "gold standard" but is not practical in most cases, because serious toxicity might be produced, especially if the reaction was life threatening, the pulmonary reaction has not fully reversed (e.g., pulmonary fibrosis), or there are alternate choices for the treatment of the basic disease. In addition, with cytotoxic and antiinflammatory agents, multidrug regimens are often used, and it can be difficult to ascribe the reaction to any specific drug. The underlying diseases, particularly some autoimmune diseases, may themselves cause pulmonary effects, which makes the diagnosis of a drug effect more difficult. Compounding factors, such as intercurrent infection or progression of tumor, may also affect the lung, which may complicate the diagnosis of drug toxicity. Indeed, the effect of some drugs on the immune system may be directly associated with the development of pulmonary infections. This is the case with several immune suppressants, including TNF antibody therapy, which may induce reactivation of tuberculosis or histoplasmosis.

Unfortunately, radiographic findings are usually nonspecific for drug toxicity, and pathology can be supportive but not pathognomonic of drug-induced injury. Whether to obtain tissue and, if so, whether a transbronchial biopsy will suffice or a VATS open biopsy is needed depend on the individual situation and is guided by benefit to the patient. In cases in which the differential diagnosis is broad, invasive procedures help eliminate other entities and indicate pulmonary toxicity. In cases in which an invasive procedure may carry a high risk (e.g., in cardiac patients) and in which other means are available for diagnosis and treatment of other suspected problems (e.g., bacterial infection or congestive heart failure), a conservative approach is often taken, which includes drug therapy withdrawal with or without corticosteroid therapy.

BOX 77-1 Diagnostic Criteria for Drug-Induced Respiratory Disease

Correct identification and singularity of drug
Normalcy of chest radiograph and/or other tests (e.g., pulmonary function) before institution of treatment with the suspect drug
Temporal eligibility (exposure vs signs and symptom relationship)
Characteristic clinical, imaging, BAL, and histopathologic pattern of reaction to the specific drug
Exclusion of other possible causes
Measurable effect of drug withdrawal (without, if possible, interference of corticosteroid therapy)
In vitro tests
Rechallenge (not generally recommended)

The mainstay of diagnosis of drug-induced injury remains a strong clinical suspicion of drug toxicity and knowledge of the types of reactions seen.

PREVENTION

Although risk factors (mainly the drug relatedness) have been described for some drugs, in most cases, it is not possible to prevent drug-induced toxicity. Use of antioxidants and antifibrotic agents is being studied in animal models and may have some relevance for prophylactic use with some cytotoxic agents, such as bleomycin and mitomycin. The low incidence of toxicity and the potential side effects of these agents may hinder their use. Lung function tests, including measurements of the diffusing capacity for carbon monoxide, have been used to detect the earliest stages of toxicity of some drugs, and diffusing capacity is the most sensitive indicator of drug-induced injury. Such tests have not been found useful with methotrexate, which is understandable given the proposed immunologic mechanism and lack of dose relationship. The tests have also not been shown to be predictive in mitomycin toxicity and, although widely used, have not been proved to help prevent bleomycin or amiodarone pulmonary toxicity. Toxicity caused by bleomycin, mitomycin, carmustine, and amiodarone has been proposed to be exacerbated by use of supplemental oxygen. In anyone suspected of toxic reactions to these drugs, prudence dictates that any supplemental oxygen be avoided unless absolutely necessary. If a patient needs surgery, in which high concentrations of oxygen are routinely used during induction of anesthesia, these potential complications must be kept in mind, and the lowest possible inspired concentration of oxygen should be used.

PITFALLS AND CONTROVERSIES

Whether screening pulmonary function tests should continue to be carried out in cases of drug-induced toxicity is unclear. These tests are now performed almost exclusively for injury related to use of cytotoxic drugs, usually bleomycin and occasionally mitomycin, carmustine, and amiodarone. They are carried out regularly during therapy; a significant decrease in gas transfer or vital capacity is taken as an indication of subclinical toxicity, and the drug is stopped. Studies have not been undertaken to show the efficacy of this practice in oncology, but many oncologists believe that stopping the drug in some patients has prevented toxicity. The use of diffusing capacity as a marker is also complicated, because of its costs, its coefficient of variation, and because cytotoxic drugs are known to affect epithelial or vascular cells that line the alveolar vascular interface and can cause a decrease in the diffusing capacity without indicating the onset of significant interstitial inflammation or irreversible fibrosis. More sophisticated tests separate the vascular and membrane components of the diffusing capacity, but routine use of these is not practical. Better screening tests for toxicity are needed, and if serum or bronchoalveolar biologic markers of fibrosis can be found and validated (e.g., TGF-β in radiation pneumonia), they may prove a better method than lung function tests.

One of the most difficult decisions for a clinician in some cases is whether a given drug can be continued or restarted when the diagnosis of drug-induced toxicity is suspected but not clear. In some cases, no effective substitute agent is available. Each case must be considered individually, but as a general principle, with drugs that have a high propensity for fibrosis, such as bleomycin and mitomycin, or in cases in which the initial reaction itself was severe and life threatening, the drugs should not be given again, even if toxicity is not proved. In cases of less severe toxicity or in which irreversible fibrosis is unlikely, prudent reinstitution with increasing doses of the drug can be considered if essential to the patient. In some cases, as documented with amiodarone, a lower dose or corticosteroid cover may ameliorate or eliminate the reaction.

The greatest pitfall with drug-induced injury is the failure to consider the diagnosis. Except for some cytotoxic agents that have a well-recognized potential for fibrosis, drug-induced lung disease is uncommon, and often less common than many other possible pulmonary complications. A clinician may be personally familiar with only a limited number of reactions and cannot be expected to have detailed knowledge of reactions to all drugs. Once the diagnosis is considered, computerized medical searches, particularly of World Wide Web sites developed to catalog cases of drug toxicity, can be informative.

SUGGESTED READINGS

Abratt RP, Onc FR, Morgan GW, *et al:* Pulmonary complications of radiation therapy. Clin Chest Med 2004; 25:167–177.

Aldrich TK, Prezant DJ: Adverse effects of drugs on the respiratory muscles. Clin Chest Med 1990; 11:177–189.

Allen JN: Drug-induced eosinophilic lung disease. Clin Chest Med 2004; 25:77–88.

Babu KS, Marshall BG: Drug-induced airways diseases. Clin Chest Med 2004; 25:113–122.

Bonniaud Ph, Camus C, Jibbaoui A, *et al:* Drug-induced respiratory emergencies. In Fein A, Kamholz S, Ost D eds: Respiratory Emergencies, London: Edward Arnold; 2006:269–290.

Camus PH: Drug-induced respiratory disease in connective tissue diseases. In Wells AU, Denton CP, eds: Handbook of Systemic Autoimmune Diseases, Part VI: Pulmonary involvement in systemic autoimmune diseases. Vol. 2. Elsevier BV; 2004:247–294.

Camus PH, Martin WJ II, Rosenow EC, III: Amiodarone pulmonary toxicity. Clin Chest Med 2004; 25:65–76.

Camus P, Fanton A, Bonniaud PH, *et al:* Interstitial lung disease induced by drugs and radiation. Respiration 2004; 71:301–326.

Cooper JAD, White DA, Matthay RA: Drug induced pulmonary disease. Part 1: Cytotoxic drugs. Am Rev Respir Dis 1986; 133:321–340.

Cooper JAD, White DA, Matthay RA: Drug induced pulmonary disease. Part 2: Noncytotoxic drugs. Am Rev Respir Dis 1986; 133:488–505.

Dean DE, Schultz DL, Powers RH: Asphyxia due to angiotensin converting enzyme (ACE) inhibitor mediated angioedema of the tongue during the treatment of hypertensive heart disease. J Forensic Sci 2001; 46: 1239–1243.

Drug-induced pulmonary toxicity web site Pneumotox®: www.pneumotox.com.

Epler GR. Drug-induced bronchiolitis obliterans organizing pneumonia. Clin Chest Med 2004; 25:89–94.

Flieder DB, Travis WD: Pathologic characteristics of drug-induced lung disease. Clin Chest Med 2004; 25:37–46.

Higenbottam T, Laude L, Emery CJ, Essener M: Pulmonary hypertension as a result of drug therapy. Clin Chest Med 2004; 25:123–132.

Huggins JT, Sahn SA: Drug-induced pleural disease. Clin Chest Med 2004; 25:141–154.

Kopko PM, Popovsky MA: Pulmonary injury from transfusion-related acute lung injury. Clin Chest Med 2004; 25:105–113.

Kotloff RM, Ahya VN, Crawford SW: Pulmonary complications of solid organ and hematopoietic stem cell transplantation. Am J Respir Crit Care Med 2004; 170:22–48.

Lee-Chiong TLJ, Matthay RA: Drug-induced pulmonary edema and acute respiratory distress syndrome. Clin Chest Med 2004; 25:95–104.

Libby D, White DA: Pulmonary toxicity of drugs used to treat systemic autoimmune disease. Clin Chest Med 1998; 19:809–821.

Limper AH: Chemotherapy-induced lung disease. Clin Chest Med 2004; 25:53–64.

Lindell RM, Hartman TE: Chest imaging in iatrogenic respiratory disease. Clin Chest Med 2004; 25:15–24.

Looney MR, Gropper MA, Matthay MA: Transfusion-related acute lung injury: a review. Chest 2004; 126:249–258.

Myers JL, Limper AH, Swensen SJ: Drug-induced lung disease: a pragmatic classification incorporating HRCT appearances. Semin Respir Crit Care Med 2003; 24:445–454.

Pham PTT, Pham PCT, Danovitch GM, *et al:* Sirolimus-associated pulmonary toxicity. Transplantation 2004; 77:1215–1220.

Ravid D, Leshner M, Lang R, *et al:* Angiotensin-converting enzyme inhibitors and cough: A prospective evaluation in hypertension and in congestive heart failure. J Clin Pharmacol 1994; 34:1116–1120.

Rosenow EC III, Myers JL, Swensen SJ, Pisoni RJ: Drug induced pulmonary disease: An update. Chest 1992; 102:239–250.

Schwarz MI, Fontenot AP: Drug-induced diffuse alveolar hemorrhage syndromes and vasculitis. Clin Chest Med 2004; 25:133–140.

White DA. Drug-induced pulmonary infection. Clin Chest Med 2004; 25:179–188.

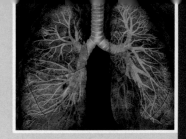

78 Lung Transplantation

LUIS G. RUIZ • EDWARD R. GARRITY, JR

INTRODUCTION

Pulmonary transplantation has become an effective and reliable means to improve survival and quality of life in carefully selected patients who have end-stage pulmonary disease. The current success in transplantation is attributed to the appropriate referral, early selection, careful evaluation, and the improving management of lung allograft donors and recipients. The multidisciplinary approach (Figure 78-1), together with meticulous care of each transplant candidate (including understanding of their disease and optimizing their psychosocial status), is of the utmost importance. The concurrent advances in surgical techniques, combined immunosuppressive regimens, surveillance for rejection and institution of prophylaxis, and early treatment of infection has resulted in the excellent survival rates and quality of life that we witness today.

The major challenges of preventing graft rejection and infection continues to impede progress. Lung transplant recipients face higher mortality rates and more frequent loss of graft function than other solid organ transplant recipients. Imbalance between organ supply and demand stresses the allocation system.

HISTORY

The pioneering experiments of numerous researchers who attempted to transplant heart, lung, and combined heart-lung blocks in different animal models laid the foundation for thoracic organ transplantation. In the 1950s, successful canine experiments performed by Demikhov, Metras, Hardin, and Kittle made lung transplantation a reality. In 1963, Dr. James Hardy and his team at the University of Mississippi Medical Center performed the first successful human lung homotransplantation. The recipient was a man with severe emphysema and a nonresectable left-sided lung cancer. His donor had recently died from a massive myocardial infarction. As with most early lung transplants, the allograft was harvested from a nonheart-beating donor, an approach that is currently re-emerging as a partial solution for the organ shortage. Immediately after the operation, which lasted less than 3 h, there was improvement in his oxygen saturation providing the first evidence of adequate allograft function. Unfortunately, the initial success would be met with failure, because the recipient died 18 days later from renal failure. Nearly 45 different transplantation attempts followed over the next 20 years. In almost all cases, failure seemed to stem from a lack of adequate bronchial perfusion to the anastomosed airways, which led to necrosis, dehiscence, and infection and to inadequate medications to prevent acute rejection.

In the early 1980s, lung transplantation would enter a new era. Dr. Bruce Reitz and the Stanford transplant group were able to achieve long-term survival with their series of combined heart-lung transplantations. Part of their success was attributed to the lack of bronchial ischemia as a result of performing the combined heart-lung approach that left the coronary circulation intact to provide collateral blood flow to the main airways after the bronchial artery had been ligated. The concurrent use of cyclosporine, the first effective T-cell suppressor drug approved for use in solid organ transplantation in the United States, helped ameliorate acute rejection episodes. Dr. Joel Cooper and the Toronto transplant group also documented success with single-lung transplants and then with en-bloc bilateral lung transplants. Improved bronchial perfusion in the Toronto group was achieved with omentopexy (i.e., wrapping omentum around the anastomosis to facilitate neovascularization). Omentopexy has now been replaced by the telescoping bronchial anastomosis technique first described by Dr. Frank Veith in 1969. In the late 1980s, the development of the bilateral sequential single-lung transplant technique, by the Toronto and San Antonio programs, would become the procedure of choice for double-lung transplantation.

Over the next two decades, the state of lung transplantation grew sporadically, but quickly, and has now stabilized. The most recent reports from multiple lung transplant centers through out the world indicate that bilateral and single-lung transplants continue to account for most procedures performed. Heart-lung transplants are now rare and reserved primarily for those patients with Eisenmenger's anomaly or severe primary pulmonary hypertension.

CURRENT TRENDS IN LUNG TRANSPLANTATION

In the United States, the United Network for Organ Sharing (UNOS) has been operating the Organ Procurement and Transplantation Network (OPTN) since 1984. The International Society for Heart and Lung Transplantation (ISHLT) in collaboration with UNOS, created a worldwide registry of all heart and heart-lung transplants in 1982. The Twenty-Third report documents that more than 21,000 lung transplants have been performed since that time, with close to 1800 lung transplants done in 2004 alone by more than 120 transplant centers worldwide. Most current transplants are bilateral sequential or double-lung transplants (Figure 78-2). Approximately 70 heart-lung transplants were done during that same year.

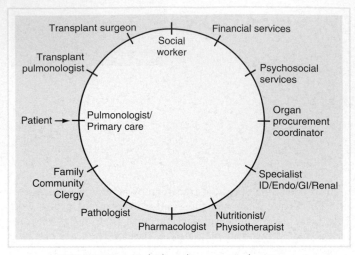

FIGURE 78-1 Multidisciplinary transplant team.

Although the number of lung transplants has increased substantially in the past two decades, the leading indications for lung transplantation remain relatively unchanged: chronic obstructive pulmonary disease (COPD), idiopathic pulmonary fibrosis (IPF), cystic fibrosis (CF), alpha$_1$-antitrypsin (A1A) deficiency with emphysema, and pulmonary arterial hypertension (PAH) (Figure 78-3). The type of transplant a patient receives is partly dictated by the recipient's underlying disease; COPD and IPF recipients tend to receive single-lung as often as double-lung transplants, whereas CF and PAH recipients usually receive bilateral lung transplants (Figures 78-4 and 78-5). Over the past 5 years, there has also been a trend toward performing double-lung transplants and transplanting older individuals in the 55–65 age range (Figure 78-6).

As of November 2006, UNOS estimates are that there are 1000 patients on the active waiting list in the United States. The median waiting time for those listed in 2003–2004 period was approximately 2 years. The most recent waiting list time is not yet known, but after the implementation of the Lung

Allocation Score (LAS), median waiting times seem to have shortened. Donors selected for lung donation are now older, mean age 35, and more donors are now accepted older than the age of 50.

SURVIVAL

Achieving successful outcomes and maximal survival in the lung transplant population starts with the proper selection of transplant candidates. This entails an understanding of the natural history of the recipient's lung disease and the projected survival with optimal medical and surgical therapy. Identifying potential candidates must be based on their current quality of life and the potential for improvement with and without transplantation. The median survival for lung transplant recipients has improved dramatically over the past several years. Transplants performed from 2000–2004 reach a median survival of 5 years, significantly higher than previous years (Figure 78-7). The survival curve is not linear, however, because approximately 20% of all recipients die in the first year after transplantation, with most occurring in the first 90 days. This rapid decline in survival then stabilizes and follows a more linear trajectory, with an estimated 6% mortality rate per year. First year mortality is attributed to postoperative graft complications, infection, cardiac failure, rejection, and early toxicity from immunosuppressive medications (Figure 78-8).

Several independent factors also seem to affect survival, including older age, higher body mass index (BMI), severe pulmonary hypertension, the type of transplant procedure performed, and recipient's native pulmonary disease. In recipients older than 65, the expected 5-year median survival is 3.4 years, considerably lower than the overall average 5-year median survival. This is one reason why age >65 is considered to be a relative contraindication.

Bilateral-lung transplant (BLTx) has a median survival of 5.6 years compared with single-lung transplant (SLTx), which has a median survival of 4.3 years (Figure 78-9). Although heart-lung transplants (HLTx) have the lowest median survival

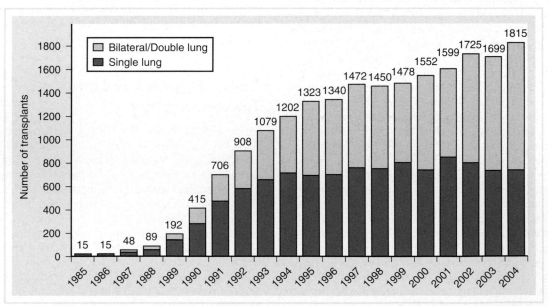

FIGURE 78-2 Number of lung transplants reported by year and procedure type.

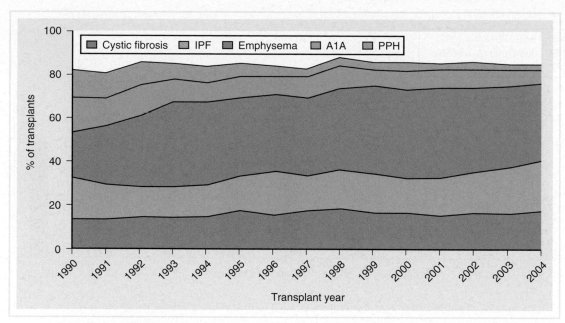

FIGURE 78-3 Adult lung transplantation indications by year (%).

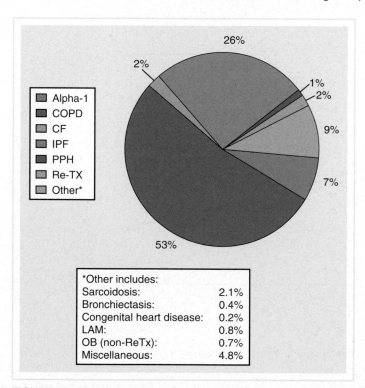

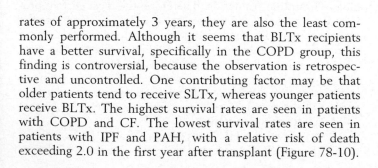

*Other includes:
Sarcoidosis:	2.1%
Bronchiectasis:	0.4%
Congenital heart disease:	0.2%
LAM:	0.8%
OB (non-ReTx):	0.7%
Miscellaneous:	4.8%

FIGURE 78-4 Adult lung transplantation: indications for single lung transplants (transplants: January 1995–June 2005).

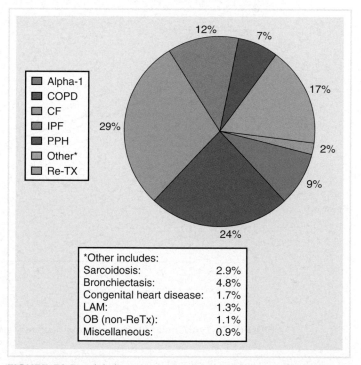

*Other includes:
Sarcoidosis:	2.9%
Bronchiectasis:	4.8%
Congenital heart disease:	1.7%
LAM:	1.3%
OB (non-ReTx):	1.1%
Miscellaneous:	0.9%

FIGURE 78-5 Adult lung transplantation: indications for bilateral/double lung transplants (transplants: January 1995–June 2005).

rates of approximately 3 years, they are also the least commonly performed. Although it seems that BLTx recipients have a better survival, specifically in the COPD group, this finding is controversial, because the observation is retrospective and uncontrolled. One contributing factor may be that older patients tend to receive SLTx, whereas younger patients receive BLTx. The highest survival rates are seen in patients with COPD and CF. The lowest survival rates are seen in patients with IPF and PAH, with a relative risk of death exceeding 2.0 in the first year after transplant (Figure 78-10).

GENERAL SELECTION CRITERIA (Table 78-1)

The international consensus guidelines for referral and selection of transplant candidates was published in 1998 as a joint effort from the American Society of Transplant Physicians, the American Thoracic Society, the European Respiratory Society, and the International Society for Heart and Lung Transplantation to facilitate the appropriate timing of referral and proper selection of candidates most likely to benefit from transplantation while ensuring a fair allocation of limited organs. These guidelines were updated in 2006. In all

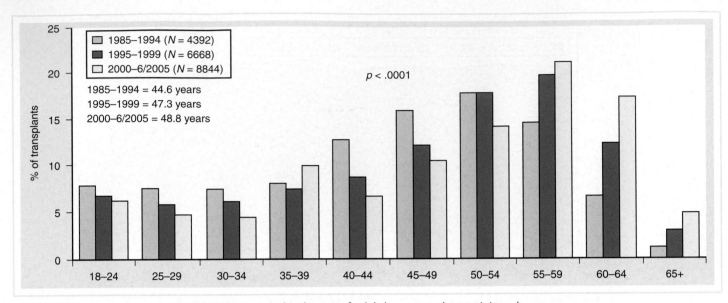

FIGURE 78-6 Age distribution of adult lung transplant recipients by era.

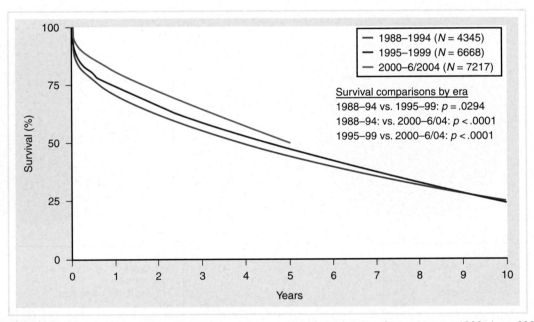

FIGURE 78-7 Adult lung transplantation Kaplan–Meier survival by era (transplants: January 1988–June 2004).

instances, selected patients with end-stage pulmonary disease should have declining and irreversible lung function despite optimal medical and surgical management. To justify the risk of transplantation, individuals should have an estimated survival of less than 2 years.

Two issues regarding this 2-year survival recommendation merit clarification. First, unique to lung transplantation, their survival differs as a function of the recipient's primary disease. Within the first 2 years, survival rates stabilize and allow a more accurate prediction of subsequent survival. Second, the average waiting time for transplantation is close to 2 years. Patients listed for transplant with a higher expected survival

may lower their survival benefit and keep more terminal candidates from transplantation. Therefore, the most current projected prognosis of lung diseases, the average time on the waiting list, and the median survival post lung transplantation should be considered when determining timing for selection. The new Lung Allocation System in the United States also affects this planning, in that the time to transplant seems to be shorter, but a median waiting time for patients has not yet been determined. In essence, there is a moving target that will take more time to define.

The typical age for HLTx is younger than 55, BLTx younger than 60, and SLTx younger than 65. Medical conditions

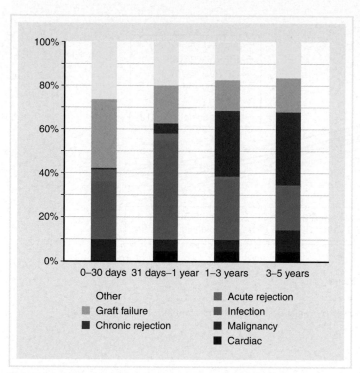

FIGURE 78-8 Cause of death in time periods after transplantation. Most strikingly, chronic rejection becomes the most common cause of death from 1 year posttransplantation. (Data from The International Society for Heart and Lung Transplantation and the United Network for Organ Sharing [Ishlt/Unos] Registry Report, 2002, Available at: www.Ishlt.Org.)

Legend: Other / Graft failure / Chronic rejection / Acute rejection / Infection / Malignancy / Cardiac

aggressive. Renal impairment is considered an absolute contraindication to transplant if the creatinine clearance is less than 50 mg/mL/min.

Cancer screening includes mammography, Papanicolaou smear, prostate screen, and colonoscopy as medically indicated. A history of cancer is not an absolute contraindication. Eligibility is determined by cancer type and requires documentation of cure without evidence of recurrence or metastasis. Lymphoma, breast, colon, renal, and prostate cancer should have a 5-year cancer-free period, because these cancers tend to have a longer recurrence period. Less aggressive skin cancers, such as squamous and basal cell, should be in remission for greater than 2 years.

Osteopenia and osteoporosis should be sought with bone densitometry measurements. Bone demineralization should be treated before transplantation by proper nutrition, calcium supplementation, vitamin D, bisphosphonates, and/or hormone replacement. Medications that increase bone resorption should be discontinued. Symptomatic osteoporosis is considered a relative contraindication. The future need for chronic steroid and immunosuppressive therapies will worsen bone loss. This can result in impaired ambulation, suboptimal rehabilitation, and limit posttransplant quality of life.

Nutritional state also affects outcome and postoperative rehabilitation. Candidates should weigh more than 70%, but less than 130% of their ideal body weight. For patients who are outside of these limits, a weight gain or weight loss program should be instituted with subsequent reevaluation for candidacy. Percutaneous enteral feeding may be necessary to achieve the desired nutritional goal. Total parenteral nutrition is an option but is not recommended enthusiastically because of the attendant risk of infection.

Dependence on tobacco, alcohol, or drugs must be treated, and patients should be substance-free for greater than 6 months. Disabling psychoaffective disorders, noncompliance, and lack of proper social support are relative contraindications. In our institution, social workers assess the support systems to maximize compliance with postoperative interventions and medications.

associated with damage to other organs are considered absolute contraindications. The exception is in rare selected cases with potential for combined heart-lung, lung-kidney, or lung-liver transplantation. For this reason, diagnosis and management of hypertension, diabetes mellitus, gastroesophageal reflux, peptic ulcer disease, and osteoporosis should be

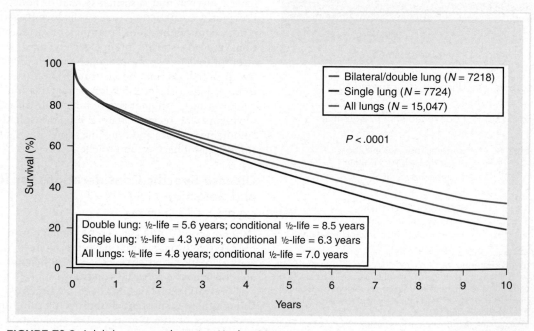

Bilateral/double lung (N = 7218)
Single lung (N = 7724)
All lungs (N = 15,047)
P < .0001

Double lung: ½-life = 5.6 years; conditional ½-life = 8.5 years
Single lung: ½-life = 4.3 years; conditional ½-life = 6.3 years
All lungs: ½-life = 4.8 years; conditional ½-life = 7.0 years

FIGURE 78-9 Adult lung transplantation Kaplan–Meier survival (transplants: January 1994–June 2004).

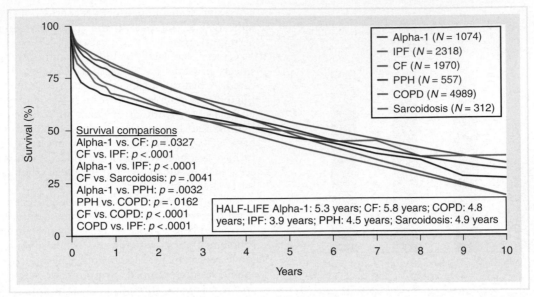

FIGURE 78-10 Adult lung transplantation Kaplan–Meier survival by diagnosis (transplants: January 1994–June 2004).

Financial issues, including supplemental aid from hospital programs, insurance companies, government agencies, and family/community support, must be explored preoperatively.

Invasive mechanical ventilation is considered a relative contraindication. Retrospective analyses suggest that acutely ventilated patients have a very high risk of perioperative complication and a mortality surpassing 50%. On the other hand, chronically ventilated patients without other contraindications may have acceptable survival rates.

Musculoskeletal disease that limits ambulation and breathing is an absolute contraindication. Less severe disease is acceptable if the recipient can undergo adequate rehabilitation and have a meaningful quality of life after transplant. Restrictive anatomic deformities of the thorax and skeleton are considered relative contraindications.

Chronic active infection with HIV, hepatitis B, and hepatitis C are considered absolute contraindications. Recipients colonized with multidrug-resistant *Burkholderia cepacia*, especially genomovar III, have an extremely high rate of mortality and graft failure. *Burkholderia* is often found in patients with CF, and many centers consider this is an absolute contraindication. Recipients with multidrug-resistant *Pseudomonas aeruginosa* have a survival that is similar to that of noncolonized patients. Previously treated infection with *Mycobacterium tuberculosis* is not a contraindication. Treatment of various pulmonary infections may be started preoperatively in some patients in an attempt to decrease the pathogen burden. In others, postoperative prophylaxis may be instituted for those who are deemed to be at high risk for infection or reactivation (e.g., *Aspergillus* colonization). A higher risk of infection still exists in colonized recipients who receive bilateral lung transplants, because many colonizing bacteria and fungi may spill down into the lung from sinuses, nasopharynx, and trachea.

TABLE 78-1 General Contraindications: Lung Transplantation

Absolute	Relative
Malignancy within 5 years (except SCC and BCC)	Age older than 65
Untreatable multiorgan dysfunction	Unstable clinical condition
Active hepatitis B, C and HIV	Poor rehabilitation potential
Severe spinoskeletal deformity	Panresistant colonization (Burkholderia cepacia genomovar III)
Current substance addiction	BMI > 30 kg/m^2 Severe osteoporosis Mechanical ventilation Poor social support and medical adherence

Adapted from Orens JB, Estenne M, Arcasoy SM, et al: International Guidelines for the Selection of Lung Transplant Candidates: 2006 Update-A Consensus Report From the Pulmonary Scientific Council of the International Society of Heart and Lung Transplantation. J Heart Lung Transplant 25: 745–55; 2006.
SCC, Squamous cell cancer; *BMI*, body mass index; *BCC*, basal cell cancer.

Disease-Specific Considerations for Referral and Selection (Table 78-2)

COPD

Patients with COPD (i.e., emphysema, chronic bronchitis, and obliterative bronchiolitis) have the highest survival rates after transplantation (patients with A1A deficiency and emphysema are considered a separate condition).

Survival benefit has not been documented in COPD, even though there is substantial improvement in functional capacity and quality of life. One potential explanation for this discrepancy is that the forced expiratory volume in 1 sec (FEV$_1$) may

TABLE 78-2 International Guidelines for the Selection of Lung Transplant Candidates: 2006 Update

Pulmonary Disease	COPD	CF and Other Bronchiectasis	IPF	PPH
Guidelines for referral	BODE index > 5	FEV1 < 30% predicted—particularly in young women Exacerbation requiring ICU stay Increasing exacerbations requiring antibiotics Refractory and/or recurrent pneumothorax Recurrent hemoptysis refractory to embolization	Histologic or radiographic evidence of UIP irrespective of FVC Histologic fibrotic NSIP	NYHA class III or IV, irrespective of therapy Rapidly progressive disease
Guidelines for transplant	BODE index of 7 to 10 or at least 1 of the following: Hospitalization for exacerbation with acute hypercapnia (Pco_2 > 50 mmHg) Pulmonary hypertension or cor pulmonale, or both, despite oxygen therapy FEV_1 < 20% and either DL_{CO} of < 20% or homogeneous distribution of emphysema	Oxygen dependent respiratory failure Hypercapnia Pulmonary hypertension	Histologic or radiographic evidence of UIP and any of the following: DL_{CO} < 39% predicted 10% or greater decline in FVC during 6 months of follow-up Pulse oximetry < 88% during a 6-MWT Honeycombing on HRCT (fibrosis score > 2) NSIP and DL_{CO} < 35% NSIP and 10% decline in FVC or 15% decline in DL_{CO} during 6 months of follow-up	Persistent NYHA class III or IV on maximal therapy Low (< 350 meter) or decline in 6-MWT Failing therapy with IV epoprostenol or equivalent CI < 2 L/min/m^2 RAP > 15 mmHg

Adapted from Orens JB, Estenne M, Arcasoy SM, et al. International Guidelines for the Selection of Lung Transplant Candidates: 2006 Update—A Consensus Report From the Pulmonary Scientific Council of the International Society of Heart and Lung Transplantation. J Heart Lung Transplant 2006; 25: 745–755.

TABLE 78-3 BODE Index Computation

BODE Points by variables	0	1	2	3
Airflow obstruction (FEV_1% predicted)	≥65	50–64	36–49	≤35
6 Minute Walk Test (Distance in meters)	≥350	250–349	150–249	≤149
Modified Medical Research Council Dyspnea Scale (Range 0–4)	0–1	2	3	4
Body-mass Index	>21	≤21		

Adapted from Celli BR, Cote CG, Marin JM, et al. The Body-Mass Index, Airflow Obstruction, Dyspnea, and Exercise capacity Index in Chronic Obstructive Pulmonary Disease. NEJM 2004; 350: 1005–1012.

not be as reliable of a referral parameter as, for example, the BODE index (Table 78-3). Patients with a BODE index between 7 and 10 should be selected for transplant. Other criteria for selecting COPD candidates includes severe worsening in pulmonary function, shorter 6-min walking distance capacity (<100 yards), weight loss (BMI <20 kg/m²), need for hospital admission (ICU in particular), and homogeneous emphysema. More severe patients will show chronic hypoventilation (i.e., $PaCO_2$ ≥55 mmHg and evidence of pulmonary hypertension despite oxygen therapy). All patients with COPD should be referred to pulmonary rehabilitation, treated with oxygen therapy, and have considered or failed potential options such as lung volume reduction surgery.

Pulmonary Fibrosis

Idiopathic pulmonary fibrosis (IPF) is the most progressive of the fibrotic diseases and is defined by the radiohistologic diagnosis of usual interstitial pneumonitis (UIP). No treatment for IPF is known to be effective and, accordingly, patients can only be supported with supplemental oxygen, pulmonary rehabilitation, and close clinical surveillance. Prompt referral of appropriate candidates for lung transplantation is essential, because it is the only measure that will prolong survival in those at highest risk of death. IPF has a median survival of 3 years from the time of diagnosis, consistent with the 30% mortality rate documented for IPF patients awaiting transplant. Lung function parameters are used to decide when patients should be referred (i.e., a forced vital capacity [FVC] <60–70% of predicted, a diffusion capacity for carbon dioxide [DLCO] <50–60% of predicted). Many, however, feel that these cutoffs are too low, because they underestimate mortality. Other variables indicating higher mortality rates include hypoxia developing during a 6-min walk test (pulse oximetry <88%), a resting PaO_2 level <50 mmHg while breathing room air, classic roentgenographic or histologic findings of UIP, and a decline in lung function within 6 months of the initial diagnosis.

Other etiologies of pulmonary fibrosis tend to have a better prognosis. Nonspecific interstitial pneumonia (NSIP), particularly the cellular variant of NSIP, has a 5-year survival rate of 75%. Other fibrotic diseases that may lead to lung transplantation include sarcoidosis, scleroderma, rheumatoid arthritis, mixed connective tissue disorders, asbestosis, histiocytosis X, and lymphangioleiomyomatosis. In general, the same criteria for referral should be used with all of these, because more disease-specific criteria have not yet been developed.

Cystic Fibrosis

Patients with CF frequently have multiorgan involvement and comorbid conditions, including malnutrition, chronic infections of the upper respiratory tract, and colonization with resistant pathogens. Current referral guidelines are inadequate,

because good prognostic models for survival in CF do not exist, but those with an FEV_1 <30% predicted or with declining pulmonary function should be referred early. This is most important in females younger than the age of 20, who seem to have a worse prognosis. Severity of disease may also be indicated by an increase in the frequency of hospital admissions, specifically, if ICU care is required. Similar to COPD, the ability to identify those with a better prognosis will likely depend on assessing multiple factors such as the degree of hypoxia and hypercapnia, evidence of cor pulmonale, and limited functional capacity. Colonization with multidrug-resistant *Pseudomonas aeruginosa*, *Staphylococcus aureus*, *Stenotrophomonas maltophilia*, and *Aspergillus fumigatus* are not contraindications for transplantation, because they have not been shown to affect posttransplant survival. The exception is *Burkholderia cepacia* genomovar III, which is associated with an unacceptably high risk of posttransplant mortality. Patients with multidrug-resistant pathogens should undergo frequent evaluation for changes in their colonizing microflora and resistance patterns. This will guide early prophylaxis and treatment in the immediate postoperative period. Complicated pneumothorax and hemoptysis are other indications for early referral.

Patients with CF have excellent survival rates similar to those with COPD. Although other causes of bronchiectasis are also amenable to transplantation, there are insufficient data to develop specific guidelines. For the most part, guidelines recommended for patients with CF are used.

Pulmonary Arterial Hypertension

Idiopathic pulmonary hypertension is a progressive and rapidly fatal disease, with an estimated median untreated survival of less than 3 years from the time of diagnosis. Current pulmonary vasodilator therapy (e.g., epoprostenol, treprostinil, and bosentan) has substantially increased survival. Transplantation is, accordingly, reserved for those who do not respond to medical management. NYHA/WHO functional class 3 and 4 patients are at highest risk of death and the most likely to benefit from transplant. Diminished exercise capacity can be measured by use of a standard 6-min walk test. Inability to walk a distance of 332 m and degree of right heart failure are important predictors of mortality.

DONOR SELECTION AND MANAGEMENT

The Lung Allocation Score (LAS) assigns donor lungs to transplant candidates by use of a scoring system determined by medical urgency and net transplant benefit (predicted posttransplant survival minus predicted wait list survival). Since its implementation in the United States in 2005, median waiting times seemed to have shortened markedly. Unfortunately, a scarcity of donated organs remains a limiting problem, leading to a consideration of use of non-heart beating donors (Table 78-4) and developing different types of lung grafts (Table 78-5).

Currently, the Ideal Donor Selection Criteria are more stringent than those used for selecting other solid organs. In light of the scarcity of available lung grafts, many are suggesting that the donor criteria be made more flexible to expand the existing donor pool. Alternate criteria include donors being older than 55, having an initial PaO_2/FiO_2 ratio <300, the presence of pulmonary infiltrates on chest imaging, purulent secretions, and a positive history of tobacco or other inhalant drug history (Tables 78-6 and 78-7). Retrospective studies suggest

TABLE 78-4 Maastricht Classification for NHBD

I	Uncontrolled	Brought in dead
II	Uncontrolled	Unsuccessful resuscitation
III	Controlled	Awaiting cardiac arrest
IV	Controlled	Cardiac arrest after brain death
V	Controlled	Cardiac arrest in a hospital inpatient

*Controlled non-heart beating donors may be eligible for lung donation.

TABLE 78-5 Types of Lung Grafts

Living donor	Donor donates single lower lobe. Recipient receives two lower lobes from two separate donors.
Heart beating donor	Whole brain death. Donor may donate one or both lungs depending on selection criteria.
Non-heart beating donor (NHBD)	Donor has sustained cardiac arrest. Resuscitated to unacceptable state and deemed suitable for organ donation.
Xenotransplantation	Porcine, bovine and primate lungs. Still under investigation.
Artificial lung	Intracorporeal or paracorporeal devices that oxygenate venous blood. Still under investigation

TABLE 78-6 Donor Selection Guidelines

	Ideal Donor	Extended Donor
Age	<55	>55
ABO	Identical or compatible	Compatible
CXR	Clear	Unilateral or focal infiltrate
*PaO_2	>300	<300 on initial assessment; must be >300 after optimization
Tobacco	<20 pack years	>20 pack years
Trauma	Absence of chest trauma	Trauma without significant abnormality
Sputum	No purulent secretions	May be considered, therapeutic suctioning can be performed
Gram stain	Absence of organisms	Certain organisms may be considered (see Table 78-5)

*Partial pressure of arterial oxygen tension (PaO_2) is measured on a fraction of inspired oxygen of 1.0 and a positive end-expiratory pressure of 5 cmH_2O.

TABLE 78-7 Donor Related Infections That May be Considered Eligible

- Gram-positive bacteremia
- Mycobacterial infection outside chest
- Fungal airway colonization
- Hepatitis B core antibody
- Herpesviruses (HHV6–8, varicella)
- CMV (high risk if donor+/recipient–)
- EBV (high risk if donor+/recipient–)

HHV, Human herpes virus.

similar outcomes for ideal and extended lung allograft recipients, specifically with respect to perioperative complications, ICU stay, requirements for mechanical ventilation, and 1-year survival (both >80%). Improved donor management is also under careful investigation, because it may help improve marginal donors and optimize them into ideal candidates. Optimizing the donor with reversal of any limiting physiologic insults is becoming the standard of care in most transplant centers (Figure 78-11). Common respiratory insults are caused by aspiration, atelectasis, infection, pulmonary edema, and the hemodynamic instability associated with neurologic dysfunction. Ventilatory strategies to improve alveolar ventilation may be implemented along with therapeutic bronchoscopy to suction excess secretions and reexpand atelectatic lung. Small-volume BAL can minimize the amount of alveolar flooding. Adequate tissue perfusion and cardiac function should be aided with vasoactive medications when needed. Repletion of cortisol, vasopressin, and thyroid hormone may also be of benefit (Figure 78-12).

DONOR GRAFT MANAGEMENT

Graft ischemic time begins after the lungs have been extracted from the donor. The lungs are flushed with a cold heparinized preservation solution—modified Euro-Collins, low potassium dextran solution (LPD), or University of Wisconsin solution are the most commonly used—and hypothermic preservation is maintained during transport at 4° C. These solutions have helped reduce the severity of ischemic injury. Additives such as surfactant, platelet and thrombin inhibitors are still under investigation. Donor lungs are matched according to compatibility in size and ABO blood group. Lymphocyte, CMV, and EBV cross matching are not routine, because these are often impractical. Each matching procedure has its supporters for certain situations, however.

LUNG ALLOGRAFT IMPLANTATION
(Figure 78-13)

The implantation depends on the planned procedure, surgical experience, and the previous surgical history of the recipient. Before all transplants, the recipient's pulmonary function should be maximized, and management should continue through surgery (i.e., continuing pulmonary vasodilators).

A single-lung transplant is often placed through an anterolateral or posterolateral thoracotomy. Bilateral lung implantation may be performed by means of a transverse sternotomy "clamshell" incision, at the level of the fourth or fifth intercostal spaces, whereas HLTx is usually done through a

Collaborative Practice	Phase I Referral	Phase II Declaration of Brain Death and Consent	Phase III Donor Evaluation	Phase IV Donor Management	Phase V Recovery Phase

The following professionals may be involved to enhance the donation process.
 	
Check all that apply.
† Physician
† Critical care RN
† Organ Procurement Organization (OPO)
† OPO coordinator (OPC)
† MedicalExaminer (ME)/ Coroner
† Respiratory
† Laboratory
† Pharmacy
† Radiology
† Anesthesiology
† OR/Surgery staff
† Clergy
† Social worker
	† Notify physician regarding OPO referral
	† Contact OPO ref: Potential donor with severe brain insult
	† OPC on site and begins evaluation
	   Time _____ Date _____
	† Ht_____ Wt _____ as documented
	† ABO as documented _____
	† Notify house supervisor/ charge nurse of presence of OPC on unit
		† Brain death documented
		   Time _____ Date _____
		† Pt accepted as potential donor
		† MD notifies family of death
		† Plan family approach with OPC
		† Offer support services to family (clergy, etc)
		† OPC/Hospital staff talks to family about donation
		† Family accepts donation
		† OPC obtains signed consent & medical/social history
		   Time _____ Date _____
		† ME/Coroner notified
		† ME/Coroner releases body for donation
		† *Family/ME/Coroner denies donation—stop pathway— initiate post-mortem protocol—support family.*
			† Obtain pre/post transfusion blood for serology testing (HIV, hepatitis, VDRL, CMV)
			† Obtain lymph nodes and/or blood for tissue typing
			† Notify OR & anesthesiology of pending donation
			† Notify house supervisor of pending donation
			† Chest & abdominal circumference
			† Lung measurements per CXR by OPC
			† *Cardiology consult as requested by OPC (see reverse side)*
			† *Donor organs unsuitable for transplant—stop path- way—initiate post-mortem protocol—support family.*
				† OPC writes new orders
				† Organ placement
				† OPC sets tentative OR time
				† Insert arterial line/ 2 large- bone IVs
				† Possibly insert CVP/Pulmonary Artery Catheter
				† See reverse side
					† Checklist for OR
					† Supplies given to OR
					† Prepare patient for transport to OR
					   † IVs † Pumps
					   † O₂ † Ambu
					   † Peep valve
					† Transport to OR
					   Date _____
					   Time _____
					† OR nurse
					   † reviews consent form
					   † reviews brain death documentation
					   † checks patient's ID band

Labs/Diagnostics		† Review previous lab results
		† Review previous hemody- namics
			† Blood chemistry
			† CBC + diff
			† UA † C & S
			† PT, PTT
			† ABO † A Subtype
			† Liver function tests
			† Blood culture X 2 / 15 minutes to 1 hour apart
			† Sputum Gram stain & C & S
			† Type & Cross Match _____# units PRBCs
			† CXR † ABGs
			† EKG † Echo
			† Consider cardiac cath
			† Consider bronchoscopy
				† Determine need for additional lab testing
				† CXR after line placement (if done)
				† Serum electrolytes
				† H & H after PRBC Rx
				† PT, PTT
				† BUN, serum creatinine after correcting fluid deficit
				† Notify OPC for
				   ___ PT >14___ PTT > 28
				   ___ Urine output
				      ___ < 1 mL/Kg/hr
				      ___ > 3 mL/Kg/hr
				   ___ Hct < 30 / Hgb <10
				   ___ Na >150 mEq/L
					† Labs drawn in OR as per surgeon or OPC request
					† Communicate with pathology: Bx liver and/ or kidneys as indicated

Respiratory	† Pt on ventilator
	† Suction q 2 hr
	† Reposition q 2 hr
		† Prep for apnea testing: set FiO₂ @ 100% and antici- pate need to decrease rate if PCO₂ < 45 mm Hg	† Maximize ventilator settings to achieve SaO₂ 98 - 99%
			† PEEP = 5cm O₂ challenge for lung placement FiO₂ @ 100%, PEEP @ 5 X 10 min
			† ABGs as ordered
			† VS q 1°
				† Notify OPC for
				   _____ BP < 90 systolic
				   _____ HR < 70 or > 120
				   _____ CVP < 4 or > 11
				   _____ PaO₂ < 90 or
				   _____ SaO₂ < 95%
					† Portable O₂ @ 100% FiO₂ for transport to OR
					† Ambu bag and PEEP valve
					† Move to OR

Treatments/ **Ongoing Care**		† Use warming/cooling blanket to maintain temperature at 36.5° C - 37.5 °C † NG to low intermittent suction	† Check NG placement & output † Obtain actual Ht _____ & Wt _____ if not previ- ously obtained		† Set OR temp as directed by OPC † Post-mortem care at conclusion of case
Medications			† Medication as requested by OPC	† Fluid resuscitation—con- sider crystolloids, colloids, blood products † DC meds except pressors & antibiotics † Broad-spectrum antibiotic if not previously ordered † Vasopressor support to maintain BP > 90 mm Hg systolic † Electrolyte imbalance: consider K, Ca, PO₄, Mg replacement † Hyperglycemia: consider insulin drip † Oliguria: consider diuretics † Diabetes insipidus: con- sider antidiuretics † Paralytic as indicated for spinal reflexes	† DC antidiuretics † Diuretics as needed † 350 U heparin/kg or as directed by surgeon
Optimal Outcomes	The potential donor is iden- tified & a referral is made to the OPO.	The family is offered the option of donation & their decision is supported.	The donor is evaluated & found to be a suitable candi- date for donation.	Optimal organ function is maintained.	All potentially suitable, con- sented organs are recovered for transplant.

Shaded areas indicate Organ Procurement Coordinator (OPC) Activities.

FIGURE 78-11 Critical pathway of organ donor management. Critical pathway for the organ donor. 2006. http://www.Unos.Org/Resources/ Pdfs/Criticalpathwayposter.pdf. Reprinted with permission of the United Network for Organ Sharing, Richmond, VA.

Cardio-Thoraic Donor Management

1. Early echocardiogram for all donors—Insert pulmonary artery catheter (PAC) to monitor patient management (placement of the PAC is particularly relevant in patients with an EF < 45% or on high dose inotropes).
   - † use aggressive donor resuscitation as outlined below

2. Electrolytes
   - † Maintain Na < 150 meq/dl
   - † Maintain K+ > 4.0
   - † Correct acidosis with Na Bicarbonate and mild to moderate hyperventilation (pco_2 30–35 mmHg)

3. Ventilation — Maintain tidal volume 10–15 mL/kg
   - † keep peak airway pressures < 30 mmHg
   - † maintain a mild respiratory alkalosis (pco_2 30–35 mmHg)

4. Recommend use of hormonal resuscitation as part of a comprehensive donor management protocol — Key elements
   - † <u>Tri-iodothyronine</u> (T3): 4 µg bolus; 3 µg/hr continuous infusion
   - † <u>Arginine Vasopressin</u>: 1 unit bolus: 0.5–4.0 unit/hour drip (titrate SVR 800–1200 using a PA catheter)
   - † <u>Methylprednisolone</u>: 15 mg/kg bolus (Repeat q 24° PRN)
   - † <u>Insulin</u>: drip at a minimum rate of 1 unit/hour (titrate blood glucose to 120–180 mg/dL)
   - † <u>Ventilator</u>: (See above)
   - † <u>Volume Resuscitation</u>: Use of colloid and avoidance of anemia are important in preventing pulmonary edema
       - † albumin if PT and PTT are normal
       - † fresh frozen plasma if PT and PTT abnormal (value ≥ 1.5 × control)
       - † packed red blood cells to maintain a PCWP of 8–12 mmHg and Hgb > 10.0 mg/dL

5. When patient is stabilized/optimized repeat echocardiogram. (An unstable donor has not met 2 or more of the following criteria.)
   - † Mean Arterial Pressure ≥ 60
   - † CVP ≤ 12 mmHg
   - † PCWP ≤ 12 mmHg
   - † SVR 800-1200 dyne/sec/cm^5
   - † Cardiac Index ≥ 2.5 L/min/M^2
   - † Left Ventricular Stroke Work Index > 15
   - † Dopamine dosage < 10 µg/kg/min

FIGURE 78-12 Critical pathway of organ donor management. Critical pathway for the organ donor. 2006. http://www.Unos.Org/Resources/Pdfs/Criticalpathway-poster.pdf. Reprinted with permission of the United Network for Organ Sharing, Richmond, VA.

midsternotomy. Bilateral sequential lung transplantation (BSLT) can also be performed through bilateral anterior thoracotomies, which is the preferred procedure because it does not split the sternum and is associated with less chest wall instability. The surgical history of the recipient is important, because previous pleurodesis or cardiothoracic surgery results in fibrous bands and adhesions. This makes resection difficult and may alter the anatomy. When a single-lung transplant is to be performed, the intact side is preferred.

In most instances, the cold ischemic time for an SLTx is approximately 4 h and for a BLTx is less than 6 h. Pleural tubes are placed before closure and maintained in place until drainage is less than 200 mL/day. Bronchoscopic evaluation of the airway mucosa, anastomotic sites, and therapeutic suctioning of secretions is performed to document graft viability and optimize function.

Intraoperative and postoperative management of patients with end-stage pulmonary diseases is challenging because of poor pulmonary gas exchange, elevated pulmonary vascular resistance, and right ventricular overload. Analgesia is controlled with multiple medications, trying to avoid narcotics for their effects of decreased respiratory drive and sedative properties. A thoracic epidural is often placed in preparation for surgery to adequately control pain and optimize postoperative lung function. Endotracheal intubation is performed with the largest-diameter dual lumen tube possible to facilitate clearance of secretions. Mechanical ventilation can increase pulmonary vascular resistance and decrease venous return leading to systemic hypotension. This is important, because anesthetics used during rapid sequence induction and surgery should be administered cautiously to avoid a precipitous drop in systemic vascular resistance. In most cases, infusions with propofol and fentanyl are used and combined with a neuromuscular blocker such as pancuronium. A fraction of inspired oxygen at 1.0 is used initially to reduce hypoxic pulmonary vasoconstriction and limit right heart afterload. Cardiopulmonary bypass (CPB) is not used routinely and should generally be avoided unless hemodynamic instability arises or simultaneous cardiac surgery is necessary. If CPB is used, aprotinin (which slows fibrinolysis) may be administered to help control the coagulopathic disturbance created by the activation of multiple cytokines from the bypass procedure (although

Types of lung transplant				
	Heart-lung	**Bilateral sequential**	**Single lung**	**Live donor lobar**
Incision	Midline sternotomy	Horizontal "clam shell" Bilateral anterior thoracotomies preferred Horizontal "clam shell" less frequently used	Lateral thoracotomy	Horizontal "clam shell"
Anastomoses	Tracheal Right atrial Aortic	Left and right bronchial "Double" left atrial Right and left pulmonary artery	Bronchial Left atrial Pulmonary artery	Lobar bronchus to bronchus Lobar vein to superior pulmonary vein Lobar artery to main pulmonary artery
Advantages	Airway vascularity All indications	Access to pleural space No cardiac allograft Less cardiopulmonary bypass	Easiest procedure Increases recipients	Increases donors Can be done "electively"
Disadvantages	Cardiac allograft Organ "consumption"	Airway complications Postoperative pain	Airway complications Poor reserve	Complex undertaking Donor morbidity
Common indications	Congenital heart disease with pulmonary hypertension Heart and lung disease Primary pulmonary hypertension	Cystic fibrosis (CF) Bullous emphysema Primary pulmonary hypertension Bronchiectasis	Emphysema Pulmonary fibrosis Primary pulmonary hypertension	Cystic fibrosis (CF) Pulmonary fibrosis Primary pulmonary hypertension

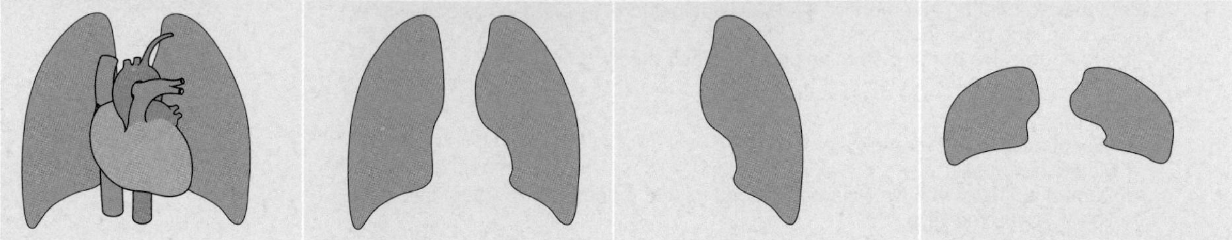

FIGURE 78-13 Comparison of the four standard lung replacement techniques, including their common indications.

recent studies have suggested aprotinin may be associated with increased thrombotic complications). When single-lung ventilation commences, hypoxia and hypoventilation may ensue. Capnography, along with serial arterial blood gases, can help detect signs of failing single-lung ventilation. This may be corrected with independent dual-lung ventilation and tolerance of moderate respiratory acidosis as long as hemodynamics and oxygenation remain stable.

Pulmonary vasodilators such as inhaled nitric oxide (iNO) are used commonly in the perioperative setting. The effects of iNO at relatively low levels (<20 parts per million) are not completely understood, but it is preferred because of the selective pulmonary vasodilation at sites receiving adequate alveolar ventilation. iNO also seems to inhibit endothelial dysfunction and capillary leak, suppress oxygen radical formation, and ameliorate ischemia-reperfusion injury to the lung allograft. These benefits could then extend to improvement in early graft function. The adverse effects of iNO at higher concentration levels includes methemoglobinemia, pulmonary edema, and cardiac contractile dysfunction. Prostacyclin, in either intravenous or aerosolized form, is also used as a direct pulmonary vasodilator.

The goal of hemodynamic management is to reach a negative fluid balance and limit pulmonary edema. The pulmonary artery occlusion pressure is kept under 10 mmHg to ensure adequate preload. In most cases, immediate normalization of pulmonary arterial pressures and right ventricular function is expected after transplantation. To prevent alveolar damage, hyperinflation, pulmonary vascular hypertension, and anastomotic dehiscence, peak airway pressures are kept under 40 cmH$_2$O, with a positive end expiratory pressure close to 5 cmH$_2$O. Liberation from mechanical ventilation is usually accomplished in the first 1–3 days after transplantation.

NONINFECTIOUS COMPLICATIONS

The most common problems in the immediate posttransplant period are the same as those occurring in most postsurgical patients. Hypoxemia may stem from poor cardiac output, endotracheal tube displacement, or obstruction of uncleared secretions, leading to lobar atelectasis. Additional complications that are unique to lung transplantation include hyperacute rejection, graft dysfunction, and cardiac failure; each may be difficult to differentiate from the others (Table 78-8). A suggested reading by Ahya and Kawut has been listed.

HYPERACUTE REJECTION (HAR)

HAR results from a recipient antibody directed against donor endothelial and human leukocyte (HLA) antigens. This immediately triggers the classic complement cascade with

TABLE 78-8 Early Non-Infectious Pulmonary Complications

Diagnosis	HAR	PGD	AR	HPE
Onset	Immediate (<2 days)	2–3 days	1 week to 3 months	Immediate (<2 days)
Etiology	Recipient antibodies to donor antigens ABO blood group antigens HLA antigens (DR and B)	Multi-injury: Donor illness, surgical harvest, ischemia, preservation, hypothermia, reperfusion	Cell-mediated reaction against donor endothelial and epithelial antigens	Pulmonary venous obstruction Cardiogenic shock LV outflow obstruction Fluid overload
Pathology	Alveolar hemorrhage Intravascular fibrin/thrombi Neutrophil interstitial infiltration Capilliritis IgG deposition	DAD Graded by level of hypoxemia	Graded by extent of parenchymal and vascular lymphocytic infiltration T cell infiltration CD8+ predominant	Alveolar edema
Treatment	• Removal of allo-antibodies • Plasmapheresis • IVIG	• Negative fluid balance • Lung protective ventilation • Nitric oxide • Prostaglandins • ECMO • Re-transplantation	• Cell-mediated immunesuppression • High-dose steroids • Anti-thymocyte globulin • Photopheresis • Radiation	• Negative fluid balance • Diuresis • Renal replacement therapy • Correction of underlying cause

HAR, Hyperacute rejection; *PGD*, primary graft dysfunction; *AR*, acute rejection; *HPE*; high-pressure pulmonary edema; *LV*, left ventricle; *DAD*, diffuse alveolar damage; *ECMO*, extracorporeal mechanical oxygenation.

reperfusion of the graft and leads to cell injury and cell death. HAR is extremely rapid in onset, occurring often within minutes of reperfusion and can be seen intraoperatively as a dusky pallor and swelling of the transplanted lung. Endothelial injury leads to capillary leak, and leukocyte injury leads to microvascular inflammation, thrombosis, and coagulopathy. This is manifested as diffuse alveolar infiltrates, low PaO_2/FiO_2 ratio, and increased plateau pressures.

HAR can be avoided by preoperatively performing a leukocyte cross-match test, where the recipient's blood is tested against the donor's cells seeking the presence of leukocyte sensitization and donor cell lysis. The plasma reactivity antibody (PRA) test is another way of checking the recipient's serum against a panel of commonly found human leukocyte antigens (HLA) and measuring the degree of sensitization. Patients with a PRA >10% are considered to be at greater risk for rejection and posttransplant mortality. In our institution, patients with high PRA levels are treated with plasmapheresis followed by intravenous immunoglobulin (IVIg) on the day of transplant. This combination treatment seems to provide outcomes comparable to those of recipients without high levels of anti-HLA antibodies. Other methods involve pulse administration of cyclophosphamide or methotrexate along with IVIg to reach a high level of immunosuppression.

PRIMARY GRAFT DYSFUNCTION (PGD)
(Table 78-9)

PGD is the current name for the syndrome of acute lung injury (ALI) after reperfusion of the lung allograft. This entity was previously referred to as ischemia-reperfusion injury, reimplantation edema, and early graft dysfunction. PGD occurs 48–72 h after transplantation and is characterized by development of bilateral diffuse alveolar infiltrates on chest radiography coupled with hypoxemia resulting from capillary leak and alveolar flooding and is associated with prolonged ischemic time (i.e., >550 min). In approximately 15% of patients,

TABLE 78-9 Recommendations for Grading of Primary Graft Dysfunction (PGD) Severity

Grade	PaO_2/FiO_2	Radiographic Infiltrates Consistent with Pulmonary Edema
0	>300	Absent
1	>300	Present
2	200–300	Present
3	<200	Present

From: Christie, JD, Carby M, Bag R, *et al*. Journal of Heart Lung Transplantation. Vol 24; Issue 10:1454–1459.

the degree of hypoxemia reaches ALI criteria (PaO_2/FiO_2 <200) with an accompanying mortality >60%. Exclusion of other causes of alveolar infiltrates, including high-pressure pulmonary edema, is necessary.

Immediate management is supportive and similar to management of patients with ALI /ARDS, including generating a negative fluid balance in an attempt to prevent further alveolar flooding by use of low tidal volume ventilation (4–6 mL/kg of predicted body weight) to limit ventilator-associated lung injury and providing hemodynamic support with vasoactive drugs to maintain adequate perfusion to major organs and the bronchial anastomoses. Renal replacement therapy is generally recommended for oliguric renal injury, because it may facilitate achieving negative fluid balance. Anecdotal evidence suggests that nitric oxide may lower pulmonary arterial pressures, improve ventilation-perfusion mismatch, and protect endothelial cells. Similarly, prostaglandins may also have protective effects in this setting and are often added to the preservation solution as a means of preventing PGD. Extracorporeal membrane oxygenation as a bridge to urgent retransplantation has been used anecdotally with little success.

HIGH-PRESSURE PULMONARY EDEMA

High-pressure pulmonary edema (i.e., a pulmonary arterial occlusion pressure >18 mmHg) can develop as a result of several problems. Fluid overload may occur from blood product transfusion and/or crystalloid infusions. Cardiogenic shock can occur as result of CPB or from previously untreated myocardial disease. Pulmonary vascular anastomoses may undergo dehiscence or become thrombosed or stenosed. Diagnosis of pulmonary venous obstruction can be made with transesophageal echocardiography with careful inspection of the PV anastomotic sites. Thrombus formation in the pulmonary outflow track and left atrium can lead to systemic embolization and may require immediate thrombectomy or anticoagulation.

ACUTE REJECTION (AR)

AR is a cell-mediated event activated by donor antigens. It occurs in 40% of transplant recipients in the first year alone, irrespective of specific induction treatment (Figures 78-14 and 78-15), but the incidence is highest in the first 6 months after transplant. It presents as alveolar infiltrates, hypoxemia, and fever, but many patients may be asymptomatic. Histologic examination is required to diagnose AR as the clinical presentation mimics pulmonary infection and increasing immunosuppression empirically can lead to toxicity, infection, and malignancy.

AR is associated with an increased risk of developing chronic rejection. For this reason, serial surveillance with fiberoptic bronchoscopy, BAL, and transbronchial biopsies is often routine during the first year after transplant. Current recommendations are to obtain at least five separate samples that contain both alveolated lung and bronchioles (because both are necessary to grade the level of AR). Treatment revolves around increasing the level of immunosuppression by administration of high-dose corticosteroids, azathioprine, or cyclosporine. In addition, antithymocyte globulin, photochemotherapy, and lymphoid irradiation may be used.

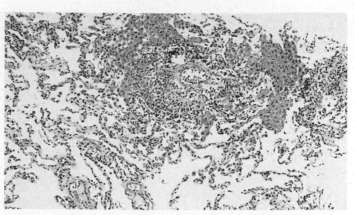

FIGURE 78-15 Transbronchial lung biopsy specimen showing acute rejection. The lymphocytes surround an arteriole and the infiltrate spreads into surrounding alveolar walls (grade A3).

BRONCHIAL ANASTOMOTIC COMPLICATIONS

Bronchial anastomotic dehiscence may result from ischemic injury, infection, or poor healing. Bronchial artery interruption during transplant disrupts perfusion to the large airways. High doses of corticosteroids impair wound healing and can lead to bronchomalacia and stenosis (Figure 78-16). Dehiscence may present as pneumomediastinum, pneumopericardium, and/or pneumothorax (Figure 78-17). Fiberoptic bronchoscopy is necessary to ensure that all bronchial anastomoses are intact. Correction consists of treating any underlying infection and

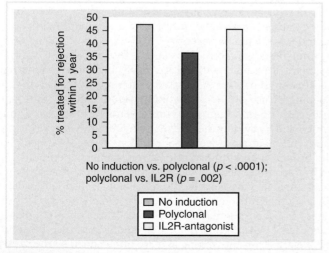

FIGURE 78-14 Percentage of adult lung transplant recipients treated for rejection in first year stratified by type of induction (transplants: January 1, 2000–June 30, 2004).

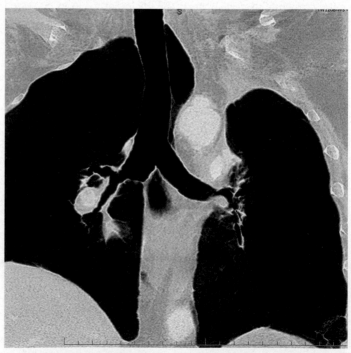

FIGURE 78-16 Bilateral bronchial stenosis (distal main bronchi) after bilateral sequential lung transplantation. Poor anastomotic perfusion from septic shock and bacterial pneumonia complicated the immediate postoperative course.

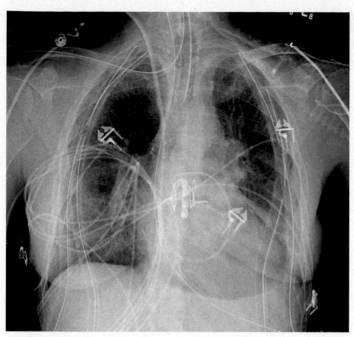

FIGURE 78-17 Pneumopericardium as a manifestation of bronchial dehiscence after lung transplant.

maintenance of adequate tissue perfusion. Bronchial stent placement, laser ablation, and balloon dilatation are often used in management.

PHRENIC NERVE INJURY

Phrenic nerve injury occurs from trauma during intraoperative manipulation of the mediastinum and pericardium. Phrenic nerve dysfunction can occur as a result of hypothermic cardioplegia and stretch injury. Both may complicate weaning. Diagnosis should be suspected in patients who have a paradoxical breathing pattern. An elevated hemidiaphragm may not be obvious on radiography or on fluoroscopic or ultrasound evaluation of diaphragmatic motion if the injury is bilateral. In these instances, a phrenic nerve conduction study would be the definitive diagnostic study of choice.

HYPERINFLATION

Hyperinflation of the native lung may be seen in patients with COPD and unilateral lung transplantation as a result of the higher lung compliance, more severe airway obstruction, and air trapping that occurs in the remaining emphysematous lung. Hyperinflation can compress the transplanted lung and/or the mediastinal structures and can cause a substantive reduction in function (Figure 78-18).

INFECTIOUS COMPLICATIONS

Infectious complications in the immediate postoperative period are the same as those associated with other major cardiothoracic surgeries. Bloodborne infections from indwelling catheters, urinary track, and wound complications are common. Pneumonia in the acute posttransplant phase requires careful assessment of the donor's and recipient's microbiologic and clinical histories, including previous bacterial colonization or recent infections. Clinical history is relevant, because it may

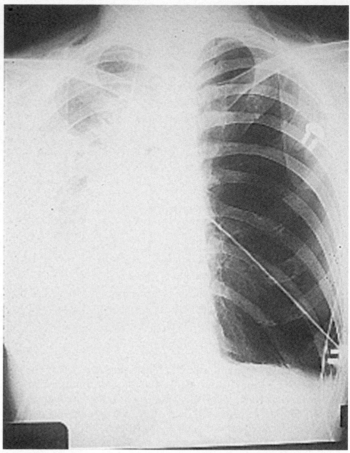

FIGURE 78-18 Chest radiograph showing right single-lung transplant for emphysema. Severe hyperinflation with mediastinal shift caused by overinflation of the native lung and compression of the transplanted right lung is shown.

detect risks for aspiration, nosocomial, and ventilator associated pathogens (Table 78-10). Physiologic abnormalities in the transplanted lung also predispose to infection. Impaired mucociliary clearance, denervation of the cough reflex, and disruption of the pulmonary lymphatic and vascular outflow all may act in combination. Infection of the allograft results in inflammation and graft damage. Although prophylaxis seems logical in preventing future infection, strong clinical evidence to support universal use of prophylaxis does not exist and varies among different transplant centers worldwide.

COMMUNITY-ACQUIRED PNEUMONIA

Pneumonia presenting in the first month after transplant is usually bacterial in origin. Community- or hospital-acquired gram-positive and gram-negative bacteria are the most common pathogens. Aspiration is another cause, as donors are at risk from emergent intubations as of neurologic impairment or critical illness. In donors who have been intubated for more than 48 h, pneumonia should be considered as ventilator associated. A history of bacterial colonization must be treated and guided by the sensitivity and resistance patterns previously documented. Identification of bacterial infection in the donor should be covered accordingly. Early fiberoptic bronchoscopy with bronchoalveolar lavage (BAL) and transbronchial biopsy (TBB) is the standard of care in

TABLE 78-10 Infectious Pulmonary Complications

Diagnosis	Community Aquired	Donor/Recipient Acquired	Hospital Acquired	Opportunistic	Reactivation
Onset	<1 month *may occur late as well	<1 month	<1 month	>1 month	>1 month
Common Organisms	Staphylococcus Streptococcus Haemophilus Chlamydia Mycoplasma Klebsiella Legionella Listeria **Community Acquired Viruses** • RSV • Adenovirus • Parainfluenza • Influenza	Pseudomonas Stenotrophomonas Burkholderia cepacia • **genomovar III most virulent** MRSA Aspergillus MTB Atypical Mycobacteria Toxoplasma	MRSA Pseudomonas Acinitobacter	CMV EBV VZV PCP Nocardia Aspergillus Candida	CMV EBV VZV MTB
Late complications	• Bronchial anastomosis • Rejection	• Bronchial anastomosis • Rejection	• Bronchial anastomosis • Rejection	• CMV and BOS • EBV and PTLD	• CMV and BOS • EBV and PTLD

the early posttransplant period. Specimens are routinely sent for bacterial, fungal, and viral analysis. Methicillin-resistant *Staphylococcus aureus* (MRSA) and resistant *Pseudomonas aeruginosa* should be suspected in those at risk for nosocomial infection or colonization, such as in patients with CF. Prophylaxis with nebulized antipseudomonal drugs such as tobramycin and colistin may be useful.

OPPORTUNISTIC INFECTIONS (OI)

OIs are uncommon before the first month after transplant. They are directly related to the immunosuppressed state that leads to the reactivation of latent infections and an inadequate response to otherwise nonvirulent pathogens. Prophylaxis against *Pneumocystis*, herpes family viruses, and *Aspergillus* reduce the frequencies of these infections; however, OI is a common cause of posttransplant morbidity.

CYTOMEGALOVIRUS (HUMAN HERPES VIRUS 5)

CMV is found in latent stage in nearly 60% of all adults. Routine screening of donor and recipient for CMV IgG allows stratification of those at highest risk of CMV reactivation and pneumonitis. Primary CMV infection (PCI) occurs when a CMV-seronegative recipient becomes infected from a CMV-positive graft or blood product. Because PCI carries the highest risk of severe infection and mortality, matching CMV-negative recipients to CMV-negative donors is preferred, but sometimes is impractical. In cases in which CMV naïve recipients receive a CMV-positive graft, passive immunization with IV CMV IgG can be given, followed by inhibition of viral replication with ganciclovir. Other anti-CMV treatments include valganciclovir, cidofovir, foscarnet, and leflunomide. These may be used in refractory or resistant cases. Secondary CMV infection and CMV superinfection can cause reactivation pneumonitis in CMV-seropositive recipients; however, these types of infections are not as severe as PCI.

CMV pneumonitis can be diagnosed by the presence of intranuclear viral inclusion bodies on histologic examination. This condition may be an indirect cause of rejection and the bronchiolitis obliterans syndrome (Figure 78-19). CMV prophylaxis is often given routinely and may delay acute infection (Table 78-11). This may result in the evolution of resistant strains, predispose to antiviral toxicity, as well as increasing the current cost of care. Alternatively, preemptive monitoring and treatment of infection can be implemented. CMV replication can be detected early by rising serum CMV antigen levels or quantitative CMV PCR assay results.

EPSTEIN–BARR VIRUS (HUMAN HERPES VIRUS 6)

EBV is also routinely screened for in both recipients and donors. Similar to CMV, it carries a high risk for reactivation and can lead to posttransplant lymphoproliferative disorder (PTLD). PTLD is believed to occur in almost half of the patient who are EBV seronegative and receive an EBV-seropositive graft. Matching EBV negative status is, therefore, extremely important, but often difficult. PTLD may present as a pulmonary nodule, mass, or infiltrate and requires tissue biopsy for diagnosis. Unfortunately, commonly used chemotherapy directed against lymphoproliferative malignancies has not been very successful in treating PTLD. EBV prophylaxis in those at highest risk is covered by antiviral treatment directed against CMV and HSV. As with all other opportunistic complications, reduction in the level of immunosuppression remains the single most important management strategy.

ASPERGILLUS SPECIES

Aspergillus is a common infection in solid organ transplants. It may present in a variety of ways, including a bronchial inflammatory disorder, necrotizing airway infection (pseudomembrane), and invasive pulmonary parenchymal aspergillosis. Invasive fungal infection is difficult to diagnose, because it is

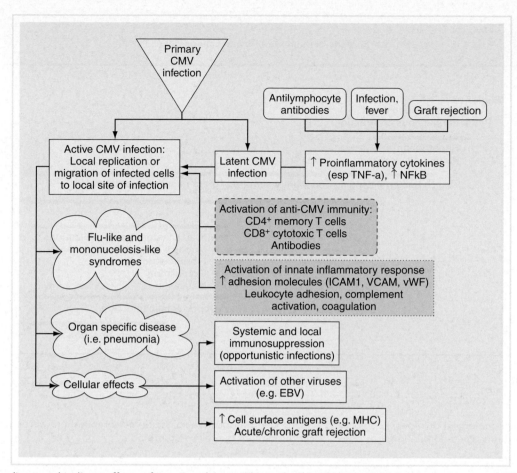

FIGURE 78-19 The direct and indirect effects of cytomegalovirus. The activation of latent CMV alters many aspects of the innate and adaptive immune response. The indirect effects include predisposition to opportunistic infections, activation of other latent viruses, and graft rejection or graft-versus-host disease. (From Ison MG, Fishman, JA: Clin Chest Med 2005; 26[4]:691–705, Viii [Fig. 1]).

TABLE 78-11 Suggested CMV Prophylaxis Post-Transplant

CMV IgG Status	Recipient (–)	Recipient (+)
Donor (–)	1. Day 1–14 Ganciclovir 5 mg/kg IV Q12h 2. Day 15–90 Valganciclovir 450 mg PO QD	1. Day 1–14 Ganciclovir 5 mg/kg IV Q12h 2. Day 15–90 Valganciclovir 450 mg PO QD
Donor (+)	1. Day 1–14 Ganciclovir 5 mg/kg IV Q12h 2. Day 15–90 Valganciclovir 450 mg PO QD	1. Day 1–90 Acyclovir 400 mg PO TID or Valacyclovir 500 mg PO QD

- Ganciclovir must be adjusted for renal function.
- CMV PCR is followed routinely if prophylaxis not given.
- Cytogam (CMV immunoglobulin) 150 mg/kg can be added for treatment.

angiocentric and not detected by routine BAL or TBB. Surgical biopsy is often necessary to make a definite diagnosis. Prophylaxis with oral amphotericin B, itraconazole, or IV liposomal amphotericin may be administered to those at highest risk of infection. The azoles must be used carefully, because they can interact with the metabolism of calcineurin inhibitors.

A figure that combines the common infectious and non-infectious complications posttransplantation over time is provided (Figure 78-20).

Chronic Rejection

Bronchiolitis Obliterans Syndrome (BOS)

BOS is a clinicopathologic common syndrome of progressive and irreversible airway obstruction with a declining DLco that occurs as a late complication in graft function with an incidence of almost 50% by the fifth year after transplantation (Figure 78-21). Pathologically, BOS is represented by bronchiolitis obliterans (BO; i.e., fibrosis of the small airways with

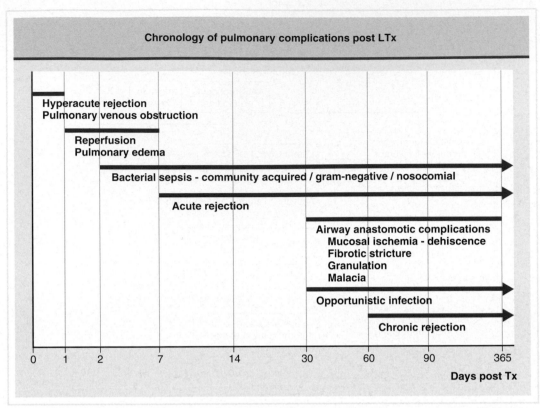

FIGURE 78-20 The chronology of pulmonary complications in the lung transplant recipient. Some complications occur during a defined time span in the early posttransplantation period, but others occur throughout the follow-up period.

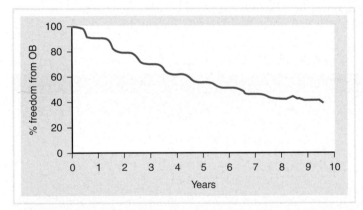

FIGURE 78-21 Freedom from bronchiolitis obliterans for adult lung recipients (follow-ups: April 1994–June 2005) conditional on survival to 14 days.

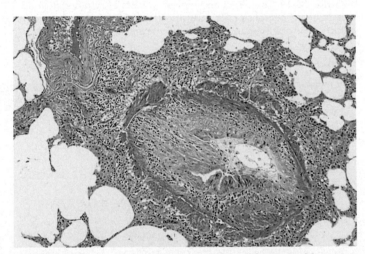

FIGURE 78-22 Open lung biopsy specimen showing obliterative bronchiolitis. The bronchiolar lumen is obliterated by organizing fibrin, myofibroblasts, and lymphocytes.

intimal thickening and sclerosis of its accompanying vessel that lead to near complete occlusion of the bronchiolar lumen and small airway obstruction) (Figure 78-22). Chest imaging should be normal in the early stages of BOS, and it remains a diagnosis of exclusion at that time. Acute rejection, infection, drug-induced pneumotoxicity, and bronchial anastomotic obstruction must be excluded. Advanced BOS may appear as peripheral bronchiectasis with a loss of vascularity and atelectasis. A staging system has been created to aid in the diagnosis

of BOS by the International Society of Heart and Lung Transplantation (Tables 78-12 and Table 78-13).

BOS is believed to be caused by alloimmune-driven tissue injury. Risk factors are a previous history of rejection episodes, viral infections, and the presence of lymphocytic bronchitis. Unfortunately, some patients with severe clinical BOS may not show histologic evidence of obliterative bronchiolitis on biopsy, whereas others with significant histologic evidence of BO may be asymptomatic. There is no effective treatment

TABLE 78-12 Histologic Classification and Grading of Pulmonary Allograft Rejection

Acute rejection

Grade 0 — none	No significant abnormality
Grade 1 — minimal	Infrequent perivascular mononuclear cell infiltrates mainly surrounding venules that are 2–3 cells deep
Grade 2 — mild	More frequent infiltrates, 5 cells or more deep, involving venules and arterioles
Grade 3 — moderate	More exuberant mononuclear cell infiltrate that extends from the perivascular space into the alveolar interstitium
Grade 4 — severe	Infiltrate extending into the alveolar space with pneumocyte damage and at times necrosis of vessels and lung parenchyma
Airway inflammation	Lymphocytic bronchitis/bronchiolitis; pathologist may grade
Chronic ariway rejection Active Inactive	
Chronic vascular rejection - accelerated graft vascular sclerosis	

Immunosuppression

The goal of immunosuppression in all solid organ transplantation revolves around a two-phase host against donor rejection model. In the initial acute posttransplant period, donor antigen presenting cells (APCs) activate T cells to react against graft antigens. B cells are also activated by graft antigens and form antibodies directed against them. This first phase must be counteracted with a high level of immunosuppression termed induction. Induction is directed against blocking the APC to T-cell interaction, preventing T-cell proliferation, and B-cell alloimmunization. The second phase of immunosuppression is termed maintenance. During the maintenance phase, the host apparently adapts to the graft. Doses of immunosuppressants can be lowered to avoid toxicity and infectious complications while stabilizing the adaptive immune response.

Induction is accomplished with antibodies directed against human lymphoid cells. Antithymocyte globulin and monoclonal antibodies directed against specific CD receptors found on human lymphocytes are used, including muromonab-CD3, alemtuzumab, basiliximab, and daclizumab. Of these, basiliximab and daclizumab have gained favor as they target activated T cells and have fewer, less-severe side effects. Depleting antibodies are used in combination with high-dose methylprednisolone, a calcineurin inhibitor, and antiproliferative drug such as an antimetabolite or a mammalian target of rapamycin inhibitor.

Maintenance therapy is based on a triple-drug regimen that includes a calcineurin inhibitor, an antimetabolite, and a corticosteroid. This triple therapy has been chosen on the basis of studies performed on other solid organ transplants showing improved survival and lower graft rejection episodes over alternate regimens.

Calcineurin Inhibitors (CIs)

CIs block the signal of activation between APCs and T cells. The classic CI is cyclosporine A, because it was the first effective immunosuppressant used in transplantation medicine. Tacrolimus is the second CI most commonly used and is now

for BOS. Slowing of further progression may be possible with a trial of increased immunosuppression. This may be warranted in those with an inflammatory predominant stage of BOS. Retransplantation remains a potential option in a few selected cases.

TABLE 78-13 Comparison of Acute Rejection and Bronchiolitis Obliterans Syndrome

Feature	Acute Rejection	Bronchiolitis Obliterans Syndrome
Peak frequency	First 6 mo	Years > 3 mo
Onset	Abrupt to subacute	Usually subtle
Symptoms	Tightness in chest (immediate postoperative period) Cough (usually not productive) Dyspnea	Dyspnea with heavy exertion Cough (often productive)
Physiologic	Restrictive impairment Desaturation of arterial blood	Obstructive impairment Normoxia until late
Radiologic	Diffuse interstitial inflitrates Pleural effusions	No abnormality until disorder is far advanced Computed tomographic evidence of bronchiectasis and mosaic pattern
Hematologic	Leukocytosis	Normal white blood cell count
Histologic	Perivascular mononuclear cell infiltrates Airway inflammation is variable	Obliterative bronchiolitis Atherosclerosis of pulmonary and bronchial arteries Pleural scarring
Response to treatment	Majority of cases improve rapidly with intravenous corticosteroid	Forced expiratory volume in 1 second at best stabalized Majority of recipients have progressive decline in allograft function

preferred in most transplant centers. CI toxicity side effects include nephrotoxicity, neurotoxicity, hemolytic uremic syndrome, and posttransplantation diabetes mellitus.

Antimetabolites

The antimetabolites inhibit the proliferation of lymphocytes. They include inhibitors of purine synthesis such as mycophenolate mofetil and azathioprine. Mycophenolate mofetil is generally preferred because of its lower side effect profile than azathioprine (AZA). Recent studies suggest, however, that the two agents have a similar effectiveness. Accordingly, AZA is still preferred at some centers because of its relatively low cost.

MAMMALIAN TARGET OF RAPAMYCIN (mTOR) INHIBITORS

The mTOR inhibitors act by inhibiting the cell cycle and preventing T-cell proliferation. Rapamycin, also known as sirolimus, is the classic mTOR inhibitor. Newer mTOR inhibitors include everolimus and temsirolimus. mTOR inhibitors used in conjunction with CIs increase the incidence of nephrotoxicity and hemolytic uremic syndrome events. mTOR inhibitors have antineoplastic properties and are used as treatment in several different types of cancers. Accordingly, these agents may have a potential role in treating PTLD.

PITFALLS OF IMMUNOSUPPRESSIVE THERAPY (Table 78-14)

Common complications from the chronic use of these drugs varies, depending on the specific agent being used and the recipient's predisposing characteristics. Toxicities may be severe and irreversible, as is evident in cases of posttransplant malignancy. Frequent checks for metabolic derangements and end organ toxicity are critical. Unfortunately, serum drug levels do not correlate with the dosage of administered drugs and are not predictive of the potential toxic effects, because these factors vary from individual to individual.

Reaching and maintaining an adequate level of immunosuppression is difficult and has led some to consider individual analysis of specific genetic polymorphisms that affect drug metabolism to tailor specific treatments to the individual patient. Adjunct testing of immune activity by the measurement of ATP levels may be a more accurate way to adjust dosing. These basic issues warrant further investigation, because they will likely affect the future of immunosuppressive management.

There is a current trend toward the use of tacrolimus, MMF, and sirolimus (Figure 78-23). A recent study comparing azathioprine to MMF in lung transplant recipients failed to show a significant difference in prevention of BOS. Although there are multiple reasons why a difference was not observed, there is still no definitive evidence to suggest superior outcomes with these newer drugs.

MEDICAL COMPLICATIONS IN LUNG TRANSPLANT SURVIVORS

Lung transplant survivors are at risk of multiple medical complications related to their predisposing illness and toxicities resulting from chronic immunosuppression. The aim of long-term care in the posttransplant patient revolves around prevention and early detection of commonly described posttransplant medical illnesses.

Neuromuscular

Neuromuscular toxicity is a well-described complication of the calcineurin inhibitors (CI). This complication is thought to be dose-dependent and presents with symptoms ranging

TABLE 78-14 Maintenance Immunosuppresive Drugs			
Drug	Dose	Adverse Effects	Interactions
Cyclosporine (Calcineurin inhibitor)	Whole blood level 250–350 ng/mL	Nephrotoxicity, HUS, neurotoxicity, post-transplant DM, hirsutism, gingival hyperplasia, gastroparesis, HTN, and electrolyte disturbances	Increased by macrolides, azoles, calcium channel blockers, gastric motility agents. Decreased by anticonvulsants, rifampin.
Tacrolimus (Calcineurin inhibitor)	Whole blood through level 10–20 ng/mL	Nephrotoxicity, HUS, neurotoxicity, post-transplant DM, hyperlipidemia, HTN, and electrolyte disturbances	Fatty meals decrease absorption. Increased by macrolides, azoles, calcium channel blockers, gastric motility agents. Decreased by anticonvulsants, rifampin.
Azathioprine (Anti-metabolite)	2–2.5 mg/kg per day Adjust for WBC 4–6k/mm^3	Leukopenia, anemia, thrombocytopenia, pancreatitis	Allopurinol in combination has higher bone marrow toxicity
Mycophenolate Mofetil (Anti-metabolite)	1000–1500 mg BID	GI symptoms can be improved if given Q 6 h or lower total dose	Anatacids, iron and magnesium decrease absorption. Increases levels of acyclovir and gangciclovir.
Sirolimus (mTOR inhibitor)	Load 6 mg then 2 mg/day (goal 10–20 ng/mL level)	Anemia, thrombocytopenia, leukopenia, HTN, electrolyte abnormalities, GI symptoms	Increased by macrolides, azoles, calcium channel blockers, gastric motility agents

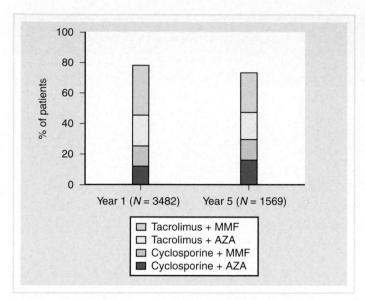

FIGURE 78-23 Adult lung recipients' maintenance immunosuppression drug combinations at time of follow-up for follow-ups between January 2002 and June 2005. Conventional combinations analysis limited to patients receiving prednisone.

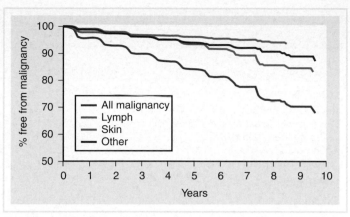

FIGURE 78-24 Freedom from malignancy for adult lung recipients (follow-ups: April 1994–June 2005).

from headache and tremors to seizures and confusion. The posterior leukoencephalopathy syndrome can result in cortical blindness from microvascular injury and encephalopathy. Myopathies are common, especially when the CIs are used in combination with corticosteroids, presumably caused by direct mitochondrial toxicity. This is an important complication, because the major limiting factor in posttransplant exercise capacity seems to be related to muscular dysfunction and inadequate mitochondrial activity rather than to cardiopulmonary deficiency. In patients with seizures, treatment should start with reducing the dose of CI and adding an antiepileptic that does not interact with the immunosuppressant regimen.

Osteoporosis

As discussed earlier, osteoporosis is a relative contraindication to transplantation. Fractures occur commonly after transplantation and can be severely debilitating. Advanced age, poor nutrition, immobility, and smoking all contribute to bone demineralization. Corticosteroids and CIs are known to increase bone resorption and further the development of severe osteoporosis. Many centers will treat patients at risk before transplantation with exercise, calcium supplementation, vitamin D, and antiresorptive agents such as the bisphosphonates to reduce the posttransplant risk.

Malignancy (Figure 78-24)

Posttransplant malignancy is frequently seen after solid organ transplantation. The calcineurin inhibitors and azathioprine have been associated with a higher risk of cancer. Currently, there is a 10% incidence of tumor development in 5-year survivors, with lymphoid and skin cancers being the majority. Newer immunosuppressive agents, such as the mTOR

inhibitors, seem to have antineoplastic properties; there is no evidence that these agents lead to lower cancer risk or mortality.

OTHER MEDICAL COMPLICATIONS POSTTRANSPLANTATION (Figure 78-25)

Acute and chronic nephrotoxicity is well described with the calcineurin inhibitors and is characterized by hyalinosis of afferent arterioles, vacuolization of proximal tubules, and focal areas of interstitial and glomerular fibrosis. Although renal dysfunction is rather common in 1-year survivors, renal failure requiring dialysis remains rare. Calcineurin inhibitors as well as corticosteroids can also lead to diabetes mellitus, hypertension, and dyslipidemia (Table 78-15).

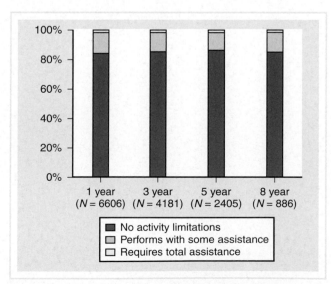

FIGURE 78-25 Adult lung recipients' functional status of surviving recipients (follow-ups: April 1994–June 2005).

TABLE 78-15 Post-Lung Transplant Morbidity for Adults

Outcome	Follow-ups: April 1994 – June 1999		Follow-ups: July 1999 – June 2005	
	Within 1 Year	Total Number with Known Response	Within 1 Year	Total Number with Known Response
Hypertension	48.3%	(N = 3162)	53.2%	(N = 4735)
Renal Dysfunction	22.2%	(N = 3088)	27.4%	(N = 4870)
Abnormal Creatinine < 2.5 mg/dl	12.5%		18.9%	
Creatinine > 2.5 mg/dl	8.0%		6.7%	
Chronic Dialysis	1.7%		1.8%	
Renal Transplant	0.0%		0.1%	
Hyperlipidemia	11.0%	(N = 3280)	23.9%	(N = 5064)
Diabetes	16.10%	(N = 3129)	26.9%	(N = 4800)
Bronchiolitis Obliterans	10.7%	(N = 2817)	7.3%	(N = 4460)

Cumulative Prevalence in Survivors within 1 Year Post-Transplant (Follow-ups: April 1994 – June 2005)

SUGGESTED READINGS

Ahya VN, Kawut SM: Noninfectious pulmonary complications after lung transplantation. Clin Chest Med 2005; 26:613–622.

De Soyza A, McDowell A, Archer L, et al: Burkholderia cepacia complex genomovars and pulmonary transplantation outcomes in patients with cystic fibrosis. Lancet 2001; 358:1780–1781.

Estenne M, Maurer JR, Boehler A, et al: Bronchiolitis obliterans syndrome 2001: An update of the diagnostic criteria. J Heart Lung Transplant 2002; 21:297–319.

Kowalski R, Post D, Schneider MC, et al: Immune cell function testing: An adjunct to therapeutic drug monitoring in transplant patient management. Clin Transplant 2003; 17:77–88.

McNeil K, Glanville AR, Wahlers T, et al: Comparison of mycophenolate mofetil and azathioprine for prevention of bronchiolitis obliterans syndrome in de novo lung transplant recipients. Transplantation 2006; 81:998–1003.

Orens JB, Boehler A, Perot MD, et al: A review of lung transplant donor acceptability criteria. J Heart Lung Transplant 2003; 22(11):1183–1200.

Orens JB, Estenne M, Arcasoy SM, et al: International Guidelines for the Selection of Lung Transplant Candidates: 2006 Update—A Consensus Report From the Pulmonary Scientific Council of the International Society of Heart and Lung Transplantation. J Heart Lung Transplant 2006; 25:745–755.

Shargall Y, Guenther G, Ahya VN, et al: Report of the ISHLT Working Group on Primary Lung Graft Dysfunction Part VI: Treatment. J Heart and Lung Transplant 2005; 24:1489–1500.

Steen S, Sjoberg T, Pierre L, et al: Transplantation of lungs from a non-heart beating donor. Lancet 2001; 357:825–829.

Trulock EP, Edwards LB, Taylor DO, et al: Registry of the International Society for Heart and Lung Transplantation: Twenty-third Official Adult Lung and Heart-Lung Transplantation Report. J Heart Lung Transplant 2006; 25:880–892.

Index

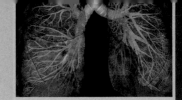

Note: Page numbers followed by 'f' indicate figures 't' indicate tables 'b' indicate boxes.

Chronic lung disease, sleep-disordered
breathing in *(continued)*
diagnosis, 936
epidemiology, 936
pitfalls/controversies, 936
risk factors, 936
treatment, 936
Chronic mucus hypersecretion, 497–498
Chronic necrotizing pulmonary aspergillosis
(CNPA), 375
chest radiograph, 376*f*
Chronic nonpolyp rhinosinusitis, 421*f*
Chronic obstructive pulmonary disease
(COPD), 145–146, 247, 523.
See also Acute exacerbations of COPD
acute dyspnea, 293, 295, 296–299
air pollution, 496–497
airway, cholinergic control of, 478*f*
antioxidants imbalance, 504
asthma and, 499–500, 573, 573*t*
asthma *v.*, 509*t*, 515
BODE index, 502*f*
bronchodilator response, 149
bronchodilator reversibility, 512*b*
CAP and, 334
chronic airway disease and emphysema,
HIV and, 467–468
chronic dyspnea, 307–309
cigarette smokers, 496
clinical features, 503*t*, 510
closing volume and, 152
combination inhalers, 473–474
comorbidities in, 492, 492*b*
differential diagnosis, 509
epidemiology, 500*f*, 501
etiology and risk factors, 499
exacerbations, pathophysiology of, 508
exhaled nitric oxide, 154–155
future trends, 481–482
genetic disorders and, 81
inflammation in, 494*b*
inflammatory cells, 494*b*
lung cancer and, 606
lung transplantation for, 960–962
mediators in, 494*b*
natural history and prognosis, 501
negative-pressure ventilation, 259–260
noninvasive ventilation, 260
long-term application, 263
NPPV, 266
pathogenesis of, 504
pathology, 495
pathophysiology, 492
postoperative pulmonary
complications, 276
pulmonary hemodynamics in, oxygen
therapy and, 539
spirometric classification of, 511*t*
systemic effects, 507–508
testing, 154
theophylline, 475
ventilating patients with, 246
Chronic respiratory acidosis, 129
Chronic respiratory alkalosis, 129
Chronic respiratory failure
NPPV, initiation guidelines, 264*t*
O₂, 541
Chronic responses, 146
increased load, 145–146

Chronic rhinosinusitis, 412, 420
Chronic thromboembolic pulmonary
hypertension (CTEPH), 778–779,
778*f*, 786
Churg-Strauss syndrome, 685–686, 685*f*
asthma and, 570
histopathology of, 570*f*
vasculitis component of, 800
Chylothorax, pleural effusions and, 861–862
Cicatrization collapse, lung and, 22
Cidofovir, CMV pneumonia, 373–374, 454
Cigarette smoking, 491, 493*f*
asthma, 555–556
COPD and, 81, 491–492, 495, 496
FEV₁ decline, 501, 501*f*
FEV₁ values, 499*f*
lung function in, 524*f*
peripheral airways, 497*f*
postoperative pulmonary
complications, 275–276
Cilia
dysfunction, COPD, 504
electron micrograph, 427*f*
respiratory system defense, 167
Ciprofloxacin
bacterial pneumonia, 370–372
pneumonia, 345
Circulatory physiology, 111–113
Circulatory structure, 111
CIs. *See* Calcineurin inhibitors
CL. *See* Lung compliance
Clarithromycin, 452–453
Clindamycin-Primaquine, HIV infected and, 449
Clinical Pulmonary Infection Score
(CPIS), 380, 380*t*, 384
Clinical studies
genetics, asthma, 555
pulmonary rehabilitation, 544
Clinical test of diffusing capacity, 152
Clofazimine, TB, 401
Closed pleural biopsy
anesthesia, 197
biopsy techniques, 200*f*
complications, 200*f*
incision, 199
indications and contraindications, 197
patient positioning, 197
pitfalls/controversies, 200
procedure, 198*f*
technique, 197–199
choice of, 200
thoracentesis and, introduction, 197
Closing capacity, 153
Closing volume, intraparenchymal airways, 153
Clubbing, 614*f*
CMV. *See* Cytomegalovirus
CNPA. *See* Chronic necrotizing pulmonary
aspergillosis
CNS. *See* Central nervous system
Coagulation, pulmonary circulation, 114
Coal nodule, 811*f*
Coal worker's pneumoconiosis (CWP), 62,
647–648, 649*t*, 809
BAL, 814
chest radiology, 812–814
chest X-ray, 813*f*
clinical course/treatment/prevention, 815
clinical features, 814
diagnosis, 811–814

Coal worker's pneumoconiosis (CWP)
(continued)
epidemiology, 809
exposure sources, 809
genetics, 810
ILOR classification, 811*t*
macular lesion of, 810*f*
management, 815
pathology, 810–811
pathophysiology, 809–810
prevention, 815
prognosis, 814
serologic/immunologic features, 814
Co-amoxiclav, *Nocardia*, 372
Cobb angle, calculation method for, 896*f*
Coccidioides, 377
Coccidioidomycosis, 357–358
HIV, 443
treatment, 453
Cochrane review, asthma, 556
Codeine, chronic cough, 290
Codominant alleles, 80
Cognitive behavioral therapy (CPT),
dyspnea, 307
Cold. *See* Common cold
Cold agglutinins, bacterial pneumonia,
341
Collagen vascular diseases, clinical
features, 804
Collapse. *See also specific collapse*
lung and, 30
Collectins, 174
Combination antimycobacterial therapy,
MAC infection, 452–453
Combination antiretroviral therapy.
See Highly active antiretroviral
therapy
Combination therapy, AEs of COPD, 521
Combined Cardiopulmonary Risk Index
(CPRI), 279
Combined lobar collapses, 28–29, 29*f*, 30
Combined primary disorders, acid-base
disorders and, 130
Common cold (Acute coryza), 412,
415–416, 420, 421
diagnosis, 416
Community-acquired MRSA, 338
Community-acquired pneumonia
(CAP), 331, 342*f*. *See also* Bacterial
pneumonia; Pneumonia
age, 333
alcoholism, 333
antibiotics for, 346*t*
aspiration pneumonia *v.*, 335
associated diseases, 334
clinical course and prevention,
345–346
clinical features, 341
diagnosis, 348
diagnostic approach, 331*f*, 341–342
empirical antibiotic therapy, 344–345
epidemiology/risk factors/
pathogenesis, 334
institutionalization, 333
lung transplantation and, 969–970
microbial etiology in, 329*t*
miscellaneous factors, 334
nutrition, 333–334
recurrent, 347